The Encyclopedia
of Elder Care

Elizabeth A. Capezuti, PhD, RN, FAAN, is the William Randolph Hearst Foundation Chair in Gerontology and associate dean for research at Hunter College School of Nursing of the City University of New York (CUNY). She teaches in Hunter's DNP program and is a professor in the PhD program in nursing science of the CUNY Graduate Center. The coeditor of five books and more than 100 scientific articles, she is known for her work in improving the care of older adults via interventions and models that positively influence health care providers' knowledge and work environment. She is part of a research team that is developing and testing an educational and technological model to improve sleep regulation among persons receiving palliative care. She is also part of an academic–community partnership in East/Central Harlem, New York City, utilizing a community-based participatory research framework that aims to improve access to palliative care in underserved communities.

Michael L. Malone, MD, is the medical director of Aurora Health Care—Senior Services and the Aurora at Home. He is a clinical adjunct professor of medicine at the University of Wisconsin School of Medicine and Public Health. He also serves as the director of the Geriatrics Fellowship Program at Aurora Health Care. He received his undergraduate and medical degrees from Texas Tech University in Lubbock, Texas; he completed his internal medicine residency and geriatric fellowship training at Mt. Sinai Medical Center in Milwaukee, Wisconsin. His Aurora Health Care practice is for homebound older persons in inner-city Milwaukee.

He is the chairman of the Public Policy Committee for the American Geriatrics Society and the section editor–Models of Geriatric Care, Quality Improvement and Program Dissemination for the *Journal of the American Geriatrics Society*. He led the development of the first acute care for elders (ACE) unit in Wisconsin. He and his colleagues have developed innovative strategies for disseminating geriatrics models of care, including the ACE Tracker software for identifying vulnerable hospitalized elders and the e-Geriatrician telemedicine program for bringing geriatrics expertise to rural hospitals with no geriatrician on staff. He has developed innovative teaching tools, including ACE Cards and the Geriatrics Fellows' Most Difficult Case Conferences. He has joined his colleagues at the Medical College of Wisconsin to implement Geriatric Fast Facts on mobile devices and tablets. In May 2015, he released a book with Elizabeth A. Capezuti and Robert Palmer, MD, titled, *Geriatrics Models of Care—Bringing "Best Practice" to an Aging America*. He recently joined Drs. Robert Kane (deceased), Joseph Ouslander, and Barbara Resnick as a coauthor of *Essentials of Clinical Geriatrics*, eighth edition.

Daniel S. Gardner, PhD, LCSW, is an associate professor at the Silberman School of Social Work at Hunter College, City University of New York (CUNY). He has more than 30 years of clinical, administrative, and research experience in health and mental health, specializing in social work practice and policy with individuals, families, and groups living with chronic and advanced illness. His areas of scholarship include aging, psychosocial oncology, palliative and end-of-life care, family decision making, and health disparities affecting underserved older adults and families. His research focuses on exploring and developing interventions to reduce disparities in pain management and palliative care among low-income minority elders. He has authored or coauthored many peer-reviewed articles, book chapters, and monographs, and his work has been funded by grants from the American Cancer Society, the John A. Hartford Foundation, the Fan Fox & Leslie R. Samuels Foundation, the National Institute of Aging (NIA), and the Health Resources and Services Administration (HRSA). He is a Hartford Faculty Scholar in Geriatric Social Work, a founding board member of the Social Work in Hospice & Palliative Care Network (SWHPN), research director of the Hartford Silberman Center of Excellence in Gerontological Social Work at Hunter College, and a Fellow at the Gerontological Society of America (GSA).

Ariba Khan, MD, MPH, is a geriatrician with Aurora Health Care (Milwaukee, Wisconsin) and clinical adjunct associate professor of medicine at the University of Wisconsin School of Medicine and Public Health. She serves as the cochair of the International Special Interest Group for the American Geriatrics Society and member of the Health Systems Innovation—Economics and Technology Committee. While serving as medical director of Aurora Sinai acute care for elders (ACE) programs, she led the Project BOOST team with the Society of Hospital Medicine on transitions of care and development of senior-friendly hospitals. She has served as associate program director of geriatrics fellowship and led the ACGME accreditation for fellowship. She led the development of several innovations in medical education, such as an interactive educational program for hospital employees recently published in the *Wisconsin Medical Journal*. She has presented internationally at the International Association of Gerontology and Geriatrics in Seoul, South Korea. Her interests include electronic health records and outcomes to improve the care of older hospitalized patients. She provides remote geriatrics services (e-Geriatrician) to outlying Aurora hospitals. She has served as community columnist for the *Milwaukee Journal Sentinel*.

Steven L. Baumann, PhD, GNP-BC, PMHNP-BC, is a professor at Hunter College School of Nursing of the City University of New York (CUNY). He teaches in Hunter's GNP/ANP and PMHNP programs and is a professor in the PhD program in nursing science of the CUNY Graduate Center. The global perspectives column editor for *Nursing Science Quarterly* for the past 10 years and the first author of 30 peer-reviewed articles and 70 other publications, he has an active practice as a nurse practitioner for the Department of Medical Psychiatry at Huntington Hospital, Northwell Health System. He has also taught GNP practice in Haiti, in the first FNP program in that country, a program he helped create, operate, and fund.

The Encyclopedia
of Elder Care
The Comprehensive Resource on Geriatric Health and Social Care

Fourth Edition

Elizabeth A. Capezuti, PhD, RN, FAAN

Michael L. Malone, MD

Daniel S. Gardner, PhD, LCSW

Ariba Khan, MD, MPH

Steven L. Baumann, PhD, GNP-BC, PMHNP-BC

Editors

SPRINGER PUBLISHING COMPANY

Springer Publishing Company, LLC
11 West 42nd Street
New York, NY 10036
www.springerpub.com

Acquisitions Editor: Joseph Morita
Compositor: Newgen KnowledgeWorks

ISBN: 978-0-8261-4052-4
ebook ISBN: 978-0-8261-4053-1

17 18 19 20 21 / 5 4 3 2 1

The author and the publisher of this Work have made every effort to use sources believed to be reliable to provide information that is accurate and compatible with the standards generally accepted at the time of publication. Because medical science is continually advancing, our knowledge base continues to expand. Therefore, as new information becomes available, changes in procedures become necessary. We recommend that the reader always consult current research and specific institutional policies before performing any clinical procedure. The author and publisher shall not be liable for any special, consequential, or exemplary damages resulting, in whole or in part, from the readers' use of, or reliance on, the information contained in this book. The publisher has no responsibility for the persistence or accuracy of URLs for external or third-party Internet websites referred to in this publication and does not guarantee that any content on such websites is, or will remain, accurate or appropriate.

Library of Congress Cataloging-in-Publication Data
Names: Capezuti, Liz, editor. | Malone, Michael L., editor. | Gardner, Daniel S., editor. |
  Khan, Ariba, editor. | Baumann, Steven L. (Professor of nursing), editor.
Title: The encyclopedia of elder care : the comprehensive resource on
  geriatric health and social care / Elizabeth A. Capezuti, Michael L. Malone,
  Daniel S. Gardner, Ariba Khan, Steven L. Baumann, editors.
Description: Fourth edition. | New York, NY : Springer Publishing Company,
  LLC, [2018] | Includes bibliographical references and index.
Identifiers: LCCN 2017039903 | ISBN 9780826140524 (paper back)
Subjects: | MESH: Health Services for the Aged | Geriatrics | Geriatric Nursing | Encyclopedias
Classification: LCC RC954 | NLM WT 13 | DDC 362.19897003—dc23
LC record available at https://lccn.loc.gov/2017039903

Contact us to receive discount rates on bulk purchases.
We can also customize our books to meet your needs.
For more information please contact: sales@springerpub.com

Printed in the United States of America by Publishers' Graphics.

CONTENTS

PREFACE

The aim of *The Encyclopedia of Elder Care* is to provide a convenient reference for the latest advances in gerontology and geriatrics. Similar to previous editions, this fourth edition is meant to bridge the information gap between research and practical application. This edition represents the combined efforts of 254 authors on 263 topics. Each entry provides a concise overview of the essential elements of elder care.

Approximately 60 years ago, gerontology was an emerging field. Now, there is considerable evidence to support the approaches and interventions described in this book. As editors, we have made decisions regarding content as we represent the major practice fields: social work, psychiatry, medicine, and nursing. We are fortunate to draw from a wide range of contributors who exemplify their special knowledge, including researchers, practitioners, and clinical educators who are leaders in advancing evidence-based practice. We have not only revised entries, but also added entries representing palliative care and social issues.

The complex and interrelated health, social, and psychological problems of older adults delivered in community-based and institutional settings frequently require input from multiple health care providers. As in previous editions, the target audience is not a single discipline, but rather any direct-care clinician or administrator of such services. Our intent is that the entries be written for such generalists rather than specialists in the individual topics. It is also our intent to serve as a vehicle for communication across disciplines and roles.

Each entry is meant to serve as a gateway to our field with inclusion, at the end of each entry, of the most relevant published or online sources for those interested in pursuing a topic in greater detail. The indexing and cross-referencing lead the reader to other related areas. We aim to present a multifaceted perspective of aging that will inspire our readers to gain beneficial insight that can be applied to their practice in the care of older adults.

We are grateful to the incredible contributions of the entry authors of this and the previous editions who dedicated their time and expertise to provide high-quality content. We are particularly grateful to our colleagues at Springer Publishing Company: Joseph Morita (Acquisitions Editor), Rachel X. Landes (Assistant Editor) and Joanne Jay (Vice President of Production and Manufacturing) for their stewardship of the project, and special thanks to Margaret Zuccarini who has shepherded this project for several editions. We are grateful to Ashita Shah for her valuable assistance in coordinating the contents of this edition.

Elizabeth A. Capezuti, PhD, RN, FAAN
Michael L. Malone, MD
Daniel S. Gardner, PhD, LCSW
Ariba Khan, MD, MPH
Steven L. Baumann, PhD, GNP-BC, PMHNP-BC

ACKNOWLEDGMENTS

The editors would like to acknowledge the following authors, who contributed to the third edition of *The Encyclopedia of Elder Care*:

Robert C. Abrams, MD

Hyochol Ahn, PhD, ARNP, ANP-BC

Mary Guerriero Austrom, PhD

Susan C. Ball, MD, MPH

Virginia W. Barrett, RN, DrPH

Teresa Belgin, BA

Susan I. Bernatz, PhD

Clara Berridge, MSW

Jeffrey Blustein, MD

Mathias P. Bostrom, MD

Abraham A. Brody, PhD, RN

Chaim E. Bromberg, PhD

Linda Bub, MSN, RN, GCNS-BC

Vivian Burnette, MS

Mary E. Byrnes, PhD, MUP

Brook Calton, MD, MHS

Thomas Caprio, MD, MPH, CMD, FACP

Deborah H. Chestnutt, MSN, RN

Erin Murphy Colligan, MPP

Angela L. Curl, PhD, MSW

JoAnn Damron-Rodriguez, LCSW, PhD

Linda Lindsey Davis, PhD, RN, FAAN

Heather E. Dillaway, PhD

Carole Ann Drick, PhD, RN, AHN-BC

Mary (Kelly) Dunn, RN, PhD, PHCNS-BC

Lois K. Evans, PhD, RN, FAAN

Eleanor E. Faye, MD

Donna M. Fick, PhD, APRN-BC, FGSA, FAAN

Kellie L. Flood, MD

Marquis Foreman, RN, PhD, FAAN

James F. Fries, MD

Daphna Gans, PhD

Miriam M. George, PhD

James Golomb, MD

Carmen Green, MD

Barry J. Gurland, MD, FRC Physicians, FRC Psychiatry

J. Taylor Harden, PhD, RN, FGSA, FAAN

Beth L. G. Hollander, PhD

Sophia Hu, PhD, RN

Mily Kannarkat, MD

Linn Katus, DO, MSc

David M. Keepnews, PhD, JD, RN, FAAN

Alan Kluger, PhD

Rosalind Kopfstein, LCSW, DSW

B. Josea Kramer, PhD

Amanda J. Lehning, MSW, PhD

Amy L. Lightner, MD

Adrianne Dill Linton, PhD, RN, FAAN

John Lung, MD

Kevin J. Mahoney, PhD

Marianne Matzo, PhD, FCPN, FAAN

Jane A. McDowell, MSN, APRN-BC

Elizabeth F. McGann, DNSc, RN

Lynne Morishita, GNP, MSN

Catherine O'Keefe, MEd, CTRS

Hamid R. Okhravi, MD

Anna Ortigara, RN, MS

Patti Pagel, MSN, RN, GCNS-BC

Gregory J. Paveza, MSW, PhD

Allison M. Pelger, BS, RN

Paul B. Perrin, PhD

Sandra J. Picot, PhD, CLNC, FAAN, FGSA

Sarah Piper, MD

Margaret R. Puelle, BS

Barbara Resnick, PhD, CRNP

Sandra L. Reynolds, PhD

Benjamin F. Ricciardi, MD

Danielle Richards, PhD

Anne Rohs, MD

Efi Rubinstein, PhD, JD

Alessandra Scalmati, MD, PhD

Andrew E. Scharlach, PhD

Shubhi Sehgal, MD

Andrea Sherman, PhD

Hilary C. Siebens, MD

Margaret Spain, MN, FNP, BC, CDE

Gwen K. Sterns, MD

Annie Stroup, BSW

Anchal Sud, MD

David Sutin, MD

Karen Amann Talerico, RN, PhD

Anne C. Thomas, PhD, ANP-BC, GNP, FAANP

Colin Torrance, RN, DLScN, BSc, PhD

Rachael Watman, MSW

Eric Widera, MD

Jennifer L. Wolff, PhD

Donna L. Yee, MSW, PhD

Andrea M. Yevchak, PhD, GCNS-BC, RN

CONTRIBUTORS

Kathleen Abrahamson, PhD, RN
Associate Professor
School of Nursing
Purdue University
West Lafayette, Indiana

Ronke E. Adawale, RN, MPH, CPH
Doctoral Student
Health Science Administration Department
School of Public Heath
University of Maryland
Baltimore, Maryland

Ronald D. Adelman, MD
Emilie Roy Corey Professor of Geriatrics and
    Gerontology
Division of Geriatric and Palliative Medicine
Weill Cornell Medical College
New York, New York

Aboud Affi, MD
Gastroenterologist
Aurora Health Care
Milwaukee, Wisconsin

Saima Ajmal, MD
Section Chief, Geriatric Medicine
Bellevue Hospital Center
Division of Geriatric Medicine and Palliative Care
NYU School of Medicine
New York, New York

Saima T. Akbar, MD
Geriatric Consult Service
St Lukes Hospital
Milwaukee, Wisconsin;
Assistant Professor of Clinical Medicine
University of Wisconsin
Madison, Wisconsin

Azmaa Albaroudi, MSG, NPA
Manager of Quality and Policy Initiatives
National PACE Association
Alexandria, Virginia

Robert Applebaum, MSW, PhD
Professor of Gerontology
Scripps Gerontology Center
Miami University
Oxford, Ohio

Mary Guerriero Austrom, PhD
Associate Dean of Diversity Affairs
Wesley P. Martin Professor of
    AD Education
Professor of Clinical Psychology in
    Clinical Psychiatry
Department of Psychiatry
Leader, Outreach and Recruitment Core
Indiana Alzheimer Disease Center
Indiana University School of Medicine
Indianapolis, Indiana

**Elizabeth A. Ayello, PhD, RN, ACNS-BC,
    CWON, MAPWCA, FAAN**
Faculty
Excelsior College School of Nursing
Albany, New York

Ronet Bachman, PhD
Professor
Department of Sociology and Criminal Justice
University of Delaware
Newark, Delaware

Ariunsanaa Bagaajav, MPH
Doctoral Fellow
Silberman School of Social Work
Hunter College, City University of New York
New York, New York

Janet M. Bairardi, PhD, RN
Associate Dean and Professor
University of Detroit Mercy
Detroit, Michigan

Saffia Bajwa
Student
Loyola University Chicago
Brookfield, Wisconsin

Tanvir K. Bajwa, MD, FACC, FSCAI
Medical Director
Cardiac/Peripheral Intervention;
Clinical Director
Vascular Center
Aurora Cardiovascular Services—Aurora
    Medical Group
Milwaukee, Wisconsin

Amy E. Z. Baker, PhD, BHlthSc (Hons) (OccTh)
    BAppSc (OccTh)
Lecturer
School of Health Sciences
University of South Australia
Adelaide, Australia

Joshua F. Baker, MD, MSCE
Assistant Professor of Medicine
Division of Rheumatology and Epidemiology
University of Pennsylvania;
Michael C. Crescent VA Medical Center
University of Pennsylvania
Philadelphia, Pennsylvania

Rosemary Bakker, MS, NCIDQ
Certified Interior Designer
Age-Friendly Design, Inc.
New York, New York

Mary C. Ballin, GNP-BC, CDE
Gerontological NP at the Wright Center on Aging
New York Presbyterian Hospital
New York, New York

Thomas Bane, LMSW
Research Assistant
Silberman School of Social Work at Hunter College
New York, New York

Anthony R. Bardo, PhD, MGS
Postdoctoral Associate
Department of Sociology
Duke University
Durham, North Carolina

Melissa Batchelor-Murphy, PhD, RN-BC, FNP-BC
Policy Fellow
Duke University School of Nursing
Fairfax, Virginia

Daniel R. Bateman, MD
Assistant Professor of Psychiatry
Indiana University School of Medicine
Indiana University Center for Aging Research
Carmel, Indiana

Steven L. Baumann, PhD, GNP-BC, PMHNP-BC
Professor and Co-Coordinator of the
    GNP/ANP Program
Hunter College, City University New York
New York, New York

Angela Beckert, MD
Assistant Professor of Medicine
Division of Geriatrics
Department of Medicine
Medical College of Wisconsin
Milwaukee, Wisconsin

Judith L. Beizer, PharmD, GCP, FASCP, AGSF
Clinical Professor
College of Pharmacy and Health Sciences
St. John's University
Queens, New York

Keith A. Bender, PhD
SIRE Professor of Economics
Department of Economics
University of Aberdeen
Aberdeen, Scotland

David E. Biegel, PhD
Henry L. Zucker Professor of Social Work Practice
Professor of Psychiatry and Sociology
Case Western Reserve University
Cleveland, Ohio

April Bigelow, PhD, ANP-BC, AGPCNP-BC
Clinical Associate Professor
Department of Health Behavior and Biological
    Sciences
University of Michigan School of Nursing
Ann Arbor, Michigan

Michel H. C. Bleijlevens, PhD
Assistant Professor
Faculty of Health Medicine and
    Life Sciences
Care and Public Health Research Institute
Department of Health Services Research
Maastricht University
Maastricht, Netherlands

Shawn M. Bloom
President and CEO
National PACE Association
Alexandria, Virginia

R. Bennett Blum, MD
Director
Geriatric Division—Park Dietz and Associates
Newport Beach, California;
Clinical Associate Professor
Department of Psychiatry
University of Arizona College of Medicine
Tucson, Arizona

Marie Boltz, PhD, GNP-BC, FGSA, FAAN
Associate Professor
College of Nursing
Pennsylvania State University
University Park, Pennsylvania

Patricia Booth, MS, RDN, FADA
Director, Nutrition Services
Department of Nutrition & Food Services
University of California, San Francisco,
    Medical Center
San Francisco, California

Enid A. Borden BA, MA
Chief Executive Officer
National Foundation to End Senior Hunger
Alexandria, Virginia

Ella H. Bowman, MD, PhD, AGSF, FAAHPM
Associate Professor of Medicine
Division of Gerontology, Geriatrics, and
    Palliative Care
University of Alabama at Birmingham;
Section Chief of Geriatrics—Acute and Specialty
    Care
Birmingham Veterans Administration Medical
    Center
Birmingham, Alabama

**Mary M. Brennan, DNP, AGACNP-BC,
    ANP, FAANP**
Clinical Associate Professor
Director, Adult and Gerontology Acute Care Nurse
    Practitioner Program
Rory Meyers College of Nursing
New York University
New York City, New York

Ellen Broach, EdD, CTRS
Associate Professor, Therapeutic Recreation
Department of Health, Kinesiology and Sport
University of South Alabama
Mobile, Alabama

Colette V. Browne, DrPH, MSW
T. Rose and Richard S. Takasaki Endowed Professor
    in Social Policy
Myron B. Thompson School of Social Work
University of Hawaii
Honolulu, Hawaii

Barbara L. Brush, PhD, ANP-BC, FAAN
The Carol J. and F. Edward Lake Professor in
    Population Health
University of Michigan
Ann Arbor, Michigan

Cary Buckner, MD
Vice Chairman
Department of Neurosciences
New York Presbyterian—Brooklyn Methodist
    Hospital
Brooklyn, New York

Sarah Greene Burger, RN, MPH, FAAN
Senior Advisor
Hartford Institute for Geriatric Nursing
New York University Rory Meyers College of
    Nursing
New York, New York

David Burnes, PhD
Assistant Professor
University of Toronto
Toronto, Ontario, Canada

Billy A. Caceres, PhD, RN, AGPCNP-BC
Post-Doctoral Research Fellow
Columbia School of Nursing
New York, New York

Margaret P. Calkins, PhD
Executive Director
Fellow of the Gerontological Society
    of America
The Mayer-Rothschild Foundation
Chicago, Illinois

Theresa M. Campo, DNP, FNP-C, ENP-BC, FAANP
Codirector
FNP Track Drexel University
Philadelphia, Pennsylvania;
Nurse Practitioner
Atlanticare Regional Medical Center
Atlantic City, New Jersey

Elizabeth A. Capezuti, PhD, RN, FAAN
Chair in Gerontology and Professor
William Randolph Hearst Foundation
Hunter College, City University New York
New York, New York

Kathleen M. Capitulo, PhD, RN, FAAN, IIWCC
Chief Nurse Executive
James J. Peters Veterans Affairs Medical Center
Bronx, New York

Sylvester Carter, PT, MHS, PhD
Physical Therapist
Physical Therapy Department
Monroeville Rehabilitation and Wellness Center
Pittsburgh, Pennsylvania

Suzanna Waters Castillo, PhD, MSSW
Distinguished Faculty Associate
Division of Continuing Studies
University of Wisconsin–Madison
Madison, Wisconsin

Mirnova Ceïde, MD
Assistant Professor
Department of Psychiatry and Behavioral Science
Montefiore Medical Center
Bronx, New York

Ching-Wen Chang, PhD
Assistant Professor
Department of Social Work
The Chinese University of Hong Kong
Hong Kong, China

Jonathan T. L. Cheah, MBBS
Rheumatology Fellow
Division of Rheumatology, Hospital for Special Surgery
Department of Medicine
Weill Cornell Medical College
New York, New York

Tracy L. Chippendale, PhD, OTR/L
Assistant Professor
Department of Occupational Therapy
Steinhardt School of Culture, Education, and Human
  Development
New York University
New York, New York

**Carolyn K. Clevenger, DNP, AGPCNP-BC,
  GNP-BC, FAANP**
Associate Dean for Clinical and Community
  Partnerships
Nell Hodgson Woodruff School of Nursing
Emory University
Atlanta, Georgia

Daniel D. Cline, PhD, RN, ANP-BC, CEN
Assistant Professor
School of Nursing
Samuel Merritt University
Oakland, California

Ann E. Cornell, MD
Gynecologist
Aurora Health Care
Milwaukee, Wisconsin

Valerie T. Cotter, DrNP, AGPCNP-BC, FAANP
Assistant Professor
Johns Hopkins School of Nursing
Baltimore, Maryland

Lynda Crandall, RN, GNP
Executive Director
Pioneer Network
Salem, Oregon

Christine Cutugno, PhD, RN, NEA-BC
Clinical Professor
Hunter College, School of Nursing
New York, New York

Chin Hwa (Gina) Dahlem, PhD, FNP-C, FAANP
Clinical Assistant Professor
University of Michigan School of Nursing
Ann Arbor, Michigan

Irene Rosner David, PhD, ATR-BC, LCAT, HLM
Director of Therapeutic Arts
Bellevue Hospital Center
New York, New York

Heather Davila, MPA
Research Fellow
School of Public Health
University of Minnesota
Minneapolis, Minnesota

Karen Davis, PhD
Eugene and Mildred Lipitz Professor
Director, Roger C. Lipitz Center for Integrated
  Health Care
Johns Hopkins Bloomberg School of Public Health
Baltimore, Maryland

Sabina M. De Geest, PhD, RN, FAAN, FRCN, FEANS
Professor of Nursing
Institute of Nursing Science
University of Basel
Basel, Switzerland

Eddy Dejaeger, MD, PhD
Head of Clinic
Department of Geriatric Medicine
University Hospitals Leuven
Leuven, Belgium

Marian C. Devereaux, RDN, CNSC
Senior Clinical Dietician
Department of Nutrition & Food Services
University of California, San Francisco, Medical Center
San Francisco, California

Marla DeVries, BA
Director of Resource Development
The Green House Project
Linthicum, Maryland

Michele Diaz, RN, MS
Doctoral Student
University of California
San Francisco, School of Nursing
San Francisco, California

Stefanie DiCarrado, PT, DPT, MSCS, CPT, CES, PES
Physical Therapist
Aspire Center for Health and Wellness
Ossining, New York;
Assistant Professor
Dominican College
Orangeburg, New York

Rose Ann DiMaria-Ghalili, PhD, RN, CNSC, FASPEN, FAAN
Associate Professor of Nursing
College of Nursing and Health Professions
Drexel University
Philadelphia, Pennsylvania

Vidita Divan, MD
Chief Resident
Internal Medicine Department
Aurora Health Care
Milwaukee, Wisconsin

Meredith Doherty, LCSW
American Cancer Society Doctoral Scholar
Hunter College, City University of New York
Graduate Center
Silberman School of Social Work at Hunter College
New York, New York

Caroline Dorsen, PhD, FNP-BC
Assistant Professor
Rory Meyers College of Nursing
New York University
New York, New York

Sarah L. Dowal, LICSW, MPH
Project Director
Hospital Elder Life Program
Aging Brain Center
Hebrew SeniorLife
Boston, Massachusetts

Carole Ann Drick, PhD, RN, AHN-BC
Immediate Past President
American Holistic Nurses Association
Youngstown, Ohio

Edmund H. Duthie, Jr., MD
Professor of Medicine (Geriatrics/Gerontology)
Chief Division of Geriatrics/Gerontology
Medical College of Wisconsin
Froedtert Health & Clement J Zablocki VAMC
Milwaukee, Wisconsin

Barbara J. Edlund, PhD, ANP, BC retired
Professor
College of Nursing
Medical University of South Carolina
Charleston, South Carolina

Nancy Eng, PhD, CCC-SLP
Associate Professor/Chair
Department of Speech/Language Pathology and Audiology
Hunter College
New York, New York

Ronald L. Ettinger, BDS, MDS, DDSc, DDSc (hc), DABSCD
Professor Emeritus
Department of Prosthodontics and Dows Institute of Dental Research
College of Dentistry
University of Iowa
Iowa City, Iowa

Gerald L. Euster, DSW
Distinguished Professor Emeritus
College of Social Work
University of South Carolina
Columbia, South Carolina

Jonathan Fahler, DO
Gastroenterologist
The Iowa Clinic
West Des Moines, Iowa

Alfred G. Feliu, JD
Principal
Feliu Neutral Services, LLP
New Rochelle, New York

Barbara L. Fischer, PsyD
Psychologist
William S. Middleton Memorial Veterans Hospital
Madison, Wisconsin

Christine G. Fitzgerald, RRT, PhD
Director of Health Science Studies
Quinnipiac University
Hamden, Connecticut

Barbara Frank, MPA
Cofounder
B&F Consulting
Warren, Rhode Island

Jaclyn R. Freshman, BA
Research Assistant
Hospital Elder Life Program
Aging Brain Center
Hebrew SeniorLife
Boston, Massachusetts

Terry T. Fulmer, PhD, RN, FAAN
President
The John A. Hartford Foundation
New York, New York

Raphael Gaeta, MSW, PhD
Research Analyst
JBS International, Inc.
Fairfax, Virginia

Marissa Galicia-Castillo, MD
Geriatrician
Sentara Healthsystem
Fairfax, Virginia

Sandy B. Ganz, PT, DSc, GCS
Director of Rehabilitation
HSS satellite emeritus
Boca Raton, Florida

Daniel S. Gardner, PhD, LCSW
Associate Professor
Silberman School of Social Work
New York, New York;
Interim Director
Brookdale Center for Healthy Aging
Hunter College, City University of New York
New York, New York

Linda K. George, PhD
Arts and Sciences Professor of Sociology
Department of Sociology and Center for the Study of
Aging
Duke University
Durham, North Carolina

Angela Ghesquiere, PhD, MSW
Program Manager
Brookdale Center for Healthy Aging
Hunter College, City University of New York
New York, New York

Ihab Girgis, PhD, LCSW-R
Program Manager
New York State Department of Health
Home Health Care and Hospice
New York, New York

Sarah E. Givens, PhD, RN
Research Associate
Frances Payne Bolton School of Nursing
Case Western Reserve University
Cleveland, Ohio

Toni L. Glover, PhD, GNP-BC, ACHPN
Assistant Professor
Department Biobehavioral Nursing Science
University of Florida
College of Nursing
Gainesville, Florida

Rebekah Glushefski, MSW
Progam Manager
Silberman School of Social Work
Hunter College, City University of New York
New York, New York

Ann Goeleven, MSc, SLP
Speech Language Pathology Therapist
Department of ENT Head and Neck Surgery
Department of Speech Language Pathology
University Hospitals Leuven;
Laboratory for Experimental
Otorhinolaryngology
University of Leuven
Leuven, Belgium

Susan M. Goodman, MD
Professor of Clinical Medicine
Division of Rheumatology
Hospital for Special Surgery
Department of Medicine
Weill Cornell Medical College
New York, New York

Esperanza L. Gómez-Durán, MD, PhD
Professor
Universitat Internacional de Catalunya
Hestia Alliance
Barcelona's Official College of Physicians
Barcelona, Spain

Marianthe D. Grammas, MD
Assistant Professor of Medicine
Division of Gerontology, Geriatrics, and Palliative Care
University of Alabama at Birmingham;
Physician Advisor, Care Transitions Department
University of Alabama at Birmingham Hospital
Birmingham, Alabama

Michele G. Greene, DrPH
Professor
Department of Health and Nutrition Sciences
Brooklyn College
Brooklyn, New York

Margaret M. Grisius, DDS
Clinical Dentist
National Institute of Dental and Craniofacial
　Research
Salivary Gland Dysfunction and Sjögren's Syndrome
　Unit
Molecular Physiology and Therapeutics Branch
　National Institutes of Health
Bethesda, Maryland

Laura E. Gultekin, PhD, FNP-BC
Assistant Professor
University of Michigan School of Nursing
Ann Arbor, Michigan

Satya Gutta, MD
Geriatric Psychiatry Fellow
Department of Psychiatry
Medical College of Wisconsin
Milwaukee, Wisconsin

Kevin E. Hansen, PhD, JD, LLM
Assistant Professor
Health Care Administration Program
University of Wisconsin—Eau Claire;
Director
National Emerging Leadership Summit
Eau Claire, Wisconsin

Laila M. Hasan, RN, BS
Student Nurse
Center for Senior Health and Longevity
Aurora Health Care
Milwaukee, Wisconsin

Arthur E. Helfand, DPM
Professor Emeritus
Temple University, School of Podiatric
　Medicine
Retired Chair
Department of Community Health, Aging, and
　Health Policy
Philadelphia, Pennsylvania

Claire Henchcliffe, MD, DPhil
Vice Chair for Research
Division Chief Parkinson's Disease and Movement
　Disorders Institute
Weill Cornell Medicine/New York Presbyterian
　Hospital
New York, New York

Hugh C. Hendrie, MB, ChB, DSc
Professor
Department of Psychiatry
Indiana University School of Medicine
Regenstrief Institute, Inc.
Indiana University Center for Aging Research
Indianapolis, Indiana

Mary T. Hickey, EdD, FNP, WHNP-BC
Clinical Professor
Associate Dean, Graduate Programs
　Coordinator
Primary Care AGNP Program
Hunter College School of Nursing
New York, New York

Renita Ho, DO, MA
Physician
Team Health
New York, New York

David R. Hoffman, JD, FCPP
President
David Hoffman & Associates
Philadelphia, Pennsylvania

Mara A. G. Hollander, DrPH, RPT, RD
Physical Therapist
Whole Health Medicine Institute
Redlands, California

Janella Hong, MD
Psychiatrist
Kaiser Permanente
Walnut Creek, California

Timothy Howell, MD
Adjunct Clinical Associate Professor
Wisconsin Geriatric Psychiatry Initiative
Geriatric Research, Education, and Clinical Center
Madison Veterans Administration Hospital;
Geriatrics Division, Department of Medicine
University of Wisconsin School of Medicine and
    Public Health
Madison, Wisconsin

Ann L. Horgas, PhD, RN, FGSA, FAAN
Associate Professor and Chair
Department of Biobehavioral Nursing Science
College of Nursing
University of Florida
Gainesville, Florida

Tammy T. Hshieh, MD, MPH
Associate Physician
Brigham and Women's Hospital
Harvard Medical School
Brookline, Massachusetts

Richard Hsu, BS, MS(c)
Medical Doctor Candidate Student
Wayne State University School of Medicine
Detroit, Michigan

Jené M. Hurlbut, RN, MSN, MS, PhD, CNE
Professor
College of Nursing
Roseman University of Health Sciences
Professor, VBSN Project Director/Principal
    Investigator-Henderson
Henderson, Nevada

Ellen Idler, PhD
Samuel Candler Dobbs Professor
Department of Sociology
Emory University
Atlanta, Georgia

Margaret B. Ingraham, BA, MA
Executive Vice President
National Foundation to End Senior Hunger
Alexandria, Virginia

Sharon K. Inouye, MD, MPH
Professor of Medicine
Beth Israel Deaconess Medical Center
Harvard Medical School;
Director
Aging Brain Center
Hebrew SeniorLife
Boston, Massachusetts

Laura Isham, PT, DPT
Doctor of Physical Therapy
Cottage Rehabilitation PT
Cottage Rehabilitation Hospital
Santa Barbara, California

Stephanie A. Jacobson, PhD, MSW, LCSW
Associate Department Chair and
    Assistant Professor
Department of Social Work
MSW Program
School of Health Sciences
Quinnipiac University
Hamden, Connecticut

Nancy S. Jecker, PhD
Professor
Department of Bioethics and Humanities
University of Washington School of Medicine
Seattle, Washington

Rebecca A. Johnson, PhD, RN, FAAN, FNAP
Millsap Professor of Gerontological Nursing and
    Public Policy
Sinclair School of Nursing
University of Missouri
Columbia, Missouri

Evanne Juratovac, PhD, RN (GCNS-BC)
Assistant Professor
School of Nursing;
Assistant Professor
School of Medicine;
Faculty Associate
University Center on Aging and Health
Case Western Reserve University
Cleveland Ohio

Ruta Kadonoff, MA, MHS
Executive Director
Pioneer Network
Belfast, Maine

Michelle Kaplan, MD
Geriatric Psychiatric Fellow
Division of Geriatric Psychiatry
Montefiore Medical Center
Albert Einstein College of Medicine
New York, New York

Richard L. Kaplan, JD
Guy Raymond Jones Chair in Law
University of Illinois at Champaign–Urbana
Champaign, Illinois

Marshall B. Kapp, JD, MPH
Director
Center for Innovative Collaboration in Medicine
    and Law
Florida State University College of Medicine and
    College of Law
Tallahassee, Florida

Arun S. Karlamangla, MD
Professor of Medicine
Department of Geriatrics
University of California, Los Angeles/Sepulveda
    Veterans Administration Medical Center
University of California, Los Angeles Med Geriatric
    Research Education and Clinical Center
San Fernando Valley, California

Herbert Karpatkin, PT, DSc, NCS, MSCS
Assistant Professor
Program in Physical Therapy
Hunter College, City University of New York
New York, New York

Jeanie Kayser-Jones, RN, PhD, FAAN
Professor Emerita
Department of Physiological Nursing & Medical
    Anthropology
University of California
San Francisco, California

Gary J. Kennedy, MD
Vice Chair for Education, Professor, and Director
Division of Geriatric Psychiatry
Montefiore Medical Center
Albert Einstein College of Medicine
New York, New York

Ariba Khan, MD, MPH, AGSF
Clinical Adjunct Associate Professor
University of Wisconsin School of Medicine and
    Public Health
Aurora Health Care
Milwaukee, Wisconsin

Jayant Khitha, MD
Interventional Cardiologist
Associate Program Director
Interventional Cardiology Fellowship
    at Aurora St. Luke's Medical Center
Milwaukee, Wisconsin

Anneline Kingsley, MD
Psychiatrist
Baptist Behavioral Health
Baptist Hospital
Jacksonville, Florida

Ashley B. Kinnaman, BSW
Case Manager
Multnomah County Long Term Care Services
Portland, Oregon

Marc B. Kramer, PhD
Otorhinolaryngologist
Department of Otorhinolaryngology
Weill Cornell Medical College
New York, New York

Joan Kreiger, EdD, RRT
Assistant Professor
School of Health and Human Services
Southern Connecticut State University
New Haven, Connecticut

Melissa Kurtz, MSN, MA
Registered Nurse/PhD Candidate
John Hopkins Hospital
Intrastaff/Johns Hopkins School of Nursing
Department of Acute and Chronic Care
Johns Hopkins Children's Center/Johns Hopkins
    School of Nursing
Baltimore, Maryland

Mark Lachs, MD, MPH
Co-Director, Division of Geriatrics and Palliative
    Medicine
Weill Cornell School of Medicine
Director of Geriatrics
New York Presbyterian Health System
New York, New York

William T. Lawson, III, JD
Principal
Law Offices of William T. Lawson, III
Philadelphia, Pennsylvania

Chungsup Lee, PhD
Post-Doctoral Researcher
Department of Recreation, Sport, and Tourism
University of Illinois at Urbana-Champaign (UIUC)
Champaign, Illinois

Susan D. Leonard, MD
Assistant Clinical Professor
University of California, Los Angeles, Department of
    Medicine
Division of Geriatrics
Los Angeles, California

Amy L. Lightner, MD
Assistant Professor of Surgery
Department of Colon and Rectal Surgery
Mayo Clinic
Rochester, Minnesota

Fidelindo Lim, DNP, CCRN
Clinical Assistant Professor
Rory Meyers College of Nursing
New York University
New York, New York

Mimi Lim, MPA, MS, RN, CIC,
NEA-BC, CNL
Clinical Director of Patient Care Services
The Graduate Center
City University of New York
New York, New York

Yvonne Lu, PhD, RN, FGSA
Associate Professor
Adult Health Nursing, Indiana University
School of Nursing
Indianapolis, Indiana

James Lubben, DSW/PhD, MPH, MSW
Louise McMahon Ahearn Professor in
    Social Work
Director of University Institute on Aging
Boston College
School of Social Work
Chestnut Hill, Massachusetts

Paula Lueras, MD
Advanced Geriatric Medicine Fellow
Division of Geriatrics and Gerontology
Department of Medicine
University of Wisconsin School of Medicine and
    Public Health
Madison, Wisconsin

Theresa L. Lundy, MS, RN, FNP
Lecturer
Department of Nursing
Lehman College of City University of
    New York
Bronx, New York

Jonny A. Macias Tejada, MD
Medical Director
Acute Care for Elders
Hospital Elder Life Program
Aurora St. Luke's Medical Center;
Clinical Adjunct Associate Professor
University of Wisconsin School of Medicine and
    Public Health
Milwaukee, Wisconsin

Michael L. Malone, MD
Medical Director
Aurora Senior Services & Aurora at Home
Director of Geriatric Medicine Fellowship Program,
    Aurora Health Care;
Clinical Adjunct Professor of Medicine
University of Wisconsin School of Medicine and
    Public Health
Milwaukee, Wisconsin

Brian Marquez, BSN, RN
Staff Nurse
University of California
Irvine Medical Center
Brea, California

Karen S. Martin, RN, MSN, FAAN
Health Care Consultant
Martin Associates
Omaha, Nebraska

Christina Matz-Costa, PhD, MSW
Assistant Professor
Boston College
School of Social Work
Chestnut Hill, Massachusetts

Yael Mauer, MD
Internist
Cleveland Clinic
Cleveland, Ohio

Caitlin McAfee, MSW
Research Associate
Brookdale Center for Healthy Aging at Hunter
    College
Austin, Texas

Donna E. McCabe, DNP, APRN-BC, GNP
Clinical Assistant Professor
Rory Meyers College of Nursing
New York University
New York, New York

Elizabeth M. Miller, RN, MSN, MBA
State President
Wellcare of Florida
Wellcare Health Plans, Inc.
Tampa, Florida

Carol M. Musil, PhD, RN, FAAN, FGSA
Professor of Nursing
Frances Payne Bolton School of Nursing
Case Western Reserve University
Cleveland, Ohio

Matthias J. Naleppa, MSW, PhD
Professor
School of Economy, Health and Social Work
Bern University of Applied Science
Grafing, Germany

Nicholas R. Nicholson, Jr., PhD, MPH, RN, PHCNS-BC
Associate Professor
School of Nursing
Quinnipiac University
Hamden, Connecticut

Christine E. Niekrash, DMD, MDSc
Associate Professor of Medical Sciences
Frank H. Netter MD School of Medicine
Quinnipiac University
Hamden, Connecticut

Uchechukwu Nnamdi, MD
Attending Physician
Montefiore Health System
Bronx, New York

Jill Nocella, PhD, APRN-BC
Associate Professor of Nursing
William Paterson University of New Jersey
Wayne, New Jersey

Lynda Olender, PhD, RN, ANP, NEA-BC
Associate Dean
Graduate Program
Hunter-Bellevue School of Nursing
City University of New York
New York, New York

Christina Oros, MSc, SLP
Speech Language Pathology Therapist
City Sounds of NY–Speech-Language Development Center, Inc.
New York, New York

Carol L. B. Ott, MD, FRCPC
Geriatrician
Women's College Hospital
Baycrest Hospital
University of Toronto
Toronto, Ontario, Canada

Karen Padua, DO
Assistant Clinical Professor of Family Medicine & Geriatrics
UCLA Geriatrics
Santa Monica, California

Robert M. Palmer, MD, MPH
Director
Glennan Center for Geriatrics and Gerontology;
Professor of Internal Medicine
Department of Internal Medicine
Eastern Virginia Medical School
Norfolk, Virginia

Michelle Pardee, DNP, FNP-BC
Clinical Assistant Professor
University of Michigan School of Nursing
Ann Arbor, Michigan

Melinda Perez-Porter, JD
Director
The Relatives as Parents Program (RAPP)
The Brookdale Foundation Group
Teaneck, New Jersey

Noralyn Davel Pickens, PhD, OT
Professor
School of Occupational Therapy
Texas Woman's University
Dallas, Texas

Carol Podgorski, PhD
Associate Professor of Psychiatry
Department of Psychiatry
University of Rochester
School of Medicine and Dentistry
Scottsville, New York

Marcella Pomeranz, DNP, APRN, BC-AGNP, CCRN, CDE
Adult Geriatric Nurse Practitioner in GI
Digestive Associates
Las Vegas, Nevada

Dominica Potenza, DNP, RN, AGPCNP-BC
Adjunct Assistant Professor
Graduate Program
Hunter-Bellevue School of Nursing
City University of New York
New York, New York

Tia Powell, MD
Director
Montefiore Einstein Center for Bioethics
Bronx, New York

Karis Pressler, PhD
Research Associate
School of Nursing
Purdue University
West Lafayette, Indiana

Nicholas G. Procter, PhD, MBA
Professor
School of Nursing and Midwifery
University of South Australia
Adelaide, Australia

Rolanda Pyle, LMSW
Assistant Director
CARE NYC Caregiver Support Services
Sunnyside, New York

Lauretta Quinn, PhD, RN, FAAN, CDE
Clinical Professor
Department of Biobehavioral Nursing
College of Nursing
University of Illinois at Chicago
Chicago, Illinois

Barrie L. Raik, MD
Associate Clinical Professor of Medicine
Division of Geriatric and Palliative Medicine
Weill Cornell Medical College
New York, New York

Nancy S. Redeker, PhD, RN, FAHA, FAAN
Beatrice Renfield Term Professor of Nursing
Yale School of Nursing
West Haven, Connecticut

Susan M. Renz, DNP, RN, GNP-BC
Director
Adult–Gerontology Primary Care Nurse Practitioner
   Program
University of Pennsylvania School of Nursing
Philadelphia, Pennsylvania

Carol Getz Rice, MS, OTR
Adjunct Faculty Member
Occupational Therapy Program
Indiana Wesleyan University
Marion, Indiana

Sara E. Rix, PhD, FRSA
Senior Fellow
National Academy of Social Insurance
Washington, DC

Jeffrey M. Robbins, DPM
Director Podiatry Service
Department of Veterans Affairs
Louis Stokes Cleveland VAMC
Cleveland, Ohio;
Clinical Assistant Professor
Department of Surgery Case Western Reserve
   University School of Medicine
Cleveland, Ohio

Marie-Claire Rosenberg Roberts, PhD, MS, MPA, RN
Assistant Professor
Pace University
New York, New York

Anissa T. Rogers, PhD, MSW, MA, LCSW
Professor and Director
Dorothy Day Social Work Program
University of Portland
Portland, Oregon

Geoffrey Rogers, BA
Director of Learning and Development
Brookdale Center for Healthy Aging
Hunter College
New York, New York

Lisa Ravdin Rosenberg, PhD, ABPP
Associate Professor, Director
Weill Cornell Medicine
Neuropsychology
New York, New York

Peri Rosenfeld, PhD
Director
Outcomes Research and Program Evaluation
Director
Center for Innovations in the Advancement of Care;
Professor (Adjunct)
New York University College of Nursing
Department of Nursing
NYU Langone Medical Center
New York, New York

Anne Steinfeld Rugova, BA
Patient Safety Coordinator
Eugene Lang College The New School University
NYC Health + Hospitals/Bellevue
New York, New York

Todd Ruppar, PhD, RN, FAHA
John L. and Helen Kellogg Professor of Nursing
Rush University College of Nursing
Chicago, Illinois

Linda A. Russell, MD
Director
Osteoporosis and Metabolic Bone Health Center
Hospital for Special Surgery
Assistant Professor of Medicine
Weill Cornell Medical School of Medicine
New York, New York

Marcia M. Russell, MD
Assistant Professor of Surgery
Division of General Surgery, Section of Colon and
    Rectal Surgery
David Geffen School of Medicine at University of
    California, Los Angeles;
Veterans Administration Greater Los Angeles
    Healthcare System
Los Angeles, California

Debra Saliba, MD, MPH, AGSF
Anna & Harry Borun Chair in Geriatrics and
    Gerontology
Los Angeles Veterans Administration Geriatrics
    Research Education and Clinical Center and
    Health Services Research & Development Center
    of Innovation
University of California, Los Angeles;
Senior Natural Scientist
R and Health
Santa Monica, California

Margaret Salisu, LMSW, M.Phil
Adjunct Professor
Hunter College
City University of New York
Graduate Center
Silberman School of Social Work at Hunter College
New York, New York

Harini Sarva, MD
Clinical Director
Parkinson's Disease and Movement Disorders Institute
Weill Cornell Medical Center/New York
    Presbyterian Hospital
New York, New York

Lorry Schoenly, PhD, RN, CCHP-RN
Visiting Professor
Graduate Nursing Program
Chamberlain College of Nursing
Genesee, Pennsylvania

Sandra Schönfeld, MSc
Graduate Student
Institute of Nursing Science
University of Basel
Basel, Switzerland

**Robert A. Schulman, MD, FAAPMR, FAAMA,
    RH(AHG), ABOIM**
Integrative Medicine Specialist
West County Integrative Medicine
Santa Rosa, California

Edna P. Schwab, MD
Associate Professor of Clinical Medicine
Geriatric Fellowship Program Director
Hospital of the University of Pennsylvania;
Chief
GEC, Interim ACOS Education, CMCVAMC
Philadelphia, Pennsylvania

Kenneth Schwartz, MD, FRCPC
Assistant Professor of Psychiatry
Department of Psychiatry
Baycrest
University of Toronto
Toronto, Ontario, Canada

Michael Schwartz, MD
Clinical Associate Professor of Psychiatry
Stony Brook University School of Medicine
Stony Brook, New York

Mary Shelkey, PhD, RN, ARNP
Clinical Educator
United Health/OptumCare
Seattle, Washington

Juliette Shellman, PhD, RN
Associate Professor
School of Nursing
University of Connecticut
Storrs, Connecticut

Lori Simon-Rusinowitz, MPH, PhD
Associate Professor and Acting Director
Health Services Administration and Center on Aging
School of Public Health
University of Maryland
College Park, Maryland

William Shapiro, PsyD, CGP
Program Director, Outpatient Services
Einstein Healthcare Network
Philadelphia, Pennsylvania

Tara J. Sharpp, RN, PhD
Assistant Professor
California State University
Sacramento School of Nursing
Sacramento, California

Kanwardeep Singh, MD
Geriatrician
Center for Senior Health and Longevity
Aurora Healthcare
Milwaukee, Wisconsin

Larry Z. Slater, PhD, RN-BC, CNE
Director of the Undergraduate Program
Clinical Associate Professor
Rory Meyers College of Nursing
New York University
New York, New York

Robert Smeltz, RN, MA, NP, ACHPN
Assistant Director, Palliative Care Program
University School of Medicine
Bellevue Hospital Center
New York, New York

Nicholas Sollom, MDiv
Palliative Care Chaplain
New York Health + Hospitals/Bellevue
New York, New York

Soryal A. Soryal, MD
Clinical Adjunct Associate Professor of Medicine
University of Wisconsin School of Medicine and
    Public Health
Madison, Wisconsin Geriatric Medicine
Center for Senior Health and Longevity
Milwaukee, Wisconsin

Jill Spice, MD
Chief Psychiatry Resident
University of Arizona College of Medicine
Tucson, Arizona

Anita Steliga, RN, MS, GNP
Nurse Practitioner
Center for Senior Health and Longevity
Aurora Health Care
Milwaukee, Wisconsin

Kathryn A. Stokes, PhD, CPsych
Psychologist
Neuropsychology and Cognitive Health Program
Baycrest
Toronto, Ontario, Canada

Leroy O. Stone, PhD
Adjunct Professor
Department of Demography
University of Montreal
Ottawa, Ontario, Canada

Melvin E. Stone, Jr., MD, FACS
Associate Professor of Clinical Surgery
Albert Einstein College of Medicine
Bronx, New York

Robyn Stone, DrPH
Senior VP for Research
LeadingAge LTSS Center @U Mass Boston
Washington, DC

Emily C. Stout, MSN, RN, AGPCNP-BC
Nurse Practitioner
Oncology, Massachusetts General Hospital
Boston, Massachusetts

Jeanette C. Takamura, MSW, PhD
Dean and Professor
Columbia University School of Social Work
New York, New York

Vidette Todaro-Franceschi, PhD, RN, FT
Professor
The College of Staten Island, of the City
    University of New York
Staten Island, New York

John A. Toner, EdD, PhD
Associate Professor and Senior
    Research Scientist
Columbia University;
Department of Psychiatry
New York State Psychiatric Institute
New York, New York

Hong-Phuc T. Tran, MD
Assistant Clinical Professor
UCLA Division of Geriatrics
Los Angeles, California

Angela K. Troyer, PhD, CPsych
Program Director and Professional Practice Chief of
    Psychology
Neuropsychology and Cognitive
    Health Program
Baycrest
Toronto, Ontario, Canada

Kathy VanRavenstein, PhD, APRN, FNP-BC
Assistant Professor
College of Nursing
Medical University of South Carolina
Charleston, South Carolina

Angel L. Venegas, MA
Assistant Director of Senior Services
Bridge Street Development Corporation
Brooklyn, New York

Maria L. Vezina, EdD, RN, NEA-BC
Chief Nursing Officer/Vice President, Nursing
Mount Sinai St. Luke's Hospital
New York, New York

Donald A. Vogel, AuD, CCC-A
Director
Hunter College, Center for Communication Disorders
Assistant Professor
Department of Speech-Language Pathology &
    Audiology
New York, New York

Marsha Vollbrecht, MS, CSW
Assistant Professor
Department of Speech-Language Pathology &
    Audiology
Center for Communication Disorders
New York, New York
Director of Senior Services
Aurora Health Care
Plymouth, Wisconsin

Laura M. Wagner, PhD, RN, GNP, FAAN
Associate Professor
Director, Adult Gerontology Primary Care NP Program
San Francisco School of Nursing
University of California
San Francisco, California

Lara Wahlberg, DNP, AGPCNP-BC, ACHPN, OCN
Nurse Practitioner
Palliative Care, Bellevue Hospital Center
New York University School of Medicine
New York, New York

Camille B. Warner, PhD, MA
Assistant Professor
Frances Payne Bolton
School of Nursing
Case Western Reserve University
Cleveland, Ohio

Sharon Stahl Wexler, PhD, RN, GCNS-BC, FNGNA
Associate Professor
Pace University Lienhard School of Nursing
New York, New York

Peter J. Whitehouse, MD, PhD
Professor
Department of Neurology
Case Western Reserve University
Cleveland, Ohio
Department of Medicine University of Toronto
Toronto, Ontario, Canada

Dorothy Wholihan, DNP, AGPCNP-BC, GNP-BC, ACHPN
Director
Palliative Care NP Specialty Program
Rory Meyers College of Nursing
New York University
New York, New York

Tim J. Wilkinson, MBChB, MClinEd, PhD, MD, FRACP, FRCP, FANZAHPE
Professor of Medicine
University of Otago
Christchurch, New Zealand

Amber Willink, PhD
Assistant Scientist
Roger C. Lipitz Center for Integrated
    Health Care
Department of Health Policy and Management
Johns Hopkins Bloomberg School of
    Public Health
Baltimore, Maryland

Peter C. Wolf, MD, LMSW, ACSW
Clinical Social Worker
Heron Ridge Associates
Clarkston, Michigan

Donna L. Yee, MSW, PhD
Chief Executive Officer
ACC senior Services
Sacramento, California

Chin Suk Yi, MD
Family Practice Specialist
Belleville, Michigan

LIST OF ENTRIES

A

ACCESS TO CARE

The social responsibility to provide essential health and social services relies on equitable access to care. Access to care is a multidimensional concept involving availability and affordability, timeliness and frequency, and appropriateness and acceptability, as well as quality and satisfaction. Availability simply means that the services exist and there is a possibility of use. Access implies that the available services are approachable and that the means to use them is reachable. In addition, the services must be available in a timely manner at the required frequency and should be presented in a cultural and linguistic manner acceptable to the receiver. Finally, quality of care and consumer satisfaction are related to acceptability and accessibility. The professional quality of an acceptable service may be technically very high but yield low consumer satisfaction if provided in an unacceptable manner. Despite its accessibility, a service may not be acceptable or preferred. Acceptability connotes the perceived usefulness as well as *user-friendliness* of the service to the targeted population.

ACCESS EQUITY AND DISPARITY

Differentials in access to health care by race/ethnicity and geographic location have been well documented. Racial/ethnic disparity in access to care is most accurately defined by the Institute of Medicine (2003) as "difference in access or treatment provided to members of different racial and ethnic groups that is not justified by underlying health conditions or treatment preferences of individuals" (p. 129).

BARRIERS TO EQUITABLE ACCESS

A predominant determinant of access to care is health insurance coverage. The majority of older persons (94% of persons older than 65 years) have basic health care coverage and benefits through Medicare; 54% of persons older than 65 years have additional supplementary coverage through private insurance, and 10% (or 4.6 million) receive only Medicaid (Medicaid.gov, n.d.). About 1%, or 690,000, of older persons are uninsured (The Kaiser Commission on Medicaid and the Uninsured, 2012). Moreover, as a group, elderly persons older than 65 years spent 46% more out-of-pocket on health care than their counterparts did a decade ago (The Henry J. Kaiser Family Foundation, 2012). Overall, 60% of older adults' costs are covered by Medicare, only 7% by Medicaid, 15% by other than public payers, and 18% by out-of-pocket payment (Federal Interagency Forum on Aging Related Statistics, 2011). Prescription drug costs make up a large portion of these out-of-pocket expenses. The Patient Protection and Affordable Care Act (PPACA) specifically targets prescription drug coverage by providing a monetary rebate for beneficiaries who reach the coverage limit, helping to close the coverage gap, known as the *donut hole*. Although the number of elders who have Medicaid coverage is small, the numbers vary greatly when broken down by race. Only 6% of White elders qualify as low income and have Medicaid in addition to Medicare, yet 19% of African American elders, 24% of Hispanic elders, and 21% of Asian American and Pacific Islander elders are covered by Medicaid (The Henry J. Kaiser Family Foundation and Urban Institute, 2012). In addition, approximately one third of the cost of long-term care in nursing care facilities and continuing-care retirement communities is covered by Medicaid (The Henry J. Kaiser Foundation, 2012).

A

Other determinants of access equity include low education, low socioeconomic status, and limited English proficiency. In addition, geographic proximity to services affects access as older adults residing in isolated rural areas experience access barriers to health care (Durazo et al., 2011).

Low utilization rates by minority older persons raise questions about preference for, availability of, and access to other forms of family- and community-based care for ethnic elders. Structural barriers associated with costs of care, intensity and duration of service, and location preclude drawing the conclusion that preference alone determines underserved groups' utilization of care settings. Even a public managed-care system such as the Veterans Health Administration can work nationally and regionally to address structural barriers such as rural access and acceptability based on veteran preference.

MEASURING ACCESS AND EQUITY

Measurement of access and equity access is equally complex. The rate of utilization is an essential element of measurement of access. However, the quality of services may affect utilization rates. Poor-quality services may generate high utilization rates when care is urgently needed. Still, for less needed services, low patient satisfaction may lead to low utilization of available and otherwise accessible services. The measurement of equity to access can be constructed by asking two questions: (a) What is the utilization rate as measured by the number of encounters of a particular service? and (b) What is the estimate of prevailing need within the target population differentiated by age, gender, and racial/ethnic group? Unmet needs or inequities in access are measured by subtracting the number of encounters, or utilization rate, from the estimate of the condition in the given population. Access evaluation relies on agency documentation of encounters and claims and regional or national estimates of need.

Access and health disparities must be measured by the type and level of care. Primary care providers as a usual source of care are the predominant measures of equitable access. Access must be defined in a specific relationship to a type of service. For older adults, important components of access to care include physicians, hospitals; rehabilitation, nursing home, and other therapeutic programs; skilled/nonskilled home care; specialized living arrangements; and other social services. Accessibility within a community is measured by utilization rates in relationship to the total population in need. Preventive, acute, and chronic care services for older adults present different challenges of both availability and accessibility.

CONSEQUENCES OF ACCESS DISPARITY

Differential access must be considered as a contributing factor in health status, service utilization rates and costs of care, treatment trajectories, and intervention outcomes. Race/ethnicity is an important predictor of poor health-care access for older persons. The result is often higher morbidity and mortality rates among minority populations. In addition, gender differences in chronic disease prevalence increase the need for long-term care services for older women. As an example of double jeopardy, diabetes is at least two to four times as high among African American, Hispanic, American Indian, and Asian Pacific Islander women as it is among White women (Agency for Healthcare Research and Quality [AHRQ], 2010).

IMPROVING EQUITABLE ACCESS

Further population characteristics that must be considered in relation to the accessibility of appropriate service include immigration status, neighborhood, level of disability, and living arrangements. Program characteristics include affordability, desired hours of operation, accommodating location or available transportation, timeliness of service provided, minimal intake procedures and paperwork, and outreach and information. Failure to consider population characteristics can lead to structural barriers that can significantly limit access.

Cultural barriers can make an accessible program or service unacceptable. Population characteristics to consider when creating acceptable services include ethnicity, language, family support systems, education (specifically, health literacy), number of generations since a family immigrated to the United States, and acculturation. Program characteristics include cultural and language competence and family enabling policies.

Access maximization means providing the right services for the right population at the right time and place in a manner that ensures quality and satisfaction. Underlying what providers can do to create better access locally are regional, state, and federal policy initiatives needed to ensure equitable access through adequate health care coverage.

See also Future of Care; Medicaid; Medicare; Risk Assessment and Identification in Older Adults.

Elizabeth A. Capezuti

Agency for Healthcare Research and Quality. (2010). Health care for minority women: Recent findings. Retrieved from https://www.ahrq.gov/research/findings/factsheets/minority/minorfind/index.html

Durazo, E. M., Jones, M. R., Wallace, S. P., Van Arsdale, J., Aydin, M., & Stewart, C. (2011). *The health status and unique health challenges of rural older adults in California*. Los Angeles: University of California, Los Angeles Center for Health Policy Research.

Federal Interagency Forum on Aging Related Statistics. (2011). Older Americans 2012: Key indicators of well-being. Retrieved from https://agingstats.gov/docs/PastReports/2012/OA2012.pdf

Institute of Medicine. (2003). *Unequal treatment: Confronting racial and ethnic disparities in health care*. Washington, DC: National Academies Press.

Medicaid.gov. (n.d.). Seniors & Medicare and Medicaid enrollees. Retrieved from https://www.medicaid.gov/medicaid/eligibility/medicaid-enrollees/index.html

The Henry J. Kaiser Family Foundation. (2012). Health care costs: A primer. Retrieved from http://www.kff.org/health-costs/issue-brief/health-care-costs-a-primer

The Kaiser Commission on Medicaid and the Uninsured. (2012). *The uninsured: A primer*. Menlo Park, CA: The Henry J. Kaiser Family Foundation. Retrieved from https://kaiserfamilyfoundation.files.wordpress.com/2013/01/7451-08.pdf

Web Resources
Agency for Healthcare Research and Quality: Advancing Excellence in Health Care: http://www.ahrq.gov
Robert Wood Johnson Foundation: http://www.rwjf.org
The Henry J. Kaiser Family Foundation: http://www.kff.org
U.S. Centers for Disease Control and Prevention, National Center for Health Statistics: http://www.cdc.gov/nchs

ACCESS TO HOSPICE CARE

Hospice is an approach to the care of patients and families at the end of life. Hospice care shares the same philosophy as palliative care, focusing on quality of life. Palliative care includes hospice care but can be offered to patients at all points in an illness trajectory, whereas hospice care is more strictly regulated in that a patient must have a prognosis of 6 months or less. Hospice does not incorporate curative care but instead focuses on quality of life as death approaches, and comfort is the goal. Hospice care addresses pain and symptom management, family support, and patient-centered goals in the time frame of the past 6 months of life (American Cancer Society, 2016).

Hospice is a philosophy, not a place. This end-of-life care is provided in a wide range of settings. Initially developed within a framework of home care, hospice care is now provided anywhere a patient can call home: long-term care settings, assisted-living facilities, prisons, and freestanding hospice residences. Originally provided to mostly cancer patients, it is now provided to anyone in the final stages of their illnesses. In 2014, 63.4% of hospice patients had noncancer diagnoses (National Hospice and Palliative Care Organization [NHCPO], 2015).

In addition, the number of patients who die in hospice was steadily increasing. In 2014, an estimated 1.6 to 1.7 million patients received services from hospice (NHPCO, 2015).

Although these numbers are encouraging, patients are often referred to hospice late in their disease, limiting the benefits of this multidisciplinary care (Yamagishi et al., 2014). Identifying

A

patients who can benefit from hospice and facilitating earlier referral is key to improving end-of-life care.

OPEN AND HONEST COMMUNICATION

One factor in effective end-of-life care is keeping patients and their families informed about the disease and its progression and giving everyone involved ample opportunity to ask questions and bring up unresolved issues. Open and honest communication can result in realistic goals and a plan of care that best suits the needs and wishes of the patient and family. Anyone involved in caring for patients who may be in need of hospice—physician, social worker, chaplain, family, even patients themselves—can contact a hospice program, which will then visit the patient and family, explain the services, and if appropriate, contact the primary physician enroll the patient.

EARLY REFERRALS

The patient and family should be given enough time to absorb and accept the idea of hospice. Early referral gives the hospice team more time to understand and anticipate the patient's needs. Delayed access to hospice and palliative care services is a considerable barrier in the provision of excellent end-of-life care. According to the NHPCO, an estimated 35.5% of hospice patients died or were discharged within 7 days of hospice admission. The median (50th percentile) length of service in 2014 was 17.41 days, a decrease from 18.51 days in 2013 (NHPCO, 2015).

The average time spent in hospice is frequently short because there is a lack of understanding of the services comprehensive hospice programs offer and hospice eligibility criteria (Torres, Lindstrom, & Hannah, 2016). More timely referrals are necessary for patients and families to reap the full benefits of hospice and palliative care services.

ADDRESS FINANCIAL AND CULTURAL BARRIERS

Issues regarding access to care, insurance coverage, and the potential need to hire a caregiver from outside the family contribute to financial barriers to care (NHPCO, 2013). Today, most patients in hospice are receiving care through the Medicare Hospice Benefit (NHPCO, 2015). However, families with limited social or economic resources may still have limited support to allow patients to remain at home. Clinicians must educate patients and families about alternative settings for hospice: nursing homes, assisted-living facilities, or any residential facility that patients may call home. However, several racial groups are underserved by; the NHPCO reports that 76% of hospice patients are White/Causcasian (NHPCO, 2015). Hospice services and benefits must be explained in a culturally sensitive manner to meet the needs of our increasingly diverse population (Drisdom, 2013).

Hospice provides patient- and family-focused care for diverse life-threatening illnesses. Care providers with knowledge of the services offered, awareness of barriers to access, and sensitive communication skills can increase the usage of these valuable services.

See also Hospice; Palliative Care; Primary Palliative Care.

Dorothy Wholihan

American Cancer Society. (2016). What is hospice care? Retrieved from https://www.cancer.org/treatment/finding-and-paying-for-treatment/choosing-your-treatment-team/hospice-care/what-is-hospice-care.html

Drisdom, S. (2013). Barriers to using palliative care: Insights into African American culture. *Clinical Journal of Oncology Nursing, 7*, 376–382.

National Hospice and Palliative Care Organization (2013). NHPCO's facts and figures. Retrieved from https://www.nhpco.org/sites/default/files/public/Statistics_Research/2013_Facts_Figures.pdf

National Hospice and Palliative Care Organization. (2015). NHPCO's facts and figures: Hospice care in America. Retrieved from http://www.nhpco.org/sites/default/files/public/Statistics_Research/2015_Facts_Figures.pdf

Torres, L., Lindstrom, K., & Hannah, L. (2016). Exploring barriers among primary care providers in referring patients to hospice. *Journal of Hospice and Palliative Nursing, 18*, 167–172.

Yamagishi, A., Morita, T., Kawagoe, S., Shimizu, M., Ozawa, T., & An, E.,…Miyashita, M. (2014). Length of home hospice care, family-perceived timing of referrals, perceived quality of care, and quality of death and dying in terminally ill cancer patients who died at home. *Supportive Care in Cancer*. Retrieved from http://www.mascc.org/assets/Pain_Center/2014_September/september2014-16.pdf

Web Resources

American Academy of Hospice and Palliative Medicine: http://www.aahpm.org
American Cancer Society: What is hospice care? https://www.cancer.org/treatment/finding-and-paying-for-treatment/choosing-your-treatment-team/hospice-care/what-is-hospice-care.html
Growth House, Inc.: Guide to improving care for the dying: http://www.growthhouse.org
Hospice and Palliative Nurses Association: http://www.hpna.org
Hospice Foundation of America: https://hospicefoundation.org
Hospice Network: http://www.hospicenet.org
Medicare.gov: How Hospice Works: https://www.medicare.gov/what-medicare-covers/part-a/how-hospice-works.html
National Cancer Institute: Fact sheet on hospice care: http://www.cancer.gov/cancertopics/factsheet/Support/hospice
National Hospice and Palliative Care Organization: http://www.nhpco.org

ACTIVE LIFE EXPECTANCY

The terms *active life expectancy* (ALE) and *healthy life expectancy* (HLE) are used interchangeably to refer to the average number of years from birth a person is expected to live without significant disability. ALE has become an important research focus for helping meet the medical, social, and monetary demands of the aging population. There is a global effort to maximize the health and well-being among all ages, as the number of older adults is increasing more rapidly than any other age group (United Nations Department of Economic and Social Affairs, Population Division, 2015).

It has been estimated that 15% of the U.S. population is 65 years of age and older (Population Reference Bureau [PRB], 2016), with a projected increase to 20% in the year 2030 (Ortman, Velkoff, & Hogan, 2014). According to Ortman et al. (2014), by 2050, the U.S. older adult population will nearly double to an estimated 83.7 million people compared with an estimated 43.1 million in 2012, due to increasing life expectancy and aging Baby Boomers. Many factors—including better medical technology, public health campaigns, and lifestyle changes—have led to an improved survivorship rates, thus increasing the average U.S. life expectancy (Ortman et al., 2014). At birth, the 2015 average life expectancy in the United States was calculated to be 79.3 years compared with 71.4 years globally (World Health Organization [WHO], 2015). Furthermore, the 2015 average HLE in the United States was calculated to be 69.1 years compared with 63.1 years globally (WHO, 2016). In 2013, people worldwide lost, on average, 9 years of healthy life when accounting for disability (United Nations Department of Economic and Social Affairs, Population Division, 2015). Several factors have contributed to global versus national differences in HLE, including (but not limited to) infrastructure, environment, income, lifestyle behaviors, and access to health care services. HLE in the United States increased by 1.9 years between 2000 and 2015 (WHO, 2015). With many of the nation's Baby Boomers aging and life expectancy significantly increasing over the past century, it will be important for research to emphasize strategies to maintain quality of life (QOL) and prevent substantial disability in older adults. This will help decrease caregiver and economic burden while implementing adequate social and health programs to provide the best care practices for the aging population.

Many older adults suffer from multiple chronic illnesses (MCLs) and disabilities that often lead to dependency. Therefore, prior to the inevitable process of aging, it is necessary to target population health in the younger age groups with health-promotion and disease-prevention initiatives that may preserve good health, independence, and QOL. In 2010, the fourth-generation government initiative *Healthy People 2020* was released by the United States

A

Department of Health and Human Services (USDHHS) as a 10-year agenda guiding national health-promotion and disease-prevention efforts to improve the overall health of all Americans. *Healthy People 2020* includes four overarching goals:

1. Attain high-quality, longer lives free of preventable disease, disability, injury, and premature death.
2. Achieve health equity, eliminate disparities, and improve the health of all age groups.
3. Create social and physical environments that promote good health for all.
4. Promote QOL, healthy development, and healthy behaviors across all life stages.

More specifically, two subcategories of the goals in *Healthy People 2020* target ALE from a measurable standpoint. The first subcategory is *General Health Status.* This subcategory focuses on, among other measures in progress, life expectancy (at birth and at age 65 years); HLE (expected years of life in good health, expected years of life free of limitation of activity, and expected years of life free of selected chronic diseases); and international comparisons when available. Limitation of activity is measured by the National Health Interview Survey (NHIS), examining people's ability to carry out activities of daily living (ADLs) and instrumental activities of daily living (IADLs), remember, to play, and to go to school or work, as well as an assessment of any other activity in which they may be limited (USDHHS, 2010). The second subcategory is *Health-Related Quality of Life* (HRQOL) *and Well-Being*, which focuses on all individuals and includes the multi-dimensional concepts of physical, mental, emotional, and social functioning (USDHHS, 2010). *Healthy People 2020* monitors and evaluates HRQOL measures with use of the Patient-Reported Outcomes Measurement Information System (PROMIS) Global Health Items (self-rated health), well-being measures (healthy and satisfied with life), and participation measures (education, employment, civic, social, and leisure activities).

To emphasize the importance of life satisfaction among older adults, more recent research has focused on *subjective well-being.* The findings of this research may help determine the need for innovative social programs, health policies, and treatments to enhance QOL, and help limit disability in this population. According to Scommegna (2015), researchers are examining subjective well-being by measuring life satisfaction (judgment about a satisfying life), eudaimonic well-being (sense of purpose in life), and experienced well-being (emotional quality of daily life). Higher levels of self-reported well-being have been recorded in older adults who lead active lifestyles (exercising, working, volunteering, and socializing). Lower levels of self-reported well-being have been linked with an increased risk for disease (Scommegna, 2015).

Physical inactivity, obesity, poor nutrition, excessive alcohol consumption, and smoking in older adults are some of the modifiable risk factors that have been studied and found to lead to increased rates of disability, hospitalization, morbidity, and mortality. Many studies have been conducted and several more are underway to help identify and implement health programs and interventions to reduce the disability and chronic illnesses that often result from poor lifestyle behaviors. One study reported by Pahor et al. (2014) found that a long-term, moderate-intensity physical activity program (aerobic, resistance, and flexibility training) for older adults at risk for disability reduced major mobility disability (ability to walk 400 m) over 2.6 years. A study of four European cohorts (England, Finland, France, and Sweden) examining modifiable risk factors revealed that both men and women who did not engage in risk-related behaviors (smoking, physical inactivity, and obesity) could expect to live an average of 6 years longer free from chronic illnesses and 8 years longer in good health between the ages of 50 and 75 years old when compared with their counterparts who engaged in at least two risk-related behaviors (Stenholm et al., 2016). Older adults who limit or refrain from poor health behaviors while participating in positive health behaviors may also reduce their risk for disability and improve QOL.

Older adults are the fastest growing global population, making it necessary to implement social programs, best-practice protocols, and disease prevention initiatives to promote wellness and to maintain independence in this population. The promotion of ALE continues to be at the forefront of national and global agendas to limit health expenditures, morbidity, mortality, and disability while improving QOL, longevity, and productivity of the older adult population. The ongoing focus of research in this population should be the implementation of health-promotion and health-prevention measures. However, it is also important to extend ALE by promoting healthy lifestyles among younger age groups, thus limiting many of the ill effects that may be manifested in later age but are, in large part, due to early risk-related behaviors.

See also African Americans and Health Care Disparities; Aging Prisoners; American Indian Elders; Demography of Aging; Employment; Hispanic and Latino Elders; Immigrant Elders, Rural Elderly.

Dominica Potenza

Ortman, J. M., Velkoff, V. A., & Hogan, H. (2014). An aging nation: The older population in the United States. Retrieved from https://www.census.gov/prod/2014pubs/p25-1140.pdf

Pahor, M., Guralnik, J. M., Ambrosius, W. T., Blair, S., Bonds, D. E., Church, T. S.,…Williamson, J. D. (2014). Effect of structured physical activity on prevention of major mobility disability in older adults: The LIFE study randomized clinical trial. *Journal of the American Medical Association, 311*(23), 2387–2396.

Population Reference Bureau. (2016). World population data sheet. Retrieved from http://www.prb.org/pdf16/prb-wpds2016-web-2016.pdf

Scommegna, P. (2015). Research on health and well-being aims to improve quality of life in later years. *Today's Research on Aging: Program and Policy Implications* (31), 1–7. Retrieved from http://www.prb.org/Publications/Reports/2015/todays-research-aging-wellbeing.aspx

Stenholm, S., Head, J., Kivimaki, M., Kawachi, I., Aalto, V., Zins, M.,…Vahtera, J. (2016). Smoking, physical inactivity and obesity as predictors of healthy and disease-free life expectancy between ages 50 and 75: A multicohort study. *International Journal of Epidemiology, 45*(4), 1260–1270. doi:10.1093/ije/dyw126

United States Department of Health and Human Services. (2010). Office of Disease Prevention and Health Promotion. Healthy People 2020 (ODPHP Publication No. B0132). Retrieved from https://www.healthypeople.gov/sites/default/files/HP2020_brochure_with_LHI_508_FNL.pdf

United Nations Department of Economic and Social Affairs, Population Division. (2015). World Population Ageing (ST/ESA/SER.A/390). Retrieved from http://www.un.org/en/development/desa/population/publications/pdf/ageing/WPA2015_Report.pdf

World Health Organization (2015). World Report on Ageing and Health. Retrieved from http://apps.who.int/iris/bitstream/10665/186463/1/9789240694811_eng.pdf

Web Resources
Healthy People 2020: https://www.healthypeople.gov
Population Reference Bureau: http://www.worldpopdata.org
World Health Organization: Global Health Observatory Data: http://www.who.int/gho/mortality_burden_disease/life_tables/hale/en

ACTIVITIES OF DAILY LIVING

Activities of daily living (ADLs) are broadly defined as basic everyday tasks that are required to take care of one's body for the maintenance of health and independent living. Health professionals also refer to ADLs as "basic activities of daily living (BDL)" or "personal activities of daily living (PDL)" (Roley et al., 2008). The six activities usually included in an ADL examination are bathing, dressing, toileting, transferring, continence, and eating. The ability to perform these six activities are theorized to represent the attainment of self-care independence in children—a precursor to independent living. With the proliferation of ADL assessment tools, more diverse activities such as sexual activity, locomotion, and personal hygiene were included. The assessment of ADL in the older adult provides a means of quantifying functional ability that can be used diagnostically and for outcomes assessment (Crabtree, 2007). In addition, ADL status is predictive of nursing home admission and the use of health services, making its assessment potentially useful for screening purposes.

A

Instrumental activities of daily living (IADLs) are commonly assessed in conjunction with ADLs. These activities are more complex than ADLs and require physical, cognitive, memory, attention, decision-making, and problem-solving abilities. Examples include activities such as home establishment and management, meal preparation and cleanup, shopping, the care of pets, communication, financial management, safety, community living skills, health management and maintenance, caring for others, and religious observance (Roley et al., 2008). ADLs and IADLs are thought to be hierarchically related, with dysfunctions in IADLs representing less severe functional disabilities. Examining IADL in older adults provides information about their ability to adapt to the environment, information not gathered by examining ADLs alone.

Rogers, Meyer, Neff, and Fisk (1998) introduced another category of activates that older adults need to be able to perform; these are referred to as *enhanced activities of daily living* (EADLs). EADLs examine an older adult's ability to adapt to a changing environment and include keeping up with technology, communicating with family and friends, and performing hobbies or leisure activities. The cognitive demands of EADLs are thought to be greater than either ADLs or IADLs. EADLs assessments are carried out primarily in ergonomic studies in which considerations of how older adults keep up with technological and communicative development are pertinent in the design of spaces where they live.

EXAMINATION OF ADL AND IADL

The central reason for performing ADL and IADL examinations is to obtain information about the older adult's functional ability. Obtaining information about functional ability is important because function is linked to an individual's health and well-being. Philosophically, the assessments should be patient centered—that is, the patient's goals are central to the evaluation process. Examinations should, when possible, be performed within the patients' normal living environments to better understand how they functions within their own context. The information gained from the examination of

ADLs and IADL may then be used to diagnose functional deficits, quantify changes in function, provide a guide for intervention and discharge planning, screen for deficits in function, guide the planning of major elective surgeries and procedures, provide data for evidence-based practice, and assist in determining the need for nursing home care. However, it should be noted that examination decisions may also be driven by reimbursement considerations. For example, in the United States, third-party payers may dictate what is to be examined.

With an aging population, the already prohibitive cost of institutionalizing older adults is expected to increase. Therefore examinations that assist in identifying markers to predict institutionalization may be useful in developing programs geared toward preventing institutionalization. As noted, one of the considerations for nursing home admission is limitations in ADLs. Fong, Mitchell, and Koh (2015) examined which of the six ADLs (bathing, dressing, eating, walking, transferring, and toileting) were more predictive of nursing home admission. The bathing limitation was found to be the only ADL that was significantly predictive of nursing home admission. Thus programs geared toward facilitating older adults aging-in-place may use limitations in the bathing ADL as a marker of possible institutionalization once these findings are confirmed in future studies.

The International Classification of Functioning, Disability and Health (ICF) model, proposed by the WHO, provides a useful theoretical framework under which ADL and IADL examinations may be performed. Part of the utility of this classification system is that it is universal and not limited to any specific grouping. The ICF classification system defines the dynamically related health and health-related domains: body function and structure, activities, and participation. The ICF system also considers body, individual, social, and environmental perspectives. This classification system is useful for categorizing, understanding, and measuring health outcomes.

In keeping with the ICF model, the examination of each individual should be a multipart process that involves determining the physical or physiological capacity for change, analyzing the task to be performed, and examining the influence of the individual's environment. In this three-point assessment, ADL and IADL measures are used to assess activity limitation and participation restriction. When this analysis is performed, care should be taken to distinguish between what individuals want to do, what they can do, and what they actually do (Quinn et al., 2011). Information is also needed on the way that an ADL or IADL task is performed, the time when it is performed, the quality of performance, the amount of assistance needed, and the use of any assistive technology and devices.

TOOLS USED TO EXAMINE ADL AND IADL

When an examination tool is selected, consideration should be given to the type of examination tool, the context in which the examination is to be performed, and the psychometric properties of the tool. For example, in a validation study of a 15-item ADL/IADL scale, the authors concluded that the tool was poorly targeted toward older adults living in the community and should not be used to compare older adults residing in residential care facilities and those dwelling in the community (Lutomski et al., 2016). Examination tools for ADLs and IADLs may be classified as self-reported or caregiver reported, interview based, or observation based. In addition, assessment tools can also be described broadly as qualitative (based on subjective assessment) or quantitative (based on objective measures). The type of examination tools chosen may also be dependent on contextual issues such as cultural and reimbursement differences internationally. Irrespective of the type, the tool chosen should be reliable, valid, sensitive, and responsive to changes in the patient.

Each type of examination tool has different strengths and weaknesses. The report- and interview-based examinations tend to be qualitative and depend on the subjective assessments of the patient, caregiver, or health care provider. These subjective assessments can be affected by cognitive status, mood, and/or bias of the reporters. They are, however, easier to administer but may give a snapshot representation of the patient (Lowe et al., 2013). The observation-based

assessments can be quantitative, for example, providing an exact measure of the distance walked. However, they are less easy to administer and may represent the performance of the individual only at the time of assessment.

A variety of examination tools measures the older adult's ADL and IADL performance, but to date there is no established gold standard for such assessment because few have been comprehensively evaluated (Lowe et al., 2013). Along with the proliferation of functional assessment tools Lowe et al. (2013) describe the evolution of three new categories of tools referred to as combination, global assessment, and performance based. The combination tools include ADL and IADL assessments; global assessment tools include assessments of ADL, IADL, psychological, and social ability; and performance-based assessments generate performance measures. Examples of each of the five categories of tools are: ADL assessment tools (the Barthel Index and Katz Scale); IADL assessment tools (Frenchay Activities Index [FAI] and Lawton Instrumental Activities of Daily Living Scale [IADL]; combination tools (Functional Independence Measure [FIM] and Groningen Activity Restriction Scale [GARS]); global assessment tools (Health Assessment Questionnaire [HAQ] and the Short Form 36 [SF-36]); and performance tools (the Physical Performance Test [PPT] and Short Physical Performance Battery [SPPB]).

INTERVENTION

ADL and IADL intervention strategies include restoring function and compensating or adapting for performance limitations (Christiansen, Haertl, & Robinson, 2009). Restoration strategies are designed to correct pathologies at the body function and structure level, such as strength and balance, that contribute to impairments in the performance of ADL and IADL (Vermeulen, Neyens, van Rossum, Spreeuwenberg, & de Witte, 2011). Compensatory strategies may involve the use of assistive devices, environmental modifications, and/or task modifications. Choosing restoration or compensation as an intervention strategy depends on clinical judgment, prognosis, and the expectations for physiological improvement (Christiansen et al., 2009).

A

Intervening involves establishing realistic goals based on consideration of the individual's and caregiver's needs, the demands of the task, and the environment. Intervention approaches that are relevant and medically necessary are available from a variety of health care providers, including occupational therapists, physical therapists, nurses, and trained caregivers. ADL and IADL interventions should consider the individual's ability to learn or relearn the needed tasks; the complexities of the tasks; and the techniques, equipment, or technology needed. ADL and IADL interventions consider the value of the task to the individual, the level of performance, and overall safety. Assistive technology or devices may be used, depending on input from the individual, the ability to use such equipment, financial resources, and the outcome. Intervention outcomes are determined by postintervention examinations that include discharge planning, safety assessments, and caregiver education. The ability to perform ADL and IADL tasks is critical to the older adult's level of independence, safety, and quality of life.

A burgeoning front into understanding disability in ADLs among older adults is investigation into sedentary behavior. Traditionally, sedentary behavior was thought to be mitigated with activity; however, under this new conceptualization sedentary behavior is viewed as an independent risk factor for disability in ADLs. That is, the amount of time spent in sedentary behavior is driving disability in ADLs irrespective of the amount of time spent engaging in activity. Dunlop et al. (2015) investigated this hypothesis using a sample of older adults participating in The National Health and Nutrition Examination Survey (NHANES). The authors reported that the odds of having a disability in ADLs were approximately 50% greater for every hour increase in sedentary time independent of time spent engaged in moderate-vigorous activity. Although this finding warrants further investigation, the amount of time spent engaging in sedentary behaviors should also be considered when interventions aimed at improving ALDs are devised for older adults.

See also Assistive Technology; Cognitive Changes in Aging; Occupational Therapy Assessment and Evaluation; Physical Therapy Services; Rehabilitation; Rheumatoid Arthritis.

Sylvester Carter

Christiansen, C. H., Haertl, K., & Robinson, L. (2009). Self-care. In B. R. Bonder, V. Dal Bello-Haas, & M. B. Wagner (Eds.), *Functional performance in older adults* (3rd ed., Vol. 3, pp. 265–289). Philadelphia, PA: F. A. Davis.

Crabtree, J. L. (2007). Assessing activities of daily living. In C. A. Emlet, V. A. Condon, & J. L. Crabtree (Eds.), *In-home assessment of older adults: An interdisciplinary approach* (pp. 101–116). Gaithersburg, MD: Aspen.

Dunlop, D. D., Song, J., Arnston, E. K., Semanik, P. A., Lee, J., Chang, R. W., & Hootman, J. M. (2015). Sedentary time in US older adults associated with disability in activities of daily living independent of physical activity. *Journal of Physical Activity and Health, 12*(1), 93–101. doi:10.1123/jpah.2013-0311

Fong, J. H., Mitchell, O. S., & Koh, B. S. (2015). Disaggregating activities of daily living limitations for predicting nursing home admission. *Health Services Research, 50*(2), 560–578. doi:10.1111/1475-6773.12235

Lutomski, J. E., Krabbe, P. F. M., den Elzen, W. P. J., Olde-Rikkert, M. G. M., Steyerberg, E. W., Muntinga, M. E.,...Melis, R. J. F. (2016). Rasch analysis reveals comparative analyses of activities of daily living/instrumental activities of daily living summary scores from different residential settings is inappropriate. *Journal of Clinical Epidemiology, 74*, 207–217. doi:10.1016/j.jclinepi.2015.11.006

Rogers, W. A., Meyer, B., Neff, W., & Fisk, A. D. (1998). Functional limitations to daily living tasks in the aged: A focus group analysis. *Human Factors, 40*(1), 111.

Roley, S. S., DeLany, J. V., Barrows, C. J., Brownrigg, S., Honaker, D., Sava, D. I.,...Youngstrom, M. J. (2008). Occupational therapy practice framework: Domain & process, 2nd edition. *American Journal of Occupational Therapy, 62*, 625–628.

Web Resources

American Occupational Therapy Association, Inc.: http://www.aota.org

American Physical Therapy Association: http://www.apta.org

Assistive Technology: http://www.resna.org/resna/webres.htm

Centers for Medicare & Medicaid Services: http://www.cms.hhs.gov

ADULT DAY SERVICES

Adult day services (ADS) are community-based, long-term care group programs that provide elderly individuals and their caregivers with out-of-home support for part of the day. These programs give older adults an opportunity for socialization through peer support and supervised activities. They may also offer specialized services such as nursing, speech therapy, physical therapy, and counseling (Dabelko-Schoeny & King, 2010; Valadez, Lumadue, Gutierrez, & de Vries-Kell, 2006). ADS providers work with elderly individuals to maintain their physical and mental functioning and well-being longer than if they were in an institutional setting (Gitlin, Reever, Dennis, Mathieu, & Hauck, 2006). Another important function of ADS is to provide respite to prevent caregiver burnout and enhance family functioning. It allows caregivers time to work, run errands, or perform other tasks that might not be completed if they were supervising their elderly relatives. According to a national study of ADS (MetLife, 2010), more than 4,600 ADS programs nationwide provide services for approximately 260,000 participants. Most ADS participants attend all day (81%) for 5 days a week (46%). The average length of stay in a program is 24 months (MetLife, 2010).

TYPES OF PROGRAMS

ADS programs usually fit one of three models: social, medical, or a combination of the two. Social ADS programs provide socialization, creative and educational activities, meals and nutritional monitoring, and supervision by professional staff, as well as medication management in some programs. This program type usually offers little or no personal care. Medical ADS programs, also referred to as adult day health care (ADHC), are for individuals requiring more intensive levels of personal and medical care. Typically, ADHC programs offer medical, nursing, and personal care as well as physical, occupational, and other forms of therapy. Participants at medical adult day centers require physician orders to receive medical treatment. The Programs of All-Inclusive Care for the Elderly (PACE) is a well-known example of medical ADS. PACE uses multidisciplinary case-management teams and delivers services through adult day health facilities to assist nursing home–eligible older adults to remain in the community. A key aspect of PACE is the integration of various funding sources, including Medicare and Medicaid capitation payments, to coordinate services that foster the health, well-being, and independence of program participants (Hirth, Baskins, & Dever-Bumba, 2009; National PACE Association, 2016).

The combined or mixed ADS model incorporates concepts that fall under the social and medical models. In addition to these three options, some programs focus on narrowly defined patient populations. Such population-specific ADS centers provide targeted services to individuals with unique health needs, such as persons with dementia or rehabilitation patients. Some ADS centers include intergenerational programming and joint activities with child day care or other community programs. Two thirds of ADS providers offer caregiver support groups, 40% provide individual counseling, and 70% incorporate educational programs (MetLife, 2010).

POLICIES AND STANDARDS

Although organizations such as the National Adult Day Services Association (NADSA) and the Commission on Accreditation of Rehabilitation Facilities (CARF) created standards and guidelines for ADS programs, there are currently no mandatory national standards (NADSA, 2016). Significant regulatory variations exist from state to state. Approximately half of states require a license to operate an adult day facility (U.S. Department of Health and Human Services (USDHHS), 2016). Medicaid certification is required for programs using this funding source. The USDHHS provides a regularly updated overview of programs by state and geographic region (HHS, 2016).

PROGRAM CHARACTERISTICS AND STAFFING

A national survey of adult day centers found that programs are generally open 8 hours a day, Monday to Friday, with few ADS providers offering weekend services (RWJF, 2003). A majority of programs are nonprofit (78%) and operate under the purview of larger parent organizations (70%) such as hospitals, nursing homes, or religious organizations (RWJF, 2003). A typical ADS program enrolls approximately 57 patients, with an average daily attendance of 34 persons (Anderson, Dabelko-Schoeney & Johnson, 2012). Most adult day centers offer transportation services to program participants.

Because there are no uniform requirements for providers, staffing may vary significantly among programs. According to the MetLife (2010) survey, 80% of ADS centers have nursing staff, 50% have social workers, 60% have case managers, and 50% have physical, occupational, or speech therapists. Many states spell out participant-to-staff ratios. They vary from 8:1 for regular ADS to 3:1 for programs specializing in dementia services (USDHHS, 2006). In medical programs, the nurses administer medications, and manage or monitor the personal and medical care of patients as directed by an individual's physician. Licensed social workers assist with accessing social services, offer caregiver support groups, and provide counseling to patients and caregivers. Their tasks may also include outreach, intake and assessment, advocacy, care management, crisis intervention, and assistance with Medicaid applications (Johnson, Sakaris, Tripp, Vroman, & Wood, 2004). Specialized therapies are provided by physical, occupational, and speech therapists. Social workers, nurses, recreational therapists, aides, or volunteers may be responsible for the social, creative, and educational activities of an ADS program.

The costs of ADS vary greatly, depending on the type of program and the services used. Public funding through the Medicaid home and community-based waivers, the Veterans Administration, and state programs accounts for 55% of ADS provider revenue. An additional 13% of costs are covered by grants, donations, and fundraising. Approximately 26% of program costs are covered through participant fees (Anderson, Dabelko-Schoeney & Johnson, 2012). The average full day participant fee is $70.00 (MetLife, 2010). Depending on the state and region, the costs range from $9,000 to $30,000 annually, being on average one-third less expensive than home health care or assisted-living programs (Genworth, 2015).

ACCESS TO SERVICES

The first step in accessing ADS is to obtain the most current information about programs in the geographic area. Next, the practitioner and patient should review the options and discuss which programs would best fit the patient's needs. In nonurban and rural areas, there might be few or no program options available. A visit to the program site should be planned before enrollment, and if possible, a practitioner should accompany patient and caregiver on this visit. If the patient is considering an ADHC program, it is helpful to speak with members of the medical staff and inquire about the appropriateness of the medical-care options. Other areas to take into account are the social and recreational activities offered.

Although it is difficult to judge the quality of a program based on one visit, interactions between staff and program participants may be a good indicator of the facility's overall atmosphere. Many programs let potential patients spend some time and attend group activities to find out whether they like the program. Other factors to appraise are personnel and physical environment. Do qualified personnel provide the services? What is the patient–staff ratio? What are the overall condition and physical environment of the facility? Are there enough handrails, signs, and adequate lighting? Does the program offer or coordinate transportation services? Will program personnel come into the home to pick up patients? Once a decision is made, the patient may need assistance completing the application. An important role for the practitioner is to review and educate the patient about the contractual terms of the adult day center.

RECOMMENDATIONS

Research indicates continued regional gaps in the availability and utilization of ADS. These gaps in service delivery are influenced by program costs, inadequate funding, transportation availability, the fit between locally available services and patient needs, and patient refusal to participate in such programs (Anderson, Dabelko-Schoeny, & Tarrant, 2012). Suggestions for increasing availability and utilization include increased public awareness, improved transportation, provision of more counseling services, and establishment of quality-of-care standards (Anderson, Dabelko-Schoeney, & Johnson, 2012; Anderson, Dabelko-Schoeney, & Tarrant, 2012; RWJF, 2003). As with other services, cultural differences exist in the way older adults utilize ADS programs. The heavy reliance on participant fees may pose a financial barrier for older adults from lower economic backgrounds. Additional emphasis should be placed on evaluating service utilization and potential access barriers for individuals from different cultural and economic backgrounds.

See also Caregiver Burnout; Programs of All-Inclusive Care for the Elderly (PACE).

Matthias J. Naleppa

Anderson, K., Dabelko-Schoeney, H., & Johnson, T. D. (2012). The state of adult day services: Findings from the MetLife National Study of Adult Day Services. *Journal of Applied Gerontology, 32,* 729–748.

Anderson, K., Dabelko-Schoeney, H., & Tarrant, S. (2012). A constellation of concerns: Exploring the present and the future challenges of adult day services. *Home Health Care Management & Practice, 24,* 132–139.

Dabelko-Schoeny, H., & King, S. (2010). In their own words: Participants' perceptions of the impact of adult day services. *Journal of Gerontological Social Work, 53*(2), 176–192.

Genworth. (2015). Genworth 2015 financial cost of care survey. Retrieved from http://www.genworth .com/dam/Americas/US/PDFs/Consumer/corporate/130568_040115_gnw.pdf

Gitlin, L., Reever, K., Dennis, M., Mathieu, E., & Hauck, W. (2006). Enhancing quality of life of families who use adult day services: Short- and long-term effects on the adult day service plus program. *The Gerontologist, 46*(5), 630–639.

Hirth, V., Baskins, J., & Dever-Bumba, M. (2009). Program of all-inclusive care (PACE): Past, present, and future. *Journal of the American Medical Directors Association, 10*(3), 155–160.

Johnson, J., Sakaris, J., Tripp, D., Vroman, K., & Wood, S. (2004). The role of social work in adult day services. *Journal of Social Work in Long-Term Care, 3*(1), 3–13.

MetLife Mature Market Institute. (2010). The MetLife National Study of adult day services. Retrieved from https://www.metlife.com/assets/cao/mmi/publications/studies/2010/mmi-adult-day-services.pdf

National Adult Day Services Association. (2016). About adult day services. Retrieved from http://www.nadsa.org/learn-more/about-adult-day-services

National PACE Association. (2016). About NPA. Retrieved from http://www.npaonline.org/about-npa

Robert Wood Johnson Foundation. (2003). The role of adult day services. Retrieved from http://www.rwjf.org/en/library/articles-and-news/2003/04/the-role-of-adult-day-services.html

U.S. Department of Health and Human Services. (2006). Adult day services: A key community service for older adults. Retrieved from https://aspe.hhs.gov/basic-report/adult-day-services-key-community-service-older-adults

U.S. Department of Health and Human Services. (2016). Overview of adult day service regulations. Retrieved from https://aspe.hhs.gov/sites/default/files/pdf/109701/adultday1.pdf

Valadez, A., Lumadue, C., Gutierrez, B., & de Vries-Kell, S. (2006). Las Comadres and adult day care centers: The perceived impact of socialization on mental wellness. *Journal of Aging Studies, 20,* 39–53.

Web Resources

Commission on Accreditation of Rehabilitation Facilities: http://www.carf.org

National Adult Day Services Association: http://www.nadsa.org

State Regulations for Adult Day Services: http://www.nadsa.org/providers/state-regulations

A

ADULT FOSTER CARE HOMES

Since the 1980s, alternative housing options for the elderly have been proliferated in the United States. These alternative settings provide

A

varying degrees of assistance. The adult foster care (AFC) home is among the oldest forms of such housing options available to older adults who have difficulty living alone due to physical and mental disabilities (Mollica et al., 2009). AFC homes are known by different names (i.e., board and care or group homes) and may operate under varying licensure requirements (Piche, 2012). Despite the lack of national standards and regulation, AFCs share an underlying philosophy of aging-in-place. More specifically, AFC homes provide long-term personalized care and supportive assistance to older adults in a home-like environment so that they can remain in their communities (Reinhard et al., 2014; Wardrip, 2010).

A defining feature of AFCs is that they serve a smaller number of residents than assisted-living residences. With a few exceptions, most states limit the number of residents, and differentiate between foster care and assisted living, to no more than six residents (Piche, 2012). In New York and Arizona, for example, homes with fewer than four care recipients are considered AFC homes, whereas those serving more than four are adult homes or assisted-living facilities. In New Jersey, single adult foster homes are allowed, and those who have two or more adults are licensed as an assisted-living facility. California and Illinois, on the other hand, do not differentiate between AFC and assisted living based on the number of residents. Therefore the same program that can be used for assisted living can be used for AFC.

SERVICES

In general, an AFC home can be an operator's private home, part of a two-family house, or part of an apartment building that is residentially zoned with an unrelated, live-in caregiver (Piche, 2012). The home must be maintained by the operator in a safe and comfortable environment. AFCs can provide a wide range of services, somewhat dependent on whether the AFC is associated with a medical center or social services agency, including room, board, housekeeping, personal care, case management, and supervision. AFC caregivers may also supervise medications, including injections, and provide

specialized nutrition, bladder training, catheter irrigations, and dressing changes (Piche, 2012). Residents are not confined to the home and can attend senior centers, sheltered workshops, and other supportive and social activities. During the preadmission process, potential residents are interviewed and screened to determine that their needs can be met safely in the AFC environment. Older adults who require a higher level of care, such as continuous skilled medical or nursing services, are referred to appropriate residential services.

COSTS

The cost of AFC varies by geographic location and level of care or services provided to the resident. Residential services and supportive care are included in a monthly charge and, varying by state, payment may be arranged through private-pay or government assistance. For low-income residents, Supplemental Security Income (SSI) covers some of the room and board portion of services. Medicaid programs typically pay for personal care provided in AFC. Covered services differ by state and program and may include Medicaid, Medicaid-managed long-term care, and home and community-based waivers that provide personal care benefits as an alternative to nursing home care.

In New York, for example, SSI pays a congregate care rate for the older adult's room, board, and services. The resident receives a portion of the rate as a personal-needs allowance, and the balance is paid to the operator (Piche, 2012). All services and fees are set out in a written admission agreement that is signed by the operator and the resident prior to the date of admission. This agreement describes all provisions and requirements of residency, including the resident's rights and responsibilities, house rules, admission, discharge, and transfer procedures, the range of services provided, and financial arrangements (e.g., personal-needs allowance, refunds, and security deposits).

OPERATORS AND CAREGIVERS

AFC operators include non-for-profit or for-profit corporations, individual home owners, and public agencies. Employees must comply with hiring standards regulated by state licensure requirements, including required education, work experience, certification and formal training commensurate with AFC titles or roles. Formal training of caregivers is designed to teach the skills and knowledge required to meet the residents' needs, such as nutrition services, assistance with personal care, supervision, medication assistance, and physical environment. Employees of AFCs may also be required to complete an orientation pertinent to the characteristics of residents served—such as residents' rights, mental health, abuse and neglect, physical environment, and psychosocial aspects of aging and illness—before employment or placement of the first resident following initial licensure (Mollica et al., 2009).

CHOOSING AN AFC HOME

Like any housing option, AFCs vary widely in the qualifications and capabilities of the operators, quality of care, and environment. Older adults and their family members who are considering an AFC home should thoroughly research potential homes and caregivers. If the AFC home is certified or licensed by the state, potential residents can review public records such as the AFC's most recent survey report, making note of any deficiencies. Older adults should visit potential AFCs to evaluate safety and physical considerations, such as safe entries and exits, well-lighted entry and parking areas, wheelchair access, maintenance of grounds and building, presence of smoke detectors and handrails, and availability of a private bedroom. The environment should be clean and free of odors with good ventilation and comfortable temperatures. The AFC should also be easily accessible to family and friends and near the older adult's doctor or hospital. Caregivers should be evaluated to ensure they are able to provide residents with the necessary services to live comfortably in their environment, hire and maintain qualified staff members, treat residents with respect and dignity, uphold residents' rights, and address allegations or incidents of abuse or neglect (Reinhard et al., 2014). Minimal caregiver training should include first

aid skills, safety and fire prevention, and prevention and containment of communicable diseases.

Financial considerations are, of course, critical for the selection process because not all AFCs accept Medicaid. Families should determine whether a basic fee covers all services or additional fees are required for services such as laundry or amenities such as telephone, cable television, or Internet access. Families should know how and under what circumstances they can terminate the contract (e.g., a change in the resident's medical or mental health condition).

The nation's aging population and longer life expectancies will increase demand for alternative residential care environments and for caregivers able to support the complex, evolving needs of older adults. AFC homes offer a viable alternative to institutionalization for older adults with a range of functional and cognitive impairments and psychosocial needs. Implications for future research and policy in AFCs include addressing the lack of a shared definition or regulations that standardize services provided and qualifications of AFC caregivers and employees.

Ihab Girgis

Mollica, R. L., Simms-Kastelein, K., Cheek, M., Baldwin, C., Farnham, J., Reinhard, S., & Accius, J. (2009). Building adult foster care: What states can do (AARP Research Report, AARP Public Policy Institute). Retrieved from http://www.aarp.org/ppi

Piche, R. (2012). Livable New York resource manual: Family types home for adults. Retrieved from http://www.aging.ny.gov/LivableNY/ResourceManual/Index.cfm

Reinhard, S. C., Kassner, E., Houser, A., Ujvari, K., Mollica, R., & Hendrickson, L. (2014). *Raising expectations: A state scorecard on long-term services and supports for older adults, people with physical disabilities, and family caregivers* (2nd ed.). Washington, DC: AARP Public Policy Institute, The Commonwealth Fund, The SCAN Foundation. Retrieved from http://www.longtermscorecard.org

Wardrip, K. (2010, March). Adult foster care: Fact sheet 174 (AARP Public Policy Institute). Retrieved from http://www.aarp.org/ppi

ADULT PROTECTIVE SERVICES

A

Adult protective services (APS) is the primary social services provided by state and local governments nationwide to vulnerable adults with cognitive or physical impairments who are at risk or in need of assistance. APS workers often serve as first responders in cases of elder abuse, neglect, or exploitation, collaborating with family members, physicians, nurses, social workers, case managers, paramedics, firefighters, and law enforcement professionals to identify and address problems in the community.

Many adults with functional or cognitive impairments live independently without assistance. Some are abused or neglected by formal or informal caregivers and need someone to advocate on their behalf. Other adults have difficulties performing activities of daily living and may benefit from support services to maintain their health and independence in the community. APS workers investigate reports of physical abuse, sexual abuse, emotional or psychological abuse, caregiver neglect and self-neglect, or financial exploitation and assess each adult's biopsychosocial functioning, needs, and resources. If APS evaluates the adult to be at risk and in need of assistance, they develop a service plan to address and resolve vulnerabilities and help maintain the person safely while preserving the adult's right to self-determination and maximizing independence.

Although regulations vary widely, APS is generally provided to adults who are 18 years of age and older who, because of mental or physical impairments, are unable to meet their essential needs for food, shelter, clothing, or medical care; need to secure services or supports or protect themselves from physical or emotional injury, neglect, maltreatment, or financial exploitation; need protection from actual or threatened harm, neglect, or hazardous conditions caused by the action or inaction of themselves or others; and have no one available who is willing and able to assist them responsibly. APS is one of the few social services that initiate involuntary interventions when a patient is deemed to be in critical need of assistance. These interventions include involuntary financial management, access to a patient's home to make an assessment, and application for legal guardianship to protect a patient from elder abuse or neglect.

Some 90% of states provide protective services to vulnerable adults, covering risks that include physical abuse, sexual abuse, emotional abuse, financial exploitation, caregiver neglect and self-neglect. Definitions vary, but the operational definitions of mistreatment are similar. The primary activities covered by most state statutes include receiving reports; conducting investigations; evaluating patient risk and capacity to agree to services; performing voluntary and involuntary interventions depending on the person's risks or needs; developing and implementing a case plan; counseling the patient; arranging for a large variety of services and benefits; and monitoring ongoing service delivery.

In 1974, Title XX of the Social Security Act empowered states to use Social Services Block Grant (SSBG) funds for the protection of adults as well as children. All states have independently created laws and regulations to govern APS, and most have implemented similar models of service delivery. Services include social casework with a coordinated, multi-disciplinary system of social and health services. The services are designed to enable elderly and/or vulnerable adults to continue living independently in the community and to protect them from abuse.

How does the APS process work?

1. A referral is made to APS to report concerns about the welfare of a vulnerable adult who is at risk.
2. The referral is screened by an APS worker to evaluate whether it meets the statutory requirements for APS.
3. If the situation meets criteria for abuse, neglect, or exploitation, APS initiates an investigation with the goal of face-to-face contact with the adult needing assistance.
4. An APS worker assesses the adult's safety and need for assistance to determine what services should be in place to address the risks and develops a service plan that is the least restrictive and tries to preserve the patient's right to self-determination.

5. Some cases may require longer-term case management for the provision of services, such as guardianship, financial management, and home care.

The goal of APS is to develop service plans that are least restrictive and, where possible, respect a person's right to self-determination. The focus should not be on involuntary interventions. Essential services should not be denied because a person lacks the ability to consent to such services. Involuntary interventions are contemplated as a last resort.

In most states, APS resides in the Department of Social Services. Other agencies where APS resides include the Department for the Aging and Departments of Health and Rehabilitation. Most states empower APS with the responsibility of investigating abuse reports in long-term care facilities. Sometimes, this role is shared with the long-term care ombudsman and/or other regulatory agencies (APWA Report, 1994). Regardless of location, there are certain basic principles that are fundamental to APS and guide the delivery of services (National Adult Protective Services Association [NAPSA], 2004). They include the following:

• Every action taken by APS must balance the duty to protect the safety of the vulnerable adult with the adult's right to self-determination.
• Adults have the right to be safe.
• Adults retain all their civil and constitutional rights unless some of these rights have been restricted by court action.
• Adults have the right to make decisions that do not conform with societal norms as long as these decisions do not harm others.
• Adults are presumed to have decision-making capacity unless a court adjudicates otherwise.
• Adults have the right to accept or refuse services.
• Practice tends to be pragmatic.

Each state has some form of legislation addressing APS for vulnerable adults, but statutes vary widely. To know when, where, and what to report to whom, familiarity with a state's APS laws is essential. A listing of state APS statutes is on the Elder Justice Coalition website (www .elderjusticecoalition.com).

Given that the problem affects an estimated 10% of older adults (Lachs & Pillemer, 2015), elder abuse and mistreatment remains a hidden problem. Often, victims are reluctant to self-report due to shame, fear, or the physical or mental inability to do so. In most states, a range of professionals, including physicians, health care professionals, law enforcement officers, social workers, staff in long-term care facilities, and mental health professionals, are mandated to report incidents of suspected abuse. Many state statutes include protections for "good-faith reporting," as well as penalties for failure to report.

The ongoing casework relationship provides essential emotional support to the victim. Once services have been initiated, the APS professional may monitor the service delivery or turn over that responsibility to an ongoing case manager. Prevention of the mistreatment of vulnerable people is highly dependent on social connection and individual and community awareness. Mistreatment is most likely committed by a family member, usually an adult child or a spouse. The job of an APS worker can be very challenging because they are often dealing with older adults with complex medical problems as well as difficult family situations (Csikai, 2011). For this reason, APS agencies provide support to prevent APS worker burnout (Bourassa, 2012).

Geoffrey Rogers

Bourassa, D. (2012). Examining self-protection measures guarding adult protective services social workers against compassion fatigue. *Journal of Interpersonal Violence, 27*, 1699–1715.

Csikai, E. L. (2011). Adult protective service workers' experiences with serious illness and death. *Journal of Elder Abuse & Neglect, 23*(2), 169–189.

Lachs, M., & Pillemer, K. (2015). Elder abuse. *New England Journal of Medicine, 373*, 1947–1956.

National Adult Protective Services Association. (2004). *Ethical principles and best practice guidelines.* Boulder, CO: Author. Retrieved from http://www.napsa-now.org/about-napsa/code-of-ethics

A

Web Resources

National Center on Elder Abuse: http://www.elder abusecenter.org

National Committee for the Prevention of Elder Abuse: http://www.preventelderabuse.org

National Council on Crime and Delinquency: http://www.nccdglobal.org

The Elder Justice Coalition: http://www.elderjustice coalition.com

The National Adult Protective Services Association: http://www.apsnetwork.org

The National Adult Protective Services Resource Center: http://www.napsa-now.org/resource -center

ADVANCE DIRECTIVES

Older persons, as well as their families and health care professionals, often face difficult decisions and conflicts regarding starting, continuing, or stopping life-sustaining medical treatments (LSMTs; Shepherd, 2014). The situation is especially complex when providers and families have little knowledge of which LSMTs a patient would want or when no one has been appointed (or is presently available) to make health care decisions for an incapacitated patient. Advance health care planning, although not a panacea for difficulties that may arise in this arena, helps maintain some degree of control over future medical treatment when a person becomes physically and/or mentally unable to make and express important LSMT decisions. Advance planning also may help individuals and their families avoid court involvement in LSMT decisions, conserve limited health care resources in a way that is consistent with patient self-determination, and reduce emotional stress on families in crisis circumstances.

Although an advance directive (AD) may be oral, it is much more likely to be followed if it is a written document. An instruction (living will)–type AD contains an individual's instructions about wanted, limited, or unwanted LSMTs in case a person becomes incapacitated or is unable to communicate. These instructions may be detailed (e.g., relate to specific medical treatments in specific situations), general (e.g., "no

extraordinary measures"), or phrased in terms of a patient's personal values (e.g., "keep me alive forever no matter what pain or expense" or "avoiding suffering is my main concern").

In contrast, a proxy directive (usually a durable power of attorney [DPOA]) is an AD that permits an individual to designate another person—called a *health care agent, surrogate, proxy,* or *attorney-in-fact*—to make health care decisions if the principal (i.e., the person who delegates away decision-making authority) loses decision-making capacity. In states that have default surrogate consent laws (i.e., statutes that designate a legal hierarchy of family members and others who may make decisions on behalf of incapacitated patients when there is no guardian appointed or instruction directive present), a DPOA can clarify which person has authority to decide when two persons have equal status (e.g., siblings) in the hierarchy. In addition, a DPOA is very valuable when a person prefers a nonrelative as the future decision maker. For example, when a person is in a committed but unmarried relationship with a significant other, it is common for the individual to appoint that significant other rather than a family member as the health care agent. Some AD documents combine the instruction and proxy elements.

Only a presently capable person may execute a valid AD. The AD becomes effective only when that individual subsequently lacks decision-making capacity regarding a particular medical treatment issue. Various states have enacted detailed statutes that outline conditions under which an AD is legally valid. In practice, however, health care providers are often unclear about when a living will applies and are uncomfortable about deciding when a patient is on a dying trajectory that warrants triggering a living will's instructions. Furthermore, health care providers sometimes find a living will's directions either too broad or too narrow to provide useful guidance in a particular situation. Thus appointing a proxy with power to make medical choices in the present, based on up-to-date information, may be more useful.

The Patient Self-Determination Act (PSDA) became effective in 1991. The PSDA mandates that hospitals, nursing homes, home health agencies, hospices, health maintenance organizations, and preferred provider organizations participating in Medicare or Medicaid (a) provide written information to individuals about their right to participate in medical decision making as provided in applicable state law; (b) ask patients whether they have completed an AD already and, if the answer is affirmative, have a system for recording the patient's AD; (c) offer decisionally capable residents an opportunity to execute an AD if the document does not already exist; (d) not discriminate in the provision of care based on the presence or absence of an AD; (e) have a system to comply with applicable state laws on medical decision making; and (f) educate staff and the community about medical decision-making rights.

Despite substantial public attention, psychological resistance to the contemplation of illness and death, coupled with inertia and legal complexities complicating the execution of an AD, keeps the rate of AD completion low among the general public, including older people (Gamertsfelder, Seaman, Tate, Buddadhumaruk, & Happ, 2016). Personal characteristics may influence AD completion rates among members of different population groups. Although nursing home residents are more likely to complete an AD than community-dwelling older persons, the PSDA expressly forbids any health care provider from requiring a patient/resident to execute an AD as a condition of admission or receipt of services.

Health care providers should attempt to discuss end-of-life preferences and complete ADs with older individuals. Many older persons want to talk about end-of-life care and are willing to fill out an AD if given the opportunity. Discussions may focus on specific LSMTs and/or an individual's remaining life and health care goals and priorities. Although physicians should be centrally involved in the communication process, the active participation of nurses, physician assistants, and social workers in this context may also be highly valuable (Nedjat-Haiem et al., 2016).

Timing of communication about end-of-life care is key. Discussions should ideally occur before a medical crisis, during regularly scheduled appointments with primary care providers, or at the time of elective procedures. A change in Medicare regulations effective in 2016 provides a mechanism under the Healthcare Common Procedural Coding System (HCPCS) for paying physicians to counsel patients about end-of-life planning (Sorrel, 2016). Periodically, and following significant health events, health care providers should review with patients who retain decision-making capacity in their AD to ascertain the accuracy of their listed preferences and other information. Patients should be advised to give copies of the AD to their designated health care agents, family members, and close friends, as well as make sure that the primary care provider has a copy in the medical records, thus ensuring easy accessibility in an emergency. In emergency situations outside of health care institutions (e.g., a cardiac arrest in the patient's own home), emergency medical service providers may not recognize and follow an AD unless it takes the form of a physician's order made in conformity with the state's applicable out-of-institution treatment statute.

No person, whether living in the community or temporarily or permanently in an institution, is legally or ethically required to execute an AD. Individuals (and their families) should be informed—and providers must understand—that the person will not be abandoned, ignored, or otherwise discriminated against regarding treatment because of failure to execute an AD.

For patients with advanced, irreversible illness who may become decisionally incapacitated, growing frustration with the inherent limitations of existing instruments (Noah, 2013) has led many attorneys, health care providers, and commentators to advocate, as the next step in health care advance planning law and policy, the use of physician orders for life-sustaining treatment (POLST) forms; the exact nomenclature varies among different jurisdictions. From a variety of perspectives, the POLST paradigm offers several opportunities for going beyond the status quo, including our present strong reliance on ADs, to potentially improve the care of individuals with advanced, irreversible illness (Wolf, Maag, & Gallant, 2014).

A

Unlike a traditional AD executed by a patient while still decisionally capable, POLST entails a medical order written by a physician (with the concurrence of the patient or surrogate) instructing other health care providers such as emergency medical squads about the treatment of a patient with advanced, irreversible illness under specific factual circumstances. "The POLST form is a more uniform, comprehensive, and portable method of documentation of patients' end-of-life treatment desires. Although the POLST form is not intended to replace ADs executed by patients, it corrects many of the inadequacies of current forms and intends to lessen the discrepancy between a patient's end-of-life care preferences and the treatment(s) eventually provided by the patients' health care providers." (Spillers & Lamb, 2011)

At least 16 states have formally implemented the POLST paradigm, with national coordination efforts being administered through the National POLST Paradigm Task Force. Many more states are in the process of developing and implementing their own versions of POLST.

See also Palliative Care; Substitute Decision Making.

Marshall B. Kapp

Gamertsfelder, E. M., Seaman, J. B., Tate, J., Buddadhumaruk, P., & Happ, M. B. (2016). Prevalence of advance directives among older adults admitted to intensive care units and requiring mechanical ventilation. *Journal of Gerontological Nursing, 42*, 34–41.
Nedjat-Haiem, F. R., Carrion, I. V., Gonzalez, K., Ell, K., Thompson, B., & Mishra, S. I. (2016). Exploring health care providers' views about initiating end-of-life care communication. *American Journal of Hospice & Palliative Medicine, 34*, 308–317. doi:10.1177/1049909115627773
Noah, B. A. (2013). In denial: The role of law in preparing for death. *Elder Law Journal, 21*, 1–31.
Shepherd, L. (2014). The end of end-of-life law. *North Carolina Law Review, 92*, 1693–1748.
Sorrel, A. L. (2016). Medicare pays for end-of-life consults. *Texas Medicine, 112*, 31–36.
Spillers, S. C., & Lamb, B. (2011). Is the POLST model desirable for Florida? *Florida Public Health Review, 8*, 80–90.
Wolf, R. B., Maag, M. J., & Gallant, K. B. (2014). The physician orders for life-sustaining treatment (POLST) coming soon to a health care community near you. *Real Property, Probate, Trusts & Estate Law Journal, 49*, 71–161.

Web Resources
American Bar Association Commission on Law and Aging: http://www.americanbar.org/groups/law_aging.html
Caring Connections (National Hospice and Palliative Care Organization): http://www.caringinfo.org
Centers for Medicare & Medicaid Services: http://www.cms.gov
Compassion & Choices: http://www.compassionandchoices.org
National Healthcare Decisions Day: http://www.nhdd.org
National POLST Program: http://www.polst.org

ADVANCED PRACTICE NURSING

In 1965, the shortage of primary care physicians, particularly in rural areas, encouraged nurse Loretta Ford and physician Henry Silver to create the first nurse practitioner (NP) certification program at the University of Colorado, allowing registered nurses to expand their education and provide a range of higher level services to a variety of patient populations (O'Brien, 2003). Advanced practice registered nurses (APRNs) have advanced education, training, and skills to provide a full range of services to patients and populations. One of the key components of advanced practice nursing (APN) is the comprehensive focus on the whole person. APRNs address health and wellness, as well as management of illness, incorporating patient education and counseling. The function of APRNs has expanded over the past decades, and registered nurses may now receive a master's or doctorate level of education in one of four roles: nurse anesthetist, nurse midwife, clinical nurse specialist, and NP. There are currently more than 267,000 APRNs in the United States (National Council of State Boards of Nursing [NCSBN],

2017), providing services in these various specialties.

REQUIREMENTS FOR PRACTICE

APRNs are licensed by each state, and must practice within the scope, rules and regulations of that state. The APRN Consensus Model is in place for regulation of APRN licensure, accreditation, certification, and education (American Nurses Association, 2016). Endorsed by more than 41 nursing organizations, it outlines the roles, population foci, and definition of APRNs. Bachelor's-prepared registered nurses may obtain a master's or doctoral degree as a nurse anesthetist, nurse-midwife, clinical nurse specialist, or NP. APRNs have a population focus on family, adult-gerontology, neonatal, pediatrics, women's health, or psychiatric (APRN Consensus Work Group, 2008) and typically concentrate in either acute care (inpatient) or primary care (outpatient). APRNs may further specialize within a clinical area, such as oncology, palliative care or gero-focused mental health. Because of the changing population demographics and the increased life expectancy, inclusion of geriatric-focused content was incorporated into adult APRN programs beginning in 2008. By 2010, APRN organizations developed competencies for a combined adult-geriatric focus; this new, combined population was further adopted by credentialing agencies (American Association of Critical-Care Nurses [AACN], 2015; APRN Consensus Work Group, 2008; National Organization of Nurse Practitioner Faculties [NONPF], 2010).

Once registered nurses have obtained a graduate nursing education from an accredited school, they may obtain national board certification by taking a standardized examination. Two organizations provide NP certification: American Nurses Credentialing Center and American Association of Nurse Practitioners. Not every state requires certification to practice. However, each APRN must obtain licensing and registration in the state where they practice and abide by the rules and regulations defined by the state. For example, an APRN may have privileges for narcotic prescription in one state but not another.

SCOPE OF PRACTICE

APRNs provide health promotion, disease prevention, education, and counseling to a variety of populations in various settings. They can provide direct patient care, order tests, diagnose and treat acute and chronic illnesses, and prescribe medications in all 50 states and the District of Columbia (American Association of Nurse Practitioners, 2016). They work in a variety of settings, including primary care offices, home care, assisted-living facilities, nursing homes, community health centers, and hospitals. A total of 22 states and the District of Columbia allow NPs full practice authority, which means that they do not have to consult with a physician to evaluate, diagnose, order tests, interpret test results, or initiate and manage treatment. States require collaboration to prescribe; other states with restricted practice privileges require supervision to diagnose, treat, and prescribe medications (American Association of Nurse Practitioners, 2016). The Institute of Medicine (2010) has urged states to release practice restrictions on APRNs and permit them to practice to the full extent of their education and training. Given the increasing need for providers in both urban and rural settings, utilizing the skill set of APRNs is warranted.

The literature supports that NPs provide comparable or improved quality care to patients in the primary care setting compared with physicians and may have better patient satisfaction (Jennings, Clifford, Fox, O'Connell, & Gardner, 2015; Naylor & Kurtzman, 2010; Paradise, Dark, & Bitler, 2011). States that have less restrictive regulations for practice have larger increases in the number of patients seen by NPs than more restrictive states, which may assist with addressing the shortage of primary care physicians and improve access to care (Kuo, Loresto, Rounds, & Goodwin, 2013). The Institute of Medicine's (2010) *The Future of Nursing* recommends that nurses practice to their full education and training to ensure quality of care delivered and reduce health care costs. Efforts to reduce regulation and allow NPs to practice to their full potential are being made on an individual state level. For example, Delaware, Maryland, Nebraska, and

New York made significant progress toward full practice authority in 2015 by eliminating collaboration models of practice after an NP has completed a supervisory period (Phillips, 2016). However, much progress is still required to meet the goals of the Institute of Medicine's report and standardize the scope of practice of NPs nationwide.

QUALITY OUTCOMES

There is strong evidence to support that NPs and APNs specializing in geriatrics provide quality care to older patients in a variety of settings equal to or lower cost, including primary care settings, long-term facilities, hospitals, and emergency rooms (Donald et al., 2013; Stanik-Hutt et al., 2013; Tolson, Morley, Rolland, & Vellas, 2011). In the primary care setting, NP have better or equivalent care for a number of diseases and outcomes, including hyperlipidemia, blood glucose, blood pressure, rheumatoid arthritis, and chronic kidney disease (Allen, Himmelfarb, Szanton, & Frick, 2014; Ndosi et al., 2014; Peeters et al., 2014). Satisfaction with care, functional and health association status, number of emergency room visits, number of hospitalizations, and mortality have documented improvements when care is provided by APRNs (Allen et al., 2014; Ndosi et al., 2014; Peeters et al., 2014).

Long-term care facilities that utilize APNs have improved outcomes in rates of depression, incontinence, use of restraints, pressure ulcers, and aggressive behavior, as well as improved patient and family satisfaction and ability to obtain personal goals (Donald et al., 2013). Adult-geriatric nurse practitioners (AGNPs) have also been integral providers in mature capitated model programs for the frail elderly, such as Programs of All-Inclusive Care for the Elderly (PACE) projects, Social/Health Maintenance Organizations (SHMOs), and programs that encourage home care agencies to offer managed care options (Newhouse et al., 2011).

In hospitals, geriatric clinical nurse experts significantly reduce morbidity, including preventing or reducing clinical syndromes common to the elderly, such as delirium; shorten hospital length of stay; reduce morbidity following discharge; and reduce emergency room use and readmission after discharge (Newhouse et al., 2011). These outcomes are evident throughout several hospital-based geriatric nurse practice models, such as Nurses Improving Care for Healthsystem Elders (NICHE; Capezuti et al., 2012). NPs have also demonstrated improved outcomes, including improved quality of care, reduced wait times, and increased patient satisfaction, in emergency room settings but may not reduce cost in this setting (Jennings et al., 2015).

GROWING DEMAND FOR GERIATRIC NURSE PRACTITIONERS

The demand for primary care providers will continue to increase with the increasing aging population, and more than 16 million are newly insured since the Patient Protection and Affordable Care Act was adopted in 2010 (American Association of Nurse Practitioners, n.d.; Blumenthal, Abrams, & Nuzum, 2015). Approximately 222,000 NPs are practicing in the United States, with two thirds serving in primary care and 22% in adult-geriatrics (American Association of Nurse Practitioners, n.d.). NPs are choosing to specialize in primary care more than physicians: 80% of NPs compared with 14.5% of physicians (American Association of Nurse Practitioners, n.d.). It is projected that by 2025, there will be 244,000 NPs (American Association of Nurse Practitioners, n.d.). One of the major health care challenges of the 21st century will be the provision of quality, comprehensive, and cost-effective care for a rapidly increasing number of older adults. Despite the recent increased emphasis on gerontology in medical and nursing curriculum, the emergence of specialized care units in hospitals, and the development of alternative long-term care options, the demand will still overwhelm the supply of qualified providers. NPs can help bridge this gap and improve access to and quality of care delivered to the geriatric population. To meet this goal, efforts to standardize the scope of practice and allow NPs to practice to their full education and training nationwide must continue.

Marcella Pomeranz and Mary T. Hickey

Advanced Practice Registered Nurse Consensus Work Group. (2008). Consensus model for APRN regulation: Licensure, accreditation, certification, and education. Retrieved from https://www.ncsbn.org/Consensus_Model_for_APRN_Regulation_July_2008.pdf

Allen, J. K., Himmelfarb, C. R. D., Szanton, S. L., & Frick, K. D. (2014). Cost-effectiveness of nurse practitioner/community health worker care to reduce cardiovascular health disparities. *Journal of Cardiovascular Nursing, 29*(4), 308.

American Association of Colleges of Nursing. (2015). APRN education. Retrieved from http://www.aacnnursing.org/Teaching-Resources/APRN

American Association of Nurse Practitioners. (n.d.). Nurse practitioners. Retrieved from https://www.aanp.org/images/about-nps/npgraphic.pdf

American Association of Nurse Practitioners. (2016). State practice environment. Retrieved from https://www.aanp.org/legislation-regulation/state-legislation/state-practice-environment/66-legislation-regulation/state-practice-environment/1380-state-practice-by-type

American Nurses Association. (2016). APRN consensus model. Retrieved from http://www.nursingworld.org/consensusmodel

Blumenthal, D., Abrams, M., & Nuzum, R. (2015). The affordable care act at 5 years. *New England Journal of Medicine, 372*(25), 2451–2458.

Capezuti, E., Boltz, E., Cline, D., Dickson, V., Rosenberg, M., Wagner, L.,…Nigolian, C. (2012). NICHE—A model for optimizing the geriatric nursing practice environment. *Journal of Clinical Nursing, 21*, 3117–3125.

Donald, F., Martin-Misener, R., Carter, N., Donald, E. E., Kaasalainen, S., Wickson-Griffiths, A.,…DiCenso, A. (2013). A systematic review of the effectiveness of advanced practice nurses in long-term care. *Journal of Advanced Nursing, 69*(10), 2148–2161.

Institute of Medicine. (2010). The future of nursing: Leading change, advancing health. Retrieved from http://www.nationalacademies.org/hmd/Reports/2010/The-Future-of-Nursing-Leading-Change-Advancing-Health.aspx

Jennings, N., Clifford, S., Fox, A. R., O'Connell, J., & Gardner, G. (2015). The impact of nurse practitioner services on cost, quality of care, satisfaction and waiting times in the emergency department: A systematic review. *International Journal of Nursing Studies, 52*(1), 421–435.

Kuo, Y. F., Loresto, F. L., Rounds, L. R., & Goodwin, J. S. (2013). States with the least restrictive regulations experienced the largest increase in patients seen by nurse practitioners. *Health Affairs, 32*(7), 1236–1243.

National Council of State Boards of Nursing. (2017). APRNs in the U.S. Retrieved from https://www.ncsbn.org/aprn.htm

National Organization of Nurse Practitioner Faculties. (2010). Consensus model for APRN regulation. Retrieved from http://www.nonpf.org/?page=26

Naylor, M. D., & Kurtzman, E. T. (2010). The role of nurse practitioners in reinventing primary care. *Health Affairs, 29*(5), 893–899.

Ndosi, M., Lewis, M., Hale, C., Quinn, H., Ryan, S., Emery, P.,…Hill, J. (2014). The outcome and cost-effectiveness of nurse-led care in people with rheumatoid arthritis: A multicentre randomised controlled trial. *Annals of the Rheumatic Diseases, 73*(11), 1975–1982.

Newhouse, R. P., Stanik-Hutt, J., White, K. M., Johantgen, M., Bass, E. B., Zangaro, G.,…Weiner, J. P. (2011). Advanced practice nurse outcomes 1990–2008: A systematic review. *Nursing Economic$, 29*(5), 1–21.

O'Brien, J. M. (2003). How nurse practitioners obtained provider status: Lessons for pharmacists. *American Journal of Health-System Pharmacy, 60*(22), 2301–2307.

Paradise, J., Dark, C., & Bitler, N. (2011). *Improving access to adult primary care in Medicaid: Exploring the potential role of nurse practitioners and physician assistants.* Menlo Park, CA: The Henry J. Kaiser Family Foundation.

Peeters, M. J., van Zuilen, A. D., van den Brand, J. A., Bots, M. L., van Buren, M., ten Dam, M. A.,…Wetzels, J. F. M. (2014). Nurse practitioner care improves renal outcome in patients with CKD. *Journal of the American Society of Nephrology, 25*(2), 390–398.

Phillips, S. J. (2016). 28th annual APRN legislative update: Advancements continue for APRN practice. *The Nurse Practitioner, 41*(1), 21–48.

Stanik-Hutt, J., Newhouse, R. P., White, K. M., Johantgen, M., Bass, E. B., Zangaro, G.,…Weiner, J. P. (2013). The quality and effectiveness of care provided by nurse practitioners. *Journal for Nurse Practitioners, 9*(8), 492–500.

Tolson, D., Morley, J. E., Rolland, Y., & Vellas, B. (2011). Advancing nursing home practice: The International Association of Geriatrics and Gerontology recommendations. *Geriatric Nursing, 32*(3), 195–197.

Web Resources

American Association of Nurse Practitioners, definition: https://www.aanp.org/all-about-nps/what-is-an-np

A

American Association of Nurse Practitioners: https://www.aanp.org

American Nurses Credentialing Center: http://www.nursecredentialing.org

Gerontological Advanced Practice Nurses Association: http://www.gapna.org

National Organization of Nurse Practitioner Faculties: http://www.nonpf.org/?page=26

The Barbara and Richard Csomay Center for Gerontological Excellence: https://nursing.uiowa.edu/csomay/

The Consensus Model for APRN Regulation, Licensure, Accreditation, Certification and Education: https://www.ncsbn.org/736.htm

AFFORDABLE HEALTH CARE FOR THE ELDERLY

Although patients may pay some out-of-pocket costs for health services and health care, most payments are substantially, if not fully, covered by health insurance. In the United States, the government partially funds health care under the umbrella of Medicare, Medicaid, the Children's Health Insurance Program, Federally Qualified Health Centers, public hospitals, Veteran's Affairs hospitals.

Medicare is federally funded and regulated health insurance for those who are aged 65 or older, those who meet disability requirements, or those who have certain chronic illnesses regardless of age. Consumers are required to enroll and select a plan that works best for their personal health care needs and situation. Part A covers traditional hospital services (sometimes also called "major medical insurance"). Part B covers other medical services, including preventive care and well visits. Medicare Advantage (formally called Medicare Part C) and MediGap can be purchased and provide coverage for services and treatments that may not be covered in Parts A or B. Medicare Part D covers specific pharmaceuticals that are listed on a formulary (www.medicare.gov).

Although Medicare is federally regulated, many older patients find that they still lack coverage for simple preventive services,

medications to treat specific problems, physical therapy after a fall or an accident, or time in skilled nursing facilities. The most recent form of federal involvement in health care coverage is in the form of the Patient Protection and Affordable Care Act (PPACA). The PPACA aims to reform health care over a period of several years with goals of filling the current gaps in coverage for the poorest Americans, many of whom are elderly.

Although most of the benefits of PPACA impact nonelderly patients in the form of Medicaid coverage, PPACA had several provisions that enhanced care and coverage for elderly patients who previously lacked essential care or services through Medicare coverage. One option offered by PPACA was the inclusion of Early Retiree Reinsurance Programs (ERRPs). The PPACA provided tax relief to small businesses, unions, and other organizations to offer affordable health care plans for employees who were able to take early retirement. This program officially closed in 2014 when similar health insurance options began to be offered through private health insurance exchanges. The Pre-Existing Condition Insurance Plan (PCIP) provided coverage to patients with a significant or chronic illness that previously led to denial of insurance. Like ERRP, PCIP closed in early 2014 when insurance companies were no longer able to discriminate based on pre-existing conditions. The Community Care Transitions Program (CTTP) implements a model for improved care transitions for those enrolled in Medicare. Launched in 2012, the program will run for 5 years. There are 27 participating sites in the program. The goal will be to provide quality care at a decreasing cost while coordinating hospital discharge planning in an effort to decrease readmission rates. In addition to these changes, the PPACA aims to increase the number of community-based health centers that will allow more home- or community-based elderly patients to seek care, specifically preventive care and screenings, so they don't have to travel to large health centers.

One of the most anticipated changes to emerge from this health care reform is the coverage of preventive care and screenings. Although not covered by many medical insurances historically, patients now receive well visits, preventive care, and screenings (such as colonoscopies, mammography, and ultrasounds) without being charged a co-pay or incurring additional personal cost. In addition, certain programs or conditions such as smoking cessation and obesity have no additional charge to the patient.

Of particular interest to many elderly consumers are the changes surrounding Medicare Part D. Under the current model, once a predetermined dollar amount has been utilized for prescription drugs, patients must pay the full cost of any additional prescription medications. Although it has an upper limit, the greater out-of-pocket cost is far too expensive for most patients to absorb. The PPACA awards patients an automatic discount on prescription medications from the Medicare formulary list after the predetermined amount has been achieved. This coverage gap is expected to close by 2020 (U.S. Centers for Medicare & Medicaid Services, 2016).

Finally, the ACA instituted an Insurance Exchange program to simplify the purchase of insurance, as well as to increase competition between companies. This program may even the playing field and decrease insurance premiums for elderly patients who choose to purchase insurance supplemental to Medicare (Health Care Marketplace, 2013). The government is also initiating specific programs and incentives aimed at decreasing waste or misuse of Medicare and Medicaid dollars, as well as health care fraud, launching accountable care organizations to help coordinate health care and streamline quality improvement from a systems perspective. The use of electronic medical records are required for all health care facilities.

Elderly patients are at particular risk for under-management of chronic disease and lack of preventive care and screening services. Although almost all older adults (e.g., U.S. citizens) are covered by Medicare, supplemental insurance is often needed to bridge the health care gaps. These additional costs, high premiums, and copays for pharmaceuticals may force some older adults to make choices between which care to seek or which medications to take. The goal of the PPACA is to provide quality, affordable, and accessible health care to all Americans.

April Bigelow

Health Care Marketplace. (2013). What is the Health Insurance Marketplace? Retrieved from https://www.healthcare.gov/what-is-the-health-insurance-marketplace

U.S. Centers for Medicare & Medicaid Services. (2016). The Affordable Care Act and Medicare. Retrieved from http://www.medicare.gov

Web Resources

AARP ACA: Fact sheets (broken down by age group): http://www.aarp.org/health/health-care-reform/health_reform_factsheets

General Information on ACA: http://www.HealthCare.gov

Medicare: http://www.medicare.gov

AFRICAN AMERICANS AND HEALTH CARE DISPARITIES

The Centers for Disease Control and Prevention (CDC) categorize racial/ethnic minority populations in the United States as Asian American, Black or African American, Hispanic or Latino, Native Hawaiian and Other Pacific Islander, and American Indian and Alaska Native (CDC, 2012). Eventually settled in the United States, Black and/or African Americans constitute a group of individuals of ethnic cohesion tracing their genealogy to Black tribes of Africa and tempered by hundreds of years of racialism and acculturation in the United States (Brown et al., 2014). (*Note*: The words "Black and/or African American" will be used throughout this entry to signify individuals of the African Diaspora, or those who are descendants of Africans dispersed from the continent of Africa.)

According to the U.S. Census Bureau (2017), in 2015, approximately 38% of the population belonged to a racial/ethnic minority group and approximately 13% identified as Black or African American. Most suffer significant health disparities that are associated with a broad, complex, and interrelated array of factors. The diagnosis, progression, response to treatment, caregiving, and overall quality of life may each be affected by race/ethnicity, gender, socioeconomic status (SES), age, education, occupation, and other genetic and lifestyle differences. For example, prevalence rates for Alzheimer's disease are higher for African Americans than for other ethnic groups, and there is a remarkable relationship between SES and health and longevity (National Institute on Aging [NIA], 2013). Persistent health disparities in the United States are unacceptable, and the need to raise awareness of these inequities remains critical.

All of the conditions discussed in this article (Alzheimer's disease, diabetes, and chronic pain) are linked and are expected to increase among African Americans. In 2003, the Institute of Medicine, a part of the National Academy of Sciences, in its report *Unequal Treatment*, reported evidence that "bias, prejudice and stereotype on the part of health care providers may contribute to differences in care" (p. 178). In 2011, the CDC released its *Health Disparities and Inequalities Report* (Meyer, Yoon, & Kaufmann, 2013), which demonstrated that people living in lower socioeconomic circumstances are at increased risk for serious disease and premature death, have reduced access to health care, and receive an inadequate quality of care. In 2012, Institute of Medicine committee member, Dr. David Williams took a historical perspective to highlight the importance of life expectancy as an indicator of health. Another way to document health disparities is to look at life expectancies for African Americans and Whites. In 1950, the life expectancy for Whites was 69.1 years. However, the life expectancy for African Americans reached 69.1 years only in 1990, four decades later (Williams, 2012). More needs to be done to redress these chronic disabling conditions.

ALZHEIMER'S DISEASE

Several NIA-funded studies have reported a higher prevalence of Alzheimer's disease among African Americans compared with non-Hispanic Whites. A team led by University of Pennsylvania, Philadelphia, researchers studied more than 1,300 people who had been either diagnosed with Alzheimer's disease or deemed cognitively normal at their initial visit to the University of Pennsylvania Alzheimer Disease Center to better understand comparative differences (Livney et al., 2011). African Americans had a slightly older age at disease onset than non-Hispanic Whites. However, African Americans had higher levels of cognitive impairment and dementia at their initial clinic visit than non-Hispanics Whites. According to researchers, reduced access to clinical facilities did not appear to play a role in this disparity. Researchers concluded that the disparities could reflect differing perspectives of African American family members regarding age-related cognitive decline or that primary caregivers may lack the knowledge to detect symptoms earlier. Findings from this research highlight some of the factors—from stress to educational levels—to be considered in future research.

A team led by University of Indiana, Indianapolis, researchers studied the incidence of cognitive impairment, no dementia (CIND) and mild cognitive impairment (MCI) in a group of older African Americans, aged 65 or older, in Indianapolis (Unverzagt et al., 2011). About 1 in 20 study participants developed CIND/MCI each year during the 5-year follow-up period. These rates are similar to those reported for other groups in the United States and abroad. Age was an important risk factor; among the oldest old (aged 85 years or older), 1 in 10 developed the condition every year. Those with a history of depression or head injury were also at greater risk of developing CIND/MCI. The investigators found that education was a strong protective factor; people with more years of school were at reduced risk.

Researchers at Rush University in Chicago studied a large sample of more than 9,500 older African Americans and Whites to see if educational levels affected health disparities (Barnes et al., 2011). They found that African American participants with lower levels of education had poorer cognitive function and physical function (leg strength, balance, and walking speed) compared with similarly educated Whites. More years of education were associated with better physical and cognitive health in both groups, and the positive effect of 12 years of education was similar for both groups. Interestingly, additional years of education beyond high school had a significantly greater positive impact on physical and cognitive health in old age for African Americans than for Whites. Those with the highest levels of education enjoyed similar levels of cognitive health and physical function in old age. The study suggests that for African Americans achieving greater levels of higher education might be helpful in reducing risk for cognitive impairments.

DIABETES

More than 23 million people in the United States have been diagnosed with diabetes mellitus (DM), the seventh leading cause of death. African American older adults are at risk of undiagnosed DM. DMs, or "sugar" as some older adults call it, lowers life expectancy by up to 15 years; increases the risk of heart disease by two to four times; and is the leading cause of kidney failure, lower limb amputations, and adult-onset blindness.

Researchers in the Intramural Research Program of the NIA in the Health, Aging, and Body Composition (Health ABC) Study conducted a prospective study of changes in weight and body composition, with a total of 58.5% of individuals with diabetes self-identifying as Black. Glycemic control was poor in all participants with diabetes, with a hemoglobin A1c greater than or equal to 7% in 73.7% of subjects; however, Black participants had worse glycemic control than Whites (age- and sex-adjusted mean A1c, 8.4% in Blacks and 7.4% in Whites; $p < .01$). Race differences in glycemic control remained significant even after adjusting for current insulin therapy, cardiovascular disease, higher total cholesterol, and lack of a flu shot in the previous year, all of which were associated with higher A1c concentrations, although controlling these risk factors reduced the association by 27%. Race remained an important factor in glycemic control, even when results were stratified by education or income.

It is likely that these results would not surprise investigators at the University of Michigan's Institute for Social Research, who seek to advance theoretical reasoning and discourse in addressing an omission in existing behavioral science and intervention models (Jackson, Herman, & Abelson, 2013; Jackson, Knight, & Rafferty, 2010). The investigators offer an interesting and perhaps radical view of health disparities among Blacks in the United States. According to the investigators, there is a robust literature that indicates Blacks in the United States are more likely to engage in poor health behaviors (i.e., tobacco smoking, diets high in fat and carbohydrates, excessive alcohol use) and, expectedly, experience disproportionate burdens of common physical health conditions associated with these behaviors, such as cardiovascular disease and DM, relative to non-Hispanic Whites. Paradoxically, population-based and clinical studies have consistently found that Blacks, compared with Whites, have the same or lower rates of most mental disorders, even while experiencing higher rates of psychological distress. The investigators, led by Dr. James Jackson, theorize that a defined set of health-related stress-coping strategies (e.g., tobacco smoking, diets high in fat and carbohydrates, excessive alcohol use) have a binary effect that helps account for this patterning. They hypothesize that the effects of poor health behaviors on pathophysiology, combined with direct effects of stressful living conditions over the life-course, contribute to the disproportionate burden of chronic physical health problems, such as DM, among Blacks (Jackson et al., 2013; Mezuk et al., 2013).

The Diabetes Prevention Program (DPP) is large and ethnically diverse. During the 2.8 years of observation of a three-arm trial, both metformin and intensive lifestyle interventions effectively delayed or prevented the development of DM in a cost-effective manner. The observation of the troglitazone intervention was limited to a mean of 10 months; it also effectively delayed the onset of DM. In this study, only the lifestyle intervention modified the development of cardiovascular risk factors (Ratner et al., 2005). The results from this and many other research studies provide evidence that changes in lifestyle are effective in preventing DM. Achieving more than 4 hours of exercise per week was associated with a significant reduction in the risk of DM. Any type of physical activity, whether walking, sports, household work, gardening, or work-related physical activity, is similarly beneficial.

CHRONIC PAIN IN OLDER ADULTS

African Americans with chronic pain have significantly more symptoms than Whites when they first seek pain treatment, including more pain, depression, and impairment in physical, emotional, and social health. In an aging society, chronic pain increasingly has a significant impact on successful aging. Chronic pain may further differentially affect racial/ethnic minorities while diminishing their health and quality of life. In a study to address the potential differential effects of chronic pain cross-culturally in older Americans, a retrospective analysis of a group of subjects presenting for chronic pain management in a tertiary care multidisciplinary pain center was performed. The comparative study of Black and White American adults was performed to determine whether there were differences in (a) psychological functioning, (b) pain characteristics, (c) pain disability, and (d) comorbidities. The Black Americans had more depressive symptoms and symptoms of posttraumatic stress disorder compared with the White Americans. The results suggest that chronic pain adversely affects the quality of life and health status of Black Americans to a greater extent than White Americans. This study showed significant differences in pain and health status based on race (Green, Baker, Smith, & Sato, 2003).

ENHANCING CULTURAL INCLUSIVITY AND COMPETENCE

Efforts to reduce significant health disparities between African Americans and White Americans are increasingly seen as part of the unfinished business of the fight for racial equality. Dr. Martin Luther King stated, "Of all the forms of inequality, injustice in health care is the most shocking and inhumane" (Moore, 2013). Among efforts to reduce health disparities in Blacks are strategies to improve cultural competence in health care providers. The following are a few strategies that can help reduce bias and promote cultural competence in addressing African Americans in health care.

- *Heighten self-awareness:* Any biases and stereotypical thinking patterns (e.g., older African American women are not "girls") should be acknowledged and eliminated.
- *Individualize:* Eliminate stereotypical generalizations. For example, even though educational opportunities were limited (particularly for those who are currently age 75 years and older), it should not be automatically assumed that elderly African Americans are illiterate. Many who had very little formal education can read, write, and count well, but some cannot. Recognizing individuality is important because African American older adults are not a monolithic group.
- *Be genuine, respectful, and courteous:* African American older adults should be properly addressed as Mr., Mrs., or Ms. (as a means of showing respect and appropriate regard), and a sense of caring and concern should be demonstrated. These qualities can be perceived and accurately interpreted even by poorly educated recipients of health and mental health services and can influence their willingness to return for subsequent care.
- *Actively listen:* Health care providers should be sensitive to possible language barriers and should seek cultural and linguistic interpretations where uncertainty exists in understanding and relating to the language or dialect. They should obtain an understanding of certain pronunciations and meanings of various concepts; for example, DM may be referred to as "sugar," and Alzheimer's and dementia may be characterized as "old timers' disease." Practitioners should seek accurate interpretations as needed from relatives and family friends. They should also withhold diagnostic assessment until a clear understanding of the articulated problem is certain.

See also Cultural Assessment; Cultural Competence and Aging.

Theresa L. Lundy

Barnes, L. L., Wilson, R. S., Hebert, L. E., Scherr, P. A., Evans, D. A., & Mendes deLeon, C. F. (2011). Racial differences in the association of education with physical and cognitive function in older Blacks and Whites. *Journals of Gerontology, Series B: Psychological Sciences and Social Sciences, 66*(3), 354–363.

Brown, C., Baker, T., Mingo, C., Harden, J. T., Whitfield, K. E., Morgan, A.,…Washington, T. (2014). A review of our roots: Blacks in gerontology. *The Gerontologist, 54*(1), 108–116.

Centers for Disease Control and Prevention. (2012). Racial and ethnic minority populations—Definitions. Retrieved from http://www.cdc .gov/minorityhealth/populations/REMP/ definitions.html

Green, C. R., Baker, T., Smith, E. M., & Sato, Y. (2003). The effect of race in older adults presenting for chronic pain management: A comparative study of Black and White Americans. *Journal of Pain, 4*(2), 82–90.

Jackson, J., Herman, W. H., & Abelson, J. L. (2013). Understanding health disparities in the progression of type 2 diabetes. Retrieved from http:// micda.psc.isr.umich.edu/project/detail/34972

Jackson, J. S., Knight, K. M., & Rafferty, J. A. (2010). Race and unhealthy behaviors: Chronic stress, the HPA axis, and physical and mental health disparities over the life course. *American Journal of Public Health, 100,* 933–939.

Livney, M. G., Clark, C. M., Karlawish, J. H., Cartmell, S., Negrón, M., Nuñez, J.,…Arnold, S. E. (2011). Ethnoracial differences in the clinical characteristics of Alzheimer's disease at initial presentation at an urban Alzheimer's disease center. *American Journal of Geriatric Psychiatry, 19*(5), 430–439.

Meyer, P. A., Yoon, P. W., & Kaufmann, R. B. (2013). Introduction: CDC health disparities and inequalities report—United States, 2013. *MMWR Supplements, 62*(3), 3–5.

Mezuk, B., Johnson-Lawrence, V., Lee, H., Rafferty, J. A., Abdou, C. M., Uzogara, E. E., & Jackson, J. S. (2013). Is ignorance bliss? Depression, antidepressants, and the diagnosis of prediabetes and type 2 diabetes. *Health Psychology, 32*(3), 254–263.

Moore, A. (2013). Tracking down Martin Luther King, Jr.'s words on health care. *The Blog.* Retrieved from http://www.huffingtonpost.com/amanda -moore/martin-luther-king-health-care_b_ 2506393.html

National Institute on Aging. (2013). Minority health and health disparities update. Retrieved from http://www.nia.nih.gov/about/minority -aging-and-health-disparities

Ratner, R., Goldberg, R., Haffner, S., Marcovina, S., Orchard, T., Fowler, S.,…Diabetes Prevention Program Research Group. (2005). Impact of intensive lifestyle and metformin therapy on cardiovascular risk factors in the Diabetes Prevention Program. *Diabetes Care, 28,* 888–894.

Unverzagt, F. W., Ogunniyi, A., Taler, V., Gao, S., Lane, K. A., Baiyewu, O.,…Hall, K. S. (2011). Incidence and risk factors for cognitive impairment no dementia and mild cognitive impairment in African Americans. *Alzheimer Disease and Associated Disorders, 25*(1), 4–10.

U.S. Census Bureau. (2017). 2010 census population and housing tables. Retrieved from https://www .census.gov/population/race/data/cen2010.html

Williams, D. R. (2012). *How far have we come in reducing health disparities? Progress since 2000: Workshop summary.* Washington, DC: National Academies Press.

Web Resources
Healthy People 2020: http://www.healthypeople .gov/2020/default.aspx

National Hartford Centers of Gerontological Nursing Excellence: http://www.geriatricnursing.org

National Institute on Aging: http://www.nia.nih.gov

National Institute on Aging, Minority Aging and Health Disparities: http://www.nia.nih.gov/ about/minority-aging-and-health-disparities

Program for Research on Black Americans at the University of Michigan: https://www.icpsr .umich.edu/icpsrweb/ICPSR/series/164

The Michigan Center on the Demography of Aging: http://micda.psc.isr.umich.edu/project/ theme/102

AGEISM

Ageism, a concept made popular by Robert Butler (1969), is a way to describe prejudice and discrimination against individuals who occupy a specific chronological age. *Ageism* is therefore an

A

all-encompassing concept that refers to negative beliefs, thoughts, and practices that disadvantage individuals who are defined by chronological age. Although typically used in reference to older individuals, the concept is applicable when prejudice and/or discrimination are practiced against any individual or group of individuals who are defined by chronological age. Just as an individual's sex or race can be a marker for negative attitudes and unfair or discriminatory treatment, one's chronological age or even a perception of one's chronological age can be a marker for such attitudes and treatment. Furthermore, ageism can be individual or institutional, implicit or explicit (Levy & Macdonald, 2016).

Individual ageism occurs when a person feels or acts in a discriminatory way because of chronological age. For example, a person could tell an ageist joke, publicly espouse the myth that older individuals are "all bad drivers," or avoid talking to an elderly individual because of ideas about what that individual might be like because of age. An individual employer might also avoid hiring or promoting an individual once after seeing an individual's age. Institutional ageism is more complex than individual ageism. Institutional ageism is practiced through the enactment and adherence to laws, rules, policies, and practices that systematically disadvantage older individuals. For example, a mandatory retirement age would be considered institutional ageism. Widespread denials of mortgage or credit card applications, grandparents' rights to gain custody of grandchildren, or teenagers' rights to make personal medical decisions, if based on the implementation of ageist policies, could all be considered clear-cut and explicit examples of institutional ageism.

Institutional ageism is not always clear-cut or even purposeful, however. Ageism may also refer to the practice of rendering older individuals as useless, a drain on economic resources and a social and economic threat to society. It could also be exemplified by a lack of attention to widespread abuses, such as the lack of attention to elder abuse in state policy. This is the difference between explicit and implicit ageism. Whether ageism is implicit or explicit depends on the perpetrator's intentions, whether that perpetrator is an individual, law,

or policy. When an individual expresses ageism with awareness to actions, thoughts, or feelings, it is considered *explicit* ageism. That is to say, the individual purposefully behaves, feels, or acts in an ageist way. *Implicit* ageism, on the other hand, is an expression of prejudice or discrimination in which the perpetrator does not intend to discriminate. Implicit ageism is not only more typical, but also it is more likely to be expressed in a negative way. For example, a common negative and implicitly ageist behavior is to use an overly accommodating or condescending tone (even *baby talk* or elderspeak) when interacting with older adults. Individuals who use such tones with older individuals do not always intend to be ageist; in fact, they might view their actions as helpful or well intentioned. This type of speech, however, is buried in a negative stereotype that older adults are incapable individuals who are child-like in their capacities.

Ageism may be more acceptable than other *isms* in society because of the many stereotypes that exist in the United States and elsewhere about older individuals. Older adults are often constructed in popular culture as sad, lonely, impoverished, greedy, frail, dependent, and stupid, as well as unable to handle important decisions. Similar judgments are made about teenagers and young adults, reminding us that ageism affects multiple age cohorts simultaneously. For example, in June 2009, Pixar Animation Studios released the animation film *Up*, in which a newly widowed "curmudgeon," Mr. Wilkinson, attaches his long-lived-in home to hundreds of colorful balloons and floats toward Paradise Falls, Venezuela, instead of being forced by court order, by two aides in medical scrubs, and a "paddy wagon" to move to a retirement community. Although well intentioned as a feel-good movie, the underlying message of this film is that older adults are incapable of making their own decisions, and children, the "do-gooders" of society, are victims to older adults' choices.

Most older adults claim to have experienced ageist treatment. The most prevalent type of ageist incidents is initiated by a general disrespect for older persons and assumed (yet false) connections about sickness and growing old. For example, it might be assumed that people walk with a limp because they are old, instead of merely injured. In other words, once they reach a certain age individuals are equated with their medical conditions and illnesses rather than viewed as the individuals they still are. In addition, older individuals' desires are overridden by younger family members and medical providers at times, simply because an assumption is made that they do not have their own best interests at heart. Although most incidents of ageism occur at an individual level, ageism is also addressed at the policy level to protect older individuals' civil rights.

In 1967, President Lyndon B. Johnson signed the Age Discrimination in Employment Act (ADEA) to address ageism in the work environment. It promotes the employment of older persons based on their ability rather than their age, prohibits arbitrary age discrimination in employment, and helps employers and workers find ways of meeting problems arising from the impact of age on employment (Age Discrimination in Employment Act of 1967, 2017). The ADEA protects individuals older than 40 years from ageist hiring practices (e.g., when a company refuses to hire a worker older than 50 years). Before the ADEA, employers could discriminate in hiring practices, working conditions, and termination practices for employment (e.g., stating a person is too young or old for a job). In addition, the ADEA prohibits forced retirement and guarantees reinstatement of employment or retroactive pay if the ageist offense is found to be intentional. However, most acts of ageism are not explicit or intentional; they are implicit, or unintentional. ADEA is a policy that protects older workers and individuals, the result of which has been increased employment of older workers. However, it has not eradicated personal ageist feelings. Approximately 64% of older persons have been, or have seen someone else be, the victim of ageism at work (Fleck, 2014). Yet, age discrimination cases are nearly impossible to prove because employers can find other reasons to discriminate against older adults in the workforce.

Perhaps one of the reasons ageism is such a widely accepted social phenomenon is because of the negative language associated with growing old. For example, we express ageism when we say, "Don't be an old maid!" or, "Stop acting like an old geezer!" Negative language extends beyond what words we choose to use personally as well. In the 1980s, older adults were characterized as "greedy geezers" as initial cuts in Social Security were made, and those sentiments are still housed within debates about Social Security and Medicare today. There is also negative language situated around the Baby Boomers, a generation of individuals born between 1946 and 1964 that is just now entering old age. Baby Boomers are being blamed for creating an economic and social "crisis" in American society because of a shift in the demographics of the population.

Students, practitioners, and scholars of age and aging should pay close attention to both structural and personal instances of ageism in everyday interactions, studies, and work. Many scholars of aging have suggested that ageism is even buried within the discipline and practice of gerontology; thus practitioners should be especially careful when considering the theories used and the sociopolitical contexts of growing old that surround research projects and gerontological practice. While working to solve societal and individual issues and problems related to aging, it is also necessary to check whether the theories used, the studies constructed, and the policies influenced and enacted are not unintentionally ageist.

See also Elderspeak; Employment.

Elizabeth A. Capezuti

Age Discrimination in Employment Act of 1967, 29 U.S.C. § 623 (2017).

Butler, R. N. (1969). Age-ism: Another form of bigotry. *The Gerontologist, 9,* 243–246.

Fleck, C. (2014). Forced out, older workers are fighting back. *AARP Bulletin.* Retrieved from http://www.aarp.org/work/on-the-job/info-2014/workplace-age-discrimination-infographic.html

Levy, S. R., & Macdonald, J. L. (2016). Progress on understanding ageism. *Journal of Social Issues, 72,* 5–25. doi:10.1111/josi.12153

AGING AGENCIES: CITY AND COUNTY LEVEL

Most older adults wish to remain in their own homes, but they may need assistance,

A

particularly from local resources, to do so. There are many options for older adults. A variety of private and governmental services are available to older adults at the city and county level. Because local services vary greatly, however, it is important for providers to contact the local government for details. Three sources of support for older adults are typically available in most areas of the United States: senior centers, area agencies on aging (AAAs), and the Eldercare Locator. Programs and services specifically designed for older persons who are actual or potential victims of abuse and neglect are provided by adult protective services.

SENIOR CENTERS

Senior centers, in some form, are typically available at the local level even in rural areas. According to the National Institute of Senior Centers (administered by the National Council on Aging [NCOA], 2017), approximately 11,000 senior centers exist throughout the United States, serving close to 10 million older adults annually. Every day, more than 1 million older adults use the services of a senior center. Senior centers are an integral part of the aging network, serving community needs, assisting other agencies in serving older adults, and providing opportunities for older adults to develop their potential as individuals. Centers may offer activities and programs for seniors to enjoy recreation and socialize with their peers. Many senior centers also offer programs to allow seniors to congregate for meals. Some centers have day programs and many provide outreach services through on-site visits from various health care providers (e.g., nurses, podiatrists, nutritionists).

The NCOA also examines senior centers and issues National Senior Center Accreditation to centers that offer exceptional standards of excellence. As of 2016, 119 senior centers have received accreditation.

Senior centers are based on the belief that aging is a normal developmental process, that peer interaction providing encouragement and support is important, and that adults have the right to actively participate in determining matters in which they have a vital interest. The centers attempt to provide an environment where older adults can continue to develop and grow while forming relationships with others. A variety of formal and informal classes and clubs are offered at centers. Even if the senior center does not provide a needed service, the center may be a resource for referrals to other community services. For many older adults and their families, the senior center serves as the *front door* to community-based services for both well and functionally impaired older adults. Senior centers may be operated by a local board of directors; may be part of local, municipal government; or may be operated as a nonprofit agency. The NCOA provides information on senior centers.

AREA AGENCIES ON AGING

AAAs are responsible for planning, coordinating, evaluating, and monitoring home- and community-based care programs for older adults. Approximately 650 AAAs are run by state, county, or city governments or as nonprofit or public agencies designated by the state. Each AAA is responsible for a designated geographical area known as a *planning and service area* (PSA). Each AAA creates a plan for its PSA to ensure that the needs of local older persons are being addressed. AAAs can be an excellent source of information to service providers and health professionals because they are familiar with most, if not all, programs serving the needs of older persons in the local community.

Many health care professionals, especially physicians, are unfamiliar with AAAs and their importance to the continuum of care. AAA staff can provide elders and their families with information and suggestions for local resources based on their specific needs. Through this service, AAAs can act as advocates for local elders at either the individual or the policy level. AAAs have financial responsibility to administer federal, state, and local funds to support locally specific services in their PSA. These services can varywidely by region but may include case-management services, transportation, counseling, adult day-care programs, health screening and education, nutritional education, meals, legal assistance, residential repair, physical fitness, recreation, home care, respite care, telephone reassurance, and volunteer services, among others. AAAs monitor the programs they support to ensure that high-quality services are being provided effectively and efficiently. The number of AAAs varies greatly from state to state. Rhode Island has only 1, whereas New York has approximately 60.

ELDERCARE LOCATOR

The Eldercare Locator provides the names, contract information, and service information for agencies throughout the United States. This service is staffed by trained professionals who provide the information needed to contact a care provider or agency in the designated area. They provide information on services such as meal programs, home care, transportation, housing alternatives, home repair, recreation, and social activities, as well as legal and other community services. The National Association of Area Agencies on Aging administers the Eldercare Locator as a public service of the U.S. Administration on Aging. They receive more than 200,000 calls a year. It can be accessed on the Internet (www.eldercare.gov), which includes an online chat feature, or by phone. The toll-free number is 1-800-677-1116, and it is operational Monday–Friday, 9 a.m. to 8 p.m., Eastern Standard Time. One value of the Eldercare Locator is its ability to research services for family members whose older relatives live far from them.

See also Adult Protective Services; Aging Agencies: Federal Level; Aging Agencies: State Level; Home Health Care; Meals on Wheels; Medicare; Older Americans Act; Retirement; Senior Centers; Veterans and Veteran Health.

William T. Lawson, III

National Council on Aging. (2017). Senior center facts. Retrieved from https://www.ncoa.org/news/resources-for-reporters/get-the-facts/senior-center-facts

Web Resources
Eldercare Locator: http://www.eldercare.gov/Eldercare.NET/Public/Index.aspx
National Association of Area Agencies on Aging: http://www.n4a.org
National Council on the Aging: http://www.ncoa.org
National Institute of Senior Center: http://www.ncoa.org/national-institute-of-senior-centers

AGING AGENCIES: FEDERAL LEVEL

In April 2012, the U.S. Department of Health and Human Services created the Administration for Community Living (ACL), a new federal agency that brought together the Administration on Aging (AoA), the Office on Disability, and the Administration on Developmental Disabilities into a single agency. This agency supports both crosscutting initiatives and efforts focused on the unique needs of individual groups, such as children with developmental disabilities or seniors with dementia. The goal of the ACL is to increase access to community supports and achieve full community participation for people with disabilities and seniors.

Within the ACL, the AoA functions as the federal focal point and advocacy agency for older persons. The official federal agency dedicated to policy development, planning, and the delivery of supportive home- and community-based services to older persons and their caregivers, the AoA administers federally funded programs established under the Older Americans Act (OAA).

Passed by Congress and signed into law by President Lyndon B. Johnson in 1965, the OAA has been amended several times and was last reauthorized in 2016. Congress intended the act to improve the lives of all older Americans in areas such as income, health, housing, employment, in-home and community services, research, and education. Anyone 60 years of age or older qualifies for programs funded by the Act, even though services tend to be targeted to elders in greatest social and economic need, with particular attention to low-income minority elders, Native Americans, persons

A

with Alzheimer's disease and related disorders (and their families), and rural older adults. The act's various titles form the foundation for a broad spectrum of services and providers that have become known as the Aging Network. Implementation of the network in the past 50 years has resulted in an impressive system of services on both the national and local levels that strives to promote independent living, create opportunities for active older persons, and meet the needs of older persons at risk of losing their independence.

The AoA has overall responsibility for administering the OAA and distributing federal funds in accordance with the Act's requirements. In addition, it sets policy for the Aging Network at the state and local levels and funds national grantees that provide research, training, support, and demonstration programs for the Aging Network. The AoA is responsible for numerous functions specified in the Act, including effective and visible advocacy for the elderly within the federal government, coordination of research and implementation of programs, provision of technical assistance to states and communities, collection and dissemination of information, and monitoring and evaluation of programs developed pursuant to the act.

The AoA oversees a network of some 56 state units on aging (SUAs); 629 area agencies on aging (AAAs); 244 tribal organizations and two Native Hawaiian organizations; 5,000 senior centers; and more than 27,000 local service providers. The AoA has 10 regional offices throughout the country that provide technical assistance to the states, communicate AoA national policies, and review and monitor SUA plans. The AoA distributes funds authorized by the act to the SUAs on the basis of state plans and according to a formula that considers the number and percentage of older persons in each state. The SUAs then distribute the funds to AAAs, which contract with local service providers.

The majority of services provided throughout the Aging Network are supported by funds authorized under Title III of the Act. Each community offers different services, depending on available resources. Title III funds can be used for information and referral services; supportive services and centers; disease prevention and

health promotion; nutrition services, including food distribution and both congregate and home-delivered meals; homemaker, home health aide, and other in-home services for the frail elderly; senior centers and day-care programs; caregiver support programs; transportation; ombudsman programs for residents of long-term care facilities; crime prevention and victim assistance programs; translation services for non–English-speaking elders; protective services for abused, neglected, and exploited elders; and legal services.

In addition to services and programs funded under Title III, the AoA administers funds under Title IV of the Act, earmarked for its own operations and for providing direct grants and contracts for research, training, and demonstration programs on a national level through the Discretionary Funds Program. The Title IV mandate is aimed, generally, at building knowledge, developing innovative model programs, and training personnel for service in the field of aging.

Title V of the Act authorizes funds to subsidize part-time community-service jobs and training opportunities for unemployed, low-income persons aged 55 years and older. Established under Title V, the Senior Community Services Employment Program is administered by the U.S. Department of Labor.

Title VI awards annual grants directly to tribes and tribal organizations and Native organizations for nutrition services (including congregate and home-delivered meals), information, and access; transportation; and in-home supportive services. Training and technical assistance are provided to Title VI grantees both electronically and through onsite, telephone, and written consultation; national meetings; and newsletters. The AoA funds three National Resource Centers on Older Indians, Alaska Natives, and Native Hawaiians to serve as focal points for the development and sharing of technical information and expertise to Indian organizations, Title VI grantees, Native American communities, educational institutions, and professionals and paraprofessionals in the field. Since 2000, Title VI grants support programs for caregivers of Native Americans.

Title VII oversees the protection of vulnerable elder rights. These activities include state long-term care ombudsman programs; programs for the prevention of elder abuse, neglect, and exploitation; and state elder rights and legal assistance development. Long-term care ombudsmen advocate on behalf of individuals and groups of residents in nursing homes, board and care homes, assisted-living facilities, and other adult care facilities. They also work to effect system changes on local, state, and national levels. The Office of Elder Justice and Adult Protective Services manages the operation, administration and assessment of elder abuse prevention. In addition, this office provides legal assistance and pension counseling programs.

The AoA supports the National Legal Resource Center (NLRC), which serves as a centralized access point for a national legal assistance support system serving professionals and advocates working in legal and aging services networks. The NLRC also funds organizations that support national legal support projects and centers that provide training and technical assistance to advocates in the field. The support centers collaborate in their efforts through information exchange, training, and liaison with field advocates. Support centers currently funded by the AoA are the National Consumer Law Center, the nation's consumer law expert; the National Senior Citizens Law Center, which provides consultation to senior legal services providers and substantive training sessions; the Center for Social Gerontology, a nonprofit research, training, and social policy organization dedicated to promoting the autonomy of older persons and advancing their well-being in society; and the American Bar Association Commission on Law and Aging, which examines law-related concerns of older persons.

Other public services supported by AoA funds include the Eldercare Locator, the National Aging Information Center, the National Center on Elder Abuse, and the Pension Rights Center. The Eldercare Locator is administered by the AoA, together with the National Association of Area Agencies on Aging and the National Association of State Units on Aging. It is a nationwide directory-assistance service designed to help older persons and caregivers locate local support resources. The National Aging Information Center serves as a

central source for a wide variety of programs and policies, related materials, and demographic and other statistical data on the health, economic, and social status of older Americans. Its services are free of charge and include access to information, databases, printed materials, statistical information, and a reading room and reference collection. The National Center on Elder Abuse provides information to professionals and the public, offers technical assistance and training to elder abuse agencies and related professionals, conducts short-term research, and assists with elder abuse program and policy development.

Caregivers, service providers, and others involved with the needs, protection, and advocacy of older persons should be familiar with the vast array of services and programs supported or administered by the AoA and the agencies and organizations with which it collaborates.

See also Aging Agencies: City and County Level; Aging Agencies: State Level; Older Americans Act; Social Security.

William T. Lawson, III

Web Resources
Administration for Community Living: https://www.acl.gov/about-acl
Centers for Medicare & Medicaid Services: http://www.cms.hhs.gov
Eldercare Locator: http://www.eldercare.gov
Justice in Aging: http://www.nsclc.org
Older Americans Act: http://www.ncpssm.org/PublicPolicy/OlderAmericans/Documents/ArticleID/1171/Older-Americans-Act
Social Security Administration: http://www.ssa.gov

AGING AGENCIES: STATE LEVEL

State services are designed to assist the elderly and their caregivers in maintaining health and adequate finances and remaining safely in the community for as long as possible. Many state services developed pursuant to passage of the federal Older Americans Act (OAA). The act

A

charges states to provide services for those who are 60 years and older and to remove economic, physical, and social barriers to their remaining in the community and out of institutions. Many federally funded services administered by the states have federal guidelines to ensure uniform eligibility nationwide. However, with trends for increased local and state control over the allocation of funds and creation of alternate delivery systems, the same service can vary among states. The state's role in care for the elderly falls into four categories: research, information dissemination, investigation and licensing, and services. How these functions are provided varies within and among states and state agencies.

RESEARCH

States conduct research on topics that affect quality of life and services for their citizens, such as quality of care in nursing homes, cost-effectiveness of managed long-term care and the effect of taxes, and new services such as assisted living. Several states are planning services for the projected increase in the number of elderly in the 21st century.

DISSEMINATION OF INFORMATION

Many state agencies have toll-free telephone services and websites to provide information for the elderly and their caregivers on topics such as finding state services, obtaining preventive services, and contacting investigatory agencies to report fraud and abuse. Almost all states offer a federally funded state health insurance program that provides information and counseling on health insurance, including Medicare and Medicaid, long-term care insurance, and Medigap insurance policies. State veterans' agencies provide information regarding veterans' benefits (state and federal), such as tax reductions, home care services, and health care.

INVESTIGATION AND LICENSING

State governments investigate fraud and abuse and control the licensing and certification of individuals (i.e., physicians, nurses, social workers, and dentists) and organizations that provide care to elderly residents of the state. Nursing homes and adult homes are licensed, certified, regulated, and surveyed by state agencies. In many states, the office of the long-term care ombudsman investigates charges of institutional abuse, mistreatment, and neglect.

SERVICES

All states provide adult protective services that investigate reports of and protect older adults from financial, sexual, physical, and mental abuse. Some states have programs and services for older residents that may not be replicated in other states, such as prescription drug programs that subsidize pharmaceuticals, special school and property tax breaks, and recreational benefits. The services may have eligibility criteria based on medical need, age, and income.

In general, services for older adults are administered and monitored by state agencies that receive and pass federal and state funds to localities. The agencies that administer these federal funds may differ in different states; programs and jurisdictions vary. Some states provide direct services to senior citizens; others monitor locally delivered services. A local area agency on aging or the state unit on aging can provide information on which services are available in communities and how they can be accessed by clinicians, older adults, and family members.

Several state-operated services support health care needs or provide preventive health programs such as health screening and well-patient clinics. Preventive and rehabilitative mental health services offered at the community level may be state funded and operated.

Many states offer property, sales, and school tax breaks for senior citizens or low-income older adults. Senior citizens may pay reduced admission fees at state parks and recreational sites. Some states also provide recreational or sport events—*senior games* or *Senior Olympics*—designed to help older adults remain healthy and competitive.

Many support services provided locally, such as home care to assist older adults with personal hygiene, light housekeeping, meals, and chores, are monitored by the state. A case-management or care-management professional assigned by the state or local agency assesses the needs of the older person and establishes a plan of care.

Services that may be available outside the home (i.e., community-based services) include nutrition education and counseling; transportation for medical appointments, shopping, and visiting; and other activities. Lunchtime or evening meals can be provided in group (congregate) settings at community sites. Senior centers in urban and rural areas offer support services, such as meals, counseling, recreation, and visiting. Social-model adult day centers offer support, management, and nutrition services. Medical-model centers provide rehabilitation and therapy as well as support and nutrition services.

Financial assistance is available through state-monitored programs that help with the costs of housing or home renovation, health care (i.e., Medicaid), and prescription drugs and provide state-funded employment opportunities for low-income older adults. The maze of services can be overwhelming to older adults, particularly those for whom English is a second language, and their families. Thus it is critical that health care professionals be aware of the services and benefits elders need to maintain a quality life.

The National Association of States United for Aging and Disabilities (formerly known as the National Association of State Units on Aging, or NASUA), a nonprofit association representing the officially designated state and territorial agencies on aging, provides general and specialized information, consultation, training, technical assistance, and professional-development support on the full range of policy, program, and management issues of concern to states.

See also Adult Day Services; Aging Agencies: City and County Level; Aging Agencies: Federal Level; Meals on Wheels; Veterans and Veteran Health.

William T. Lawson, III

Web Resources

Administration for Community Living, Aging and Disability: https://www.acl.gov

National Conference of State Legislatures Committee on Aging: http://www.ncsl.org/state-federal -committees.aspx?tabs=855,25,669#Aging
The National Association of State United for Aging and Disabilities: http://www.nasuad.org

AGING PRISONERS

The elderly inmates are one of the fastest growing segments of incarcerated individuals. Between 2000 and 2009, the number of older prisoners in U.S. state and federal prisons grew to 79% (Williams, Stern, Mellow, Safer, & Greifinger, 2012). The proportion of aging prisoners is increasing because of stricter sentencing and parole requirements, the aging of the Baby Boom generation, and a greater number of serious crimes committed by older adults (Williams, Goodwin, Baillargeon, Ahalt, & Walter, 2012). A major difficulty in describing prison-residing elderly is the lack of clarity on the age limit of the population. There is no standard among correctional systems for categorizing inmates as elderly—anywhere from 50 to 70 years can be considered a starting age. This variability may come from the commonly held belief that inmates age rapidly in the correctional system. Poor prior health care, increased physical and psychological trauma, and other life event stressors push the physiological age of inmates 10 to 15 years beyond their biological age (Maschi, Gibson, Zgoba, & Morgen, 2011; Williams, Stern, et al., 2012). However, correctional health care experts and the Bureau of Justice Statistics are settling on age 55 years as the start of the older inmate category (Williams, Stern, et al., 2012).

The overall annual cost of older prisoners is estimated to be three times higher than that of their younger counterparts (Williams, Stern, et al., 2012). Inmates aged 55 years and older carry a greater burden of chronic illness and greatly increase the costs of prison management. A research review found that jail and prison inmates have higher rates of chronic conditions such as hypertension, asthma, and arthritis than the general population (Binswanger, Krueger, & Steiner, 2009). Higher rates of disability of

A

aging inmates increases housing costs due to the need for special accommodation for decreased functionality.

Nearly 60% of inmates older than 50 years have at least one disability, with the most common being declines in ambulation and cognition (Bronson & Maruschak, 2015). Cognitive and sensory decline can affect the elderly inmate in several ways. Although inmates are relieved of cognitively complex activities such as financial management, other prison-specific activities such as locating the right cell or avoiding victimization arise as challenges. The aging inmate may be inappropriately disciplined for not following officers' directions due to deafness, declining judgment, or growing dementia. Inmates may be manipulated by younger or predatory criminals. Incarcerated older adults are isolated from possible family and community support during a critical time of declining functionality (Maschi et al., 2011).

Elderly female inmates have additional concerns. Although this is a much smaller segment of the inmate population, female incarceration, particularly of women older than 55 years, is on the increase. The smaller number of elderly female inmates, coupled with the unique needs of this population, often means that resources are not available to meet requirements. Yet female inmates use significantly more health care resources and report more chronic medical conditions, psychiatric disorders, and drug dependence than male inmates (Binswanger, Merrill, et al., 2010). These differences may be exacerbated with age.

Correctional officers, who are in contact with the prisoner population on a continual basis are a liaison between the elderly inmate and health care services. Yet correctional officers have little understanding of the needs of geriatric prisoners (Masters, Magnuson, Bayer, Potter, & Falkowski, 2016). More training is needed for prison staff to be aware of age-related inmate impairments, such as the potential for falls, growing confusion, incontinence, and declining mobility. State and federal correctional systems are moving to protect the older inmate population through the addition of geriatric housing, dementia units, and palliative care programs.

More is needed in developing reentry programs that identify and resolve the postincarceration transition issues of elderly prisoners (Williams, Stern, et al., 2012).

Lorry Schoenly

Binswanger, I. A., Krueger, P. M., & Steiner, J. F. (2009). Prevalence of chronic medical conditions among jail and prison inmates in the USA compared with the general population. *Journal of Epidemiology and Community Health, 63*(11), 912–919. doi:10.1136/jech.2009.090662

Binswanger, I. A., Merrill, J. O., Krueger, P. M., White, M. C., Booth, R. E., & Elmore, J. G. (2010). Gender differences in chronic medical, psychiatric, and substance-dependence disorders among jail inmates. *Journal Information, 100*(3). doi:10.2105/AJPH.2008.149591

Bronson, J., & Maruschak, L. M. (2015). Bureau of Justice Statistics (BJS)—Disabilities among prison and jail inmates, 2011–12. *Bureau of Justice Statistics*. Retrieved from https://www.bjs.gov/index.cfm?ty=pbdetail&iid=5500

Maschi, T., Gibson, S., Zgoba, K. M., & Morgen, K. (2011). Trauma and life event stressors among young and older adult prisoners. *Journal of Correctional Health Care, 17*(2), 160–172. doi:10.1177/1078345810396682

Masters, J. L., Magnuson, T. M., Bayer, B. L., Potter, J. F., & Falkowski, P. P. (2016). Preparing corrections staff for the future: Results of a 2-day training about aging inmates. *Journal of Correctional Health Care, 22*(2), 118–128. doi:10.1177/1078345816634667

Williams, B. A., Goodwin, J. S., Baillargeon, J., Ahalt, C., & Walter, L. C. (2012). Addressing the aging crisis in U.S. criminal justice health care. *Journal of the American Geriatrics Society, 60*(6), 1150–1156. doi:10.1111/j.1532-5415.2012.03962.x

Williams, B. A., Stern, M. F., Mellow, J., Safer, M., & Greifinger, R. B. (2012). Aging in correctional custody: Setting a policy agenda for older prisoner health care. *American Journal of Public Health, 102*(8), 1475–1481.

Web Resources
Academy of Correctional Health Professionals: http://www.correctionalhealth.org
CorrectionalNurse.Net: https://correctionalnurse.net
National Commission on Correctional Health Care: https://www.ncchc.org

ALZHEIMER'S ASSOCIATION

Alzheimer's disease, the most common form of dementia, is a progressive degenerative disease of the brain. An estimated 5.4 million Americans have Alzheimer's disease and an estimated 15 million family members consider themselves *caregivers* for persons with Alzheimer's disease. Alzheimer's care takes a unique physical, emotional, and financial toll on families (Alzheimer's Association, 2016). Family caregivers of people with dementia may experience greater risk of chronic disease, physiological impairments, increased health care utilization and mortality than those who are not caregivers (McCabe, You, & Tatangelo, 2016).

Alzheimer's disease is officially listed as the sixth-leading cause of death in the United States (Alzheimer's Association, 2016). One in nine persons older than 65 years and 32% to 44% of persons older than 85 years have Alzheimer's disease. Alzheimer's disease progresses over an average of 4 to 8 years—for some, as many as 20 years—from the onset of symptoms. In later stages, persons are vulnerable to developing other medical conditions and dying before they would if they did not have Alzheimer's disease. The disease knows no social or economic boundaries, and more women than men have Alzheimer's disease and other dementias. Risk factors include advancing age and a strong family history, although rare familial Alzheimer's disease can begin in the 30s, 40s, or 50s.

More than 70% of persons with Alzheimer's disease live at home, where family and friends provide almost 80% of their care. More than 60% of persons living in nursing homes and up to 40% of persons living in assisted-living and non–nursing home residential care have Alzheimer's disease. Alzheimer's disease is devastating to patients and to families, with annual economic value of informal family care estimated at $216.4 billion in 2012. Alzheimer's disease costs American businesses more than $61 billion annually, primarily attributable to lost productivity of family caregivers. The average lifetime cost per patient is estimated to be $174,000, with paid care at home averaging $61,000 per year per patient and nursing home care averaging $90,520 per year (Alzheimer's Association, 2016).

RESEARCH

The Alzheimer's Association is the only national voluntary health organization dedicated to research for the causes, cures, treatment, and prevention of Alzheimer's disease and to the provision of education and support services to affected individuals and their families. The national Alzheimer's Association, headquartered in Chicago and with a public policy office in Washington, DC, operates through a network of more than 200 local and area chapters. Chapters sponsor support groups, publish newsletters, run volunteer telephone helplines, and provide education and support to patients, families, and health and social service professionals caring for those with Alzheimer's disease.

Funding biomedical research through both the Alzheimer's Association and the National Institutes of Health is at the top of the association's federal agenda. Since 1990, the Association has been successful in boosting federal research funding from $146 million to about $647 million, and the association itself has funded more than $185 million in research grants since 1982.

The association's vision is to create a world without Alzheimer's disease while optimizing quality of life for individuals and their families. The organization has moved over time from a sole focus on family support to a broader focus on individuals with Alzheimer's. There is now good evidence that a long latent or preclinical phase of Alzheimer's disease occurs before symptoms develop and new evidence that persons with mild cognitive impairment are at high risk of converting to Alzheimer's disease in 3 years. Such persons are diagnosed at a point of insight, and their families are looking for support programs that focus on the patient as well as the family.

PUBLIC POLICY

Other goals of the Alzheimer's Association are to promote, develop, and disseminate educational

A

programs and guidelines for health and social service professionals; to increase public awareness and concern for the impact of Alzheimer's disease on individuals and families in a diverse society; and to expand access to services, information, and optimal care techniques. Current programs focus on personalized knowledge services through toll-free lines, the Internet, and publications, as well as care-coordination services on the local level.

Perhaps the greatest success of this voluntary organization has been its public policy coalitions and extensive federal, state, and local advocacy networks that promote legislation responsive to the needs of individuals with Alzheimer's disease and their families. Nearly a quarter of a million Americans signed the Association's petition to President Obama, calling for a strong national Alzheimer's plan to help all Americans affected by this disease. An annual public policy conference provides opportunities for family advocates from the entire country to meet with elected representatives to discuss a national program to conquer Alzheimer's disease. A state-policy clearinghouse tracks long-term care and other legislation at the state and local level that affects Alzheimer's families.

The Chicago office of the national Alzheimer's Association houses the Green-Field Library, publishes research and practice updates for physicians and consumers, coordinates the Walk to End Alzheimer's as a national fundraising and awareness program, and hosts an annual educational conference for care professionals. A national toll-free hotline (800-272-3900) and website (www.alz.org) link families and professionals to local and area chapters and support groups.

See also Cognitive Changes in Aging; Cognitive Instruments; Dementia: Special Care Units; Wandering and Elopement.

Elizabeth A. Capezuti

Alzheimer's Association. (2016). Alzheimer's disease facts and figures. Retrieved from http://www.alz .org/documents_custom/2016-facts-and-figures .pdf

McCabe, M., You, E., & Tatangelo, G. (2016). Hearing their voice: A systematic review of dementia family caregivers' needs. *The Gerontologist, 56*(5), e70–e88. doi:10.1093/geront/gnw078

Web Resource
Alzheimer's Association: http://www.alz.org

AMDA—THE SOCIETY FOR POST-ACUTE AND LONG-TERM CARE MEDICINE

AMDA—The Society for Post-Acute and Long-Term Medicine (formerly known as the AMDA—Dedicated to Long-Term Care Medicine as well as the American Medical Directors Association) is the professional association of medical directors, physicians, and other health care providers in long-term care, dedicated to excellence in patient care by providing education, advocacy, information, and professional development.

Founded in 1975, the AMDA is a national organization representing more than 5,500 medical directors and other physicians who practice in long-term care settings. AMDA is committed to the continuous improvement of the quality of patient care by providing education, advocacy, information, and professional development for medical directors and other health care professionals. The Society has two affiliate organizations. The American Board of Post-Acute and Long-Term Care Medicine oversees a certification program for medical directors in post-acute/long-term care, credentialing certified medical directors (CMDs). The Foundation for Post-Acute and Long-Term Care Medicine oversees awards, community outreach, education, and research with the mission to advance the quality of life for persons in post-acute and long-term care by educating future and current health care professionals.

Among AMDA's many accomplishments are its public policies for improved care. These policies include the establishment of the Certified Medical Director Program to demonstrate competence in both clinical medicine and medical direction and administrative responsibilities. It has also worked to improve standards in federal nursing facilities, contributing to the passage of the 1987 Nursing Home Reform Act. To help clinicians more directly, AMDA develops information kits and organizes national symposia to aid in the efforts to improve long-term care.

Elizabeth A. Capezuti

Web Resource
American Medical Directors Association: http://www.amda.com

AMERICAN FEDERATION FOR AGING RESEARCH

The American Federation for Aging Research (AFAR) is a national nonprofit organization dedicated to biomedical research into the fundamental processes of aging, which holds out the promise of extending healthy life and finding cures for diseases that accompany old age. This hope is based on the accelerating pace of scientific discovery and the commitment of new scientists, such as those funded by AFAR, who dedicate their career to answering the fundamental questions of how and why we age. Since 1981, AFAR, through its own privately funded grants and other administered programs, has granted more than $150 million to more than 3,000 talented researchers to help them begin and further careers in aging research and geriatric medicine.

Elizabeth A. Capezuti

Web Resources
American Federation for Aging Research: http://www.afar.org
Foundation for Health in Aging: http://www.healthinaging.org

AMERICAN GERIATRICS SOCIETY

The American Geriatrics Society (AGS) is a leading professional organization of health care providers dedicated to improving the health and well-being of all older adults. With an active membership of nearly 6,000 health care professionals, the AGS has a long history of effecting change in the provision of health care for older adults. In the past decade, the society has become a pivotal force in shaping attitudes, policies, and practices regarding health care for older people.

In 1942, a group of physicians interested in advancing medical care for older adults met with the intention of forming a specialty society dedicated to geriatric medicine. At this inaugural meeting, the founding membership of the AGS decided that any physician with an interest in geriatrics who had graduated from a recognized medical school and was a member in good standing of a state medical society would be eligible to join the society. The AGS promotes high-quality, comprehensive, and accessible care for America's older population, including those who are chronically ill and disabled. The work is done at the national level as well as through state affiliates and special interest groups of the organization. Their objectives are:

- Expanding the geriatrics knowledge base through initiatives that promote basic, clinical, and health services research regarding the health of older adults.
- Increasing the number of health care professionals employing the principles of geriatric medicine when caring for older persons by supporting the expansion of geriatric education in all applicable health professions and promoting the development of systems of care and practice redesign that facilitate the provision of quality geriatric care.
- Recruiting physicians and other health care professionals into careers in geriatrics through efforts to ensure that geriatrics is a viable, attractive, and rewarding career choice.
- Guiding public policy through advocacy so policy supports improved health and health care for seniors.
- Raising public awareness of the need for high-quality, culturally sensitive geriatric health care so an empowered, proactive public can help drive improvements in the quality of care that older persons receive (AGS, n.d., "Strategies for Achieving Our Vision").

The organization provides leadership to health care professionals, policy makers, and the public by developing, implementing, and advocating programs in patient care, research, professional and public education, and public policy. In response to the many challenges that a rapidly aging population poses, the AGS has established the Foundation for Health in Aging (FHA). The FHA's goals are to build a bridge between geriatrics health care professionals and the public and to advocate on behalf of older adults and their special needs: wellness and preventive care, self-responsibility and independence, and connections to family and community.

Elizabeth A. Capezuti

American Geriatrics Society. (n.d.). Who we are. Retrieved from https://www.americangeriatrics.org/about-us/who-we-are

Web Resources
American Federation for Aging Research: http://www.afar.org
American Geriatrics Society: http://www.americangeriatrics.org

AMERICAN HEALTH CARE ASSOCIATION

The American Health Care Association (AHCA) is a nonprofit federation of affiliated state health organizations, together representing more than 13,000 nonprofit and for-profit assisted-living, nursing-facility, developmentally disabled, and post-acute care providers that care for more than 1 million older and disabled individuals each day. At its Washington, DC, headquarters, the association maintains legislative, regulatory, and public affairs and member services staffs that work both internally and externally to assist the interests of government and the general public, as well as member providers.

The AHCA provides educational, informational, and administrative tools to consumers of long-term care, providers, health care professionals, regulators, and policy makers. Daily and monthly electronic updates on the AHCA Website and *Provider Magazine* distill current clinical and health services research and issues, proposed legislation, and statistical data for all members of its public, professional, and industry constituency.

The annual national conference invites participants to special seminars, presentations, and poster sessions on issues affecting long-term care. Many of the sessions are approved for continuing-education credit. Regulators and policy makers participate in many of the informational sessions, describe new initiatives, and hear the concerns of providers.

Research is supported, conducted, and disseminated through the Research and Information Service and includes impact assessments of current and proposed public policy; regulatory compliance reports; publication of *Facts and Trends*, an annual compilation of data about residents in assisted living, nursing-home, and post-acute care facilities; utilization and expenditure reports; and quality initiatives.

AHCA and collaborating organizations provide a large number of resources such as clinical practice guidelines. A scholarship program is specifically maintained for student nurses in registered nursing or licensed practical or vocational training programs. The National Council of Assisted Living (NCAL) is a program affiliate of AHCA dedicated to representing the needs and interests of residents of assisted-living facilities and their owner-operators. NCAL is a resource for legislative updates and quality guidelines for assisted living, model consumer agreements, and state listings of providers and has an active informational and advocacy role in assisted living.

AHCA is committed to developing necessary and reasonable public policies that balance economic and regulatory principles to support quality care and quality of life, and it is dedicated to professionalism and ethical behavior among all who provide long-term care.

Elizabeth A. Capezuti

Web Resource
American Health Care Association: http://www.ahca.org

AMERICAN INDIAN ELDERS

According to the U.S. Census Bureau, approximately 5 million individuals, or about 1.5% of the U.S. population, identified themselves in 2010 as American Indian or Native Alaskan (AINA; Norris, Vines, & Hoeffel, 2012). The U.S. Office of Management and Budget (OMB, 1970) defined *AINA people* as descendants of "any of the original peoples of North and South America (including Central America) and who maintain tribal affiliation or community attachment." Although most use the terms *Native American* and *American Indian* interchangeably, there has been controversy around how to represent this population; some American Indians prefer to be called *Indian* rather than *Native American*, based on the belief that the term *Indian* reflects the language used in treaties with the federal government. Others have used *First Nations, indigenous peoples*, or specific tribal designations (e.g., Lakota) as more culturally sensitive nomenclature (Wilkins, 2006).

In 2010, approximately 20% of AINA people resided in designated American Indian areas (i.e., federal reservation and/or off-reservation trust land, Oklahoma tribal statistical area, state reservation, or federal- or state-designated American Indian statistical areas). There are more than 561 federally recognized tribes, with each sovereign tribe having established its own standards of membership. All federal agencies are obligated by executive orders to actively engage in tribal consultations on affairs that affect AINA peoples living on or near federally recognized reservations. The federal responsibility to the tribes includes health care, education, and public health.

Despite their diversity in terms of traditional culture and lifestyle, most Native Americans honor and respect their elders in their families and communities; older adults are widely valued for their wisdom and spiritual leadership. Being an "elder" is not necessarily tied to chronological age; rather, it is a symbol of social or physical status. Native American elders are valued members of their communities, who most often prefer to remain and grow old in their own home and community settings. Accordingly, family caregiving is an extended tradition that is strongly tied to cultural preferences and expectations.

SPIRITUALITY AND HEALTH

Spiritual beliefs are intrinsic to AINA culture and form the basis of understanding about diseases and healings. Some tribes or nations explain the causes of illness as an "imbalance" between the spiritual, mental, physical, and social interactions of the individual with the family or clan. Illnesses that are considered nonindigenous such as diabetes, cancer, and gallbladder disease, are often treated with "white man's medicine," whereas indigenous Indian problems such as physical pain, family relationship problems resulting in physical symptoms, or "sickness of the spirit" (what Western providers often diagnose as mental illness or alcoholism) are treated primarily with Indian medicine (Hendrix, 2001).

HEALTH AND ACCESS TO HEALTH CARE

Although health information about urban AINA populations is limited to cross-sectional studies, the available research indicates that these communities have poorer health and functional status, in virtually all respects, than the general population or their reservation-based counterparts. AINAs are more likely than non-Hispanic whites to report that they have no usual source of health care or health insurance coverage. The leading causes of death among AINAs aged 65 years or older are cardiovascular diseases and cancer, and their likelihood of contracting diabetes is more than double that of the general population. The incidence of Alzheimer's disease appears to be lower in this population than in the US population in general for all races (USDHHS, 2014).

Native Americans are less likely to use services such as in-home supportive services for personal care, respite, and adult day care because of language and cultural barriers. Native American elders lack access to and have low participation rates in age-specific federal programs, such as Social Security, Medicare, and Medicaid, for which they are eligible. Access to health care varies according to residential

A

location and government recognition of tribal status. The Indian Health Service (IHS), an agency within the U.S. Department of Health and Human Services (USDHHS), provides health care for approximately 2 million eligible AINAs through a system of programs and facilities located on or near Indian reservations and through contractors in certain urban areas. However, more than half of the total American Indian population, including elders, lives in urban areas where IHS operates few clinics.

Access to both institutional and non-institutional long-term care is also limited in rural areas, where most federally recognized reservations are located. IHS does not directly provide long-term care, and contract funds are limited. To partially remediate this, the Veterans Health Administration (VHA) and IHS have executed a number of agreements and initiatives to improve access and health care outcomes for AINA veterans who are eligible to receive health care from both federal agencies. The results of these efforts, including noninstitutional long-term care programs, are regularly reported to standing Congressional committees on Indian and veterans' affairs. Although younger veterans may use IHS services exclusively, reliance on the VA for health care increases with age and co-morbidity (Kramer et al., 2011).

Health-promotion and disease-prevention programs targeted to AINA populations have focused on risk-reduction strategies (such as education on exercise and dieting) that take into account tribal-specific variations in health-related risks and behaviors. Successful methods often invoke traditional values of respect and authority for older role models and spokespersons, oral transmission of knowledge, non-intrusive guidance, and the importance of family and community continuity. Although scant literature has focused on AINA elders, an online bibliography of peer-reviewed health research for this special population is available the U.S. National Library of Medicine (americanindian health.nlm.nih.gov).

IMPLICATIONS FOR TREATMENT

Providers should perform a comprehensive cultural assessment when offering care to Native American elders. Traditional etiquette may call for avoidance of eye contact, firm handshakes, and shunning of direct questions and responses; these behaviors indicate respect in Indian cultures and should not be mistaken for furtiveness. Silence may indicate responsiveness rather than avoidance or hostility. Conversational pauses allow the older person and their family to absorb information and formulate a thorough response; they denote respect for the serious nature of the business at hand. A calm, accepting, nonjudgmental approach is appreciated when establishing a trusting relationship, which may take more than one visit.

End-of-life treatment decisions tend to favor natural approaches in which the inevitability of death is accepted. Clinicians should be aware of spiritual healing, which patients and families may wish to use as an accompaniment to treatment. When elders can no longer speak for themselves, a family proxy (whose role may reflect the indigenous social structure) usually emerges to express what should be accepted as the authentic wishes of the patient, if these have not been previously determined with the provider. For elders seeking surgery, it is not unusual for patients to request return of any removed body tissues after surgery, based on the belief that the body must be whole to transition into the next world (Hendrix, 2001). Clinicians providing pain management to an elder should be aware that most AINAs regard expression of pain as unacceptable, whereas being able to withstand discomfort is a survival skill. As such, older AINAs may be less likely to request pain medication and more likely to use internal resources to manage their suffering (Hendrix, 2001).

Margaret Salisu

Hendrix, L. R. (2001). Health care of American Indian and Alaska Native elders. In G. Yeo (Ed.), *Curriculum in ethnogeriatrics* (2nd ed.). Palo Alto, CA: Stanford Geriatric Education Center. Retrieved from http://www.stanford.edu/group/ethnoger

Kramer, B. J., Jouldjian, S., Wang, M., Dang, J., Mitchell, M. N., & Saliba, D. (2011). Do correlates of dual use by American Indian and Alaska Native Veterans operate uniformly across the Veterans

Health Administration and the Indian Health Service? *Journal of General Internal Medicine, 26,* 662–668.

Norris, T., Vines, P. L., & Hoeffel, E. M. (2012). *The American Indian and Alaska Native Population: 2010* (pp. 1–32). Washington, DC: U.S. Department of Commerce, Economics and Statistics Administration, U.S. Census Bureau.

Office of Management and Budget. (1970). Revisions to the standards for the classification of federal data on race and ethnicity. Retrieved from https://www.whitehouse.gov/omb/fedreg_1997standards

U.S. Department of Health and Human Services, Indian Health Service, Office of Public Health Support, Division of Program Statistics. (2014). *Trends in Indian health,* 2014 edition. Retrieved from https://www.ihs.gov/dps/publications/trends2014

Wilkins, D. (2006). *American Indian politics and the American political system.* New York, NY: Rowman & Littlefield.

Web Resources

Centers for American Indian and Native Alaska Mental Health: http://www.ucdenver.edu/academics/colleges/PublicHealth/research/centers/CAIANH/NCAIANMHR/Pages/ncaianmhr.aspx

Library of Medicine: http://www.americanindianhealth.nlm.nih.gov

National Indian Council on Aging: http://www.nicoa.org

National Legal Resource Center, Older Native Americans: https://nlrc.acl.gov/Legal_Issues/Older_Native_Americans/Native_Americans.aspx

National Resource Center on Native American Aging: http://www.med.und.nodak.edu/depts/rural//nrcnaa

U.S. Deptartment of Health & Human Services, Indian Health Service: http://www.ihs.gov

U.S. National Library of Medicine, American Indian Health: https://americanindianhealth.nlm.nih.gov

AMERICAN NURSES ASSOCIATION

The American Nurses Association (ANA) is the only full-service professional organization representing the interests of the nation's 3.6 million registered nurses through its constituent and state nurses associations, as well as its organizational affiliates. The ANA advances the nursing profession by fostering high standards of nursing practice, promoting the rights of nurses in the workplace, projecting a positive and realistic view of nursing, and lobbying Congress and regulatory agencies on health care issues affecting nurses and the public. The mission statement of ANA is "nurses advancing our profession to improve health for all."

The ANA comprises itself, its constituent members, associate organizational members, organizational affiliates, individual members, individual affiliate members, and related entities. The ANA's affiliates are nursing organizations that belong to ANA as organizations. Working together, ANA and these organizational affiliates seek to share information and collaborate in finding solutions to issues that face the nursing profession, regardless of specialty. Affiliates each hold a voting seat in both ANA's House of Delegates and ANA's Congress of Nursing Practice and Economics.

The three ANA-affiliated organizations are the American Nurses Foundation (ANF), the American Academy of Nursing (AAN), and the American Nurses Credentialing Center (ANCC). The ANF was founded in 1955 as the research, education, and charitable affiliate of the ANA. The foundation complements the work of the ANA by raising funds and developing and managing grants to support advances in research, education, and clinical practice. The AAN is an organization of distinguished leaders in nursing who have been recognized for their outstanding contributions to the profession and to health care. The AAN consists of approximately 2,400 Fellows who are leaders in academia, practice, research, and management.

The mission of the ANCC is to promote excellence in nursing and health care globally through credentialing programs. ANCC's internationally renowned credentialing programs certify and recognize individual nurses in specialty practice areas; recognize health care organizations for promoting safe, positive work environments (Magnet Recognition Program®); and accredit continuing nursing

A

A

education organizations. The ANA established its certification program in 1973 to provide tangible recognition of professional achievement in defined functional or clinical areas of nursing. The ANCC bases its programs on the standards set by the ANA Congress for Nursing Practice.

The ANA also publishes *American Nurse, American Nurse Today,* and *OJIN: The Online Journal of Issues in Nursing.*™

Elizabeth A. Capezuti

Web Resources
American Academy of Nursing: http://www.aannet
.org
American Nurses Association: http://www.nursing
world.org
American Nurses Credentialing Center: http://www
.nursecredentialing.org
American Nurses Foundation: http://www.anfon
line.org

AMERICAN SOCIETY ON AGING

The American Society on Aging (ASA) was founded in 1954. It is an association of individuals bound by a common goal: to support the commitment and enhance the knowledge and skills of those who seek to improve the quality of life of older adults and their families. No other organization in the field of aging represents the diversity of settings and professional disciplines reached by ASA.

The ASA is founded on the premise that the complexity of aging in our society can be addressed only as a multidisciplinary whole. The membership of ASA is an array of researchers, practitioners, educators, businesspeople, and policy makers who are concerned with the physical, emotional, social, economic, and spiritual aspects of aging. Throughout the country, 5,000 professionals rely on ASA to keep them on the cutting edge in an aging society. Through educational programming, publications, and state-of-the-art and training resources, ASA members tap into the knowledge and experience

of the largest and most dynamic network of professionals in the field of aging.

ASA publications offer current information and research to help professionals stay on the cutting edge in the field of aging: *Aging Today* is newspaper-format bimonthly coverage of all the issues facing professionals in aging today; *Generations* is a scholarly quarterly journal; and *AgeBlog* is an on-line blog of issues facing the ASA and the field of aging. ASA hosts a variety of award programs honoring individuals and organizations that are making a difference in the lives of older adults. See ASA Awards (asaging .org/more-40-years-asa-awards) for more information.

Elizabeth A. Capezuti

Web Resource
American Society on Aging: http://www.asaging.org

AMERICANS WITH DISABILITIES ACT

Legal protection for older persons takes many forms, including protection from discrimination in employment and housing and elder abuse in nursing homes and other settings, as well as the provision of public benefits. One less obvious source of legal protection for older persons is the Americans with Disabilities Act (ADA) of 1990 and its sister federal, state, and local disability–discrimination–protection statutes.

Of course, being older is not synonymous with being disabled. Nonetheless, many needs of older persons are touched and perhaps addressed by the ADA and related statutes. For that reason, a working knowledge of the disability laws is essential for those working in the field of elder care.

The ADA prohibits discrimination in private employment and in public accommodations settings. The rights that the ADA affords disabled persons in each setting are quite distinct.

ADA APPLICATION TO THE EMPLOYMENT SETTING

The ADA applies to employers with 15 or more employees as well as to state and local governments, employment agencies, and labor unions. The statute protects a qualified individual with a disability. To be a qualified individual, the applicant or employee must have the skills, experience, and education necessary to perform the essential functions of the job with or without a reasonable accommodation.

Definition of Disability

Disability is defined as a mental or physical impairment that substantially limits a major life activity or the record or perception by the employer of the individual having such an impairment. A record of an impairment could be, for example, a history of cancer. An example of a perception could be the assumption that a homosexual employee has or will be exposed to the AIDS virus.

Major life activities, for purposes of the ADA, include caring for oneself, performing manual tasks, walking, seeing, hearing, speaking, breathing, learning, working, sitting, standing, thinking, concentrating, and interacting with others. The determination of whether an impairment substantially limits a major life activity, which is required under the ADA for the statute's protection to be triggered, depends on a number of factors, including the severity and expected duration of the impairment and its long-term impact on the individual. The helpful effects of mitigating measures (e.g., medication to address or ameliorate manifestation of the disability) are not to be considered in determining whether the employee is substantially limited in a major life activity. The interpretation of the term "substantially limited" is to be broadly interpreted in favor of coverage.

Exclusions from the definition of disability under the ADA include (a) temporary illnesses or injuries (e.g., broken bones) because the temporary nature of the condition is deemed not to substantially limit a major life activity, (b) current users of illegal drugs, and (c) compulsive gambling or sexual behavioral disorders.

Duty to Accommodate

One of the key elements of the ADA is the duty it imposes on employers to reasonably accommodate a disabled applicant or employee. An employer's duty to reasonably accommodate the needs of qualified applicants and employees can be quite substantial. Examples of reasonable accommodations include (a) making existing facilities readily accessible to and usable by disabled individuals; (b) acquiring or modifying equipment and devices; (c) providing ergonomically correct furniture; (d) adjusting and modifying tests, training materials, and policies; (e) restructuring jobs to reallocate marginal job functions; (f) modifying work schedules; (g) providing leaves of absence; (h) reassigning disabled employees to vacant positions; and (i) providing qualified readers with interpreters and personal assistants.

The ADA requires that the process of determining the appropriate accommodation be interactive and with the employee's full participation. An employer is not obligated, however, to necessarily adopt a specific accommodation proposed by the applicant or employee but must merely implement a reasonably effective option among viable alternatives that permits the individual to perform satisfactorily the essential functions of the position. In providing an accommodation, an employer is not obligated to eliminate an essential function of the job. For example, an employer would not be required to eliminate the obligation for a truck driver to drive to accommodate that employee's visual impairment.

The duty to accommodate is often straightforward when the disability is physical. A more difficult issue is posed when the disability is mental or emotional. For example, must an employer excuse the erratic behavior of a clinically depressed employee? The answer is, as with many issues arising in the disability area, fact intensive and dependent on a number of factors, including whether the employee's condition rises to the level of a disability, the severity of the condition, and the employee's ability (with or without an accommodation) to perform the essential functions of the job.

A

Medical Examinations

A The ADA prohibits employers from requiring or giving medical examinations before making an offer of employment. Once a job offer has been made, an employer may condition actual employment on the passing of a medical examination. To be lawful, the postoffer examination must be required of all entering employees in the same job category. The ADA also prohibits employers from inquiring into the physical or mental condition of a job applicant whether by questionnaire, application, or interview.

An employer's discretion in requiring that existing employees submit to medical examinations is also limited to situations in which the examination is necessary to determine fitness for duty or in which there is evidence of a performance or safety problem. A fitness-for-duty test, such as lifting and carrying a heavy weight for a firefighter, measures the employee's ability to perform the essential functions of the position. Postemployment medical examinations are also permitted when the examination is performed to monitor compliance with federal, state, or local laws. Medical examinations may also be conducted as part of a voluntary health program as long as the information obtained is not used in violation of the ADA. Information obtained from a postoffer medical examination must be maintained in a separate medical file and must be treated as a confidential medical record.

RELATED FEDERAL, STATE, AND LOCAL LAWS

In addition to the ADA, many other federal, state, and local laws provide significant protections against disability discrimination. The Rehabilitation Act of 1973 applies to employers receiving federal contracts in excess of $2,500 and to participants in federally funded programs. It provides many of the same protections for disabled employees as the ADA.

Many states have human rights or civil rights laws that provide the same and often additional protections for disabled individuals. For example, many of those state laws apply to smaller employers with fewer employees (e.g., 4 in contrast to the 15 employees required by the ADA), protect a broader range of disabilities (e.g., include temporary disabilities), and provide a wider range of damages (e.g., unlimited compensatory and punitive damages). Some localities, such as New York City, have equivalent laws.

ADA APPLICATION TO PUBLIC ACCOMMODATIONS

The ADA also prohibits covered entities from discriminating against individuals with disabilities in the provision of services and access to their facilities. This means that entities must provide to disabled and nondisabled customers, patients, and clients the same type and quality of care, services, and access to their facilities. Covered entities deemed to be public accommodations include, but are not limited to, hotels, restaurants, theaters, retail stores, medical and professional offices, hospitals and nursing homes, schools, and sports and entertainment venues.

Covered entities must make reasonable modifications in policies, practices, and procedures as needed so that individuals with disabilities can make full use of the services provided or the facilities. For example, a visually impaired individual must be permitted to be accompanied by a guide dog even if animals are not normally permitted on the premises. Covered entities must also furnish aides and services to ensure effective communication with the disabled individual. For example, schools may be required to provide and pay for a sign-language interpreter or to translate a document into Braille. The entities cannot charge the users of these auxiliary aides and services to cover their added costs.

Covered entities must remove structural, architectural, and communications barriers in their facilities where such removal is "readily achievable," which means that the removal can be easily carried out without much difficulty or expense. Examples of such efforts include installing wheelchair ramps, widening doorways, installing grab bars near toilets, replacing sink handles, installing flashing emergency alarm lights, and providing special seating areas in theaters and sports arenas.

DISABILITIES LAWS AND THE OLDER ADULT

The goal of the ADA is to fully integrate disabled people into the general sweep of society. This goal is particularly applicable and noble with the older adult in mind.

An older applicant or employee is entitled to the full protection afforded by the ADA. An older employee whose medical condition limits the ability to perform tangential, nonessential tasks may call on the ADA for protection if the employer seeks to terminate that employee's employment as a result of the inability to perform these nonessential tasks. An applicant with a medical history of a disabling condition may not be judged on that history but rather must be evaluated on current ability to perform the essential functions of the job.

Older persons may not be denied access to public accommodations because of a disabling condition. Restaurants and theaters must be fully accessible to disabled individuals. Public transportation also must be accessible.

Anyone seeking to assert rights under the ADA and its sister laws may do so in court or before the Equal Employment Opportunity Commission or its state and local equivalent agencies.

The ADA's far-reaching goals for American society have yet to be fully realized in the employment and public accommodations settings. There are many reasons for this, with ignorance of its mandates as the most prominent. Resorting to legal proceedings may not always be required. The first step in any effort to seek the protection of the ADA should be notification of the offending employer or entity of the ADA issue and a request for relief or an accommodation. It is only after voluntary, cooperative efforts fail that resorting to legal remedies is warranted.

See also Environmental Modifications: Home.

Alfred G. Feliu

Web Resources
ADA Amendments Act—United States Department of Labor: https://www.dol.gov/odep/topics/ADA.htm

ADA Project: http://www.adaproject.org
A Guide to Disability Rights Law: https://www.ada.gov/cguide.htm
Americans with Disabilities Act: http://www.ada.gov

ANEMIA

Anemia in an elderly person (i.e., hemoglobin less than 12 g/dL in women and less than 13 g/dL in men; Nierodzik, Sutin, & Freedman, 2002) should be viewed as a sign, not a disease. Anemia is not a part of normal aging. Normal parameters for complete blood count (CBC) indices can be used. The first step in treatment is to find the underlying disease that is causing the anemia. The main causes of chronic anemia in the elderly are iron deficiency, vitamin B_{12} or folate deficiency, myelodysplastic syndromes (MDS), and anemia of chronic disease.

DIAGNOSIS

Presenting symptoms of anemia may include fatigue, exertional shortness of breath, anginal chest pain, palpitations, dizziness, syncope, or a change in mental status (Table A.1). The physical signs of anemia include pallor (especially in the mucous membranes), tachycardia, systolic ejection murmur, and a widened pulse pressure. The speed at which the signs and symptoms develop is often a clue to the acuteness of the condition. To rule out an acute gastrointestinal bleed, a stool examination must be done to characterize the nature of the stool; a guaiac test should be done to check for occult blood. Clinicians should try to elicit a history of melena or other change in bowel habits. Follow-up may include monitoring vital signs and stools for occult blood (on three or more separate occasions). Evaluation of the patient's nutritional status is also essential in the initial evaluation of anemia in the older adult. Issues such as alcohol use, *Helicobacter pylori* infection, reduction of cobalamin absorption secondary to atrophic gastritis, adequacy of dietary folate, and use

A

Table A.1
DIAGNOSIS OF ANEMIA

Microcytic Anemia (MCV <80 fL)	Normocytic Anemia (MCV: 80–100 fL)	Macrocytic Anemia (MCV >100 fL)
Iron deficiency anemia	Acute blood loss	Ethanol abuse
Thalassemic disorders	Iron deficiency (early)	Folate deficiency
Anemia of inflammation/anemia of chronic disease (late, uncommon)	Anemia of inflammation/anemia of chronic disease (e.g., infection, inflammation, malignancy)	Vitamin B_{12} deficiency
Sideroblastic anemia (e.g., congenital, lead, alcohol, drugs; uncommon)	Bone marrow suppression (may also be macrocytic)	Reticulocytosis
Copper deficiency, zinc poisoning (rare)	• Bone marrow invasion	• Hemolytic anemia
	• Acquired pure red blood cell aplasia	• Response to blood loss
	Aplastic anemia	• Response to appropriate hematinic (eg, iron, B_{12}, folic acid)
	Chronic renal insufficiency	Acute myeloid leukemias
	Endocrine dysfunction	Myelodysplastic syndromes
	• Hypothyroidism	Drug-induced anemia
	• Hypopituitarism	• Hydroxyurea
		• AZT
		• Chemotherapy
		Liver disease
		Hypothyroidism (less common)

AZT, azidothymidine (also called zidovudine); MCV, mean corpuscular volume.

of agents that suppress gastric acid production need to be assessed (Carmel, 2008).

The initial laboratory test is a CBC that not only reports the hemoglobin and hematocrit levels, but also provides information on the size and shape of the red blood cells (RBCs). Additional tests that may be helpful in the initial workup are ferritin, iron, total iron-binding capacity, vitamin B_{12} and folate levels, lactate dehydrogenase, indirect bilirubin, serum protein electrophoresis, and reticulocyte count. Methylmalonic acid (MMA) may be tested if results of B_{12} and folate levels are borderline low. Erythrocyte sedimentation rate and C-reactive protein may also be helpful if anemia of inflammation (formerly classified as anemia of chronic disease) is suspected.

Classically, anemia is characterized by the size and appearance of the RBCs seen on the peripheral smear (i.e., microcytic, normocytic, macrocytic) and by the rate of RBC production, as indicated by the reticulocyte count and reticulocyte production index. After the anemia is classified by these indices, the differential diagnosis identifies the disease behind the anemia. Bone-marrow examination may be necessary if the diagnosis is not clear from patient history, physical examination, and standard blood tests, and it is required when the anemia is secondary

to a malignancy such as leukemia, lymphoma, and multiple myeloma. A bone-marrow examination is also usually necessary to establish the diagnosis of myelodysplasia.

Microcytic Anemias

A mean corpuscular volume (MCV) less than 80 fL indicates microcytic anemia. Iron deficiency, thalassemia, sideroblastic anemia, and some cases of anemia of inflammation present in this fashion.

Normocytic Anemias

An MCV of greater than 80 and less than 100 fL falls within the normocytic range. The differential diagnosis in this category includes anemia of inflammation, intrinsic marrow disease (e.g., aplasia or malignancy), and acute blood loss or hemolysis. The finding of a normal MCV may be a confounding factor because it may represent a combination of microcytic and macrocytic processes or an early stage in the development of the anemia. The range distribution width can be a clue in this situation; for example, a range distribution width greater than 15 indicates that the RBC population is heterogeneous and that a combination of factors may be at work.

Table A.2
TREATMENT OF ANEMIA

Type of Anemia	Preferred Treatment
Iron deficiency	Iron tablets (ferrous sulfate 325 mg) orally, once a day
Thalassemia minor	None
Myelodysplasia	Varies depending on prognostic score
Vitamin B$_{12}$ deficiency	Maintenance: vitamin B$_{12}$ 1,000 mcg intramuscularly every month
Folate deficiency	Folic acid 1 mg orally once a day
Anemia of inflammation	If refractory and severe, erythropoietin

Macrocytic Anemias

Anemias that present with an MCV greater than 100 fL include megaloblastic anemia (i.e., vitamin B$_{12}$ or folate deficiency), chronic liver disease, alcoholism, hypothyroidism, some cases of MDS, and conditions with increased reticulocytes.

TREATMENT

Acute Gastrointestinal Bleed

If an acute bleed is discovered, the patient should be admitted to the hospital; a patient with signs of shock, tachycardia, or orthostatic hypotension should be in a closely monitored setting, such as an intensive care unit (Table A.2). In general, an elderly patient with a hemoglobin less than 8 g/dL or hematocrit less than 25% should be considered a candidate for a blood transfusion of packed RBCs. Similarly, if the patient has obvious signs of hemorrhage or end-organ damage, such as chest pain, dyspnea, or hypotension, with hemoglobin less than 10 g/dL, an immediate transfusion should be considered. In the very aged (i.e., those older than 85 years) and those with a history of congestive heart failure, transfusions should be administered as half units (i.e., 125 mL) to run over 3 to 4 hours. In addition, 10 mg of furosemide may be given intravenously with each unit to prevent fluid overload.

Iron Deficiency

Iron deficiency anemias are characterized by microcytosis, low ferritin level (i.e., less than 30 ng/mL), low iron, high total iron-binding capacity, high RBC distribution width (i.e., greater than 15), and low reticulocyte production index. Iron deficiency in the elderly can be caused by malnutrition, malabsorption, achlorhydria, or most commonly, chronic blood loss. In a study of 100 patients with iron deficiency anemia, endoscopic examination of the upper gastrointestinal tract found a lesion in 36 patients (19 peptic ulcers); colonoscopy showed a lesion in 25 (colon cancer in 11; Rockey & Cello, 1993). The finding of iron deficiency, therefore, warrants a workup of the gastrointestinal tract, including upper and lower-tract endoscopy.

Treatment consists of iron supplements taken orally; when continued blood loss exceeds the gastrointestinal tract's ability to absorb oral iron, which is equivalent to about 60 mL of whole blood loss a day (Schrier & Auerbach 2013), or when iron cannot be given orally, parenteral iron (e.g., iron dextran or ferric gluconate complex) may be given. Oral iron is available in several formulations: ferrous sulfate (usually 325 mg once a day, which is equivalent to 65 mg of elemental iron), ferrous gluconate, ferrous fumarate, and ferrous polysaccharide. Because ferrous sulfate is constipating, a stool softener such as docusate is recommended. Vitamin C, or a half glass of orange juice, administered with the iron can help maintain the iron in its reduced state and improve absorption.

Thalassemias

The thalassemias are hereditary disorders characterized by low MCV (often less than 70 fL); target cells on peripheral smear; low reticulocyte index; normal range distribution width; and normal iron, ferritin, and total iron-binding capacity. The form most likely to be encountered in the elderly population is thalassemia minor. No treatment is usually required, and iron therapy is contraindicated because it may produce iron overload.

Myelodysplastic Syndromes

The MDSs are a group of stem cell disorders that may result in anemia, neutropenia, and thrombocytopenia. In MDSs, the bone marrow does not function effectively to produce blood cells. MDS has been associated with environmental factors (e.g., exposure to chemicals, radiation), genetic abnormalities, and other hematological diseases. Some people with MDS have no symptoms, whereas others seek medical care due to symptoms of anemia. MDS is diagnosed with peripheral blood testing and bone marrow aspiration and biopsy. Patients with MDS have been classified into risk groups based on prognostic scoring. They are assigned an International Prognostic Score System (IPSS) and then categorized as having high-, intermediate-, or low-risk disease. Treatment recommendations are based on patient risk groups, and may include supportive therapy, chemotherapy, and bone marrow transplantation.

Vitamin B$_{12}$ Deficiency

Vitamin B$_{12}$ deficiency is characterized by macrocytosis, high range distribution width, and low reticulocyte index. In addition to causing anemia, vitamin B$_{12}$ deficiency may also cause neurological damage, including dementia, ataxia, or peripheral neuropathy. Normal B$_{12}$ levels (but less than 350 pg/mL) are often found in B$_{12}$ deficiency and should be corroborated with elevated homocysteine and methylmalonic acid levels. B$_{12}$ deficiency may arise due to a number of conditions such as a lack of gastric acid or pepsin, so B$_{12}$ cannot be freed from its binding to dietary proteins, an autoimmune disease with production of auto antibodies against parietal cells and intrinsic factor (i.e., pernicious anemia), bacterial overgrowth, and diseases of the terminal ileum.

The most efficient way to treat vitamin B$_{12}$ deficiency due to pernicious anemia (auto antibodies to intrinsic factor) is with injections of 1,000 mcg of vitamin B$_{12}$ intramuscularly. There are a number of regimens of initial replenishment followed by maintenance therapy; a convenient one is to give the injections daily for 1 week, then weekly for 4 weeks, then monthly for life. The maintenance dose is 1,000 mcg every month. Potassium and phosphate levels must be monitored during the initial stage of therapy. B$_{12}$ may be given orally, especially if the B$_{12}$ deficiency is due to a lack of acid or pepsin, and some patients with pernicious anemia respond to a high dose (1,000 mcg/d) of oral B$_{12}$. Because the pernicious anemia form of B$_{12}$ deficiency is associated with gastrointestinal cancer, it is recommended that patients be monitored for this as well.

Folate Deficiency

Folate deficiency presents in a similar manner to vitamin B$_{12}$ deficiency. When macrocytic anemia is diagnosed and folate deficiency is suspected, it is imperative that both B$_{12}$ and folate levels, as well as homocysteine and methylmalonic acid levels, be checked. In folate deficiency, homocysteine may be elevated, but the methylmalonic acid levels are normal. Replacing only folate in a patient who is also deficient in vitamin B$_{12}$ can improve the anemia but fails to stop, and may worsen, the neurological sequelae of B$_{12}$ deficiency. Treatment is 1 mg of folic acid orally once a day.

Anemia of Inflammation

Anemia of inflammation (formerly known as anemia of a chronic disease) is normally a diagnosis of exclusion. Anemia of inflammation is characterized by increased uptake and retention of iron within the cells of the reticuloendothelial system, which leads to diversion of iron from the circulation. The acute-phase protein hepcidin plays an important role in this (Guenter & Goodnough, 2005). Erythropoietin response is also often inadequate for the degree of anemia.

The characteristic findings are low reticulocyte index, reduced iron, reduced total iron-binding capacity, and normal or increased ferritin. Implicated diseases include chronic inflammatory disease such as in the collagen-vascular diseases, malignancy, chronic infections, or chronic renal disease.

A search should be made for correctable nutritional deficiencies (i.e., iron, B_{12}, or folate). Dementia, poverty, or elder abuse can contribute to nutritional inadequacy. In the case of collagen vascular diseases and malignancy, the anemia often responds to treatment of the underlying illness. In refractory cases and in chronic renal disease, careful treatment with erythropoietin may be necessary, although there are concerns about its use in certain malignancies (Guenter & Goodnough, 2005). If erythropoietin is used, careful monitoring of the adequacy of iron stores, with supplemental iron given as necessary, is required.

Presence of Multiple Etiologies

Clinicians must be aware that older adults can also have multiple causes of anemia. For example, a prospective study of 191 hospitalized patients older than 70 years that analyzed iron deficiency anemia and anemia of chronic disease found that many subjects had other clinically important diagnoses that contributed to their anemia (Lioen, 2015). Underlying thyroid dysfunction, infection, nutritional disorder, myelodysplasia, and renal insufficiency can inhibit the ability of the patient's bone marrow to respond to blood loss or hemolysis and may also interfere with the ability of the patient to respond to appropriate treatment. Effective management of anemia in the older adult requires detection and correction of any treatable underlying etiology (Steensma & Tefferi, 2007). Therefore, full evaluation of anemia in an elderly patient may take multiple visits, which may include monitoring for response to nutrient supplementation to bone marrow biopsy if initial workup is inconclusive.

Saima Ajmal and Renita Ho

Carmel, R. (2008). Nutritional anemias and the elderly. *Seminars in Hematology, 45*(4), 225.

Guenter, W., & Goodnough, L. T. (2005). Medical progress: Anemia of chronic disease. *New England Journal of Medicine, 352*, 1011–1024.

Lioen, J. (2015). Iron deficiency anemia and anemia of chronic disease in geriatric hospitalized patients: How frequent are comorbidities as an additional explanation for the anemia? *Geriatrics & Gerontology International, 15*(8), 931–935.

Nierodzik, M. L., Sutin, D., & Freedman, M. L. (2002). Blood disorders and their management in old age. In R. C. Tallis & H. M. Fillit (Eds.), *Brocklehurst's textbook of geriatric medicine and gerontology* (6th ed., Chapter 28). New York, NY: Churchill Livingstone.

Rockey, D. C., & Cello, J. P. (1993). Evaluation of the gastrointestinal tract in patients with iron deficiency anemia. *New England Journal of Medicine, 329*, 1691–1695.

Schrier, S. L., & Auerbach, M. (2017). Treatment of iron deficiency anemia in adults. In W. C. Mentzer, *UpToDate*. Retrieved from https://www.uptodate.com/contents/treatment-of-iron-deficiency-anemia-in-adults?source=see_link

Steensma, D. P., & Tefferi, A. (2007). Anemia in the elderly: How should we define it, when does it matter, and what can be done? *Mayo Clinic Proceedings, 82*(8), 958.

Web Resources
American Family Physician: http://www.aafp.org/afp/2000/1001/p1565.html
Mayo Clinic: http://www.mayoclinic.com/health/anemia/DS00321
WebMD: http://www.webmd.com/a-to-z-guides/understanding-anemia-basics

ANIMAL-ASSISTED HEALTH CARE

The capacity of animals to assist in the health care of young and old and acute or chronically ill patients has long been regarded as vital and powerful. Much of the literature on this topic has consisted of clinical anecdotes and case reports. Although most reports of the therapeutic effects of animal-assisted therapy (AAT) in health care are primarily anecdotal, an increasing number of empirically based studies have found that AAT or interaction with animals is

A

associated with positive physical and mental health benefits (Kamka et al., 2014).

Human–animal therapy has been shown to have a beneficial effect in mental health treatment of abused children (Dietz, Davis, & Pennings, 2012). Equine therapy has been successfully used with adolescents with mental health problems (Bachi, Terkel, & Teichman, 2012). Life quality of parents with children with ADHD was improved with animal-assisted play therapy (Motarabesoun & Tabatabaei, 2016). Animal therapies have been used extensively with older adults, demonstrating beneficial effects in those living in long-term care facilities (Mercer, 2015). Palliative-care settings provide yet another health care setting conducive for beneficial human–animal interactions (Engelman, 2013).

In modern AAT, a variety of animals are used in a multitude of health settings. Although dogs and cats are most commonly associated with these programs, many other species are used, including rabbits, birds, pigs, fish, horses, dolphins, llamas, and even snakes. Breed and species are usually not the most important criteria for such programs. Animals are often chosen for their temperament, tolerance, and energy level consistent with the health care environment and the focus of the team. The purposes and goals of the program are critical in choosing the animal. Although the risks associated with human–animal interactions are minimal, awareness of these potential problems (e.g., zoonoses [diseases transmitted from animal to human], allergies, and bites) is important when planning to use an animal in a health care environment.

PROGRAM TYPES

Diverse and overlapping terms are used to describe animal-assisted health care programs, including *pet therapy*, *AAT*, and *service animals*. Although these terms are often used interchangeably, each type is distinct and characterized by different goals. Pet therapy consists of volunteers bringing animals into health care settings. It is also called *pet visitation* or *animal-assisted activities*. Typically, the animals are not trained and institutional policies and local health care regulations govern the rules

of visitation. Health care clinicians, including nurses, have been active in advocating and instituting pet-visitation programs across health care settings, including the homebound elderly. The Eden Alternative (www.edenalt.org) is a nationally recognized model developed for using live-in pets in nursing-home environments as part of an overall goal to improve the quality of life of the residents.

AAT is more structured and goal-directed than pet therapy. People (termed *handlers*) escorting the animals are given training, and animals are screened and certified for health, obedience, sociability, and temperament. Each AAT team has specific goals, and animals are chosen for their ability to assist in accomplishing the psychosocial or physical therapeutic goals for a patient. Specific goals might include increasing rapport between a psychotherapist and a patient and maximizing mobility and muscle coordination in a physically debilitated patient. Visits are structured and therapeutic outcomes for the patient are monitored. Often, the AAT human partner is a health care professional.

Service animals are highly trained and legally defined assistance animals. The Americans with Disabilities Act (ADA) of 1990, a federal civil rights law, defines a *service animal* as any animal individually trained to do work or perform tasks for the benefit of a person with a disability. The law defines a *disabled person* as an individual whose physical or mental impairment substantially limits one or more major life activities. The tasks that service dogs can perform include guiding persons with impaired vision, alerting persons with hearing impairments to various sounds, pulling wheelchairs, pulling a person into a lying or sitting position, turning switches on or off, retrieving objects, and summoning help. Certain dogs are able to detect an impending seizure and alert the victim before the seizure occurs.

Federal laws protect the rights of disabled individuals to be accompanied by their service animals into public places. These animals are closely partnered with their owners, who rely on them to provide vital services. Laws do not restrict the type of service the animals perform, and owners are not required to disclose their disability. Service animals usually wear an identifying harness or vest, but this is not required by law. The rules for interacting with human–animal teams vary when dealing with pet visitation, AAT teams, and service-animal teams.

Care Guidelines

Guidelines are available that govern all types of animal-assisted health care programs. Health care facilities are required to adhere to state or federal guidelines regarding the use of animals. Animals require health screening and immunizations by a veterinarian prior to entering a health care facility. For animals that live in a facility, there are regulations outlining the care of the animal. Pet visitation and AAT programs follow the institutional guidelines for dealing with persons who may be allergic or phobic. Staff and residents should be notified in advance of animal visits, or visits may be restricted to discrete areas of the health facility. Those who are phobic or allergic or do not wish to participate can then remove themselves from the vicinity. Caution should be exercised when animals are exposed to patients who have disabilities that may cause them to handle the animal roughly or frighten the animal unexpectedly.

Institutional and other regulatory systems (local or state) also regulate infection control. Handwashing, before and after handling, is standard when there is contact with an animal. People with open wounds or active infectious processes are typically excluded from such programs. Pet visitation and AAT programs have recorded thousands of visits without any substantial risk of zoonoses being substantiated in the literature.

Strangers, including health care professionals, should always speak to the person before interacting with the animal partner and should not grab the elbow of visually disabled persons or assist without permission. Such actions may confuse the dog or prevent it from doing its job. Strangers should not talk to, pet, or feed a service animal because these activities also may distract the animal from its work. It is often necessary to explain to others who complain about an animal's presence that the animal is medically necessary and that federal law protects the right of the person to be accompanied in public places. If a service animal/dog barks or growls, it may be necessary to find out what happened (e.g., the dog may have been stepped on). The owner of the service animal/dog may be asked to have the dog lie down, as long as this does not interfere with the animal's work. Federal law requires that animals acting in a vicious or destructive manner be excluded from a public setting.

The needs of the animal (e.g., adequate water, toileting, and exercise) must be scheduled. Noise, sanitation, staff concerns about the appropriateness of service animals, and cost issues all must be considered before instituting animal-assistance programs in a health care setting. Costs for the animals vary widely. Pet therapy and AAT team animals are often owned by the handler. Service dogs are the most costly because of their extensive training, and public funds do not typically reimburse these costs. Service animals are often provided at a nominal fee to disabled individuals by nonprofit animal organizations, but waiting lists can be as long as 2 years. Many organizations provide information, training, publications, and videos. Pet Partners (formerly Delta Society; www.petpartners.org) is an international organization for promoting the human–animal bond. It serves as a valuable resource for information about the various types of animal programs.

The use of animals to assist with the care of older adults offers numerous opportunities. Benefits include well-described improvements in psychological well-being and social acceptance, as well as decreased need for paid and unpaid assistance. Animals may be utilized purely as companions for social support, and their usefulness extends from home assistance to facilitation of community activities. The use of animals across health settings is an increasingly valuable strategy and continues to demonstrate the many positive uses of the human–animal bond.

Mary Shelkey

Bachi, K., Terkel, J., & Teichman, M. (2012). Equine-facilitated psychotherapy for at-risk adolescents: The influence on self-image, self-control and trust. *Clinical Child Psychology & Psychiatry, 17*(2), 298–312.

Dietz, T. R., Davis, D., & Pennings, J. (2012). Evaluating animal-assisted in group treatment for child sexual abuse. *Journal of Child Sexual Abuse, 21*(6), 665–683.

Engelman, S. R. (2013). Palliative care and use of animal-assisted therapy. *OMEGA: Journal of Death and Dying, 67*(1–2), 63–67.

Kamka, H., Okada, S., Tsutan, K., Park, H., Okuum, H., Handa, S.,...Mutoh, Y. (2014). Effectiveness of animal-assisted therapy: A systematic review of randomized controlled trials. *Complementary Therapies in Medicine, 22*(2), 371–390.

Mercer, K. A. (2015). Animal-assisted therapy and application to older adults in long-term care. *Advances in Bioscience and Clinical Medicine, 4*(3), 26–37.

Motarabesoun, N., & Tabatabaei, S. M. (2016). The effect of animal-assisted play therapy on improving the life quality of parents having children with ADHD treated with methylphenidate. *Advances in Bioscience and Clinical Medicine, 4*(3), 26–37.

Web Resources
Eden Alternative: http://www.edenalt.com
Pet Partners: http://www.petpartners.org

ANXIETY DISORDERS, TRAUMATIC AND STRESSOR-RELATED DISORDERS, AND OBSESSIVE-COMPULSIVE DISORDERS IN LATE LIFE

Anxiety at any age has many manifestations—it can vary from transient minor worry to full-blown panic attacks. However, familiarity with the experience of anxiety may obscure understanding of the kinds of anxiety experienced by older adults, resulting in failure to adequately assess and treat late-life anxiety disorders. In an effort to appreciate older adults' experiences in anxiety-provoking situations, health care practitioners may fail to understand their experiences, perspectives, and values. In the process, practitioners may often err in their estimation of the nature and degrees to which older adults are experiencing stress. In the face of what may seem to be a relatively minor surgical procedure, such as arthrocentesis (removal of fluid from a joint), a younger person might have few concerns, whereas an older adult, perhaps one who had a friend who went through the same procedure and suffered significant complications from a subsequent infection, might be exceedingly apprehensive.

The prevalence rate of anxiety disorders in older adults may be higher than that of depressive disorders, but they are often undiagnosed and can be just as disabling (Schuurmans & van Balkom, 2011). Also, individuals vary in the degree to which they manifest the symptoms of anxiety. Thus it is important not to trivialize what might appear to be a degree of apprehension as normal for a given situation. Adults in late life constitute a heterogeneous population, and their organ systems decline in function at different rates, making for high levels of physiological variability. Hence, it is important to have an objective familiarity with anxiety and to remember that discovering the meaning of the situation for an older adult is crucial to an effective outcome.

Anxiety can be construed nonpathologically as part of the natural response to stressors, whether internal or external. It alerts people to pay attention and be prepared for challenging situations. Analogous to pain, anxiety becomes problematic when it is excessive. The extent to which anxiety is experienced can vary with the perceived gap between what individuals perceive as challenges versus resources. The traditional way of understanding the stress response has been in terms of "fight, flight, or freeze." However, in recent years, this approach has been found to be wanting in terms of its generalizability. It is not readily applicable, for example, to situations in which a parent is stressed by a fussy child. Hence it is helpful to add "engage" to the list of categorical stress responses. This is especially the case with older adults, who, for various reasons, develop functional changes that compromise their abilities to engage effectively in response to stressors.

SIGNS AND SYMPTOMS OF ANXIETY

Anxiety has two sets of biological manifestations: the signs and symptoms of heightened autonomic nervous system activity and psychomotor changes. The former includes light-headedness/dizziness, dry mouth, difficulty swallowing, stomach "butterflies," nausea, gastrointestinal distress, increased heart rate, palpitations, shortness of breath, hyperventilation, flushing, perspiration, tingling sensations (in the fingers and toes and around the mouth), and frequent urination. Psychomotor symptoms include muscle tension/tightness, tremulousness, achiness/soreness, and easy fatigability.

The psychological features of anxiety are also twofold, involving apprehension and vigilance. Apprehension is marked by uncomfortable expectations and sometimes associated with avoidance of anxiety-provoking stimuli. Indicators of vigilance include feelings of being on edge, exaggerated startle responses, poor concentration, irritability, and insomnia. Cognitive ideations that are part of the experience of anxiety may include misappraisals that overestimate the challenges of and/or underestimate the available resources or options for a specific set of circumstances. The behavioral manifestations of anxiety include angry outbursts (fight), avoidance of anxiety-provoking situations (flight), immobilization (freeze), and problem solving (engage). None of these responses are dysfunctional per se because their effectiveness is determined by the context. One needs to consider cultural factors and personal beliefs that may contribute to the anxiety experienced by an older adult.

Appreciation of the burdens of anxiety and anxiety disorders has been gradually growing. Patients with higher levels of anxiety report lower quality of life. They may be also more prone to developing cardiovascular disorders, such as hypertension, cardiac arrhythmias, and myocardial infarction, and at greater risk for impaired recovery or death from these problems. Older adults in general tend to underreport mental health issues, as well as prefer to obtain health services from their primary care providers, rather than mental health practitioners, because busy practitioners in clinical settings are focused on addressing medical treatments for the anxiety. Anxiety disorders, not unlike depressive disorders, tend to be underrecognized and undertreated.

PREVALENCE AND RISK FACTORS

One of the problems in determining the prevalence of anxiety and anxiety disorders in late life is that many of these signs and symptoms may stem, at least in part, from concurrent medical problems. Medical illnesses themselves cause some of the same biological signs and symptoms. As internal stressors (e.g., apprehension over being ill), they may not only generate their own psychological symptoms of anxiety, but also amplify other biological symptoms of anxiety. The experience of anxiety, in turn, may also exacerbate some of the biological signs and symptoms of concurrent medical problems (e.g., pain, shortness of breath). Anxiety also frequently accompanies other co-occurring psychiatric disorders, such as depression and dementia, although some data seem to show that approximately three-fourths of older adult's experience anxiety disorders without co-occurring depression (Beekman et al., 2000; Schuurmans & van Balkom, 2011).

Given these considerations, it can be appreciated why epidemiological studies yield variable rates for the prevalence of different kinds of anxiety disorders in late life. Nonetheless, some patterns have emerged. The rate of clinically significant anxiety symptoms can be up to 20% in community-dwelling older adults and up to 40% in those in long-term care (LTC) settings. The prevalence of diagnosable anxiety disorders in geriatric populations also varies by setting: up to 10% in community samples and up to 20% in LTC facilities. The most common anxiety disorders in late life are generalized anxiety disorder (GAD) and simple phobias. Panic disorder and agoraphobia have been observed less frequently in older adults, as have posttraumatic stress disorder (PTSD) and obsessive-compulsive disorder (OCD). These last two disorders have recently been recategorized in the American Psychiatric Association's *Diagnostic and Statistical Manual of Mental Disorders* (5th ed.; *DSM-5*; American

A

Psychiatric Association, 2013) into separate sections: traumatic and stressor-related disorders, and OCDs.

ANXIETY DISORDER DUE TO SUBSTANCES

The diagnosis of anxiety disorder due to a substance is made when there are clear-cut connections between the anxiety symptoms and intoxication with, or withdrawal from, a substance being used or misused. Medications used by older adults that can sometimes be associated with increased anxiety include cardiovascular drugs (e.g., for heart failure or hypertension), stimulants, steroids, decongestants, bronchodilators (e.g., for asthma or emphysema), agents with significant anticholinergic side effects, and excessive thyroid supplements. Substances commonly causing anxiety in older adults include caffeine and alcohol; the extent to which these are used by older adults is frequently overlooked or underestimated. It is estimated that more than 50% of older adults (above 60 years of age) with a diagnosis of GAD consume an average of 5+ alcoholic drinks per week (Ivan, 2014).

ANXIETY DISORDER DUE TO A MEDICAL PROBLEM

The diagnosis of an anxiety disorder due to a medical problem is warranted by a direct connection between a medical problem and the signs and symptoms of anxiety. Many medical problems in late life can generate significant anxiety, especially cardiovascular, respiratory, endocrine, and neurologic disorders, as well as acute and chronic pain. These may warrant further workup with appropriate screening and testing to determine whether the anxiety stems directly from the medical condition, an emotional response to the medical problem, and/or a separate, unrelated anxiety problem.

ANXIETY ASSOCIATED WITH ANOTHER PSYCHIATRIC DISORDER

Anxiety signs and symptoms frequently occur to a significant degree in most other major psychiatric disorders (e.g., cognitive, mood, psychotic, somatoform). According to the *DSM-5*, the presence of significant anxiety is a complicating factor that can be appended to the primary diagnosis. Depression and anxiety frequently occur together in late-life mood disorders, and the combination can make both diagnosis and treatment more difficult.

The remaining types of anxiety disorders are those that cannot be primarily attributed to medical problems, problems with substances, or other psychiatric disorders. They are distinguished by the types of stressors that provoke somatic sensations of fear/anxiety and generate cognitive appraisals that together result in ineffective responses.

SITUATIONAL ANXIETY

Situational anxiety in older adults is usually generated by the prospect of having to engage in unfamiliar activities or in familiar ones but under unfamiliar conditions. Patients with dementia who have lost their ability to cope with previously familiar situations (e.g., due to cognitive deficits in executive functioning and memory) are prone to catastrophic reactions. These are characterized by sudden, intense, and usually transient emotional and behavioral responses to tasks or situations that were previously handled with little or no distress.

PHOBIAS

Phobias involve anxiety that is recurrently precipitated by exposure to certain objects or situations and subsequently results in avoidant behaviors to the degree that functioning is compromised. The prevalence of phobias in late life ranges from 3.1% to 10% (Flint, 1994). In the National Comorbidity Survey Replication, the estimated 12-month prevalence of specific phobia was 4.7% in people aged 65 years and older (Gum, King-Kallimanis, & Kohn, 2009). Per the *DSM-5*, individuals with phobias may or may not have insight into the degree to which their fears are irrational. Phobias are one of the most common types of anxiety found in surveys of community-dwelling older adult populations. The prevalence of fear of falling has been estimated to be up to 65% in those who have never fallen and up to 90% in those who have. Elderly individuals not infrequently attribute their phobic symptoms to a distressing social or medical problem. Hence, it is important to not discount these as "just phobias," especially in cases of new (late-onset) phobias, but to assess them carefully. Some, traumatized earlier in life, may exhibit phobic anxiety when exposed to a situation reminiscent of that earlier painful experience (see "Posttraumatic Stress Disorder").

SEPARATION ANXIETY DISORDER

The cardinal feature of separation anxiety disorder is anxiety driven by inordinate fear of losing an attachment figure, either through physical separation or because of "something bad" happening to that person. This disorder, usually associated with children, can occur in older adults who have become very dependent on others for assistance because of physical and/or mental decline. A patient with dementia, for example, may be reluctant to be left alone or left with someone with whom they are unfamiliar or no longer recognize.

ELECTIVE MUTISM

Elective mutism is a persistent failure to speak in certain limited situations, but not generally in others in which there is normally an expectation to speak. In elective mutism, normal social communication is interrupted.

SOCIAL ANXIETY DISORDER

Individuals affected by social anxiety disorder are characteristically distressed by situations that they feel would subject them to the scrutiny of others. Because of thoughts that they would be judged critically and/or rejected by others, be embarrassed, or offend others, older adults with this disorder tend to avoid situations that would involve performing tasks in front of other people, especially those with which they are less familiar. This may become an issue in later life, for example, for those who restrict their social activities because they have developed urinary incontinence or because, in the early stage of a dementia, they have lost the ability to follow conversations that involve multiple speakers.

GENERALIZED ANXIETY DISORDER

GAD is characterized by the experience of persistent, frequent anxiety that is deemed to be either excessive or unrealistic and that the affected individual finds difficult to control. Compared with older adults who do not have GAD, those who do have been found to have greater amounts of disability (especially in social functioning), poorer quality of life (QOL), and higher rates of health care utilization. Interestingly, recent functional MRI (fMRI) studies conducted to evaluate neuronal and cognitive functions in the setting of known GAD have shown hypofunctional and hypoconnected areas in the prefrontal and anterior cingulated cortexes and the amygdala, leading to the emotional dysregulation seen in GAD (Mochcovitch, da Rocha Freire, Garcia, & Nardi, 2014). Thus greater degrees of anxiety in GAD have been found to be associated with higher levels of disability and lower levels of QOL, even when controlling for medical burden and depressive symptoms.

PANIC DISORDER

Panic attacks occur when individuals experience sudden surges, whether unexpected or expected, of the autonomic, psychomotor, psychological, and cognitive symptoms of anxiety. They typically peak within several minutes and are relatively transient in nature. The diagnosis of panic disorder can be made when an affected individual, having experienced a number of panic attacks, typically develops vigilant and behavioral symptoms of anxiety, becoming quite worried about further panic attacks and avoiding situations similar to those in which the prior attacks occurred. The latter behavior can lead to agoraphobia. Panic disorder has been found to typically be a chronic problem, usually with an onset earlier in life and with symptoms that gradually decrease over the years. Late-onset panic disorder is rare. Hence onset of panic attacks for the first time in an

A

older patient can be challenging, since panic symptoms can be precipitated by medical problems involving cardiovascular (e.g., myocardial infarction), pulmonary (e.g., pulmonary embolus), neurological (e.g., transient ischemic attack or stroke), or other organ systems. The prevalence and incidence of panic disorder decreases with age and usually presents with fewer and less intense symptoms compared with those in young adults (Flint & Gagnon, 2003; Katerndahl & Talamantes, 2000).

AGORAPHOBIA

Agoraphobia can also arise independently of panic disorder. It is typically characterized by signs and symptoms of increased anxiety in circumstances experienced as extremely distressing because of a lack of either an easy escape or of readily available help. Per the *DSM-5*, individuals with agoraphobia may or may not have insight into the degree to which their fears are irrational. Situations that tend to become associated with agoraphobia include being alone outside of home, in a crowd, and in wide-open or confined spaces. In late life, agoraphobia frequently occurs in the context of other anxiety problems.

TRAUMATIC AND STRESSOR-RELATED DISORDERS

Adjustment disorders and PTSD have been placed in a different category and allocated a separate section in the *DSM-5*. This was done because mood signs and symptoms, rather than those of anxiety, predominate in most individuals whose disorders stem from experiences that range from moderately to extremely stressful.

ADJUSTMENT DISORDERS

Adjustment disorders with anxiety occur acutely in the context of known stressors. They may become chronic when the signs and symptoms of anxiety become ongoing because the stressor persists and efforts to adapt to it fall short.

POSTTRAUMATIC STRESS DISORDER

PTSD is characterized by a cluster of signs and symptoms that emerge from psychologically painful experiences. Precipitating events typically involve exposure to actual or threatened violence, injury, and/or death. PTSD can emerge from being directly subjected to such experiences or witnessing them happening to others (e.g., in war, disasters, accidents, crimes), learning that they have occurred to close relatives or friends, or being repeatedly exposed to the distressing details about them (e.g., the collection of body parts by first responders or of information about abuse by child or adult protective service workers).

The signs and symptoms of PTSD cluster into four categories pertaining to the traumatic event: reexperiences of it, avoidance of reminders about it, distressing moods and thoughts concerning it, and increased levels of anxiety. Reexperiencing symptoms is recurrent and both physiologically and emotionally distressing. It may include intrusive thoughts, memories, nightmares, or dissociative episodes (e.g., flashbacks) in which the traumatic event is relived. These may occur spontaneously or in response to everyday situations reminiscent of, or associated with, the traumatic event. Affected individuals typically try to minimize these painful recollections by trying not to talk about them and avoiding reminiscent situations. As a consequence, they may become quite withdrawn from their previously usual activities. Distressing moods may include persistently feeling estranged, guilty, ashamed, sad, irritable, or disinterested, along with a diminished ability to have positive feelings. Distressing thoughts can involve inordinately negative perceptions of oneself, others, or the world at large (e.g., as unworthy or unsafe); self-blame; and undue pessimism. The signs, symptoms, and behaviors of PTSD-related anxiety include angry outbursts, hypervigilance, exaggerated startling, poor concentration, insomnia, and engagement in reckless or self-destructive activities.

OBSESSIVE-COMPULSIVE DISORDERS

Obsessions are images, ideas, or impulses that persistently recur and are experienced by individuals as unwanted and intrusive. The involuntary nature of their occurrence makes them seem senseless and morally repugnant, especially when they involve sexual or aggressive themes. Because obsessions are frequently difficult to ignore or suppress, they can be very distressing to those afflicted with them. The most common themes of obsessions in late life OCD involve fear of contamination, pathological doubting, concern about bodily functioning, aggression, a need for symmetry, and sexual images or impulses.

Compulsions consist of repetitive behaviors driven by obsessions and usually consist of actions aimed at somehow relieving the anxiety caused by the obsessions. Compulsions may seem to represent purposeful repetitive behaviors, enacted according to specific rules or in a stereotypic fashion, but actually are efforts to cause or prevent something else. They typically afford the sufferer temporary relief from anxiety that has been building, but the increasing anxiety soon recurs, thereby establishing repetitive, reinforcing pattern. In older adults with OCD, the most common compulsions involve checking, counting, and washing. Less frequent are those involving the need to ask or confess something, arrange items precisely, and hoarding.

According to the *DSM-5*, although individuals with OCD may and usually do have insight into the irrational nature of their symptoms and behaviors, the lack of such insight no longer precludes the diagnosis. Ruminations occurring in the context of depression, delusions in psychotic depression, and dementia-associated repetitive behaviors can sometimes mimic OCD. The onset of OCD for the first time in late life is rare, but the combination of certain personality traits (e.g., meticulousness, rigidity) with late life stressors can sometimes lead to OCD.

HOARDING DISORDER

A new addition to the *DSM-5* is the diagnosis of hoarding disorder. The diagnosis requires that specific cognitive, emotional, and behavioral criteria be met. The cognitive criterion consists of a perceived need to save certain items and the emotional criterion of significant distress when those items are discarded. The behavioral criterion is the consequent persistent problem of failing to dispose of those belongings to the point where living spaces can no longer be used as intended. With older adults, hoarding-like phenomena can occur in the context of other psychiatric disorders, stemming from a lack of energy in depression, delusions or hallucinations in psychosis, neglect, lack of initiative in dementia, or obsessions in OCD. Likewise, physical disabilities may interfere with the ability of some older adults to prevent an overaccumulation of items.

MANAGEMENT AND TREATMENT

Both psychotherapeutic and pharmacotherapeutic interventions can be effective for older adults with anxiety disorders (Tampi & Tampi, 2014). Effective management and treatment requires both comprehensively assessing for contributing factors, which in late life are more apt to be multiple, and systematically addressing each identified factor. The same rules of thumbs apply to subsyndromal anxiety symptoms, as they are also common and disabling. Initial steps include efforts to eliminate or minimize the use of medications and/ or substances that cause or exacerbate the signs and symptoms of anxiety; to adequately treat concurrent medical and psychiatric problems, whether chronic or acute; and to begin to modify or eliminate social and environmental stressors as much as possible. Determining what the anxiety symptoms and the anxiety-provoking situations mean to patients can often provide valuable clues to guide interventions that are more sensitive and specific to the unique needs of the individual.

For older adults whose subsyndromal anxiety, specific anxiety disorders, or signs and symptoms of anxiety persist despite initial interventions, the next steps involve non-pharmacological interventions to enhance individuals' coping abilities. Examples found to be effective, to varying degrees, for anxiety disorders in late life include psychoeducation as well as a number of different kinds of therapies—supportive psychotherapy, cognitive

A

A

behavioral therapy, and interpersonal therapy. Systematic desensitization (exposure therapy) can be helpful for agoraphobia and phobias, thought stopping can be helpful for OCD, and progressive relaxation techniques can be helpful for anxiety marked by significant muscle tension.

Treatment with antianxiety medications is best reserved for situations in which the nonpharmacological interventions have not afforded adequate relief in terms of the intensity, frequency, and/or duration of signs and symptoms. Although benzodiazepines continue to be commonly prescribed to older adults with anxiety, their use is apt to be associated with adverse side effects, particularly with increasing age and/or longer duration of treatment. Elderly patients are more susceptible to side effects such as impaired cognition, sedation, unstable gait (with increased risk of falling), and slower reaction time (e.g., when driving, using machinery, or trying to recover from a stumble to prevent a fall). For these reasons, antidepressants, including both selective serotonin reuptake inhibitors (SSRIs) and serotonin-norepinephrine reuptake inhibitors (SNRIs), have come to replace the benzodiazepines as the first choice for treating anxiety in geriatric patients. Although the number of studies on the use of antidepressants for anxiety, PTSD, and OCD in late life has been limited, such research has found them to be generally effective and fairly well tolerated. In older adults with GAD, either venlafaxine or citalopram seems to be effective (Flint, 2005; Katz, Reynolds, Alexopoulos, & Hackett, 2002), and in those with panic disorder, SSRI is the first line of treatment (Flint & Gagnon, 2003).

In addition to these general therapeutic approaches, the cultivation of ad hoc teams can help considerably with the clinical tasks of assessing complex situations, developing and implementing care plans, and monitoring results of interventions. Ongoing education and communication with both patients and caregivers (family and professional) is critical to achieving effective outcomes. Using concrete visual and written aids (e.g., lists) can facilitate learning through multisensory

pathways, and thereby enhance treatment outcomes.

See also Psychosis in Late Life.

Paula Lueras and Timothy Howell

American Psychiatric Association. (2013). *Diagnostic and statistical manual of mental disorders* (5th ed.). Arlington, VA: American Psychiatric Publishing.

Beekman, A., de Beurs, E., van Balkom, A., Deeg, D., van Dyck, R., & van Tilburg, W. (2000). Anxiety and depression in late life: Co-occurrence and communality of risk factors. *American Journal of Psychiatry, 157,* 89–95.

Flint, A. (1994). Epidemiology and comorbidity of anxiety disorders in the elderly. *American Journal of Psychiatry, 151,* 640–649.

Flint, A. (2005). Generalized anxiety disorder in elderly patients: Epidemiology, diagnosis and treatment options. *Drugs & Aging, 22*(2), 101–114.

Flint, A., & Gagnon, N. (2003). Diagnosis and management of panic disorder in older patients. *Drugs & Aging, 20*(12), 881–891.

Gum, A. M., King-Kallimanis, B., & Kohn, R. (2009). Prevalence of mood, anxiety, and substance-abuse disorders for older Americans in the National Comorbidity Survey-Replication. *American Journal of Geriatric Psychiatry, 17,* 69–781.

Ivan, M., Amspoker, A., Nardorff, M., Kunik, M., Cully, J., Wilson, N.,…Stanley, M. (2014). Alcohol use, anxiety, and insomnia in older adults with generalized anxiety disorder. *American Journal of Geriatric Psychiatry, 22*(9), 875–883.

Katerndahl, D., & Talamantes, M. (2000). A comparison of persons with early- versus late-onset panic attacks. *Journal of Clinical Psychiatry, 61,* 422–427.

Katz, I., Reynolds, C., Alexopoulos, G., & Hackett, D. (2002). Venlafaxine ER as a treatment for generalized anxiety disorder in older adults: pooled analysis of five randomized placebo-controlled clinical trials. *Journal of the American Geriatrics Society, 50*(1), 18–25.

Mochcovitch, M., da Rocha Freire, R., Garcia, R., & Nardi, A. (2014). A systematic review of fMRI studies in generalized anxiety disorder: evaluating its neural and cognitive basis. *Journal of Affective Disorders, 167,* 336–342.

Schuurmans, J., & van Balkom, A. (2011). Late-life anxiety disorders: a review. *Current Psychiatry Reports, 13*(4), 267–273.

Tampi, R., & Tampi, D. (2014). Anxiety disorders in late life: a comprehensive review. *Healthy Aging Research, 3*(14), 1–8.

AORTIC STENOSIS

Aortic stenosis is rapidly emerging as the most prevalent valvular heart pathology in older adults. In symptomatic patients who do not receive treatment, severe aortic stenosis causes high mortality. Through ongoing research, a new minimally invasive, catheter-based valve treatment has emerged that provides hope for patients at high risk but not eligible for surgical repair.

EPIDEMIOLOGY

In the Cardiovascular Health Study, the prevalence of aortic valve stenosis, which involves thickening or calcification of the valve without obstruction, was reported at 26% and was noted predominately in men. The prevalence of aortic stenosis in those 65 and older was reported at 2% to 4% (Fried et al., 1991).

ETIOLOGY

Calcific Aortic Stenosis

Calcific aortic stenosis is the most common form of aortic stenosis in patients older than 65. The pathophysiology of calcific aortic stenosis has been controversial. Previously, stenosis was considered the result of a degenerative process; atherosclerosis is now widely accepted as the underlying pathology leading to aortic stenosis, a process that similarly leads to coronary artery disease. In fact, most patients with aortic stenosis also tend to have underlying coronary artery disease. Both diseases tend to be more prevalent in men and are associated with higher incidences of dyslipidemia and elevated inflammation markers. Calcium deposition in the cusps of the aortic valve results in stenosis with some commissural fusion. This process leads to variable shapes of the valve orifice, resulting in altered hemodynamic response to conditions that increase cardiac output.

Congenital Aortic Stenosis

The majority of patients with congenital aortic stenosis are diagnosed in early childhood. It is often associated anatomically with a unicommissural unicuspid valve. Symptomatic patients without treatment have a poor prognosis. Biscuspid aortic valve is the most common adult congenital aortic valve disease, with a prevalence of 2% in the general population, predominantly in men. It typically presents early, in the third decade of life. The underlying pathology of bicuspid aortic stenosis also is atherosclerosis and calcium deposition. It is believed that altered hemodynamics in the bicuspid valve may accelerate the process of valve stenosis.

Rheumatic Valve Disease

Rheumatic valve disease, a form of aortic stenosis, is more prevalent in developing countries and invariably is associated with concomitant mitral valve disease. Diagnosis is generally made by echocardiography, with features of commissural fusion being a hallmark of the disease.

SYMPTOMS

Symptomatic patients with aortic stenosis have a mortality rate of 25% per year or approximately 2% a month. Asymptomatic patients with severe aortic stenosis also carry a risk of sudden cardiac death of 2% per year (Carabello, 2002).

Hallmark symptoms are angina, syncope, and congestive heart failure. Symptomatic patients with aortic stenosis presenting with angina have a mortality risk of 50% in 5 years. Those with syncope have a mortality risk of 50% in 3 years, whereas those with heart failure have a mortality risk of 50% in 2 years (Carabello & Paulus, 2009).

Progressive valve stenosis results in increased left ventricular (LV) pressure afterload or wall stress, resulting in compensatory

A

concentric LV hypertrophy. As a result, impairment of coronary blood flow reserve and diastolic filling of the left ventricle occur, leading to diastolic dysfunction. Blood flow to the heart occurs mainly in diastole, and normal coronary reserve is approximately eight times resting flow. However, in concentric LV hypertrophy, blood flow is diminished by 50% to 60% of baseline, possibly due to incomplete capillary growth in the hypertrophied myocardium. In addition, increased filling pressures could compress the endocardium, further impairing blood flow, resulting in angina and congestive heart failure.

Syncope in aortic stenosis usually occurs during exercise as a result of multiple mechanisms. It could be a result of decreased cardiac output, increased LV pressure resulting in vasoplegic syncope, a reflex depressor response, or ischemia causing malignant ventricular arrhythmias.

PHYSICAL EXAMINATION

Auscultation reveals a crescendo-decrescendo murmur, often radiating to the neck. In severe aortic stenosis, the murmur is diminished in intensity with reduction in stroke volume, peaks later in systole, and is associated with a thrill. Carotid upstrokes are diminished in volume and rate of rise (pulsus parvus et tardus). The apical impulse is prominent and displaced.

DIAGNOSTIC TESTS

Electrocardiogram abnormalities, including LV hypertrophy with left atrial abnormality, are nonspecific for aortic stenosis. X-ray may show a boot-shaped heart suggestive of concentric hypertrophy with aortic calcification. Echocardiography is the mainstay of diagnosis. It is used to assess LV function, the extent of hypertrophy and calcification, transvalvular gradient, and valve area. The criteria for diagnosing aortic stenosis in patients with normal LV function are outlined in Tables A.3 and A.4 and Figure A.1.

Cardiac MRI and CT are evolving as useful adjunct modalities for assessing the severity of aortic stenosis. The heavy calcific burden seen with CT suggests aortic stenosis. In particular situations, such as depressed LV function, dobutamine stress echocardiography is recommended to resolve discrepancies between symptoms and severity of aortic stenosis. Asymptomatic patients with severe aortic stenosis and elevated baseline brain natriuretic peptide (BNP) and pro-BNP levels have a worse prognosis.

All patients with severe symptomatic stenosis should undergo cardiac catheterization for evaluation of concomitant coronary artery disease. When there is a discrepancy between symptoms and severity of aortic stenosis as determined by noninvasive testing, cardiac catheterization is recommended to obtain an invasive transvalvular gradient.

TREATMENT

No medical treatment has shown any benefit in chronic aortic stenosis. Statin therapy may slow the progression of aortic stenosis if started early in mild disease. Balloon valvuloplasty has not been shown to be superior to medical therapy, but is being increasingly used as a temporizing measure for patients who are ultimately candidates for valve replacement therapy or as a palliative procedure for symptom relief. Surgical aortic valve replacement (SAVR) has been the standard therapy for low- and intermediate-risk patients with aortic stenosis; it is associated with a periprocedural mortality rate of 1% to 3% and periprocedural stroke risk of 1.5% to 4%.

Recently, percutaneous transcatheter aortic valve replacement (TAVR), or catheter-based valve, has emerged as a viable option for inoperable and high-risk patients with aortic stenosis. All patients are seen by a heart team consisting of cardiothoracic surgeons and cardiologists and are risk stratified by their Society of Thoracic Surgeons (STS) score and frailty index. The STS score takes into account a patient's age and other comorbid conditions such as renal failure, previous bypass or valve replacement surgery, and pulmonary disease. The frailty index is a measure of a patient's functional capacity such as mental status, activities of daily living, nutritional assessment, and strength and balance. Patients with an STS score of greater than 10% or a score of predicted risk

Table A.3

CRITERIA FOR AORTIC STENOSIS IN PATIENTS WITH NORMAL LEFT VENTRICULAR FUNCTION

Severity	Valve Area (cm²)	Mean Gradient (mmHg)	Velocity (m/s)	Indexed Valve Area (cm²/m²)
Mild	>1.5	<20	2.6–2.9	>0.85
Moderate	1.0–1.5	20–40	3.0–4.0	0.60–0.85
Severe	<1.0	>40	>4.0	<0.6
Very severe	—	>50	>5	—

Source: Data from Baumgartner et al. (2008).

of death by 30 days after surgery of greater than or equal to 15% are considered high-risk patients. Inoperable patients are characterized by a score of greater than or equal to 50% for predicted mortality or serious irreversible complication 30 days postsurgery.

Data from the recently published PARTNER trial demonstrated that in inoperable patients randomized to either standard therapy or TAVR, the 1-year all-cause mortality was 50.7% for standard therapy versus 30.7% for TAVR (Leon et al., 2010). It also demonstrated that in high-risk patients who had severe symptomatic aortic stenosis and STS score greater than 10% and who were randomized to TAVR or SAVR, the overall 1-year mortality was similar postprocedure (24.2% TAVR vs. 26.8% SAVR). Death rates from cardiovascular causes were equivalent at 1 year (14.3% TAVR vs. 13% SAVR; Leon et al., 2010), with significant reduction in repeat hospitalizations and improvement in cardiac symptoms. These benefits were sustained at 5-year follow-up with a significant absolute reduction in mortality. Similar results were seen in the CoreValve U.S. Pivotal Trial using a self-expanding prosthesis; it showed a reduction in all-cause mortality at 1 and 2 years, respectively, when compared with SAVR. Based on the results of the PARTNER and CoreValve trials, the U.S. Food and Drug Administration approved TAVR for inoperable (STS score greater than 15), high-risk (STS score greater than 8), and intermediate-risk (STS score: 4–8) patients in the United States.

CONCLUSION

Symptomatic severe aortic stenosis is a lethal disease if not treated in a timely manner. Surgery is still the first treatment option for low- and intermediate-risk patients. Catheter-based valve replacement is the treatment of choice for high-risk and inoperable patients with severe aortic stenosis. It likely may become the preferred treatment option in suitable surgical patients. This procedure is becoming more widely available in the United States. Different valves with improved designs and lower profile also are being evaluated, which may reduce complications and increase procedural success.

Jayant Khitha and Tanvir K. Bajwa

Baumgartner, H., Hung, J., Bermejo, J., Chambers, J. B., Evangelista, A., Griffin, B. P.,...Quiñones, M. (2008). Echocardiographic assessment of valve stenosis: EAE/ASE recommendations for clinical practice. *European Journal of Echocardiography*, 22(1), 1–23. doi:10.1016/j.echo.2008.11.029

Carabello, B. A. (2002). Evaluation and management of patients with aortic stenosis. *Circulation, 105*, 1746–1750.

Carabello, B. A., & Paulus, W. J. (2009). Aortic stenosis. *Lancet, 373*, 956–966.

Fried, L. P., Borhanim, N. O., Enright, P., Furberg, C. D., Gardin, J. M., Kronmal, R. A.,...O'Leary, D. H. (1991). The Cardiovascular Health Study: Design and rationale. *Annals of Epidemiology, 1*(3), 263–276.

Leon, M. B., Smith, C. R., Mack, M., Miller, D. C., Moses, J. W., Svensson, L. G.,...Brown, D. L. (2010). Transcatheter aortic-valve implantation for aortic stenosis in patients who cannot undergo surgery. *New England Journal of Medicine, 363*(17), 1597–1607.

Nishimura, R. A., Otto, C. M., Bonow, R. O., Carabello, B. A., Erwin, J. P., III, Guyton, R. A.,... Thomas, J. D.; American College of Cardiology/ American Heart Association Task Force on Practice Guidelines. (2014). AHA/ACC guideline for the management of patients with valvular heart disease: A report of the American College

Table A.4

NEWER CLASSIFICATIONS FOR STAGES OF VALVULAR AORTIC STENOSIS

Stage	Definition	Valve Anatomy	Valve Hemodynamics	Hemodynamic Consequences	Symptoms
A	At risk of AS	• Bicuspid aortic valve (or other congenital valve anomaly) • Aortic valve sclerosis	• Aortic V_{max} <2 m/s	• None	• None
B	Progressive AS	• Mild-to-moderate leaflet calcification of a bicuspid or trileaflet valve with some reduction in systolic motion or • Rheumatic valve changes with commissural fusion	• Mild AS: Aortic V_{max} = 2.0–2.9 m/s or mean ΔP <20 mmHg • Moderate AS: Aortic V_{max} = 3.0–3.9 m/s or mean ΔP = 20–39 mmHg	• Early LV diastolic dysfunction may be present • Normal LVEF	• None

C: Asymptomatic severe AS

Stage	Definition	Valve Anatomy	Valve Hemodynamics	Hemodynamic Consequences	Symptoms
C1	Asymptomatic severe AS	• Severe leaflet calcification or congenital stenosis with severely reduced leaflet opening	• Aortic V_{max} ≥4 m/s or mean ΔP ≥40 mmHg • AVA typically is ≤1.0 cm² (or AVAi ≤0.6 cm²/m²) • Very severe AS is an aortic V_{max} ≥ 5m/s or mean ΔP ≥60 mmHg	• LV diastolic dysfunction • Mild LV hypertrophy • Normal LVEF	• None: Exercise testing is reasonable to confirm symptom status
C2	Asymptomatic severe AS with LV dysfunction	• Severe leaflet calcification or congenital stenosis with severely reduced leaflet opening	• Aortic V_{max} ≥4 m/s or mean ΔP ≥40 mmHg • AVA typically ≤1.0 cm² (or AVAi ≤ 0.6 cm²/m²)	• LVEF <50%	• None

D: Symptomatic severe AS

Stage	Definition	Valve Anatomy	Valve Hemodynamics	Hemodynamic Consequences	Symptoms
D1	Symptomatic severe high-gradient AS	• Severe leaflet calcification or congenital stenosis with severely reduced leaflet opening	• Aortic V_{max} ≥4m/s or mean ΔP ≥40 mmHg • AVA typically ≤1.0 cm² (or AVAi ≤0.6 cm²/m²) but may be larger with mixed AS/AR	• LV diastolic dysfunction • LV hypertrophy • Pulmonary hypertension may be present	• Exertional dyspnea or decreased exercise tolerance • Exertional angina • Exertional syncope or presyncope
D2	Symptomatic severe low-flow/low-gradient AS with reduced LVEF	• Severe leaflet calcification with severely reduced leaflet motion	• AVA ≤1.0 cm² with resting aortic V_{max} <4 m/s or mean ΔP <40 mmHg • Dobutamine stress echocardiography shows AVA ≤1.0 cm² with V_{max} ≥4 m/s at any flow rate	• LV diastolic dysfunction • LV hypertrophy • LVEF <50%	• HF • Angina • Syncope or presyncope
D3	Symptomatic severe low-gradient AS with normal LVEF or paradoxical low-flow severe AS	• Severe leaflet calcification with severely reduced leaflet motion	• AVA ≤1.0 cm² with aortic V_{max} <4 m/s or mean ΔP <40 mmHg • Indexed AVA ≤0.6 cm²/m² • Stroke volume index <35 mL/m² • Measured when patient is normotensive (systolic BP <140 mmHg)	• Increased LV relative wall thickness • Small LV chamber with low stroke volume • Restrictive diastolic filling • LVEF ≥50%	• HF • Angina • Syncope or presyncope

AR, aortic regurgitation; AS, aortic stenosis; AVA, aortic valve area; AVAi, aortic valve area indexed to body surface area; BP, blood pressure; HF, heart failure; LV, left ventricular; LVEF, left ventricular ejection fraction; ΔP, pressure gradient; V_{max}, maximum aortic velocity.

Source: From Nishimura et al. (2014), with permission of Elsevier.

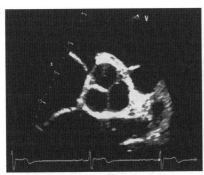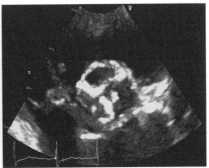

FIGURE A.1 Echocardiography demonstrating (left) a normal aortic valve and (right) a stenotic aortic valve.

of Cardiology/American Heart Association Task Force on Practice Guidelines. *Journal of American College of Cardiology, 63,* e57–e185.

Asian American and Pacific Islander Elders

In the United States, Asian Americans and Pacific Islanders (AAPI) are a diverse population who immigrated from or whose ancestors are from various countries in Asia and the Pacific Islands. Numbering 1.6 million, or 10% of the total AAPI population in 2010, the population of those 65+ is expected to grow 352%, to 7.3 million by 2060, when they will be about 21% of the total AAPI population in the United States. The older Asian population is among the fastest growing older populations in the United States. As many as 40 different languages and dialects are spoken. With only 15% of AAPI elders reporting that they speak English at home, 60% have limited English proficiency (Barker, 2013). The larger Asian American groups include Chinese, Filipinos, Japanese, Asian Indians, Koreans, and Vietnamese. The larger Pacific Islander groups include Native Hawaiians, Fijians, Tongans, and Guamanians. The life experiences of AAPIs are affected by economic, political, and social policies in areas of the government as diverse as justice, defense, labor, education, and foreign relations. As with all populations, their life experiences have an impact on access to and participation in health and social service programs.

HISTORICAL CONTEXT

Each AAPI ethnic community in the United States has a rich and varied history linked to the wave or cohort in which community members arrived. Initial waves of Chinese immigrants were bound by historic policies and practices of segregation: specific streets and schools in many California towns; mining claims in California, Wyoming, and Nevada; low-paid, high-risk jobs building the transcontinental railroad; and later, restaurant, laundry, and other service-sector jobs unlikely to compete with White jobs. Initial waves of Japanese, Filipinos, and Koreans were allowed limited social and economic roles as farmworkers, domestic or food service workers, and day laborers. In the 1960s, relatively large numbers of older adult Chinese, Filipinos, Koreans, Asian Indians, Tongans, and others arrived as U.S. laws supported family reunification. By the early 1970s, other U.S. policies supported the immigration of Vietnamese, Cambodians, Hmong, Laotians, and Chinese seeking refuge from political unrest and war.

In the past 40 years, life for many AAPI and other elders of color in the United States has been affected by major social, economic, and political change: reparations paid to Japanese Americans in recognition of their unfair incarceration during World War II; statutes permitting AAPIs to own property and businesses; affirmative efforts to ensure fair access to housing, public schools and public accommodations; and drivers' tests, election ballots, and health information in languages other than English. In some instances, relations within ethnic groups of AAPI have undergone as much change as those between each AAPI ethnic group and "Americans."

DEMOGRAPHICS

AAPI older adults are more likely to be foreign born (i.e., 70% compared with 9% for non-AAPI elders) and more likely to speak a language other than English at home (i.e., 85% for AAPI compared with 12% for non-AAPI). Yet aggregated data for all AAPI hide significant group differences. For example, almost all elders from Bangladesh, Cambodia, Vietnam, Indonesia, India, and Sri Lanka were born outside the United States, whereas 66% of Japanese American and Samoan American elders were born in the United States. Perhaps more startling is that about two thirds of foreign-born Asian American elders are naturalized U.S. citizens, including more than 70% of Indians, Thais, Filipinos, Sri Lankans, Laotians, Hmong, Koreans, and Vietnamese elders (Barker, 2013). Nativity, language, and citizenship differences among AAPI elders are the types of indicators that could help service providers better understand AAPI patients. Among Japanese, Chinese, and Cambodians, for example, differences are pronounced and are further affected by the length of time individuals have been in the United States (e.g., arrival as children or young adults) and U.S. school attendance.

PROGRAM PARTICIPATION

In community capacity-building assessment meetings, elders stated that they were uninformed about, ignored by, and at times unwelcome at mainstream programs for older adults in their communities (Yee, Sanchez, & Shin, 1999). Although many AAPI elders (especially in Western states) have resided in the same place for decades, paid taxes, and participated in the economic growth of their communities, they are often not visible and did not participate in social and health service programs in their

communities, even though data lead to expectations that they would need such help.

Nearly all AAPI elders live in urban and suburban areas, and in 2017, most AAPI lived in Hawaii and California (U.S. Department of Commerce, 2017). Yet, few microdata sources on AAPIs overall or on any specific AAPI ethnic group in the United States are maintained. Considered too small a population to include in analyses of national survey data, AAPI elders are also less likely to participate in national mailed or telephone surveys that are in only English: Many AAPI elders have also learned from life experience that talking about problems or personal situations to "government" representatives can result in oppressive and retaliatory actions, such as having benefits curtailed or denied or having family members investigated. Efforts by service providers to understand and respond to the needs of AAPI elders are often problematic and are unsuccessful in establishing rapport, identifying possible interventions that meet stated needs, and achieving successful referrals to available service programs.

CHALLENGES FOR SERVICE PROVIDERS

Recent work consistently indicates that service providers and AAPI elder communities must jointly take steps to address critical needs to improve the quality of life for AAPI older persons. Since the late 1970s, community-wide outreach programs and service-delivery strategies for infants and young children, AIDS or HIV-infected individuals, the unemployed, and frail older adults have met with mixed results and have been largely ineffective and unsuccessful in reaching target populations such as AAPI elders.

Several voluntary community-based organizations that serve specific AAPI ethnic groups have had long-term success with service delivery in their geographic areas. At the same time, many public health and social service programs appear to have abandoned efforts to systematically reach and appropriately serve AAPI elders. Increasing complexity within service systems, scarcity of resources, and a lack of leadership to effectively serve newer, smaller, harder-to-reach communities are among the reasons given for the lack of effort and success in serving AAPI elders. Gathering in forums that promote community capacity-building by eliciting community issues, listening to elders' perspectives, and enjoining problem solvers to sustain dialogue until new solutions are developed can be an effective intervention (Yee et al., 1999).

Addressing language and information barriers is a first step toward increasing understanding among AAPI elders and indicating that service systems want to be responsive to their social, health, and other human service needs. Quick fixes, such as the use of "black box" communications (i.e., conferencing-in a language service into medical examination rooms and government offices), may be better than nothing in some cases but could be more harmful in other situations. Anyone who has been frustrated while trying to decipher literally translated instructions (from Japanese or German into English) to assemble furniture or to operate electronic equipment can understand why literal translations from English into an AAPI language cannot be assumed to work. Cultural translation is also needed to ensure communication and rapport between doctor and patient, provider and consumer, and outsider and family. Literal interpretation might not be enough to facilitate the breadth and depth of communication needed when exchanges are about complex issues. At the same time relying on adult children can be fraught with limitations. Children may not have the same skill and fluency in English as they do in their first language: A child's vocabulary may be limited to parent–child interactions unrelated to cognitive conditions, chronic disease, or emotional conditions.

The literature on the nature and impact of disparities among marginal populations across the United States has been replete with examples of how poor access to health care and poor health literacy are correlated with disparate health outcomes at the individual and population levels. Indifference and ignorance about the nature and extent of differences among AAPI groups result in prevalence data that average the experiences of Hmong and Japanese elders when the risks and need for treatment might be evident and compelling if data were disaggregated. Elders need explanations of how service programs and service systems work in ways that make sense to them. Concepts such as prepaid health care or home- and community-based care are not likely to be part of the vocabulary or life experience of most AAPI elders. Practitioners must be willing to recognize differences in cultural assumptions about private and public roles. Understanding family roles in decision making among many AAPI may mean asking about and being open to ways in which an eldest son, a husband, or a brother-in-law can make decisions rather than the elder patient herself. An AAPI family may not understand that "Americans" place importance on end-of-life, preventive care, or insurance issues and that care decisions are usually made by the individual patient. Concurrently, service providers may need to recognize that an AAPI elder may have different priorities, such as "going out the way I came in," "not dying among strangers," or refusing costly care to ensure that adequate resources are available for a grandchild's education. A mutual understanding of differences and a mutual willingness to communicate in the context of such differences can be what defines person-centered care for many AAPI elders.

BEST PRACTICES AND LESSONS LEARNED

Fadiman's account (1997) of harrowing mismatches between the "American" health system and a Hmong family and Ariyoshi's novel (1984) of a woman's relationship with her frail in-laws in postwar Japan are two excellent portrayals of how help-seeking behavior, problem identification, and problem solving between a care receiver, family caregiver(s) and service provider(s) are only the first steps in providing appropriate and good care in cross-cultural situations. Attending to the cross-cultural aspects of each mini-episode of the caregiving relationship is critical to identifying appropriate interventions that address the initial problem (Yee, 1999).

Contact between those whose mission it is to provide services and meet needs and those who need assistance is critical in building relationships. Communication with one another about shared and differing cultural assumptions

A

can build a bridge of cultural competence and make significant differences in the quality of life and health outcomes for AAPI elders.

See also Cultural Assessment; Cultural Competence and Aging.

Donna L. Yee

Ariyoshi, S. (1984). *The twilight years.* New York, NY: Kodansha America.

Barker, K. (2013). *Asian Americans and Pacific Islanders in the United States aged 65 years and older: Population, nativity, and language* (Vol. 1). Seattle, WA: National Asian Pacific Center on Aging.

Fadiman, A. (1997). *The spirit catches you and you fall down.* New York, NY: Noonday Press.

U.S. Department of Commerce. (2017). U.S. Census Bureau releases key statistics in honor of Asian-American and Pacific Islander Heritage Month. Retrieved from https://www.commerce.gov/news/blog/2017/05/us-census-bureau-releases-key-statistics-honor-asian-american-and-pacific-islander

Yee, D. L. (1999). Preventing chronic illness & disability: Asian Americans. In M. L. Wykle & A. B. Ford (Eds.), *Serving minority elders in the 21st century* (pp. 37–50). New York, NY: Springer Publishing.

Yee, D. L., Sanchez, Y. N., & Shin, A. (1999). *Establishing information infrastructure for API elders: A roadmap for assuring rights and protections of HCFA beneficiaries (final recommendations on the vulnerable populations project).* Seattle, WA: National Asian Pacific Center on Aging.

Web Resources

AARP-Health of AAPI: http://www.aarp.org/content/dam/aarp/research/surveys_statistics/health/2015/The-Health-and-Healthcare-of-Asian-Americans-and-Pacific-Islanders-Age-50-Plus-AARP-res-health.pdf

AARP-Family Issues AAPI: http://www.aarp.org/content/dam/aarp/home-and-family/asian-community/2016/04/2016-aaaj-report-aarp.pdf?intcmp=AE-ASIANCOMM-NEWS

AARP-Caregiver Guide AAPI: http://www.aarp.org/content/dam/aarp/home-and-family/caregiving/2014-11/report_caregiving_aapis_english.pdf

National Asian Pacific Center on Aging: http://www.napca.org

ASSESSING NEEDS OF FAMILY CAREGIVERS

An estimated 43.5 million adults in the United States provide unpaid care to an adult or a child each year, and approximately 10% of those who provide care are older than 75 years (National Alliance for Caregiving and AARP, 2015). Although many family members assume caregiving responsibilities willingly and derive great satisfaction and meaning from the role, others report feeling isolated, burdened, underappreciated, and overwhelmed. Whether caring for a loved one after surgery, after a life-altering medical event, or throughout the course of a protracted chronic illness, there is no question that caregiving alters the lives of those providing care and their families.

Caregiving is complex and embraces varied tasks, including locating, accessing, and coordinating services; filling out forms; managing medications; providing direct care; managing roles; preserving dignity; and prioritizing competing needs. Because of shorter hospitalizations, family caregivers are increasingly assuming responsibility for tasks that were formerly performed by nurses. About 57% of caregivers assist with these *medical/nursing tasks*, which include skilled activities such as injections, tube feedings, and catheter and colostomy care (Reinhard, Levine & Samis, 2012). Because they rarely feel comfortable or equipped to serve these functions, family caregivers commonly face emotional strain, mental disorders, workplace challenges, financial burdens, retirement insecurity, health risks, and lost opportunities. Burgeoning needs of caregivers have contributed to an expanded marketplace of community-based services and to an increase in disease-specific services such as cancer and dementia. Although an extensive array of services is beneficial, caregivers are often confused about how to choose, access, and pay for services, thus adding to their burden.

Although, family caregivers are acknowledged as the premier providers of long-term care, their needs often remain unaddressed and overshadowed by those of the care recipient.

Caregiver neglect of self-care and compromised quality-of-life have been linked to poor health outcomes and higher care costs for both caregivers and care recipients. This discussion describes the guiding principles and domains of assessment involved in the process of identifying and addressing the needs of family caregivers.

What Is Caregiver Assessment? The term *caregiver assessment* is generally used to describe a systematic process of gathering information about a caregiving situation and identifying the problems, needs, resources, and strengths of the family. It considers the family context, including the quality of the relationship between the caregiver and care receiver, other resources, and family dynamics. It approaches issues from the caregiver's perspective and culture, focuses on what assistance the caregiver may need, and strives to maintain the caregiver's own health and well-being. It also addresses the caregiver's regard for the care receiver's wishes and preferences and ways that those concerns influence decision making. The goal of the assessment is to develop a care plan that identifies appropriate, available, and affordable services that meet the needs and priorities of the caregiver without compromising the quality of life of the care receiver or other family members.

Why Assess Family Caregivers? Although it is critical to meet the needs and preserve the dignity and autonomy of the care receiver, it is also essential to recognize, respect, assess, and address the needs of the caregiver. Family members often, but not always, undertake caregiving willingly. The best predictor of the caregiver–care receiver relationship is the quality of the relationship prior to the need for care. In addition to the nature of the relationship, the family member's motivation for caregiving also influences the caregiving experience. Caregiving motivated by feelings of attachment is more often associated with favorable outcomes than caregiving motivated by feelings of obligation or expectations of reward.

The success of most care plans, from hospital discharge to home-based care, often rests on the family caregiver's shoulders. Strain and health risks can impede the caregiver's ability to provide care, lead to higher health care costs, and affect the quality of life for caregivers and

their loved ones. A systematic assessment of needs captures information on the caregiver's everyday experience and legitimizes the process of listening to them. Assessment is a first step toward helping caregivers obtain the information and services they need to maintain their well-being (Bradley, 2003). Acknowledgment of the impact that caregiver well-being has on patient care outcomes led the American Medical Association to participate in the development and promotion of the Caregiver Self-Assessment Questionnaire (American Psychological Association, 2012; Epstein-Lubow, Gaudiano, Hinckley, Salloway, & Miller, 2010).

What Are the Components of a Family Caregiver Assessment? Although the purpose of caregiver assessment differs by setting, the components are generally the same across care venues. Experts from the 2005 National Consensus Project for Caregiver Assessment (Family Caregiver Alliance, 2006a, 2006b, 2006c) recommended the following domains of assessment:

- *Context.* Context refers to the background on the caregiver and the caregiving situation. What is the caregiver's relationship to the care recipient? What is the nature and quality of their relationship? How long has he or she been in the caregiving role? Is the caregiver currently employed? What is known about the care recipient's diagnosis and related care needs?
- *Caregiver's Perceptions of Function.* Can the care recipient carry out activities of daily living (ADLs), such as bathing or dressing, without assistance? Can the care recipient carry out instrumental activities of daily living (IADLs) such as managing finances or using the telephone without assistance? Does the care recipient have any behavioral problems, such as wandering, and how frequently do they occur? How does the caregiver respond to behaviors perceived as problematic?
- *Caregiver Values and Preferences.* Is the caregiver willing to assume the caregiving role? What types of care arrangements are culturally acceptable for this family? How do the caregiver's and care recipient's values and preferences differ?

- *Caregiver Well-being.* How does the caregiver perceive personal health? What types of emotional reactions does the caregiver experience while spending time with the care recipient? What types of activities does the caregiver engage in to promote well-being?
- *Consequences of Caregiving—Perceived Challenges/ Benefits.* Does the caregiver suffer any work-related difficulties due to the caregiving role? How much does the caregiver's health stand in the way of doing things he or she wants to do? How does caregiving impact other members of the caregiver's family such as a spouse or children? What are the benefits of being a caregiver?
- *Caregiver Skills/Knowledge.* How knowledgeable does the caregiver feel about the care recipient's condition? What are the skills and abilities needed to provide care? How confident and competent does the caregiver feel in these areas? What type of assistance or support does the caregiver enjoy providing?
- *Caregiver Resources.* What are the caregiver's coping strategies? What is going well? What other community resources, such as caregiver support groups or religious organizations, is the caregiver utilizing or aware of? How do finances impact the caregiver's ability to provide for the care recipients' basic needs and affect access to local resources?

The following tasks, adapted from the Family Caregiver Alliance (2006c), are generally accepted standards of practice for a caregiver assessment:

- Identify the primary caregiver and other family/friends involved in arranging, coordinating, and providing care.
- Approach issues and priorities from the caregiver's perspective.
- Assess the availability of resources (e.g., financial, transportation).
- Discuss the caregiver's understanding of the role.
- Identify what the caregiver needs to know to carry out the required tasks.
- Address services available for the caregiver and provide appropriate and timely referrals.
- Assess only essential information so that the process is no longer than necessary.

Who Is Qualified to Perform Assessments? Various health and social service providers can assess caregivers, including physicians, social workers, marriage and family therapists, mental health counselors, psychologists, care managers, nurses, and rehabilitation professionals. These professionals work in primary care, behavioral health, hospitals, long-term care facilities, specialty clinics, disease-focused nonprofit agencies, and organizations within the aging services network. In addition, professionals assuming the emerging roles of transition coaches in hospitals and care managers in primary care medical homes, both of whom focus on chronic disease management, are also well positioned to assess caregivers.

Professionals conducting caregiver assessments need to have specialized knowledge and skills, including an understanding of how the assessment process guides and informs their work with families. It is essential to understand the caregiving process; have a working knowledge of various aspects of illnesses, treatments, and disease progression; and familiarity with community resources, eligibility criteria, and costs. Because cultural, ethnic, and religious influences help define family roles and affect the use of services, cultural competence is critical.

Other Considerations. Caregiving assessment is the foundation for the development of mutually agreed on, affordable, and accessible goals and interventions. Resources and services identified in the plan need to be readily available and accessible. Similarly, it is good practice to avoid focusing on issues that the assessing professional is not equipped or trained to address, as well as on needs that may require referral to other providers. In an effort to avoid overwhelming families with decisions they are not yet prepared to make, it is often useful to focus on caregiving assessment as an ongoing process with plans consisting of both short- and long-term goals and a built-in opportunity for periodic reassessment to monitor changes in needs over time.

See also Caregiver Burnout; Caregiver Stress; Caregiving Relationships.

Carol Podgorski and Ann Cornell

AARP. (2015). AARP report. Retrieved from http:// www.aarp.org/content/dam/aarp/ppi/2015/ caregiving-in-the-united-states-2015-report -revised.pdf

Bradley, P. (2003). Family caregiver assessment: Essentials for effective home health care. *Journal of Gerontological Nursing, 29*, 29–36.

Epstein-Lubow, G., Gaudiano, B. A., Hinckley, M., Salloway, S., & Miller, I. W. (2010). Evidence for the validity of the American Medical Association's Caregiver Self-Assessment Questionnaire as a screening measure for depression. *Journal of the American Geriatrics Society, 58*(2), 387–388.

Family Caregiver Alliance. (2006a). *Caregiver assessment: Principles, guidelines and strategies for change. Report from a National Consensus Development Conference* (Vol. I). San Francisco, CA: Author. Retrieved from https://www .caregiver.org/national-consensus-report-care giver-assessment-volumes-1-2

Family Caregiver Alliance. (2006b). *Caregiver assessment: Voices and views from the field. Report from a National Consensus Development Conference* (Vol. II). San Francisco, CA: Author. Retrieved from https://www.caregiver.org/ national-consensus-report-caregiver-assessment -volumes-1-2

Family Caregiver Alliance. (2006c). Caregivers count too! A toolkit to help practitioners in assessing the needs of family caregivers. Retrieved from https://www.caregiver.org/caregivers -count-too-toolkit

National Alliance. (2015). Caregiving in the U.S. Retrieved from http://www.caregiving.org/ caregiving2015

Reinhard, S. C., Levine, C., & Samis, S. (2012). *Home alone: Family caregivers providing complex chronic care*. Washington, DC: AARP Public Policy Institute & United Hospital Fund. Retrieved from http://www.aarp.org/home-family/care giving/info-10-2012/home-alone-family-care givers-providing-complex-chronic-care.html

Web Resources

Administration on Aging, National Family Caregiver Support Program: http://www.aoa.acl.gov/AoA _Programs/HCLTC/Caregiver

Aging and Disability Resource Center: https:// www.adrc-tae.acl.gov/tiki-index.php?page= ADRCHomeTest

Alzheimer's Association: 2016 Alzheimer's disease facts and figures: https://www.alz.org/documents_ custom/2016-facts-and-figures.pdf

American Psychological Association, Caregiver Self-Assessment Questionnaire: http://www.apa .org/pi/about/publications/caregivers/practice -settings/assessment/tools/self-assessment.aspx

Caregiver Action Network: http://caregiveraction .org

Family Caregiver Alliance: http://www.caregiver.org

Family Caregiver Alliance, Selected Caregiver Assessment Measures: https://www.caregiver .org/sites/caregiver.org/files/pdfs/SelCG AssmtMeas_ResInv_FINAL_12.10.12.pdf

National Alliance for Caregiving: 1-301-718-8444; http://www.caregiving.org

National Alliance for Caregiving (2015): Caregiving in the U.S., 2015: http://www.caregiving.org/ caregiving2015

National Family Caregivers Association: http:// www.nfcacares.org

ASSISTED LIVING

Assisted living (AL) is a congregate residential setting for six or more adults that provides or coordinates housekeeping and personal services, 24-hour supervision and assistance, activities, and health-related services, primarily for older adults (Stevenson & Grabowski, 2010). AL is known by several names—residential care, home for the aged, housing with services, board and care, personal care, enriched housing—and the distinctions lie in state regulations, certification, or licensing; type of housing unit (e.g., shared room or apartment); and the needs that a particular setting can meet. Today all types of group residential care are commonly referred to as *assisted living* (Assisted living, 2011). In contrast, state-licensed adult foster or family care is for four to six people residing in the provider's home. In 2012, the federal government released data from the first nationally representative survey of AL/residential care facilities. The latest study demonstrated that in 2014, there were a total of 835,200 residents in AL/residential care facilities. Some 62% of residents required assistance with bathing, the most common functional limitation, and 4 in 10 were diagnosed with Alzheimer's disease or other dementias (Centers for Disease Control and Prevention [CDC], 2015).

A

Although some federal laws apply, AL is regulated and monitored by the state. The number, nature, and scope of AL regulations continue to increase, particularly because AL residents are frailer, sicker, and older than when AL first appeared as a residential-care option. AL is generally defined as an environment that offers and/or provides assistance with ADLs and instrumental activities of daily living (IADLs) such as meals and assistance with medications. The goal of AL is to promote "aging-in-place," the ability to live in a residence of one's own choice, safely and comfortably, as one ages.

A vexing problem for states as well as providers is the balance between resident autonomy (and risk taking) and safety needs. In some facilities, residents or their family surrogates can sign "negotiated risk" contracts that allows them to remain in the assisted-living residences (ALRs) despite functional and/or cognitive decline. A negotiated risk agreement was considered an important topic several years ago, but few states address the topic in regulations because of liability risk with residents with cognitive impairment (U.S. Department of Health and Human Services [USDHHS], 2015). Also known as "managed risk" or "shared responsibility," potential consequences of the resident's actions must be described, as do options to limit risk and honor the resident's wishes, such as requiring the resident or family to hire extra help if needed. The agreement process and areas of disagreement must be documented. Some states (e.g., Oregon) do not permit a risk agreement if the resident is unable to comprehend the consequences associated with actions.

The consumer-centered philosophy of AL, as defined by the National Center for Assisted Living (Assisted living, 2013), promotes wellness and maximizes quality of life, independence, privacy, choice, safety, decision making, and "aging in place" in a homelike environment. Private living units, including private baths (in an estimated 80% of ALRs), are a critical feature of AL; residents may lock their doors. Forty-one states have at least one residential category that allows three or more residents to share a room and/or toilets and bathing facilities (USDHHS, 2015). At least 30 states allow two people to share a unit (i.e., apartment) or bedroom but, in

some states, only if the two parties choose to do so (e.g., Washington). Depending on the licensing category, some states allow as many as four people to share a unit and up to eight residents to share a toilet (USDHHS, 2015). Regulations in 21 states contain a statement of AL philosophy, in greater or lesser detail (e.g., aging in place), as well as describe services that may or may not be offered. Given the likelihood of increasing needs and frailty and the ALRs' obligation to provide appropriate care, many ALRs feel they will evolve into a kind of "nursing home lite" environment—something they did not intend philosophically, operationally, or fiscally. Although state regulations set boundaries for the scope of services, providers (i.e., operators) nevertheless have considerable latitude in deciding what will be offered and which residents (i.e., tenants) will be admitted, retained, or discharged.

An occupancy, service, "contract," or "residency" agreement, executed before or immediately on admission to an ALR, is based on an assessment of the person's need for services and how they can best be met. In 2014, Centers for Medicare & Medicaid Services (CMS) clarified that residential settings serving individuals under Medicaid provide a residency agreement and/or follow applicable landlord/tenant laws that reference eviction processes and appeals as well as rights and responsibilities (USDHHS, 2015). Thirty-nine states require that ALRs disclose the services that will be provided to meet reasonable care needs. More than half of states require disclosure of costs and services beyond the basic rate, discharge criteria, grievance processes, resident rights, and retention and relocation criteria in case the ALR is unable to meet the resident's health and safety needs. In some states, ALRs must disclose their staffing pattern and staff training. Forty-four states have special regulations for ALRs that claim they provide dementia care, including specific disclosure regarding services provided, programming, staff training, the environment, and security provisions.

States can have a single level of AL or a two- or three-level model stipulating the services that can be provided or needs that can be met. It is illegal for an ALR to refuse to admit an individual whose health care needs can be met in the ALR as stipulated in the state's regulation and as protected by the Americans with Disabilities Act (ADA). The most compelling reason for discharge, permitted by most states, is when the ALR cannot provide the services needed or care needs exceed what the ALR license permits. Hence, the nature, frequency, duration, and intensity of health-related and nursing care permitted by regulation determine the feasibility of aging in place. A resident can be at risk of discharge for reasons unrelated to licensure but rather for financial reasons (i.e., inability to privately purchase the additional care and services needed from a home health agency). The worst-case scenario is a resident who remains too long in an ALR where the staff is not trained for complex health care management and provisions are not made to secure the health and safety of the resident.

The number and type of staff vary with the number of residents, their needs, and the services provided. Personal-care staff can be employed by the facility or contracted from an outside agency (e.g., licensed home care agency). Thirty-eight states require the ALR to employ or contract with a licensed nurse (i.e., RN or licensed practical nurse) to either be available or on staff at least some hours per week. Only one state, Alabama, requires a physician medical director. Every ALR must have an administrator (i.e., manager, director, or operator) who has overall responsibility for staff performance and resident well-being. Administrators must be specially trained in 72% and specially licensed in 46% of states. National Study of Long-Term Care Providers (NSLTCP) found that less than half of all ALFs employ an RN. Some ALRs employ an advanced practice nurse (i.e., geriatric or adult nurse practitioner) to conduct admission assessment, develop a plan of care, and provide health maintenance oversight and medication management.

Forty-two states have specific staffing standards based on resident needs; 32 states that use flexible or as-needed staffing also have minimum staffing ratios. In all ALRs, there must be at least one person available during the night hours. Most states (98%) require that direct-care staff be trained at the time of or prior to employment, but the curriculum varies: resident rights (required in 80% of states); emergency procedures (including CPR), first aid, and fire/safety/disaster preparedness (60%); infection control and abuse/neglect prevention (42%); dementia and behavior management (35%); special needs of resident/elderly (36%); and the aging process (18%). Few states develop the curriculum; the ALR or a staff-development enterprise can create the content with scant state review for quality. Few states require an examination or trainer standards—training can vary from 1 to 25 hours or more—and 40 states require continuing education.

All ALRs monitor residents' well-being and provide daily supervision and assistance with IADLs and ADLs; three meals a day, including therapeutic diets; housekeeping and laundry services; medication management; transportation for recreational and shopping trips; and an emergency call system. Thirty-six states permit nonlicensed staff to administer medications and 18 states allow unlicensed staff to assist with medications. Residents who are temporarily incapacitated or recuperating from surgery, injury, or illness or those who are dying can remain in the AL facility if it can provide the necessary services and care. Health care is supervised by a physician of each resident's choosing.

Admission and retention criteria vary widely among states. In the 10 states with broad criteria and flexible rules (e.g., Maine, Oregon, and Minnesota), ALRs are most likely to support aging in place. However, the ALR is not required to retain the resident. Some states simply require that a prospective resident be in stable health and not need 24-hour nursing care; other states' criteria screen out those who are bedbound, are incontinent, have deep pressure ulcers, need artificial feeding or hydration, or are ventilator-dependent. States may have criteria relating to independent ambulation, ability to use the toilet unassisted, and stage of dementia. New Jersey ALRs may admit and retain residents who are continuously dependent in four ADLs, have impaired decision-making capacity, are bedbound more than 14 days, are medically unstable, are a danger to self or others, and require treatment for severe pressure sores. Almost all states require discharge if the resident is no longer independently mobile, a requirement linked to fire safety and ability to evacuate the premises.

Exceptions to a state's discharge criteria, approved by the state, include temporary conditions (associated with remaining in bed for as many as 10 days); the resident's ability to independently perform or direct another in performing a medical procedure (e.g., oxygen administration, tube feeding, changing of sterile dressings, and insulin injection); consent by the resident, facility, and physician; state approval on a case-by-case basis; and family assistance with care. Some states allow home health care or third-party provider assistance for "skilled nursing care" if it is short term, temporary, or for an acute illness. Home health is permitted in more than two thirds of states as a component of AL, unrelated to admission or retention. Residents can contract directly with the agency or third-party provider for desired services.

Home care can be provided in ALRs for Medicare beneficiaries who meet eligibility criteria. An RN from a certified home-care agency supervises and monitors the care. Hospice care as a home care service can also be provided in ALRs. This decision is made by the facility and the resident or family, is not contingent on state regulations, and constitutes an exception from the discharge requirement. The USDHHS Office of the Inspector General (OIG) assessed Medicare hospice care in ALs between 2007 and 2012, finding that Medicare payment for hospice care in ALs more than doubled. Consequently, the OIG recommended hospice care payment reforms, with agreement by the CMS, and the role of hospice in these settings may change in the future (USDHHS, 2015).

More than 70% of AL residents are women. More than 50% are 85 years and older, with 10% younger than 65 years. Approximately 75% of residents receive some type of assistance with ADLs. Although most residents come to AL facilities from their own homes, slightly fewer than 20% come from nursing homes. Studies indicate that AL residents are taking more medication, in general, than nursing home residents and receive more psychotropic medications than their nursing home and community-residing peers. In addition, many of their medications are inappropriate for their age, unrelated to a diagnosis or condition, and poorly monitored. After an average stay of 26 months, approximately 45% of residents are discharged to nursing homes and 26% die. Approximately 5% of residents leave AL facilities for financial reasons.

The AL market is predominantly private pay; there is no ALR entry fee. In 2011 and 2014, the CMS issued proposed regulations to better define community settings where Medicaid recipients could receive services that are covered by Section 1915(c) Home and Community-Based Service (HCBS) waiver programs. The regulation requires that AL services (24-hour on-site supervision, safety, and social and recreational programming) be provided in settings that are home and community based, are integrated into the community, and provide access to the community (Mollica, Houser, & Ujvari, 2011). The 2014 regulations focused on person-centered planning, privacy, choice of roommate, access to food, and other issues related to autonomy and choice (USDHHS, 2015).

Forty-three states pay for some components of AL for Medicaid-eligible ALR residents (estimated at 121,000) under the Medicaid state plan, the HCBS waiver (Section 1915c; www.payingforseniorcare.com/medicaid-waivers/assisted-living.html), or some combination thereof. Under the waiver (36 states), states can provide home and community services to nursing home–eligible Medicaid beneficiaries; such services include personal care and homemaker services, medication management, home-delivered meals, and staffing for supervision and services. Because room and board cannot be covered by the waiver, some states assist Medicaid AL residents by fixing the room and board cost that the ALR can charge the resident, supplementing the resident's Supplemental Security Income (SSI) payment to use for this cost, or offering housing subsidies. State Medicaid policy determines the type of unit (i.e., single or shared) for Medicaid beneficiaries in ALRs (Washington permits shared units only by choice). Long-term care insurance is infrequently used or available among AL residents.

Average monthly fees are about $3,000; this is higher than the typical board-and-care fee but lower than nursing home costs (Argentum,

2016). The fee paid by the resident depends on the type of housing (i.e., shared vs. private room) and the kind and number of services included in the contract. Medicaid reimbursement can be an all-inclusive, flat-rate monthly price; tiered pricing based on the package of services needed (or desired) by the resident; tiered rates based on the resident's acuity level; fee-for-service pricing based on the resident's "a la carte" selection of services; or some combination of these models.

Several states are developing innovative financing mechanisms to assist developers in constructing affordable AL housing. A growing number of nonprofit and for-profit nursing homes are converting beds and wings to AL. Many continuing-care retirement communities offer AL either in the tenant's current domicile or by relocation to an AL facility on the premises. Medicare-capitated managed-care organizations view AL as being well suited for managing rehabilitation and providing a supportive environment for frail managed-care enrollees.

Virtually every state is studying or promulgating regulations and licensure requirements that distinguish AL from other long-term care and residential models. States have the authority to set provider standards; many have done so with respect to food preparation and fire safety. There is wide variability across facilities in services offered and across states in the degree of government involvement as a regulator of these services (Stevenson & Grabowski, 2010).

Medication management, staffing, qualifications and quality, adequacy of care, and plans of care are the major sources of complaints and deficiencies in ALRs. Twenty-four states use different surveyors for AL and nursing home quality-of-care inspections. Federal quality-of-care standards probably will not be promulgated in the near future because it is unlikely that the federal government will become a major AL payor. The state role in monitoring and licensure will continue to grow, especially as Medicaid assumes greater responsibility for the costs of care and services.

A growing body of scholarly research, much of it multidisciplinary, is engaging the AL industry as well as state legislative bodies, advocacy groups, professional associations, and academia (Grabowski, Stevenson, & Cornell, 2012). In-depth information is needed about AL users: their expectations and preferences, finances, functionality, conditions and illness trajectories, relocation, and outcomes. Research is needed regarding dementia care services and outcomes. Comparisons with other kinds of long-term health and social services and settings might help sharpen the focus and future of AL. An examination of the lack of uniformity among states in quality standards and regularity expectations is needed to meet the needs of our aging population.

See also Continuing Care Retirement Communities; Nursing Homes.

Susan M. Renz and Emily C. Stout

Argentum Excecutive Report. (2016). Getting to 2025: A senior living roadmap. Retrieved from https://www.argentum.org/images/Argentum2025.pdf

Assisted living state regulatory review. (2013). Washington, DC: National Center for Assisted Living. Retrieved from https://www.ahcancal.org/ncal/advocacy/regs/Documents/2016%20State%20AL%20Regulatory%20Review.pdf

Centers for Disease Control and Prevention. (2015). National survey of residential care facilities. Retrieved from https://www.cdc.gov/nchs/nsrcf/index.htm

Grabowski, D., Stevenson, D., & Cornell, P. (2012). Assisted living expansion and the market for nursing home care. *Health Services Research, 47*(6), 2296–2315.

Mollica, R., Houser, A., & Ujvari, K. (2011). Assisted living and residential care in the states in 2010. Retrieved from http://www.aarp.org/content/dam/aarp/research/public_policy_institute/ltc/2012/residential-care-insight-on-the-issues-july-2012-AARP-ppi-ltc.pdf

Stevenson, D. G., & Grabowski, D. C. (2010). Sizing up the market for assisted living. *Health Affairs, 29*(1), 35–43.

U.S. Department of Health and Human Services, Assistant Secretary for Planning and Evaluation, Office of Disability, Aging and Long-Term Care Policy. (2015). Compendium of residential care and assisted living regulations and policy. Retrieved from https://aspe.hhs.gov/sites/default/files/pdf/110391/15alcom.pdf

A

ASSISTIVE DEVICES

The Administration on Aging projects that 19% of adults aged 65 years and older will have some limitations in performing activities of daily living and 4% will have severe disability associated with aging. More than 75% of older adults with disabilities use some type of assistive device. Seniors with disabilities need to adapttheir lifestyle and their surrounding environment in response to their disability. Likewise, tools, often called *assistive devices*, are used to compensate for their disabilities.

Assistive devices are great resources for improving quality of life, improving mobility, helping independence, and communicating with surroundings. Appropriately selected assistive technology also may help seniors stay in their own home for a longer time. Tools, most often used to help seniors walk, bathe, and use the toilet, may prevent the need to move to higher level of care. Assistive devices also help prevent falls and injuries, which could be serious or life-threatening. Thus assistive devices provide a potential savings in formal care services.

NUANCES IN PRESCRIBING ASSISTIVE DEVICES

It is important to identify the underlying cause of disability before prescribing an assistive device. Medical and/or surgical evaluation should be completed in collaboration with rehabilitation experts. The use of assistive devices varies widely by age, race/ethnicity, education, income, and type and severity of disability. Many older persons choose to avoid social interactions rather than being seen using a device. This social isolation may lead to a further decline in independence. Older adults with disability who use assistive technology require fewer hours of personal assistance compared with individuals who refuse these devices. This observation adds to the economic case for prescribing assistive devices to seniors who need them.

WHAT ASSISTIVE DEVICES ARE AVAILABLE AND FOR WHICH INDICATIONS

Assistive technology is defined as any item, piece of equipment, or product system, whether acquired commercially, modified, or customized, that is used to increase, maintain, or improve functional capabilities of individuals with disabilities. The most common assistive devices used for ambulation are walkers, canes, wheelchairs, and motorized scooters.

Orthotics (such as ankle–foot orthotics, called AFOs) are designed to assist, align, and stimulate function. Feeding aids (e.g., light-weight utensils, utensils with easy-to-hold/rubber handles, plates with sides, and cups with antisplash lids) are available based on occupational therapy recommendation. Bathing devices such as transfer benches, bath sponges, long-handled brushes, handheld showers, and bath chairs are designed to improve hygiene and quality of life. Other assistive devices include a reacher, a shoe horn, a sock aid, toilet tongs, and walker tray/bags/baskets.

Environmental modification used in bathrooms include handrails, grab bars, and elevated toilet seats. Assistive devices for communications are low-vision kits and sound amplifiers. Low-vision kits may include a magnifying glass, talking clocks, a tablet computer with large font, a phone with large buttons, and a large communication board. Many of these devices are available from low-vision stores. Assistive devices for older persons who are at risk of wandering include alarms, monitors, locks, and advanced devices using Bluetooth signals. Community-dwelling persons with dementia may also benefit from safety devices such as automatic turn-off switches for stove burners, and automatic timers for lights.

"Smart home" technology is becoming more affordable for seniors. These systems connect household devices to a personal computer, and with voice recognition, lights, music, and alarm systems can be activated. Life Alert buttons can also be important for seniors' safety and independence. Self-driving cars also sound promising for seniors' independence

COLLABORATING WITH OCCUPATIONAL THERAPY AND PHYSICAL THERAPY TO IMPROVE CARE

Rehabilitation experts can make recommendations about the appropriate use of assistive devices. They work as a part of an interdisciplinary team to identify and address seniors' needs. The process of recommending assistive device includes patient assessment, evaluation of the patient's motivation to use the device, determination of the proper type of device needed, and training of the patient on how to use the device.

Therapists can use the WHO's International Classification of Function, Disability and Health (ICF) and the Occupational Therapy Practice Framework to guide them in determining assistive technology needs. The ICF is structured around three broad components: (a) body functions and structure, (b) activities and participation, and (c) additional information on severity and environmental factors. In essence, therapists integrate the medical and social aspects of the patient's health condition. An occupational therapist (OT) evaluates older persons' self-care skills, recommends appropriate assistive devices, and challenges them to provide care for themselves. An OT further provides home assessments of patient safety and optimal use of assistive devices. OTs also assess patients' cognitive ability to manage physical limitations.

MEDICARE COVERAGE OF ASSISTIVE DEVICES

Medicare covers most basic tools for mobility, including canes, walkers, and orthotics. Motorized wheelchairs and scooters may be covered, but only after specific criteria have been met. Recent abuse of these expensive items has been noted by the Centers for Medicare &

Medicaid Services. Additional assistive devices are covered by Medicare including buttonhooks, grab loops, footwear with Velcro closures, a bath bench, rubber mats, and hydraulic lifts, and bath seats. Eating tools covered include nonslip mats, rocker knives, and two-handled, spouted cups. Medicare does not cover installation expenses for devices. Furthermore, medication-dispensing tools, reachers, and accessories for walkers are not covered. All durable medical equipment (DME) is covered under Medicare Part B plan. In most states, equipment must be ordered from contract suppliers only.

Soryal A. Soryal and Michael L. Malone

ASSISTIVE TECHNOLOGY

Defined as assistive, adaptive, and rehabilitative services or tools that facilitate performance of functional activity, assistive technology encompasses a wide range of devices and services used to help individuals who are older or live with disabilities. With age, certain tasks and daily routines become more difficult and sometimes impossible to complete independently because of changes in vision, hearing, strength, memory, dexterity, and mobility. As these tasks become more challenging, it may be necessary to employ interventions to improve functioning. Assistive technology is associated with improved activity performance, satisfaction with activity performance, and reduced caregiver burden (Mortenson et al., 2012, 2013).

ASSISTIVE TECHNOLOGY DEVICES

The Technology-Related Assistance for Individuals with Disabilities Act of 1988 first described an assistive device as "any item, piece of equipment or product system whether acquired commercially off the shelf, modified, or customized that is used to increase, maintain or improve functional capabilities of individuals with disabilities." More than 25,000 of these devices can be used in all facets of life, including daily care, work, and mobility. Such

A

devices are considered either high or low tech. High-tech devices, such as powered wheelchairs, electronic communication systems, or computers, are considered more expensive and difficult to obtain or create. Low-tech devices such as paper communication boards, simple writing aids, and modified eating utensils are generally inexpensive, simple to make, and easy to obtain. Within the growing industry of assistive technology, such items are getting easier to obtain and can be purchased at general stores, pharmacies, and medical-supply stores, through mail-order catalogs, and online. It is common to find assistive devices such as a large-button phone for vision loss or a cane for mobility in an elderly person's home.

DEVICE TYPES

- Devices that aid an individual with visual impairments include closed-captioning televisions; talking devices such as a talking calculator, watch, or scale; screen readers for the computer; audio books; tactile markings on important items; magnifiers; items labeled with large print; increased lighting; and transparency sheets to change the contrast on printed material.
- Devices used for hearing impairments include hearing aids, cochlear implants, vibrating or light-up alarm clocks, flashing smoke detectors, captioned TVs, assistive listening devices, and TTY telephones.
- Speech impairments, temporary and permanent, may require aids such as text-to-speech interfaces, computers with scanning, picture boards, dry-erase boards, paper and pencils, pointing, finger spelling, and signing.
- Mobility aids include both high- and low-tech devices such as wheelchairs, scooters, adapted vehicles, seating and positioning systems, canes, walkers, and hand controls for driving.
- An increasing number of products have been designed to enhance memory function, including products such as the FINDIT Key Finder that beeps when a person claps; a keychain recorder that fits on the keychain and records short voice memos; Talking Rx that tells the patient how many pills to take,

when to take them, and what they are for; handheld computers to record appointment dates and times; voice recorders to record reminders; a pill box, a notepad, and a pencil that are kept in a pocket; a chain that attaches keys to the body; and Post-It Notes placed around the home as reminders of when to do certain activities.

- Activities of daily living (ADLs) such as feeding, dressing, and self-care may also become challenging as a person ages due to decreased strength, mobility, and dexterity. Aids for dressing include reachers, long-handled shoehorns, sock aids, zipper pulls, trouser pulls, and buttonhooks. For food preparation and eating, an elderly person may use a suction-cup plate, bowl, and pan holders; enlarged rims on plates for easier scooping; removable plate rims; capped cups; nose cutouts for cups; and built-up handles for utensils. Self-care assistive devices include tub benches, grab bars, bath lifts, nonslip bathmats, walk-in shower units, handheld shower sprays, long-handled sponges, sponge holders, curved-handle brushes, built-up or modified rush handles, universal cuffs for brushing teeth or hair and shaving, lever-handled faucets, and raised toilet seats.
- Older adults may also have a difficult time manipulating their environment easily. There are a few aids that can be of assistance in these instances. Environmental control units operate a variety of home electronics, from telephones and lights to appliances and window coverings. In addition, robotic systems are increasingly being used. For example, mounting a robotic system on a desktop can help control the working environment, or one can be installed on a track system to manipulate throughout the entire home, as well as to assist in feeding, self-care, and object movement.
- Many assistive-technology devices and home modifications may be used to increase the safety of individuals in their homes. Some examples include installing flashing smoke detectors, adding ramps, widening doorways, using tub benches and grab bars, removing loose rugs, increasing lighting in dark hallways, eliminating the constant use

of stairs, and adding levered or gripped door handles for easy exit in case of emergency.

ASSISTIVE TECHNOLOGY SERVICES

The Assistive Technology Act of 2004 (29 U.S.C. Sec 2202(2)) defines assistive technology service as "any service that directly assists an individual with a disability in the selection, acquisition or use of an assistive technology device." This includes evaluating an individual's needs and skills for assistive technology; selecting, designing, repairing, and fabricating assistive-technology systems; coordinating therapy services; and training both individuals using the device and their caregivers in its proper use.

Included in assistive-technology services is the evaluation of a patient's needs and skills for the use of assistive technologies. The individual must have an established need for assistive technology and be referred for it, which can be done by the consumer, nurse, caregiver, rehabilitation professional, or physician. Then the service provider gathers information regarding the individual's background and perceived need for assistive technology. Evaluation of the individual follows, which entails the service provider completing a needs-identification assessment. This is a key aspect of the evaluation because it guides how the remainder of the evaluation is completed. Components included in the needs assessment are the patient's life roles, activities, difficult tasks to perform, contexts, and prior technology history. A needs assessment is most effective and comprehensive when completed by a team working with the older adult in the setting where the assistive technology will be used. The service provider then completes an evaluation to determine the skills of the individual in terms of sensory, physical, cognitive, and language systems.

Once the evaluation has been completed, the service provider makes recommendations and helps the individual make optimal decisions regarding assistive technology by providing information about the cost, funding available, and use of the item. If assistive technology is needed, the service provider orders, delivers, and installs it, if necessary. Training

is then provided to help the individual use the assistive device independently and safely.

FUNDING

Funding for assistive technology depends on the state in which one lives. For individuals 65 years old and older, the primary source of funding is Medicare. Medicare is federally administered; however, each state also has its own rules governing the use of its funds. Medicare may cover durable medical equipment and supplies, which include wheelchairs, grab bars, hospital beds, lifts, walkers, and prosthetic devices; however, the decision is based on how that device is medically necessary for assisting the individual in the home. Federal and local grants may also provide additional funding. The Veterans Health Administration is another source of funding for veterans with disabilities. The Veterans Health Administration funds driving and transportation aids, medical equipment, wheelchairs, hearing aids, prosthetics, speech aids, and assessment services, among others. However, although a variety of funding sources are available for assistive technology, most often the primary payor is the consumer.

See also Americans with Disabilities Act; Environmental Modifications: Home.

Sharon Stahl Wexler and Marie-Claire Rosenberg Roberts

Assistive Technology Act of 1998, as amended (P.L. 108–364). (2004, October 2004). Retrieved from http://www.gpo.gov/fdsys/pkg/PLAW-108publ364/html/PLAW-108publ364.htm

Mortenson, W. B., Demers, L., Fuhrer, M. J., Jutai, J. W., Lenker, J., & DeRuyter, F. (2012). How assistive technology use by individuals with disabilities impacts their caregivers: A systematic review of the research evidence. *American Journal of Physical Medicine & Rehabilitation, 91*(11), 984–998.

Mortenson, W. B., Demers, L., Fuhrer, M. J., Jutai, J. W., Lenker, J., & DeRuyter, F. (2013). Effects of an assistive technology intervention on older adults with disabilities and their informal caregivers: An exploratory randomized controlled trial. *American Journal of Physical Medicine & Rehabilitation, 92*(4), 297–306.

A

ASSOCIATION FOR GERONTOLOGY IN HIGHER EDUCATION

The Association for Gerontology in Higher Education (AGHE), an educational unit of the Gerontological Society of America, was established in 1972 as a membership organization of colleges and universities that provides research, education, training, and service programs in the field of aging. Its basic goal is to provide an organizational network to assist faculty and administrators in developing and improving the quality of gerontology and geriatric programs in institutions of higher education. The current membership of AGHE consists of more than 280 institutions throughout the United States, Canada, and abroad.

The purpose of AGHE is to foster the commitment of higher education to the field of aging through education, research, and public service. AGHE offers an annual meeting, the *AGHExchange* newsletter, the National Directory of Educational Programs in Gerontology, the Online Directory of Educational Programs in Gerontology and Geriatrics, a consultation service that provides technical assistance in the development and expansion of academic gerontology programs, research on gerontology education and workforce needs for the field of aging, and the advocacy of public and private support for aging education and research. Each is available to AGHE members as a free service.

Elizabeth A. Capezuti

WEB RESOURCE

AUTONOMY

Autonomy is the first of three major principles guiding medical ethics and sets the tone for those principles through its respect for personhood. The two other principles are beneficence/nonmaleficence and justice. Advance care planning and preserving elders' decision making are important ways to honor autonomy. In the clinical setting, this can be challenging because providers often do not trust elder patients' capacity to make decisions and elders are often reticent to discuss difficult medical issues, to assert their autonomy, or do both.

Autonomy was best defined in a 1914 landmark case by Justice Benjamin Cardozo: "Every human being of adult years and sound mind has a right to determine what shall be done with his own body" (*Schloendorff v. Society of New York Hospital*, 1914). This definition, acknowledging the autonomy of the patient, was the basis for Cardozo's ruling that if surgery is performed without the patient's consent, the surgeon commits a battery and the patient may sue for damages (*Schloendorff v. Society of New York Hospital*). In short, every adult of sound mind has the right to self-determination, meaning that the patient can consent to or refuse treatment, provided that the patient is capable of making the decision.

Autonomy and self-determination also encompass the patient's right to make decisions for the future when he or she is no longer capable. Signing an advance directive (AD) such as a living will or a health care proxy documents these future wishes. As such, autonomy lies at the very root of medical care and the provider–patient relationship (Tonelli & Misak, 2010).

Autonomy applies not only to medical decision making, but also to the degree to which an individual is able to exercise control, personal choice, and responsibility in general. Seminal literature from the 1970s to 1980s by Ellen Langer and Judith Rodin changed the field of geriatrics. Their research showed that older adults who perceived themselves as having greater control over their environments, schedule, and relationships had improved health outcomes (Mallers, Claver, & Lares, 2014).

Autonomy recognizes that each person is unique and possesses a personal set of religious or other values, traditions, and sense of what life is about. Relational autonomy recognizes that people are not simply isolated rational beings but that their existence within a social context has bearing on decision making and personhood (Sherwin & Winsby, 2011). A medical recommendation is only one consideration—albeit an important one—in making a health care decision. For the physician, nurse, or other clinician, the major consideration is which treatment is most likely to be beneficial. The patient, for personal reasons, may decide against the recommended treatment even though this decision may not be in the patient's best interest. The provider may encourage patients to change their mind, but ultimately it is their life and their decision.

Establishing autonomy as the centerpiece of medical ethics and each person's right to informed consent has not been easy. In clinical settings, providers often fail to elicit or, worse yet, ignore a patient's wishes. A French study of patients older than 80 years who came to the emergency room likely to need intensive care found that only 12% were asked their opinion about whether they would want intensive care unit (ICU) level care (Le Guen et al., 2016).

Autonomy is often thought of in clinical scenarios as a patient's right to refuse unwanted treatments. It may also be difficult to honor autonomy when someone is requesting an inappropriate treatment, intervention, or medication. Autonomy is not the same as having the final authority in all care decisions. Although patients may wish to live independently because of advancing illness or declining functional status, they may not be able to go home if it is deemed unsafe. The patient must choose among reasonable options, which may include discharge to home with home care or placement in a long-term care facility. One way of dealing with requests that conflict with standard or safe practice is to use the four-box method, which considers not only medical indications and treatment preferences, but also when these are in conflict, quality of life and contextual features to help resolve the conflict (Ho, Spencer, & McGuire, 2014). When a patient makes a decision that runs counter to the provider's values, the patient's wishes prevail, but the provider does not have to compromise personal beliefs. The provider is obligated to honor the patient's wishes but can do so by referring the patient to another provider.

Attempts to honor a patient's autonomy should continue even when a person loses the capacity to make medical decisions. A family member or health care agent should not be able to overturn a decision made by the patient, even if the patient has lost decisional capacity. The patient's professed preferences supersede anyone else's decision, even when the proxy or surrogate is authorized to act. For individuals who retain the capacity to make decisions, autonomy empowers patients to remain in control of their lives by being able to consent to or reject a medical treatment or intervention, even if such treatment or intervention may be life sustaining (Tonelli & Misak, 2010).

Maintaining autonomy allows the full range of options: to take full responsibility for decision making or to abdicate that role by designating a family member or a named representative to make the decision. Some cultures favor this decision-making style, and it is important to honor the person's choice to defer decision making to someone else. In the best-case scenario, a full discussion of medical preferences would be desirable, but if patients rely on representatives to interpret their wishes, that too is up to the patient and need not be considered a breach of autonomy by physicians or other providers.

A person's capacity to make a particular decision is critical to autonomy. To make an informed decision, a person must have the ability to understand the nature and consequences of that decision (Tonelli & Misak, 2010). The patient should be able to repeat previously expressed statements, indicate an understanding of the specific decision, and articulate a choice. The level of capacity needed to make decisions increases with the degree of difficulty in understanding the information required to make the decision, as well as with the risks associated with its consequences.

Patients can manifest "waxing and waning" capacity. Older, ill persons people may "sundown"—that is, they can be clear and lucid in the morning but lose clarity as the day progresses, so they should be consulted and asked to make decisions in the morning. If not convinced that the patient has made a conscious, deliberate decision, the provider should ask a second and even a third and fourth time. A consistent response indicates that the patient understands the decision made. Capacity may also be temporarily lost due to delirium, which is common in hospitalized elders. All attempts should be made to reverse delirium, or any other temporary incapacitating state, to include the patient in medical decision making.

For an incapacitated patient who has no AD and no surrogate decision maker, beneficence/ nonmaleficence becomes the prevailing principle. This means that a clinician who is unable to establish the patient's preferences should be guided in making treatment decisions in the best interest (i.e., beneficence) of the patient and, as always, is charged to do no harm (i.e., nonmaleficience; Tonelli & Misak, 2010).

Confidentiality of information is another component of patient autonomy (Gaertner et al., 2011). Family members are not entitled to information without the patient's consent. Truth-telling in the interest of patient autonomy prevails. A family's desire to shield the patient from a difficult diagnosis or a provider's reluctance to share bad news with the patient may violate the patient's right to keep information private and obstruct the ability to make personal decisions. Only if permission is sought from the patient, or if the patient asks the provider to consult with or inform a family member, may the clinician reveal the information.

Part of honoring personhood means having empathy for older patients' experience and understanding the fear experienced when they are admitted to a medical facility, especially in an emergency. Providers should not shy away from giving older patients encouragement and assistance in making decisions that require expertise and medical knowledge. Honoring autonomy does not absolve the clinician of the responsibility of making a recommendation based on training, experience, and evidence. By deeply listening to patients' values and preferences about quality of life, getting to know them, and, understanding them within their social and relational context, the provider will be more likely to make recommendations that are truly in their best interest.

Respecting autonomy contributes to the health and welfare of older patients, allows maintenance of self-esteem, and may reduce fears regarding the loss of control common among elders.

See also Advance Directives; Cultural Assessment; Patient–Provider Relationships; Substitute Decision Making.

Lara Wahlberg

Gaertner, J., Vent, J., Greinwald, R., Rothschild, M. A., Ostgathe, C., Kessel, R., & Voltz, R. (2011). Denying a patient's final will: Public safety vs. medical confidentiality and patient autonomy. *Journal of Pain and Symptom Management*, 42(6), 961–966.

Ho, A., Spencer, M., & McGuire, M. (2015). When frail individuals or their families request nonindicated interventions: Usefulness of the four-box ethical approach. *Journal of the American Geriatrics Society*, 63(8), 1674–1678.

Le Guen, J., Boumendil, A., Guidet, B., Corvol, A., Saint-Jean, O., & Somme, D. (2016). Are elderly patient's opinions sought before admission to an intensive care unit? Results of the ICE-CUB study. *Age and Ageing 45*, 303–309. doi:10.1093/ageing/afv191

Mallers, M., Claver, M., & Lares, L. (2014). Perceived control in the lives of older adults: The influence of Langer and Rodin's work on gerontological theory, policy, and practice. *The Gerontologist*, 54(1), 67–74.

Schloendorff v. Society of New York Hospital, 105 N.E. 92. (N.Y. 1914).

Sherwin, S., & Winsby, M. (2011). A relational perspective on autonomy for older adults residing in nursing homes. *Health Expectations, 14*(2), 182–190. doi:10.1111/j.1369-7625.2010.00638.x

Tonelli, M. R., & Misak, C. J. (2010). Compromised autonomy and the seriously ill patient. *Chest, 137*(4), 926–931.

Web Resources

American Society of Bioethics and Humanities: http://www.asbh.org

American Society of Law, Medicine, and Ethics: http://www.aslme.org

The Hastings Center: http://www.thehastingscenter.org

A

B

Balance

Approximately 75% of older adults are known to have balance problems or unsteadiness when walking or changing positions (Dillon, Gu, Hoffman, & Ko, 2010). The goal of "balancing" is to maintain the body's center of gravity, which is located anterior to the second sacral vertebra, over the body's base of support. The requirements of balance are specific to the task being performed and change according to the demands of the task and the environment in which the task occurs. Balance can be maintained statically over a nonchanging base of support (as in standing tasks) or dynamically, with a changing base of support (as occurs during walking). Balance is a necessary component of all movement. Assessing for balance deficits requires a comprehensive subjective and objective evaluation starting with defining how the individual is affected by a balance disorder. Balance is multifactorial, so all related physical impairments must be identified. From there, the clinician can determine whether the impairment is remediable (via physical therapy or medication) or if it requires compensation (i.e., an assistive device). To achieve balance during activity, coordination is required among afferent mechanisms or sensory systems (i.e., visual, vestibular, and proprioceptive), efferent mechanisms or motor systems (i.e., muscle strength and flexibility), cognitive systems (i.e., mood and attention), and automatic processes of the cerebellum and basal ganglia (i.e., movement coordination and initiation). When the center of gravity extends beyond the body's base of support, the resulting imbalance is detected by the sensory system, relayed to the brain, and fixed via motor systems in an attempt to realign the body.

EFFECTS OF AGING ON BALANCE

As individuals age, they commonly experience decreases in muscle size, strength, and power with a sedentary lifestyle (Bougea et al., 2016; Nilwik et al., 2013). Decreased muscle strength complicates the execution of postural strategies because of compensations from other muscles or a decreased ability to move as quickly and with the correct range. Hence it may be more difficult for older adults to adjust their center of gravity in response to changing task demands. This may increase an individual's risk of falling by creating a delayed or incorrect response to a loss of balance and an increase in unsteadiness under both static and dynamic conditions. Because of diminished function in the vestibular, visual, and sensory systems (particularly proprioception) and in neuromuscular coordination, older adults tend to exhibit greater postural sway compared with younger individuals (Manchester et al., 1989, as cited in Donath, Kurzm, Roth, Zahner, & Faude, 2015; Motoki & Masani, 2012). This may result in larger displacements of the center of mass past the base of support and can lead to a fall.

In some older adults, there is a reversal of the normal distal-to-proximal sequence of muscle activation following a change in balance. Older adults tend to utilize a hip strategy, rather than the typical ankle strategy, when trying to correct a loss of balance (Freitas & Duarte, 2012, as cited in Donath et al., 2015), presumably due to increased co-contraction of anterior and posterior ankle muscles that increase the overall stiffness of the ankle (Donath et al., 2015). Older adults also attempt to compensate by using visual input when proprioceptive feedback is reduced, unreliable, or absent. (Dillon et al., 2010). For example, older adults may look down to view the correct placement of their feet when walking. Diverting one's gaze downward can pull bodyweight

Table B.1
EFFECTS OF VARIOUS PATHOLOGIES ON BALANCE

Pathology	Typical Presentation
Parkinson's disease (PD)	Findings may begin unilaterally and progress to bilaterally as Parkinson's disease progresses. Individuals have a high falls risk because of the festinating gait in which their upper body moves further than their legs, also due to decreased initiation of any recovery strategy. Postural balance reactions are delayed, and there is reduced motion of the trunk and extremities.
Cerebral vascular accident (CVA)	Individuals lean away from the hemiplegic side, which increases the risk of falling, and may not have intact postural reactive timing on the affected side.
Multiple sclerosis (MS)	Individuals can fall for numerous reasons: foot drag, poor vision, cerebellar dysfunction, and sensory loss. Falls are more likely when the individual is fatigued, so balance testing should occur in a fatigued and an unfatigued condition.
Cerebellum dysfunction	Individuals are at risk of falling because of a lack of control over their limbs, which can throw them off balance and impair their ability to recover from a loss of balance. People overcompensate when attempting to correct a loss of balance and put themselves even further off balance.
Sensory loss (peripheral neuropathy vs. central dysfunction)	Decreased awareness of position leads to a delay in reaction time, with a loss of balance increasing fall risk. Falls are likely to occur when vision is impaired.
Vestibular dysfunction	Vestibular dysfunction may be either peripheral or central. Loss of balance often occurs with rapid changes in head position, rapid head motions, or conflicting visual input.

forward leading to possible anterior loss of balance. This may cause the individual to walk into nearby objects and may lead to increased risk of developing a fixed thoracic kyphosis. Pathological conditions associated with aging can further complicate balance (Table B.1).

The subjective portion of the evaluation should include a thorough medical history, report of falls history, and fear of falling (Table B.2). The Activities-Specific Balance Confidence (ABC) Scale can provide an objective means of classifying a patient's subjective perception of balance and safety during various tasks (Rolenz & Reneker, 2016). Pertinent medical history information includes alcohol consumption and ingestion of medications that might cause blood pressure changes or impact stability such as cardiovascular medications, benzodiazepines, antidepressants, anticonvulsants, hypnotic sedatives, neuroleptic agents, antihypertensives, and vasodilators. Further relevant assessment includes surgical history and previous orthopedic injuries. A falls history includes information on onset of falls, frequency of loss of balance, frequency of hitting the ground or other nearby objects, related injuries, direction of the loss of

balance, activity at the time of the fall, footwear, and ability to get up independently. It is important to further investigate claims of dizziness to determine whether the individual is experiencing lightheadedness, which might be a result of problems in blood pressure regulation, or vertigo, which indicates vestibular system involvement. Vertigo creates a sensation of movement for the individual and can be differentiated from dizziness by asking if an individual is experiencing movement of the self or the environment.

The objective portion of the examination identifies functional limitations (via functional assessments that provide objective scores based on task performance) and the underlying impairments (via system evaluation). Functional assessments, such as the Berg Balance Scale (BBS), Tinetti Falls Efficacy Scale (FES), Function in Sitting Test (FIST), Mini-BESTest, and the Timed Up and Go (TUG) Test not only can indicate the risk of falls, but also can help identify tasks in which the individual has struggled (see Table B.3). These tasks can be incorporated into the treatment plan.

A comprehensive systems evaluation should be conducted to determine whether there is a reversible cause of the balance problem, with

B

Table B.2
Components of Balance Assessment

Assessment Components	Specific Aspects to Include
Patient history	Ask about age, height, weight, diagnosis, prognosis, history of falls, mechanism of falls, date of onset of the problem, goals, use of an assistive device, medications, usual activity level, past medical problems.
Muscular and neurological evaluation	Determine motor deficits, strengths/weaknesses, muscle tone, sensory deficits, proprioceptive deficits, range of motion limitations, coordination limitations, cognitive limitations, safety awareness.
Static alignment	Ask patient to stand in a relaxed, comfortable position with equal weight on both lower extremities and observe for malalignments.
Dynamic alignment	Observe the patient balancing in double and single stance.
Balance	Have patients hold three different stances for at least 10 seconds: – Stand with feet together. Test with eyes open and closed. – Take a semi-tandem stance, with the heel of one foot touching the side of the big toe of the other foot. Test with eyes open and closed. – Do a full-tandem stance with the heel of one foot directly in front of the other foot's toes. Test with eyes open and closed. Abnormalities indicate a need for therapeutic interventions (therapy) and/or exercise. Perform an objective functional balance assessment (BBS, Mini-BESTest, Tinetti Falls Efficacy Scale)

BBS, Berg Balance Scale.

special focus on the cardiac, neurological, sensory, and musculoskeletal systems. Cardiac evaluation should include arrhythmias, bruits, valvular disorders, and postural hypotension. Neurological evaluation should include mental status (cognition, attention, movement disorders, tremor, and stiffness), sensation testing (vision, hearing, light touch, and position and vibration sense), deep tendon reflexes and hypertonicity/spasticity, and cerebellar and vestibular testing (vestibulo-ocular reflex [VOR], dysmetria, dysdiadochokinesia). Musculoskeletal evaluation should include range of motion (foot, ankle, knee, hip, and spine) and muscle strength (in midrange and fully lengthened and shortened positions). Any musculoskeletal impairment must be further evaluated to identify the cause of decreased range of motion (pain, swelling, joint instability, or subluxation) and to determine whether muscle weakness is related to decreased core stability or a peripheral or central nerve disorder. Subjective reports of vertigo or observations of nystagmus should be further explored. Episodes of vertigo may be caused by a peripheral or central vestibular disorder. Benign paroxysmal positional vertigo (BBPV) is the most frequent cause of vertigo in the elderly and can often be quickly and effectively treated

with the Epley maneuver. Other peripheral vestibular issues include unilateral or bilateral damage to the vestibular nerve via trauma, disease, or inflammation. Central vestibular dysfunction can be related to central nervous system disorders such as stroke (cerebrovascular accident [CVA]), traumatic brain injury, cancer, and multiple sclerosis. A skilled clinician can differentiate between central and peripheral vestibular disorders based on the behavior of the vertigo and the nystagmus.

TREATMENT

A comprehensive treatment plan is built from the functional limitations and impairments discovered during the evaluation. If the impairment is remediable, then the plan addresses the impairments and limitations found in the evaluation via targeted exercise regimens. This may include strengthening lower extremity muscles, improving joint flexibility, and engaging in task-specific balance training (Clemson, 2012; Lee, Hale, Hemingway, & Woolridge, 2012; Nardone, Godi, Artuso, & Schieppati, 2010; Newell, Shead, & Sloane, 2012). Activities such as the use of Wii Fit games (Toulotte, Toursel, & Olivier, 2012), tai chi (Lee, Hale, Hemingway, & Woolridge, 2012),

Table B.3
BALANCE ASSESSMENT TOOLS

Functional Test	Indications	Summary	Norms
Berg Balance Scale (BBS)	Brain injury Geriatric Multiple sclerosis Orthopedic surgery Osteoarthritis Parkinson's disease Spinal cord injury Stroke Vestibular disorders	14 items graded 0–4 Assess static balance May have ceiling affect Individual must be able to transfer from sitting to standing Max score of 56	For community-dwelling healthy adults: 60–69 years old M: 55; F: 55 70–79 years old M: 54; F: 53 80–89 years old M: 53; F: 50
Tinetti Falls Efficacy Scale (FES)	Brain injury Geriatric Multiple sclerosis Parkinson's disease Stroke Spinal cord injury	10-item questionnaire regarding confidence to perform specific tasks without falling 1 = very confident 10 = not confident at all	Geriatric: 91.85 SCI: 30.7 Parkinson's disease: 24–39
Function in Sitting Test (FIST)	Stroke Adults with sitting balance disorder	14 items graded 0–4 0 = requires complete assistance 1 = needs assistance 2 = needs upper extremity support 3 = needs cues 4 = independent	Not established
Timed Up and Go (TUG) Test	Acute medical patients (on inpatient units) Alzheimer's disease Arthritis (before and/or after joint arthroplasty Cerebral palsy Community-dwelling Older adults Frail individuals Low back pain Lower extremity amputations Multiple sclerosis Osteoarthritis Parkinson's disease Rheumatoid arthritis Spinal cord injury Stroke Vestibular disorders	Rise from a chair, walk 3 m turns, walks back to the chair, and sits down. Timing begins at "go" and stops when the patient is seated. Assistive device okay to use, using the same each trial.	Cut-off scores for falls risk: Community-dwelling adults in general >65 years old: >13.5 seconds Frail elderly: >32.6 seconds 60–69 years old: M: 8 seconds F: 8 seconds 70–79 years old: M: 9 seconds F: 9 seconds 80–89 years old: M: 10 seconds F: 11 seconds
Mini-BESTest	Age-related balance disorders Ataxia Cervical myelopathy CNS neoplasm Multiple sclerosis Neuromuscular disease Brain injury Parkinson's disease Peripheral vascular disease Stroke	14-item dynamic balance assessment Max score = 28 Includes anticipatory postural correction, reactive postural correction, sensory orientation, dynamic gait	≤19/28 = high fall risk ≤21 = postural response deficits

CNS, central nervous system; SCI, spinal cord injury.

Source: Rehabilitation Measures Database (www.rehabmeasures.org). The contents of this database were developed under a grant from the United States Department of Education, National Institute on Disability, Independent Living, and Rehabilitation, research grant number H133B090024 (PI: Allen Heinemann, PhD, awarded to the Shirley Ryan AbilityLab, formerly the Rehabilitation Institute of Chicago).

B

Pilates (Newell et al., 2012), and platform exercises (Nardone et al., 2010) have been shown to improve balance in older individuals and can be more fun than typical exercise programs (Clemson, 2012; Howe, Rochester, Jackson, Banks, & Blair, 2007; Orr, Raymond, & Fiatarone Singh, 2008).

If the individual's impairment is not remediable via physical therapy, a compensatory approach is indicated. This individual should be evaluated for an assistive device. Remediation of impairments should be initiated first to avoid learned compensation and disuse atrophy that can occur when an assistive device is used. Canes, crutches, and walkers increase stability by providing a wider base of support and additional sensory input, and they supplement muscle activity by assisting with propulsion and deceleration during ambulation (Bradley & Hernandez, 2011). A cane, the least restrictive of the gait aids, is fitted properly if its handle is near the level of the ulnar styloid process. Walkers provide the most stable base of support and are indicated for patients requiring maximal mechanical assistance for ambulation.

See also Activities of Daily Living; Gait Assessment Instruments; Gait Disturbances.

Stefanie DiCarrado

Bradley, S. M., & Hernandez, C. R. (2011). Geriatric assistive devices. *American Family Physician, 84*(4), 405–411.

Bougea, A., Papadimas, G., Papadopoulos, C., Paraskevas, G. P., Kalfakis, N., Manta, P., & Kararizou, E. (2016). An age-related morphometric profile of skeletal muscle in healthy untrained women. *Journal of Clinical Medicine, 5*(11), 97.

Clemson, L. (2012). Integration of balance and strength training into daily life activity to reduce rate of falls in older people (the LiFE study): Randomized parallel trial. *British Medical Journal, 345*, e4547. doi:10.1136/bmj.e4547

Dillon, C. F., Gu, Q., Hoffman, H. J., & Ko, C. W. (2010). Vision, hearing, balance, and sensory impairment in Americans aged 70 years and over: United States, 1999–2006. *NCHS Data Brief.* Retrieved from http://www.cdc.gov/nchs/data/databriefs/db31.htm

Donath, L., Kurzm, E., Roth, R., Zahner, L., & Faude, O. (2015). Different ankle muscle coordination patterns and co-activation during quiet stance between young adults and seniors do not change after a bout of high intensity training. *BMC Geriatrics, 15*, 19–28.

Howe, T. E., Rochester, L., Jackson, A., Banks, P. M., & Blair, V. A. (2007). Exercise for improving balance in older people. *Cochrane Database of Systematic Reviews, 2007*(4), CD004963. doi:10.1002/14651858.CD004963.pub3

Lee, H. Y., Hale, C. A., Hemingway, B., & Woolridge, M. W. (2012). Tai chi exercise and auricular acupressure for people with rheumatoid arthritis: An evaluation study. *Journal of Clinical Nursing, 21*(19/20), 2812–2822.

Motoki, K., & Masani, K. (2012). Postural sway during quiet standing is related to physiological tremor and muscle volume in young and elderly adults. *Gait & Posture, 35*(1), 11–17.

Nardone, A., Godi, M., Artuso, A., & Schieppati, M. (2010). Balance rehabilitation by moving platform and exercises in patients with neuropathy or vestibular deficit. *Archives of Physical Medicine & Rehabilitation, 91*(12), 1869–1877.

Newell, D., Shead, V., & Sloane, L. (2012). Changes in gait and balance parameters in elderly subjects attending an 8-week supervised Pilates programme. *Journal of Bodywork & Movement Therapies, 16*(4), 549–554.

Nilwik, R., Snijders, T., Leenders, M., Groen, B. B., van Kranenburg, J., Verdijk, L. B., & van Loon, L. J. (2013). The decline in skeletal muscle mass with aging is mainly attributed to a reduction in type II muscle fiber size. *Experimental Gerontology, 48*(5), 492–498.

Orr, R., Raymond, J., & Fiatarone Singh, M. (2008). Efficacy of progressive resistance training on balance performance in older adults: A systematic review of randomized controlled trials. *Sports Medicine, 38*(4), 317–343.

Rolenz, E., & Reneker, J. C. (2016). Validity of the 8-foot up and go, timed up and go, and activities-specific balance confidence scale in older adults with and without cognitive impairment. *Journal of Rehabilitation Research & Development, 53*(4), 511–519.

Toulotte, C., Toursel, C., & Olivier, N. (2012). Wii Fit® training vs. adapted physical activities: Which one is the most appropriate to improve the balance of independent senior subjects? A randomized controlled study. *Clinical Rehabilitation, 26*(9), 827–835.

Web Resources

Balance exercises from the Mayo Clinic: http://www.mayoclinic.com/health/balance-exercises/SM00049

Eldergym Elderly Balance Exercises for Seniors to Help Prevent Falls: http://www.eldergym.com/elderly-balance.html

Exercise and Daily Living: Your Everyday Guide from the National Institute on Aging: http://www.nia.nih.gov/health/publication/exercise-physical-activity-your-everyday-guide-national-institute-aging-1

International Council on Active Aging. Balance exercises. *The Journal on Active Aging*: http://www.icaa.cc/2_Individual_member/member_client handouts/bandsandbalance.pdf

Medline Plus Exercise for Seniors: http://www.nlm.nih.gov/medlineplus/exerciseforseniors.html

Rehabilitation Measures Database: http://www.rehabmeasures.org

BEHAVIORAL AND PSYCHOLOGICAL SYMPTOMS OF DEMENTIA

Neuropsychiatric symptoms—problems stemming from dysfunctional perceptions, thoughts, feelings, and behaviors—are extremely common in dementia. They have come to be referred to collectively as the *behavioral and psychological symptoms of dementia (BPSDs)*. BPSDs are problematic not only for older adults with dementia but also for their family and professional caregivers. Symptoms include physical and/or verbal aggression, yelling, resisting cares, wandering, tearfulness, neglect of personal hygiene, and apathy or withdrawal, as well as behaviors that are distressingly repetitive, sexually or socially inappropriate, and reckless or careless. These problems can be conveniently categorized in terms analogous to the major psychiatric syndromes—disturbances involving cognition, mood, psychosis, personality, anxiety, and sleep (Gitlin, Kales, & Lyketsos, 2012). About 60% to 90% of patients with dementia experience one or more BPSDs over the course of their illness. BPSDs are associated with further functional impairment and tend to be much more troubling and distressing to the caregivers of dementia patients than memory problems. BPSDs are often exacerbated during acute hospitalization (White et al., 2016).

They also raise the risk of institutionalization and hospitalization (White et al., 2016).

COGNITIVE IMPAIRMENTS AND BPSDS

Cognitive problems underlie most BPSDs. These consist of not only impairments in short- and long-term memory for facts and procedures, but also difficulties with aphasia (decline in the ability to communicate through the capacity to express oneself with words as well as understand the language of others), agnosia (diminished ability to recognize familiar people and places), and/or apraxia (loss of ability to perform simple tasks such as buttoning a shirt that cannot be attributed to other problems such as severe arthritis or stroke-related weakness or paralysis).

Deficits in executive functioning are often underappreciated as cognitive factors contributing to BPSDs. These include problems with attention, inhibition of responses to distractions, and diminished working memory (the amount of information one can keep in mind at any one time). For someone whose working memory is significantly impaired, absorbing information can be like drinking from a hose. Other executive deficits include a decrease in the ability to think abstractly (reflected in concrete thoughts and a tendency to take things too literally) and to plan for the future (living in the moment versus remembering issues in the future that require attention and generating options to address them). Difficulties with implementing plans represent another category of executive deficits and include problems with making decisions, initiating actions, sustaining those actions, and stopping them once complete. It can sometimes be confusing and frustrating to caregivers how a patient with such executive deficits can know what task needs to be done, and even demonstrate it, but then not do it (unless prompted). A consistent lack of follow-through with tasks that is inconsistent with how a patient used to perform before developing cognitive impairment (i.e., an impaired ability to initiate) is often a "red flag" for this type of executive deficit.

Executive problems with organizing and sequencing adversely affect communication

B

and the ability to carry out tasks, as can difficulties with novel problem solving. Impaired ability to set-shift (to move smoothly from one type of task to another) is another executive deficit that frequently contributes to BPSDs. This issue arises frequently when patients with dementia are expected to perform multistep tasks too quickly. The abilities to monitor oneself—how one is personally doing (e.g., track the quality of one's performance at tasks)—and to monitor others—how one is doing interpersonally (e.g., track the quality of one's interactions with other people)—decline with the progression of dementia, thereby contributing to BPSDs. The latter is frequently perceived as the loss in the ability to empathize. The decline in the abilities to modulate how one is thinking, feeling, and acting represent additional kinds of executive deficits that frequently contribute to the emergence of the other kinds of BPSD described below.

MOOD PROBLEMS AND BPSDs

Patients with BPSD also need to be assessed for mood problems. Sudden, usually transient episodes of tearfulness, irritability, or laughter that are out of proportion to the circumstances and/or inconsistent with the patient's usual responses to such circumstances may represent affective lability (i.e., decreased ability to modulate overt expressions of feelings). Patients still able to communicate may report that they are at a loss to explain these outbursts because they are not having any feelings of sadness or anger that would account for them. Lability of affect in the absence of other diagnostically characteristic symptoms or signs is sometimes mistaken for clinical depression, when it is actually caused by the dementia itself or a superimposed delirium.

Studies of depression in dementia have revealed that the mood disturbance is associated with an increased risk for aggression. The following suggest clinical depression occurring in the context of the dementia: sustained periods of low or irritable mood and/or decreased ability to enjoy usually pleasurable activities, accompanied by social withdrawal and disturbances in appetite, sleep, energy level, and concentration. Because some of these biological symptoms of depression can stem from concurrent medical problems, it is important to also look for psychological symptoms, including expressions of feeling helpless, hopeless, worthless, undue pessimism about the future; a wish to be dead; or even suicidal ideation.

Assessing for the presence of depressive disorders in dementia is a challenging task, particularly when patients have lost much of their ability to communicate effectively. Symptoms of depression may be a side effect of a medication, a direct or indirect consequence of a medical problem, an episode of previously recurrent depression or bipolar disorder, a component of another psychiatric disorder, and/or a reaction to a social stressor. In clinically ambiguous situations, an empirical trial with an antidepressant medication and monitoring of any response in the patient's moods can be a reasonable diagnostic strategy. The Cornell Scale for Depression in Dementia (Reus et al., 2016) can sometimes be helpful.

A common form of a BPSD is the development of a pronounced lack of interest and participation in activities that used to be enjoyable. In this situation, caregivers frequently express concern that the patient has developed depression. In the absence of additional characteristic signs of depression, however, this change more likely represents an apathy syndrome stemming from a loss in the ability to initiate and sustain activity. One way to clarify such a situation is for the caregiver to arrange for the patient to participate in some previously enjoyable activity. If the patient enjoys this activity, and is not manifesting other signs or symptoms of depression, it most likely represents the development of problem with apathy. This can be addressed by coaching the caregivers to be more proactive in encouraging the patient, through prompting and/or assisting, to participate in meaningful activities.

PSYCHOSIS AND BPSDs

Dysfunctional perceptions and thoughts represent another set of problems that occur over the course of dementing illnesses. Up to 70% of patients with Alzheimer's disease (AD) may develop psychotic symptoms over the course of their illness. Delusional ideas are more common than hallucinations in AD and usually are paranoid in nature. Common kinds of delusions are that misplaced items have been stolen, that there are intruders in the house (which may also be accompanied by corresponding visual hallucinations), that spouses are being unfaithful, or that familiar people are impostors. Dementia patients may try to leave the house under the delusion that they still need to go to work and become agitated with attempts to redirect them. Because of visual agnosia, they may no longer recognize their own reflections in a mirror and believe that someone is trapped in the walls the house. Prominent visual hallucinations are one of the hallmarks of Lewy body dementia.

Such delusions or hallucinations can be significantly distressing to both patients and their caregivers. Some psychotic symptoms, however, may be benign and not require treatment because they do not cause subjective distress or impair functioning. For example, a retired farmer with AD might see (nonexistent) cows outside his window and find this experience pleasant. All that might be required in such an instance is reassuring patient's family as to the benign nature of this visual hallucination.

PERSONAL FACTORS AND BPSDs

Personal factors are almost invariably the key to understanding BPSD. The brain is the neurobiological base from which personality emerges within an individual's environment. Changes in personality, however subtle, are sometimes the earliest signs of developing dementia. Although usually a separate diagnosis of personality change is not made in instances of dementia (as it is considered a part of the dementia), understanding how neurocognitive disorders can affect personality traits can be extremely helpful in deciphering BPSDs. Problems involving lability of affect, apathy, aggression, (nondelusional) paranoia, and social disinhibition, which are out of character for the person prior to the onset of the dementia, are some of the cardinal signs of personality change.

Evidence-based research has demonstrated that the criteria used to diagnose personality disorders in younger adults does not work with the elderly. A more useful approach is to appreciate how all human beings have all the personality traits that a person can have, albeit to different degrees of intensity and flexibility. Rather than using psychiatric jargon that is stigmatizing and off-putting, one can think about personality traits in terms of everyday language (e.g., independent, autonomous, shy, sensitive, self-important, scrupulous, tidy, suspicious). From this perspective, personality traits can be problematic when they are, for example, too strong or too weak or too rigid or too flexible for a given context. For example, it can be risky to not be sufficiently paranoid in dangerous environments such as certain neighborhoods after dark but quite problematic to maintain the same degree of paranoia when with trustable family members.

Asking family members and friends who have known persons with dementia for a long time to describe how they used to be as people can generate significant clues for solving problems. Once one has a grasp on a patient's salient personality traits (e.g., independence and autonomous), one can then assess whether the BPSD is causing a significant degree of stress in a patient with those traits (e.g., the prospect of losing independence and control). It can be especially helpful to consider what the particular situation means to the patient.

In addition to personality traits, other components, such as situational awareness, past experiences, and personal values, and loyalties, can be used to cope with and guide behavior. For example, the spouse of a retired military officer was better able to understand her husband's suddenly getting up during dinner to do the laundry after she learned that this behavior stemmed from her inadvertent statement that this task needed to be done. Her casual remark triggered with his awareness of the task, his altruistic values, his loyalty to her, and his rule of thumb of being prompt in doing tasks. Because of his dementia, he was not able to inhibit his response or adequately monitor its emotional impact on his wife.

ANXIETY AND BPSDs

Anxiety is a frequent component of most BPSDs. In nonpathological terms, anxiety is a part of

B

our natural responses to stressors, whether internal or external. As such it, alerts us to situations that are likely to be challenging—to pay attention and be prepared. Analogous to pain, anxiety becomes problematic when it is disproportionate to the circumstances. The extent to which one experiences anxiety varies with how one perceives a challenge and the resources available to address that challenge. The greater the perceived gap, the more likely that the intensity of the anxiety will be higher. The stress response has traditionally been formulated in terms of "fight, flight, or freeze." None of these is intrinsically dysfunctional; the effectiveness of each depends on the context. However, this approach falls short in understanding many situations that do not fit this paradigm (e.g., a parent stressed by a fussy infant). This can be remedied by adding "engage" to the list of categorical stress responses. This is especially helpful when assessing BPSDs.

With increasing executive deficits reducing their abilities to engage effectively in situations previously managed with minimal stress, individuals with dementia become more prone to ineffective responses. Individuals very dependent on others for assistance with activities of daily living because of their dementia, for example, may become quite anxious when left alone even briefly, become angry or tearful, or try to follow their caregivers. Such sudden outbursts are commonly referred to as *catastrophic reactions*. Other examples include (a) "fight," angry outbursts, often manifested as resistance to care; (b) "flight," avoidance of anxiety-provoking situations; (c) "freeze," passive refusal to cooperate; and (d) dysfunctional "engagement," ineffective problem solving. An instance of wandering in a patient with moderate dementia, for example, might represent a (conscientious) effort to obtain (misplaced) important items by making a trip to the store (but resulting in getting lost on the way back home).

Individuals' knowledge, experiences, personality traits, values, rules of thumb, and cultural factors may all contribute to anxiety-driven BPSDs. Attending to each set of factors can help caregivers, whether family or professional, more fully understand their meaning, respond with greater sensitivity and specificity, and thereby

themselves cope more effectively. Indeed, these same principles can also be applied to the stress of caregivers having to care for family members or patients with BPSDs (Howell, 2015).

SLEEP DISTURBANCES AND BPSDs

The adverse effects of dementia on the brain also disrupt its sleep mechanisms. Normal aging is associated with more shallow sleep, accompanied by more frequent awakenings.

These changes in "sleep architecture" are often accelerated and intensified in dementia and can generate major changes in sleep patterns, including a complete reversal in usual sleep-wake cycles. Individuals with dementia may awaken during the night and have trouble distinguishing between their dreams and reality. Lewy body dementia is sometimes associated with rapid eye movement (REM) sleep disorders (e.g., recurrent episodes of verbal and behavioral arousal while still asleep). Daytime dozing or napping, which can be fostered by the combination of decreased initiative with lack of an optimal amount of stimulation, can contribute to episodes of nocturnal agitation.

ASSESSMENT OF BPSDs

The successful management of BPSDs begins with a careful differential diagnosis to determine the factors that may be contributing to them. This not infrequently requires some detective work and collaboration between all those involved in the care of the person with dementia. Because these factors are usually not only multiple, but also interacting, this task may seem daunting, especially when multiple BPSDs occur simultaneously or fluctuate in frequency, intensity, or duration. Using behavioral logs to track BPSDs can help objectify otherwise subjective global impressions.

Cultivation of an ad hoc team—with a diversity of members, both professional and family, each with different knowledge of the patient and different perspectives—can be very helpful. Ad hoc team members, by sharing their current and past experiences with the patient, can contribute to developing a fuller, more sensitive and specific picture of the BPSDs (Howell, 2015). For example, while mopping the floor, the janitor might notice a change in the color of a dementia patient's sputum, thus providing a clue as to the likelihood of a lung infection contributing to the BPSD. Likewise, a family member might recall a traumatic experience that patient had in childhood that could be contributing as well.

Medications, concurrent medical problems, comorbid psychiatric problems, personal issues, and environmental stressors all represent factors potentially contributing to BPSDs. The addition of a new medication with new potential side effects or a change in the dosage of an ongoing medication could adversely affect any of these cognitive abilities. Even medications that a patient has been taking for a long time may be suspect because of age-related changes in how the body absorbs, distributes, metabolizes, and excretes a medication and can gradually lead to changes in how the body responds to it. For example, over time, the gradual decline in kidney function associated with increasing age results in higher serum levels of digoxin in patients who take this medicine for congestive heart failure. Higher drug levels in such situations can cause toxic side effects, which may include adverse changes in cognition and/or mood, thereby precipitating BPSDs.

Similarly, the development of a new medical problem or a change in a chronic medical problem could be factors in an individual's BPSDs. Medical problems occurring in older adults often do not manifest the usual, characteristic signs and symptoms that make their cause readily apparent. The absence of usual diagnostic indicators and/or the presence of atypical ones can be misleading (e.g., acute bronchitis without fever or cough or urinary tract infection with only changes in mental status and behavior as symptoms). Any significant increase in pain or discomfort (e.g., shortness of breath due to an upper respiratory infection, joint pain due to arthritis or a bone fracture, abdominal bloating from constipation, or a simple toothache) can contribute to BPSDs, especially when individuals have difficulty communicating the source of their distress (Hodgson, Gitlin, Winter, & Czekanski, 2011).

The introduction of something new in the patient's physical environment (e.g., relocation to a new living situation) or a physical change (e.g., in the usual level of temperature or noise) in an otherwise familiar living situation (e.g., a move from an upstairs to a downstairs bedroom) can also trigger BPSD. Likewise, changes in the social environment, especially interpersonal relationships (e.g., role reversals), frequently play a role in the genesis of BPSDs.

There are two basic approaches to BPSDs: the ABC method and the unmet needs method. Both of these approaches require carefully detailed descriptions of the problematic behavior, preferably from eyewitnesses. BPSDs are often described in terms of agitation, but this nebulous term is not specific enough for developing effective interventions. It is also important that these descriptions not inadvertently contain overt or subtle implications about causes; for example, "Mr. A won't (or can't) cooperate," versus "Mr. A isn't cooperating." Such implications can lead to premature closure in the problem-solving process (e.g., incorrectly assuming that Mr. A has the capacity to cooperate with a given task when he does not, or vice versa).

The ABC method involves looking for one or more Antecedent circumstances that could be causing the problematic Behavior, along with one or more Consequences that may be (inadvertently) reinforcing the problematic behavior. An example is determining why some with moderate dementia become resistive with caregivers during bathing. Possible antecedent causes might include (a) cognitive factors (e.g., progression of the dementia to the point where they no longer appreciate the need for bathing and/or have developed a dressing apraxia [no longer have the capacity to get dressed or undressed]); (b) medical factors (e.g., a new or worsening medical problem, such as arthritis causing pain when climbing into the tub); (c) mood factors (e.g., the development of a new depression and associated irritability); (d) psychotic factors (e.g., the development of a delusion that the caregiver is an imposter); (e) anxiety factors (e.g., development of a catastrophic reaction to the bathing situation because of loss of the ability to tolerate frustration and/or symptoms of panic because bathing reminds them of childhood incidents of abuse); (f) sleep factors (e.g., a reversed normal sleep/wake cycle clashing with the scheduled bath time); (g) personality factors (e.g., intensification of a long-standing personality trait of being independent and not needing help); and (h) discomfort from the physical environment (e.g., chilly room temperature because of the air conditioning). Potential reinforcing consequences might include the caregiver "rewarding" completion of the bath by providing some special food and extra companionship time.

The unmet needs method involves determining what the BPSDs might mean to the persons with dementia. This is a particularly helpful approach when individuals have lost the ability to adequately describe their perspectives on what is troubling them. An example of applying this method is determining possible causes for a distressing repetitive behavior such as yelling "Help me! Help me!" This may represent unsuccessful attempts to communicate feelings arising from factors like those in the ABC method: cognitive (e.g., confusion), medical (e.g., pain), mood (e.g., sadness/helplessness), psychotic (e.g., frightening visual hallucinations), anxiety (e.g., feeling abandoned), sleep (e.g., nightmare), personality (e.g., loss of control), and/or environmental (e.g., relocation) factors.

The ABC and unmet needs methods ideally are used together, taking advantage of how they can complement each other. Their use can generate plausible hypotheses that can then be tested by determining whether specific interventions are effective. BPSDs frequently have multifactorial causes. Hence it is important to not come to premature closure, which can be challenging when one is under pressure to deal with an acute situation. Likewise, it is more effective to think of the possible causes of BPSD in terms of "both/and" and avoid slipping into overly simplistic "either/or" thinking.

More recently, an effective, evidence-based set of nonpharmacological strategies—the DICE approach—have been developed to assess BPSDs in a manner that incorporates most of the concepts of the ABC and unmet needs methods. DICE stands for "Describe, Investigate, Create, and Evaluate" the neuropsychiatric symptoms (NPS) of dementia. With this approach, the immediate caregiver describes the problematic behavior(s) to the provider in terms of context, environment, patient perspective, and degree of

stress. The team, in turn, investigates the possible underlying causes. Having developed working hypotheses about the likely root cause(s), the caregiver and team collaborate to create and implement a management plan, followed by evaluating the implementation of interventions, the extent of their effectiveness, and the degree to which they were safely tolerated (Reus et al., 2016). This allows for real-time application of nonpharmacological and, if warranted, pharmacological treatments for specific BPSDs.

A further hazard in addressing BPSD arises when solutions to problematic behaviors have been effective for a while but then recur. It can be tempting to fall back on old ways of dealing with these kinds of problems, especially when they have been effective in the past. In the medical journal literature, this is known as "anchoring." However, if these ways no longer work, it is important to start the process over and approach BPSDs with a fresh perspective, again using the ABC, unmet needs, and/or DICE methods.

TREATMENT AND MANAGEMENT

Nonpharmacological Interventions

It is generally more effective to begin to address BPSDs with nonpharmacological interventions (NPIs). The foundation of NPIs is a nonjudgmental, nonconfrontational approach, combining empathic listening with redirection or diversion to a different activity that is not stressful. This is followed by reducing or eliminating the significant internal or external stressors identified in the assessment. An exception might be when individuals' BPSD constitutes a significant imminent danger to themselves and/or others. Even then, instituting pharmacotherapy requires incorporating the principles of NPI into the approach.

Once the specific instance of a BPSD has been adequately addressed, the focus of the NPIs shifts to the prevention of recurrences. For each individual this involves addressing medication issues, such as needless polypharmacy, previously underappreciated medication side effects, and problems with adherence. Likewise, attending to medical problems judged to be contributing factors is also crucial. This includes not overlooking any sensory losses and providing appropriate remedies (e.g., hearing aids, corrective lenses) to optimize individuals' interactions with their social and physical environments. When psychiatric factors are significant, implementation of an appropriate behavioral health care program may be necessary (e.g., cognitive behavioral therapy for depression).

Psychosocial interventions vary according to the severity of the dementia, as well as the unique issues for each individual. Learning how to prevent catastrophic reactions is critical. Validation therapy may help. It involves focusing on the meaning that may be hidden in a confused person's impaired communication. This can be facilitated by implementing verbal and nonverbal principles for enhancing communication with individuals with dementia, based on their residual abilities: speaking clearly and distinctly in sentences that are short and simple; actively listening, with attention to nonverbal gestures or posturing and provision of enough time for a response (i.e., not interrupting); maintaining eye contact and appropriate nonverbal gesturing; and paraphrasing what has been heard to ensure that the communication has been correctly understood. Caregivers can learn to become more flexible regarding rules and expectations, as long as safety is ensured, and to not get caught in distressing, ineffective arguments when differences of opinion arise (Gitlin et al., 2012).

Controlled multisensory stimulation (Snoezelen therapy) and music therapy can sometimes be helpful. Especially important is maintaining routines for persons with dementia that are not only familiar but also meaningful and engaging, based on which skills they still retain (Gitlin et al., 2008). (These can be identified through a meaningful skills evaluation by an occupational therapist.) Modulating environmental stimuli (e.g., noise, activity) to a level that fits what an individual tolerates can minimize confusion and thereby decrease frustration.

Environmental interventions for unsafe wandering include alarms to alert caregivers, methods for camouflaging exits or deploying visual barriers (e.g., horizontal or crosshatched lines on the floor), and the provision of pleasant, safe areas in which to wander. The use of physical restraints for managing BPSDs can lead to demoralization and increase agitation, as well as result in eventual physical deconditioning, falls, fractures, and even blood clots. Hence they need to be avoided, except briefly in emergency situations.

For caregivers, ongoing education and coaching/mentoring is necessary for understanding and addressing BPSD, both in terms of general principles and in ways specific to the individuals for whom they are caring (Gitlin et al., 2012). Managing sexually inappropriate behaviors, for example, requires caregivers to understand that these actions usually stem from misconceptions (e.g., mistaking a stranger for a spouse) or the person's executive deficits (e.g., needing to use the toilet but then disrobing in public). Caregivers need to plan for sexually inappropriate behaviors, being mindful of their own personal and cultural expectations regarding the sexual behavior of older adults. At the system level, care facilities also need to develop humane policies that respect the human needs for intimacy at all ages.

Other system-level interventions that may assist both individuals with dementia and their caregivers include collaborative care teams, community support groups, and provision of in-home assistance, as well as adult day care services and respite admissions.

Pharmacological Interventions

Pharmacotherapy for BPSDs is a complex issue. Situations that call for the initiation of pharmacotherapy include (a) when BPSDs fail to respond to NPIs; (b) when BPSDs significantly interfere with the ability of individuals with dementia to participate in NPIs; and (c) when BPSDs, together with NPIs, involve significant depression, psychosis, or aggression that puts individuals with dementia or others at risk of harm. In keeping with general principles of geriatric psychopharmacology, medications for BPSD should be started at low doses, titrated gradually, and monitored for effectiveness and tolerability.

Many studies and reports on the use of psychotropic medications for BPSDs have,

B

in general, demonstrated relatively little significant benefit from any particular medication. Hence the use of all the following classes of medications is, per the U.S. Food an Drug Admistration, "off-label" (i.e., neither clinically approved not clinically contraindicated; see entry on Psychotropic Medication Use in Nursing Homes). It is also important to note that the applicability of these evidence-based reviews to any individual with BPSDs is quite limited because of the very high levels of biopsychosocial variability among individuals with dementia (Reus et al., 2016).

The initial choice of medication is guided by the predominant nature of the BPSDs (e.g., antidepressants for depression and/or anxiety and antipsychotics for psychotic symptoms; Reus et al., 2016). Antiseizure medications (e.g., valproate, gabapentin), normally used as mood stabilizers (e.g., in bipolar affective disorder), are sometimes utilized, generally, as a second choice for nonspecific agitation.

The establishment of an effective pharmacological regimen for BPSDs may require a series of therapeutic trials. These trials can be developed through close collaboration with caregivers, carefully making periodic adjustments in the amounts and timing of administration to determine the most effective dosage and dosing schedule. Because of concerns about the potential side effects of antipsychotic medication in the context of dementia (Reus et al., 2016), the use of medications in this class of psychotropic drugs warrants careful discussion with patients and their families regarding the potential trade-offs between benefits and risks. (See sections on Psychosis in Late Life and on the Use of Psychotropic Medications in Nursing Homes.) For patients with Lewy body dementia, who are especially sensitive to side effects from antipsychotic medications, cholinesterase inhibitors may sometimes be effective.

The use of benzodiazepines (e.g., lorazepam) for anxiety or nonspecific agitation should be limited to only brief periods because of the high likelihood of adverse reactions in elderly patients, especially those with dementia. Adverse effects include increased confusion, unsteady gait, prolonged reaction times, and behavioral disinhibition.

The effectiveness of medication for BPSDs guides the duration of its use. Although periodic trials for the discontinuation of antipsychotic medications for BPSD in nursing homes are federally mandated by the Centers for Medicare & Medicaid Services, very few studies have focused on the ideal time to discontinue such medications, as well as on the outcomes from doing so (Reus et al., 2016). Guidance regarding the duration, titration, or tapering and discontinuation of medication stems from expert opinion and best-practices guidelines. For example, if there is no response to an antipsychotic medication after a 4-week trial, that medication should be tapered and withdrawn per the American Psychiatric Association practice guideline (Reus et al., 2016).

The likelihood of BPSD recurrence is lower if full remission has been achieved for a few months. Otherwise BPSDs are likely to worsen following discontinuation of a medication that has been only partially effective. In a recent randomized, double-blind study of the discontinuation of an antipsychotic (risperidone) for psychosis or agitation in patients with Alzheimer's disease, the medication reduced the severity of these BPSD over a 4-month period. When it was then discontinued, the risk of relapse was nearly twice as high in the placebo group (60%) versus in those who continued the risperidone (33%) and nearly three times higher (48% vs. 15%) when discontinued after 8 months (Reus et al., 2016).

As previously mentioned, despite the many studies on groups of patients with BPSD not experiencing significant benefit in general from any psychotropic agents, individual patients may and do respond well to one or another judiciously chosen medication. The limited applicability of these studies to any individual is because people with dementia vary so much in terms of their physical constitutions, their psychological makeups, and their social experiences over lifetimes.

It has sometimes been said that "if you have seen one individual with dementia, you have seen one individual with dementia." The treatment and management of BPSDs for any individual often involves some trial and error. The more specific and sensitive the interventions, both nonpharmacological and pharmacological, to the particular contributing factors for each individual's BPSDs, the more likely they are to be effective. Mobilizing an ad hoc team of caregivers, both personal and professional, can be extremely helpful with developing, implementing and adjusting interventions, monitoring the responses, and supporting one another.

See also Anxiety Disorders, Traumatic and Stressor-Related Disorders, and Obsessive-Compulsive Disorders in Late Life; Psychosis in Late Life; Psychotropic Medication Use in Long-Term Care; Validation Therapy; Vascular and Lewy Body Dementias.

*Satya Gutta, Paula Lueras,
and Timothy Howell*

Gitlin, L. N., Kales, H. C., & Lyketsos, C. G. (2012). Nonpharmacologic management of behavioral symptoms in dementia. *Journal of the American Medical Association, 308*(19), 2020–2029.

Gitlin, L. N., Winter, L., Burke, J., Chernett, N., Dennis, M. P., & Hauck, W. W. (2008). Tailored activities to manage neuropsychiatric behaviors in persons with dementia and reduce caregiver burden: a randomized pilot study. *American Journal of Geriatric Psychiatry, 16*(3), 229–239.

Hodgson, N., Gitlin, L. N., Winter, L., & Czekanski, K. (2010). Undiagnosed illness and neuropsychiatric behaviors in community-residing older adults with dementia. *Alzheimer Disease and Associated Disorders, 24*(4), 603–609.

Howell, T. (2015). The Wisconsin Star Method: Understanding and addressing complexity in geriatrics. In M. L. Malone, E. Capezuti, & R. M. Palmer (Eds.), *Geriatrics models of care: Bringing 'best practice' to an aging America* (pp. 87–94). Cham, Switzerland: Springer International.

Reus, V., Fochtmann, L., Eyler, A., Hilty, D., Horvitz-Lennon, M., & Jibson, M. (2016). The American Psychiatric Association practice guideline on the use of antipsychotics to treat agitation or psychosis in patients with dementia. *American Journal of Psychiatry, 173*, 543–546.

White, N., Leurent, B., Lord, K., Scott, S., Jones, L., & Sampson, E. (2016). The management of behavioural and psychological symptoms of dementia in the acute general medical hospital: a longitudinal cohort study. *International Journal of Geriatric Psychiatry, 32*(3), 297–305.

Web Resources
Alzheimer's Association: http://www.alz.org
Alzheimer's Disease Education and Referral Center: http://www.alzheimers.org
Canadian Academy of Geriatric Psychiatry (Resources Section: Guidelines and Clinical Tools): http://www.cagp.ca
Hartford Institute for Geriatric Nursing (1): http://www.hartfordign.org (2) http://www.nursingcenter.com (series on "How to try this")
Music & Memory: http://www.musicandmemory.org
National Family Caregivers Association: http://www.nfcacares.org

BEHAVIORAL EXPRESSIONS OF DISTRESS IN PEOPLE WITH NEUROCOGNITIVE DISORDERS

Behavioral expression is the primary language for as many as 90% of the 5.4 million Americans with neurocognitive disorders, which is how *the Diagnostic and Statistical Manual of Mental Disorders* (5th ed., *DSM-5*; American Psychiatric Association, 2013) categorizes Alzheimer's disease and other dementias. Behavioral expressions of distress, such as restlessness, vocalizations, hitting, pacing, and disinhibition (e.g., cursing, disrobing), often lead to care partner frustration, burnout, and injury and increase the risk of elder abuse. They contribute greatly to the cost of caring for people with neurocognitive disorders (PWNCD), resulting in hospitalization and long-term care placement. What is known about the behavioral expressions of distress in PWNCD is that they often occur in the context of personal grooming; untreated or undertreated pain and depression; and impairments in communication, function, and cognition. Although the search for effective ways to prevent and cure Alzheimer's disease remains disappointing, efforts to provide safe and effective care for PWNCD and their care partners remains critically important. Evidence-based strategies for enhancing the well-being of PWNCD who communicate distress through behavioral expressions are a major part of this work.

Historically, and still today, various pejorative terms are used to describe these behaviors, including *problematic, obstreperous,* and *disruptive,* but such labeling result in attempts to control the behavior to minimize disruption in care partner tasks. Widespread use of physical and chemical restraints and oversedation was common. More recently, person-centered care practices, focused on promoting autonomy and making sense of behavior from the perspective of PWNCD, have enjoyed wider use. Behaviors are better understood, and responded to, as expressions of perceived danger, unmet needs, and/or desires of the individual. These expressions are influenced by the diminished language, cognition, and emotional resources associated with dementia.

The importance of perceiving behavioral expressions as a form of communication cannot be overemphasized. This paradigm shift has facilitated the development of humane interventions that take into account basic knowledge about what drives behavior, continuity over a lifetime, and care partner actions that may unintentionally trigger distress. Thus, throughout this entry the term *behavioral expression of distress* is used to represent behaviors previously referred to as *disruptive* to remind care partners of their meaning and to avoid biased labeling. Furthermore, the term *care partner* is used to refer to paid and unpaid individuals who support and assist PWNCD in their daily lives. Care partner emphasizes the centrality of autonomy and personhood of PWNCD and the interactive nature of these relationships.

SYSTEMATIC ASSESSMENT

Assessment is the cornerstone of care and support for PWNCD who communicate their feelings, needs, and desires through behavioral expressions. A critical first step in this process is evaluation for delirium, an acute confusional state due to a medical instability. Many behavioral expressions are eliminated when delirium is treated, and function often improves. A delirium assessment adapted for PWNCD includes a full physical examination by a provider armed with accurate information about their baseline function and mental status, together with in-depth information obtained from someone with knowledge of their usual behavior, communication style, previous preferences, current daily pattern, and past potentially pain-causing illnesses and injuries. Studies support that pain is often missed or undertreated in PWNCD; thus, nonverbal manifestations of pain provide critical assessment information (McAuliffe, Brown, & Fetherstonhaugh, 2012). After delirium, medical conditions and pain have been considered and optimally treated; remaining behavioral expressions of distress require further systematic assessment. This includes a detailed history of preferred daily patterns and pleasurable activities. Neuropsychiatric testing and/or occupational therapy assessments can help identify treatable mental health disorders and preserved abilities (e.g., ability to recognize icons such as stop signs or to perform oral care with verbal prompts only).

Collecting clues is essential for identifying precipitating events or contexts. Care partners should be encouraged to describe nonjudgmentally the behavioral expression observed (e.g., *hitting* or *biting* rather than *agitation*). Care partners who are most familiar with PWNCD should be encouraged to keep a behavior log, typically for 3 to 7 days, to track each occurrence of the most distressing or potentially dangerous behavioral expressions by recording the time of occurrence, environment, person(s) present, and other relevant information. The log is invaluable in identifying patterns, triggers, early warning signs, fears, and unmet needs and is essential for effectively targeting strategies. Because of their more intimate longitudinal knowledge of the pre-illness personality and behavioral style, family and friends are critical in interpreting these logs. The process of keeping a log can also mitigate the anger, helplessness, and frustration experienced by care partners when behavioral expressions of distress occur. A history of anxiety, depression or psychosis may also influence interpretation of the behavioral expressions, but when such mental health issues are present, caution must be taken not to miss other targets for intervention. Careful attention to facial affect, vocal tone, and gestures yields much information about unmet needs. Finally, vision or hearing loss may contribute to misperceptions by PWNCD that normal caregiving activities are threatening.

PERSON-CENTERED STRATEGIES

The specific strategies selected to respond to behavioral expressions must stem directly from the assessment. The process involves forming a hypothesis regarding the meaning of the behavioral expression, testing the strategies in a systematic and consistent manner, and making modifications based on the response. This section outlines overarching themes and issues for consideration; specific psychosocial and environmental, pain management, and medication strategies are detailed elsewhere.

Nonpharmacological Strategies

Nonpharmacological strategies include focusing on altering the emotional and social environment for PWNCD and their care partners and should be the initial and mainstay of support in response to behavioral expressions of distress. Psychosocial strategies include social contact; behavioral shaping; care partner training focusing on the well-being, comfort, choice, and needs of PWNCD rather than the speed of task completion; hand massage; personalized recreational activities; and environmental changes, such as memory care units or bright light therapy (Forbes et al., 2009).

Pain-Management Strategies

Recognizing pain, and managing it with routine rather than "as needed" analgesics, is important in treating acute and chronic pain in older PWNCD. Care partner barriers to appropriate treatment include lack of knowledge and skill in the assessment of pain as a factor in behavioral expressions of distress and in analgesics use, as well as fear of and reluctance to use narcotic analgesia for chronic pain in frail PWNCD. Regularly scheduled analgesia avoids some barriers to proper pain management and often results in reduced behavioral expressions of distress (McAuliffe et al., 2012). Altering personal

care activities, such as using an in-bed towel bath, can reduce pain activation, as can altering clothing type or size to limit movement of painful areas during dressing. Simple approaches to avoiding discomfort from constipation, such as providing raised support for feet during bowel movements to facilitate natural evacuation, providing adequate and consistent time to move bowels, and including natural laxatives such as fiber and dried fruit in the daily diet can help immeasurably with little risk. A wide variety of strategies for addressing pain is available but beyond the scope of this chapter.

Physical Restraints and Antipsychotic Drugs

A large body of research on physical restraints (including wrist ties and vests, locked tray tables, and restrictive bedrails) demonstrates not only lack of efficacy for behavioral expressions of distress, but also multiple adverse consequences, even death, from their use. Physical restraints have been associated with increased behavioral expressions of distress, which declined following restraint removal. The high value that American society places on autonomy results in some restrained PWNCD experiencing a sense of imprisonment, with consequent psychological trauma from the fear and assault on their independence. Federal regulations for hospitals and long-term residential settings have placed significant restrictions on physical restraint use because of lack of efficacy and public and professional outcries about their associated dangers and deaths.

Reviews of psychoactive drug trials to control behavior in older PWNCD have found moderate effectiveness for antipsychotic agents but also high adverse event rates and deaths (Greenblatt & Greenblatt, 2016). The American Psychiatric Association (APA, 2016) guidelines on the use of antipsychotics to treat agitation and psychosis in patients with dementia provides strict recommendations on their use; these include that they should be used not as a first-line treatment but only after nonpharmacological strategies have failed, when symptoms are severe or dangerous, and as part of a comprehensive individualized approach. Then they should be used at the minimal dosage and gradually titrated upward so that the minimal effective dose can be established. Their use needs to be continually monitored, at least every 4 weeks, for effectiveness and tolerability, followed by a trial to reduce the dose after 4 months. The risks and benefits need to be discussed with the individual, if possible, and the surrogate decision maker, if relevant, as well as the care partners. Except for acute delirium, haloperidol (Haldol) is not recommended (APA, 2016).

Understanding behavioral expressions of distress is a significant issue for PWNCD and their care partners. Evidence suggests that unmet needs and, potentially, the inflexible, task-focused systems established to provide care and support for PWNCD may be causative factors. Preliminary evidence supports efforts to humanize long-term care with a focus on meaningful activity and small, homelike environments rather than the mere absence of behavioral expressions of distress; this model is epitomized by the Eden Alternative and the Pioneer Network. Dissemination of the evolving science regarding behavioral expression promises relief and increased quality of life and well-being for PWNCD and their care partners.

See also Constipation in the Elderly; Nursing Homes; Restraints.

Steven L. Baumann

American Psychiatric Association. (2013). *Diagnostic and statistical manual of mental disorders* (5th ed.). Arlington, VA: American Psychiatric Publishing.
American Psychiatric Association. (2016). *The American Psychiatric Association practice guideline on the use of antipsychotics to treat agitation or psychosis in patients with dementia*. Arlington, VA: American Psychiatric Association. Retrieved from https://www.guideline.gov/summaries/summary/50334/the-american-psychiatric-association-practice-guideline-on-the-use-of-antipsychotics-to-treat-agitation-or-psychosis-in-patients-with-dementia?q=American+Psychiatric+Association+use+of+antipsychotics+in+the+treatment+of+agitation+and+psychosis+in+patients+with+dementia
Forbes, D., Culum, I., Lischka, A. R., Morgan, D. G., Peacock, S., Forbes, J., & Forbes, S. (2009). Light therapy for managing cognitive, sleep, functional, behavioral, or psychiatric disturbances in dementia. *Cochrane Database of Systematic Reviews, 2009*(4), CD003946. doi:10.1002/14651858.CD003946.pub3
Greenblatt, K. H., & Greenblatt, D. J. (2016). The use of antipsychotics for the treatment of behavioral symptoms of dementia. *Journal of Clinical Pharmacology, 56*(9), 1048–1057. doi:10.1002/jcph.731
McAuliffe, L., Brown, D., & Fetherstonhaugh, D. (2012). Pain and dementia: An overview of the literature. *International Journal of Older People Nursing, 7*(3), 219–226.

Web Resources
Alzheimer's Disease Education and Referral (ADEAR) Center of the National Institute on Aging (NIA), U.S. National Institutes of Health: http://www.nia.nih.gov/alzheimers
American Health Care Association (nonprofit federation representing many nonprofit long-term residential facilities) downloadable brochure for "making the business case to residential facilities to reduce antipsychotic drug use": http://www.ahcancal.org/quality_improvement/quality initiative/Pages/default.aspx
Bathing Without a Battle: Creating a Better Bathing Experience for Persons with Alzheimer's Disease and Related Disorders: CD and video package that teaches person-centered methods for making the bathing experience more enjoyable for both caregivers and the people they are bathing: http://www.bathingwithoutabattle.unc.edu

BEREAVEMENT

The loss of a significant other, especially a spouse or partner, can be one of the most stressful experiences in a person's life. More than 900,000 people are widowed each year; the majority are 65 years old and older. Older adult conjugal loss tends to be particularly stressful. This loss of a longtime companion and confidant comes at a time in life when support networks are becoming more diminished with each passing year.

In this discussion, the term *bereavement* refers to a specific type of loss—the death of a significant person in one's life. Grief or grieving is a universal multidimensional human experience with intensely personal physical, behavioral, and meaning/spiritual components. *Grieving* refers to the emotional reactions that follow loss. Mourning is the expression of social cultural rituals used to express grief.

THE COURSE OF BEREAVEMENT

The scarcity research is noteworthy because elderly bereavement can lead to psychological illness, although most elderly widowed are able to adjust without interventions (Hashim et al., 2013). Because one in five (20%) Americans will be older than 65 years by 2030 (Keegan & Drick, 2011), elderly bereavement research is expected to increase dramatically. Unexpected bereavement in older couples appears to increase mortality more than bereavement after chronic illness (Shah et al., 2013). This points to the importance of preparing individuals for the death of a spouse with a chronic illness, as well as providing extra support for those who experience sudden unexpected bereavement.

With late-life widowerhood, resilience was seen in those who had a positively viewed history, participated in relationships and activities, and returned to a life of meaning and satisfaction (Bennett, 2010). Influencers in achieving resilience included personal characteristics and both informal and formal social support. Gender did not appear to be a factor in differentiating older adult normal grievers and complicated grievers. Most studies reveal that more women were grievers than nongrievers, although this appears largely because of longer lifespan of women and their usually higher social contacts (Newson, Boelen, Hek, & Hoffman, 2011).

COMPLICATED GRIEF

In general, the majority of bereaved spouses experience a progressive decrease in distress within the first 12 months after a loved one's death. For a minority, the loss results in lengthy adjustment challenges extending well beyond the commonly accepted postbereavement period. Commonly called *complicated grief*, it includes disbelief, anger, painful emotion, and preoccupation with thoughts of the deceased. An estimated 7% of 75- to 85-year-olds are more vulnerable to experiencing complicated grief

than other older adults (Newson et al., 2011). Two of the many coexisting features are particularly noteworthy: depression/anxiety and sleep disruption (Monk, Pfoff, & Zarotney, 2013). Sleep disruption correlated significantly with depression and with the intensity of grief. There was no correlation between sleep measures and days since the death.

Elderly complicated grief responses are fairly common following the death of a spouse and may qualify as a traumatic stressor (O'Connor, 2010). Emerging elder spousal research is exploring posttraumatic stress disorder (PTSD) as a possible effect of the loss. O'Connor's findings indicate that PTSD frequency is 4 times higher (16%) in the spousal bereavement group in contrast to the comparison group (4%) and remained stable over time. This highlights the importance of considering PTSD as part of complicated grief. For those for whom symptoms persist, ongoing assessment and intervention would most likely be beneficial to support appropriate ongoing care, intervention, and treatment.

Complicated grief is a serious mental health problem (Bryant, 2014), including negative health outcomes, functional impairment, and increased suicide (Szanto et al., 2006). The *Diagnostic and Statistical Manual of Mental Disorders* (5th ed., *DSM-5*; American Psychiatric Association, 2013) defines *complicated grief* as a "persistent complex bereavement disorder" and lists it among conditions in need of further study. In addition, a diagnosis of "prolonged grief disorder" has been proposed for inclusion in the *International Classification of Diseases*, 11th Revision, 2018 (Maercker, 2013). Until the criteria are finalized, persons with complicated grief can still be reliably identified using the Inventory of Complicated Grief (ICG), a 19-item, self-report questionnaire (Prigerson, Maciejewski, & Reynolds, 1995).

RISK AND PROTECTIVE FACTORS

Diverse factors have been identified as either risk factors for adverse grief reactions or protective/psychological resources that may lower such risk. Elder bereavement risk factors include old age, caregiver stress, low socioeconomic status, and poor social support. These factors can

B

B

be identified before the pending death. Active intervention by primary caregivers and quality end-of-life care assist in minimizing both the burden of care and caregivers' feelings of regrets. This expedites the caregiver's psychological recovery. During the early bereavement period, a call is recommended to assess the widow's or widower's coping abilities as well as determining the need for intervention (Hashim et al., 2013).

Individual bereavement differences can be categorized into four patterns: *resilience* (66.3%), *chronic grief* (9.1%), *pre-existing chronic depression* (14.5%), and *depressed-improved* (10.1%). Health, financial stress, and emotional stability are strong predictors of variability in depression for some patterns. Bereavement depression levels do not have a shared etiology. Identifying distinct predictors informs both the course and etiology of bereavement depression (Galatzer-Levy & Bonnano, 2012).

A United Kingdom study found a marked increase in the incidence of cardiovascular events in older individuals in the months after spousal death. This connection was found separately for myocardial infarction (MI), stroke, acute coronary syndrome (ACS), and pulmonary embolism (PE) (Carey et al., 2014). In 2016 a study conducted in New York demonstrated that recently bereaved were more likely than nonbereaved to have depression symptoms and financial strain (Ghesquiere et al., 2016). It is evident that risk factors are very diverse and individualized.

A key protective factor in elderly spousal bereavement is trait resilience, with marital status and gender as important indicators (Spahni, Bennett, & Perrig-Chiello, 2016). Marital history and context of death appear to be secondary factors. Good social support, emotionally and practically, is found to promote greater resilience and inner strength. Being older with previous life experiences also enables the older widow or widower to cope with death as mostly an "expected" event. Family and friends play a fundamental role supporting older bereaved adults, as do existing community-based/religious organizations. In New Zealand many question the role, need, and value of formal bereavement support services. Consider the value in adopting

a public, health-based approach to optimizing bereavement support via use of community organizations previously known to older people. In countries with limited provisions for bereavement supports due to resource constraints, this is especially important (Bellany, Gott, Waterworth, McLean, & Kesse, 2014).

Biopsychosocial resilience is evident in the older adult as caregiver when significant stress is buffered by cognitive reframing and acceptance of interpersonal limits. Prior terminal caregiving provides a framework and difficult family dynamics added a layer of complexity. During stressful times cortisol levels rose outside normal boundaries (Ewen, Chahal, & Fenster, 2015).

HELPING THE BEREAVED ELDERLY COPE WITH LOSS

In helping the bereaved elderly, one first needs to understand what is happening to them. Listening to what they are saying, not saying anything at first, is quite possibly the best indicator of how or where to start in effectively assisting the bereaved. There is a fine balance between support and intruding, helping and pushing, to fit another's expectations.

The first year of life after the loss of a loved one is quite possibly the most difficult and the most challenging time in a person's life. In the elderly, this can be even more challenging because of decreasing mobility, loss of hearing, increasing acute and chronic symptoms, decreasing social support systems, and the realization, conscious or unconscious, that life is coming to an end, probably sooner than later. In one breath, the spouse has become a widow or widower. Unfortunately, American culture generally does not speak to death, much less bereavement. As a result, the first year after a loss becomes monumental in "How can I live without…?" and "Now what do I do about…?" Everyone has a choice to "go through" or "grow through" this adjustment period known as bereavement. "Going through" suggests reluctance and resistance, which everyone has at times, whereas "grow through" suggests a directness to moving through this time of both ending and beginning with as much grace and understanding as possible. Here is where we can begin to determine how to assist the grieving elderly (Keegan & Drick, 2013).

During the first year after the loss, there are many rites of passage that, once recognized, can give clear direction about the type of support needed. These include, but are not limited to, allowing the presence of grief, letting go of tears and anger, giving away and reorganizing, celebrating first holidays without the deceased, remembering, maintaining hope and faith, and getting stuck and unstuck (Keegan & Drick, 2013).

Bereaved individuals sometimes direct their anger regarding the deceased or the loss toward health care professionals. Compassion and understanding is essential at this time because this is part of the personal grieving process. We need to meet them where they are and gently guide them through this time.

Although there is often adequate support for bereaved spouses immediately following the loss and at the time of the funeral, family and friends tend to withdraw quickly after the first few months. Americans are generally uncomfortable with people in mourning. After the funeral, we often do not have the words, time, or understanding to assist them. The bereaved often find themselves alone as they struggle to assume new tasks and responsibilities. Bereavement support groups may offer a mutual support system, share coping strategies, and calm insecurities about living alone. Whether depressed bereaved individuals should be treated with medications after the first few months following a loss is debatable. Is bereavement a normal process or does depression distort grief work and increase poor adaptation?

Older individuals move through bereavement in many ways. Clinicians are realizing through both evidenced- and experience-based research that meeting widows and widowers where they are remains the key.

See also Hospice; Palliative Care.

Carole Ann Drick

American Psychiatric Association. (2013). *Diagnostic and statistical manual of mental disorders* (5th ed.). Arlington, VA: American Psychiatric Publishing.

Bellany, G., Gott, M., Waterworth, S., McLean, C., & Kesse, N. (2014). "But I do believe you've got to accept that that's what life's about": Older adults living in New Zealand talk about their experiences of loss and bereavement support. *Health and Social Care in the Community, 22*(1), 96–103.

Bennett, K. M. (2010). How to achieve resilience as an older widower: Turning points or gradual change? *Aging and Society, 30*(3), 369–382.

Bryant, R. A. (2014). Prolonged grief: Where to after *Diagnostic and Statistical Manual of Mental Disorders,* 5th edition? *Current Opinion Psychiatry, 27*(1), 21–26.

Carey, I. M., Shah, S. M., DeWilde, S., Harris, T., Victor, C. R., & Cook, D. G. (2014). Increased risk of acute cardiovascular events after partner bereavement: A matched cohort study. *JAMA Internal Medicine, 174*(4), 598–605.

Ewen, H., Chahal, J. K., & Fenster, E. (2015). A portrait of resilience in caregiving. *Research in Gerontology Nursing, 8*(1), 29–38.

Galatzer-Levy, I. R., & Bonnano, G. A. (2012). Beyond normality in the study of bereavement: Heterogeneity in depression outcomes following loss in older adults. *Social Science and Medicine, 74*(12), 1987–1994.

Ghesquiere, A. R., Bazelain, K. N., Berman, J., Greenberg, R. L., Kapland, D., & Bruce, M. L. (2016). Associations between recent bereavement and psychological and financial burden in homebound older adults. *OMEGA: Journal of Death and Dying, 73*(4), 326–339.

Hashim, S. M., Eng, T. C., Tohit, N., & Wahab, S. (2013). Bereavement in the elderly: The role of primary care. *Mental Health in Family Medicine, 10*(3), 159–162.

Keegan, L., & Drick, C. A. (2011). *End of life: Nursing solutions for death with dignity* (pp. 20–21). New York, NY: Springer Publishing.

Keegan, L., & Drick, C. A. (2013). *The golden room: A practical guide for death with dignity.* North Charleston, SC: Create Space.

Maercker, A., Brewin, C. R., Bryant, R. A., Cloitre, M., Reed, G. M., . . . Saxena S. (2013). Proposals for mental disorders specifically associated with stress in the *International Classification of Diseases-*11. *Lancet, 381*(9878), 1683–1685.

Monk, T. H., Pfoff, M. K., & Zarotney, J. R. (2013). Depression in the spousally bereaved elderly; corrections with subjective sleep measures. *Depression, Research and Treatment, 2013,* 409–538.

Newson, R. S., Boelen, P. A., Hek, L., & Hoffman, A. (2011). The prevalence and characteristics of complicated grief in older adults. *Journal of Affective Disorders, 132*(1–2), 231–238.

O'Connor, M. (2010). A longitudinal study of PTSD in the elderly bereaved: [corrected] prevalence and predictors. *Aging and Mental Health, 14*(3), 310–318.

Prigerson, H. G., Maciejewski, P. K., Reynolds, C. F., III, Bierhals, A. J., Newsom, J. T., Fasiczka, A., . . . Miller, M. (1995). Inventory of complicated grief: A scale to measure maladaptive symptoms of loss. *Psychiatry Research, 59*(1-2), 65–79.

Shah, S. M., Carey, I. M., Harris, T., DeWilde, S., Victor, C. R., & Cook, D. G. (2013). The effect of unexpected bereavement on mortality in older couples. *American Journal of Public Health, 103*(6), 140–145.

Spahni, S., Bennett, K. M., & Perrig-Chiello, P. (2016). Psychological adaptation to spousal bereavement in old age: The role of trait resilience, marital history, and context of death. *Death Studies, 40*(3), 182–190.

Szanto, K., Shear, M. K., Houck, P. R., Reynolds, C. F., III, Frank, E., Caroff, K., & Silowash, R. (2006). Indirect self-destructive behavior and overt suicidality in patients with complicated grief. *Journal of Clinical Psychiatry, 67*(2), 233–239.

Web Resources
AARP: http://www.aarp.org/families/grief_loss
GoldenRoomAdvocates.org
HealthyPlace.com: http://www.healthyplace.com/communities/depression/related/loss_grief.asp
National Library of Medicine/National Institutes of Health: http://www.nlm.nih.gov/medlineplus/bereavement.html

BIPOLAR DISORDER IN LATER LIFE

Bipolar disorder (BD), sometimes referred to as *manic-depressive illness*, refers to a variety of mood disorders. The average age for the beginning of early-onset (i.e., before the age of 50–60 years) BD is 25 years. Over the course of a lifetime, an elderly patient with early-onset BD may have experienced intermittent episodes of both depression and mania, of just mania, or of just depression. In addition, in some, initial manic episodes are of late onset. About 10% of older adults admitted to the hospital with mood disorders are diagnosed with BD, even though they have no earlier history of mood swings. Episodes of manic symptoms, which are mild to moderate, are referred to as *hypomania*. A careful history from relatives may reveal hypomanic episodes that were not seriously impairing but in retrospect were clear signs of an early onset.

SYMPTOMATOLOGY

Previously, the symptoms of mania occurring in late life were considered distinctively different from those occurring earlier in life. Mania occurring in late life has been found to be generally similar, except for higher degrees of associated cognitive dysfunction and of complications resulting from age-related physiological changes, concurrent medical problems, and medications.

Older adults with BD frequently experience cognitive deficits as well, which may include impairments in problem solving, inhibitory control, sustained attention, processing speed abstract thinking, and verbal memory. Cognitive dysfunction is thought to reflect a distinct neurobiological origin from neurodegenerative diseases and may represent the cumulative effects of neurodevelopmental factors, disease burden, long-term exposure to antipsychotic medications and comorbid disease processes exacerbated by aging (Sajatovic, Forester, Gildengers, & Mulsant, 2013; Valiengo, Stella, & Forlenza, 2014).

In addition, the concept of BD has broadened from one that is purely psychiatric to a multisystem model that includes both medical comorbidities and functional disability (Gildengers et al., 2013). Relative to age-matched peers, older bipolar patients are more likely to carry diagnoses of diabetes mellitus, hypertension, thyroid disorders, and cancer and to experience earlier mortality (Rise, Haro, & Gjervan, 2016). Also, individuals with BD often contend with functional impairments such as difficulty managing medications or finances and trouble maintaining personal relationships. Evidence suggests that higher levels of mood disturbance, medical comorbidities, and cognitive impairment are all associated with worsening functional decline (Gildengers et al., 2013).

A recent report from the International Society for Bipolar Disorders Task Force (Sajatovic et al.,

2015) summarizes that cognitive impairment in multiple functional domains leads to blunted social, occupational, and cognitive functions (Baune & Malhi, 2015). Although the nature of cognitive dysfunction remains controversial—normal aging versus mood disorder—it has been suggested that the number of recurrent mood episodes may serve as a strong clinical marker for neuroprogression of BD, as reflected in decreased cortical neuronal density, glial cell counts, and number of oligodendrocytes, as well as increased rates of neuronal apoptosis seen in various parts of the brain of older adults with BD (Gildengers et al., 2014; Passos, Mwangi, Vieta, Berk, & Kapenzinski, 2016).

Concurrent problems with anxiety and substance use appear to be less common in older patients. Characteristic features of manic episodes include sustained periods of elevated, expansive, or irritable mood associated with racing thoughts, which may manifest in pressured (hard-to-interrupt) speech; hyperactivity; distractibility; grandiose thoughts; or decreased sleep without corresponding fatigue.

The hyperactivity can become dangerous when it leads to driven, reckless behaviors such as spending too much money, driving carelessly or too fast, drinking too much alcohol, or engaging in hypersexual activity. Sometimes, these manic symptoms are interspersed with symptoms of depression, including sadness, tearfulness, and suicidal ideation. Such mixed episodes can be confusing to others and the source of misdiagnosis. Acute episodes of BD in late life, whether manic or mixed, can look like delirium, agitated depression, schizophrenia, schizoaffective disorder, or even dementia, especially in the presence of co-occurring medical problems, age-related structural changes in the brain, and/or increased sensitivity to medication side effects.

Episodes of sustained low mood occurring over the course of BD are characterized by the signs and symptoms of depression and are typically associated with disturbances of appetite, sleep, and energy level; diminished capacity for enjoyment; and psychological symptoms such as feeling helpless, hopeless, worthless, unduly pessimistic about the future, and/or suicidal. Depressive episodes in BD significantly raise the risk for suicide.

ASSESSMENT AND TREATMENT

Individuals older than 50 years who experience an episode of mania for the first time, whether as part of a long-standing history of early-onset BD or as the beginning of late-onset BD, require careful consideration. They warrant a comprehensive medical evaluation, since manic symptoms occurring for the first time at this point in the life cycle are often secondary to underlying medical problems (e.g., strokes, brain tumors, endocrine disorders, dementia) or untoward effects of medications (e.g., steroids, antidepressants, anti-Parkinson medications that increase levels of dopamine in the brain).

As with other psychiatric disorders, effective treatment of BD in late life is predicated on the establishment of a sound therapeutic alliance. Establishing an effective working relationship with patients suffering from BD can be particularly challenging because the elevated mood and hyperactivity in manic episodes are frequently accompanied by lack of insight and poor judgment, especially about the nature of the illness, the need for treatment, and the adverse consequences of reckless behaviors. During a hypomanic phase prior to full-blown mania, patients may feel that their moods are quite good, they are in fact getting a lot accomplished, and hence there is no cause for treatment. Sometimes, it is not until they engage in activities dangerous to themselves or others that they receive treatment, albeit on an involuntary basis. Sometimes, it is not until they have gone through repeated episodes of mania that they come to appreciate the need to avoid the adverse consequences of foregoing treatment. Cultivating ad hoc teams of the patient and all those who are or may become involved with the patient can be quite helpful (Howell, 2015). Networking with and educating these team members about the nature and treatment of BD in late life is important. Counseling and supporting them to deal patiently with the ethical and medical-legal issues of both voluntary and involuntary treatment are additional key components for effective outcomes. These issues require a careful balancing between patient autonomy and safety in what can become very stressful situations.

B

There have been few published reports from randomized, controlled trials for older adults experiencing episodes of either mania or depression in the context of BD. One exception is the GERI-BD trial (Young et al., 2010). One finding was that manic symptoms were less severe at the initiation of treatment for patients who had more social interaction within their community, but the duration of the manic episode for these patients took longer to resolve (Beyer et al., 2014). Having psychotic symptoms, having higher Young Mania Rating Scale scores, and being a non-Hispanic White were associated with admission to inpatient treatment but the degree of depression was not (Al Jurdi et al., 2012). Further considerations include age-related changes in the effects of medications on different organ systems, co-occurring medical problems, and medications. All these factors require consideration when selecting mood stabilizers to ensure, as much as possible, that their use will be not only effective, but also safe and tolerable.

Although limited data are available to support the effectiveness of lithium, divalproex, quetiapine, and lamotrigine, newer studies suggest the safety and effectiveness of lithium for older adults with BD (Rej et al., 2015). Lamotrigine augmentation in older adults with bipolar depression also seems to be effective (Sajatovic et al., 2011). More recently, a post hoc analysis on use of lurasidone, an atypical antipsychotic, demonstrated this medication to be safe and effective, both as monotherapy and as adjunctive therapy, in older adults with BD. This is one of only a few studies that look at treatment efficacy of newer medications among geriatric patients (Sajatovic et al., 2016). Nonetheless, judicious use of medication involves starting pharmacotherapy at a low dose, gradually increasing the dosage, and carefully monitoring for medication response and side effects. Which medication to start with depends on patients' prior experiences (i.e., response to medications and any side effects), any concurrent medical illnesses and medications (e.g., potential drug interactions), patients' preferences, and cost.

Lithium thus remains the gold standard for the treatment of BD, and it can be continued into late life as treatment for early-onset BD

as long as attention is paid to the diminishing margin of safety with increasing patient age. The use of lithium requires periodic measurements of its level in the bloodstream. Generally, the older the patient, the narrower the effective blood level range that can be tolerated without untoward side effects. Because of the delay in lithium and other mood stabilizers becoming adequately effective, acute episodes of mania typically require antipsychotic medication on a short-term basis (i.e., up to a few weeks). Long-term continuous lithium treatment may be neuroprotective against the neurodegenerative changes seen in dementia because of its inhibitory effect on glycogen synthase kinase-3 as part of the metabolic dysfunction seen in dementia (Gildengers et al., 2015; Gerhard, Devanand, Huang, Crystal, & Olfson, 2015). Compared with older adults who use valproate or an antipsychotic medication, those who use lithium do not seem to develop more comorbidities or higher utilization of health care services (Rej et al., 2015). Although there is no real consensus yet, lithium seems to be a fairly safe choice for older adults with BD.

Acute episodes of or depression or mania may become highly risky because of intense psychomotor symptoms (severe hypoactivity or hyperactivity) in the face of increasing physical frailty (e.g., inadequate oral intake of food and/or fluids), imminent suicidality, or intense psychotic features. In such situations, electroconvulsive therapy (ECT) can be very effective. ECT may also be an effective recourse in instances in which medications are ineffective (e.g., after three to four or more adequate trials) or their side effects are not tolerable.

Because BD is a highly recurrent illness, maintenance treatment between episodes (usually with the same initially effective medication regimen), rather than no treatment, is recommended; psychotherapy is also recommended. Most older patients with BD require maintenance treatment for years, and some require it for their remainder of their lives. This is especially true for patients with early-onset BD, residual symptoms (e.g., suicidal ideation), and/or ongoing psychosocial stressors. Those with a history of suicide attempts or of more frequent, longer, or more severe episodes are also more likely to need maintenance treatment. Although elderly patients usually recover from each mood episode, they are at higher risk of cognitive decline and compromised psychosocial functioning. The higher rate of suicide with BD persists into late life, and mortality (independent of suicide) is elevated compared with the general population.

The complexity of the management and treatment of BD in older patients means that follow-up appointments and tracking of relevant laboratory and electrocardiogram studies need to be more frequent than with younger patients. It is also important to recognize specific care needs of older adults with BD, particularly engagement in the social functioning realm to maintain the benefits and quality of life associated with social activities exposure (Dautzenberg, 2016). Caregiver burden also needs to be taken into consideration as more than 50% of caregivers of older adults with BD experience substantial burden. Because caregiver burden can impact the optimal care of older adults with BD, brief, two-session group psychoeducation for caregivers has been shown to be effective in alleviating caregiving burden (Hubbard, McEvoy, Smith, & Kane, 2016) and should be considered as part of the overall treatment plan by providers who identify this as a problem.

Barbara L. Fischer and Timothy Howell

Al Jurdi, R. K., Schulberg, H. C., Greenberg, R. L., Kunik, M. E., Gildengers, A., Sajatovic, M.,… Young, R. C. (2012). Characteristics associated with inpatient versus outpatient status in older adults with bipolar disorder. *Journal of Geriatric Psychiatry & Neurology, 25*(1), 62–68. doi:10.1177/0891988712436684

Bailine, S., Fink, M., Knapp, R., Petrides, G., Husain, M. M., Rasmussen, K.,… Kellner, C. H. (2010). Electroconvulsive therapy is equally effective in unipolar and bipolar depression. *Acta Psychiatrica Scandinavica, 121*, 431.

Baune, B., & Malhi, G. (2015). A review on the impact of cognitive dysfunction on social, occupation, and general functional outcomes in bipolar disorder. *Bipolar Disorder, 17*(2), 41–55.

Beyer, J. L., Greenberg, R. L., Marino, P., Bruce, M. L., Al Jurdi, R. K., Sajatovic, M.,… Young, R. C. (2014). Social support in late life mania: GERI-BD.

International Journal of Geriatric Psychiatry, 10, 1028–1032. doi:10.1002/gps.4093

Chen, P., Korobkova, I., Busby, K., & Sajatovic, M. (2011). Managing late-life bipolar disorder: An update. *Aging Health, 7*, 557.

Dautzenberg, G., Lans, L., Meesters, P., Kupka, R., Beekman, A., Stek, M.,…Dols, A. (2016). The care needs of older patients with bipolar disorder. *Aging & Mental Health, 20*(9), 899–907.

Gerhard, T., Devanand, D. P., Huang, C., Crystal, S., & Olfson, M. (2015). Lithium treatment and risk for dementia in adults with bipolar disorder: Population-based cohort study. *British Journal of Psychiatry, 207*, 46–51.

Gildengers, A. G., Butters, M., Aizenstein, H., Marron, M., Emanuel, J., Anderson, S.,… Reynolds, C. F., III (2015). Longer lithium exposure is associated with better white matter integrity in older adults with bipolar disorder. *Bipolar Disorder, 17*(3), 248–256.

Gildengers, A. G., Butters, M. A., Chisholm, D., Rogers, J. C., Holm, M. B., Bhalla, R. K.,…Mulsant, B. H. (2007). Cognitive functioning and instrumental activities of daily living in late-life bipolar disorder. *American Journal of Geriatric Psychiatry, 15*, 174.

Gildengers, A. G., Chung, K., Huang, S., Begley, A., Aizenstein, H., & Tsai, S. (2014). Neuroprogressive effects of lifetime illness duration in older adults with bipolar disorder. *Bipolar Disorder, 16*(6), 617–623.

Gildengers, A. G., Tatsuoka, C., Bialko, C., Cassidy, K. A., Dines, P., Emanual, J.,… Sajatovic, M. (2013). Correlates of disability in depressed older adults with bipolar disorder. *Cutting Edge Psychiatry Practice, 1*, 332–338.

Goldstein, B. I., Herrmann, N., & Shulman, K. I. (2006). Comorbidity in bipolar disorder among the elderly: Results from an epidemiological community sample. *American Journal of Psychiatry, 163*, 319–321.

Howell, T. (2015). The Wisconsin Star Method: Understanding and addressing complexity in geriatrics. In M. L. Malone & E. A. Capezuti (Eds.), *Geriatrics models of care: Bringing 'best practice' to an aging America* (pp. 87–94). Cham, Switzerland: Springer International.

Hubbard, A., McEvoy, P., Smith, L., & Kane, R. (2016). Brief group psychoeducation for caregivers of individuals with bipolar disorder: A randomized controlled trial. *Journal of Affective Disorders, 200*, 31–36.

Passos, I., Mwangi, B., Vieta, E., Berk, M., & Kapenzinski, F. (2016). Areas of controversy in neuroprogression in bipolar disorder. *Acta Psychiatrica Scandinavica, 134*, 1–13. doi:10.1111/acps.12581

Prabhakar, D., & Balon, R. (2010). Late-onset bipolar disorder: A case for careful appraisal. *Psychiatry (Edgmont), 7*, 34–37.

Rej, S., Yu, C., Shulman, K., Hermann, N., Fischer, H., Fung, K., & Gruneir, A. (2015). Medical co-morbidity, acute medical care use in late-life bipolar disorder: A comparison of lithium, valproate, and other pharmacotherapies. *General Hospital Psychiatry, 37*(6), 528–532.

Rise, I. V., Haro, J. M., & Gjervan, B. (2016). Clinical features, comorbidity, and cognitive impairment in elderly bipolar patients. *Neuropsychiatric Disease and Treatment, 12*, 1203–1213.

Sajatovic, M., & Chen, P. (2011). Geriatric bipolar disorder. *The Psychiatric Clinics of North America, 34*, 319–333.

Sajatovic, M., Forester, B. P., Gildengers, A., & Mulsant, B. (2013). Aging changes and medical complexity in late-life bipolar disorder: Emerging research findings that may help advance care. *Neuropsychiatry, 3*(6), 621–633. doi:10.2217/npy.13.78

Sajatovic, M., Forester, B., Tsai, J., Kroger, H., Pikalov, A., Cucchiaro, J.,…Loebel, A. (2016). Efficacy of lurasidone in adults aged 55 years and older with bipolar depression: Post-hoc analysis of 2 double-blind, placebo-controlled studies. *The Journal of Clinical Psychiatry, 77*(10), e1324–e1331.

Sajatovic, M., Gildengers, A., Al Jurdi, R., Gyulai, L., Cassidy, K., Greenberg, R.,…Young, R. C. (2011). Multisite, open-label, prospective trial of lamotrigine for geriatric bipolar depression: A preliminary report. *Bipolar Disorder, 13*(3), 294–302.

Sajatovic, M., Strejilevich, S., Gildengers, A., Dols, A., Al Jurdi, R., Forester, B.,…Shulman, K. L. (2015). A report on older-age bipolar disorder from the International Society for Bipolar Disorders Task Force. *Bipolar Disorder, 17*(7), 689–704.

Valiengo, L., Stella, F., & Forlenza, O. (2014). Mood disorders in the elderly: Prevalence, functional impact, and management challenges. *Neuropsychiatric Disorders and Treatment, 12*, 2105–2114. doi:10.2147/NDT.S94643

Young, R. C., Schulberg, H. C., Gildengers, A. G., Sajatovic, M., Mulsant, B. H., Gyulai, L.,…Alexopoulos, G. S. (2010). Conceptual and methodological issues in designing a randomized, controlled treatment trial for geriatric bipolar disorder: GERI-BD. *Bipolar Disorders, 12*, 56–67.

Web Resources

Depression and Bipolar Support Alliance: http://www.DBSAlliance.org

National Alliance on Mental Illness: http://www.nami.org

National Institute of Mental Health: http://www.nimh.nih.gov

C

CANCER TREATMENT

Cancer is a common disease in the elderly. The median age of new cancer diagnosis is 65 years and of cancer-related death is 72 years (National Cancer Institute, 2013). By 2030, an estimated 70% of all cancer diagnoses will occur in patients older than 65 years. The most prevalent types of malignancies in women older than 60 years of age are breast, colorectal, and uterine cancer. In men older than 60 years, the most prevalent cancers are prostate, colorectal, and transitional cell carcinoma of the bladder (National Cancer Institute, 2013). There is an increasing incidence of thyroid cancer, melanoma, and liver cancer in adults 65 years and older (National Cancer Institute, 2013). Cancer still accounts for more deaths than heart disease in people younger than 85 years, but after age 85 years, heart disease becomes the number one cause (Magnuson & Mohile, 2016).

CANCER BIOLOGY AND AGING

Aging and its role in cancer development is complex, and multiple factors likely contribute to the increased incidence and prevalence of malignancy in old age. Many cancers tend to develop over a long time. For example, colon cancer starts with an intermediate precursor, the adenomatous polyp, which progresses into cancer because of an accumulation of mutations in tumor suppressor genes and additional genetic defects in oncogenes. It takes 8 to 10 genetic lesions to develop into a malignancy (Magnuson & Mohile, 2016). Another reason for increased prevalence is the decline of DNA repair mechanisms, which allows endogenous oxygen free radicals and exogenous stresses to cause genomic damage. Autophagy—a process that allows the cell to eliminate defective

structures—is also less effective with aging, resulting in an accumulation of damaged proteins and mitochondria that eventually become carcinogenic (Kilari & Mohile, 2012). Furthermore, telomeres—DNA structures that provide genomic stability—become progressively shorter with aging, thus exponentially increasing the rate of DNA mutations (Kilari & Mohile, 2012). The immune system can recognize and control certain cancers. Because its function declines with aging, a malignancy that was previously controlled can eventually emerge in old age (Magnuson & Mohile, 2016).

MANAGEMENT OF OLDER ADULTS WITH CANCER

The management of geriatric cancer patients can be challenging for various reasons. First, only 3% of older adults are treated in clinical trials, and participants are typically healthier older patients. Hence, little evidence exists regarding cancer treatment efficacy and tolerability in older patients. Moreover, older adults may not have classic signs of malignancy such as hemoptysis in lung cancer patients and rectal bleeding in colon cancer patients, which may cause delayed or missed diagnoses. An older person with lung cancer could present with a persistent pneumonia, and an older person with colon cancer may simply be anemic.

Once an older adult is diagnosed with cancer, the provider needs to obtain a full history and complete physical examination. Depending on the cancer, evaluation of the tumor size, grade, histology, margins, lymph nodes, and presence of hormone receptors may be appropriate. Imaging studies (bone scan, CT, PET) and biopsies may also be indicated. Older adults also have age-related needs that require additional assessment before making treatment recommendations.

C

The National Comprehensive Cancer Network (NCCN) provides a comprehensive guideline for geriatric oncology. The key elements in the approach to geriatric cancer care are to determine (a) the likelihood of dying or suffering from cancer given remaining life expectancy, (b) the patient's decision-making capacity, and (c) the patient's goals and values regarding cancer management (Hurria et al., 2016). Life expectancy calculators (available at www.eprognosis.com) are useful in the shared decision-making process. If a patient's life expectancy is poor and/or if the risk of dying or suffering from the cancer is high, palliative care/symptom management may be the most appropriate treatment option. If anticancer treatment is chosen, the next step is to determine whether the patient can tolerate treatment. The clinician assesses for risk factors for adverse outcomes, treats any modifiable factors, or pursues alternate treatments to lower the risk of treatment toxicity. Common risk factors include medical comorbidities, geriatric syndromes, and socioeconomic issues.

Comprehensive Geriatric Assessment (CGA) addresses these risk factors and there is growing evidence supporting CGA, or a variation of it, in the management of geriatric cancer. Key components to CGA in oncology are (Dale, Chow, & Sajid, 2016; Li, de Glas, & Hurria, 2016; Magnuson & Mohile, 2016):

- Physical function assessment (e.g., Katz's Index of Activities of Daily Living [ADL], Lawton's Instrumental Activities of Daily Living [IADL] Scale). Dependence in ADL and IADL has been predictive of mortality in geriatric cancer patients.
- Nutritional status evaluation (e.g., Mini Nutritional Assessment). There is an approximately twofold increased risk of mortality in patients with a weight loss of 5% of body weight.
- Social support assessment (e.g., available caregivers, transportation and financial concerns, spiritual needs). Older patients who lack social support are less likely to adhere to medical treatment, whereas social isolation carries an increased mortality risk.
- Cognitive evaluation (e.g., Mini-Cog, Mini-Mental State Examination (MMSE), St. Louis University Mental Status [SLUMS] examination, or Montreal Cognitive Assessment [MoCA]). Cognitive impairment may limit life expectancy in more advanced cancer and increase risk of delirium with cancer treatment.
- Polypharmacy identification, which increases risk of treatment complications and adverse events from chemotherapy.
- Psychological evaluation using the Geriatric Depression Scale (GDS) or Patient Health Questionnaire-9 (PHQ-9). Studies have found that depression is a significant prognostication factor in patients undergoing cancer treatment.
- Identifying and treating comorbidities which can affect survival and treatment tolerance.

CGA evaluates global health and stratifies an older adult as "fit/robust," "vulnerable," or "frail." This assessment provides meaningful information to guide the shared decision-making process, potentially avoiding both overtreatment and undertreatment of malignancy in older patients. Incorporating CGA into oncological management of older adults has been shown to predict toxicity, morbidity, and mortality; prevent disability; reduce hospitalizations; and uncover problems relevant to cancer care that would otherwise go unrecognized (Dale et al., 2016; Kilari & Mohile, 2012).

TREATMENT MODALITIES

Multiple treatment modalities are available to cancer patients. Because tumors are not resistant to treatment by virtue of age alone, therapies that are effective in younger patients can also be successful in older adults. Furthermore, the data suggest that cancer aggressiveness may decline with age, exhibiting slower growth, more favorable histologies, fewer metastases, and longer survival. In selecting an appropriate treatment, cancer site, stage, histology, the patient's overall health, and goals of care are considered. Notably, older adults who are *fully informed* about treatment options often choose life-extending treatments despite the risk of toxicity. In addition, other studies have shown that older patients with good performance status are often able to tolerate and benefit from the same therapies compared with younger patients (Li et al., 2016). Hence, advanced age alone should not preclude offering cancer treatment with either curative or palliative options. Thus comprehensive geriatrics assessment is important for making treatment decisions.

Surgery

The primary concerns related to major tumor resections in older adults are safety and rehabilitation potential. Although age itself is not a risk factor for elective cancer surgery, longer hospital stay and time to full recovery are associated with older age. Improvements in anesthesia, the availability of less invasive surgical procedures such as endoscopy, and the use of initial neoadjuvant chemotherapy before surgery in select cancers have made surgery a more effective option for palliation and/or cure (Magnuson & Mohile, 2016).

Chemotherapy

The normal physiological, anatomical, and structural changes associated with aging can alter the efficacy of chemotherapy drugs, as well as increase susceptibility to treatment-related toxicities. For example, a diminished glomerular filtration rate in an older adult can increase the half-life of chemotherapeutic agent excreted by the kidneys, leading to more severe toxicities and therefore necessitating dose reduction. Changes in the mucosal protective mechanism with aging cause increased susceptibility to mucositis. Gastrointestinal motility alterations can lead to reduced or increased toxicity. Changes in arterial pressure, cerebral blood flow, and disequilibrium lead to increased risk of confusion, syncope, and falls (Magnuson & Mohile, 2016). Chemotherapy can also induce peripheral neuropathy. On the other hand, acute toxicities such as nausea, vomiting, and hair loss may be less likely to occur in older adults, and with certain chemotherapy agents, the age-related changes can confer specific advantages, making them particularly suitable for treating older patients (Magnuson & Mohile, 2016).

Radiation

Radiation therapy is generally safe and effective in older patients. It provides palliation for nearly all cancers and often is part of the treatment of lymphomas and cancers of the prostate, bladder, cervix, esophagus, breast, head, and neck. It has long been used as an alternative to surgery in poor surgical candidates (Magnuson & Mohile, 2016).

Biological Therapy

Immunotherapy, or modulation of the immune response, is particularly beneficial when treating older patients because immune defenses are often impaired with aging. Over the last decade, options for biological therapies have increased significantly. Some examples include monoclonal antibodies targeting growth factors and cytotoxic T cells or B cells. Dose-dependent toxicity can occur with various agents, resulting in severe hypertension or hypotension, respiratory distress, myelosuppression, and liver, cardiac, and/or renal impairment.

Hormonal Therapy

Hormone therapy can be effective in the treatment of breast, prostate, and uterine cancers and is usually well tolerated. Older women with breast cancer are more likely to exhibit estrogen and progesterone receptor–positive histologies, which allows for selective estrogen-receptor modulators such as tamoxifen to be effective. Tamoxifen can increase bone density and decrease cardiovascular risk factors without increasing risk of uterine cancer, but it can increase the risk of blood clots. Hormonal therapy is the first line in systemic prostate cancer, but its use is associated with metabolic syndrome, cardiovascular disease, osteoporosis/fractures, and physical performance issues in men (Magnuson & Mohile, 2016).

Yael Mauer, Michael L. Malone, and Karen Padua

Dale, W., Chow, S., & Sajid, S. (2016). Socioeconomic considerations and shared-care models of cancer care for older adults. *Clinics in Geriatric Medicine, 32*, 35–44.

Hurria, A., Wides, T., Blair, S. L., Browner, I. S., Cohen, H. J.,…Sundar, H. (2016, August 31). National

C

comprehensive cancer network. *Clinical practice guidelines in oncology: Older adult oncology, Version 2.2016.* Retrieved from https://www.nccn.org/professionals/physician_gls/f_guidelines.asp#age

Kilari, D., & Mohile, S. G. (2012). Management of cancer in the older adult. *Clinics in Geriatric Medicine, 28*(1), 33–49. doi:10.1016/j.cger.2011.10.003

Li, D., de Glas, N., & Hurria, A. (2016). Cancer and aging. *Clinics in Geriatric Medicine, 32*, 1–15.

Magnuson, A., & Mohile, S. (2016). Oncology and hematologic malignancies. In A. Medina-Walpole & J. T. Pacala (Eds.), *Geriatrics review syllabus* (9th ed.). [Online]. New York, NY: American Geriatrics Society.

National Cancer Institute. (2013, July 10). SEER cancer statistics review, 1975–2010. Retrieved from http://seer.cancer.gov/csr/1975_2010/results_merged/sect_01_overview.pdf

CARE MANAGEMENT

THE MANY FACES OF CASE MANAGEMENT

Health and human service programs have been consistently criticized for poor quality (Applebaum, Straker, & Geron, 2000). Inadequate information for consumers, confusing eligibility rules, an uncoordinated array of providers, and limited monitoring of services are universal concerns across settings. In response, the concept of case management has emerged as a popular strategy for helping individuals navigate the fragmented health and human services system. Such diverse service areas as corrections, unemployment, child welfare, mental health, substance abuse, and acute health care have all used case management as a technique to fix a troubled system (Ackerly & Grabowski, 2014; Barman-Adhikari & Rice, 2014; Chinman et al., 2015; Dauber, Neighbors, Dasaro, Riordan, & Morgenstern, 2012; McDonald & Arlinghaus, 2014; Rapp, Noortgate, Broekaert, & Vanderplasschen, 2014).

LONG-TERM SERVICES CARE MANAGEMENT

Although there are many faces of case management, the focus here is on one area, long-term services and supports for older people experiencing disability. Most give little thought to tasks of daily living, such as taking a shower, getting dressed, or cooking breakfast. However, it is the need for continual help because of physical or cognitive limitations that results in older people receiving long-term services and supports. Dramatic changes in how long-term services are provided in the United States has occurred in the last two decades, with virtually every state in the nation now operating a home- and community-based Medicaid-waiver program. In many states, the proportion of older people receiving long-term services at home, compared with in a facility, reached 50%, and this trend has continued to grow (Eiken, Sredl, Burwell, & Saucier, 2016).

The initial efforts to expand home- and community-based services in the United States were driven by a desire to control Medicaid expenditures and limit the growth of nursing home use (Kemper, Applebaum, & Harrigan, 1987). A second push for the expansion of in-home services was inspired in large part by the U.S. Supreme Court's Olmstead decision (1999), which highlighted the rights of individuals with disability to live in the setting of their choice. One shift that occurred as a result of this decision was a new emphasis on helping nursing home residents return to the community. More than 44 states have participated in a federal initiative (i.e., the Money Follows the Person Demonstration Grant) that provides an incentive to transition long-term nursing home residents back into the community (Watts, Reaves, & Musumeci, 2015).

Using case managers to coordinate community-based long-term services was first tested in the United States in the early 1970s as part of a search for cost-effective alternatives for people with complex needs that required long-term services and supports (Davies & Challis, 1986; Kemper et al., 1987). At least six factors have been linked to the significant growth of case management: (a) the shift from institutionalized care to home and community-based care, (b) the growing number of individuals living at home with complex needs, (c) the growing awareness of the importance of social support and informal caregivers, (d) the decentralized nature of the community-based service network, (e) the fragmented nature of community-based services, and (f) the need for cost containment (Moxley, 1989; Reilly, Hughes, & Challis, 2010).

COMPONENTS

The provision of services and supports in a community setting, typically in a person's home, often requires a complex set of decisions by the individual, family members and, in many instances, a service professional. What type of assistance does an individual need? What can be provided by the informal support system? What needs to be provided by formal service providers? How much monitoring and support are needed by the individual? How much will the necessary services cost? These and other questions shape the core elements of long-term care management, as the service is now known.

Outreach is used to identify persons in need of care management. Target populations are defined and specified in policy and program regulations, and care managers are typically instructed to focus on high-risk populations. Standardized protocols are used in screening, which is a preliminary assessment of an individual's circumstances and resources to determine presumptive eligibility. However, such standardized protocols are becoming more complex. For example, care managers are spending considerable effort targeting long-term nursing home residents who want to return home (Arling, Kane, Cooke, & Lewis, 2010). Such efforts often require a varied approach to care management, which can have an impact on assessment, care planning, care coordination, and evaluation (Bardo, Applebaum, Kunkel, & Carpio, 2013).

Comprehensive assessment focuses on a multitude of domains: physical health, cognitive functioning, emotional status, ability to perform activities of daily living, social supports, physical environment, and financial resources. A multidimensional assessment using a standardized instrument to collect in-depth information about a person so that a care plan can be developed is considered a best practice (Reilly et al., 2010). Sometimes, because of the multidimensional breadth of a comprehensive assessment, a team of health care and social service professionals (e.g., nurse, social worker, physician, psychologist) assist case managers in this process.

Care planning is a key resource-allocation process that uses information collected during the assessment process to specify services, providers, frequency of service delivery, and costs. Care planning requires the participation of individuals and caregivers because a balance between formal and informal services is a major consideration in the care-planning process.

Service arrangement and care coordination involves contacting formal and informal providers to arrange services specified in the care plan. This process can be limited by the availability of providers and community resources, which tend to vary by geographic location (e.g., urban vs. rural). Although it is a case manager's responsibility to arrange for the needed services and supports, the selection of providers should be driven by the participant themselves; in some new self-directed programs, it is the primary responsibility of the consumer to do so (De Milto, 2015). In these programs, the case manager's role shifts to one of consultant rather than manager.

Monitoring and evaluation involve determining whether the participant is receiving the most appropriate long-term services and supports to meet their needs. This process includes monitoring and evaluating the quality of service providers, as well as the individual's status. Systematic and regularly scheduled reassessments are necessary for identifying possible changes in a patient's situation and for assisting in the evaluation of care plan outcomes.

ISSUES

Is case management even necessary? The rationale for care management is that the current system of care is fragmented to such a degree that typical older persons and their families cannot negotiate the confusing maze of services. Care management has thus been seen as the strategy for helping consumers navigate a complex system. Some have argued that a better and less costly alternative would be to simply design a better long-term services system, one that would not require a professional to manage care. The argument from a quality-management perspective is that we would be better off spending resources on fixing the broken system than using a vast amount of professional staff time for incrementally fixing large system imperfections. Despite the appealing logic of this argument, thus far no country has been able to develop such an efficient system, and some have suggested that such a goal may not be achievable.

Another issue of concern surrounds the specific role of case managers and the term that describes their work. For many years advocates have argued that people are not cases and they do not need to be managed. Accompanying this concern is the question of the balance between consumer choice and empowerment and professional direction and expertise. Long-term services are often very personal, and advocates have argued that the consumer needs to be more in charge of their services (Stone, 2011). Care managers, typically trained as nurses or social workers, have a professional orientation that values technical expertise, health and safety, and cost controls, which are not necessarily the top values of the consumer. Questions about how to use the professional expertise of care managers while maintaining consumer autonomy still present an enormous challenge to case management.

A third issue focuses on the changing nature of long-term services and supports systems. Nursing homes and even home care services are often used for much shorter durations than in the past. How will the shorter time frame of enrollment impact the nature of case-management practice? Will assessment and monitoring approaches need to be modified?

A fourth area involves the role of caregivers. Working with family members is increasingly acknowledged as a critical component of case management. How should case managers best assess the ongoing needs of caregivers? How does the case manager balance the needs of the older person with the needs of the caregivers? How will the case manager acknowledge and address conflicts?

Finally, it is critical to examine the role of case management in a long-term services system that is moving into managed care. For example, more than half of states are exploring integrated long-term care demonstrations to combine Medicaid and Medicare coverage for individuals with disabilities. Although case managers have also had a role in controlling participant expenditures, it traditionally was balanced by the fact that most care managers were employed in private nonprofit or public community agencies. Under the current proposal for integrated care, the majority of plans will be for-profit entities, which this could place care managers in a very different position when it comes to consumer advocacy and cost controls.

Although these and other issues make the future uncertain, it is clear that the world of long-term services will continue to rely on care managers to help consumers navigate the complex systems of care. That system is getting more complicated each day, as is the job of care manager.

Robert Applebaum and Anthony R. Bardo

Ackerly, D. C., & Grabowski, D. C. (2014). Post-acute care reform—beyond the ACA. *New England Journal of Medicine, 370*(8), 689–691.

Applebaum, R. A., Straker, J. K., & Geron, S. (2000). *Assessing satisfaction in health and long-term care: Practical approaches to hearing the voices of consumers.* New York, NY: Springer.

Arling, G., Kane, R. L., Cooke, V., & Lewis, T. (2010). Targeting residents for transitions from nursing home to community. *Health Services Research, 45*(3), 691–711.

Bardo, A. R., Applebaum, R. A., Kunkel, S. R., & Carpio, E. A. (2013). Everyone's talking about it, but does it work? Nursing home diversion and transition. *Journal of Applied Gerontology, 33*(2), 205–224.

Barman-Adhikari, A., & Rice, E. (2014). Social networks as the context for understanding employment services utilization among homeless youth. *Evaluation and Program Planning, 45*, 90–101.

Chinman, M., Oberman, R. S., Hanusa, B. H., Cohen, A. N., Salyers, M. P., Twamley, E. W., & Young, A. S. (2015). A cluster randomized trial of adding peer specialists to intensive case management teams in the Veterans Health Administration. *Journal of Behavioral Health Services & Research, 42*(1), 109–121.

Dauber, S., Neighbors, C., Dasaro, C., Riordan, A., & Morgenstern, J. (2012). Impact of intensive case management on child welfare system involvement for substance-dependent parenting women on public assistance. *Children and Youth Services Review, 34*, 1359–1366.

Davies, B., & Challis, D. (1986). *Matching resources to needs in community care*. Aldershot, UK: Gower.

De Milto, L. (2015). *Cash & Counseling: This national program introduced or expanded participant-directed personal assistance services in Medicaid*. Princeton, NJ: Robert Wood Johnson Foundation.

Eiken, S., Sredl, K., Burwell, B., & Saucier, P. (2016). *Medicaid long-term services and supports (LTSS) in FY 2014*. Bethesda, MD: Truven Health Analytics.

Kemper, P., Applebaum, R. A., & Harrigan, A. (1987). Community care demonstrations: What have we learned? *Health Care Financing Administration Review, 8*(4), 87–100.

McDonald, D., & Arlinghaus, S. L. (2014). The role of intensive case management services in reentry: The northern Kentucky female offender reentry project. *Women & Criminal Justice, 24*(3), 229–251.

Moxley, D. (1989). *The practice of case management*. Newbury Park, CA: Sage.

Olmstead v. L.C., 527 U.S. 581 (1999).

Rapp, R. C., Noortgate, W. V. D., Broekaert, E., & Vanderplasschen, W. (2014). The efficacy of case management with persons who have substance abuse problems: A three-level meta-analysis of outcomes. *Journal of Consulting and Clinical Psychology, 82*(4), 605–618.

Reilly, S., Hughes, J., & Challis, D. (2010). Case management for long-term conditions: Implementation and processes. *Ageing & Society, 30*, 125–155.

Stone, R. (2011). *Long-term care for the elderly*. Washington, DC: Urban Institute Press.

Watts, M. O., Reaves, E. L., & Musumeci, M. (2015). *Money follows the person: A 2015 state survey of transitions, services, and costs*. Washington, DC: The Henry J. Kaiser Family Foundation.

CAREGIVER BURDEN

In 2015, an estimated 34.2 million Americans cared for loved ones or friends aged 50 years and older (National Alliance for Caregiving [NAC] & AARP, 2015). Unpaid family or informal caregivers, most often female partners/wives or adult children, provide support and assistance to community-dwelling older adults in activities of daily living (ADL), IADL, or medical tasks (Family Caregiver Alliance, 2017). Family caregivers provide approximately 37 billion hours of care each year, averaging 18 hr/wk in 2013. With an estimated economic value of $470 billion (Reinhard et al., 2015), spending on informal caregiving has surpassed the costs of formal home and institutional long-term care (Arno, Levine, & Memmott, 1999).

A preponderance of research over the past 40 years supports the negative physiological, behavioral, and psychosocial effects of family caregiving, which exposes caregivers to chronic stress, often for extended periods (Adelman, Tmanova, Delgado, Dion, & Lachs, 2014; Bevans & Sternberg, 2012; Pinquart & Sörensen, 2007). Although family caregiving is often associated with personal fulfillment and satisfaction, self-efficacy, and other rewards (Kramer, 1997; Zarit, 2012), caregivers experience significantly higher rates of cardiovascular disease, hypertension, social isolation, and depression and face greater mortality risks (NAC & AARP, 2015; Schulz & Beach, 1999) than non-caregiving peers. The negative health and mental health effects of caregiving thus pose a critical public health concern as the population of older adults needing assistance grows.

Caring for loved ones and family members demands a wide range of coping skills and the ability to manage multiple tasks, responsibilities, interpersonal challenges, and adaptations, often for many years. Caregivers must often balance the evolving needs of the care recipient with their own health and mental health needs and with concurrent role demands (i.e., work or other caregiving responsibilities) while navigating a fragmented, complex system of health and social care resources on behalf of care recipients. As the health care system continues to shift from hospital-based to ambulatory and community-based care, the needs of an aging population with multiple chronic conditions have progressively increased the burden of care on families. Moreover, informal caregivers are increasingly responsible for providing complex medical care (e.g., infusions, wound care) that were in the past provided by formal providers (NAC & AARP, 2015; Reinhard, Levine, & Samis, 2012).

Gerontologists use the term *caregiver strain* to describe the adverse perceptions or emotions (e.g., anxiety, frustration, helplessness) that people experience as a result of significant caregiving demands. *Caregiver burden* refers to

C

the negative impact on emotional and physical health that occurs when care demands exceed the caregiver's ability to cope or access support (Elliott, Burgio, & Decoster, 2010). Caregiver perceptions and coping skills and care recipient characteristics such as psychoneurobehavioral difficulties (e.g., agitation, confusion) and ability to perform ADL are common determinants of level of caregiver burden (Hughes et al., 2014; Pearlin, Mullan, Semple, & Skaff, 1990; Pinquart & Sörensen, 2007).

Much of the empirical literature on informal caregiving focuses on providing care to older adults with dementia, a role that is highly associated with caregiver burden (Cheng, 2017; Cooper, Balamurali, & Livingston, 2007; Torti, Gwyther, Reed, Friedman, & Schulman, 2004). Other caregivers particularly vulnerable to burden include those whose loved ones have cancer (Kim & Schulz, 2008; Raveis, Karus, & Siegel, 1998); those who have illnesses associated with stigma, such as AIDS and mental illness (Bevans & Sternberg, 2012); and those from rural areas or regions with little access to caregiving resources (Perrin et al., 2013).

ASSESSMENT

Identifying individuals vulnerable to caregiver burden can be difficult because each person and each caregiving context is different (NAC & AARP, 2015). To determine whether caregiver burden is an issue, health care professionals should assess for (a) background or contextual factors, (b) primary and secondary stressors, (c) mediators of stressors to outcomes, and (d) caregiving outcomes. Background and contextual factors include race/ethnicity, cultural justifications for caregiving, socioeconomic status (education, income, purchasing power), gender, age, familial relationship of caregiver to care recipient, past quality of relationship, geographic distance between the caregiver and care recipient, and quantity and quality of community resources.

Understanding the cultural meaning of caregiving for individuals and families is important because culture influences expectations and perceptions among caregivers and care recipients, caregiving demands, coping responses,

outcomes of caregiving, and acceptable interventions (Cox, 1999; Dilworth-Anderson et al., 2005). Female caregivers or caregivers of African (Dilworth-Anderson et al., 2005), Asian (Kong, 2007), Native American, or Hispanic descent have been found to express stronger cultural justifications for caregiving than Whites and men (Jervis & Manson, 2002). Thus their caregivers express more guilt—and their care recipients, more disappointment—when these expectations are unmet (Dong, Chang, Wong, Wong, & Simon, 2011). In addition, the size of caregiving networks and tendency to include extended family members and neighbors in caregiving also vary as a function of the levels of individualism or collectivism in the caregivers' ethnic group, with African American, American Indian, and Hispanic caregivers involving more family and nonfamily members in care than Whites (Dilworth-Anderson, Williams, & Gibson, 2002; Jervis & Manson, 2002). Also, despite commonalities among caregivers within these ethnic groups, there is still heterogeneity among the socioeconomic statuses within each ethnic group, greatly affecting access to interventions.

Primary stressors originate from the functional and behavioral challenges of the care recipient (Perrin, Heesacker, Stidham, Rittman, & Gonzalez-Rothi, 2008). Particular attention must be given to the number, duration, frequency, and unrelenting nature of care demands. Care demands can be quickly assessed using a standard measure of the care recipient's physical ADL such as the Katz Index of Independence in Activities of Daily Living (Katz, 1983) or instrumental activities of daily living (IADL) such as the Lawton Instrumental Activities of Daily Living (Lawton, & Brody, 1969). Researchers and health care professionals with more time for assessment may want to use the Resources for Enhancing Alzheimer's Caregiver Health (REACH) II study modification of these two measures and assess the care recipient's need of caregiver help and associated caregiver burden (i.e., bother or upset; Gitlin et al., 2005). The Revised Memory and Behavior Problems Checklist (Teri et al., 1992) can be used to assess the range of behavioral problems exhibited by patients with dementia and without nondementia living in private homes and the corresponding responses of caregivers. Researchers who study Native Americans express concern regarding the lack of culturally relevant measures to assess both care recipient and caregiver (Goins et al., 2011; Jervis & Manson, 2002). Nevertheless, American Indians tend to have many of the chronic diseases of other ethnic minority groups, especially diabetes, liver disease, and mental illness. The lack of culturally relevant measures makes dementia assessment challenging.

Secondary stressors consist of role and intrapsychic strains. Caregiver role strains often arise from other competing roles within the context of the family (e.g., spouse, parent, employee/breadwinner). Using knowledge of the disease and associated diagnostic and treatment trajectories, health professionals must anticipate periods of increased care demands and intrapsychic strains. Intrapsychic strains include lowered perceptions of mastery, gain, and self-esteem. Caregivers who have competing roles; who are young, female, and White; and who perceive intrapsychic strains with little knowledge of the condition contributing to the care recipient's disability appear to be most at risk for caregiver burden and declining health resulting from secondary stressors. Social isolation accentuates caregiver burden and depression, placing the care recipient at risk for mistreatment and elder abuse (Dong et al., 2011; Jervis & Manson, 2002). Thus health care professionals must assess the extent of the caregiver's social and recreational activities.

Mediators of stress outcomes include coping and social support. The coping measure suggested by Pearlin et al. (1990) offers strategies related to the meaning of the caregiving situation and management of stress. In assessing social support, it is crucial to avoid assuming that the availability or size of a social support network translates into caregiver satisfaction and therefore the absence of burden. Depending on the social support quality and effectiveness of coping strategies, caregivers may experience varying effects on their health. One very important form of social support is the quality of family functioning, which has been shown to be a very powerful buffer of the

influence of care recipient deficits on caregiver burden, especially among Hispanic caregivers (Coy et al., 2013).

Global assessment of the caregiver's self-perceived health—physical, mental, social, and spiritual—can be assessed with the Caregiver Strain Index (Robinson, 1983). As care demands change, health care professionals should periodically reassess the caregiver's health status. Global assessment of the self-perceived health of caregivers compared with their peers' health is important. Also important is attention to chronic stress indicators, such as increasing hair and salivary cortisol, blood pressure, blood glucose, and compromised immune system responses. Also important is increased doctor visits, medication use, and substance abuse. Measures that include symptoms of specific organ systems (e.g., respiratory, cardiovascular), such as the Cornell Medical Index, help health care professionals target specific areas for monitoring and intervention.

Mental health evaluations should include symptoms of stress with the Perceived Stress Scale (Cohen, Kamarck, & Mermelstein, 1983). However, symptoms lasting at least 2 weeks may suggest depression; these include low or irritable mood; feelings of worthlessness, self-reproach, or excessive guilt; suicidal thinking or attempts; motor retardation, agitation, or disturbed sleep; fatigue and loss of energy; loss of interest or pleasure in usual activities; difficulty focusing; and changes in appetite or weight. The most commonly used community measure of depression is The Center for Epidemiologic Studies Depression Scale (Radloff, 1977).

The social health of the caregiver can be evaluated by asking who is available and reliable, in the caregiver's social support network, to provide respite, empathic listening, help with care tasks, or resources (Pearlin et al., 1990). Social support, social engagement, and spiritual health can help buffer the development of other adverse health consequences for caregivers. Spiritual distress can occur when caregivers are unable to leave the home, or the caregiving situation and the care recipient's suffering challenge their spiritual beliefs (Picot, Debanne, Namazi, & Wykle, 1997). In addition to the role and importance of spirituality in

C

C

their lives, questions about caregivers' ability to attend religious services, receive visits from fellow parishioners or clergy, and have time for contemplation or prayer help gauge spiritual health. After identifying caregivers at risk for stress, burden, and health problems, health care professionals should identify and link the caregiver with community services and resources to assist with providing care to the care recipient, reducing caregiver stress and burden, and promoting health in the caregiver–care recipient dyad.

SUPPORTS AND INTERVENTIONS

Although many psychosocial interventions for caregivers have been conducted irrespective of caregivers' ethnic backgrounds, a growing body of research supports the importance of health care professionals performing these interventions in a culturally sensitive manner. For example, a telehealth intervention for Hispanic stroke caregivers encompassing caregiver skill development, education about the mental health effects of being a caregiver, and problem-solving training reduced caregiver strain (Perrin et al., 2010). Also, a telephone-based, cognitive behavioral therapy intervention for African American caregivers who care for those with dementia and who have depression was found to be equally effective as face-to-face interventions in reducing caregiver burden and depression (Glueckauf et al., 2012). Telehealth interventions like these overcome obstacles such as transportation to health care facilities and may be more culturally concordant, given that caregivers remain in their own home and community when participating in the intervention. In addition, given that greater numbers of family members within the same family take on the caregiving role in some ethnic groups, interventions may be needed by more than just the primary caregiver.

Caregivers may benefit from assistance in identifying and coordinating acceptable family and professional care providers and in planning for anticipated changes, including transferring care of the care recipient to others. Caregivers may also need support or counseling to accept that transferring care responsibilities can have positive consequences for both the caregiver and care recipient (Fink & Picot, 1995). Even though American Indian caregivers prefer to care for their care recipients in the home, few culturally competent, acceptable, or affordable community resources exist for them. Despite some inconsistency in the literature, psychosocial interventions (e.g., counseling, problem solving) have been shown to promote effectively healthy changes in caregiver mastery, stress, burden, and depression levels (Brodaty, Green, & Koschera, 2003; Sörensen, Pinquart, & Duberstein, 2002).

Caregivers who are experiencing burden often do not seek assistance for themselves while accompanying care recipients during health care visits, and health care professionals rarely inquire about their health status and concerns. Providers may not recognize the distinct needs of caregivers or refer them to culturally acceptable or feasible resources (Dilworth-Anderson et al., 2005). Thus caregivers are often referred to as the *hidden* or *secondary patients*. To address caregiver burden, health care professionals must be empathic listeners and prepared referral sources as they conduct careful assessments of caregivers' backgrounds, stressors, mediators, and outcomes. Effective strategies for avoiding or minimizing caregiver burden should be planned with the caregiver and care recipient (when feasible) and should be responsive to each caregiver's unique situation.

See also Caregiver Burnout; Caregiving Relationships; Cultural Competence and Aging.

Daniel S. Gardner

Adelman, R. D., Tmanova, L. L., Delgado, D., Dion, S., & Lachs, M. S. (2014). Caregiver burden: A clinical review. *Journal of the American Medical Association, 311*(10), 1052–1060.

Arno, P. S., Levine, C., & Memmott, M. M. (1999). The economic value of informal caregiving. *Health Affairs, 18*(2), 182–188.

Bevans, M., & Sternberg, E. M. (2012). Caregiving burden, stress, and health effects among family caregivers of adult cancer patients. *Journal of the American Medical Association, 307*(4), 398–403.

Brodaty, H., Green, A., & Koschera, A. (2003). Meta-analysis of psychosocial interventions for caregivers of people with dementia. *Journal of the American Geriatrics Society, 51*(5), 657–664.

Cheng, S. T. (2017). Dementia caregiver burden: A research update and critical analysis. *Current Psychiatry Reports, 19*(9), 64.

Cohen, S., Kamarck, T., & Mermelstein, R. (1983). A global measure of perceived stress. *Journal of Health and Social Behavior, 24*(4), 385–396.

Cooper, C., Balamurali, T. B., & Livingston, G. (2007). A systematic review of the prevalence and covariates of anxiety in caregivers of people with dementia. *International Psychogeriatrics, 19*(2), 175–195.

Cox, C. (1999). Race and caregiving: Patterns of service use by African American and White caregivers of persons with Alzheimer's disease. *Journal of Gerontological Social Work, 32*(2), 5–19.

Coy, A. E., Perrin, P. B., Stevens, L. F., Hubbard, R., Díaz Sosa, D. M., Espinosa Jove, I. G., & Arango-Lasprilla, J. C. (2013). Moderated mediation path analysis of Mexican traumatic brain injury patient social functioning, family functioning, and caregiver mental health. *Archives of Physical Medicine and Rehabilitation, 94*(2), 362–368.

Dilworth-Anderson, P., Brummett, B. H., Goodwin, P., Williams, S. W., Williams, R. B., & Siegler, I. C. (2005). Effect of race on cultural justifications for caregiving. *Journals of Gerontology. Series B, Psychological Sciences and Social Sciences, 60*(5), S257–S262.

Dilworth-Anderson, P., Williams, I. C., & Gibson, B. E. (2002). Issues of race, ethnicity, and culture in caregiving research: A 20-year review (1980–2000). *The Gerontologist, 42*(2), 237–272.

Dong, X., Chang, E. S., Wong, E., Wong, B., & Simon, M. A. (2011). How do U.S. Chinese older adults view elder mistreatment? Findings from a community-based participatory research study. *Journal of Aging and Health, 23*(2), 289–312.

Elliott, A. F., Burgio, L. D., & Decoster, J. (2010). Enhancing caregiver health: Findings from the resources for enhancing Alzheimer's caregiver health II intervention. *Journal of the American Geriatrics Society, 58*(1), 30–37.

Family Caregiver Alliance. (2017). *Caregiver statistics: Demographics.* National Center on Caregiving. Retrieved from https://www.caregiver.org/caregiver-statistics-demographics

Fink, S. V., & Picot, S. F. (1995). Nursing home placement decisions and post-placement experiences of African-American and European-American caregivers. *Journal of Gerontological Nursing, 21*(12), 35–42.

Gitlin, L. N., Roth, D. L., Burgio, L. D., Loewenstein, D. A., Winter, L., Nichols, L., … Martindale, J.

(2005). Caregiver appraisals of functional dependence in individuals with dementia and associated caregiver upset: Psychometric properties of a new scale and response patterns by caregiver and care recipient characteristics. *Journal of Aging and Health, 17*(2), 148–171.

Glueckauf, R. L., Davis, W. S., Willis, F., Sharma, D., Gustafson, D. J., Hayes, J., … Springer, J. (2012). Telephone-based, cognitive-behavioral therapy for African American dementia caregivers with depression: Initial findings. *Rehabilitation Psychology, 57*(2), 124–139.

Goins, R. T., Spencer, S. M., McGuire, L. C., Goldberg, J., Wen, Y., & Henderson, J. A. (2011). Adult caregiving among American Indians: The role of cultural factors. *The Gerontologist, 51*(3), 310–320.

Hughes, T. B., Black, B. S., Albert, M., Gitlin, L. N., Johnson, D. M., Lyketsos, C. G., & Samus, Q. M. (2014). Correlates of objective and subjective measures of caregiver burden among dementia caregivers: Influence of unmet patient and caregiver dementia-related care needs. *International Psychogeriatrics, 26*(11), 1875–1883.

Jervis, L. L., & Manson, S. M. (2002). American Indians/Alaska natives and dementia. *Alzheimer Disease and Associated Disorders, 16*(Suppl. 2), S89–S95.

Katz, S. (1983). Assessing self-maintenance: Activities of daily living, mobility, and instrumental activities of daily living. *Journal of the American Geriatrics Society, 31*(12), 721–727.

Kim, Y., & Schulz, R. (2008). Family caregivers' strains: Comparative analysis of cancer caregiving with dementia, diabetes, and frail elderly caregiving. *Journal of Aging and Health, 20*(5), 483–503.

Kong, E. H. (2007). The influence of culture on the experiences of Korean, Korean American, and Caucasian-American family caregivers of frail older adults: A literature review. *Taehan Kanho Hakhoe chi, 37*(2), 213–220.

Kramer, B. J. (1997). Gain in the caregiving experience: Where are we? What next? *The Gerontologist, 37*(2), 218–232.

Lawton, M. P., & Brody, E. M. (1969). Assessment of older people: Self-maintaining and instrumental activities of daily living. *The Gerontologist, 9*(3), 179–186.

National Alliance for Caregiving & AARP. (2015). *Caregiving in the U.S.* Washington, DC: Authors.

Pearlin, L. I., Mullan, J. T., Semple, S. J., & Skaff, M. M. (1990). Caregiving and the stress process: An overview of concepts and their measures. *The Gerontologist, 30*(5), 583–594.

Perrin, P. B., Heesacker, M., Stidham, B. S., Rittman, M. R., & Gonzalez-Rothi, L. J. (2008). Structural equation modeling of the relationship between caregiver psychosocial variables and functioning of individuals with stroke. *Rehabilitation Psychology, 53,* 54–62.

Perrin, P. B., Johnston, A., Vogel, B., Heesacker, M., Vega-Trujillo, M., Anderson, J., & Rittman, M. (2010). A culturally sensitive Transition Assistance Program for stroke caregivers: Examining caregiver mental health and stroke rehabilitation. *Journal of Rehabilitation Research and Development, 47*(7), 605–617.

Perrin, P. B., Stevens, L. F., Villaseñor Cabrera, T., Jimenez-Maldonado, M., Martinez-Cortes, M. L., & Arango-Lasprilla, J. C. (2013). Just how bad is it? Comparison of the mental health of Mexican traumatic brain injury caregivers to age-matched healthy controls. *NeuroRehabilitation, 32*(3), 679–686.

Picot, S. J., Debanne, S. M., Namazi, K. H., & Wykle, M. L. (1997). Religiosity and perceived rewards of black and white caregivers. *The Gerontologist, 37*(1), 89–101.

Pinquart, M., & Sörensen, S. (2007). Correlates of physical health of informal caregivers: A meta-analysis. *Journals of Gerontology. Series B, Psychological Sciences and Social Sciences, 62*(2), P126–P137.

Radloff, L. S. (1977). The CES-D scale: A self-report depression scale for research in the general population. *Applied Psychological Measurement, 1,* 385–401.

Raveis, V. H., Karus, D. G., & Siegel, K. (1998). Correlates of depressive symptomatology among adult daughter caregivers of a parent with cancer. *Cancer, 83*(8), 1652–1663.

Reinhard, S. C., Feinberg, L. F., Choula, R., & Houser, A. (2015). Valuing the invaluable: 2015 update. *Insight on the Issues, 104,* 1–25. Retrieved from http://www.aarp.org/content/dam/aarp/ppi/2015/valuing-the-invaluable-2015-update-new.pdf.

Reinhard, S. C., Levine, C., & Samis, S. (2012). *Home alone: Family caregivers providing complex chronic care.* Washington, DC: AARP Public Policy Institute.

Robinson, B. C. (1983). Validation of a Caregiver Strain Index. *Journal of Gerontology, 38*(3), 344–348.

Schulz, R., & Beach, S. R. (1999). Caregiving as a risk factor for mortality: The Caregiver Health Effects Study. *Journal of the American Medical Association, 282*(23), 2216–2219.

Sörensen, S., Pinquart, M., & Duberstein, P. (2002). How effective are interventions with caregivers? An updated meta-analysis. *The Gerontologist, 42*(3), 356–372.

Teri, L., Truax, P., Logsdon, R., Uomoto, J., Zarit, S., & Vitaliano, P. P. (1992). Assessment of behavioral problems in dementia: The revised memory and behavior problems checklist. *Psychology and Aging, 7*(4), 622–631.

Torti, F. M., Gwyther, L. P., Reed, S. D., Friedman, J. Y., & Schulman, K. A. (2004). A multinational review of recent trends and reports in dementia caregiver burden. *Alzheimer Disease and Associated Disorders, 18*(2), 99–109.

Zarit, S. H. (2012). Positive aspects of caregiving: More than looking on the bright side. *Aging & Mental Health, 16*(6), 673–674.

Web Resources
AARP: Caregiving Resource Center: http://www.aarp.org/home-family/caregiving/?intcmp=HP-BANNERD

AARP: Health and Wellness and Explore Health: http://www.aarp.org/indexes/health.html#caregiving

American Psychological Association Assessment Instruments for Caregivers: http://www.apa.org/pi/about/publications/caregivers/practice-settings/assessment/tools/index.aspx

Family Caregiver Alliance: National Center on Caregiving: http://www.caregiver.org/caregiver/jsp/home.jsp

National Caregiver Support Program: http://www.aoa.gov/prof/aoaprog/caregiver/caregiver.asp

National Family Caregivers' Association: http://www.nfcacares.org/about_nfca

USA Government: Caregiver Resources: http://www.usa.gov/Citizen/Topics/Health/caregivers.shtml

CAREGIVER BURNOUT

Burnout is a multifaceted syndrome that develops gradually over time and manifests with physical, mental, and emotional exhaustion (Maslach & Leiter, 2016; Schaufeli, Leiter, & Maslach, 2009). Equated with the extinguishing of a candle, *burnout* implies a draining of energy related to the demands of one's work. Originally thought to only affect those working in human services, it is now known to affect people in all walks of life (Schaufeli et al., 2009). When associated with work that involves caring for people, it is frequently referred to as caregiver burnout. Teachers, police officers, social workers, mental health workers, health care professionals, and informal caregivers may develop burnout over time. For all instances of caregiver burnout, whether it is related to professional or informal caregiving, the demanding nature of caring for others—physical, mental, and emotional—plays a part in its development.

Burnout results in widespread apathy; the caregiver develops a disinterest in work and relationships that ultimately affects quality of life (Todaro-Franceschi, 2013). In the past decade, it has become evident that burnout is a global issue in the caring professions (Todaro-Franceschi, 2013). In various European countries, burnout is an established medical diagnosis (Schaufeli et al., 2009).

INFORMAL CAREGIVER BURNOUT

Informal caregivers, usually loved ones or family members who routinely care for chronically ill, disabled, or elderly persons are at risk for burnout related to caregiver burden or stress (Kim, Chang, Rose, & Kim, 2012). Because of increasing longevity, it is expected that more family members will find themselves in the role of caregiver for aging loved ones. People are not only living longer, but are also living with chronic illnesses. The complexity of care needed for those who are chronically ill, often with more than one condition, puts additional burden on informal caregivers. For instance, evidence suggests that caregivers of loved ones with cancer or dementia are at increased risk for negative health consequences associated with their caring work (Kim, Carver, Shaffer, Gansler, & Cannady, 2015; Lilly, Robinson, Holtzman, & Bottorff, 2012).

The functional status of the caregiver, who is often an older adult, as well as the functional status of the care-recipient, also plays a part in caregiver burden. Elderly abuse, diminished social life, poor health, and lack of positive outlook on caring, along with depression, have been shown to be associated with caregiver burden (Cooper, Blanchard, Selwood, Walker, & Livingston, 2010). However, burden alone is

not sufficient for predicting whether someone will develop burnout or whether negative consequences will ensue. Other variables, such as one's relationship with the person being cared for, feelings about caregiving, and perception regarding being adequately supported to provide the care, are all important factors (Cooper et al., 2010).

PROFESSIONAL CAREGIVER BURNOUT

In the caring professions, workforce issues, such as heavy case load, staffing mix, inadequate communication among staff, insufficient resources, poor leadership, and less than optimal physical working environments can contribute to the development of burnout (Todaro-Franceschi, 2013). A related syndrome is compassion fatigue (sometimes referred to as *secondary traumatic stress*) in which caregivers co-suffer with the people they are caring for and internalize the anguish to such a degree that it affects their own quality of life (Todaro-Franceschi, 2013). Compassion fatigue is sudden in onset and is often not recognized by the caregiver; thus it may continue for a time and, if not adequately addressed, can spiral into burnout, which is known to develop gradually and is more difficult to heal without intervention.

Another issue that can add to the development of compassion fatigue and burnout in the health care professions is a lack of preparedness to care for the dying and their loved ones (Todaro-Franceschi, 2013). Professional caregivers may feel compelled to cure at all costs and when they are unable to do so, it results in dissatisfaction with their work.

Manifestations

With an imbalance of demand and resources, along with the fact that the ideal and the real regularly differ significantly, burned-out people often feel hopeless to create change, so over time, they flick a shutoff switch (Todaro-Franceschi, 2013). Three core dimensions of burnout have been identified: (a) an overwhelming feeling of exhaustion, (b) feelings of cynicism and detachment from the job, and (c) a sense of ineffectiveness and lack of accomplishment (Maslach &

Leiter, 2016; Schaufeli et al., 2009). Thus burnout manifests in negative ways that not only are detrimental to the caregiver, but also affect the quality of care provided to others. Some of the things to look for include feeling overwhelmed, fatigued, listless, ineffectual, angry, anxious, and depressed and distancing oneself from things one normally enjoys.

Burnout often impairs the control and coping mechanisms used to regulate emotional expression. Burned-out caregivers may turn away from their depression, anger, and/or anxiety by using alcohol and drugs (Todaro-Franceschi, 2013). They tend to isolate themselves rather than interact with others. Although burnout appears to be a defense mechanism of sorts, similar to the flight-or-fight response, all aspects of one's life may be negatively affected if measures are not taken to heal from burnout.

Healing Interventions

Caregivers can do many things to heal from burnout, but first, they need to be able to acknowledge that there is a problem. Anyone involved with caring for others should be aware of the physical and psychological signals indicating that some kind of intervention is needed. It can be very rewarding to care for others, but to do it well, caregivers must first take care of themselves. It is also important to recognize that how one goes about providing care is crucial to the well-being of both caregivers and the individuals entrusted to their care.

Burnout develops over time, and it cannot be expected to go away without attention to changing life circumstances or perspectives. Key to healing from caregiver burnout is to realize that what one does, when caring for another, is meaningful and can make a difference.

Mindful Awareness and the ART Model

Mindful awareness (also known as *mindfulness*) is an ancient Buddhist practice, a form of meditation that entails being aware of how one is moving through life from moment to moment (Todaro-Franceschi, 2013). Focusing on the present and feeling at a specific time while going about caregiving can help in the recognition of trouble. A therapeutic model called ART, created to help those suffering from compassion fatigue and burnout, offers a framework for guiding mindful awareness (Todaro-Franceschi, 2013, 2015). ART is an acronym for Acknowledging feelings, Recognizing choices and choosing to take purposeful action, and Turning toward the self and others. ART is ongoing and steps may overlap.

To acknowledge that there is a problem, people must first work through how they are feeling while going about day-to-day caregiving activities. Journaling or speaking with friends, family, or a counselor can be helpful. It is also necessary to identify negative coping behaviors such as overeating, increased alcohol intake, or drug use—all indicative of turning away from problems rather than facing them and addressing them in a healthy way.

The second step of ART is the *recognition* that a person always has choices and then, after identifying what choices are available, choosing actions that reaffirm purpose. Our lives are full of choices; not only do they shape the path of each person's present and future, but they also inform and transform the lives of others.

The third step of ART is *turning* toward the self and others, encouraging reconnection with the self and others. Once one is aware of negative feelings and coping behaviors, it is easier to see where to reconnect with positive, rather than negative, things—such as making time to appreciate what is here right now, finding the beauty and sometimes the humor in things (Todaro-Franceschi, 2013, 2015).

Coping Strategies

Relaxation techniques such as breathing exercises, meditation, and yoga are useful for achieving a feeling of well-being. Making some time for oneself every day, seeing the things one might not normally notice, can lift spirits (Todaro-Franceschi, 2013). Connecting with friends, family, and nature on a regular basis can also help. Eating and sleeping well are important, and it is crucial to identify whether one needs help with addictive behaviors such as overeating, alcohol, or drug use.

Counseling therapy for either the individual or the family can assist the burned-out caregiver to find ways to renew well-being. Individual therapy may be warranted for anger and depression. Family therapy that focuses on context, relationships, and meaning can be helpful. Family members can be guided by therapists to explore their resources and draw on the strengths of their relationships. Therapists can also help facilitate better communication among family members and create a context in which family members gain a different perspective of themselves and their world.

Support Groups

In-person, online, and even telephone support groups can provide an opportunity to speak with others who are caregivers. Many people find solace by sharing feelings with others who understand the challenges of caregiving. For professional caregivers, there are many workshops and programs on compassion fatigue and burnout, along with a growing body of literature on the subject.

Resources

For informal caregivers who are feeling overwhelmed, there are resources to help with caregiving, such as home and adult day care, nursing homes, and assisted living. Local houses of worship may also have volunteer services to assist with tasks associated with caregiving. Other information can be found through local agencies on aging and the health department.

Caregiver's Bill of Rights

According to the Family Caregiver Alliance's Caregiver's Bill of Rights, caregivers have the right to seek information about providing better caregiving activities as well as to protect their own quality of life. Advocating for caregivers' rights from the beginning and bringing awareness of the need for taking care of oneself, and getting adequate support to ensure that one can do so, can prevent burnout and encourage effective caregiving.

See also Caregiving Relationships; Elder Mistreatment: Overview; Elder Neglect; Support Groups.

Vidette Todaro-Franceschi

Cooper, C., Blanchard, M., Selwood, A., Walker, Z., & Livingston, G. (2010). Family carers' distress and abusive behavior: Longitudinal study. *British Journal of Psychiatry, 196*(6), 480–485.

Kim, Y., Carver, C. S., Shaffer, K. M., Gansler, T., & Cannady, R. S. (2015). Cancer caregiving predicts physical impairments: Roles of earlier caregiving stress and being a spousal caregiver. *Cancer, 121*(2), 302–310.

Kim, H., Chang, M., Rose, K., & Kim, S. (2012). Predictors of caregiver burden in caregivers of individuals with dementia. *Journal of Advanced Nursing, 68*(4), 846–855.

Lilly, M. B., Robinson, C. A., Holtzman, S., & Bottorff, J. L. (2012). Can we move beyond burden and burnout to support the health and wellness of family caregivers to persons with dementia? Evidence from British Columbia. *Health and Social Care in the Community, 20*(1), 103–112.

Maslach, C., & Leiter, M. P. (2016). Understanding the burnout experience: Recent research and its implications for psychiatry. *World Psychiatry, 15,* 103–111.

Schaufeli, W. B., Leiter, M. P., & Maslach, C. (2009). Burnout: 35 years of research and practice. *Career Development International, 14*(3), 204–220.

Todaro-Franceschi, V. (2013). *Compassion fatigue and burnout in nursing: Enhancing professional quality of life.* New York, NY: Springer Publishing.

Todaro-Franceschi, V. (2015). The ART of maintaining the "care" in healthcare. *Nursing Management, 46*(6), 53–55.

Web Resources
AARP Caregiver Resource Center: http://www.aarp.org/home-family/caregiving
Caregiver Action Network: http://caregiveraction.org
Compassion Fatigue Awareness Project: http://www.compassionfatigue.org
Family Caregiver Alliance: http://www.caregiver.org/caregiver/jsp/home.jsp
Figley Institute: http://www.figleyinstitute.com
National Alliance for Caregiving: http://www.caregiving.org
Quality Caring: http://www.qualitycaring.org

C

CAREGIVER SUPPORT GROUPS

Caregiver support groups are an important source of information, guidance, and peer support for adults who provide assistance to frail or disabled older relatives or friends. Support groups provide social support and emotional reassurance, education about illnesses and disability, strategies for coping with the physical and emotional demands of providing care, and information about community services for older adults and their caregivers. Typically provided by social service agencies or disease-specific organizations, support groups can be led by peers, paraprofessionals, or professionals such as social workers or psychologists, depending on the goals and structure of the group. Caregiver support groups can be divided into two major types: (a) mutual support and (b) psychoeducational groups, although groups typically combine aspects of both.

Support groups are one of the basic services authorized under the National Family Caregiver Support Program (NFCSP), established in 2001 as Title III-E of the reauthorized Older Americans Act. Surveys indicate that approximately 10% of caregivers participate in support groups. Support group participation is most likely among caregivers who are older, more highly educated, have higher incomes, and provide assistance to care recipients with the greatest physical or cognitive disabilities (Alzheimer's Association & National Alliance for Caregiving, 2004; Scharlach et al., 2003).

MUTUAL SUPPORT GROUPS

Mutual support groups provide a supportive and understanding context within which caregivers can discuss common concerns about providing assistance to an impaired family member or friend. The primary focus is on the development of a social support network within which participants can give and receive emotional support, exchange proven strategies for managing elder care, and share concrete information about community resources (Chien, 2010; Sörensen, Pinquart, & Duberstein, 2002; Toseland & Smith,

2001). Mutual support groups tend to have less structure than psychoeducational groups: Content typically is determined on an ad hoc basis at each group meeting; leaders may be peers or paraprofessionals; membership often is flexible, with participants attending as desired; and groups typically are ongoing, frequently lasting for months or years.

PSYCHOEDUCATIONAL GROUPS

Psychoeducational groups involve a structured program aimed at improving participant knowledge and skills to cope more effectively with care-related stresses and provide better care to elderly care recipients. Psychoeducational groups frequently focus on enhancing a particular caregiver skill, such as managing care recipient problem behaviors, coping with perceived stress, or improving interpersonal relations. Group leaders, for example, may educate caregivers about empowerment techniques, teach specific coping strategies and relaxation techniques, or offer behavioral strategies for increasing participants' positive affective experiences between group meetings.

Psychoeducational groups tend to be more structured than mutual support groups: Content is predetermined in accordance with a conceptually based curriculum outline; leaders almost always are professionals trained in particular psychoeducational techniques; membership is fixed, with members expected to attend every session if possible; and groups typically are time limited. One type of psychoeducational group, for example, uses cognitive behavioral principles to train caregivers in depression and anger management using highly structured 2-hour workshops (Coon, Thompson, Steffen, Sorocco, & Gallagher-Thompson, 2003). Each session begins with a review of homework assigned during the previous meeting, followed by a 20- to 30-minute lecture on a specific skill. The didactic part of anger-management sessions might focus on recognizing thoughts that lead to feelings of frustration, whereas depression-management sessions might teach participants about the relationship between pleasant events and mood. The rest of each group session is then spent personalizing the specific skills for group participants through discussion, practice, and homework exercises. Another type of psychoeducational caregiver group, designed for caregivers of persons with early stage memory loss and conducted by volunteers trained by the Alzheimer's Association, involves weekly 90-minute structured sessions that provide information about treatment options, research, and coping mechanisms for caregivers dealing with loss, grief, and challenging behaviors (Logsdon et al., 2010). Caregivers and persons with early stage dementia meet together in the first part of each session and then meet separately during the rest of the session.

BENEFITS OF CAREGIVER SUPPORT GROUPS

Existing empirical evidence suggests that support groups can improve the well-being of both caregivers and care recipients. For caregivers, support groups can enhance problem-solving skills, decrease stresses related to caregiving, expand knowledge about available services, and improve social and psychological well-being (Chien et al., 2011; Logsdon et al., 2010; Signe & Elmståhl, 2008; Toseland & Smith, 2001). In addition, there is some evidence that caregiver support groups can delay nursing home placement of care recipients and decrease care recipients' use of other health care services (Mittelman, Haley, Clay, & Roth, 2006; Reinhard, Feinberg, Choula, & Houser, 2015). Despite the success of large-scale research on caregiver support interventions (Belle et al., 2006; Mittelman, Roth, Coon, & Haley, 2004), effect sizes reflected in the literature are generally small to moderate and depend on the particular type of support group being studied. Moreover, although group interventions are more effective at enhancing social support than are individual caregiver interventions, there is substantial evidence that individual counseling and case management may be more effective at improving caregiver well-being than support groups (Parker, Mills, & Abbey, 2008; Pinquart & Sörensen, 2006; Selwood, Johnston, Katona, Lyketsos, & Livingston, 2007).

Mutual support groups and psychoeducational groups generally have been found to effect distinct advantages for caregivers. Mutual support groups appear to be effective at enhancing social support, expanding social networks, and helping caregivers to reassess their interpretations of the caregiving situation, thereby potentially leading to more positive evaluations of their caregiving role. Psychoeducational groups demonstrate a greater impact on caregiver well-being, as measured by reduced emotional distress and depressive symptoms, increased self-efficacy, and more effective responses to care-recipient disruptive behaviors (Gallagher-Thompson et al., 2000; Signe & Elmståhl, 2008). Whereas psychoeducational interventions and mutual support groups both have been found to produce significant positive effects on caregiver burden and care-related knowledge and skills, only psychoeducational interventions also consistently produce gains in subjective well-being, decreases in self-rated depression, and reductions in care-recipient symptoms (Sörensen et al., 2002). Caregivers in psychoeducational groups experience a larger decline in depression, greater use of positive coping strategies, less use of negative coping strategies, and fewer negative social interactions than those in peer support groups. Psychoeducational groups also have been found to produce greater improvements in depression and psychological well-being than do purely educational groups (Chien et al., 2011). Research suggests that multicomponent intervention strategies, including respite care and resource referral for caregivers, are most likely to reduce burden and increase well-being in caregivers (Belle et al., 2006; Gallagher-Thompson & Coon, 2007).

CAREGIVER SUPPORT GROUPS AND RACE/ETHNICITY

Support group participation is higher for non-Hispanic White caregivers than for African American, Asian American, Native Hawaiian, Pacific Islander, or Hispanic caregivers (Chow, Auh, Scharlach, Lehning, & Goldstein, 2010). Differential participation rates have been attributed to a lack of personal contact by support group organizers, geographically inconvenient locations for group meetings, inconvenient scheduling, transportation barriers, lack of care for

C

recipients during group meetings, taboos against discussing problems in public groups, and reluctance to attend a group composed primarily of White caregivers (Bank, Argüelles, Rubert, Eisdorfer, & Czaja, 2006; Henderson, Gutierrez-Mayka, Garcia, & Boyd, 1993). Proactive efforts to overcome these barriers through targeted recruitment and culturally appropriate intervention strategies have shown substantial promise. Improved support group participation and outcomes among Latina caregivers, for example, can result from strategies such as recruiting participants at local senior centers serving Latino communities, creating advertisements printed in both Spanish and English, utilizing bilingual or bicultural group leaders, and adjusting group content to address cultural expectations. Hispanic caregivers, more so than non-Hispanic caregivers, consider sessions that teach caregiving skills to be the most helpful support service (Evercare, 2008); by including homework assignments and chalkboards, it is possible that Latino participants may view group participation as educational and avoid the cultural stigma associated with psychotherapy.

Evidence regarding the differential impact of support groups on caregivers from diverse racial/ethnic or socioeconomic groups is sparse, although there is some evidence that culturally appropriate psychoeducational groups can result in the same benefits for White and Latina female caregivers. There are few large, randomized, controlled trials of caregiver interventions with ethnically diverse participants (Schulz, Martire, & Klinger, 2005). Although relatively little is known about support group interventions for Asian American caregivers, a randomized controlled study of mutual support groups for caregivers of family members with dementia in Hong Kong revealed significant improvements in quality of life and distress levels (Wang, Chien, & Lee, 2012). A multicomponent psychosocial caregiver intervention that included telephone-based support groups in Spanish and English was found to reduce isolation and improve quality of life for Hispanic and White participants caring for persons with dementia (Bank et al., 2006). As with in-person support groups, participants valued the emotional support, social contact, and information provided

by other participants. This intervention was implemented at multiple sites, and results varied according to participants' ethnic and cultural backgrounds. Among African American participants, for example, these improvements were realized only for spousal caregivers. Further analysis revealed that the greatest benefit was experienced by older caregivers and those with low levels of religious coping, perhaps because younger caregivers had more access to information and those with high levels of religious coping had less need for alternative caregiving resources (Lee, Czaja, & Schulz, 2010). Findings such as these may have important implications for designing in-person, telephonic, and technology-assisted support groups that reflect the differential needs of caregivers from diverse backgrounds and populations.

Overall, support groups appear to provide caregivers with skills and social support that can increase their caregiving capabilities as well as their personal well-being. Additional research is needed to identify the particular components of support groups that might lead to the greatest benefits for particular groups of caregivers and care recipients. Furthermore, researchers and practitioners need to address racial/ethnic disparities in service utilization, designing caregiver support groups that reflect the differential needs and sensibilities of an increasingly diverse caregiver population.

See also Alzheimer's Association; Caregiver Burden; Caregiving Relationships; Support Groups.

Daniel S. Gardner

Alzheimer's Association, & National Alliance for Caregiving. (2004). *Families care: Alzheimer's caregiving in the United States.* Chicago, IL: Alzheimer's Association and Bethesda, MD: National Alliance for Caregiving.

Bank, A. L., Argüelles, S., Rubert, M., Eisdorfer, C., & Czaja, S. J. (2006). The value of telephone support groups among ethnically diverse caregivers of persons with dementia. *The Gerontologist, 46*(1), 134–138.

Belle, S. H., Burgio, L., Burns, R., Coon, D., Czaja, S. J., Gallagher-Thompson, D., ... Zhang, S.; Resources for Enhancing Alzheimer's Caregiver Health

(REACH) II Investigators. (2006). Enhancing the quality of life of dementia caregivers from different ethnic or racial groups: A randomized, controlled trial. *Annals of Internal Medicine, 145*(10), 727–738.

Chien, W. T. (2010). An overview of mutual support groups for family caregivers of people with mental health problems: Evidence on process and outcome. In L. D. Brown & S. Wituk (Eds.), *Mental health self-help: Consumer and family initiatives* (pp. 7–152). New York, NY: Springer.

Chien, L. Y., Chu, H., Guo, J. L., Liao, Y. M., Chang, L. I., Chen, C. H., & Chou, K. R. (2011). Caregiver support groups in patients with dementia: A meta-analysis. *International Journal of Geriatric Psychiatry, 26*(10), 1089–1098. doi:10.1002/gps.2660

Chow, J., Auh, E. Y., Scharlach, A. E., Lehning, A. J., & Goldstein, C. (2010). Types and sources of support received by family caregivers of older adults from diverse racial and ethnic groups. *Journal of Ethnic and Cultural Diversity in Social Work, 19*(3), 175–194.

Coon, D. W., Thompson, L., Steffen, A., Sorocco, K., & Gallagher-Thompson, D. (2003). Anger and depression management: Psychoeducational skill training interventions for women caregivers of a relative with dementia. *The Gerontologist, 43*(5), 678–689.

Evercare. (2008). Hispanic family caregiving in the U.S.: Findings from a national study. Evercare in collaboration with National Alliance for Caregiving. Retrieved from http://www.care giving.org/data/Hispanic_Caregiver_Study_ web_ENG_FINAL_11_04_08.pdf

Gallagher-Thompson, D., & Coon, D. W. (2007). Evidence-based psychological treatments for distress in family caregivers of older adults. *Psychology and Aging, 22*(1), 37–51. doi:10.1037/ 0882-7974.22.1.37

Gallagher-Thompson, D., Lovett, S., Rose, J., McKibbin, C., Coon, D., Futterman, A., & Thompson, L.W. (2000). Impact of psychoeducational interventions on distressed family caregivers. *Journal of Clinical Geropsychology, 6*, 91–110.

Henderson, J. N., Gutierrez-Mayka, M., Garcia, J., & Boyd, S. (1993). A model for Alzheimer's disease support group development in African-American and Hispanic populations. *The Gerontologist, 33*(3), 409–414.

Lee, C. C., Czaja, S. J., & Schulz, R. (2010). The moderating influence of demographic characteristics, social support, and religious coping on the effectiveness of a multicomponent psychosocial caregiver intervention in three racial ethnic groups.

Journals of Gerontology. Series B, Psychological Sciences and Social Sciences, 65B(2), 185–194. doi:10.1093/geronb/gbp131

Logsdon, R. G., Pike, K. C., McCurry, S. M., Hunter, P., Maher, J., Snyder, L., & Teri, L. (2010). Early-stage memory loss support groups: Outcomes from a randomized controlled clinical trial. *Journals of Gerontology. Series B, Psychological Sciences and Social Sciences, 65*(6), 691–697. doi:10.1093/ geronb/gbq054

Mittelman, M. S., Haley, W. E., Clay, O. J., & Roth, D. L. (2006). Improving caregiver well-being delays nursing home placement of patients with Alzheimer disease. *Neurology, 67*(9), 1592–1599. doi:10.1212/01.wnl.0000242727.81172.91

Mittelman, M. S., Roth, D. L., Coon, D. W., & Haley, W. E. (2004). Sustained benefit of supportive intervention for depressive symptoms in caregivers of patients with Alzheimer's disease. *American Journal of Psychiatry, 161*(5), 850–856. doi:10.1176/ appi.ajp.161.5.850

Parker, D., Mills, S., & Abbey, J. (2008). Effectiveness of interventions that assist caregivers to support people with dementia living in the community: A systematic review. *International Journal of Evidence-Based Healthcare, 6*(2), 137–172. doi:10.1111/ j.1744-1609.2008.00090.x

Pinquart, M., & Sörensen, S. (2006). Helping caregivers of persons with dementia: Which interventions work and how large are their effects? *International Psychogeriatrics, 18*(4), 577–595. doi:10.1017/ S1041610206003462

Reinhard, S. C., Feinberg, L. F., Choula, R., & Houser, A. (2015). Valuing the invaluable 2015 update: Undeniable progress, but big gaps remain. *Insight on the Issues, 104*, 1–25.

Scharlach, A., Sirotnik, B., Bockman, S., Neiman, M., Ruiz, C., & Dal Santo, T. (2003). *A profile of family caregivers: Results of the California statewide survey of caregivers.* Berkeley: University of California, Center for the Advanced Study of Aging Services.

Schulz, R., Martire, L. M., & Klinger, J. N. (2005). Evidence-based caregiver interventions in geriatric psychiatry. *Psychiatric Clinics of North America, 28*(4), 1007–1038. doi:10.1016/j.psc.2005.09.003

Selwood, A., Johnston, K., Katona, C., Lyketsos, C., & Livingston, G. (2007). Systematic review of the effect of psychological interventions on family caregivers of people with dementia. *Journal of Affective Disorders, 101*(1–3), 75–89. doi:10.1016/ j.jad.2006.10.025

Signe, A., & Elmståhl, S. (2008). Psychosocial intervention for family caregivers of people with dementia reduces caregiver's burden: Development and effect after 6 and 12 months. *Scandinavian Journal of Caring Sciences, 22*(1), 98–109. doi:10.1111/j.1471-6712.2007.00498.x

Sörensen, S., Pinquart, M., & Duberstein, P. (2002). How effective are interventions with caregivers? An updated meta-analysis. *The Gerontologist, 42*(3), 356–372.

Wang, L. Q., Chien, W. T., & Lee, I. Y. (2012). An experimental study on the effectiveness of a mutual support group for family caregivers of a relative with dementia in mainland China. *Contemporary Nurse, 40*(2), 210–224. doi:10.5172/conu.2012.40.2.210

Web Resources

AARP: Caregiving Resource Center: http://www.aarp.org/home-family/caregiving

Alzheimer's Association: http://www.alz.org/apps/we_can_help/support_groups.asp

Family Caregiver Alliance: http://www.caregiver.org/caregiver/jsp/home.jsp

National Alliance for Caregiving: http://www.caregiving.org

National Family Caregiver Support Program (Administration for Community Living): https://www.acl.gov/node/314

Older Adult and Family Center, Stanford University: http://oafc.stanford.edu

CAREGIVING RELATIONSHIPS

An estimated 43.5 million American adults are in an unpaid caregiving relationship in the United States, with the majority of those providing care to the elderly (National Alliance for Caregiving [NAC] & AARP, 2015). Caregiving consists of a variety of actions one does for another person who is unable to do the action themselves (Hermanns & Mastel-Smith, 2012). This can manifest in many ways, such as in the relationship between a medical professional and a patient, a parent and child, or a well family member caring for an ill family member. Caregiving can vary in length of time and frequency and encompasses a wide variety of tasks, from assistance with everyday tasks to medical care (Schulz & Eden, 2016). Caregiving relationships fall within several domains, including

relationships between the caregiver and the care recipient, those among different caregivers, and those between formal (paid provider, physician, nurse, therapist, social worker) and informal family-based care providers. Elder care is the most prevalent of caregiving relationships, with an estimated 17.7 million people in the United States engaged in a caregiving role for an older adult (Schulz & Eden, 2016).

When a family becomes involved in the care of one of its older members, it takes on a new, supportive function. Consequently, a number of structural and functional changes occur within the larger family system that affects many aspects of family life, including family relationships. Structural aspects of family relationships refer to the composition of the family social network and the participation of its members, whereas functional aspects refer to the family's ability to garner different types of support for specific needs (Li, Seltzer, & Greenberg, 1997). Several factors contribute to making a decision to undertake family-based care. This includes tangible resources, such as money or available space in the caregiver's home, and social resources, such as the number and proximity of family members who can help. Prior relationships among the caregivers and care recipient also play a role in the decision to provide care. A less tangible resource, but equally important, is the family's ability to discuss and negotiate a plan of family-based care among its members. To promote successful caregiving relationships, the care recipient and caregivers must acknowledge the perspectives of each person and work to honor the needs, rights, and wishes of all concerned. Decision making and the delegation of caregiving tasks often require negotiation and compromise among family members to develop a "care plan" or course of action.

Family caregiving often brings to the forefront prior issues and unresolved conflicts with a backdrop of stress and emotional reactivity, particularly if the decision about family-based caregiving is sudden. In contrast, watching the gradual deterioration of a family member because of a debilitating illness is difficult, but it allows the family to begin considering options for the care of that member. Because family caregiving is a time of change for all involved, it is also an opportunity for families to strengthen relationships and develop new ways to solve problems. The caregiving relationship often results in a time of bonding for family members and an opportunity to appreciate life and feel useful and needed by family (Tarlow et al., 2004).

Women are significantly more likely to take on the role of primary caregiver. As women generally outlive men, more women than men may expect to provide family-based care to their spouses. Adult children generally recognize that caregiving responsibility is likely; their chances of doing so are increased if they are married. The adult child with the fewest competing responsibilities (e.g., career, spouse, children) may be the designated caregiver in a family of multiple siblings, although sometimes, the most able family member emerges to assume the caregiver role. Work and school schedules and competing family demands affect the type of care given and the person providing care. In some instances, the care recipient nominates a caregiver or expresses preference for specific types of assistance from one or more family members. Parents are less likely to anticipate caregiving to their older children, but as life spans increase, more parents outlive their children and help in their care when they are ill. Such caregiving to adult children may be extremely burdensome, both physically and emotionally. Caregiving among siblings is somewhat less common, in part because individuals are likely to turn to their children first for caregiving help.

A number of background factors influence the type of care and the extent to which family-based care is offered to older persons. The gender of the caregiver likely influences the types of caregiving help provided. Women tend to assist with housekeeping, meal preparation, and personal care, whereas men tend to offer transportation assistance, make household repairs, and manage financial affairs. Factors such as racial/ethnic background, family traditions and history, and religion also influence decisions to care for family members at home and the degree to which family caregivers feel burdened. Historically, persons of color have been more likely to care for family members at home because of a strong sense of family, extended

networks of helpers made up of family and friends, financial considerations, and past discrimination by formal health services. There is a higher incidence of caregiving among Asian American, African American, and Hispanic households than White, non-Hispanic households (NAC & AARP, 2015), and minority families are more likely to care for more than one person. In addition, family caregivers in these groups are more likely to live with the care recipient and to receive help from others.

Caregiving for older persons is not universally distressing, particularly if it is considered a culturally acceptable, rewarding, or expected event. Other family-based care relationships reflect nontraditional family structures, such as friends, domestic partners, and extended families. Recent social changes have made domestic partners eligible for health care and other benefits that extend the support base to many individuals. Single persons—divorced, widowed, or never married—must rely on their extended families and broader social network, as well as paid help, to provide assistance.

Informal caregivers in the immediate family may have more stress and depressive symptoms than other caregivers who are more distant relations (Paulson & Lichtenberg, 2011). Providing practical and social support to family caregivers through sharing of the workload is conventionally understood to be a positive way of helping the caregiver. However, family caregivers may experience that a certain amount of perceived effort in caregiving is always present and that is not reduced with the availability of other family or formal caregiving supports (Juratovac, Morris, Zauszniewski, & Wykle, 2012).

One form of family-based caregiving that has gained recent attention focuses on grandparents and grandchildren. Increasing numbers of children live in homes maintained by grandparents, with or without one or more parents present; according to U.S. Census data, the number of children being raised by their grandparents has nearly doubled from the years 2000 to 2010 (U.S. Census Bureau, 2010). These grandparents' involvement in the daily care of grandchildren is markedly different from that of grandparents who provide day care or babysitting or have more traditional grandparenting roles. In situations in which the grandparents take on parenting responsibilities and become surrogate parents to grandchildren, they are likely to have complex relationships with the children's parents. In addition, grandchildren may directly assist with caregiving to their grandparents.

Where caregiving falls in the life course has an impact on the effects of caregiving. In addition to the relationships with those directly involved in caregiving, other aspects of the caregiver's life are affected (Moen & Chermack, 2005). The type of care necessary and the available supports influence the degree to which caregiving demands spill over into other settings, such as one's work. The Family and Medical Leave Act of 1993, which provides up to 3 months of leave for the care of family members, recognizes and provides support for such caregivers. In some circumstances, such as debilitating diseases of long duration such as Alzheimer's or Parkinson's disease, the caregiving relationship may be extensive and long-standing; in other cases, caregiving may not extend beyond several months or a year. Maintaining existing relationships with family and friends is important to the caregiver's health, yet the activities of caregiving deplete the time and energy necessary to sustain these relationships. Caregiving over time can lead to increased stress for caregivers (Musil, Morris, Warner, & Saied, 2003). People who report caregiving roles to a child, an elder, or both report higher levels of stress and worse psychosocial functioning compared with those in noncaregiving roles (DePasquale et al., 2015). Family caregivers must therefore be assisted to find time and respite to engage in rewarding noncaregiving activities that can prevent burnout and alleviate the burden of caregiving responsibilities.

Since the start of the new millennium, caregiving relationships have begun to include robots, particularly "social robots," in which a robot provides therapeutic social interaction for a human and fulfills a human need to provide care for another (Pfadenhauer & Dukat, 2015), particularly within the context of elder care. Robot caregiving is a newer area of research and is subject to ethical debates, although it is also recognized as having immense potential in various applications of caregiving (Borenstein & Pearson, 2010; Pearson & Borenstein, 2013).

Because of the importance of family caregiving, health care professionals should work to establish partnerships with family caregivers. Nurses, physicians, social workers, and other health professionals can collaborate with informal caregivers and the care recipient to achieve their mutual goal in caring for the care recipient. Professionals must also take the lead in supporting the caregiver, the relationship between the caregiver and the care recipient, and the relationships among the other caregivers as well.

See also Caregiver Burnout.

Sarah E. Givens, Carol M. Musil,
Camille B. Warner, and Evanne Juratovac

Borenstein, J., & Pearson, Y. (2010). Robot caregivers: Harbingers of expanded freedom for all? *Ethics and Information Technology, 12*(3), 277–288. doi:10.1007/s10676-010-9236-4

DePasquale, N., Polenick, C. A., Davis, K. D., Moen, P., Hammer, L. B., & Almeida, D. M. (2015). The psychosocial implications of managing work and family caregiving roles: Gender differences among information technology professionals. *Journal of Family Issues.* doi:10.1177/0192513X15584680

Hermanns, M., & Mastel-Smith, B. (2012). Caregiving: A qualitative concept analysis. *The Qualitative Report, 17*(38), 1–18.

Juratovac, E., Morris, D. L., Zauszniewski, J. A., & Wykle, M. L. (2012). Effort, workload, and depressive symptoms in family caregivers of older adults: Conceptualizing and testing a work-health relationship. *Research and Theory for Nursing Practice: An International Journal, 26*(2), 74–94.

Li, L., Seltzer, M., & Greenberg, J. (1997). Social support and depressive symptoms: Patterns in wife and daughter caregivers. *Journals of Gerontology: Psychological Sciences and Social Sciences, 52B*, S200–S211.

Moen, P., & Chermack, K. (2005). Gender disparities in health: Strategic selection, careers, and cycles of control. *Journals of Gerontology: Psychological Sciences and Social Sciences, 60B*, S99–S108.

Musil, C., Morris, D., Warner, C., & Saied, H. (2003). Issues in caregivers' stress and providers' support. *Research on Aging, 25,* 505–526.

National Alliance for Caregiving & American Association of Retired Persons. (2015). *Caregiving in the U.S.* Washington, DC: Author.

Paulson, D., & Lichtenberg, P. (2011). Effect of caregiver family status on care recipient symptom severity and caregiver stress at nursing home intake. *Clinical Gerontologist*, *34*(2), 132–143. doi:10.1080/07317115.2011.539518

Pearson, Y., & Borenstein, J. (2013). The intervention of robot caregivers and the cultivation of children's capability to play. *Science and Engineering Ethics*, *19*(1), 123–137. doi:10.1007/s11948-011-9309-8

Pfadenhauer, M., & Dukat, C. (2015). Robot caregiver or robot-supported caregiving? *International Journal of Social Robotics*, *7*(3), 393–406. doi:10.1007/s12369-015-0284-0

Schulz, R., & Eden, J. (2016). *Families caring for an aging America*. Washington, DC: National Academies Press.

Tarlow, B., Wisniewski, S., Belle, S., Rubert, M., Ory, M., & Gallagher, D. (2004). Positive aspects of caregiving: Contributions of the REACH project to the development of new for Alzheimer's caregiving. *Research on Aging*, *26*, 429–453.

U.S. Census Bureau. (2010). S1001 grandchildren characteristics, American Community Survey 5-Year Estimates, 2005–2009. Retrieved from http://factfinder.census.gov

Web Resources
Family Caregiver Alliance: http://www.caregiver.org
National Alliance for Caregiving: http://www.caregiving.org
National Family Caregivers Association: http://caregiveraction.org

CATARACTS AND GLAUCOMA

CATARACTS

Cataracts remain a leading cause of blindness and vision impairment worldwide. They account for more than one third of the world's cases of blindness (Khairallah et al., 2015). In the United States, where there is greater access to refractory lenses and cataract extraction surgery, cataracts account for a smaller percentage of blindness and visual impairment (Congdon et al., 2004) but remain of significant clinical importance. Cataracts affects more than 22 million Americans aged 40 years and older. A disease of aging, by the age of 80 years, more than half of Americans have cataracts (National Eye Institute, 2016).

A cataract is an opacity of the lens of the eye. There are several types of cataracts: nuclear, cortical, and subcapsular (anterior and posterior) that have different clinical presentations and natural histories. Most commonly found in the elderly are nuclear cataracts, sometimes referred to as *age-related* or *senile cataracts*. As the human lens ages, the nucleus undergoes compression and hardening, resulting in nuclear sclerosis. Nuclear cataracts progress slowly and painlessly in a variable manner but typically progress and lead to worsened visual function with no chance of recovery (Olson et al., 2016). Distance vision is often more affected than near vision. Nuclear cataracts can also dull colors and white.

Risk factors for cataracts include age, diabetes mellitus, long-term corticosteroid use (topical, systemic, or inhaled), prior intraocular surgery and trauma, smoking, and sunlight exposure (West & Valmadrid, 1995). Most studies are observational and show association but not causation (Olson et al., 2016). To prevent progression, it may be reasonable to suggest smoking cessation, ultraviolet B–blocking sunglasses, limitation of exposure to systemic and inhaled corticosteroids if possible, and prevention and treatment of type 2 diabetes mellitus and metabolic syndrome. There is no convincing evidence that vitamin supplementation or antioxidants reduce the risk of cataracts.

The only treatment for cataract is to surgically remove and replace the opacified lens with an artificial intraocular lens. The U.S. Preventive Services Task Force reports that there is insufficient evidence to recommend routine screening (Chou, Dana, Bougatsos, Grusing, & Blazina, 2016). Instead, screening and treatment of cataracts is based on clinical presentation. There is no single objective measure or clinical tool used to determine when cataract surgery is indicated. Generally, surgery is recommended when cataracts cause vision impairment that can no longer be improved with eyeglasses and when vision impairment interferes with function. If an ophthalmologist determines that diminished vision is because of cataracts through ophthalmic evaluation and there is reported functional

C

impairment, cataract surgery is strongly recommended (Olson et al., 2016).

Cataract extraction is considered a very successful intervention, with 90% of patients achieving 20/40 acuity or better following cataract surgery (Powe et al., 1994). Cataract surgery has also been shown to lead to improvement in functional status and quality of life (Mangione et al., 1994). Cataracts have been associated with nursing home placement and poor driving ability (Olson et al., 2016). A first cataract surgery has been found to reduce the risk of falls and fracture by 34% for more than a 12-month period (Harwood et al., 2005). Similar reduction has also been confirmed for a second cataract surgery (Foss et al., 2006). In addition, cataract surgery is typically a low-risk procedure (Greenberg et al., 2010), and visual complications are also low (Powe et al., 1994). According to one study, the most common ocular complication was a posterior capsular tear, anterior vitrectomy, or both during surgery (3.5%) and posterior capsule opacity after surgery (4.2%). The rate of severe complication in the 1-year post operation was 0.5% (Stein, Grossman, Mundy, Sugar, & Sloan, 2011). Routine preoperative testing is not recommended because it has not been shown to reduce the risk of intraoperative or postoperative medical adverse events (Keay, Lindsley, Tielsh, Katz, & Schein, 2012). Surgery is usually performed in an ambulatory setting with local anesthesia and monitored intravenous sedation. Postoperative follow-up is surgeon dependent but typically includes an ambulatory appointment within 24 to 48 hours and variable regimens of topical antibiotics, topical corticosteroids, topical nonsteroidal anti-inflammatory drugs, and analgesics. This varies among practitioners, and there are no controlled investigations to establish optimal regimens (Olson et al., 2016).

Cataract surgery with intraocular lens implantation was the largest single expense for any Medicare Part B procedure, with payments equaling $2.1 billion in 2009 (Centers for Medicare & Medicaid Services, 2009). However, the cost-effectiveness of surgery has been shown to compare favorably to other medical procedures when measuring quality-adjusted life years (Busbee, Brown, Brown, & Sharma, 2002).

GLAUCOMA

Glaucoma is the second leading cause of blindness in the world after cataracts and the leading cause of irreversible blindness (Tham et al., 2014). Glaucoma is an optic neuropathy that is usually characterized by elevated intraocular pressure (IOP). The two most common types of glaucoma are primary open angle glaucoma (POAG) and primary angle closure glaucoma (PACG). Acute PACG is an ophthalmological emergency. Secondary glaucoma can have many subtypes and may result from conditions such as uveitis, trauma, glucocorticoid therapy, pseudoexfoliation (Prum, Rosenberg, et al., 2015).

Primary Open Angle Glaucoma

POAG is the most common type of glaucoma in patients of European and African descent. It is estimated that 45 million people worldwide have POAG with projections that more than 4 million people in the United States will be affected by glaucoma by 2030. It is the leading cause of blindness among African Americans (Sommer et al., 1991) and prevalence in this population is three times higher than in non-Hispanic Whites in the United States. Hispanics and Latinos may also have high prevalence rates comparable to those of African Americans (Prum, Rosenberg, et al., 2015).

Glaucoma is characterized as a chronic and progressive optic neuropathy in which peripheral visual field loss is followed by central field loss as the optic nerve atrophies in a characteristic pattern that leads to irreversible blindness when left untreated (Prum, Rosenberg, et al., 2015). It is generally bilateral but can often be asymmetric. Usually there is elevated IOP, but this is not always the case (Dielemans et al., 1994). The majority of patients have disc changes or structural abnormalities of the retinal nerve fiber layer. The optic nerve may be described as "cupped" when the optic nerve takes on a hollowed-out appearance on examination. POAG is also associated with a characteristic vision-loss pattern, adult onset, open anterior chamber angles, and lack of secondary causes (Prum, Rosenberg, et al., 2015). The pathogenesis is not clear, but many studies have demonstrated that the prevalence of POAG increases as the level of IOP increases and provide evidence that IOP may play a role in the pathogenesis of optic neuropathy. However, there appears to be great variation in the susceptibility of the optic nerve to IOP (Sommer et al., 1991). In addition to race and IOP, older age, family history, thinner central cornea, low ocular perfusion pressure (low diastolic perfusion pressure), type 2 diabetes mellitus, hypertension, and myopia are also risk factors for POAG (Prum, Rosenberg, et al., 2015).

Although screening for glaucoma in the general population is not cost-effective, screening targeted populations, such as the elderly, those with a family history, and African Americans, may be reasonable given that glaucoma is often initially asymptomatic. In general, screening is done through a combination of measuring the IOP, assessing the optic disc and retinal nerve fiber layer, and evaluating the visual field. Although IOP has been the most well-studied method of screening and diagnosis, any IOP cutoff is somewhat arbitrary and not sensitive (Dielemans et al., 1994), although, historically, cutoffs of 21 mmHg have been used. The diagnosis of POAG requires a comprehensive history and physical examination of the eye which includes visual acuity measurement, pupil examination, anterior segment examination, IOP measurement, gonioscopy (evaluation of the anterior chamber angle), examination of the optic nerve head and retinal nerve fiber layer, fundus examination, central cornea thickness, and visual fields (Prum, Rosenberg, et al., 2015).

Although the diagnosis of POAG and its relationship with IOP is variable, treatment generally focuses on lowering the IOP to prevent progression of visual field loss and optic neuropathy (Maier, Funk, Schwarzer, Antes, & Falck-Ytter, 2005). The target pressure is chosen by the eye care provider and considers pretreatment pressure, level of optic nerve damage, and additional risk factors. Treatment may include pharmacological therapy, laser therapy, or incisional glaucoma surgery. Topical medical treatment works to either increase aqueous outflow or decrease aqueous production to lower IOP. Pharmacological therapy often requires multiple medications and frequent dosing. The cost of these medications can be high, and there are potential systemic side effects. Initial treatment is typically topical prostaglandins because they

tend to be efficacious, are more well tolerated, and have once-daily dosing regimens (Prum, Rosenberg, et al., 2015). Topical beta blockers are also common but can have side effects similar to systemic beta blockers. Alpha-adrenergic agonists, carbonic anhydrase inhibitors (topical and systemic), and cholinergic agonists are other classes of medications that may be used. Follow-up is needed to determine efficacy, monitor for side effects, and reinforce adherence, which is often difficult to maintain. Although medical therapy is generally attempted first, other treatment options include laser therapy, trabeculoplasty to increase aqueous flow, or surgical therapy. Surgical therapy is indicated when other methods fail to control disease and has various success rates in different populations.

Primary Angle Closure Glaucoma

Angle closure glaucoma results from the narrowing or closure of the anterior chamber angle. Unlike open angle glaucoma, angle closure glaucoma is more common in populations of Asian descent. In 2013 there were an estimated 20 million people worldwide with angle closure glaucoma (Tham et al., 2014). This review focuses on primary angle closure, but secondary causes such as neovascular glaucoma, mass, or hemorrhage in the posterior segment are also possible.

PACG results when aqueous humor, produced in the ciliary body, cannot flow normally through the pupil because of anatomical risk factors. The pressure in the posterior chamber increases, and the iris bows forward, crowding the angle. When this occurs repeatedly or for prolonged periods, scarring and damage to the trabecular meshwork occurs, and the aqueous humor cannot drain properly, leading to increased IOP and damage to the optic nerve. This can occur acutely or chronically. A majority of cases of PACG are bilateral, but in acute cases, most are unilateral. In acute angle closure, IOP can rise rapidly and lead to symptoms of blurred vision, halos around lights, eye pain, headache, and nausea. On examination, conjunctival redness, corneal edema, and mid-dilated pupil may be found. Acute PACG may resolve spontaneously or recur. If untreated, it can lead to permanent vision loss and blindness, so it is considered an ophthalmic emergency. Conversely, chronic angle closure occurs over time as the angle becomes progressively more closed. Patients are classified as having primary angle closure when they are noted to have angle closure and increased IOP. When optic nerve damage occurs, patients are considered to have PACG. Patients who develop PACG chronically are often asymptomatic and the IOP is generally not as high as in acute cases. Risk factors include race, Asian descent, older age, female gender, and anatomical factors such as shallow anterior chamber depth and thick crystalline lens (Prum, Herndon, et al., 2015).

Any patient with symptoms of acute PACG should have emergent ophthalmic examination by an ophthalmologist. Eye examination generally includes taking a history on prior episodes of angle closure, as well as a family history, and performing a review of medications that may induce angle narrowing. Physical examination includes gonioscopy to visualize the angle, evaluation of the pupil, refractive status, visual acuity, undilated fundus examination (dilation can exacerbate the problem), slit-lamp examination, and determination of IOP.

Iridotomy is indicated for patients with primary angle closure or PACG. Iridotomy is performed by creating a tiny hole in the peripheral iris through which the aqueous humor can flow and reach the angle bypassing the pupillary block. Complications can include increased IOP, so perioperative ocular hypotensive agents are used. IOP is checked immediately before surgery and again 30 to 120 minutes after surgery. Topical steroids are prescribed postoperatively, and follow-up evaluations examine the patency of the iridotomy, measure IOP, and use gonioscopy to visualize the angle (Prum, Herndon, et al., 2015). Additional treatment after iridotomy aims to reduce IOP and is similar to what was described earlier for POAG. For acute cases, after emergency referral to an ophthalmologist, medical therapy is usually initiated first to lower IOP and reduce pain, with iridotomy performed as soon as possible.

Angela Beckert

Busbee, B. G., Brown, M. M., Brown, G. C., & Sharma, S. (2002). Incremental cost-effectiveness of initial cataract surgery. *Ophthalmology, 109*(3), 606–612.

Centers for Medicare & Medicaid Services. (2009). Medicare leading Part B procedure codes based on allowed charges: Calendar year 2009. Table V.6a. Retrieved from http://www.cms.hhs.gov/datacompendium

Chou, R., Dana, T., Bougatsos, C., Grusing, S., & Blazina, I. (2016). Screening for impaired visual acuity in older adults: Updated evidence report and systematic review for the U.S. Preventive Services Task Force. *Journal of the American Medical Association, 315*(9), 915–933.

Congdon, N., Vingerling, J. R., Klein, B. E., West, S., Friedman, D. S., Kempen, J., …. Taylor, H. R. (2004). Prevalence of cataract and pseudophakia/aphakia among adults in the United States. *Archives of Ophthalmology, 122*(4), 487–494.

Dielemans, I., Vingerling, J. R., Wolfs, R. C., Hofman, A., Grobbee, D. E., & de Jong, P. T. (1994). The prevalence of primary open-angle glaucoma in a population based study in The Netherlands: The Rotterdam study. *Ophthalmology, 101*, 1851–1855.

Foss, A. J., Harwood, R. H., Osborn, F., Gregson, R. M., Zaman, A., & Masud, T. (2006). Falls and health status in elderly women following second eye cataract surgery: A randomised controlled trial. *Age and Ageing, 35*, 66–71.

Greenberg, P. B., Liu, J., Wu, W. C., Jiang, L., Tseng, V. L., Scott, I. U., & Friedmann, P. D. (2010). Predictors of mortality within 90 days of cataract surgery. *Ophthalmology, 117*(10), 1894–1899.

Harwood, R. H., Foss, A. J., Osborn, F., Gregson, R. M., Zaman, A., & Masud, T. (2005). Falls and health status in elderly women following first eye cataract surgery: A randomised controlled trial. *British Journal of Ophthalmology, 89*, 53–59.

Keay, L., Lindsley, K., Tielsh, J., Katz, J., & Schein O. (2012). Routine preoperative medical testing for cataract surgery. *Cochrane Database of Systematic Reviews*, (3), CD007293. doi:10.1002/14651858 .CD007293.pub3

Khairallah, M., Kahloun, R., Bourne, R., Limburg, H., Flaxman, S. R., Jonas, J. B., … Taylor, H. R. (2015). Number of people blind or visually impaired by cataract worldwide and in world regions, 1990–2010. *Investigative Ophthalmology & Visual Science, 56*(11), 6762–6769.

Maier, P. C., Funk, J., Schwarzer, G., Antes, G., & Falck-Ytter, Y. T. (2005). Treatment of ocular hypertension and open angle glaucoma: Meta-analysis of randomised controlled trials. *British Medical Journal, 331*, 134. doi:10.1136/bmj.38506.594977.E0

Mangione, C. M., Phillips, R. S., Lawrence, M. G., Seddon, J. M., Orav, E. J., & Goldman, L. (1994). Improved visual function and attenuation of declines in health-related quality of life after cataract extraction. *American Academy of Ophthalmology, 112*, 1419–1425.

National Eye Institute. (2016). Statistics and data: Cataract. Retrieved from https://nei.nih.gov/eyedata/cataract

Olson, R. J., Braga-Mele, R., Chen, S. H., Miller, K. M., Pineda, R., Tweeten, J. P., & Musch, D. C. (2016). Cataract in the adult eye preferred practice pattern. *Ophthalmology*. Retrieved from http://www.aao.org/ppp

Powe, N. R., Schein, O. D., Gieser, S. C., Tielsch, J. M., Luthra, R., Javitt, J., & Steinberg, E. P. (1994). Synthesis of the literature on visual acuity and complications following cataract extraction with intraocular lens implantation. Cataract Patient Outcome Research Team. *American Academy of Ophthalmology, 112*, 239–252.

Prum, B. E., Rosenberg, L. F., Gedde, S. J., Mansberger, S. L., Steine, J. D., Moroi, S. E.,…Williams, R. D. (2015). Primary open angle glaucoma preferred practice pattern guidelines. *Ophthalmology*. Retrieved from http://www.aao.org/ppp

Prum, B. E., Herndon, L. W., Moroi, S. E., Mansberger, S. L., Steine, J. D., Lim, M. C.,…Williams, R. D. (2015). Primary angle closure preferred practice pattern guidelines. *Ophthalmology*. Retrieved from http://www.aao.org/ppp

Sommer, A., Tielsch, J. M., Katz, J., Quigley, H. A., Gottsch, J. D., Javitt, J. C.,…Ezrine, S. (1991). Racial differences in the cause-specific prevalence of blindness in east Baltimore. *New England Journal of Medicine, 325*(20), 1412–1417.

Stein, J. D., Grossman, D. S., Mundy, K. M., Sugar, A., & Sloan, F. A. (2011). Severe adverse events after cataract surgery among Medicare beneficiaries. *Ophthalmology, 118*, 1716–1723.

Tham, Y. C., Li, X., Wong, T. Y., Quigley, H. A., Aung, T., & Cheng, C. Y. (2014). Global prevalence of glaucoma and projections of glaucoma burden through 2040: A systemic review and meta-analysis. *Ophthalmology, 121*(11), 2081–2090.

West, S. K., & Valmadrid, C. T. (1995). Epidemiology of risk factors for age-related cataract. *Survey of Ophthalmology, 93*, 323.

CENTENARIANS

Centenarians are people who have lived to the age of 100 years or older. Many scientists and practitioners alike are interested in the influencing factors that contribute to the phenomenon of longevity, yet centenarians represent a largely understudied population (Jopp, Boerner, Ribeiro, & Rott, 2016). With increasing life spans, many people may be fortunate to become centenarians; therefore it is important to focus on how this population can live a more satisfying, healthier life.

The population of centenarians is on the rise. In 2010, centenarians accounted for 1 of every 5,786 people in the U.S. population (Werner, 2011). Based on more recent data from the U.S. Census Bureau's annual estimates (2015) of resident population, the number of American centenarians increased from 57,703 in 2011 to 72,197 in 2014. Mortality rates are decreasing among the *oldest old*, strongly suggesting that the number of centenarians will continue to increase.

Women account for a greater number of centenarians than men. It was estimated that in 2014, there were 58,468 female centenarians and 13,729 male centenarians (U.S. Census Bureau, 2015). According to Werner (2011), 2010 U.S. Census data revealed the largest growth in women over men occurred in the centenarian age group compared with other 5-year age groups starting at 65 years old. However, men that live long enough to become centenarians are usually more functional and healthier than their female counterparts (Boston University School of Medicine: New England Centenarian Study, n.d.).

Supercentenarians are those aged 110 years or older. There are 48 validated living supercentenarians in the world, 46 females and 2 males (Gerontology Research Group [GRG], 2016). Approximately half of these validated supercentenarians were born in Japan, where they still reside. The GRG (2016) reports that the validated number of living supercentenarians differs from the *actual* number, which has been estimated at 300 to 450 globally, with 60 to 75 residing in the United States. The oldest verified woman ever was Jeanne Calment of France, who died at 122 years old in 1997. The oldest verified man ever was Jiroemon Kimura of Japan, who died at 116 years old in 2013 (GRG, 2016).

Environmental and genetic influences, as well as their interaction, are thought to contribute to longevity. It is estimated that one third of

C

longevity can be attributed to genetic factors, whereas the remaining variation in longevity among individuals can be attributed to epigenetic and environmental factors (Govindaraju, Atzmon, & Barzilai, 2015).

There appear to be geographic clusters of centenarians throughout the world. In the United States, there is a ratio of 1.73 centenarians per 10,000 people, whereas in Japan there is a ratio of 3.43 centenarians per 10,000 people (Meyer, 2012). More specifically, on the Japanese island of Okinawa, many centenarians have been found to be astonishingly healthy with much lower rates of atherosclerotic disease and cancer (Okinawa Centenarian Study, n.d.). Although the reasons for geographic clustering are not fully understood, according to Govindaraju et al. (2015), several hundred genes influencing longevity have been found to be overrepresented in geographical areas where there are increased numbers of centenarians. Many of these genes play a role in cellular and metabolic functions such as development, oxidative stress, genome maintenance, cognitive pathways, lipid metabolism, and glucose metabolism (Govindaraju et al., 2015).

Environmental factors such as climate, surroundings, and social or cultural conditions also play a key role in longevity. A nationwide analysis with 28 million participants in 3,034 U.S. counties revealed that communities with lower levels of ambient pollution, smoking, poverty, and obesity contributed to exceptional aging (Baccarelli et al., 2016). Nutritional interventions with calorie restrictions have also been shown to increase life span in several organisms, including mammals, whereas overeating often leads to metabolic disorders, decreasing life span (Govindaraju et al., 2015). According to Boston University School of Medicine: New England Centenarian Study, the largest study of centenarians in the world, few centenarians have been found to be obese or to smoke, and there is a suggestion that many of them may be better equipped to handle stress. Furthermore, it has been found that the remarkable health and appearance of centenarians living on the Japanese island of Okinawa can, in part, be attributed to their physically active lifestyles, low-glycemic/low-calorie diets, and their ability

to maintain low body mass indexes (ranging from 18 to 22) throughout their lives (Okinawa Centenarian Study, n.d.).

The lives of centenarians remain poorly understood (Jopp et al., 2016). More recently, however, studies have been implemented to better capture the unique social, psychological, and health characteristics associated with meaningful and successful aging. Although popular belief holds that old age is a difficult time, characterized by profound disability and deficit, some studies of centenarians counter these views. Centenarians have been found to possess better health profiles compared with people of normal life span (Govindaraju et al., 2015). In addition, not all centenarians are cognitively impaired: Approximately half retain normal cognitive function or suffer only minimal impairment (Jopp et al., 2016). In contrast, one area in which centenarians commonly have a great deal of trouble is with sensation: Many have significant impairment in sight and hearing.

Many centenarians further share a "serene" personality, generally accepting what they cannot change and enjoying the life they have been given. Although longitudinal studies would be required to prove this, it is likely that this attitude is lifelong for many centenarians.

The study of centenarians can provide insight into the biology of aging, as well as the mechanisms and promotion of longevity. As research advances and a better understanding of the many factors that influence this growing population is gained, it will be important to develop both social and economic initiatives to enhance the quality of life for centenarians. Moving forward, there is much to learn from this population. Although the longevity of centenarians can, in part, be traced to genetic factors, genes are not everything. The most valuable lesson therefore may be that lifestyle significantly affects how humans age and it is never too late to make a change for the better to lead a long, healthy, happy life.

Dominica Potenza

Baccarelli, A. A., Hales, N., Burnett, R. T., Jerrett, M., Mix, C., Dockery, D. W., & Pope, C. A., III. (2016). Particulate air pollution, exceptional aging, and rates of centenarians: A nationwide analysis of the United States, 1980–2010. *Environmental Health Perspectives.* doi:10.1289/EHP197

Boston University School of Medicine: New England Centenarian Study (n.d.). Retrieved from http://www.bumc.bu.edu/centenarian/overview

Gerontology Research Group. (2016). Gerontology world supercentenarian rankings list. Retrieved from http://www.grg.org/SC/WorldSCRankingsList.html

Govindaraju, D., Atzmon, G., & Barzilai, N. (2015). Genetics, lifestyle, and longevity: Lessons from centenarians. *Applied and Translational Genomics, 4,* 23–32. doi:10.1016/j.atg.2015.01.001

Jopp, D. S., Boerner, K., Ribeiro, O., & Rott, C. (2016). Life at age 100: An international research agenda for centenarian studies. *Journal of Aging & Social Policy, 28,* 133–147. doi:10.1080/08959420.2016.1161693

Meyer, J. (2012). *Centenarians: 2010: 2010 census special reports.* Washington, DC: U.S. Government Printing Office. Retrieved from http://www.census.gov/prod/cen2010/reports/c2010sr-03.pdf

Okinawa Centenarian Study. (n.d.). Retrieved from http://www.okicent.org/index.html

U.S. Census Bureau. (2015). *Population estimates: Postcensal estimates for 2010–2014.* Washington, DC: U.S. Government Printing Office. Retrieved from http://www.census.gov/popest/data/national/asrh/2014/index.html

Werner, C. A. (2011). *The older population: 2010: 2010 census briefs.* Washington, DC: U.S. Government Printing Office. Retrieved from https://www.census.gov/prod/cen2010/briefs/c2010br-09.pdf

CHALLENGES OF HOSPITAL CARE: PREVENTABLE HOSPITALIZATION, COMPLEX CARE TRANSITIONS, AND REHOSPITALIZATION

Persons aged 65 years and older account for 14% of the U.S. population but nearly half of all hospital days. By 2060, nearly one in four residents will surpass age 65 years, and 19.7 million will be 85 years or older, many aging with complex multimorbidity, leading to increased hospitalizations (U.S. Census Bureau, 2015). Some 5% of U.S. adults, 12 million people, live with three or more chronic conditions and functional impairment (Hayes, 2016). Under-recognition of such impairment during hospitalization contributes to adverse outcomes (functional decline, delirium, medication errors), increased morbidity, higher costs, and complex care transitions (Brown, Redden, Flood, & Allman, 2009; Covinsky et al., 2003; Inouye, 2000). Traditional hospital care models focus on single acute events, not elders with multimorbidity and geriatric syndromes. In 2006, the Centers for Medicare & Medicaid Services (CMS) spent three times more per capita on seniors with chronic conditions and functional impairment than on seniors with chronic conditions alone (Scan Foundation, 2011).

The Joint Commission, CMS, and other payors now mandate quality outcomes for accreditation and reimbursement. The Patient Protection and Affordable Care Act instituted financial incentives encouraging hospitals to improve outcomes and reduce readmissions. Lower-performing hospitals now have a portion of Medicare payments withheld, and the goal is that by 2018, 90% of all Medicare fee-for-service payments will be tied to quality or value. In 2017, readmission penalties will top $525 million, and CMS controversially does not take into account the socioeconomic status of patient populations served by different hospitals. With the population of persons older than 85 years, many living with complex health conditions (expected to triple from 6.2 to 14.6 million by 2040) there is great momentum to implement evidence-based care models that improve outcomes while lowering costs (Burwell, 2015).

PREVENTABLE HOSPITALIZATION

Several interventions demonstrate comprehensive geriatric care while preventing unnecessary hospitalization. These include Hospital at Home, Programs of All-Inclusive Care for the Elderly (PACE), Geriatric Resources for Assessment and Care of Elders (GRACE), Interventions to Reduce Acute Care Transfers (INTERACT II), and palliative care programs for patients with life-limiting illness/injury.

Hospital at Home provides hospital-level, in-home care for acute illness for patients meeting medical eligibility criteria. Necessary medical equipment (oxygen, infusions, laboratory testing, and radiology testing) is provided. Patients receive nurse and physician visits daily, with additional visits as needed. Hospital at Home programs demonstrate improved patient and caregiver satisfaction and reduced costs with comparable or improved clinical outcomes (Cryer, Shannon, Van Amsterdam, & Leff, 2012; Leff et al., 2006; Scan Foundation, 2011).

PACE is a capitated CMS-managed, community-based program providing interdisciplinary team care. Persons aged 55 years and older are eligible for PACE if they live in a catchment area and meet state Medicaid nursing home eligibility criteria. PACE enables frail elders to continue community living via an interdisciplinary team that develops comprehensive, individualized care plans. PACE is associated with improved survival, quality of life, functional status, patient satisfaction, and reduced hospitalizations and nursing home placements (Grabowski, 2006).

Similar in concept, GRACE helps frail, community-dwelling elders age in place by incorporating in-home geriatric assessment of patient and caregiver(s) through a geriatric nurse practitioner (NP) and social worker (SW) team in conjunction with the primary care physician (PCP). Individualized care plans addressing geriatric syndromes developed by the GRACE team (geriatrician, pharmacist, mental health liaison, NP/SW dyad) are approved by the PCP before implementation. GRACE has demonstrated improved patient-centered care transitions and reduced hospital readmissions and nursing home placement (Counsell et al., 2007).

For patients residing in nursing facilities, INTERACT II shows promise in preventing avoidable hospitalizations through proactive identification and management of changes in resident clinical status. INTERACT II interventions are implemented through reinforced staff training led by a facility-based program champion. A quality-improvement project in 25 nursing homes over a 6-month period found that INTERACT II reduced hospital admissions by 17% (Ouslander et al., 2011).

Palliative medicine provides symptom management and interdisciplinary support for patients and families experiencing illness-related symptom burden. Not exclusively end-of-life care, palliative care provides an additional layer of support at all illness stages in which symptom burden occurs, even in conjunction with potentially "curative" therapies. Patients receiving palliative care experience improved symptom control and satisfaction, reduced emergency department and hospital costs, and greater likelihood of dying at home compared with those receiving conventional care (Brumley et al., 2007; Morrison, 2005). Caregivers also experience better short- and long-term outcomes when patients receive supportive palliative care services (Abernethy et al., 2008).

COMPLEX CARE TRANSITIONS: DIFFICULT HOSPITAL DISCHARGES

Many factors combine to often hinder patient comprehension of discharge plans, including cognitive impairment, low health literacy, care complexity, cultural barriers, absent caregivers, and physical limitations. Research demonstrates that many elders and caregivers misunderstand instructions, lack appropriate follow-up, and do not receive complete, accurate, and legible medication lists at hospital discharge. Furthermore, older patients are often discharged with unrecognized functional debilities that limit self-care. Disease-based models of inpatient care and reimbursement often lead to patients no longer "qualifying" for inpatient or rehabilitation settings. Many of these individuals are too frail to return home, which often results in unplanned readmission.

Options for an older adult requiring additional care at discharge range from home health care or outpatient rehabilitation to inpatient care, including (a) acute rehabilitation center, (b) subacute rehabilitation in a skilled nursing facility, or (c) chronic care hospital for those with the most intensive needs. All of these services require meticulous documentation and justification of level of care and payor source. Most services require physician certification of medical necessity; in some settings, documentation of face-to-face evaluation by the certifying physician is necessary. Uninsured patients have far fewer post–hospital care options. Patients with chronic or life-limiting illnesses have many post-discharge needs and are at highest risk of rehospitalization, yet will not necessarily need (or qualify for) discharge rehabilitation services; these patients are often better served with a palliative approach aligned with their goals of care.

REDUCING REHOSPITALIZATION AND IMPROVING HOSPITAL CARE TRANSITIONS

Hospital discharge transitions are an increasingly important quality and financial imperative for our health care system. A 2009 study of Medicare claims data for more than 11.8 million beneficiaries revealed that 20% of discharged beneficiaries were rehospitalized within 30 days; 34% were rehospitalized within 90 days. Half of patients discharged back to community and rehospitalized within 30 days lacked a PCP follow-up visit before rehospitalization. The authors estimated that the cost to Medicare for these unplanned readmissions in 2004 was $17.4 billion (Jencks, Williams, & Coleman, 2009). Recent models of transitional care have shown promise that specialized programs emphasizing patient/caregiver coaching, early transition planning, and meticulous medication reconciliation can reduce readmission rates. The Transitional Care Model, Care Transition Intervention, Project RED (Re-Engineered Hospital Discharge), Project BOOST (Better Outcomes for Older adults through Safe Transitions), and acute care for elders (ACE) units are five such models.

The Transitional Care Model provides comprehensive, evidence-based transitional care coordination for chronically ill, high-risk older adults. A transitional care nurse (TCN) follows enrolled patients from in-hospital planning meetings to home, focusing on caregiver and patient needs. The TCN is available 7 days/week through home visits and telephone access for 1–3 months. Findings from multisite randomized controlled trials (RCTs) demonstrate reduced readmissions, total hospital days, and costs, along with increased patient, caregiver, and provider satisfaction (Naylor et al., 1999, 2004).

The Care Transitions Intervention addresses four primary pillars of successful care transition: (a) improved communication via a portable personal health record of essential health information the patient carries across care settings, (b) medication reconciliation and self-management training, (c) patient-scheduled follow-up appointments, and (d) improved patient knowledge regarding clinical symptoms signaling worsening status (*red-flags*) and ways to respond. These components are taught by a nurse Care Transitions Coach, who provides coaching throughout hospitalization and for 4-weeks after discharge via home visits and phone calls. An RCT of the Care Transitions Intervention demonstrated significantly lower 30- and 90-day rehospitalizations, reduced mean hospital costs at 90 and 180 days, and improved patient disease self-management and increased confidence about the patient's role during care transitions (Coleman et al., 2004; Coleman, Parry, Chalmers, & Min, 2006).

Project RED seeks to engage patients through disease self-management training, medication reconciliation, matching of the discharge plan with published clinical guidelines, improvement of communication through expedited transmission of discharge summaries, and transport of patient health records to all care settings. Patient coaching is again performed by a nurse; postdischarge phone calls by a pharmacist ensure medication reconciliation and reinforcement of the discharge plan. An RCT of Project RED demonstrated significantly reduced 30-day post-hospital utilization (Jack et al., 2009).

Project BOOST is an initiative through which a multidisciplinary leadership team provides hospitals with yearlong mentoring in developing evidence-based, best-care transition practices. Preliminary aggregate outcomes from BOOST sites included reduced 30-day readmission rates from 14.2% to 11.2% (Williams et al., 2014). Qualitative analysis of six pilot hospitals demonstrated common denominators challenging the current hospital discharge process, including insufficient administrative support, inadequate understanding of the current processes, lack of protected time or dedicated resources, and lack of frontline buy-in (Williams et al., 2014).

ACE units improve outcomes in hospitalized elders by emphasizing patient-centered care, frequent interdisciplinary team rounds designed to manage geriatric syndromes, and early transition planning. Research demonstrates improved care, prescribing practices, physical functioning, restraint use, patient and provider satisfaction, reduced hospital stay and institutionalization rates, and reduced 30-day readmissions (Flood et al., 2013; Hung, Ross, Farber, & Siu, 2013; Landefeld, Palmer, Kresevic, Fortinsky, & Kowal, 1995).

Ultimately, the "perfect" hospital transitional care program improves discharge instruction adherence, prevents adverse outcomes and medication errors, facilitates reestablishment of primary care, decreases costly health care resource utilization, improves patient physical function and satisfaction, and decreases caregiver burden. Exemplary models of care should also provide means of educating medical trainees across all disciplines and settings to work as interdisciplinary teams to meet the needs of complex elders. Efforts focused on moving palliative care upstream to recognize the highly specialized needs of the chronically ill are critical with the aging population and shrinking financial resources. To date, although existing care models show promise, none succeed in achieving all these goals, fueling ongoing research.

Ella H. Bowman and
Marianthe D. Grammas

Abernethy, A. P., Currow, D. C., Fazekas, B. S., Luszcz, M. A., Wheeler, J. L., & Kuchibhatla, M. (2008). Specialized palliative care services are associated with improved short- and long-term caregiver outcomes. *Supportive Care in Cancer, 16*(6), 585–597.

Brown, C. J., Redden, D. T., Flood, K. L., & Allman, R. M. (2009). The underrecognized epidemic of low mobility during hospitalization of older adults. *Journal of the American Geriatrics Society, 57*(9), 1660–1665.

Brumley, R., Enguidanos, S., Jamison, P., Seitz, R., Morgenstern, N., & Saito, S. (2007). Increased satisfaction with care and lower costs: Results of a randomized trial of in-home palliative care. *Journal of the American Geriatrics Society, 55*(7), 993–1000.

Burwell, S. M. (2015). Setting value-based payment goals—HHS efforts to improve U.S. health care. *New England Journal of Medicine, 372*, 897–899.

Coleman, E. A., Parry, C., Chalmers, S., & Min, S. J. (2006). The care transitions intervention: Results of a randomized controlled trial. *Archives of Internal Medicine, 166*(17), 1822–1828.

Coleman, E. A., Smith, J. D., Frank, J. C., Min, S. J., Parry, C., & Kramer, A. M. (2004). Preparing patients and caregivers to participate in care delivered across settings: The care transitions intervention. *Journal of the American Geriatrics Society, 52*(11), 1817–1825.

Counsell, S. R., Callahan, C. M., Clark, D. O., Tu, W., Buttar, A. B., Stump, T. E., & Ricketts, G. D. (2007). Geriatric care management for low-income seniors: A randomized controlled trial. *Journal of the American Medical Association, 298*(22), 2623–2633.

Covinsky, K. E., Palmer, R. M., Fortinsky, R. H., Counsell, S. R., Stewart, A. L., Kresevic, D.,…Landefeld, C. S. (2003). Loss of independence in activities of daily living in older adults hospitalized with medical illnesses: Increased vulnerability with age. *Journal of the American Geriatrics Society, 51*(4), 451–458.

Cryer, L., Shannon, S. B., Van Amsterdam, M., & Leff, B. (2012). Costs for "hospital at home" patients were 19 percent lower, with equal or better outcomes compared to similar inpatients. *Health Affairs (Project Hope), 31*(6), 1237–1243.

Flood, K. L., Maclennan, P. A., McGrew, D., Green, D., Dodd, C., & Brown, C. J. (2013). Effects of an acute care for elders unit on costs and 30-day readmissions. *JAMA Internal Medicine, 173*(11), 981–987.

Grabowski, D. (2006). The cost-effectiveness of non-institutional long-term care services: Review and synthesis of most recent evidence. *Medical Care Research and Review, 63*(1), 3–28.

Hayes, S. L., Salzberg, C. A., McCarthy, D., Radley, D. C., Abrams, M. K., Shah, T., & Anderson, G. F. (2016). High-need, high-cost patients: Who are they and how do they use health care— A population-based comparison of demographics, health care use, and expenditures. Retrieved from http://www.commonwealthfund.org/publications/issue-briefs/2016/aug/high-need-high-cost-patients-meps1

Hung, W. W., Ross, J. S., Farber, J., & Siu, A. (2013). Evaluation of the mobile acute care of the elderly (MACE) service. *JAMA Internal Medicine, 173*(11), 990–996.

Inouye, S. K. (2000). Prevention of delirium in hospitalized older patients: Risk factors and targeted intervention strategies. *Annals of Medicine, 32*(4), 257–263.

Jack, B. W., Chetty, V. K., Anthony, D., Greenwald, J. L., Sanchez, G. M., Johnson, A. E.,…Culpepper,

L. (2009). A reengineered hospital discharge program to decrease rehospitalization: A randomized trial. *Annals of Internal Medicine, 150*(3), 178–187.

Jencks, S. F., Williams, M. V., & Coleman, E. A. (2009). Rehospitalizations among patients in the Medicare fee-for-service program. *New England Journal of Medicine, 360*(14), 1418–1428.

Landefeld, C. S., Palmer, R. M., Kresevic, D. M., Fortinsky, R. H., & Kowal, J. (1995). A randomized trial of care in a hospital medical unit especially designed to improve the functional outcomes of acutely ill older patients. *New England Journal of Medicine, 332*(20), 1338–1344.

Leff, B., Burton, L., Mader, S., Naughton, B., Burl, J., Clark, R., … Burton, J. R. (2006). Satisfaction with hospital at home care. *Journal of the American Geriatrics Society, 54*(9), 1355–1363.

Morrison, R. S. (2005). Health care system factors affecting end-of-life care. *Journal of Palliative Medicine, 8* (Suppl. 1), S79–S87.

Naylor, M. D., Brooten, D. A., Campbell, R. L., Maislin, G., McCauley, K. M., & Schwartz, J. S. (2004). Transitional care of older adults hospitalized with heart failure: A randomized, controlled trial. *Journal of the American Geriatrics Society, 52*(5), 675–684.

Naylor, M. D., Brooten, D., Campbell, R., Jacobsen, B. S., Mezey, M. D., Pauly, M. V., & Schwartz, J. S. (1999). Comprehensive discharge planning and home follow-up of hospitalized elders: A randomized clinical trial. *Journal of the American Medical Association, 281*(7), 613–620.

Ouslander, J. G., Lamb, G., Tappen, R., Herndon, L., Diaz, S., Roos, B. A.,…Bonner, A. (2011). Interventions to reduce hospitalizations from nursing homes: Evaluation of the INTERACT II collaborative quality improvement project. *Journal of the American Geriatrics Society, 59*(4), 745–753.

The Scan Foundation. (2011). Data brief: Medicare spending by functional impairment and chronic conditions. Retrieved from http://www.the scanfoundation.org/sites/default/files/1pg_databrief_no22.pdf

U.S. Census Bureau. (2015). Facts for features: Older Americans month: May 2015. Retrieved from https://www.census.gov/newsroom/facts-for-features/2015/cb15-ff09.html

Williams, M. V., Li, J., Hansen, L. O., Forth, V., Budnitz, T., Greenwald, J. L.,…Coleman, E. A. (2014). Project BOOST implementation: Lessons learned. *Southern Medical Journal, 107*(7), 455–465.

Web Resources
Care Transitions Intervention: https://caretransitions.org
Centers for Medicare & Medicaid Services: Hospital Value-Based Purchasing: http://www.cms.gov/Medicare/Quality-Initiatives-Patient-Assessment-Instruments/hospital-value-based-purchasing/index.html
Center to Advance Palliative Care: http://www.capc.org
Hospital at Home: http://www.hospitalathome.org
National PACE Association: http://www.npaonline.org
Project RED (Re-Engineered Discharge) Training Program: http://www.ahrq.gov/qual/projectred
Society of Hospital Medicine: Project BOOST (Better Outcomes for Older Adults Through Safe Transitions): http://www.hospitalmedicine.org/BOOST

CHRONIC ILLNESS

Chronic illnesses are treatable conditions but, by definition, cannot be completely cured. These illnesses frequently lead to disability and require ongoing management shared by the patient, health care professionals, and/or caregivers. Based on data from the 2017 National Health Interview Survey (NHIS), it was estimated that 85.8% of noninstitutionalized civilian Americans, aged 65 years and older, have at least one chronic condition and 60.8% have two or more. The Centers for Disease Control and Prevention (CDC, 2013) reports 95% of health care expenditures for older Americans are related to chronic diseases.

Hypertension (55.9%), arthritis (49.0%), heart disease (29.4%), cancer (23.4%), and diabetes (20.8%) are among the most prevalent chronic health conditions reported in older adults (Federal Interagency Forum on Aging-Related Statistics, 2016). Stroke, asthma, and chronic obstructive pulmonary disease are also prevalent conditions. The two most common chronic health condition dyads among Americans aged 65 years and older reported by the 2010 NHIS were estimated at 63% for arthritis and hypertension, followed by 25.4% for diabetes and hypertension; the two most common chronic health condition triads were estimated at 32.6% for arthritis, diabetes, and hypertension, followed by 26.9% for arthritis, cancer, and hypertension (Ward & Schiller, 2013).

In large part, clinical guidelines focus on the management and care of older adults with one chronic condition; yet many older adults suffer from multiple chronic conditions (MCCs). On January 1, 2015, a government initiative entitled Chronic Care Management (CCM) Services was implemented to target primary care outpatient management of older adults with MCC (two or more) in an effort to reduce health expenditures and provide better care coordination (Centers for Medicare & Medicaid Services [CMS], 2015). CCM allows for 20 minutes of monthly access for non–face-to-face health care coordination with a designated practitioner to implement a comprehensive care plan for adults suffering from MCC (CMS, 2015).

The U.S. Department of Health and Human Services (USDHHS) has convened a work group that developed, *Multiple Chronic Conditions: A Strategic Framework* (2010) that serves as a national-level roadmap for assisting USDHHS programs and public and private stakeholders in improving the health of individuals with multiple chronic illnesses via four major goals:

1. Strengthening the health care and public health systems
2. Empowering the individual to use self-care management
3. Equipping health care providers with tools, information, and other interventions
4. Supporting targeted research about individuals with MCCs and effective interventions

Chronic illness causes physical, mental, and functional impairment, which significantly influences an individual's independence, friends and family, social status, financial stability, physical comfort, and/or the ability to engage in meaningful pursuits. Health care professionals can help meet the needs of patients requiring chronic-illness care through a variety of approaches.

Develop a team approach. To adequately respond to the needs of those with chronic illnesses, an interdisciplinary team is required; it consists of a physician or advanced practitioner,

nurse, social worker, and specialists (e.g., occupational therapist, physical therapist, nutritionist, psychiatrist, neuropsychologist, and pharmacist) as needed. Utilization of a case (or care) manager in private practice or affiliated with a home care or social-service agency can be particularly helpful for complicated cases. Lawyers have a role in financial asset planning, navigating patients through Medicare and insurance matters, and helping with other legal and financial issues that can accompany chronic illness. Good communication, trust, and a strong partnership between the patient and individual health professionals who compose the team are crucial.

Educate health professionals. Professionals need to appreciate the multidimensional impact chronic disease has on older adults. Creative educational programs are now being integrated into graduate, doctoral, and medical school curricula throughout the United States. Web-based resources are also being developed to educate health professionals and provide practical resources for them to become more effective and efficient in working with older patients with chronic illness.

Conduct a thorough assessment. The professional team's degree of involvement with the patient, family, and/or other caregivers depends on the seriousness of the illness and its impact on the patient's function and quality of life. An assessment of the following issues serves to guide the development of intervention strategies.

MEDICAL ASSESSMENT

Disease onset, diagnosis, and certainty. Was the disease onset rapid or gradual? Was it life threatening, debilitating, or merely annoying? What impact does the diagnosis have on the patient? Is the diagnosis definitive or is there a possibility for better or worse news?

Disease course, pain, and familiarity. Will the patient's condition stabilize, improve, or worsen with time? What is the potential for the patient's increased self-reliance? Should the onset of significant pain be anticipated? What preparations do the patient and family need to make to provide future care?

Other acute and chronic illnesses. Is the patient already suffering from acute or chronic illness?

If so, what is the anticipated effect of the additional health problems on the patient's overall quality of life and well-being? Will newly prescribed medicine interfere with current prescriptions or complicate the patient's current medical condition?

Treatment and pain management. Will the patient require surgery, medications, physical therapy or other rehabilitation, a home health aide, psychotherapy, an exercise program, or a new diet regimen? Is polypharmacy an issue? Are appropriate medications being utilized at proper doses? Does the patient have the motivation, desire, and ability to proceed with the recommended interventions? Is palliative care an option?

End-of-life care. Is the end of life approaching? Are advance directives in place? Have the patient's wishes about end-of-life care been discussed? Have these wishes been communicated by the patient to the designated health care agent? How will the patient's wishes be translated into medical intervention?

FUNCTIONAL ASSESSMENT

Functional status. What is the patient's overall functional ability as determined by assessing activities of daily living (ADL) and instrumental ADL (IADL)? How does this compare to what it had been?

Restrictions. What areas of life will be changed, including mobility, diet, cognitive function, employment, and self-care?

Service site. Where will care be provided and who is willing to help? If the patient is homebound, are the needed heath care services obtainable at home?

Environmental obstacles. Would environmental modifications in the home improve the patient's function, quality of life, and safety?

Health literacy. How will the patient's level of health literacy affect the reporting of symptoms and the ability to adhere to the health professionals' recommendations?

PSYCHOSOCIAL ASSESSMENT

Cognitive and emotional status. Do the patient and caregiver understand the disease, likely progression, associated problems, and treatment recommendations? Does the patient have the cognitive capacity to adapt to lifestyle changes and restrictions and make health care decisions? Is there evidence of depression, suicidal ideation, anxiety, or alcohol/drug abuse?

Social stigma. Does the patient feel ashamed about the illness or functional impairment? Is the patient isolated because of shame about functional loss (e.g., having to rely on a wheelchair or walker?)

Community resources. Would medical day care, respite services, transportation services, friendly visitors, care management, and/or psychotherapy be helpful?

Social supports. Does the patient have a sufficient network of friends and family willing and able to provide emotional and instrumental support with the patient's daily needs? Are they experiencing caregiver stress? Is additional support needed?

Financial status. Are financial resources sufficient to cover health care needs and services? Does the patient have the cognitive capacity to manage finances? Has someone been designated power-of-attorney or guardian?

Religious, spiritual, and cultural status. Is there something the provider should know about the patient's spiritual life or health beliefs to provide the best possible care? Is there a role for pastoral care services? Is there a need for an interpreter to overcome language barriers?

Provide multipronged interventions. The following interventions should aim to optimize the patient's functional independence, improve social connections, and advance the patient's comfort and well-being.

PREVENTION INTERVENTIONS

Provide prevention and early-detection services. Primary prevention includes health-promotion practices that can delay dependency, such as nutritional support, smoking cessation, home safety modifications, exercise, and immunization. Secondary prevention is screening for diseases such as diabetes, hypertension, breast cancer, colon cancer, glaucoma, and depression. Tertiary prevention includes patient support, education, monitoring, and rehabilitation in an

C

effort to forestall further health and functional decline in individuals already diagnosed with a chronic illness.

MEDICAL INTERVENTIONS

Medical and surgical services. The intervention focus is on care—symptom management and relief, function, and quality of life—not cure. The nurse frequently has a pivotal role in caring for the patient and coordinating and monitoring medical services. Conveying an unwavering commitment to the patient of continuing quality care and concern in the face of no cure is critical.

Education and disease monitoring. Patients, family members, and other caregivers usually need education about the illness and require training in the use of equipment and medication administration. Education is frequently provided by a nurse, is usually disease-specific, and may be ongoing, requiring reminders and review. Attention must be paid to any language and literacy barriers in conveying this information.

Palliative care. Palliative care focuses on the relief of symptoms and is important at any stage of a chronic illness. Health professionals need to be clear about advance directives and to make certain there is concordance between the patient's wishes and the health care agent's understanding of these wishes. Providers should be able to offer guidance and options, including hospice care and other end-of-life options, to their patients.

FUNCTIONAL INTERVENTIONS

Rehabilitation. Based on the patient's medical problems, physical limitations, potential for rehabilitation, and participation readiness— physical therapists, occupational therapists, and speech and swallow therapists may work with the patient to set realistic short- and long-term rehabilitation goals. Rehabilitation therapy enables patients to restore function as well as prevent further deterioration.

Environmental adaptations. User-friendly environments for those with disabilities may include simple and low-cost interventions such as grab bars, improved lighting, and wheelchair-accessible counters.

PSYCHOSOCIAL INTERVENTIONS

Social services and mental health services. Social workers play a pivotal role in providing services once problems are identified. For example, social workers can help patients acknowledge the difficulties arising from a functional loss, grieve that loss, and learn to utilize remaining capabilities.

Financial and legal assistance. Clinicians need to discuss financial solutions with patients and family for whom financial problems prohibit medical adherence. Financially qualified patients may find substantial discounts through drug manufactures' Patient Assistance Programs (PAPs) or discount cards. Pharmacists and social workers are also excellent resources for finding less expensive options for medication (i.e., generic/formulary prescriptions) or helping patients make an appropriate choice for prescription coverage. Social workers and nurses are often involved in recognizing new or unresolved financial and legal problems and bringing them to the attention of team members for discussion and resolution.

Social support. Social support is crucial to preventing loneliness, depression, and premature cognitive decline. Providers should work to preserve patients' present relationships and help them expand their social networks if these have diminished. Individual and/or family counseling services may be effective interventions for helping patients relieve the emotional distress associated with social isolation and strategize ways of increasing social integration. When feasible, services offered in a group-related format may be particularly conducive to lessening social isolation. In addition, respite, counseling, and other support services should be considered for caregivers.

Dominica Potenza

Centers for Disease Control and Prevention. (2013). The state of aging and health in America 2013. Retrieved from http://www.cdc.gov/features/agingandhealth/State_of_aging_and_health_in_america_2013.pdf

Centers for Medicare & Medicaid Services. (2015). Chronic care management services. Retrieved from https://www.cms.gov/Outreach-and -Education/Medicare-Learning-Network-MLN/ MLNProducts/Downloads/ChronicCareManage ment.pdf

Centers for Disease Control and Prevention. (2017). National health interview survey. Retrieved from https://www.cdc.gov/nchs/data/factsheets/ factsheet_nhis.htm

Federal Interagency Forum on Aging-Related Statistics. (2016). *Older Americans 2016: Key indicators of well-being*. Washington, DC: U.S. Government Printing Office. Retrieved from http://www.agingstats .gov/docs/LatestReport/OA2016.pdf

U.S. Department of Health and Human Services. (2010). Multiple chronic conditions: A strategic framework: Optimum health and quality of life for individuals with multiple chronic conditions. Retrieved from http://www.hhs.gov/ash/initia-tives/mcc/mcc_framework.pdf

Ward, B. W., & Schiller, J. S. (2013). Prevalence of multiple chronic conditions among US adults: Estimates from Health Interview Survey, 2010. *Preventing Chronic Disease, 10*(120203). doi:10.5888/ pcd10.120203

Web Resources

Family Caregiver Alliance: http://www.caregiver .org

Improving Chronic Illness Care, Robert Wood Johnson Foundation: http://www.improvingchroniccare .org

National Council on Aging: https://www.ncoa.org/ healthy-aging/chronic-disease/chronic -disease-self-management-program

POGOE: Portal of Geriatric Online Education: http:// www.pogoe.org

CLINICAL PATHWAYS

Clinical pathways are structured interdisciplinary, evidence-based plans for the management of a well-defined group of patients. Clinical pathways are variously called *care pathways*, *care guidelines*, and *care maps*, among other names. These pathways define goals and key elements of care based on current best-practice evidence and detail essential steps in the daily interdisciplinary care of patients with a specific clinical problem.

Evidence-based practice and collaboration among professionals delivering care are integral to quality health care. Interdisciplinary care that is based on scientific data is an expectation of both oversight regulatory and reimbursement agencies. Collaboration and outcome-focused, interdisciplinary communication ensure that identified patient needs are addressed in a timely way by the discipline most skilled in achieving these outcomes. Use of clinical pathways is also in line with the goals of the Patient Protection and Affordable Care Act (PPACA): to control health care costs and to improve health care delivery. In line with these goals, careful and diligent adherence to clinical pathways can help minimize hospital-acquired complications, prevent unnecessary and costly long lengths of stay and decrease readmissions (Brooks, 2014).

The aim of any clinical pathway is to improve the quality of care, reduce risks, increase patient satisfaction, and improve the efficient use of resources by standardizing care. A focus on quality initiatives in health care has been evident since the influential 1999 Institute of Medicine report that faulted the health care system for preventable hospital-acquired complications that resulted in unnecessarily extended lengths of stay and loss of lives. Clinical pathways provide clear indications of the activities of the multidisciplinary care team members, the sequence and expected outcomes of these activities and the required monitoring for variances from the expected outcomes. The consistent challenge is not in the development of these guidelines, but in the diligent adherence needed for them to be effective.

The origins of clinical pathways can be found in the Centers for Medicare & Medicaid's promotion of hospital reimbursement based on diagnosis-related groupings (DRGs) in the early 1980s. The introduction of DRG-based reimbursement was one of the early attempts to hold down spiraling health care costs. DRGs allotted reimbursement monies based on patient diagnosis (or multiple diagnoses) and not on hospital days. Hospitals therefore needed to reconcile the length of stay for each diagnosis with the DRG reimbursement they would receive. They began to design plans for clinical care based

C

on what needed to be accomplished each hospitalized day so the patient could be safely discharged in the number of days that the DRG reimbursement would support. These changes in reimbursement practices gave impetus to several measures to ensure that costs would not exceed reimbursement. Case management, utilization review, and the oversight of coding and billing were expanded, and clinical pathways were developed.

Research on clinical pathways demonstrates that patient outcomes can be improved when care processes are standardized. This is particularly notable for hospitalized older adults, who are at risk for complications and extended hospitalization. A number of these pathways have been developed for elderly patients sustaining hip fractures, a too common injury in this age group with a range of associated deleterious outcomes. Hip fractures have significant adverse effects on the performance of activities of daily living and thus on independence and quality of life. Implementing clinical pathways for these patients has demonstrated reduced lengths of stay and improved mortality (Gooch et al., 2012). Additional clinical pathways for hip fractures address all stages of care from the emergency room visit through the perioperative and inpatient services to discharge from rehabilitative services. In one study, patients were notably clustered on one unit to maximize specialty nursing skills, and their care involved daily geriatric consultative services. Length of stay was found to be significantly less, 7 days in the intervention group versus 11 days in the control group (Flikweert et al., 2014).

Clinical pathways have been shown to reduce postoperative length of stay, improve management of chronic obstructive pulmonary disease (COPD) exacerbations, decrease ventilator-associated pneumonia and stroke, standardize the choice of chemotherapeutic agents and promote adherence to pneumonia guidelines (Ban et al., 2012; Beattie, Shepherd, Maher, & Grant, 2012; Ellis, 2013; Panella, Marchisio, Brambilla, Vanhaecht, & Di Stanislao, 2012). Though referred to as care bundles or protocols, not clinical pathways, interdisciplinary evidence-based management guidelines to prevent hospital-acquired complications can be found on the websites of organizations such as the Centers for Disease Control and Prevention (CDC) and the American Association of Critical-Care Nurses. These care guidelines include those for preventing catheter-related urinary tract infections, ventilator-associated pneumonia, central line–related bloodstream infections, and delirium.

Clinical pathways can serve as general guidelines for ensuring that the best standard of care is applied to all patients. Pathways should also incorporate assessments specific to the older adult, such as sensory and mobility evaluations, thus focusing all clinicians on the self-care needs of both hospitalized and community-dwelling older adults. Being alert to the possibility of confusion, unsteady gait, and incontinence may preempt these complications at any time during the care continuum. Although patients are expected to reach clinical milestones such as ambulating or being able to eat their usual diet by the time of discharge, older adults often require additional care in their homes, and the home health team can assist them in improving their self-management skills.

Discharge pathways can be essential for better preparing the patient for independence and decreasing early hospital readmissions that can result in payment denial. A continuum pathway focused on the specific needs of an older adult with heart failure (Garin et al., 2012), for example, may emphasize initial skills during hospitalization such as learning medication routines, self-managing diet, and monitoring weight daily. Discharge pathways also need to incorporate a home health assessment that includes safety awareness and education.

Clinical pathways have been associated with better teamwork, higher levels of organized care, and lower risk of burnout in acute health care teams. These pathways offer clinicians an opportunity for outlining key processes that must occur for patients to move safely through the continuum of care (Deneckere et al., 2013). Clinical pathways for older adults should address all sites at which care is delivered, from hospitalization to rehabilitation to long-term care to home. This continuum approach promotes communication and collaboration among caregivers and ensures that elder-specific care is delivered with a focus on quality.

Christine Cutugno

Ban, A., Ismail, A., Harun, R., Abdul Rahman, A., Sulung, S., & Syed Mohamed, A. (2012). Impact of clinical pathway on clinical outcomes in the management of COPD exacerbation. *BMC Pulmonary Medicine, 12*, 27.

Beattie, M., Shepherd, A., Maher, S., & Grant, J. (2012). Continual improvement in ventilator-acquired pneumonia bundle compliance: A retrospective case matched review. *Intensive & Critical Care Nursing, 28*, 255–262.

Brooks, J. (2014). The new world of health care quality and measurement. *American Journal of Nursing, 114*(7), 57–59.

Deneckere, S., Euwema, M., Lodewijckx, C., Panella, M., Mutsvari, T., Sermeus, W., & Vanhaecht, K. (2013). Better interprofessional teamwork, higher level of organized care, and lower risk of burnout in acute health care teams using care pathways: A cluster randomized controlled trial. *Medical Care, 51*, 99–107.

Ellis, P. (2013). Development and implementation of oncology care pathways in an integrated care network. *Journal of Oncology Practice, 9*(3), 171–173.

Flikweert, E. R., Izaks, G. J., Knobben, B. A., Stevens, M., & Wendt, K. (2014). The development of a comprehensive multidisciplinary care pathway for patients with a hip fracture: Design and results of a clinical trial. *BMC Musculoskeletal Disorders, 15*(1), 188.

Garin, N., Carballo, S., Gerstel, E., Lerch, R., Meyer, P., Zare, M.,...Perrier, A. (2012). Inclusion into a heart failure critical pathway reduces the risk of death or readmission after hospital discharge. *European Journal of Internal Medicine, 23*, 760–764.

Gooch, K., Marshall, D., Faris, P., Khong, H., Wasylak, T., Pearce, T.,...Frank, C. (2012). Comparative effectiveness of alternative clinical pathways for primary hip and knee joint replacement patients: A pragmatic randomized, controlled trial. *Osteoarthritis & Cartilage, 20*, 1086–1094.

Institute of Medicine. (1999). *To err is human: Building a safer health system*. Washington, DC: National Academies Press. Retrieved from http://www.nationalacademies.org/hmd/Reports/1999/To-Err-is-Human-Building-A-Safer-Health-system

Panella, M., Marchisio, S., Brambilla, R., Vanhaecht, K., & Di Stanislao, F. (2012). A cluster randomized trial to assess the effect of clinical pathways for patients with stroke: Results of the clinical pathways for effective and appropriate care study. *BMC Medicine, 10*, 71.

Web Resources
American Association of Critical Care Nurses: http://www.aacn.org

American Case Management Association: http://www.acmaweb.org

Case Management Society of America: http://www.cmsa.org

Case Manager's Resource Guide: http://www.cmrg.com

Center for Case Management: http://www.cfcm.com

Centers for Disease Control: http://www.cdc.gov

COGNITIVE CHANGES IN AGING

Cognitive changes, whether naturally arising with age or due to abnormal processes such as a neurocognitive disorder, cast a wide net of influence over virtually all areas of an elderly individual's life. Tasks such as installing new software on a computer, recalling phone conversations, or understanding a document that lists several different health insurance options may become more difficult. Some types of cognitive decline begin in young adulthood: Perceptual processing speed peaks in the 20s and numeric ability in the 30s. Other cognitive abilities, such as inductive reasoning and verbal meaning (i.e., vocabulary recognition), continue to develop into midlife (40s–60s) and then reach a plateau before beginning a modest decline. Most people in their 60s and beyond experience some degree of further cognitive decline, particularly in the domains of processing speed, working memory, inhibitory functioning, and long-term memory.

A significant decline from the cognitive function baseline of an individual before the age of 60 years is unlikely to be attributable to aging alone; instead it likely signals the development of a neurocognitive disorder. Such changes must not be assessed in comparison to a peer group or research-based averages for a certain age but should be compared only to the individual's own unique baseline. Each person has a unique

C

set of cognitive abilities based on their genetics and lifetime experiences.

The latter include both psychosocial factors (e.g., education, culture, work experience, attention to diet and exercise) and biological factors (e.g., sensory impairments, illnesses, head trauma, and environmental exposure to neurotoxic substances). Cognitive decline tends to occur earlier for individuals who suffer from chronic illnesses, such as cardiovascular disease, diabetes, and cancer, but later for those who demonstrated high levels of intelligence in childhood. Those with a lot of waist fat, midlife–onset diabetes, problems with the sense of smell, high blood pressure, or metabolic syndrome are at higher risk for developing mild cognitive impairment (MCI), as well as for that MCI later converting into dementia (Ng et al., 2016).

For all adults, changes in brain structure and function are the source of age-related declines. Recent research, however, has revealed that the human brain is by no means a static organ with a limited number of neurons that can only be lost. The discoveries that it can generate new brain cells (neurogenesis) and establish new functional networks (neuroplasticity) has opened new insights into how the brain is a dynamic organ that can respond to internal or external challenges to maintain its functioning. Functional neuroimaging has revealed how the aging brain can recruit new circuits to augment or replace aging circuits. Such reorganization may function less efficiently, however, than the previous brain structuring it has modified. This compensatory capacity, which has been referred to as *scaffolding*, may account not only for the preservation of some cognitive processes, but also for the decline in processing speed. Neurogenesis and neuroplasticity are themselves eventually susceptible to change with age. The steeper declines in cognitive functions of very late life likely reflect losses of these abilities.

COGNITIVE AGING

By middle age, many adults have begun to experience a cognitive decline in a range of domains involving memory and executive function (Turner & Spreng, 2012). Executive functions include attention, response inhibition (i.e., the ability to block out distractions), working memory, planning and implementation of tasks, task shifting, judgment, monitoring, and modulaton of activities. For most individuals in their 70s and 80s, memory performance, language comprehension, effective reasoning, and the ability to learn new things gradually become increasingly difficult. Failure to initiate or follow through on complex tasks involving multiple steps often signals a decline in executive function. By age 80, the declines for older adults are on average severe, except for accrued knowledge, reflected in verbal abilities.

Decreases in working memory—the ability to store and process a limited amount of information while actively engaging with other information and tasks—is a common consequence of age-related brain changes. Decreases in the functionality of working memory can compromise a number of other cognitive functions, including comprehension, learning, and long-term memory. For example, the ability to later recall two possible dates and times for a family reunion requires keeping them in working memory long enough to record them internally, in the long-term memory of the brain, or externally, by jotting them down on a notepad. Diminishing working memory can also adversely affect overall memory performance, particularly when the situation calls for an individual to learn or recall information under stressful circumstances. Likewise, when visual, auditory, or other informational distractions abound, decline in response inhibition can adversely affect working memory and thereby undermine comprehension, learning, and remembering. Such changes in turn can result in the deterioration of older adults' abilities to perform instrumental activities of daily living, such as meal preparation, cleaning, and shopping, as well as managing finances or medication regimens.

Not all cognitive abilities decline with age to the same degree. For instance, consistent mental activity allows many individuals to continue to maintain their knowledge base and even gain new knowledge. The accumulation of information allows individuals to successfully maneuver through day-to-day life, in part because it bolsters automatic ("second nature") processes. The ability to perform certain tasks automatically, without having to give them much, if any thought, is a major way that the brain organizes itself to be more efficient. Such "overlearned" cognitive processes are easier to rely on when experiencing cognitive changes, particularly a decline in working memory. For example, an older man may choose to whip up his famous tuna casserole that he has made for more than 30 years rather than follow a more complex recipe.

Most individuals go about their days performing tasks that are largely automatic and that require minimal conscious processing. Throughout a lifetime, these automatic activities become even more consolidated into an individual's routine. Individuals consistently return to facts and sage advice ("rules of thumb") they have picked up over the years as a means of making daily decisions and modulating their everyday thoughts, feelings, and behaviors.

Prospective memory is a domain of cognition that does not seem to be as negatively affected over time. Much of past research has focused on changes in retrospective memory, the recollection of past events, as individuals' age. Significant deficits in retrospective memory are consistently reported, including increased difficulty with the ability to remember lists of words spontaneously (free recall of a list that includes the name of a specific color), with categorical clues (cued recall; e.g., "it was a color"), and eventually, recognition memory (multiple choice; e.g., "was it red, blue, or green?"). More recently, studies have begun to explore prospective memory, or memory for future intentions. Unlike retrospective memory, older adults seem to have a relatively greater capacity for prospective memory than their younger counterparts.

SELF-REPORTS

Many patients provide self-reports to their caregivers, which can prove to be incredibly insightful and helpful. However, for these self-reports to be beneficial for both parties, the older individual must be able to do a number of things, such as comprehend a caregiver's questions and effectively articulate answers. To be effective requires an individual to follow a policy of honesty when reporting symptoms, names, medications, family histories, dietary intakes, and moods. Although many caregivers rely heavily on self-reports, they can be fairly unreliable. Critical information may be left out or overlooked, a tendency that may increase as a patient experiences more cognitive decline with age.

COMMUNICATION

To aid comprehension, caregivers can use simply phrased questions and scenarios (Harwood et al., 2012). In addition, giving the individual a chance to read the question and hear it may help. Some older individuals who have limited working memory may find a caregiver's speech too rapid to follow, thereby obstructing comprehension. Auditory presentations can also put more strain on working memory. Research has shown that, more frequently than younger adults, older adults tend to endorse the final choice of several that have been auditorily presented; this difference does not extend to visually presented choices. Although individuals of all ages struggle to recall how many times a particular event has occurred (e.g., doctor appointments), elderly individuals have more trouble with this task. To aid in the retrieval of more accurate information, caregivers can ask the older individual about the specifics of the event, such as the name of the doctor or the purpose of each visit to the doctor. In addition, providing individuals with written options rather than open-ended inquiries can increase memory regarding topics such as family medical histories.

People may forget information related to their care soon after they hear it, even though caregivers often spend significant time and resources trying to present such information. The aging process exacerbates this forgetfulness, especially when information is presented only verbally. When a caregiver speaks rapidly, avoids eye contact and thereby fails to assess understanding, does not bother to emphasize important points, uses unfamiliar or complicated jargon, or presents too much critical information at one time, the process of retaining information is made that much harder for an elderly individual. In contrast, asking individuals to take notes, encouraging them to repeat key points, and presenting them with a straightforward and concise written summary can be quite beneficial.

If there are misgivings about the patient's memory, the caregiver should invite a family member to sit in on or participate in the discussion. Basic and minimal sensory-correction modalities such as a well-lit room, a bigger font size, static web pages, hearing aids, and prescription glasses should always be encouraged. Interviewers should keep this in mind and encourage at least temporary use of a portable amplifier to engage with elderly persons who decline the use of hearing aids.

Stressful situations can make it difficult for any individual, regardless of memory ability, to fully comprehend and remember instructions. In addition, aspects of cognition can have an impact on an individual's ability to take medication consistently. Research suggests that the young to old (ages 60–75 years) tend to take medication much more consistently than the older to old (older than 75 years). Cognitive interventions can improve an individual's ability to consistently follow through on taking medications (e.g., giving an older individual a pill organizer and drafting a chart that outlines their personalized medication regimen). These interventions are likely to lessen the demands on memory and executive function that often arise with more complex regimens.

An interesting way that may improve working memory is use of day-to-day modalities such as computer-based exercises for the brain that can improve cognition (Hill et al., 2017). Aerobic exercise also has some benefits on cognition in this regard in those with normal cognition or even in those with MCI (Zheng, Xia, Zhou, Tao, & Chen, 2016). Cognitive enhancers appear to have only a very minimal role in helping elderly individuals with normal age-related slowing of brain processes (Ströhle et al., 2015).

When speaking, individuals produce two to three words per second; listeners must follow and comprehend speech at the same pace. Verbal communications can tax the working memory capacity of older individuals. When listening, an older individual is unable to retrieve words that have been spoken even a few seconds before. This is very different from written communications, in which an older individual can reread a passage as many times as desired.

When communicating with older individuals, caregivers should attempt to use syntactically simple sentences and clearly emphasize key points. To improve the quality of communication, speakers are encouraged to give examples and summarize important points. This should be done without adopting a tone of condescension toward the older listener. Respect for the elderly individual should always inform a caregiver's words and actions.

Many older individuals experience reduced auditory perception, which makes it more difficult to distinguish spoken sounds and therefore necessitates greater reliance on nonverbal components of communication. Therefore older individuals may utilize their general knowledge of interactions to fill in what they were unable to hear to a much greater extent than younger individuals. Older individuals may also focus on normal intonations and changes in pitch during spoken conversation to increase their understanding of what is being said.

Overall, difficulties in comprehending and recalling important care-related information often arise in the wake of diminished cognitive processing and more limited working memory resources. When a caregiver is aware of these difficulties and in turn presents information in ways that allow and encourage the older individual to utilize general knowledge about daily interactions to aid comprehension, most cognitive deficits associated with aging can be lessened (Harwood et al., 2012).

See also Depression in Dementia; Medication Adherence.

Satya Gutta and Timothy Howell

Harwood, J., Leibowitz, K., Lin, M., Morrow, D. G., Rucker, N. L., & Savundranayagam, M. Y. (2012). *Communicating with older adults: An evidenced based review of what really works.* Washington, DC: The Gerontological Society of America.

Hill, N. T., Mowszowski, L., Naismith, S. L., Chadwick, V. L., Valenzuela, M., & Lampit, A. (2017). Computerized cognitive training in older adults with mild cognitive impairment or dementia: A systematic review and meta-analysis. *American Journal of Psychiatry, 174,* 329.

Ng, T. P., Feng, L., Nyunt, M. S., Feng, L., Gao, Q., Lim, M. L.,...Yap, K. B. (2016). Metabolic syndrome and the risk of mild cognitive impairment and progression to dementia: Follow-up of the Singapore longitudinal ageing study cohort. *JAMA Neurology, 73,* 456.

Ströhle, A., Schmidt, D. K., Schultz, F., Fricke, N., Staden, T., Hellweg, R.,...Rieckmann, N. (2015). Drug and exercise treatment of Alzheimer disease and mild cognitive impairment: A systematic review and meta-analysis of effects on cognition in randomized controlled trials. *American Journal of Geriatric Psychiatry, 23,* 1234.

Turner, G. R., & Spreng, R. N. (2012). Executive functions and neurocognitive aging: Dissociable patterns of brain activity. *Neurobiology of Aging, 33*(4), 826.e1–826.e13.

Zheng, G., Xia, R., Zhou, W., Tao, J., & Chen, L. (2016). Aerobic exercise ameliorates cognitive function in older adults with mild cognitive impairment: A systematic review and meta-analysis of randomised controlled trials. *British Journal of Sports Medicine, 50*(23), 1443–1450.

Web Resources

Administration for Community Living: https://www.acl.gov

The Gerontological Society of America: https://www.geron.org/policy-center/resourcecenter/hot-topics

University of California, San Francisco: http://memory.ucsf.edu/Education/Topics/normalaging.html

COGNITIVE INSTRUMENTS

The prevalence of neurocognitive disorders or dementia increases with age, doubling every 5 years after the age of 65. The current demographic and epidemiological predictions are that the current 35.6 million persons worldwide with these conditions is expected to triple by the year 2050, unless effective prevention or disease-modifying interventions can be found and made widely available to all those at risk. Although such interventions remain unavailable or limited in effectiveness, increasing numbers of things can be done to slow the progression of these conditions and to reduce the exposure of cognitively vulnerable persons to factors that accelerate cognitive decline and associated behavioral problems, making early detection increasingly important. Early detection also allows families and persons with these conditions to prepare for the functional decline and safety issues that accompany neurocognitive disorders. The instruments described here remain helpful as part of the screening, detection, and monitoring of cognitive deterioration.

Neurocognitive disorders are a group of progressive, global, cognitive syndromes associated with neuronal loss or structural damage. Each instrument discussed here assesses different cognitive functions with different levels of accuracy, sensitivity, and reliability. Moreover, depending on the area of the brain most affected by the specific neuropathological process under consideration, specific illnesses, such as Alzheimer's dementia and frontotemporal dementia present with a slightly different profile of cognitive deficits and associated symptoms.

Ideally, primary care providers, or any trained health care professional involved in the care of older adults, should screen persons older than 65 years for cognitive deficits annually, even in the absence of a family history of dementia, clinical red flags, or subjective complaints. With practice, use of the instruments are sensitive, specific, valid, reliable, and relatively brief, although some take more time than others. The most commonly used instruments, indications for their use, and criteria for determining when further testing is indicated are described.

PREPARATION FOR TESTING

To interpret tests meaningfully and better estimate the underlying etiology of the neurocognitive disorder, the clinician should obtain from the patient (and, whenever possible, a family member) a detailed clinical history regarding the patient's memory and overall functioning. Any change in functioning, such as forgetting recent conversations, word-finding difficulty, or problems managing finances should prompt a more standardized assessment. It is important to identify sensory impairments that can alter test performance and the interpretation of findings. Collateral information is helpful when evaluating activities of daily living (ADL) and instrumental activities of daily living (IADL). In the absence of reliable corroborate history, the clinician should carefully observe the person's grooming, hygiene, appropriateness of clothing to the weather; state of nourishment, capacity to understand and follow medical recommendations, medication adherence, and regular attendance to appointments, tests, and follow-ups.

Accurate evaluation of a patient's performance requires understanding the patient's cultural and ethnic background, primary language, education level, employment history, and overall premorbid functioning. Education level and occupational history, for instance, can alter the cut-off points of certain instruments. Some tests display greater language and cultural biases than others, yielding uneven accuracy levels across populations.

Depression, pain and general uncooperativeness can impact test performance and render the results less reliable. Clinicians need to be careful when assessing the level of impairment because a patient can maintain social skills and present surprisingly well—at least, superficially.

SCREENING INSTRUMENTS

All cognitive-impairment screening instruments evolved with research in mind. Key attributes and limitations of the most commonly used instruments are discussed.

Mini-Mental State Examination

The Mini-Mental State Examination (MMSE) by Folstein, Folstein, and McHugh (1975) is the best known and best studied of all mental-status instruments. Since its introduction, it has served as the "gold standard" against which subsequently developed cognitive screening tools have been compared. The MMSE involves 22 questions to measure orientation, spatial ability, immediate memory, short-term recall, calculations, concentration, abstract thinking, judgment, aphasia, apraxia, agnosia, and

constructional ability. To perform the MMSE, the patient must have intact functional abilities, including motor control, vision, and hearing. If the patient is functionally impaired beyond correction, the clinician should use another test or refer the patient to a neuropsychologist. The clinician must carefully assess the patient's educational level and primary language ability before administering the MMSE, which is only valid and reliable (i.e., sensitivity of 87%, specificity of 82%) for persons whose primary language is English. With a scale from 0 to 30 points, the MMSE's cut-off score to indicate cognitive impairment drops from 24 for patients with a high school education to 18 for patients with only an eighth-grade education. To use the MMSE, a clinician should record a patient's answers verbatim, both correct and incorrect, to enable comparisons during follow-up care. Some limitations of the examination are that a relatively small proportion of points are earned for tasks that test frontal lobe functioning, and the test is not very sensitive for identifying mild cognitive impairment (MCI). The tool retains its copyright protection.

Montreal Cognitive Assessment (MoCA)

Originally designed as a tool to screen for MCI, the Montreal Cognitive Assessment (MoCA; Nasreddine et al., 2004; Zahinoor, Rajji, & Shulman, 2010) has gained popularity as a general cognitive screening tool. It is not copyright protected and therefore is more widely available. The MoCA tests multiple domains, including short-term memory, visuospatial function, executive function, attention, concentration, working memory, language, and orientation. The MoCA has demonstrated superior sensitivity compared with the MMSE for detection of both MCI (90% vs. 18%) as well as Alzheimer's dementia (100% vs. 78%). One drawback of the MoCA is that it is less specific than the MMSE (78%–87% vs. 100%). A patient can score a maximum of 30 points, with a cutoff for normal of less than 26.

Quick Mild Cognitive Impairment

The Quick Mild Cognitive Impairment (Qmci; O'Caoimh, Timmons, & Molloy, 2016) is another cognitive screening instrument that is effective in identifying MCI and differentiating MCI from normal cognitive aging and dementia (with high sensitivity and specificity). It is a little shorter and easier to administer than the MoCA, with equal or better accuracy. The Qmci has elements covering five domains: orientation, registration, clock drawing, delayed recall, verbal fluency (e.g., naming of animals), and logical memory (testing immediate verbal recall of a short story; O'Caoimh et al., 2016).

The Mini-Cog

The Mini-Cog assessment instrument (Borson, Scanlon, Brush, Vitaliano, & Dokmak, 2000) is a brief test that can be administered in approximately 3 minutes; it is relatively uninfluenced by level of education or language variations and, in at least one study, is comparable to the MMSE in a diverse population. The Mini-Cog combines an uncued three-item recall test with the clock-drawing test (CDT) that is used as a distracter during the interval for short-term recall. The main strength of this instrument is its ease of use and the combination of memory and executive function instruments. However, an uncued recall test is not particularly accurate because it screens as impaired patients who suffer only from difficulties in retrieval, and not storage, of information. Retrieval can be impaired in patients with Parkinson's disease or other neurological illnesses; deficits in learning of new information are characteristic of Alzheimer's dementia. Patients with Alzheimer's dementia will not benefit from cues; however, patients with Parkinson's disease will. Therefore, a more accurate instrument could be obtained combining a cued recall test (e.g., Memory-Impairment Screen) with the CDT.

Clock Drawing Test

The CDT (Freedman et al., 1994) is a brief, widely used, and easy-to-administer instrument for assessing executive control and temporo-parietal abilities. The CDT is reliable and less influenced by language, culture, and education, given that most people use clocks. The test's main limitation stems from its many versions,

each varying slightly in scoring criteria and instructions. Whereas each version accurately assesses certain functions, different scoring methods impede comparisons across studies. Yet the CDT's fundamental concept remains easy to understand and is sound. A clinician asks a patient to draw a clock set at a specific time. Instructions vary in setting the clock at different times, in drawing freehand versus completing a predrawn circle, and in copying a clock that the examiner has already drawn. Scoring also varies by the number of details evaluated. Practitioners should use one version of the CDT consistently to facilitate follow-up comparisons. It is unclear if the test will remain as useful with persons who grew-up relying on digital sources for the time.

Memory-Impairment Screen

The Memory-Impairment Screen (MIS; Buschke et al., 1999) is a brief, reliable, and valid test for early dementia and memory impairment. The MIS is part of a longer, more complex screening with high discriminative validity. The MIS tests only memory, proving most accurate for patients with a suspected diagnosis of Alzheimer's dementia and least accurate for persons with suspected frontal-lobe deficits, subcortical dementias, and intact memory. The MIS tests free and cued recall of four words that the patient has been asked to learn. A clinician determines the patient's score, on a scale of 0 to 8, by making the following calculation: (2 × Free Recall) + Obtained Cued Recall. The cutoff score of 4 has a sensitivity of 0.69 for mild dementia and 0.92 for moderate dementia. When analyses are restricted only to Alzheimer's dementia, the sensitivity for mild dementia is 0.79 and 0.95 for moderate impairment.

Other Tests

Several other instruments are available to test for cognitive deficits. A full battery of tests typically requires several hours to administer, score, and interpret and should be administered only by trained practitioners. Most clinicians caring for older adults need to be familiar with only a few instruments and know when to refer a patient to a specialist. Some of the more complex tests are relevant primarily for their usefulness in clinical research. Among such tests is the Dementia Rating Scale (DRS; Gardner, Oliver-Munoz, Fisher, & Empting, 1981) that consists of 36 tasks comprising five subscales that measure attention, initiation/perseveration, construction, conceptualization, and memory. The DRS's total score cut-off is 123, with separate cut-off scores for each subcategory indicating specific deficits. For example, a patient with impaired scores in the initiation/perseveration and conceptualization subscales but with intact memory would suggest a frontal-lobe deficit and make a diagnosis of Alzheimer's dementia unlikely.

The Boston Naming Test (Kaplan, Goodglass, & Weintnaube, 1983) assesses naming difficulties associated with aphasia common to cortical dementias. The Trail-Making Test (Reintan & Wolfson, 1985) measures attention capacity, with particular sensitivity to frontal-lobe deficits and early detection of subcortical dementia.

No instrument for screening cognitive deficits is perfect or complete. Some are more affected by primary language, education, and cultural background; others are less standardized or measure only specific functions. Testing with the MMSE, MIS, and CDT generates a reasonably thorough set of results. Together, these three tests require 10 to 15 minutes to complete, are easily interpreted, and facilitate screening for cortical and subcortical dementia that is superior to any single instrument. Most important, a clinician must determine when to refer a patient for further testing. If a patient with a high level of education and premorbid functioning complains of cognitive decline but scores above the cutoff threshold in a screening test, the patient should be referred for further testing. Moreover, any person showing a discrepancy between functional capacity and screening performance should see a specialist.

See also Depression Measurement Instruments; Pain Assessment Instruments.

Steven L. Baumann

Borson, S., Scanlon, J. M., Brush, M., Vitaliano, P. P., & Dokmak, A. (2000). The Mini-Cog: A cognitive "vital signs" measure for dementia screening in multilingual elderly. *International Journal of Geriatric Psychiatry, 15*(11), 1021–1027.

Buschke, H., Kuslansky, G., Katz, M., Stewart, W. F., Sliwinski, M. J., Eckholdt, H. M., & Lipton, R. B. (1999). Screening for dementia with the Memory Impairment Screen. *Neurology, 52*(2), 231–238.

Folstein, M. F., Folstein, S. E., & McHugh, P. R. (1975). "Mini-Mental State": A practical method for grading the cognitive state of patients for the clinician. *Journal of Psychiatric Research, 12*(3), 189–198.

Freedman, M., Leach, L., Kaplan, E., Winocur, G., Shulman, K. T., & Delis, D. C. (1994). *Clock drawing: A neuropsychological analysis.* New York, NY: Oxford University Press.

Gardner, R., Oliver-Munoz, S., Fisher, L., & Empting, L. (1981). Mattis Dementia Rating Scale: Internal reliability study using a diffusely impaired population. *Journal of Clinical Neuropsychology, 3,* 271–275.

Kaplan, E. F., Goodglass, H., & Weintnaube, S. (1983). *The Boston Naming Test.* Philadelphia, PA: Lea & Febiger.

Nasreddine, Z. S., Chertkow, H., Phillips, N., Whitehead, V., Collin, I., & Cummings, J. L. (2004, April). The Montreal Cognitive Assessment (MoCA): A brief cognitive screening tool for detection of mild cognitive impairment. *Neurology, 62*(7), S5.

O'Caoimh, R., Timmons, S., & Molloy, D. W. (2016). Screening for mild cognitive impairment: Comparison of "MCI specific" screening instruments. *Journal of Alzheimer's Disease, 51*(2), 619–629.

Reitan, R.M., & Wolfson, D. (1985). *The Halstead-Reitan neuropsychological battery: Theory and clinical interpretation.* Tucson, AZ: Neuropsychology Press.

Zahinoor, I., Rajji, T. K., & Shulman, R. (2010). Brief cognitive screening instruments: An update [Review article]. *International Journal of Geriatric Psychiatry, 25,* 111–120.

Web Resources
Montreal Cognitive Assessment: http://www.mocatest.org
Society of Hospital Medicine Clinical Toolbox: http://www.hospitalmedicine.org/geriresource/toolbox

---

COMMUNITY ASSESSMENT

Comprehensive geriatric assessment (CGA) in the home is a systematic, interdisciplinary evaluation identifying and describing the problems, needs, resources, and strengths of an older adult, in the physical, functional, psychosocial, and environmental domains. A CGA assesses unmet needs and proposes a focused, individualized plan for addressing these concerns, optimizing the health and well-being of the older patient (National Institutes of Health, 1988; Wieland & Hirth, 2002). A cornerstone of a successful community assessment, CGA in the home setting provides a unique picture of the older person. In addition, an innovation in the organization of patient-care communications, the CGA assists the clinician in effectively communicating among multiple providers and family caregivers (Siebens, 2001). One widely used and tested approach to CGA is the Domain Management Model (DMM), which organizes patient information related to strengths, concerns, and problems into the following four domains: medical/surgical issues, mental status/emotions/coping, physical function, and living environment (Siebens, 2001, 2002).

ASSESSMENT

A summary of what is typically covered in the comprehensive assessment of an older adult is summarized in this section, organized in the DMM format (Siebens, 2001).

Domain I: Medical/Surgical Issues

- Physical health—salient results from assessing: medical history, review of systems, self-reported chronic conditions, self-perceived health status; physical examination (body systems, nutritional status, oral health, skin, gait, and balance performance); laboratory studies; examination of home pharmacy—medication, other daily supplement use; and preventive visits and health maintenance adherence

Domain II: Mental Status/Emotions/Coping

- Psychological (mental) health and related topics—salient results from assessing: communication (hearing, vision, verbal, and nonverbal expression); mental status—cognitive screening; emotions—depression and anxiety screening; coping—self-perceived quality of life, management of stressors; spirituality—spiritual beliefs and practices; religion; and behaviors

Domain III: Physical Function

- Function—salient results from assessing: basic activities of daily living (BADL)—home mobility, self-care; instrumental activities of daily living (IADL)—community mobility, household tasks; and advanced activities of daily living (AADL)—vocational, avocational, social roles

Domain IV: Living Environment

- Environment—salient results from assessments of three main areas: physical environment, home safety/hazards, and accessibility to community
- Social issues—social support network (size, quality of relationship, family coping), social resources such as attendants, and community connections such as senior center social activities
- Financial and other community resources—health insurance, income, financial benefits such as Social Security, transportation, and financial or legal services

Results from in-home CGA studies reveal a high prevalence of suboptimally treated health problems (Stuck et al., 1995). The most common include hearing deficits (65% of patients), musculoskeletal problems (63%), arthritis (61%), hypertension (58%), cataracts (50%), and unsafe environments (46%). Less frequent, but with major potential health consequences, are vision deficits (35%), urinary incontinence (32%), osteoporosis (31%), depression (26%), anemia (23%), arrhythmia (23%), postural hypotension (23%), and gait and balance disorders (23%). The use of CGA, organized by domains, is likely to reduce the number of undertreated conditions.

RECOMMENDATIONS

Community assessment becomes an intervention only when linked with a care plan. The plan can take different forms, depending on the patient population. For frail older adults, community

CGA is the basis of medical, psychological, and functional management. This may include recommendations for placement for services for lost abilities to prevent nursing home placement. For well elders, CGA becomes a risk-appraisal method with recommendations made to the older person for what can be done to maintain or improve health and prevent functional decline. CGA and the DMM can improve posthospital outcomes, manage chronic disease, supplement regular primary care for the elderly, and prevent functional decline (Alessi et al., 1997; Barer, 2011; Kushner, Peters, & Johnson-Greene, 2015; Siebens, 2001, 2002).

As the front end of a system of care, community assessment is supported by a comprehensive set of community resources, educational materials, and negotiation strategies. Each health problem uncovered may have several alternative management responses. For example, an older adult's gait and balance disorder may need to be presented as a serious health risk (of falling). Recommendations are likely to cover several domains: discontinue the use of open-back clogs (dressing, BADL), remove throw rugs in the home (physical environment), see the podiatrist for foot care (medical-issue management), and see the primary care physician regarding the increasing pain in the hips (medical management).

ADHERENCE

The next step in the care system requires turning recommendations into action. In clinic- and hospital-based CGA, the best health outcomes result from situations in which the clinician doing the CGA also carries out the plan; this contrasts with typical community assessment in which recommendations are made to be implemented by the older person, family, or primary care provider. The DMM can be used as part of a patient-care communications protocol that includes a patient care notebook, which facilitates the organization of medical information for the patient and provider (Siebens & Randall, 2005).

One advantage of community assessment, reported by CGA program nurses, is that the relationship with the older person is on more equal terms (Stuck et al., 1995). More of a

partnership is established between the patient and the health care provider. The nurse remains the expert, and older persons are expert on their own situations. In addition, common self-care recommendations—taught, modeled, and reinforced in the home environment—have a greater likelihood of being followed. In one study, nurse practitioners made 5,694 specific recommendations to 202 patients for 3 years; 51% involved a self-care activity; 20%, referral to a nonphysician professional or community service; and 29%, referral to a physician (typically the patient's own primary care provider). Referrals to physicians had the highest level of full or partial adherence (70%), self-care recommendations were followed approximately 60% of the time, and community referrals were followed approximately 50% of the time (Alessi et al., 1997). Adherence to recommendations made to patients appeared to follow a pattern related to the degree of habit change involved, perceived seriousness of the problem, and familiarity with the recommended behavior. Moreover, according to Aminzadeh (2000), strategies for improving patient adherence to plans of care include, "developing treatment plans based on an understanding of patient beliefs and resources, using a combination of methods to communicate the plan effectively, simplifying the plan and taking early steps to facilitate implementation, and creating a continuum of formal and informal support to carry out the plan" (p. 405).

CLINICIAN COMPETENCIES

The clinician doing community assessment should have the knowledge and skill to complete all components of the CGA and know about self-care and community resources, how and when to seek consultation, when to refer to physician care (and when not to), and how to use principles of adult learning to promote behavior change for good health behaviors and outcomes. The DMM and organized, written information, such as inpatient care notebooks, are easy-to-use methods for efficient organization and communication about essential community-assessment information (Moscowitz, 2002). These methods are also critical for effective team functioning and collaboration.

Interdisciplinary clinical teams are extremely important to successful community assessment. The team may include a nurse practitioner or community nurse, with backup from a geriatrician, and consultation as needed from a social worker. Depending on the available resources and the skills of the nurse, consultation from a physical therapist, occupational therapist, nutritionist, and pharmacist can be helpful. The intervention is more cost effective if only one person is in the field (i.e., the nurse). This also improves adherence and communication because only one person interacts with the patient. Simple but comprehensive documentation and communication are essential for team collaboration and for prevention of oversight of important issues.

TIME FRAME

Behavior change and improvement in health status (or prevention of functional decline) takes place over months and years. Repeated assessments yield new problems and recommendations. Reinforcement of positive change is a continual process. In a randomized controlled trial (Stuck et al., 1995), after 3 years of annual in-home CGA and quarterly home visits by a nurse practitioner, intervention group subjects ($n = 215$) had significantly fewer permanent nursing home placements and fewer nursing home days than the control group ($n = 199$). In addition, the participants were more independent in daily chores and activities. They also had increased physician visits (which, although increasing the costs of the program, may have also led to a concomitant reduction in nursing home days) and used more community services that promoted socialization, such as senior transportation and special community college programs. There were no significant differences between the intervention and control groups in the use of in-home supportive or personal-care services. In addition, Stuck and Iliffe (2011), assert that the long-term use of CGAs will result in improved patient outcomes and possibly reduce health care costs by decreasing hospital admission rates and long-term care placements.

Community-assessment programs are slow in gaining acceptance. As for any intervention that is primarily diagnostic and preventive, payment sources are elusive and methods for enrollment sometimes complex. Nevertheless, growing evidence of the cost-effectiveness of CGAs, associated improved health outcomes, and effective communication strategies make these approaches promising for further development and wider implementation.

See also Geriatric Evaluation and Management Units; Home Health Care.

Jené M. Hurlbut

Alessi, C. A., Stuck, A. E., Aronow, H. U., Yuhas, K. E., Bula, C. J., Madison,…Beck, J. C. (1997). The process of care in preventive in-home comprehensive geriatric assessment. *Journal of the American Geriatrics Society, 45*(9), 1044–1050.

Aminzadeh, F. (2000). Adherence to recommendations of community-based comprehensive geriatric assessment programmes. *Age and Ageing, 29*(5), 401–407.

Barer, D. (2011). ACP Journal Club. Review: Inpatient comprehensive geriatric assessment improves the likelihood of living at home at 12 months. *Annals of Internal Medicine, 155*(12), JC6–JC2.

Kushner, D., Peters, K., & Johnson-Greene, D. (2015). Evaluating use of the Siebens Domain Management Model during inpatient rehabilitation to increase functional independence and discharge rate to home in stroke patients. *American Academy of Physical Medicine and Rehabilitation, 7*(4), 354–364.

Moscowitz, B. (2002). Bridging to family and community support for older adults and the Domain Management Model. *Topics in Stroke Rehabilitation, 4*, 75–86.

National Institutes of Health, Consensus Development Conference. (1988). National Institute of Health, Consensus Development Conference statement: Geriatric assessment methods for clinical decision making. *Journal of the American Geriatrics Society, 36*, 342–347.

Siebens, H. (2001). Applying the Domain Management Model in treating patients with chronic diseases. *The Joint Commission Journal on Quality Improvement, 27*(6), 302–314.

Siebens, H. (2002). The Domain Management Model: Organizing care for stroke survivors and other persons with chronic diseases. *Topics in Stroke Rehabilitation, 9*(3), 1–25.

Siebens, H., & Randall, P. (2005). The patient care notebook: From pilot phase to successful hospital-wide dissemination. *Joint Commission Journal on Quality and Patient Safety/Joint Commission Resources, 31*(7), 398–405.

Stuck, A. E., Aronow, H. U., Steiner, A., Alessi, C. A., Büla, C. J., Gold, M. N.,...Beck, J. C. (1995). A trial of annual in-home comprehensive geriatric assessments for elderly people living in the community. *New England Journal of Medicine, 333*(18), 1184–1189.

Stuck, A. E., & Iliffe, S. (2011). Comprehensive geriatric assessment for older adults. *British Medical Journal, 343,* d6799. doi:10.1136/bmj.d6799

Wieland, D., & Hirth, V. (2002). Comprehensive geriatric assessment. *Cancer Control: Journal of the Moffitt Cancer Center, 10*(6), 454–462.

Web Resources

Administration for Community Living: https://www.acl.gov

Fall Prevention Center of Excellence: http://www.stopfalls.org

Geriatrics at Your Fingertips–On-line Edition. American Geriatrics Society: http://www.geriatricsatyourfingertips.org

Merck Manual of Geriatrics: http://www.merckmanuals.com/professional/geriatrics

National Institute on Aging: http://www.nia.nih.gov

Siebens Patient Care Communications: http://www.siebenspcc.com

COMPETENCY AND CAPACITY

In 2000, Americans aged 65 years or older constituted 12.4% of the population; by 2051, this group of Americans is projected to constitute 20% of the population (Administration on Aging, 2016). It is appropriate to be concerned about disorders affecting the higher cortical brain functions in this group and the consequent effect on abilities to maintain the mental capacity for decision making (Moye, Marson, & Edelstein, 2013). Although the capacity to consent to or to refuse a medical or surgical treatment is an important consideration regardless of the patient's age, it is far more likely that higher cortical functioning will be negatively affected in older adults. The causes of impaired functioning in older adults may be attributed to central nervous system or systemic illness (e.g., dementia, delirium, heart failure, pneumonia, and urinary tract infections, schizophrenia, mood disorders, anxiety disorders), the effects of prescribed medications (e.g., anxiolytics, antihypertensives, opioid analgesics, chemotherapeutic agents), over-the-counter medications (e.g., antihistamines), and intoxicating substances (e.g., alcohol).

Theoretically, all aspects of the patient–health care provider interaction are governed by the principles of informed consent (*Schloendorff v. Society of New York Hospital*, 1914). The process of informed consent begins with a responsible member of the treatment team explaining to the patient (a) the nature and seriousness of the illness or disorder requiring treatment, (b) the nature of the medical/surgical treatment that is being recommended, (c) the risks and benefits of the medical/surgical treatment that is being recommended, and (d) reasonable treatment alternatives and their risks and benefits. Consent must be given voluntarily (not coerced), and the patient must have the mental capacity to give consent (Grisso & Appelbaum, 1998).

Among the elements of cognitive functioning required to understand the disclosures that are made in the informed-consent process are orientation, memory, attention, intelligence, abstract thinking, and problem solving. These functions contribute to intact executive functioning, defined as the mental capacity to engage in independent, purposeful, self-serving behavior (Holzer, Gansler, Moczynski, & Folstein, 1997). In the elderly patient, impairments in these abilities may have an acute (e.g., delirium, new-onset dementia) or a chronic basis (e.g., intellectual disability, chronic mental illness). Questions regarding a patient's competency/capacity most often arise in the medical setting and include decisional capacity (informed consent), capacity to volunteer for a research study, and ability to function independently in the community (including the ability to safely operate a motor vehicle).

The concepts of competency (a *legal* determination) and capacity (a *clinical* determination)

refer to the individual's mental capacity to enter into a number of legally binding decisions. In clinical practice, the legal determination of competency (*de jure* competency) is an expensive and time-consuming process, so clinical determination by a physician (*de facto* competency) is determinative in most clinical situations (Leo, 1999). In life-threatening clinical situations and in the absence of an advance directive, informed consent is assumed. In clinical situations in which an immediate decision by the patient is urgent but not critical and in which there is much at stake either in terms of risk of adverse outcome to the patient or liability to the treatment team, consultation with a psychiatric expert is advisable. Regarding formal assessment, the MacArthur Competence Assessment Tool provides a structured way of assessing and rating the patient's capacity for decision making (Grisso & Appelbaum, 1998).

Individuals are presumed to have the mental capacity to make decisions on their own behalf (*Schloendorff v. Society of New York Hospital*, 1914). Even the presence of one or more disorders of higher cognitive function does not automatically negate this presumption. When lack of capacity is suspected, the reasons must be carefully documented by the clinicians directly involved in the patient's care. The *lack of capacity/incompetence* has been defined as the presence in the individual of "functional deficits (because of mental illness, mental retardation, or other mental conditions) judged to be sufficiently great that the person currently cannot meet the demands of a specific decision-making situation weighed in light of its potential consequences" (Grisso & Appelbaum, 1998).

Capacity (and competence) is considered to be *task-specific* (Leo, 1999), so assessment of the patient should be focused on the ability to comprehend a specific clinical situation and to make a reasoned decision regarding that situation. Requests for psychiatric consultation should make explicit the clinical dilemma and the reason that the treating clinician suspects that the patient lacks decisional capacity. In many cases, decisional capacity may be restored by treating the underlying cause of impaired mentation (e.g., delirium, intoxication, acute psychosis,

severe depression), so capacity may need to be repeatedly assessed over time.

The elements of the capacity assessment are (a) the ability to make a choice, (b) the ability to understand relevant information, (c) the ability to appreciate the situation and its likely consequences, and (d) the ability to manipulate information rationally (Grisso & Appelbaum, 1998; Leo, 1999). The clinician thus determines that the patient can articulate a choice to accept or refuse treatment, that the patient has a basic understanding of the facts of the illness and the proposed treatments, that the patient appreciates the clinical dilemma and the possible outcomes, and that the patient is able to use the information in a logical fashion to arrive at a decision.

Certain conditions carry a high risk of adverse outcome if left untreated, and treatments themselves may offer a variable likelihood of success in association with a variable likelihood of adverse side or toxic effects. Assessment of capacity must take these factors into consideration (Buchanan, 2004). Capacity would be questioned for treatment refusal in the context of a serious illness that would be effective and relatively low risk (e.g., pneumonia treated with intravenous antibiotics) or treatment of marginal effectiveness and high risk of discomfort and or adverse side effects (e.g., debilitating chemotherapy for advanced metastatic carcinoma). Many difficult capacity assessments involve medical conditions and treatments that do not lie at these obvious extremes, so treatment team personnel must regard the informed consent process with utmost seriousness.

Patients bring a range of intellectual and emotional endowments with them to the treatment situation. Contemporary understandings of illnesses and treatments may be much more complicated and nuanced than may be appreciated by the older adult. Patients may have overly simplistic expectations of what can be provided by caregivers. Being ill and being in a hospital or health care-provider's clinic are stressful. There are stress-inducing and stress-related manifestations of illness, which include both physical symptoms (e.g., shortness of breath, pain, physiological and functional limitations) and emotional symptoms (e.g., anxiety and dread

C

associated with life-threatening symptoms or syndromes and the need to make decisions quickly). These factors must also be taken into consideration when assessing treatment consent or refusal when there is doubt about a patient's decisional capacity (Grisso & Appelbaum, 1998).

DECISION MAKING FOR THE INCAPACITATED PATIENT

If the patient is found to lack capacity for treatment, legal or clinical solutions are possible. Legal remedies are costly and time consuming and may be sought in only the most difficult circumstances such as withdrawing life support when there is no advance directive (*Cruzan v. Director, Missouri Department of Health*, 1990). Many individuals establish advance directives by appointing a health care proxy or creating a living will (Grisso & Appelbaum, 1998). The creation of an advance directive presumes mental capacity to do so at the time of its creation. A living will documents the patient's wishes in the event of anticipated medical crises and mental incapacity. A problem with this is that not every circumstance can be anticipated. A health care proxy allows the individual to designate the person(s) they appoint to make decisions for them (in the event of mental incapacity). Problems with this arrangement include mental incapacity on the part of the proxy or an inability or unwillingness for the proxy to act in accordance with the patient's wishes.

The legal/ethical principle guiding decision making by a surrogate (individual or court) is known as *substituted judgment* (Leo, 1999). This is judgment based on the known wishes of the patient that have been explicitly written or expressly stated. In instances in which it is not possible to apply the principle of substituted judgment, the principle of *best interest of the patient* has been applied, but this is generally considered to be an inferior standard (Leo, 1999). The *best practice* is for health care providers to assume that all of their patients will at some point face a clinical situation requiring a loss of decisional capacity and encourage them to discuss this and to prepare the appropriate advance directive. The advance directive will not cover every contingency, but a well-thought-out

advance directive should cover the most common clinical scenarios and relieve the patient, family, and health care provider of a considerable amount of stress. A combination of a living will and a health care proxy should offer the most protection for the patient. Of course, unless there has been a frank discussion or the patient's wishes with the proxy before incapacity sets in, even the advance directive may prove insufficient.

PARTICIPATION IN RESEARCH

Decisional capacity with regard to participation in a research study has garnered increased attention over the past two decades. The obvious incapacity of research subjects who would be recruited for studies of dementia, combined with the pressures on researchers to recruit a necessary cohort of research subjects and investigatory procedures that may be uncomfortable and investigatory treatments that have only a modest chance of success, creates challenges for designing an ethically sound research study. Because the cognitive abilities of Alzheimer's patients are impaired, tests of decisional capacity that rely on an understanding of the nature of research procedures and treatments may not be completely appropriate in deciding who may be included in a research protocol. In this regard the concepts of *authenticity* (Kim, 2011), which refers to the congruence between a person's values and a decision and *substituted judgment*, are highly relevant.

CAPACITY TO DRIVE

Finally, health care personnel may find themselves called on to give an opinion on the patient's capacity to operate a motor vehicle (Carr & Ott, 2010). Approximately 4% of current drivers aged 75 years and older have dementia. The consensus is that individuals with moderately severe dementia lack the capacity to drive, but the situation is more uncertain in individuals with milder degrees of dementia. The clinician must take a careful history to determine the patient's and family members' concerns about driving, the patient's recent driving record (near-misses and accidents, getting lost), and evidence of cognitive slippage (orientation, memory, attention, reaction time). Referral to a neuropsychologist who can test these areas of cognitive function may prove very helpful in making the determination about driving capacity, especially because many individuals are in denial about cognitive deterioration and their driving abilities.

Michael Schwartz

Administration on Aging, Administration for Community Living, U.S. Department of Health and Human Services: Projected future growth of the older population: http://aol.acl.gov/aging_statistics/future_growth/future_ growth.aspx

Buchanan, A. (2004). Mental capacity, legal competence and consent to treatment. *Journal of the Royal Society of Medicine, 97*(9), 415–420.

Carr, D. B., & Ott, B. R. (2010). The older adult driver with cognitive impairment. *Journal of the American Medical Association, 303*(16), 1632–1641.

Cruzan v. Director, Missouri Department of Health, 197 U.S. 261 (1990).

Grisso, T., & Appelbaum, P. S. (1998). *Assessing competence to consent to treatment: A guide for physicians and other health professionals.* New York, NY: Oxford University Press.

Holzer, J. C., Gansler, D. A., Moczynski, N. P., & Folstein, M. F. (1997). Cognitive functions in the informed consent evaluation process: A pilot study. *Journal of the American Academy of Psychiatry and the Law, 25*(4), 531–540.

Kim, S. Y. H. (2011). The ethics of informed consent in Alzheimer disease research. *Nature Reviews Neurology, 7*(7), 410–414.

Leo, R. J. (1999). Competency and the capacity to make treatment decisions: A primer for primary care physicians. *Primary Care Companion to the Journal of Clinical Psychiatry, 1*(8), 131–141.

Moye, J., Marson, D. C., & Edelstein, B. (2013). Assessment of capacity in an aging society. *American Psychologist, 68*(3), 158–171.

Schloendorff v. Society of New York Hospital, 105 N.E. 92 (N.Y. 1914).

CONSTIPATION IN THE ELDERLY

Constipation is a very common problem in the elderly. It has a huge impact on quality of life for the patient and caregivers and is an economic burden on the U.S. health care system.

DEFINITION

Constipation has been difficult to define because of the subjective nature of complaints. Bowel frequency, which may be used as objective criteria, has a wide range of normality, varying from one bowel movement (BM) in 3 days to three BMs in 1 day. Also, the symptoms of constipation are different in different patients. The revised Rome criteria of 1999 (Talley et al., 1999) defines *functional constipation* as the presence of two or more of the following symptoms lasting for at least 12 weeks (not necessarily consecutively): straining, hard or pellet stools, feeling of incomplete evacuation, sensation of anorectal obstruction or blockage, use of digital maneuvers in at least 25% of BMs, and a decrease in stool frequency to less than three BMs per week.

It is important to differentiate acute constipation (symptoms lasting less than 6 months) from chronic constipation (symptoms lasting more than 6 months) and from symptoms of constipation-predominant irritable bowel syndrome (C-IBS).

PREVALENCE AND RISK FACTORS

The prevalence of constipation is difficult to determine and varies from 10% to 18% in community-dwelling elderly to more than 74% in nursing home residents. Risk factors for constipation include increasing age, female gender, physical activity, medications, depression, and reduced intake.

ETIOLOGY

Constipation in the elderly is often multifactorial (Costilla & Foxx-Orenstein, 2014; Gallegos-Orozco, Foxx-Orenstien, Sterler, & Stoa, 2012). Age-related changes that predispose constipation in the elderly result from a delay in the defecation response because of increased rectal compliance and impaired rectal sensation. Delayed colonic transit, mostly limited to the rectosigmoid region, plays a small role in the development of constipation.

Functional chronic constipation, also known as *chronic idiopathic constipation*, is the most prevalent type. It is a functional disorder that does not meet C-IBS criteria, which is characterized by an association of abdominal pain with defecation.

Secondary causes of constipation (may accompany functional chronic constipation) are categorized as follows:

- Diet and lifestyle: Low-fiber diet, reduced dietary intake, dehydration, inactive lifestyle, immobility, and privacy to toilet
- Medications: Aluminum- or calcium-containing antacids, anticholinergics, antihistamines, tricyclic antidepressants, antipsychotics, lithium, antihypertensives (calcium channel blockers, diuretics, clonidine), digoxin, analgesics (opiates, nonsteroidal anti-inflammatory drugs), antiepileptics, antiparkinsonian medicines, anesthetics, iron supplements, barium, bismuth, and others
- Endocrine and metabolic causes: Diabetes mellitus, hypothyroidism, hyperparathyroidism, panhypopituitarism, hypercalcemia, hypokalemia, and chronic kidney disease
- Neurological diseases: Autonomic neuropathy, dementia, depression, multiple myeloma, amyloidosis, Parkinson's disease, cerebrovascular accident, spinal cord injury, paraplegia, chronic intestinal pseudo-obstruction, and paraneoplastic syndromes
- Organic causes: Pain from anal fissure and anal stricture, mechanical obstruction from colorectal cancer, extraintestinal mass, inflammatory bowel disease, proctitis, postischemic or diverticular stricture, postsurgical abnormalities, and volvulus

Constipation because of primary colorectal dysfunction is less common and can be classified pathophysiologically as slow transit constipation, dyssynergic defecation, or C-IBS, which may have overlapping symptoms.

ASSESSMENT

Constipation should be asked about at every patient visit because most patients do not bring it up until it has progressed significantly. If unchecked, it may lead to fecal impaction, fecal incontinence, mucosal ulceration, rectal bleeding, anemia, urinary infections, and urinary retention. Therefore a comprehensive history and physical examination needs to be undertaken to identify the duration and underlying causes of constipation.

History should include an evaluation of dietary intake (food and fluids), physical activity, review of medications, habitual use of laxatives, and associated comorbid conditions. Next, psychosocial aspects that contribute to patients' mental and physical state should be evaluated; these include beliefs about bowel habits, lack of independence, decreased mobility, social isolation, financial constraints, anxiety, and depression. This should be followed by an assessment of alarm symptoms that include rectal bleeding, melena, positive fecal occult blood, obstructive symptoms, change in caliber of stool, nocturnal symptoms, acute constipation, severe and persistent constipation unresponsive to treatment, weight loss of 10 pounds or more and a family history of colon cancer or inflammatory bowel disease.

Physical examination should include a rectal examination to evaluate for the presence of fecal impaction, rectal mass, anal stricture, anal fissure, hemorrhoids, sphincter tone, inappropriate contraction of the anal sphincter during simulated evacuation suggestive of dyssynergic defecation, pelvic floor dysfunction, benign prostatic hyperplasia, cystocele or rectocele, and various other signs for detecting secondary causes of constipation.

Diagnostic testing is not recommended early unless there are alarm signs. If needed, laboratory tests may include complete blood count, thyroid-stimulating hormone, calcium, comprehensive metabolic panel, and others based on the patient's comorbidities. The American College of Gastroenterology guidelines (Ford et al., 2014) indicate that data are inadequate for making recommendations about the routine use of laboratory tests in patients with chronic constipation without alarm symptoms. Colonoscopy should be performed in patients who are older than 50 years and who have never had colorectal cancer screening.

If rectal evaluation is negative and constipation is highly suspected, plain x-ray of the abdomen may be done to confirm constipation.

Invasive tests such as anoscopy, flexible sigmoidoscopy, and colonoscopy are reserved for when there is reason to suspect an organic cause of constipation. If evaluation leads to a definitive diagnosis, then the underlying cause is treated, including stopping all medicines causing constipation.

Other specialized physiological testing for colorectal function, such as anorectal manometry, colonic scintigraphy, and wireless motility capsule, are reserved for patients with chronic intractable constipation who do not respond to lifestyle and diet modification and initial treatment.

MANAGEMENT OF FUNCTIONAL CHRONIC CONSTIPATION

Lifestyle and dietary modification are the first steps in the treatment of chronic functional constipation. However, increased fluid intake and physical activity do not have evidence-based support. Elderly patients should be given adequate privacy for toileting. Patients should be encouraged to recognize and respond to the urge for defecation, especially in the morning. They should develop a regular routine for having a BM, as most people usually tend to have one about the same time of the day. Timing should preferably be within 2 hours after waking or a high-fiber breakfast, when colonic motor activity is most active. Patients should avoid prolonged straining (more than 5 minutes).

Dietary fiber intake should be gradually increased to a goal of 20 to 30 g/day by incorporating foods such as prunes, bananas, fruits, vegetables, whole grains, and bran. This increases colonic bulk, leading to colonic distention and increased motility. Sudden increase in fiber intake may cause bloating, distention, and flatulence and should be avoided. Dietary changes may take several weeks to have an impact on constipation.

If there is no response to these modifications, bulk laxatives (Fleming & Wade, 2010), such as psyllium (Metamucil), methylcellulose (Citrucel), calcium polycarbophil (FiberCon), and wheat dextran (Benefiber), should be tried, provided that fluid intake has been increased to 1,500 mL/day. Dosage should be adjusted to have a soft BM at the patient's baseline frequency and without the adverse effects of bloating and flatulence. Bulk-forming laxatives act by absorbing water in the gastrointestinal tract and increasing the fecal mass. They are not useful in managing slow transit constipation, dyssynergic defecation, and opioid-induced constipation.

If this trial is ineffective, osmotic laxatives such as polyethylene glycol (17 g daily), lactulose (20 g daily), or sorbitol (30 g daily) should be tried. Osmotic laxatives act by increasing the water content of fecal matter. Saline laxatives such as magnesium hydroxide should be used with caution because of lack of trials in the elderly and risk of hypermagnesemia in renal patients.

A recent review (Izzy, Malieckal, Little, & Anand, 2016) of laxatives use in elderly patients concluded that senna combinations and polyethylene glycol are better than other traditionally used laxatives.

Glycerin or bisacodyl rectal suppositories are often used periodically for existing or impending fecal impaction and dyssynergic defecation.

Enemas should be used only if the patient has been constipated for several days to prevent fecal impaction, but not more than twice a week. Warm tap water enemas are preferred. Soapsuds enemas are more likely to cause rectal mucosal damage. Sodium phosphate enemas should not be used in those older than 70 years because of high-risk complications, including hypotension, volume depletion, dyselectrolytemia, renal failure, and prolonged QT interval. Oil-retention enemas are reserved for constipation refractory to other enemas.

Patients taking laxatives and enemas regularly may develop a dependency on them. After a large colonic evacuation with enemas and laxatives, several days may pass before a spontaneous BM occurs, resulting in their cyclical use.

Stool softeners although widely used, have limited efficacy. They act as surfactants, thereby allowing water to enter the fecal mass easily, but do not promote colonic motility.

Newer therapies for chronic functional constipation include colonic secretagogues. Lubiprostone (24 mcg daily) activates the type-2 chloride channels in intestinal epithelial cells, and linaclotide (145 or 290 mcg daily)

C

is a guanylate cyclase-C receptor agonist; both result in increased fluid secretion and colonic transit by different mechanisms. Prucalopride is a selective serotonin (5-HT4) receptor agonist, is available for use in Europe, Canada, and Israel but not the United States. These treatments are reserved for patients with severe constipation unresponsive to other therapies. The long-term risks and benefits of these medications are unknown.

Alvimopan and methylnaltrexone are two new peripherally acting mu-opioid receptor antagonists, which may be used to treat narcotic-induced constipation and paralytic ileus, but their use in older adults has not been evaluated. These medicines do not cross the blood–brain barrier and therefore act only peripherally. This way, they do not oppose the analgesic effect of opioids.

Use of chenodeoxycholic acid (CDCA) and elobixibat are also being evaluated for treatment of constipation in elderly.

Probiotics (Lacy et al., 2016) containing *Bifidobacterium lactis* DN-173 010, *Lactobacillus casei* Shirota, and *Escherichia coli* Nissle 1917 may help improve stool frequency and consistency in patients with chronic functional constipation.

Biofeedback therapy should be considered in patients with dyssynergic defecation.

Treatment options in the elderly should be individualized, taking into account patient preferences, cardiac and renal comorbidity, drug interactions, side effects, and costs. Enemas should be used only for patients whose constipation persists for several days despite oral treatments and for patients with fecal impaction. For narcotic-induced constipation and paralytic ileus, new opioid antagonists are available.

Kanwardeep Singh

Costilla, V. C., & Foxx-Orenstein, A. E. (2014). Constipation: Understanding mechanisms and management. *Clinics in Geriatric Medicine, 30,* 107–115.

Fleming, V., & Wade, W. E. (2010). A review of laxative therapies for the treatment of chronic constipation in older adults. *American Journal of Geriatric Pharmacotherapy, 8*(6), 514–550.

Ford, A. C., Moayyedi, P., Lacy, B. E., Lembo, A. J., Saito, Y. A., Schiller, L. R.,...Quigley, E. M. M.

(2014). American College of Gastroenterology monograph on the management of irritable bowel syndrome and chronic idiopathic constipation. *American Journal of Gastroenterology, 109,* S2–S26. doi:10.1038/ajg.2014.187

Gallegos-Orozco, J. F., Foxx-Orenstien, A. E., Sterler, S. M., & Stoa, J. M. (2012). Chronic constipation in the elderly. *American Journal of Gastroenterology, 107*(1), 18–25.

Izzy, M., Malieckal, A., Little, E., & Anand, S. (2016, May 6). Review of efficacy and safety of laxatives use in geriatrics. *World Journal of Gastrointestinal Pharmacology and Therapeutics, 7*(2), 334–342.

Lacy, B. E., Mearin, F., Chang, L., Chey, W. D., Lembo, A. J., Simren, M., & Spiller, R. (2016). Bowel disorders. *Gastroenterology, 150*(6), 1393–1407.

Talley, N. J., Stanghellini, V., Heading, R. C., Koch, K. L., Malagelada, J. R., & Tytgat, G. N. (1999). Functional gastroduodenal disorders. *Gut, 45*(Suppl. 2), 1137–1142.

Web Resources
American Gastroenterologic Society: http://www.gastro.org

American Geriatrics Society: http://www.americangeriatrics.org/files/documents/beers/FHATipMEDS.pdf

Food and Nutrition: Dietary fiber: Essential for a healthy diet: http://www.mayoclinic.com/health/fiber/NU00033

International Foundation for Functional Gastrointestinal Disorders: http://www.iffgd.org

CONTINUING CARE RETIREMENT COMMUNITIES

Continuing care retirement communities (CCRCs) provide independent housing, services, and nursing care, usually in one location or campus. A CCRC may be a single-campus organization or part of a system; the majority are in the latter category. About one third have more than 300 units, and only 8% have more than 500 units. Through long-term contracts signed on admission to a CCRC, elderly individuals or couples secure a place to live, access to a range of services, and the opportunity to move to higher levels of care (i.e., assisted living/

memory care or skilled nursing) if they need a more intensive setting. At the end of 2010, the latest date for which published data are available, there were approximately 1,900 CCRCs in the United States (Zebolsky, 2014). The number of older adults living in CCRCs more than doubled over the decade between 1997 and 2007, from 350,000 to 745,000 (Tumlinson, Woods, & Avalere Health, 2007).

As of 2010, CCRCs were governed by state regulations in 38 states and were typically classified as an insurance model under the jurisdiction of the state department of insurance or another similar entity. Each component of the retirement community may also be subject to separate oversight: The independent housing units may be regulated at the local level, the assisted living is regulated by the state, and the skilled-nursing (i.e., nursing home) component is governed by state and federal regulations. Roughly, one in four CCRCs is voluntarily accredited by the Commission on Accreditation of Rehabilitation Facilities/Continuing Care Accreditation Commission.

The CCRC contract is a legal agreement between the consumer and the community. On payment of an entry fee and an ongoing monthly service charge, the agreement generally secures living accommodations and services, including long-term care and health services, over the long term. Under the Type A (i.e., extensive, full insurance model) contract, residents pay an upfront fee and an ongoing monthly fee that guarantees them lifetime occupancy in an independent-living unit, certain services and amenities, and the ability to transfer to the appropriate level of assisted living or skilled nursing while continuing to pay the same monthly fee as they paid in independent living. Under the Type B (i.e., modified) contract, residents typically pay an upfront fee and an ongoing monthly fee for the right to lifetime occupancy of an independent-living unit plus certain amenities and access to a higher level of care setting for a limited time (usually 30–60 days). For longer periods in assisted living or the nursing home, the resident pays a higher but discounted rate relative to individuals who may be directly admitted to these settings from outside the CCRC. The Type C (i.e., fee-for-service) contract may

also require an entrance fee but does not include any discounted health care or assisted-living services. Residents must pay the regular per diem rate to receive more intensive services but may receive priority admission to assisted living and the nursing home. The majority of CCRCs that require an entrance fee offer some degree of refund or repayment of this fee to the resident if the resident moves out of the community or to the resident's estate of the resident dies. Finally, admission to rental CCRCs require no upfront entrance fee and the resident pays the prevailing market rate for the level of care provided.

Ten states—Pennsylvania, Ohio, California, Illinois, Florida, Texas, Kansas, Indiana, Iowa, and North Carolina—account for 60% of the communities and two thirds of the CCRC units. Approximately 82% of the CCRCs are owned by not-for-profit organizations, often with faith-based affiliations or linked to a university, health system, or fraternal organization. Entrance fees range from about $20,000 to more than $1 million based on the geographic location, features of the living space, the additional services and amenities selected, the type of service contract, and entrance fee refundability. In 2010, the average CCRC entrance fee nationally was $248,000, a figure strongly correlated with local housing prices in the CCRC market area (Bowblis & McHone, 2013).

A 2009 study of CCRC residents (American Seniors Housing Association, 2010) found that the average age of recent move-ins was 81. The average age of a resident in independent living in a mature CCRC (older than 10 years) is between 85 and 87 years. Two thirds of residents were female, 54% were widowed, and 35% were married. New residents were twice as likely to have a college degree as the average older adult aged 65 years and older. CCRC residents were also more likely than the average older adult to be middle or upper class. More than half (53%) of respondents in entrance-fee CCRCs sold their homes for $300,000 or more And one in three residents of entrance-fee CCRCs had a net worth of $1 million or more compared with 14% of those in rental CCRCs.

A 2010 study of CCRCs by the Government Accountability Office (GAO, 2010) for the Senate Special Committee on Aging noted that although CCRCs offer long-term residence and care in the

C

same community, residents may face considerable risk, particularly if CCRC financial difficulties lead to unexpected increases in monthly fees or loss of all or part of entrance fees in the case of bankruptcies or closures. Some states directly protect the financial interests of residents by establishing escrow requirements for fees and deposits, addressing criteria for monthly fee increases, or placing liens on CCRC assets on behalf of residents in the event of liquidation. Such requirements, however, vary tremendously by states. Only 17 states require CCRCs to submit periodic actuarial studies to address risks to long-term viability (American Seniors Housing Association, 2010).

The National Continuing Care Residents' Association (NaCCRA) was organized to help ensure that residents' interests are protected. This organization has proposed a Bill of Rights for residents of CCRCs and is working on a set of model laws designed to improve the business and financial practices of CCRC management and to elevate the financial soundness of the entire CCRC industry. NaCCRA also focuses on ensuring that residents participate on CCRC boards and has been advocating for more principled accounting and auditing standards for this sector.

A 2009 survey of CCRC providers found that organizations are projecting growth in four key areas (Brecht, Fein, & Hollinger-Smith, 2009). Trends include (a) expanding wellness programs into senior living residence design; (b) providing web-based education and lifelong learning programs for residents; (c) building "small house" models for residents receiving long-term care; (d) obtaining Leadership in Energy and Environmental Design (LEED) certification to demonstrate that new construction and renovations meet "green" standards; (e) incorporating "smart home" technology and wireless connectivity into senior living residences; (f) bringing telehealth technology, geriatric assessment services, and nonmedical home care into independent living; and (g) opening services and education to the larger community beyond the campus.

A number of CCRCs struggled with vacancies in regions of the country that were hardest hit by the 2008 recession and substantial declines in housing value. The occupancy rates of CCRCs, however, continue to exceed those of free-standing assisted living homes, nursing homes, and free-standing rental independent living properties (Zarem, 2010). Many CCRCs are exploring new business lines, including providing home health and a range of home- and community-based services both to residents and to patients in the surrounding communities. Many are establishing formal partnerships with active adult communities, local colleges/universities, naturally occurring retirement communities (NORCs) and community-based senior village models, and health systems focusing on population health management. A number of CCRCs are also beginning to offer Continuing Care at Home programs, a life care membership program that provides the same kind of services as a Type A CCRC to consumers who choose to remain in their own homes or choose to live in a setting other than a traditional CCRC. An initial screening is required, and only those not in need of services and with no degenerative diagnoses may enroll. Access to services is typically triggered by a deficit in at least one in five activities of daily living (Spellman & Townsley, 2012).

See also Assisted Living; Home Health Care; Long-Term Care Policy; Naturally Occurring Retirement Communities (NORCs).

Robyn Stone

American Seniors Housing Association. (2010). *Assisted living and continuing care retirement community state regulatory handbook*. Washington, DC: Author.

Bowblis, J. R., & McHone, H. S. (2013). An instrumental variables approach to post-acute care nursing home quality: Is there a dime's worth of evidence that continuing care retirement communities provide higher quality? *Journal of Health Economics, 32*(5), 980–996.

Brecht, S. B., Fein, S., & Hollinger-Smith, L. (2009). Preparing for the future: Trends in continuing care retirement communities. *Seniors Housing and Care Journal, 16*(1), 47–62.

Government Accountability Office. (2010, June). *Continuing care retirement communities can provide benefits, but not without some risk (GAO-10-611)*. Washington, DC: Author.

Spellman, S., & Townsley, S. (2012). Continuing care at home: Evolution, innovation and opportunity.

CliftonLarsonAllen. Retrieved from http://www
.claconnect.com/-/media/files/white-papers/
whitepapercontinuingcareathome.pdf?la=en

Tumlinson, A., Woods, S., & Avalere Health. (2007,
October). *Long-term care in America: An introduc-
tion.* Washington, DC: National Commission for
Quality Long-Term Care.

Zarem, J. E. (2010). Today's continuing care retire-
ment communities. American Seniors Housing
Association and the American Association for
Homes for the Aged. Retrieved from https://
www.seniorshousing.org/filephotos/research/
CCRC_whitepaper.pdf

Zebolsky, G. T. (2014, July 28). An introduction to
continuing care retirement communities. *Milliman
Insight.* Retrieved from http://us.milliman.com/
insight/2014/An-introduction-to-continuing
-care-retirement-communities

Web Resources
Commission on Accreditation of Rehabilitation
Facilities: http://www.carf.org
LeadingAge: http://www.leadingage.org

CONTRACTURES

EPIDEMIOLOGY

Because activity and mobility are vital to the total health of older persons, musculoskeletal problems that limit functional capacity have confounding effects. Physical changes thought to be associated with normal aging are all too often because of inactivity. Aging predisposes frail older persons to development of contractures as a result of gradual but progressive loss of muscle bulk and subsequent formation of fibrous tissue. Although the clinical definition of *contractures* remains ambiguous, contractures are defined as "an alternation in viscoelastic properties of the periarticular connective tissue where the muscles potentially lead to a reduction in the range of motion (ROM) in a joint, or an increased resistance to passive joint movement, which reduces joint flexibility and mobility" (Offenbächer et al., 2014). A contracture can be the result of joint ankylosis and muscle shortening acting in concert or independently.

The development of contractures is precipitated by muscle inactivity, producing the so-called disuse syndrome that follows prolonged (more than 3 days) bed rest. The syndrome comes about because of the negative effects of an imbalance between rest and physical activity and is characterized by decreased physical work capacity, muscle atrophy, negative nitrogen and protein balance, cardiovascular deconditioning, pulmonary restrictions, and depression. Immobilization results in a 3% loss of original muscle strength each day for the first 7 days; thereafter, the process plateaus. Inactivity of any kind leads to muscle atrophy and replacement of muscle bulk with noncontractile tissue. This is primarily because of lack of usual weight-bearing forces and a decrease in the number and intensity of muscle contractions.

ETIOLOGY

Contractures are a major health concern for frail older persons and are commonly the result of immobilization and disuse during hospitalization or residence in a long-term care environment such as a nursing home. Nationally, approximately 28.9% or 386,000 nursing home residents suffer from contractures. However, precise measurement of the prevalence of contractures in frail older persons is difficult because of variation in diagnostic criteria and a lack of standard practice (Offenbächer et al., 2014; Wagner et al., 2008).

Causes of joint contractures can include immobility from illness, surgery, or neuromuscular disease. Several chronic neuromuscular and osteomuscular conditions common in older persons predispose them to the development of muscle and joint contractures, including Parkinson's disease, osteoarthritis, rheumatoid arthritis, and Alzheimer's disease. Spasticity and muscular hypertonia associated with neuromuscular conditions often precipitate muscle immobility and contracture. In some patients, however, contractures potentiate spasticity. Thus the pathophysiological mechanism creates a feedback cycle by which contractures and spasticity augment each other.

Muscular weakness, immobility, and loss of dexterity can lead to the development of

C

contractures. For example, muscle contractures are observed as early as 2 months after a cerebrovascular accident. Contracture of the shoulder joint, or frozen shoulder, is often seen in poorly rehabilitated stroke patients. Adhesive capsulitis is also responsible for poststroke arthropathies and resultant contractures of the ankles and hips.

Alzheimer's disease poses the greatest risk for contracture development. Despite late-developing motor function disturbances, nearly one quarter of patients with dementia studied had contractures in the early or middle stages of the disease. More than three quarters of patients with Alzheimer's disease who had lost the ability to walk had contractures. At the end stage of Alzheimer's disease, it was exceptionally rare to find a patient without contractures of the hips, knees, elbows, shoulders, and wrists.

Dupuytren's contracture—the most studied and discussed contracture in medical literature because it is seen across all adult ages, including 10% to 15% of older persons—is caused by fibroblastic proliferation in the fine structure of the palmar fascia, resulting in finger deformity. Of unknown etiology, it is seen in chronic alcoholism, diabetes mellitus, HIV, phenytoin therapy, and patients undergoing hemodialysis. The condition is painless and may be related to repetitive microtrauma.

Hip-flexion contracture—ambulating with the upper torso tipped forward—is more likely the result of prolonged or restrained sitting than an age-related change. Heel-cord contractures often result from the effect of gravity on an unsupported foot while in bed or a lounge-type chair. A high frequency of gait and postural abnormalities and hip-flexion contractures is observed among arthritic, ambulatory older patients who have adapted their gait to their painful hips and spines; therefore they do not report their discomfort to the clinician. Often, osteomuscular pain is accepted as an almost normal consequence of aging by both patients and their physicians. However, pain universally leads to the limitation of motion. As a painful disease progresses, the sites and intensity of joint contractures also increase. End-stage osteoarthritis of the hip results in limitation in external rotation, abduction, and flexion.

COMPLICATIONS

Older patients and their caregivers often underestimate the degree of damage and complications that can stem from immobility. Complications from contractures range from aesthetically repugnant and psychologically disturbing body disfigurement to forced immobilization, increased dependence, and predisposition to pressure injuries over affected bony prominences. Immobility itself has complications, including not only muscular atrophy, but also flexion contracture, body fluids and circulation alterations, postural hypotension, venous thrombosis, pulmonary embolus, respiratory difficulties, incontinence, and osteoporosis. When rest is recommended for an older person with functional limitations, this exacerbates disuse and initiates a downward spiral of decline.

Contractures and the ensuing immobility also increase the older adult's risk for pathophysiological complications such as pneumonia and infections of the genitourinary tract precipitated by functional incontinence. Pain is another complication from contractures; however, it is often underreported and underassessed in nursing homes, particularly for those who are cognitively or communication impaired.

IMPLICATIONS FOR HEALTH PROFESSIONALS

Functional decline is the inability to bathe, dress, toilet, and be mobile without assistance. Limitations in mobility such as contractures lend themselves directly to functional decline and loss of independence. For example, individuals who develop a contracture of an upper limb cannot feed themselves simply because they are unable to bring utensil to their mouth. Lower-limb contractures impede walking or propelling oneself in a wheelchair.

Frail older persons with limited ROM should receive appropriate treatment and services to address their functional needs or prevent further decrease. In terms of regulatory oversight, some contractures are avoidable; as such, a contracture is a negative outcome that can be measured and used to judge the standard of care provided in an institution. Contracture risk assessment and avoidance must be an integral part of community-based intake or institutional admission process.

There are also extrinsic factors (e.g., medical devices) that limit mobility and physical activity. Use of restraints, for example, is strongly associated with the consequences of immobility. In addition, the natural history of contracture is sometimes associated with learned dependence that is unknowingly "taught" by caregivers, who anticipate and expedite the functional activities of daily living for the care recipient. In turn, volitional mobility is discouraged, disuse is advanced, and contracture formation is potentiated. The development of the Restorative Care Nursing Model is based on this premise, and its goal is to optimize function for older adults and prevent sequelae of immobility (Resnick, 2012).

Effective preventive and treatment interventions for patients who have or are predisposed to contractures rely on collaboration among medical, rehabilitation, and nursing services. Medical oversight is needed for pain management and surgical consultation with regard to some forms of contractures. Patients may benefit from interventions provided by restorative nursing assistants, physical or occupational therapists, and physiatrists; these interventions include walking, passive or active ROM, soft tissue manipulation, splinting, botulinum toxin treatments, and microinvasive needle tetony (Schnitzler et al., 2016).

Most contractures appear to be preventable and, if detected in early stages, reversible. Unfortunately, once an older person develops one or more contractures, the opportunity for functional performance diminishes. Thus avoiding prolonged immobility is essential for optimal care.

See also Physical Therapists; Restraints.

> *Laura M. Wagner, Michele Diaz and*
> *Carolyn K. Clevenger*

Offenbächer, M., Sauer, S., Rieß, J., Müller, M., Grill, E., Daubner, A.,…Herold-Majumdar, A. (2014). Contractures with special reference in elderly: Definition and risk factors—A systematic review with practical implications. *Disability Rehabilitation*, 36(7), 529–538.

Schnitzler, A., Diebold, A., Parratte, B., Tliba, L., Genêt, F., & Denormandie, P. (2016). An alternative treatment for contractures of the elderly institutionalized persons: Microinvasive percutaneous needle tetony of finger flexors. *Annals of Physical and Rehabilitation Medicine, 59*, 83–86.

Resnick, B. (2012). *Restorative care nursing for older adults: A guide for all care settings* (2nd ed.). New York, NY: Springer Publishing.

Wagner, L. M., Capezuti, E., Brush, B. L., Clevenger, C., Boltz, M., & Renz, S. (2008). Contractures in frail nursing home residents. *Geriatric Nursing*, 29(4), 259–266.

Web Resources
American Academy of Physical Medicine and Rehabilitation: http://www.aapmr.org

American Occupational Therapy Association: http://www.aota.org

American Physical Therapy Association: Section on Geriatrics: http://www.geriatricspt.org

Association of Rehabilitation Nurses: http://www.rehabnurse.org

Merck Manual of Geriatrics: Overview: http://www.merckmanuals.com/professional/geriatrics.html

---

COPING WITH CHRONIC ILLNESS

Chronic illness is a common accompaniment of advancing age. Approximately 85% of people 65 years and older suffer from at least one chronic illness, the most common diseases being arthritis (49%), heart disease (30%), any cancer (24%), diabetes (21%), and hypertension (71%; Administration on Aging, 2016). Evidence suggests that older adults generally adjust better psychologically to the diagnosis of a chronic disease than do younger adults, presumably because of the acknowledgment and expectation that advanced age carries an increased risk of illness and disability (Settersten, 1997). For younger adults, serious illness and associated disability are particularly stressful because they are perceived as "off-time" events (i.e., not developmentally normative) and therefore assaults/insults to one's sense of self and social identity.

Nevertheless, for both younger and older adults, diagnosis of a chronic illness is likely to be a distressing event that inevitably disrupts their lives and elicits a range of psychological reactions (Miller, 1992). Most common is a loss of self-esteem because usual social involvements may become constricted and social roles curtailed. Patients' sense of self-worth is further undermined if the illness creates dependency on others. They may feel guilty about the demands their illness places on others or may experience fear that others will withdraw or abandon them to avoid the burden of caregiving. Guilt may also arise from having become ill, especially if their lifestyle choices (e.g., smoking, drinking, being inactive) are implicated in their disease or if it is seen as an outcome of being negligent about their health care. Physical limitations and loss of control over bodily functions may result in an increased sense of vulnerability and shame, both of which may lead to social withdrawal and isolation. Anger and depression are common psychological sequelae of having a chronic illness; however, they tend to be more pronounced among younger patients who perceive their plight as more age-inappropriate and thus unfair (Schnittker, 2005).

Whether older adults cope with stressors, including physical illness, differently from younger adults has received considerable research attention. Few differences have been found, but older adults appear to engage in less help seeking and seem to exhibit a more stoic psychological acceptance of being ill. It remains unclear whether the few age-related differences in coping strategies that have been identified are a function of changes in the coping strategies individuals use as they age or differences in the kinds of stressors people confront at different stages of life (Aldwin, Sutton, Chiara, & Spiro, 1996).

COPING STRATEGIES

Attempts to master illness-related stressors (as with most kinds of stressors) typically include both problem- and emotion-focused coping strategies. Problem-focused coping involves action directed at removing or circumventing the stressor or gathering resources to confront it, such as seeking information and eliciting social support. Emotion-focused coping involves attempts to reduce or eliminate the emotional distress associated with or cued by the stressor through, for instance, positive reappraisal, minimization, distancing, and acceptance of responsibility. Emotion-focused coping tends to be used when the situation is not alterable and thus must be tolerated or endured. Given that the course of a chronic illness is often uncontrollable, emotion-focused strategies that enable a more favorable reappraisal of the illness and restore one's sense of control over life become particularly significant (Taylor, Helgeson, Reed, & Skokan, 1991).

Cognitive emotion-focused strategies commonly used to cope with the distress of chronic illness include redefining "doing well" and "being healthy," normalizing one's plight, engaging in downward comparisons, and finding positive meaning in the experience. These strategies constitute facets of cognitive restructuring that enable one to feel less victimized by the experience of becoming ill and minimize illness-related loses and threats.

REDEFINING "DOING WELL" AND "BEING HEALTHY"

Redefining what it means to be "doing well" and "being healthy" often allows chronically ill patients to feel less ill and distressed and even contributes to their maintaining valued physical and social activities (Duke, Leventhal, Brownlee, & Leventhal, 2002). For example, patients may see themselves as healthy if their medical conditions are stable and they manage to avoid hospitalizations or unscheduled visits to the physician. Some patients may substitute a spiritual definition of well-being for a physical one. Others may construe "doing well" as staying involved in valued activities or preserving their prediagnosis daily routines. Still others who believe that physical and mental states are closely tied may be able to think of themselves as healthy by maintaining a positive mental state. In general, these strategies allow patients to experience a subjective sense of physical well-being despite the objective reality of living with a chronic or serious illness.

In an effort to promote "doing well" and lessen the feelings of being diseased, the Institute of Medicine (IOM) published a report that focused less on specific diseases, but instead emphasized living well with chronic illness (IOM, 2012). This report has a unique approach that challenges health care providers to acknowledge and address the physical and psychosocial toll of chronic illness in addition to management of the illness itself. It further states that the goal of health care should be to assist patients in living as well as possible regardless of their official diagnosis or current state of health (IOM, 2012).

NORMALIZING THEIR PLIGHT

When normalizing suffering, patients reason that suffering is an inescapable aspect of life and that everyone is confronted with adversity in life. Embracing such a worldview minimizes the difference between themselves as patients and the healthy others, thus diminishing the sense of alienation and victimization that often accompany an illness diagnosis.

Engaging in Downward Social Comparisons

Older individuals may compare their own illness to that of their peers or others with the same condition that seem to be more incapacitated, either medically or psychologically. They may even compare themselves to a hypothetical "other" patient who they deem to be worse off. Such downward social comparisons help restore one's self-esteem and sense of emotional well-being because patients feel less victimized by the illness and more in control of their situation. Self-reminders that "it could be worse" are emotionally reassuring and allow patients to view personal circumstances as less threatening.

Finding Positive Meaning in the Experience

Being able to find a positive or constructive meaning in a negative life event such as a chronic illness contributes to subsequent psychological adjustment (Park & Folkman, 1997). Patients who interpret their illness in a way that allows them to reconcile it with their worldview and value system feel less victimized and less distressed. Thus patients may claim that their illness made them appreciate the value of health and adopt a more positive lifestyle, so they feel "healthier" than before the diagnosis. Others may suggest that the illness-related challenges provided the opportunity to discover their personal strengths, thus increasing feelings of self-efficacy or for family and friends to express their support, thus enhancing feelings of being loved.

Behavioral and Cognitive Adaptive Tasks

The incurable nature of a chronic illness reduces prospects of full recovery. Successful adjustment commonly requires the mastery of a number of adaptive tasks (Miller, 1992).

Modifying Daily Routines

Living with a chronic illness typically necessitates a change in one's daily routine to accommodate symptoms (e.g., fatigue, pain) or comply with treatment regimens and medical-care appointments. Patients often reorganize their daily lives to better conserve limited energy or minimize disruption of valued activities.

Mastering the Information and Skills Required for Self-Care

Chronic illness, because of its protracted nature, often demands that patients adopt an active role in preserving their health and adhering to treatment. Patients must master considerable information and acquire competence in carrying out these self-care activities or must rely on the assistance of family and friends.

Adhering to Treatment Regimens

Treatment regimens for chronic illnesses vary in their complexity and demands on the patient. Medication and dietary nonadherence is common among patients with chronic diseases regardless of age. Although such behavior may appear self-destructive or irrational to health professionals, research typically reveals that patients have their own rationale that accounts for their nonadherence. Attempts to reassert control, test their health limits, or preserve quality of life by avoiding distressing treatment side effects are

C

often reasons patients violate physicians' orders. At times, however, these behaviors can be a form of denial regarding the illness or its severity.

Coping With Uncertainty

Chronic illnesses often follow an unpredictable trajectories, and treatment efficacy often varies by patient or over time. Patients live with considerable uncertainty regarding their conditions' stability, severity, and manageability. Uncertainty is inherently stressful and difficult to endure. Moreover, it is hard to establish an appropriate psychological and/or practical coping response when the manifestation and intensity of the stressors are unpredictable.

Maintaining a Sense of Control

Chronic illnesses can undermine patients' sense of control over health and life. Although a sense of control is viewed as a fundamental human need, there has been some debate whether this sense diminishes in late life. Common patient strategies for regaining a sense of control include acquiring knowledge about the illness, adopting alternative therapies to enhance one's health, adhering strictly to treatment regimens, construing as omnipotent one's medical provider, or turning over control of one's health to a higher power.

Preserving Self-Esteem

Latent negative self-images are often activated by chronic illness. Patients may feel vulnerable, helpless, incapacitated, and dependent on others. A lower self-esteem and even depression are common among the chronically ill elderly and often lead to social isolation and withdrawal. Patients may attempt to preserve or restore self-esteem through strategies such as downward comparisons, normalization, or minimization of their plight, as well as the search for meaning in the illness experience. Strategies that enhance patients' sense of control over their illness or its symptoms that disrupt their lives can also enhance self-esteem.

Renegotiating Social Relationships

Chronic illness has both social and physical consequences. A patient's family and friends are also affected as they witness or are called on to assist with the physical and psychological impact of the illness. Therefore illnesses have both positive and negative interpersonal consequences. Distant or estranged family members may become closer and more supportive. Alternately, the physical and emotional burden of care giving may cause family members to resent the patient, feel guilty about such feelings, and even withdraw.

Several factors associated with aging may compromise coping with chronic illness. The typically attenuated social networks of older adults may reduce the availability of informal practical and emotional support. Limited financial resources may hinder access to medical care, formal assistance, and alternative therapies not covered by health insurance. Older adults' ability to acquire new knowledge and learn new skills necessary for managing their illness may be restricted. Finally, the common perception that illness and disability are inevitable consequences of aging may completely undermine older adults' motivation to use coping strategies for preserving their health and well-being.

April Bigelow

Administration on Aging. (2016). *A profile of older Americans: 2015.* Washington, DC: U.S. Department of Health and Human Services. Retrieved from https://www.acl.gov/sites/default/files/Aging%20and%20Disability%20in%20America/2015-Profile.pdf

Aldwin, C. M., Sutton, K. J., Chiara, G., & Spiro, A. (1996). Age differences in stress, coping, and appraisal: Findings from the Normative Aging Study. *Journals of Gerontology. Series B, Psychological Sciences and Social Sciences, 51*(4), P179–P188.

Duke, J., Leventhal, H., Brownlee, S., & Leventhal, E. A. (2002). Giving up and replacing activities in response to illness. *Journals of Gerontology. Series B, Psychological Sciences and Social Sciences, 57*(4), P367–P376.

Institute of Medicine. (2012). *Living well with chronic illness: A call for public health action.* [Report Brief]. Bethesda, MD: Board on Population Health and Public Health Practice.

Miller, J. F. (1992). *Coping with chronic illness: Overcoming powerlessness* (2nd ed.). Philadelphia, PA: F. A. Davis.

Park, C. L., & Folkman, S. (1997). Meaning in the context of stress and coping. *Review of General Psychology, 1*, 115–144.

Schnittker, J. (2005). Chronic illness and depressive symptoms in late life. *Social Science & Medicine (1982), 60*(1), 13–23.

Settersten, R. A. (1997). The salience of age in the life course. *Human Development, 40*, 257–281.

Taylor, S. E., Helgeson, V. S., Reed, G. M., & Skokan, L. A. (1991). Self-generated feelings of control and adjustment to physical illness. *Journal of Social Issues, 47*, 91–109.

Web Resources
Administration for Community Living: https://www.acl.gov
American Association for Geriatric Psychiatry: http://www.aagponline.org
ElderCare Services: http://www.elderweb.com
HealthinAging.org: http://www.healthinaging.org
National Chronic Care Consortium: http://www.nccconline.org
National Institute of Health, Senior Health: http://nihseniorhealth.gov

CREATIVITY

Creativity is a powerful source of growth that is vital across the life span as we continually create and re-create ourselves. For the aging individual, creativity may be a response to the uncertainties, losses, and challenges of existence. Creativity can continue until death; it is not necessarily tied to chronological age, but rather is tied to the process of self-actualizing creative potential (Simonton, 1998).

Rollo May (1975) defined creativity as "the process of bringing something new into being" (p. 39). In addition to the creative arts, domains of creativity include social creativity, as well as what gerontologist Gene Cohen (2000) calls the distinction between creativity with a big "C" versus creativity with a little "c." Creativity with a big "C" refers to the more sweeping accomplishments that can change a community or a society, whereas creativity with a small "c" refers to accomplishments that can change a family's or individual's life course.

Creative expression can be stimulated and nurtured in older adults through their involvement in the creative arts: music, dance, theater, writing, and visual arts. This includes the folk or traditional arts, which are anchored in and expressive of shared ways of life, ethnic heritage, and religion. The arts offer possibilities for increased self-esteem, socialization, mentorship, learning, integration, mastery, joy, and self-discovery.

Participation in community-based arts programs impacts both health promotion and disease prevention, which in turn support independence. In one study, older adults who participated in arts programs over 35 weekly meetings had better health, had fewer doctor visits, used fewer medications, were less depressed and lonely, had higher morale, and were more socially active compared with a control group (Cohen, 2005). The study showed that participation in arts programs gave participants a sense of mastery and control, social engagement, and relationship building and that the engaging nature of art promoted sustained involvement.

Participation in the creative arts can optimize health outcomes. People with Parkinson's disease participating in a 13-week tango group improved on all measures of balance, falls, and gait, revealing that the tango is an effective modality for improving both mental function and balance (Hackney, Kantorovich, & Earhart, 2007). Another study demonstrated that the manipulation of clay during a 6-week group was beneficial for patients with Parkinson's, enabling an increase in their exploration of emotions and a decrease in depression, stress, obsessive-compulsive thinking, and phobias (Elkis-Abuhoff, Goldblatt, Gaydos, & Convery, 2013).

Inspiration provided by the creative arts can also increase life satisfaction and quality of life for well to frail elders. The use of collage for those with dementia has been shown to facilitate reminiscence through a nonverbal means of communication (Stallings, 2010), and in an exploration of the relationship between dementia and art making, patients benefitted by creative expression, problem solving, enhanced sense of self, and mastery (Safar & Press, 2011). The Meet Me at MoMA program for people in the early stages of dementia and their caregivers

C

presents art in a predetermined sequence. Mood changes in both the caregivers and the people with dementia suggest that arts participation enhanced the self-esteem of the caregivers and engaged the group in an imaginative experience together (Safar & Press, 2011).

Music is interwoven throughout our lives and is the most common art form studied. Lifelong music training, appreciation, and exposure have a positive impact on cognition for people with dementia, brain injury, or neurological impairment. Research in this area has demonstrated that music intervention results in decreased levels of depression and agitation, as well as improved quality of life even for people with later stages of dementia. In addition to improved emotional states, there is cognitive gain such as improved memory, word retrieval through melody, and relevance of communication (Tomaino, 2013).

Self-expression is a basic need throughout the life span that affects overall health and well-being. Jung (1971) regarded imagination and creativity as healing forces, whereby deep-seated feelings could be symbolically represented and released through the creative act. The creative arts are an opportunity for self-expression, achievement, and reengagement amid losses, voids, and uncertainty.

Clinicians must probe to find out about an older adult's interests, past work, or hobbies. A "creativity assessment" can include these questions: What makes you feel most alive? What projects have given you the most pleasure? What skills do you have that you would like to pass on? What are your sources of imagination? Are there creative issues in your life that are troubling you now? How would you like to express yourself creatively? Engaging an elder in painting, writing a poem about turning 80, working on a pottery wheel, joining a discussion, moving to the beat in a dance class, or expressing sorrow when listening to a musical piece are ways out of isolation.

The creative arts can help stimulate and compensate for sensory loss—the "thinning of life"—through one-on-one or group activities, working with each sense separately or as a total sensory experience. There is a natural pathway from sense memory to life review that

transforms sensory-inspired stories into reminiscence and art. A theater and writing project called Timeslips, which uses visual image cues to promote storytelling in people with Alzheimer's and related dementia, gives a glimpse into the experience of living with dementia. This creative process not only provides opportunities for self-expression, but also provides staff and caregivers with new vehicles to reach those with dementia. The University Without Walls is a conference-call program for homebound older adults. Taught by volunteers, the classes include a wide range of creative arts subjects to provide opportunities for stimulating conversation, discussion, friendship, and lifelong learning.

Creativity may be used as both a strategy for reducing loss and a tool for problem solving. In his later-life poetry, William Carlos Williams wrote of "an old age that adds as it takes away" (Evans & Jeste, 2004, p. 129). Loss can be a catalyst for creative expression. Matisse had diminishing vision and suffered from severe intestinal disorders; he created from his wheelchair. Monet continued painting into his 80s following two cataract operations. The Connecticut Hospice Program offers an exceptional arts program for older adults that specifically address loss through the creative arts. Art activities for hospice patients range from bedside art to evening concerts and from home-care arts to ongoing exhibits in the main gallery. Hospice-employed artists are oriented to the hospice program, are directly involved with patients and families at the bedside, and are core members of the caregiving team. The hospice program was the first to offer a model for arts in hospice care, resulting in the inclusion of arts in the Connecticut State Public Health Code—the first time that arts were integrated by law into a health care program. All arts program activities are recorded in patient charts and discussed as part of the patient assessment. The program is notable in that the arts are used as a vehicle for self-care for the health care providers; they may participate in a "musical spa" or other activities designed as antidotes to caregiver burnout.

Many older adults are the keepers of cultures and traditions. Their lives are their life stories—rich natural resources of experience and wisdom. Elders Share the Arts has created

Generating Community, a model intergenerational program that brings together older adults in nursing homes, community centers, and senior centers with youths age 5 to 18. For example, teenagers from the Dominican Republic were trained to explore turning points in life. They interviewed older adults about their work histories and how the elders felt about their jobs when they were younger. This process provided the teenagers with role models for solving problems and making decisions in their own life.

Creative rituals can be used to help mark significant events in a lifetime. Such rituals, as developed by the Transitional Keys program, acknowledge celebrations, losses, and transitions that occur as people age, such as losing a driver's license, getting a walker, losing a limb, transferring property, and entering a nursing home. The basic structure of ritual is its theme, acknowledging the turning point, marking the event, naming the losses, telling the stories, developing strategies for compensation, and sharing with a community.

The National Center for Creative Aging has launched Directory of Creative Aging Programs in America, the first of its kind. The directory reinforces the fact that the arts are applicable across health care settings and can help support transitions of care, thereby providing continuity through the continuum of care settings for all older persons.

Clinicians should strive to recognize older adults for the creative individuals they are and bring art and creativity to their practices, restoring the "art" of health care.

See also Activities of Daily Living; Intergenerational Programs; Life Review.

Lara Wahlberg and Irene Rosner David

Cohen, G. D. (2000). *The creative age*. New York, NY: Avon Books.

Cohen, G. D. (2005). *The mature mind*. New York, NY: Basic Books.

Elkis-Abuhoff, D., Goldblatt, R. B., Gaydos, M., & Convery, C. (2013). A pilot study to determine the psychological effects of manipulation of therapeutic art forms among patients with Parkinson's disease. *International Journal of Art Therapy, 18*(3), 113–121.

Evans, E., & Jeste, D. (2004). William Carlos Williams. *American Journal of Geriatric Psychiatry, 12*(2), 129–133.

Hackney, M. E., Kantorovich, S., & Earhart, G. M. (2007). A study on the effects of Argentine tango as a form of partnered dance for those with Parkinson disease and the healthy elderly. *American Journal of Dance Therapy, 29*(2), 109–127.

Jung, C. (1971). *The portable Jung.* New York, NY: Viking.

May, R. (1975). *The courage to create* (p. 39). New York, NY: W. W. Norton.

Safar, L. T., & Press, D. Z. (2011). Art and the brain: Effects of dementia on art production in art therapy. *Art Therapy: Journal of the American Art Therapy Association, 28*(3), 96–103.

Simonton, D. K. (1988). Age and outstanding achievement: What do we know after a century of research? *Psychological Bulletin, 104,* 251–267.

Stallings, J. W. (2010). Collage as a therapeutic modality for reminiscence in patients with dementia. *Art Therapy: Journal of the American Art Therapy Association, 27*(3), 136–140.

Tomaino, C. M. (2013). Meeting the complex needs of individuals with dementia through music therapy. *Music and Medicine* (4), 24–241.

Web Resources

Elders Share the Arts: http://www.estanyc.org

National Center for Creative Aging: http://www.creativeaging.org

Timeslips: http://www.timeslips.org

Transitional Keys: http://www.Transitionalkeys.org

University Without Walls: http://www.dorotusa.org/site/PageServer?pagename=seniors_programs_on_phone_D

CRIME VICTIMIZATION

PREVALENCE AND EPIDEMIOLOGY

Among all demographic groups stratified by age, older adults have the lowest prevalence of crime victimization. In 2015, the National Crime Victimization Survey (NCVS), a nationally representative sample of household residents conducted by the U.S. Bureau of Justice Statistics (2016), found an annual incidence rate of 5.2 violent crime victimizations per 1,000 individuals

C

aged 65 years or older. In contrast, the highest prevalence of violent victimization was estimated for individuals between the ages of 12 and 17 years, with an annual incidence rate of 31.3 per 1,000, representing a six-fold increase in risk over their older counterparts (Truman & Morgan, 2016). However, these findings obscure other troubling aspects of crime in older people. First, although violent crime rates have generally remained the same or declined significantly across younger age groups since 2014, older adults are the only age group to experience a significant increase (67%) in violent crimes over the same period. Second, rates of elder abuse or neglect exceed those of crime victimization. A recent review of population-based elder abuse studies found an annual elder abuse/neglect prevalence rate of 95 victimizations per 1,000 individuals among community-dwelling, cognitively intact older adults (Pillemer, Burnes, Riffin, & Lachs, 2016). An 11-year longitudinal study of 2,321 community-dwelling older people found that 393 (16.6%) were seen by police for follow-up because of reported crime victimization (M. Lachs et al., 2005). A more detailed analysis of NCVS data by gender and crime type reveals very disturbing trends.

CRIME VICTIMIZATION AMONG OLDER ADULTS: A CLOSER LOOK

Several aspects of victimization in older adults are alarming. Chu and Kraus (2004) found that elderly victims had increased risk of death from assault compared with younger victims. In the NCVS data, older victims of robbery, particularly women, were more likely than younger victims to sustain injuries, and injured elderly victims of violent crime were more likely than younger injured victims to suffer a serious medical injury that required hospitalization or other medical care. This may reflect an underlying loss of physiological reserve known to accompany normal aging, which may place the older person at greater risk for significant trauma. For example, given equivalent assault force to an extremity, an older woman with osteoporosis is more likely to sustain a fracture than her younger counterpart.

Other important differences in older crime victims point to contextual characteristics of the crime. Bachman and Meloy (2008) found that firearms are the most common method of killing for all homicides; however, older adults are more likely to be stabbed or bludgeoned to death than victims younger than 65 years. Older adults are at greater risk of being killed by strangers compared with younger homicide victims. Similarly, in nonfatal robbery victimization, elderly women are more likely to be robbed by strangers, whereas younger women are equally as likely to be robbed by a known offender. Older homicide victims are more likely to be killed in the context of another felony, whereas younger victims are more likely to be killed because of a conflict situation. Elder victims of assault are more likely to be victimized in their home and during the day compared with younger assault victims (Bachman & Meloy, 2008).

Research has also shed light on risk factors for crime victimization among older people (M. Lachs et al., 2005). The stereotype of the older crime victim as frail and impaired is simply incorrect. On the contrary, functional independence and better health status appear to be risk factors for victimization, probably because high-functioning older people are more able to venture into an environment that places them at risk.

IMPACT OF CRIME ON HEALTH IN OLDER ADULTS

Every clinician involved in the care of an older person can recall the patient who suffered a loss of physical and/or psychosocial well-being after crime victimization. Slowly emerging data now suggest that such victimization is indeed morbid. For example, in a study that followed members of the New Haven Established Populations for Epidemiologic Studies of the Elderly (EPESE) cohort (a community-based study of 2,812 older people followed for more than a decade), those who experienced violent-crime victimization were at an independent increased risk of nursing home placement (M. Lachs et al., 2006). Many of these individuals were ostensibly well compensated in all spheres (i.e., medical, functional, and psychosocial) before experiencing a crime, but victimization set in motion an inexorable spiral that ultimately resulted in loss of independence.

For people who are not well compensated, this spiral is only worse. These cases are striking not only for their trajectory, but also for how seemingly "minor" victimization can insidiously erode quality of life.

The notion that a single event might set into motion a progressive spiral of decline in many domains for an older adult has a basis in aging theory (Burnes & Burnette, 2013). Normal aging is accompanied by a loss of physiological reserve in various systems that need not lead to phenotypic decline. However, when the organism is taxed through stress, illness, or other factors, this loss of physiological reserve is unmasked. Clinicians skilled in geriatric medicine encounter the effects of this disequilibrium on a daily basis: the ostensibly high-functioning older adult who develops new incontinence with simple pneumonia; the patient with mild cognitive impairment who develops alarming confusion with the addition of a medication; or the compensated older person who declines medically after bereavement.

Crime victimization may be such a precipitating event in the life of an older person. It is a stressful experience that may impact on physical health, mental health, and functional independence.

ROLE OF MULTIDISCIPLINARY PROVIDERS

Given the paucity of research in this area, what is the clinician's role in the care of an older person who is a victim of crime? Is it simply to treat lacerations and abrasions, or should health care professionals play a more aggressive role in these situations? Or is crime simply not within the purview of the clinician?

We favor the more aggressive stance. A fundamental tenet of gerontology is that medical and social problems conspire to threaten the independence of the older person. Whether such a functional spiral is provoked by an acute medical illness such as shingles or an acute social problem such as robbery is ultimately moot. The outcome of such provocation is undeniably medical, undeniably quality-of-life depleting, and undeniably costly when independence is lost.

Besides caring skillfully for acute illnesses, clinicians should recognize that the older person who experiences crime is vulnerable in many ways. Elders with chronic diseases that have been well controlled may decompensate for physiological reasons or because psychological factors related to crime may result in noncompliance or self-neglect. Although data are lacking, older crime victims are probably at risk for psychological distress in many ways, ranging from major depressive disorders to posttraumatic stress syndrome. These should be screened for and aggressively treated if identified. Support groups for victims of crime may be useful in this regard, although the issues for older crime victims may be somewhat different from those for younger ones, and the authors are unaware of support groups geared specifically to the older individual. Social isolation because of the fear of recurrent crime victimization is also a concern. Specific inquiries should be made regarding the size and quality of social interactions (e.g., maintenance of previously cherished hobbies and activities after crime).

Clinicians should also not be lulled into complacency because victimization is perceived as "minor." For many older adults, an episode of victimization, such as burglary, seems trivial because little was stolen, there was no contact with the perpetrator, and insurance was available to replace stolen items. Yet despite an initial complacent response, a dramatic decline ensued.

FINANCIAL EXPLOITATION OF OLDER ADULTS

The subject of financial exploitation of older adults deserves special mention because it is the most prevalent form of elder abuse (Pillemer et al., 2016). Combined family-based financial abuse and stranger-perpetrated fraud/scams affect 5% to 10% of cognitively intact older adults living in the community each year (Burnes et al., 2017). Elder financial exploitation is associated with increased risks of mortality and hospitalization, poor physical and mental health, and diminished quality of life. Age-associated vulnerability to financial exploitation is rooted in exposure to neurological, cognitive, functional, and psychosocial risks and is conceptualized as a potential clinical syndrome to be screened (M. S. Lachs & Han, 2015). Older victims are more likely to have more financial resources than their younger counterparts, which in combination with the higher prevalence of social isolation, cognitive impairment, and other factors, renders them uniquely susceptible to exploitation. Clinicians may become aware of exploitation when an older person or a family member describes it frankly to them or other aspects of the clinical presentation make it clear that something is amiss in the finances of the older person (e.g., not purchasing medicines that were previously affordable).

In this situation, the clinical evaluation involves an assessment of cognitive status and may include the clinician recommending involvement in a supportive decision-making protocol or guardianship with respect to finances if decision-making capacity is impaired. Consultation with a neuropsychologist should be considered. Susceptibility to economic predation in the context of dementia itself may be linked to impaired decision-making capacity if, for example, the older person chooses to pursue sweepstakes entries rather than purchase insulin. Appropriate social service and legal authorities should be involved in accordance with state reporting laws and in concert with the older adult's self-determined notion of resolution (Burnes, 2016). Educating older citizens on how to identify culprits and resist their overtures is a role played by many senior centers and elder advocacy agencies.

See also Adult Protective Services; Elder Mistreatment: Overview; Elder Neglect; Financial Abuse.

David Burnes, Ronet Bachman and Mark Lachs

Bachman, R., & Meloy, M. L. (2008). The epidemiology of violence against the elderly: Implications for primary and secondary prevention. *Journal of Contemporary Criminal Justice*, 24, 186–197. doi:10.1177/1043986208315478

Burnes, D. (2016). Community elder mistreatment intervention with capable older adults: Towards a conceptual practice model. *The Gerontologist*. Advance online publication. doi:10.1093/geront/gnv692

Burnes, D., & Burnette, D. (2013). Broadening the etiological discourse on Alzheimer's disease to include trauma and posttraumatic stress disorder as psychosocial risk factors. *Journal of Aging Studies*, 27(3), 218–224. doi:10.1016/j.jaging.2013.03.002

Burnes, D., Henderson, C., Sheppard, C., Zhao, R., Pillemer, K., & Lachs, M. S. (2017) (revise/resubmit). Prevalence of elder financial fraud and scams in the United States: A systematic review and meta-analysis. *American Journal of Public Health*, 107(8), 1295.

Chu, L. D., & Kraus, J. F. (2004). Predicting fatal assault among the elderly using the national incident-based reporting system crime data. *Homicide Studies*, 8, 71–95. doi:10.1177/1088767903262396

Lachs, M., Bachman, R., Williams, C. S., Kossack, A., Bove, C., & O'Leary, J. R. (2005). Older adults as crime victims, perpetrators, witnesses, and complainants: A population-based study of policy interactions. *Journal of Elder Abuse and Neglect*, 16, 25–40.

Lachs, M., Bachman, R., Williams, C. S., Kossack, A., Bove, C., & O'Leary, J. R. (2006). Violent crime victimization increases the risk of nursing home placement in older adults. *The Gerontologist*, 46(5), 583–589.

Lachs, M. S., & Han, S. D. (2015). Age-associated financial vulnerability: An emerging public health issue. *Annals of Internal Medicine*, 163(11), 877–878.

Pillemer, K., Burnes, D., Riffin, C., & Lachs, M. S. (2016). Elder abuse: Global situation, risk factors and prevention strategies. *The Gerontologist*, 56, S194–S205. doi:10.1093/geront/gnw004

Truman, J., & Morgan, R. (2016, October). Criminal victimization, 2015. Bureau of Justice Statistics, U.S. Dept. of Justice (2016). NCJ 250180. Retrieved from https://www.bjs.gov/content/pub/pdf/cv15.pdf

U.S. Bureau of Justice Statistics. (2016). Data collection: National crime victim survey. Retrieved from https://www.bjs.gov/index.cfm?ty=dcdetail&iid=245

Web Resource
U.S. Bureau of Justice Statistics: http://www.bjs.gov

CULTURAL ASSESSMENT

Culturally sensitive health care can improve health care delivery to older adults and reduce continuing disparities in health outcomes. Cultural practices and beliefs have an impact on the health of individuals and the way that health is perceived (Hakim & Wegmann, 2002). In clinical settings, cultural assessment is used to determine best approaches to care, improve patient satisfaction, and optimize adherence to treatment regimens. In geriatrics care, the clinical merit of understanding psychosocial factors is well established; clinicians routinely address complex physiological, psychological, and social issues in treating older adults. Health providers need to have the ability to assess how culture and belief systems impact the health care needs of older patients to provide relevant and holistic care (Rawlings-Anderson, 2004). Culture encompasses such a broad range of beliefs, behaviors, and definitions that the notion of conducting an assessment may seem daunting. Although a symbolic construct through which social life is patterned, acted, and perceived, culture can be observed as enactment and outcome of behaviors in a changing environment and throughout the life span. There is a dynamic, adaptive quality to this "cognitive map"; cultures are not static. Texts describing cultural patterns should be used with caution. Broad, heterogeneous categories—such as Asian/Pacific Islander, which represents more than 25 ethnic groups, some from the same countries of origin—do not meaningfully reflect intragroup or individual variation in ethnicity and life experience. The cultural patterns discussed here as examples describe a range of beliefs. As in any clinical situation, the focus should be on the individual; stereotyping should be avoided.

Providers should be aware of the cultural and historical experiences of older patients when determining their health care expectations for cure, treatment, palliative care, or reassurance about particular conditions. Because practitioners and patients may not share the same beliefs and values about health and illness, their expectations for health care, treatment, and healing may also vary. Older rural African Americans, Filipinos, Mexican Americans, and Native Americans, for example, may conceive of health as an attribute of personal spirituality (Hodge & Limb, 2010). African Americans may believe that prayer and faith may be more important than preventive health measures. Filipinos and Mexican Americans may perceive poor health as punishment or as the result of malevolent witchcraft. Older adults with these cultural perceptions about health and illness may feel that symptoms should be tolerated until their impact on function is too severe for informal or community-based care. Coping skills developed over a lifetime in response to racism or other inequalities may also hinder the evaluation and diagnosis of serious disorders. Minority elders may be reluctant to divulge information, especially about alternative therapies or dissatisfaction with Western biomedicine. Whereas geriatricians typically seek information about social support for patients, patients may not envision themselves as the center of a family or community support network. Allocentrism— emphasizing the importance of the group over the individual—is a common cultural value shared by many older Hispanics and Asians. The notion of autonomy in decision making is not universal.

Culture-bound syndromes have received attention, although their significance is not well understood. Cultural norms define illness and its expression. For example, among Western Europeans, there is a higher frequency of stomach ailments among Germans, liver ailments among French, and headaches among English. Hispanics might describe shortness of breath as fatigue (*fatiga*) and back pain as a kidney pain (*dolor de los rinones*). Asian Pacific Islanders might complain of a "weak kidney" to indicate sexual dysfunction because the kidney is believed to be the site of libido. Native Americans might describe stress in their family support system as the patient having a "bad heart," indicating the lack of harmony with caregivers. Whereas patients experience illness as a cluster of symptoms that affect functioning in the social context of their daily lives, physicians embedded in Western biomedical culture often define symptoms as disease, devoid of social context. Recognition of the culturally mediated experience of poor health is a significant element in the culturally sensitive assessment and treatment of older patients.

C

CONDUCTING CULTURAL ASSESSMENT AND REDUCING ACCESS BARRIERS

Health care providers often do not have the time or the training to conduct a comprehensive assessment during a single encounter. As with other diagnostic tools, cultural assessment is linked to the level of care and professional domain. Physicians use cultural assessment to inform their evaluation of symptoms, choice of screening instruments, discussion and selection of treatment options, care plans, advance directives (ADs), and placement options. Nurses and other allied health professionals use cultural assessment to implement care plans, assess health status and pain, respond to personal-care issues, and provide appropriate emotional and spiritual support to patients and families. Psychosocial assessment of patients in the context of their families and communities is a core social-work skill. Care planning is based on an assessment of beliefs about disease, efficacy of treatment, and potential for rehabilitation, as well as the impact of disease on quality of life. The basic elements of cultural assessment, asked or observed, include personal and medical history, health practices and preferences, information needs, and communication styles.

Personal history includes place of birth, length of residence in the United States if foreign-born, economic status, major support systems, ethnic affiliation and strength of that association, and religious beliefs and importance of those beliefs to daily life. Clinicians should assess the type, depth, and complexity of information a patient wishes to be told and by whom. Dietary preferences, prescriptions, proscriptions, and lifestyle changes should be noted with respect to their potential conflict with cultural values. Differing values about the appropriateness of informal home care or institutional care for specific conditions (e.g., cognitive impairments, incontinence, advanced age) may have to be explored. Communication styles include primary and secondary language, speech and reading levels, print and oral traditions, and nonverbal expression. Patients' descriptions of symptoms using culture-bound references may need to be interpreted, even if the provider and patient speak the same language. When translators are used, clinicians should speak in short phrases and use simple, nontechnical language. To ensure the accuracy of the translation, the interpreter should report the patient's words exactly; accuracy can be checked by asking the patient to repeat the information or instructions and by monitoring nonverbal communication (e.g., facial expression, body language). When family members are used as translators, the purpose of the session should be discussed beforehand with them to ascertain their comfort level with sensitive topics (e.g., anatomical function, especially across gender and generations; bad news). In some cases, a more appropriate relative or a professional interpreter should be found.

Culturally sensitive medical histories and examinations do not differ from any thorough examination. The art of patient interviewing may diverge from the structured medical model if patients voice multiple complaints or divulge important symptoms only at the conclusion of the interview. Past medical history should be thoroughly reviewed and discussed. Foreign-born patients may have been exposed to treatment strategies that are not familiar to U.S. physicians, and patients may not have access to the same information about diseases in their countries of origin. Medications that are well controlled in the United States may be sold over the counter or prescribed with few safeguards in other countries. Histories of drug allergies may be more complex to elicit from foreign-born elders. Clinicians may need to schedule several visits before a trusting relationship is established.

Effective communication is always key to good patient care. Cross-cultural barriers to access often occur unintentionally. At a first meeting, clinicians may habitually introduce themselves, shake hands firmly, and promptly determine the reason for the patient encounter. In some cultures, this businesslike attitude would be offensive. Native Americans, for example, would likely prefer a light touch to an aggressive handshake. In other cultures, traditional (i.e., indigenous or folk) medicine incorporates the healing arts of counseling and talk therapy. Patients from diverse cultures relate that their traditional doctors "really know them as a person"; they feel distrustful of an abrupt and impersonal approach. Patients' expressions of respect may be misinterpreted by providers. Avoidance of direct eye contact is a common form of respect shown by Native Americans, Mexican Americans, and African Americans and should not be interpreted as furtiveness or untrustworthiness. Giving respect and feeling distrust may overlap, as when an African American patient avoids direct disagreement with a doctor's recommendations. Silence and failure to report adverse reactions or unsatisfactory responses to treatment may simply be a way to respectfully avoid direct confrontations, or it may be the patient's way of shielding the clinician from the humiliation associated with treatment failure. Silence may indicate respect, acknowledgment of the discourse, or an opportunity to carefully weigh a response. It does not necessarily indicate discomfort or anger and should be an expected element in pacing an interaction.

The clinician may carefully schedule patient care by the clock, but many cultures do not share a similar orientation to time. This may be because of the practical difficulties of arriving at a destination at an exact time or the irrelevance of exact timing of most activities. Clinical questions about a symptom's occurrence, intensity, and effect on the patient and social life may initiate a discussion about cultural values. In addition to avoiding harm in the physician–patient relationship, learning about cultural norms can be an enjoyable aesthetic experience for providers.

Simple forms of etiquette are often most effective. Most cultures afford respect to elders as well as to health care practitioners. Treating patients with respect may be indicated via appropriate terms of address, using a title and surname (e.g., Mrs. Brown) rather than a first name or a term of endearment. Personalized relationships are important to many cultures and are established through noncommercial transactions. Patients may offer food or other token gifts to reduce the formal barrier and create a more personal relationship; refusal would be treated with suspicion. Establishing this type of relationship may also be accomplished by the provider offering a personal disclosure, such as

initiating a conversation about a mutual interest (which may entail responding to personal questions), to reduce communication barriers. Clinicians should avoid any temptation to relate to patients of different cultures by using terms that are not in their own vocabulary, such as speaking Black English to African American elders or using putative honorifics that may be offensive, such as "chief" to a Native American. Clinicians may adjust their medical and anatomical vocabulary to the patient's education and language, but they need to check that the information provided is understood.

ADVANCE DIRECTIVES AND END-OF-LIFE CARE

In a multicultural society, concern for justice brings ethical issues to the fore. Most of the literature on cultural assessment of elderly persons in the United States relates to significant differences among ethnic and cultural groups on the completion of ADs and end-of-life decision-making strategies. For example, African Americans tend to want all possible life-sustaining treatments; they distrust ADs and see them as authorizing neglect or inferior care based on racial and socioeconomic factors. Korean Americans may voice a personal wish for a natural death (i.e., no life-prolonging technology) but expect their children to insist on all possible life-saving measures. Cultural-assessment strategies use the same principles as any other medical encounter of effective communication, recognition, and sensitivity to cultural variation and may also include assessment of family attitudes and practices (Bhat, McFarland, Keiser, Wehbe-Alamah, & Filter, 2015; Crawley, Marshall, Lo, Koenig, & End-of-Life Care Consensus Panel, 2002; Ersek, Kagawa-Singer, Barnes, Blackhall, & Koenig, 1998; Hepburn & Reed, 1995; Hornung et al., 1998; Kagawa-Singer & Blackhall, 2001; Zager & Yancy, 2011).

To set the context for ethical decision making, clinicians need to ascertain whether patients are reluctant or responsive to discussing end-of-life care. In addition, clinicians should attempt to understand beliefs about death, spiritual issues associated with dying, the nature of the social support system, and attitudes of patients

C

and their families toward the health care system. In many cultures, the direct, frank, structured discussions of death implied in ADs and end-of-life care planning are considered harmful to the patient's well-being, insinuate hopelessness, increase suffering, and hasten the inevitable outcome. Among Native Americans, for example, the issue is best addressed indirectly, talking about others who have died (using a referent term rather than the personal name) to elicit responses about what would constitute a "good death." Clinicians who can address these issues over time are more likely to reach an understanding of their patients' wishes.

Concepts of autonomy vary and imply different norms in the disclosure of information and decision making. Ethiopian and Persian immigrants believe that bad news should be conveyed to the patient by a family member or close friend, not by a health care provider. In these circumstances, physicians confront the dilemmas of concealment of information, truthfulness in diagnosis or prognosis, and protection of patient confidentiality. Some physicians manage the problem by asking patients how much information they want to know, who else should be informed, and who they want to make decisions with or for them. Another strategy is to encourage patients to ask questions over several visits to absorb information.

The role of decision maker varies with cultural norms. Daughters might be the first choice among Hispanics and African Americans, sons among Asians, and spouses among Anglo-Europeans. In general, Native American cultures strongly support autonomous decision making, and children are unlikely to interpose their wishes. However, if an elder is without capacity, a family spokesperson would likely emerge to represent the elder's authentic wishes. Clinicians should avoid directing information to and expecting decisions from the best-educated family member; this person may not necessarily be culturally empowered with decision-making authority.

See also Advance Directives; Cultural Competence and Aging; Spirituality.

Jené M. Hurlbut

Bhat, A., McFarland, M., Keiser, M., Wehbe-Alamah, H., & Filter, M. (2015). Advancing cultural assessments in palliative care using web-based education. *Journal of Hospice & Palliative Nursing, 17*(4), 348–355.

Crawley, L. M., Marshall, P. A., Lo, B., & Koenig, B. A., & End-of-Life Care Consensus Panel. (2002). Strategies for culturally effective end-of-life care. *Annals of Internal Medicine, 136*(9), 673–679.

Ersek, M., Kagawa-Singer, M., Barnes, D., Blackhall, L., & Koenig, B. A. (1998). Multicultural considerations in the use of advance directives. *Oncology Nursing Forum, 25*, 1683–1690.

Hakim, H., & Wegmann, D. (2002). A comparative evaluation of the perceptions of health of elders of different multicultural backgrounds. *Journal of Community Health Nursing, 19*(3), 161–171.

Hepburn, K., & Reed, R. (1995). Ethical and cultural issues with Native American elders: End of life decision making. *Clinics in Geriatric Medicine, 11*, 97–112.

Hodge, D., & Limb, G. (2010). Conducting spiritual assessments with Native Americans: Enhancing cultural competency in social work practice courses. *Journal of Social Work Education, 46*(2), 265–284.

Hornung, C. A., Eleazer, G. P., Strothers, H. S., Wieland, G. D., Eng, C., McCann, R., & Sapir, M. (1998). Ethnicity and decision-makers in a group of frail older people. *Journal of the American Geriatrics Society, 46*(3), 280–286.

Kagawa-Singer, M., & Blackhall, L. J. (2001). Negotiating cross-cultural issues at the end of life: "You got to go where he lives." *Journal of the American Medical Association, 286*(23), 2993–3001.

Rawlings-Anderson, K. (2004). Assessing the cultural and religious needs of older people. *Nursing Older People, 16*(8), 29–33.

Zager, B. S., & Yancy, M. (2011). A call to improve practice concerning cultural sensitivity in advance directives: A review of the literature. *Worldviews on Evidence-based Nursing/Sigma Theta Tau International, Honor Society of Nursing, 8*(4), 202–211.

Web Resources

Center for MulticulturalHealth: http://www.multi-culturalhealth.org

Henry Ford Health System Institute on Multicultural Health: http://www.henryford.com/body.cfm?id=39779

Network for Multicultural Research on Health and Healthcare: http://www.multiculturalhealthcare.net

Program for Multicultural Health (PMCH) at the University of Michigan Health System: http://www.med.umich.edu/multicultural

CULTURE CHANGE

Culture change refers to an ongoing movement to transform care and support systems so that they are organized to provide individualized care in accordance with each person's customary routines to "attain or maintain their highest practicable physical, mental, and psychosocial well-being" (Omnibus Reconciliation Act of 1987). Culture change engages staff closest to each resident, integrating quality of life and quality of care for optimal outcomes. The movement originated in nursing homes, but its principles are being adapted across the spectrum of care and support settings. Care is directed by the older adult's daily routines, needs, and preferences, whether stated directly or by observation of nonverbal communications, including reflexive responses; culture change revolves around how each person wants to live. It is person-directed, relationship-based care and produces better outcomes for individuals and the people and organizations caring for them.

Individualized care, the central theme of NHRA, requires transformation from the traditional institutional care model that facilities adapted from hospitals to one in which staff is assigned to support the same residents and coworkers and supervisors form a stable, collaborative team. In addition, operations support decentralized decision making that allows the care team closest to each resident to be flexible, nimble, and responsive in maintaining residents' customary routines and rhythms of life. The care team closest to the resident is empowered to make decisions that immediately respond to residents' choices and needs, with support from the rest of the organization to provide care and services accordingly. The approach promotes health and prevents avoidable declines (Kane, Lum, Cutler, Degenholtz, & Yu, 2007; Kane & Cutler, 2009; Sloane et al., 2004).

Through culture change, nursing homes shift from "risk prevention" to "health promotion," building on each elder's strengths, preferences, and daily routines. In this new culture, care and support are provided in the context of a mutual relationship wherein each person's routine sets the pace for tasks coordinated through interdepartmental collaboration. These language changes are more than simply cosmetic: the resident is now a "person" in a "household," "community," or "neighborhood" that replaces "nursing unit."

A hypothetical example of a nursing home that has undertaken culture change illustrates how people and their caregivers experience these changes. The nursing home administrator and RN leader, in consultation with other professionals and caregiving staff, have established a permanent neighborhood team that knows Mrs. Jones prefers to awaken around 10 a.m. Her consistently assigned certified nursing assistant (CNA) assists Mrs. Jones on arising, slowly but easily because of her painful arthritis. Breakfast is provided according to her customary routines—two eggs over medium on toast and a hot cup of coffee. The staff is able to make cook-to-order food. Well rested, Mrs. Jones walks around a little, engages with others during the day, and maintains her window-box garden. Mrs. Jones is living with dementia, but this diagnosis does not negate her ability to live with meaning and purpose and to self-direct her day to the greatest extent possible. The day starts and proceeds according to Mrs. Jones' lifelong habits and ends with a long bath that helps her sleep comfortably through the night. The staff provides care with great ease. Before culture change, two CNAs who rotated into an assignment to care for Mrs. Jones struggled to get her moving at 7 a.m. to meet the facility breakfast time. Mrs. Jones cried in pain each morning and struggled against those who helped her. In the old culture, Mrs. Jones used more pain medication, an antidepressant, and medications for agitation and developed a stage II pressure injury from being in the wheelchair too long. The medications caused constipation; suppositories were used to address this concern. Mrs. Jones was uncomfortable and sleep deprived, unable to participate with others in daily activities. She was slowly declining physically, mentally, and psychosocially, and staff struggled to provide care.

C

BACKGROUND

The notion of culture change has galvanized nursing homes for the past two decades. In a 1995 conference session organized by the National Citizens' Coalition for Nursing Home Reform (now National Consumer Voice for Quality Long-Term Care, a citizen advocacy organization), several practitioners shared new approaches: The Regenerative Community built connections between people; Resident-Directed Care restored control to each resident; Individualized Care replaced facility routines; and the Eden Alternative brought spontaneity and normalcy to life by creating social and biological diversity to break through the loneliness, helplessness, and boredom rampant in nursing homes. In 1997, an expanded "pioneering" group brought together by Lifespan, a local elder service organization, met in Rochester, New York, convened by Carter Williams, MSW, and Rose Marie Fagan, the Rochester Long-term Care Ombudsman. The group founded the Pioneer Network and articulated the vision and principles of culture change that guide this movement's evolution.

Culture change knowledge and practice build incrementally. Certain organizational practices are key to success in transforming from institutional to individualized care: consistent assignment of staff so that they develop deep relationships and come to know each resident intimately; organizational structures and processes that support open and continuing communication, such as "huddles" among staff closest to the residents to share information and problem solve together; and daily rounds or stand-up huddles with management and staff closest to the resident to support any needed adjustments to care or operations. With these practices in place, staff who know residents well recognize early signs that something is wrong and use their knowledge of each person's routines and preferences to put the right interventions in place. As with the original pioneering practitioners, these systems depend on RN presence to achieve the leadership and organization for positive outcomes of quality of life and care as evidenced by recent research (Mueller, Bowers, Burger, & Cortes, 2016).

Some homes change their physical space, whereas others work within their existing environment. Several organizations reorganize the existing physical plant into distinct neighborhoods or households. Unlike the larger nursing homes, others build small houses; some are called Green Houses, set up from the start to reflect the home instead of an institution. These smaller houses generally care for fewer than 20 people per building, with central support across a group of homes for functions such as nursing, administration, and other operations and decentralized scheduling and management at the household level so that residents maintain completely individualized routines.

In collaboration with the Pioneer Network, nursing, medical director, and administrator organizations have incorporated culture change into their standards of practice and have identified nursing competencies to support these standards (Mueller, Burger, Rader, & Carter, 2013). In national symposia on the environment and on dining practices, national stakeholder organizations and the federal government have joined with the Pioneer Network in identifying new practice standards and fire safety rules that support culture change living.

BUSINESS CASE FOR CULTURE CHANGE

Research shows that there are identifiable differences between facilities that have stable staff and good resident outcomes and those that do not. Resident, human resource, and business interests coincide when there is high-quality leadership—a *positive chain of leadership*—throughout an organization. Human resource policies and systems of care that value and engage staff and sufficient resources to properly and respectfully care for residents result in less staff turnover (Eaton, 2002). Financially, facilities with "consistent nursing and administrative leadership, use of team and group processes, and active quality improvement programs" have lower costs of care (Rantz & Flesner, 2003). Research demonstrates that consensus management lowers turnover compared with top-down management (Donoghue & Castle, 2009). Culture change adopters compared with a control group of nonadopters experienced higher occupancy rates leading, on average, to more than $500,000 added revenue per year for a 140-bed nursing home (Elliot, 2010). In a pilot study, 49 nursing homes that used systems to engage staff in individualizing care saw better outcomes for residents and their organization (Elliot, Cohen, Reed, Nolet, & Zimmerman, 2014).

OUTCOMES AND EVALUATION

Culture change practices stabilize staff, as well as reduce staff turnover, use of psychoactive medications, resident weight loss, dehydration, pain, agitation, and aggression. Furthermore, the approach is associated with increased family visits and socialization (Rantz et al., 2004; Rantz & Flesner, 2003; Sloane et al., 2002; Stone et al., 2004). After 9 months in a 2005 Medicare Quality Improvement Organization (QIO) pilot program in applying the Holistic Approach to Transformational Change (HATCh) model, 254 nursing homes in 21 states reported collective improvement in turnover rates, pain, pressure injuries for residents at high risk, activities of daily living (ADL) decline, locomotion, and restraints (Quality Partners of Rhode Island, 2005 [now known as Healthcentric Advisors]). In participating nursing homes, publicly reported quality measures (QMs) for pressure injuries in both high- and low-risk residents, as well as for depression, improved, and the use of physical restraints decreased. Falls were reduced by 8.9%, antipsychotic use by 50%, and workers compensation claims from 44 to 7 (Quality Partners of Rhode Island, 2005).

Research on the Green House Project shows a positive impact on operational efficiencies and resulting financial performance, as well as significant improvements in quality of life, family satisfaction, and staff satisfaction (Jenkens, Sult, Lessell, Hammer, & Ortigara, 2011; Kane & Cutler, 2009; Kane et al., 2007) and early promising results in reducing rehospitalizations and pressure injury incidence.

FEDERAL AND STATE SUPPORT FOR CULTURE CHANGE

In 2002, the Centers for Medicare & Medicaid Services (CMS) held a satellite broadcast for federal and state surveyors and other stakeholders focused on demonstrating that culture change practices are what the NHRA requires. A four-part broadcast, *From Institutional to Individualized Care*, based on the 2005 QIO workforce and resident-directed care projects, aired in 2006 and 2007. CMS developed the Artifacts of Culture Change Tool with measures covering the domains of care, environment, family and leadership, workplace practice, and outcomes.

The St. Louis Accord, a national meeting sponsored by the Quality Partners of Rhode Island (now Healthcentric Advisors) and the Pioneer Network in 2005 fostered the formation of state culture change coalitions. States sent teams of stakeholders to learn about culture change and coalition building. Almost every state now has a culture change coalition; they vary in structure, approaches, practices, and financing. Provider associations and other state stakeholders are partnering to bring culture-change activities to their membership (Koren, 2010).

Since 2009, the federal government has initiated several efforts to promote culture change, including revised surveyor guidelines that highlight the importance of honoring customary routines, a new resident assessment tool that includes interviews with residents about their routines and preferences, surveyor interview questions to residents and staff about how well residents' routines and preferences are followed, and a revision of the long-term care facility requirements for participation that make person-centered care a more explicit expectation. In addition, the revised guidelines fostered a nationwide collaborative campaign to improve dementia care by using individualized approaches to reduce residents' distress and use of antipsychotic medications to treat their externally (e.g., low nursing staff) or clinically (e.g., untreated pain) induced stress behaviors. National culture change demonstrations were included in the Patient Protection and Affordable Care Act of 2010.

ENFORCEMENT AND ACCREDITATION

Despite supporting language in NHRA, state and federal survey processes continue to tolerate and sometimes even endorse institutionalized approaches to care, often favoring safety

C

over practices to support resident rights and foster autonomy. However, as more evidence of the positive impact of quality of life on quality of care emerges, surveyors are beginning to evolve with the field. The CMS enforcement process required by the NHRA surveys quality of care; however, the process has been less precise for quality-of-life except for citations around physical restraint and off-label use of antipsychotic medications. Surveyors may find it more challenging to cite quality-of-life violations as they tend to be measured more subjectively than quality-of-care issues. In addition, changing some aspects of care through culture change does not guarantee that facilities become providers of good care. If residents have a choice of foods but staff are not available or do not assist with eating, poor outcomes ensue.

Private long-term care accreditation organizations are also addressing culture change. The Commission on Accreditation of Rehabilitation Facilities incorporated some culture-change practices in its standards. The Joint Commission is exploring how each standard might capture the philosophy of resident centeredness. The movement continues to grow, as does the evidence that culture change is the pathway to better results for residents and for care providers.

See also Nursing Homes; Pioneer Network.

Sarah Greene Burger and Barbara Frank

Donoghue, C., & Castle, N. (2009). Leadership styles of nursing home administrators and their association with staff turnover. *The Gerontologist, 49*(2), 166–174.

Eaton, S. C. (2002). What a difference management makes! Nursing staff turnover variation within a single labor market. In *Appropriateness of minimum nurse staffing ratios in nursing homes* (Phase II Report to Congress). Washington, DC: U.S. Department of Health and Human Services.

Elliot, A. (2010). Occupancy and revenue gains from culture change in nursing homes: A win-win innovation for a new age of long-term care. *Seniors Housing & Care Journal, 18*(1), 61–76.

Elliot, A., Cohen, L. W., Reed, D., Nolet, K., & Zimmerman, S. (2014). A "recipe" for culture change? Findings from the THRIVE survey of culture change adopters. *The Gerontologist, 54*(Suppl. 1), S17–S24.

Farrell, D., Brady, C., & Frank, B. (2011). *Meeting the leadership challenge in long-term care: What you do matters.* Baltimore, MD: Health Professions Press.

Jenkens, R., Sult, T., Lessell, N., Hammer, D., & Ortigara, A. (2011). Financial implications of THE GREEN HOUSE® Model. *Senior Housing & Care Journal, 18*(1), 3–21.

Kane, R., & Cutler, L. (2009). Promoting homelike characteristics and eliminating institutional characteristics in community based residential care settings: Insights from an 8 state study. *Senior Housing and Care Journal, 17*, 15–37.

Kane, R., Lum, T., Cutler, L., Degenholtz, H., & Yu, T. (2007). Resident outcomes in small-house nursing homes: A longitudinal evaluation of the initial Green House program. *Journal of the American Geriatrics Society, 55*(6), 832–839.

Koren, M. J. (2010). Person-centered care for nursing home residents: The culture-change movement. *Health Affairs, 29*(2), 312-317.

Mueller, C., Bowers, B., Burger, S., Cortes, T. (2016). Policy brief: Registered nurse staffing requirements in nursing homes. *Nursing Outlook.* Retrieved from http://www.sciencedirect.com/science/article/pii/S0029655416301191

Mueller, C., Burger, S., Rader, J., Carter, D. (2013). Nurse competencies for person-directed care in nursing homes. *Geriatric Nursing, 34*, 101–104.

Omnibus Budget Reconciliation Act of 1987, Pub. L. No. 100-203, Subtitle C: Nursing Home Reform (1987).

Patient Protection and Affordable Care Act of 2010. Pub. L. No. 111-148.

PHI. (2011). Best practices: Augsburg Lutheran Home, Wellspring Program. Retrieved from http://phihnational.org/training/resources/best-practices/augsburg

Quality Partners of Rhode Island. (2005). *Final project report. October: Improving nursing home culture pilot study* (Centers for Medicare & Medicaid Services contract number 7SOW-RI-INHC-102005).

Rantz, M. J., & Flesner, M. K. (2003). *Person-centered care: A model for nursing homes.* Silver Spring, MD: American Nurses Publishing.

Rantz, M. J., Hicks, L., Grando, V., Petroski, G. F., Madsen, R. W., Mehr, D. R.,…Mass, M. (2004). Nursing home quality, cost, staffing, and staff mix. *The Gerontologist, 44*(1), 24–38.

Sloane, P. D., Hoeffer, B., Mitchell, C. M., McKenzie, D. A., Barrick, A. L., Rader, J.,…Koch, G. G. (2004). Effect of person-centered showering and the towel bath on bathing-associated aggression, agitation and discomfort in nursing home residents with dementia. *Journal of the American Geriatrics Society, 52*(11), 1795–1804.

Stone, R., Reinhard, S., Bowers, B., Zimmerman, D., Phillips, C., Hawes, C., ... Jacobson, N. (2002). *Evaluation of the Wellspring Model for improving nursing home quality.* New York, NY: The Commonwealth Fund. Retrieved from http:// www.cmwf.org/programs/elders/stone wellspringevaluation550.pdf

Web Resources

The Commonwealth Fund: http://www.cmwf.org

National Consumer Voice for Quality Long-Term Care (formerly National Citizen's Coalition for Nursing Home Reform): http://theconsumervoice.org/ uploads/files/family-member/culture-change -in-nursing-homes.pdf

Pioneer Network: http://www.pioneernetwork.net

The HATCh Model: http://theconsumervoice.org/ uploads/files/family-member/culture-change -in-nursing-homes.pdf

Wellspring: http://www.lifespan-network.org

CULTURAL COMPETENCE AND AGING

Today, one of every seven Americans, or 14% of the population, is an older American. Increasingly, the older adult population is racially/ethnically diverse. As a result of differential fertility, mortality, and immigration patterns, the older ethnic minority population will grow even more rapidly in the future. The 2010 Census reports that one of every four persons now identifies as a racial/ethnic minority in the United States (U.S. Census, 2012). Demographers predict that by 2050, nearly half of Americans will be of ethnic/minority descent. Inherent in the growth rate of minority populations is an increase in the older minority population. Nearly 20% of people aged 65 years and older identify as minorities: 8.4% Black or African American, 7% Hispanic, 3.5% Asian or Pacific Islander, and less than 1% American Indian or Native Alaskan. Although diversity has primarily been associated in the United States with ethnicity, it has more recently taken on a broader definition to include the sociohistorical and sociocultural

experiences of gender and peoples of different social classes, linguistic abilities, religious and spiritual beliefs, sexual orientations and identifications, physical and mental abilities, and immigrant populations (National Association of Social Workers [NASW], 2001).

The increase in the diversity among elders and society's commitment to equal access to resources predispose a responsibility to develop and provide opportunities for economic well-being, as well as health and social services that are uniquely tailored for these populations. This responsibility is amplified when viewed in context of the economic and health disparities and the differing health care and social service utilization patterns that exist for older ethnic minority populations, women, the poor, immigrant, and other at-risk populations. To accommodate the changing needs of an increasingly older population, it is important to provide opportunities for a good life throughout the life course and design services that respond to diversity. One national agenda, as reflected in the *Healthy People 2020* report, identifies goals and strategies that seek to eliminate resource disparities among all Americans, achieve health equity, and improve health and well-being across all populations (Centers for Disease Control and Prevention/National Center for Health Statistics, 2015).

SCOPE, PARAMETERS, AND BEST PRACTICES

In the last 20 years, there has been pronounced attention to the importance of cultural competence in a nation that is increasingly diverse. In addition to acknowledgment of the heterogeneity of the aged population and the concurrent evidence of economic and health disparities, a compelling justification for a cultural-competence perspective is the promotion of social justice (Brach & Fraser, 2000). Social justice is founded on respect for human dignity and self-determination and an assurance that all members of society have the same basic rights and opportunities. Advocating for culturally competent programs and services for diverse older adults supports the goal of providing equitable access, enhanced service utilization,

C

and improved physical, social, and economic health for all Americans.

There are multiple definitions of cultural competence, but all share several common denominators, including (a) knowledge and skills that are compatible with culturally diverse groups, (b) attitudes and values that honor diversity, and (c) a dual focus on the responsibilities of the provider and institution to improve practice, policy, and research related to the culturally diverse (NASW, 2001). Implicit in these denominators is the importance of engaging continually in self-reflective activities that increase providers' awareness of their own worldviews and values regarding oppression, discrimination, and work with culturally diverse groups. The Office of Minority Health (OMH) in the Bureau of Primary Health Care provides the following definitions of culture and competence:

Culture refers to integrated patterns of human behavior that include the language, thoughts, communications, actions, customs, beliefs, values and institutions of racial, ethnic, religious or social groups. Competence implies having the capacity to function effectively as an individual and an organization within the context of the cultural beliefs, behaviors, and needs presented by consumers and their communities (U.S. Department of Health and Human Services, 2001).

The OMH (2013) published standards for cultural and linguistic competence that are viewed by many health care organizations as operating principles in the 21st century. These standards emphasize the importance of providing culturally competent, respectful care for diverse patients, access to language services (i.e., by providing bilingual staff and interpreter services), and organizational supports to maintain a demographic, cultural, and epidemiological profile of the community. Additional strategies viewed include the use of indigenous community health workers, the incorporation of culture-specific attitudes and values into health promotion, and the inclusion of family members in health care decision making.

Recognition of the importance of cultural competence and the need for culturally based interventions are a response to the serious and persistent social and health disparities documented in the nation's racial/ethnic minority populations. The literature related to cultural competence with older minority populations continues to expand. In general, this literature reflects a combination of conceptual and empirical research and seeks to improve the theoretical understanding of the relationship of aging to ethnicity, gender, social class, and other structural variables. It also broadly describes ways to reconceptualize health and social services to be more culturally appropriate for diverse elders. Social and health disparity research and the new attention to translational research—moving from the bench to bedside—offer opportunities for researchers to further test the efficacy of using evidence-based practices with diverse populations that have been neglected in prior testing.

Available findings on the effectiveness of cultural competence are mixed. Results from some studies suggest that implementing culturally competent approaches with diverse elders and their families is associated with improved health outcomes and quality of care. Culturally sensitive programs and services have benefitted those with breast cancer, for example (Mokuau, Braun, & Daniggelis, 2012) and other chronic diseases and conditions (Tomioka, Braun, Compton, & Tanoue, 2011). "Taking Steps Toward Cultural Competence," a fact sheet from The SHARE Approach, is a shared decision-making toolkit. However, a recent systematic review of interventions to improve culturally appropriate care conducted by the Agency for Healthcare Quality Research (AHQR) demonstrated limited evidence for the impact of cultural competence for people with disabilities; lesbian, gay, bisexual, and transgender (LGBT) people; and racial/ethnic minorities. The review found that many of the existing intervention studies lacked rigor and systematic study designs, which limits the generalizability of positive findings (AHQR, 2016).

Because cultural competence is also about expanding choice and opportunity for all with special needs, it also speaks to the need for policies to safeguard the rights of all. Thus a critical component of cultural competence consists of policy efforts that advocate for the rights of all Americans, respects diversity, and promotes antidiscriminatory efforts and legislation.

CULTURAL COMPETENCE AND PROFESSIONAL EDUCATION

Major professional associations in health and social services (i.e., NASW, American Medical Association, and American Nurses Association) have published standards and guidelines on cultural competence and have encouraged the development of education and training that addresses disparities and the unique characteristics, issues, and needs of the diverse racial/ethnic groups. Cultural values, practices, and traditions reflecting cultural strengths should be utilized in assessment and intervention to build on patients' strengths (i.e., talents, knowledge, capabilities, and resources) in achieving a better quality of life (NASW, 2001).

Cultural competence approaches acknowledge resiliency in the human condition and encourage social workers and other health care professionals to respect the cultural identity, values, and practices of older patients. The emphasis on culture and cultural values does not negate the very real structural problems facing racial/ethnic and other populations at risk: poverty, racism and discrimination, inaccessible care, and limited opportunities for a better life that often require legal action and advocacy. The website *Think Cultural Health* provides easy-to-use, practical tools for understanding how to provide culturally and linguistically appropriate services (CLAS). From this resource, one can:

- Track state efforts to promote and provide CLAS through legislation, policies, and practices with the Tracking CLAS map.
- Better understand the National CLAS Standards with a printable list of the Standards and The Blueprint, a technical assistance document that lists a timeline of health equity milestones and crosswalks.
- Improve communication skills via learning programs designed for a range of social service and health professionals.
- Search for more online resources, including educational videos on CLAS and a curriculum

exploring health care and civil rights, in the Resources section.

Promoting the dissemination of culturally competent services is the best strategy at present to reduce disparities among culturally diverse elders, promote understanding of health and social disparities, and improve social and health outcomes for populations at risk.

See also Cultural Assessment.

Colette V. Browne

Agency for Healthcare Quality Research. (2016). *Improving cultural competence to reduce disparities: A review of cultural competence research.* Washington, DC: Author.

Brach, C., & Fraser, I. (2000). Can cultural competency reduce racial and ethnic health disparities? A review and conceptual model. *Medical Care Research and Review, 57,* 181–217.

Centers for Disease Control and Prevention/National Center for Health Statistics. (2015). Healthy People 2020. Retrieved from https://www.cdc.gov/nchs/healthy_people/hp2020.htm

Mokuau, N., Braun, K., & Daniggelis, E. (2012). Building capacity for Native Hawaiian women with breast cancer. *Health and Social Work, 37*(4), 216–224.

National Association of Social Workers. (2001). *Cultural competence standards.* Washington, DC: Author.

Office of Minority Health, U.S. Department of Health and Human Services. (2013). National CLAS standards fact sheet. Retrieved from https://www.thinkculturalhealth.hhs.gov/content/clas.asp

Tomioka, M., Braun, K., Compton, M., & Tanoue, L. (2011). Adapting Stanford's Chronic Disease Self-Management Program for Hawaii's multicultural population. *The Gerontologist, 52*(1), 121–132.

U.S. Census Bureau. (2012). U.S. Census Bureau projections show a slower growing, older, more diverse nation a half century from now. Retrieved from https://www.census.gov/newsroom/releases/archives/population/cb1212-243.html

U.S. Department of Health and Human Services. (2001). National standards for culturally and linguistically appropriate services in health care: Final report. Retrieved from https://minorityhealth.hhs.gov/assets/pdf/checked/finalreport.pdf

C

Web Resources

Achieving Cultural Competence, the Administration on Aging (AoA): http://www.aoa.gov

Improving cultural competence to reduce disparities: https://www.effectivehealthcare.ahrq.gov/ehc/products/573/2206/cultural-competence-report-160327.pdf

National Association of Social Workers (NASW): Cultural competence in social work practice: http://www.socialworkers.org

National Center for Cultural Competence: http://www.athealth.com/Practitioner/particles/compellingneed.html

Office of Minority Health, U.S. Department of Health and Human Services (USDHHS): http://www.omhrc.gov

The National Institute on Aging (NIA): http://www.nia.nih.gov/news

DAYTIME SLEEPINESS

Excessive daytime sleepiness (EDS) is the increased propensity to fall asleep, or sleepiness in a situation in which the person would be expected to be awake and alert. It is abnormal to fall asleep unintentionally during the day, and EDS is twice as common among older adults as middle-aged adults (Bixler et al., 2005). It results from sleep deprivation. Distinct from fatigue, which is difficulty sustaining a high level of performance, EDS is the inability to maintain alertness, with characteristic hypersomnia. The common misbelief that daytime sleepiness is acceptable in older adults can complicate attempts to isolate the cause of EDS. This perception may prevent older individuals from seeking medical attention or receiving medical care for daytime sleepiness. However, sleep problems can impair daily functioning and increase caregiver burden, increasing the risk of institutionalization.

CAUSES

Age-related changes in chronobiology, sleep disorders, other medical and psychological disorders, medications, environmental factors, and altered social patterns can lead to EDS. It is unclear how much of the change in sleep patterns experienced by older adults is due to normal physiological alterations, pathological events, sleep disorders, or poor sleep hygiene. EDS can also result from medications and other conditions. Many medications such as benzodiazepines, barbiturates, some antiepileptic medications, H_1 antihistamines, beta-blockers, and dopaminergic agonists (i.e., anti-Parkinson drugs) have sedating side effects. Pain medications, alcohol, and sleeping medications (prescription or over-the-counter [OTC]) are also associated with EDS. Heart failure, asthma, and gastroesophageal reflux disrupt sleep, as do symptoms such as chronic pain, depression, and nocturia (Leigh, Hudson, & Byles, 2016; Roehrs, Carskadon, Dement, & Roth, 2005). Some 57% of persons 60 years and older have a primary sleep disturbance that increases daytime sleepiness (i.e., 24% have sleep apnea, 45% have periodic leg movements, and 29% have insomnia; Kryger, Monjan, Bliwise, & Ancoli-Israel, 2004). However, despite the objective presence of increasing severity of sleep disorders, such as sleep apnea, with advancing age, self-reports of symptoms such as insomnia and EDS appear to decrease (Vaz Fragoso, Van Ness, Araujo, Iannone, & Klar Yaggi, 2015). Long-term care and hospital settings also impair circadian rhythms and sleep quality because of noise, lack of external time cues (i.e., zeitgebers), care routines or roommates, social isolation, reduced daytime light exposure, and excessive nighttime light exposure.

CONSEQUENCES

In older adults, EDS is associated with an increased risk for cardiovascular mortality, hypertension, and stroke. EDS has been shown to have neurobehavioral consequences, such as decreased reaction time and attention span. Motor vehicle accidents occur when people with EDS fall asleep at the wheel or fail to drive defensively. Sleepy older adults experience decrements in social outcomes, general productivity, vigilance, activity level, and global assessment of functional status when compared with nonsleepy older adults (Gooneratne et al., 2003). Daytime sleepiness impairs working memory, cognitive processing, affect, and mood. Sleepiness may also, therefore, contribute to difficulty in self-managing health and daily life activities. Many of these symptoms are similar to those found in depression, delirium, and dementia. Thus when these conditions are evaluated, sleep-related causes should rank high in the differential diagnosis for older adults.

ASSESSMENT OF AN OLDER ADULT WITH EXCESSIVE DAYTIME SLEEPINESS

A comprehensive sleep history and a sleep diary should be used to assess EDS. One tool for quantifying EDS is the Epworth Sleepiness Scale (Johns, 1991), a brief, valid, reliable measure that asks how likely an individual would fall asleep during usual daily activities (e.g., watching television, riding in a car, or listening to a lecture). Clinicians should ask about risk factors for obstructive sleep apnea (OSA) such as snoring, periods of not breathing (apnea) during sleep, and upper body obesity. Restless legs symptoms should be evaluated. Any suspicion of OSA should generate a referral to a sleep specialist. Assessment of OSA and pronounced EDS may require an overnight sleep study (polysomnography) and may also require a daytime test of sleepiness (i.e., Multiple Sleep Latency Test).

SLEEP HYGIENE

In addition to treating sleep disorders, behavioral strategies are useful in improving the quality and duration of sleep and may improve EDS. These behaviors are often categorized as "sleep hygiene." Strategies that may increase sleep quantity and efficiency, strengthen circadian rhythms, and improve EDS include the following:

- Do not go to bed unless sleepy.
  The bed should be used only for sleeping (or intimacy or sex). If not sleepy, the person should do something that is relaxing but not stimulating.
- Develop a consistent and rest-promoting bedtime routine.
  One should go to bed at the same time each evening. A warm bath, a light snack, or a few minutes of reading can help one relax before bed. The bedroom should be dark, quiet, and slightly cool. One should not read, eat, watch TV, talk on the telephone, or play cards in bed.
- Get up at the same time every morning.
  On awakening, one should get out of bed, no matter what time it is. On awaking during the night, one should avoid looking at the clock; frequent time checks heighten anxiety and make sleep onset more difficult.
- Avoid naps.
  One should avoid frequent naps or naps longer than 30 minutes. One should never take a nap after 3 p.m.
- Avoid things that disturb sleep.
  Strenuous exercise should be avoided 6 hours before bedtime; it is best to time it early in the day. Caffeine should be avoided after lunch. Cigarettes and alcoholic beverages should be avoided before bedtime. Large meals and excitement should be limited before bedtime. Bedtime is a time to rest, not to worry.
- Avoid sleeping pills, if at all possible.
  Sleeping pills often cause daytime dysfunction among older adults but may be useful in the short term. OTC sleeping pills should be avoided; no alcohol should be consumed if taking sleeping pills.

SUMMARY

EDS has serious negative consequences for health, safety, and quality of life, especially in older adults. It is not a normal part of aging. Evaluation of EDS and focus on contributing factors should be included in routine patient-care interactions.

See also Sleep Disorders.

Nancy S. Redeker

Bixler, E. O., Vgontzas, A. N., Lin, H. M., Calhoun, S. L., Vela-Bueno, A., & Kales, A. (2005). Excessive daytime sleepiness in a general population sample: The role of sleep apnea, age, obesity, diabetes, and depression. *Journal of Clinical Endocrinology & Metabolism, 90*(8), 4510–4515.

Gooneratne, N. S., Weaver, T. E., Cater, J. R., Pack, F. M., Arner, H. M., Greenberg, A. S., ... Pack, A. I. (2003). Functional outcomes of excessive daytime sleepiness in older adults. *Journal of the American Geriatrics Society, 51*(5), 642–649.

Johns, M. W. (1991). A new method for measuring daytime sleepiness: The Epworth Sleepiness Scale. *Sleep, 14*(6), 540–545.

Kryger, M., Monjan, A., Bliwise, D., & Ancoli-Israel, S. (2004). Sleep, health, and aging: Bridging the gap between science and clinical practice. *Geriatrics, 59*(1), 24–30.

Leigh, L., Hudson, I. L., & Byles, J. E. (2016). Sleep difficulty and disease in a cohort of very old women. *Journal of Aging and Health, 28*(6), 1090–1104. doi:10.1177/0898264315624907

Roehrs, T., Carskadon, M. A., Dement, W. C., & Roth, T. (2005). Daytime sleepiness and alertness. In M. H. Kryger, T. Roth, & W. C. Dement (Eds.), *Principles and practice of sleep medicine* (4th ed., pp. 39–50). Philadelphia, PA: W. B. Saunders.

Vaz Fragoso, C. A., Van Ness, P. H., Araujo, K. L., Iannone, L. P., & Klar Yaggi, H. (2015). Age-related differences in sleep-wake symptoms of adults undergoing polysomnography. *Journal of the American Geriatrics Society, 63*(9), 1845–1851. doi:10.1111/jgs.13632

Web Resources

American Academy of Sleep Medicine: http://www.aasmnet.org

National Center on Sleep Disorders Research: http://www.nhlbi.nih.gov/health/public/sleep/index.htm (for the general public); http://www.nhlbi.nih.gov/health/prof/sleep/index.htm (for health care professionals)

National Sleep Foundation: http://www.sleepfoundation.org

New Abstracts and Papers in Sleep (NAPS): http://www.websciences.org/bibliosleep/NAPS

DEATH AND DYING

Death is the end of life. Experiences surrounding death and dying are influenced by many factors, including religion, culture, philosophy, and law. The universal event represents a nonnegotiable, imperative, which is an individual and communal crisis for every human being. The existential conflict of death lies in the blueprint of all living creatures. The unique anticipated experience of death creates an environment of self-reflection, value assessment, and loneliness.

Preparation for the end of life involves more than the person dying. The death event encompasses a network of relationships with the dying and the society from which that person evolves (Institute of Medicine [IOM], 2015; Sopcheck, 2016). In many cases, people facing end-of-life decisions have spent much time contemplating such choices yet are likely to encounter difficulty communicating their thoughts and decisions. Families and those linked to the dying person's end-of-life choices are also likely to avoid discussion of their views and perceptions because of social, cultural, spiritual, and religious beliefs (IOM, 2015).

In the United States, the conceptualization of death and dying is framed by a curative paradigm and a concomitant health care system that is highly technological. Epidemiological trends for causes of death and life expectancy have changed dramatically over the last century. In the early 1900s, communicable diseases accounted for nearly all deaths. Since the 1950s, chronic diseases such as cancer and heart disease have become the leading causes of death. Furthermore, life expectancy continues to increase, meaning that more Americans are likely to die from chronic conditions. Coupled with advances in treatment and technology, increased life expectancy presents significant challenges as to how we acknowledge and confront death and dying.

In 1900, most Americans died at home, frequently surrounded by multiple generations of family members. By 1950, approximately 50% of all deaths occurred in an institution, and by 1980, 75% of all Americans died in an institution, no longer cared for by family but by paid medical staff (IOM, 1997). Although the numbers of deaths occurring in acute care institutions has decreased slightly, the end of life is often fraught with frequent hospitalizations and interventions (IOM, 2015). Increases in health care funding, advances in diagnostic and treatment approaches to disease, and technology accounted for many of these changes. The medical paradigm with a curative framework provides a social imperative that death could be delayed or even avoided (Callahan, 2012). As the location of death shifted from community to institution, care of the dying has been heavily

D

influenced and delivered by health care professionals, shifting the decision making away from family and community. Often, physicians and other medical personnel, rather than the dying person and/or the family, define the dying process and assume the role of decision maker. Some of these patterns began to shift during the 1980s when Medicare, along with private insurers, began to provide reimbursement for hospice services. In addition, prospective payment systems were emphasized to decrease in-patient hospital stays. Hospice services are now considered mainstream (IOM, 2015), with increased emphasis on quality and palliative intervention.

Research indicates that health care professionals need to be better prepared to explore and guide patients and families through the risks of treatments and expected outcomes and to explore the desires/wishes of the patient. There are no simple solutions for assisting patients, families, and health care professionals with end-of-life decisions. Previous research has indicated that the dying process in the hospital was not satisfactory and providers were often unaware of family desires and wishes (Writing Group for the SUPPORT Investigators, 1995). This landmark study resulted in significant investments in the education of health care professionals surrounding end-of-life discussions (IOM, 2015). Research continues to support the need for open communication around the difficult topic of death and dying. A recent qualitative study reveals that the oldest old prefer to avoid hospitalization and are comfortable talking to others about death preferences but that these discussions, particularly with family, were infrequent (Fleming, Farquhar, Cambridge City over 75s Cohort study collaboration, Brayne, & Barclay, 2016). A meta-synthesis of family experiences of end-of-life care in long-term care settings (Jackson et al., 2012) identified the need to have conversations about dying well before the need for decision making. The evolution of palliative care provides a promising avenue toward bridging the transition to end-of-life discussions and assisting families and healthcare providers with these discussions. Palliative care programs follow the continuum of care, and open discussions about end-of-life and hospice are often standard. Palliative care and open discussions

may circumvent the issues surrounding enrollment into hospice programs late in the course of dying. One retrospective study (Riggs et al., 2016) examined the predictors of enrollment into hospice programs for persons receiving community-based palliative care and found that hospice enrollment for these participants was earlier and length of time in hospice was longer. They also noted that hospice services were less likely to be utilized by persons in underserved communities, which may be related to access and education issues.

Hospice programs debuted in the United States with the purpose of providing holistic care to dying persons and their families in the home or institution. The hospice philosophy embodies the goal of controlling pain and minimizing suffering without prolonging life. Hospice care continues to grow in the United States. The National Hospice and Palliative Care Organization (NHPCO, 2015) estimated that 1.6 million persons received hospice care in 2014. The figure demonstrates substantial growth since 1995 (IOM, 1997), with most utilizing the Medicare Health Benefit (MHB) that restricts utilization of curative and hospital services (Harrison & Connor, 2016). The evolution of hospice highlights the awareness of the transitional struggle between curative and hospice care under the restrictions of the MHB. Many prefer some degree of curative or palliative concurrent care, which has demonstrated some positive outcomes. This evolution calls for a growing need to review and adjust benefits to include an open-access hospice model that integrates concurrent care. The recent Medicare Care Choices Model is one innovative model that provides an opportunity to explore the benefits of, barriers to, and best practices of concurrent care. Harrison and Connor (2016) identify the need for policy and payment structures to address the need for coordinated care in our aging population.

Ultimately, end-of-life practitioners achieve the goals of pain control and minimization of suffering without prolonging life via medications and well-informed empathetic listening skills. The practitioner's comfort and skills with the discussion of death sets the stage for exploring the private thoughts of patients with respect and openness to their decision making about the death transition. Empathetic listening should include not only acknowledging the potential of death, but also providing as much information as possible concerning the diagnosis and care. The universal approach is to hope for the best but help prepare patients and families for the worst. This does not mean predicting death but starting with death as the final life event and working from there to the present to determine what the patient desires. The more informed a patient, the greater the potential of ensuring confidence in making end-of-life choices. Therefore interventions need to fill the gaps of knowledge, advocate for patients, and allow them as much control over their lives as possible. Some modalities of communicating with patients about end-of-life decisions include understanding their inner feelings, perceptions, and thoughts by listening to their life story. Beginning with an open-ended question such as "What do you know about your illness?" initiates the discussion, leading to more in-depth questions such as "What thoughts come to mind about death?" The use of simple nonverbal forms of media such as paper and markers provides options for communicating their story about life and death. Other forms of media, such as music, painting, and poetry, also provide windows of learning about their lives and perceptions of dying.

Even with the skills of engaging in discussions of death and dying, the health care professional may fear causing the patient increased anxiety or even fear creating and augmenting symptoms of disease progression. Yet research indicates that the ability of the practitioner to interact with patients on the topic of death and dying greatly influences their ability to share their private concerns and decision making about care. The success of meeting treatment goals lies in fundamental involvement of the patient and family in the processing of end-of-life care.

Janet M. Bairardi and Peter C. Wolf

Callahan, D. (2012). *In search of the good: A life in bioethics.* Cambridge, MA: MIT Press.

Fleming, J., Farquhar, M., Cambridge City over 75s Cohort (CC75C) study collaboration, Brayne, C., & Barclay, S. (2016). Death and the oldest old: Attitudes and preferences for end-of-life care— qualitative research within a population-based cohort. *PLOS ONE, 11*, 1–25. doi:10.1371/journal .pone.0150686

Harrison, K. L., & Connor, S. R. (2016). First Medicare demonstration of concurrent provision of curative and hospice services for end-of-life care. *American Journal of Public Health, 106*, 1405–1408. doi:10.2015/AJPH.2016.303238

Institute of Medicine. (1997). *Approaching death: Improving care at the end of life.* Washington, DC: National Academies Press.

Institute of Medicine. (2015). *Dying in America: Improving quality and honoring individual preferences near the end of life.* Washington, DC: National Academies Press.

Jackson, J., Derderian, L., White, P., Ayotte, J., Fiorini, J., Osgood Hall, R., & Shay, J. (2012). Family perspectives on end-of-life care: A metasynthesis. *Journal of Hospice and Palliative Nursing, 14*, 303–313. doi:10.1097/NJH.0b013e31824ea249

National Hospice and Palliative Care Organization. (2015). *NHPCO facts and figures: Hospice care in America.* Alexandria, VA: Author. Retrieved from http://www.nhpco.org/sites/default/files/ public/Statistics_Research/2015_Facts_Figures .pdf

Riggs, A., Breuer, B., Dhinra, L., Chen, J., Hiney, B, McCarthy, M.,…Knotkova, H. (2016). Hospice enrollment after referral to community-based specialist-level palliative care: Incidence, timing, and predictors. *Journal of Pain and Symptom Management, 52*, 170–177. doi:10.1016/j.jpainsymman.2016.02.011

Sopcheck, J. (2016). Social, economic, and political issues affecting end-of-life care. *Policy, Politics, & Nursing Practice, 17*(1), 32–42. doi:10.1177/ 1527154416642664

Writing Group for the SUPPORT Investigators. (1995). A controlled trial to improve care for seriously ill hospitalized patients. The study to improve care for seriously ill hospitalized patients. The study to understand prognoses and preferences for outcomes and risks of treatments (SUPPORT). *Journal of the American Medical Association, 274*(20), 1591–1598. doi:10.1001/jama1995.03530200027032

Web Resources
American Psychological Association: Death and Dying: http://www.apa.org/topics/death

Elisabeth Kübler-Ross Foundation: http://www .ekrfoundation.org

Hospice Foundation of America: http://www .hospicefoundation.org/endoflife

National Cancer Institute: End of Life Care for People Who Have Cancer: http://www.cancer.gov/ cancertopics/factsheet/Support/end-of-life-care

National Caregivers Library: End of Life Issues: http://www.helpguide.org/harvard/saying-goodbye.htm

National Hospice and Palliative Care Organization: End-of-Life Care Resources: http://www.nhpco.org/learn-about-end-life-care

National Institute on Aging End of Life: Helping with Comfort and Care: https://www.nia.nih.gov/health/publication/end-life-helping-comfort-and-care/introduction

National Institute on Aging Senior Health: https://nihseniorhealth.gov/endoflife/preparingfortheendoflife/01.html

Saying Goodbye: Health Guide Collaboration with Harvard: http://www.helpguide.org/harvard/saying-goodbye.htm

Understanding Death and Dying: Dying Matters: http://www.dyingmatters.org/page/understanding-death-and-dying

DEHYDRATION

Dehydration is a decrease in total body water from intracellular fluid (Thomas et al., 2008) and occurs more frequently in older adults. It is one of the Agency for Healthcare Research and Quality's Prevention Quality Indicators (Agency for Healthcare Research and Quality, n.d.) Dehydration can be categorized as isotonic, hypertonic, or hypotonic based on the quantity of sodium lost in relation to water lost. Isotonic dehydration occurs with a loss of extracellular fluid without any change in the intracellular fluid; sodium and water are lost in equal amounts (Schols, De Groot, Van Der Cammen, & Olde Rikkert, 2009). Hypertonic dehydration is characterized by greater water loss than sodium loss, with high serum sodium levels and high serum osmolarity, and is a result of excessive water loss or inadequate water intake (Schols et al., 2009). Hypotonic dehydration occurs when more sodium than water is lost (Schols et al., 2009), with low serum sodium levels and low serum osmolarity. Extracellular fluid is the lowest with hypotonic dehydration. Dehydration can be acute (a sudden loss of water and sodium from vomiting, diarrhea, sweating, or blood loss) or chronic (prolonged imbalance due primarily to insufficient fluid intake; Wakefield, Mentes, Holman, & Culp, 2008). Volume depletion is associated with loss of extracellular fluid (Thomas et al., 2008) and is different than dehydration. The focus of this chapter is on dehydration, not volume depletion.

INFLUENCE OF AGING ON DEHYDRATION

Older people have increased sensitivity to dehydration because of the normal physiological changes of aging. In normal aging, fat is increased and lean body mass is decreased corresponding to decreased total body water (Schols et al., 2009). The thirst threshold is increased in aging, so there is a decreased perception of thirst (Schols et al., 2009). Other age-related changes include decreased kidney function, leading to reduced ability to conserve water and concentrate urine, and decreased sensitivity to antidiuretic hormone (Schols et al., 2009).

RISK FACTORS

The risk factors for dehydration can be remembered with the mnemonic FLAME, which stands for Faulty fluid intake, Limited physical function, Advanced age, Medications, and Environment. A decreased fluid intake or a fluid intake that is not augmented in the presence of fluid loss is a primary risk factor (Schols et al., 2009). The decreased fluid intake can be self-imposed to avoid incontinence. Limited physical functioning resulting from decreased functional ability, use of physical restraints, immobility, diminished vision, or cognitive impairment (Mentes, 2006a) can result in limited access to fluids or failure to recognize the need for fluid intake. Whereas all elderly people are at risk for dehydration, the oldest old (i.e., 85 years of age and older) are at greatest risk (Mentes, 2013). Polypharmacy is common in the elderly and certain medications, especially diuretics, laxatives, angiotensin-converting enzyme inhibitors, and psychotropic medications that have anticholinergic effects, increase the need for fluid (Schols, De Groot, Van Der Cammen, & Olde Rikkert, 2009). Internal and external environmental conditions can also lead to dehydration. Infection, frailty, diabetes, cancer, cardiac disease, and renal disease can trigger dehydration through varied mechanisms. The external environmental temperature must also be considered because the normal fluid requirement of 1.5 L/day is increased when outside temperatures are increased or when inside temperatures are overheated (Schols et al., 2009).

DIAGNOSIS

The diagnosis of dehydration is based on patient history, biomarkers, and clinical signs. Serum osmolality is the gold standard for diagnosing dehydration (Hooper et al., 2015). An osmolality greater than 300 mmol/kg indicates impending dehydration, and an osmolality between 295 and 300 mmol/kg indicates impending dehydration (Hooper et al., 2015). Other biochemical markers include a blood urea nitrogen/creatinine ratio greater than or equal to 25 and serum sodium greater than 148 mmol/L (Wakefield et al., 2008). Urine color (dark yellow), urine specific gravity (greater than 0.029), and urine osmolality (greater than 1,050 mmol/kg) are less reliable markers of dehydration in older adults (Mentes, 2006a; Wakefield et al., 2008). Clinical signs of dehydration include altered thirst, confusion, altered speech, dry tongue with longitudinal furrows, dry axillae, mucosal dryness, fever, cardiovascular signs (e.g., orthostatic hypotension and tachycardia); light-headedness, weight loss, sunken eyes, dark concentrated urine, and decreased skin turgor (tenting of skinfolds; Schols et al., 2009; Thomas et al., 2008; Wakefield et al., 2008).

BEST PRACTICES

Recognition of Dehydration

Recognition of dehydration is the first step for ensuring adequate fluid maintenance in the older adult (Thomas et al., 2008). Initial assessment should be individualized but should focus on basic physiological measures such as vital signs, weight, height, body mass index, and review of systems. Biochemical measures (discussed previously) should be assessed for abnormalities. Other assessment parameters should include 24-hour fluid intake and urine output, determination of treatments that may cause dehydration

such as nothing-by-mouth status and tube feedings, usual pattern of fluid intake and fluid preferences, and intake behaviors or problematic behaviors associated with fluid intake. Cognitive status, functional health status, mood status, medical history, and review of current medications should also be assessed.

The Dehydration Risk Appraisal Checklist (Mentes & Wang, 2011), an assessment tool used to evaluate dehydration risk in nursing home residents, focuses on personal characteristics, significant health conditions, medications, intake, and laboratory abnormalities. Vivanti, Harvey, and Ash (2010) refined a dehydration screening tool for hospitalized older adults.

Interventions

In the United States, the recommended adequate intake for total daily water intake from food and beverages for healthy elderly women is 2.7 L/day and for elderly men is 3.7 L/day (Institute of Medicine, 2005). Most experts recommend that older adults consume between 1.5 and 2 L/day of fluid, assuming that no cardiovascular, renal, or mental disorders limit or alter fluid intake (Schols et al., 2009). A more precise formula for calculating a normal fluid goal is as follows:

100 mL/kg for the first 10 kg of weight
50 mL/kg for the next 10 kg of weight
15 mL/kg for the remaining weight (Mentes, 2006a)

The treatment plan for rehydration should consider the fluid deficit, the rate at which dehydration occurred (acute versus chronic), and the extent to which salt loss is associated with water loss (Schols et al., 2009). In acute situations, fluid repletion should occur within 24 hours in a hospital setting (Schols et al., 2009). The oral route should be used initially unless the oral administration of fluids is contraindicated or the patient's condition is unstable. In an unstable patient, intravenous rehydration is preferred. Hypodermoclysis can be implemented in the nursing home setting (Thomas et al., 2008) and may be considered if the intravenous route is difficult to obtain or not desired. Rehydration via a nasogastric or gastrostomy tube should be the last choice when selecting a route of administration (Schols et al., 2009).

Suggestions for enhancing fluid intake include providing liquids and foods high in water content throughout the day; considering an individual's previous intake pattern and individual preferences; educating the patient, staff, and informal caregivers regarding the need for water intake; assessing the patient's individual water intake goal; and recommending fluids and foods that are high in water content.

Whereas recent research has demonstrated that hydration problems in frail, older nursing-home residents can be categorized as "can drink," "can't drink," "won't drink," and end of life (Mentes, 2006b), the associated interventions for each category need further validation for the elderly in the hospital or community setting. However, the interventions do provide a logical approach to treating actual or impending dehydration in the elderly who can receive oral repletion. Whenever possible, preferred beverages should be offered. If the older adult can drink and is independent, interventions should focus on education on the importance of the amount of liquid to be ingested and the provision of tools to measure intake. If the older adult can drink but forgets to, interventions should focus on ways to increase fluid exposure. If the older adult cannot drink because of either dysphagia or physical dependency, interventions focus on enabling fluid intake, as appropriate, with the use of assistive devices, swallowing exercises, or alteration of fluid texture. If the older adult will not drink and is a sipper, then small amounts of preferred fluid are offered with contact and activities. On the other hand, if the older adult will not drink because of fears of incontinence, interventions should focus on the importance of maintaining fluid intake, Kegel exercises, urge inhibition, and last, medication (Mentes, 2006b). If hydration is an issue at the end of life, then interventions should focus on resident and family preference in accordance with advance directives.

SPECIAL CONSIDERATIONS FOR TUBE-FED PATIENTS

Dehydration is a common metabolic problem in tube-fed patients, including the elderly. Risk factors contributing to dehydration in tube-fed patients include use of concentrated enteral formula (1.5 kcal/mL or greater); decrease in fluid intake by mouth; uncontrolled hyperglycemia; formula with a high renal solute load; fever; increased activity level, particularly in warm weather; diarrhea; failure to receive the volume of formula prescribed; and insufficient free-water flushes (Worthington & Reyen, 2004). If free water is not given in addition to the enteral feeding formula, the older adult is at increased risk for dehydration. To prevent dehydration in a tube-fed older patient, additional free water should be administered throughout the day, when flushing the tube, or when giving medications. A dietician should be consulted to calculate the precise amount of additional free water required.

Rose Ann DiMaria-Ghalili

Agency for Healthcare Research and Quality. (n.d.). Prevention quality indicators overview. Retrieved form https://www.qualityindicators.ahrq.gov/modules/pqi_overview.aspx

Hooper, L., Abdelhamid, A., Ali, A., Bunn, D. K., Jennings, A., John, W. G.,…Shepstone, L. (2015). Diagnostic accuracy of calculated serum osmolarity to predict dehydration in older people: Adding value to pathology laboratory reports. *BMJ Open, 5*(10), e008846.

Institute of Medicine. (2005). *Dietary reference intakes for water, potassium, sodium, chloride and sulfate.* Washington, DC: National Academies Press.

Mentes, J. C. (2006a). Oral hydration in older adults: Greater awareness is needed in preventing, recognizing, and treating dehydration. *American Journal of Nursing, 106*(6), 40–49; quiz 50.

Mentes, J. C. (2006b). A typology of oral hydration problems exhibited by frail nursing home residents. *Journal of Gerontological Nursing, 32*(1), 13–19.

Mentes, J. C. (2013). The complexities of hydration issues in the elderly. *Nutrition Today, 48*(4S), S10–S12.

Mentes, J. C., & Wang, I. (2011). Measuring risk for dehydration in nursing home residents. Evaluation of the dehydration risk appraisal checklist. *Research in Gerontological Nursing, 4*, 148–156.

Schols, J. M., De Groot, C. P., Van Der Cammen, T. J., & Olde Rikkert, M. G. (2009). Preventing and treating dehydration in the elderly during periods of illness and warm weather. *Journal of Nutrition, Health, and Aging, 13*, 150–157.

Thomas, D. R., Cote, T. R., Lawhorne, L., Levenson, S. A., Rubenstein, L. Z., Smith, D. A.,…Dehydration Council. (2008). Understanding clinical dehydration and its treatment. *Journal of the American Medical Directors Association, 9*, 292–301.

Vivanti, A., Harvey, K., & Ash, S. (2010). Developing a quick and practical screen to improve the identification of poor hydration in geriatric and rehabilitative care. *Archives of Gerontology and Geriatrics, 50*, 156–164.

Wakefield, B. J., Mentes, J., Holman, J. E., & Culp, K. (2008). Risk factors and outcomes associated with hospital admission for dehydration. *Rehabilitation Nursing, 33*, 233–241.

Worthington, P., & Reyen, L. (2004). Initiating and managing enteral nutrition. In P. Worthington (Ed.), *Practical aspects of nutritional support: An advanced practice guide* (pp. 311–341). Philadelphia, PA: Saunders.

Web Resources

Academy of Nutrition and Dietetics: http://www.eatright.org/Public

Geriatric Nursing Resources for Care of Older Adults: https://consultgeri.org/geriatric-topics/hydration-management

Hospital Hydration Best Practices Tool Kit: http://www2.rcn.org.uk/newsevents/campaigns/nutritionnow/tools_and_resources/hydration

Hydration for Health: http://www.h4hinitiative.com/everyday-hydration/how-your-needs-change-over-time/hydration-and-elderly

DEMENTIA: SPECIAL CARE UNITS

Half of all adults living in nursing homes exhibit dementia symptoms, 42% of assisted-living residents have mild to severe cognitive impairment, and 40% of residential care facility residents have a dementia diagnosis (Alzheimer's Association, 2016a; Cadigan, Grabowski, Givens, & Mitchell, 2012; Caffrey et al., 2012; Zimmerman, Sloane, & Reed, 2014). Long-term care residents with dementia are at a greater risk for anxiety, sensory overload, aggressive behaviors, social withdrawal, and falls. Consequently, dementia special care units (SCUs) specializing in environmental modifications that promote quality of life for residents with dementia have become common fixtures within nursing homes, assisted-living, and other long-term care residential settings.

In response to the increased number of older adults diagnosed with dementia as a result of population aging, 15% of nursing homes, 17% of assisted-living facilities, and 12% of residential care units in the United States have a dementia SCU (Caffey et al., 2012; Harris-Kojetin et al., 2016; Jones & Greene, 2016; Park-Lee, Sengupta, & Harris-Kojetin, 2013; Zimmerman et al., 2015). Nursing homes pioneered dementia care through the implementation of the dementia SCU. In the past decade, specialized dementia care within assisted living has flourished because of the assisted-living model's emphasis on providing supportive care as opposed to nursing care (Zimmerman et al., 2015).

Research findings addressing the differences in care quality between SCU and traditional nursing home units are mixed. In general, research reveals that SCUs have a positive impact on some, but not all, clinical outcomes and care processes (Cadigan et al., 2012; Luo, Fang, Liao, Elliot, & Zhang, 2010). One study found that SCU residents had higher quality of life scores in the areas of autonomy, meaningful activities, comfort, and environmental modifications but lower mood scores (Abrahamson, Clark, Perkins, & Arling, 2012). The ability to assess the effectiveness of SCU care using longitudinal methods is complicated by the absence of standardized SCU structures and processes that facilitate comparisons over time and across sites, as well as the complexity of measuring outcomes, such as quality of life, among cognitively impaired populations (Beerens, Zwakhalen, Verbeek, Ruwaard, & Hamers, 2013; Hyde, Perez, & Forester, 2007; Marquardt, Bueter, & Motzek, 2014). Contributing to this complexity, people with dementia often experience multiple transfers between the home, hospital, nursing homes, and the community (Callahan et al., 2012).

Because no national standards differentiate dementia SCU care from standard nursing home care, government regulation and oversight of dementia SCUs differ across facilities and states. Similarly, dementia SCUs vary dramatically between assisted-living and other residential

D

care settings. As a result, the environmental features, staff training, and services offered in SCUs vary across settings (Parker-Oliver, Aud, Bostick, Schwarz, & Tofle, 2005). Organizations such as the Alzheimer's Association have advocated for additional regulation and oversight to clarify what services are offered within dementia SCUs.

Ideally, five features contribute to an SCUs unique purpose: (a) specific admission and discharge criteria, (b) staff selection and training according to accepted standards of care for persons with dementia, (c) activity programming designed for persons with cognitive impairments, (d) family programming and involvement, and (e) segregated and modified environments that provide reduced but appropriate sensory stimuli (Teri, Holmes, & Ory, 2000). Criteria for admission, discharge, and resident selection are key policies for an SCU. The diagnosis of dementia should be made after a comprehensive neuropsychological examination. Preadmission assessment should describe the resident's behaviors; family and resident preferences, values, beliefs, and interests (preadmission and current); family support, understanding, acceptance, and desire for continued involvement in the care of the resident; and cognitive, physical, and social function within the preadmission social milieu. Preadmission assessment should address advance directives and resident and family preferences for end-of-life care. Admission criteria should also focus on appropriate placement to prevent avoidable relocation of the resident.

Several theoretical frameworks guide programs and interventions for persons with dementia in nursing homes. Underlying the person–environment fit (P-EF), person–environment interaction (P-EI), and progressively lowered stress threshold (PLST) models is the notion that the environment must be modified to enhance function for residents with dementia and assist caregivers in coping with their behaviors. The PLST model is most often used to develop SCUs and to evaluate outcomes of residents, families, and staff. Environmental modifications found on SCUs can include, but are not limited to, camouflaged exits to reduce elopement attempts, single rooms to promote privacy, walking areas to allow for unobstructed pacing behaviors, reduction in noise and other sensory stimuli, and employment of staff members who are specially trained in the needs of residents with dementia (Zeisel et al., 2003). The social environment also plays a significant role in resident well-being as the consistent presence of familiar staff can contribute to a unit's home-like environment, reducing anxiety among residents (Abrahamson et al., 2012; Edvardsson, Sandman, & Rasmussen, 2012).

SCUs are often coordinated by RNs but may also be directed by individuals trained in the social sciences or gerontology who are not RNs. The key concern is not who coordinates the SCU program but that best-practice interdisciplinary care is provided. Adequate staffing is essential for effectively addressing the needs of residents and their families, and all administrators and staff should be thoroughly trained in dementia care (Maas & Buckwalter, 2006). Common nursing home ratios of total nursing staff to residents are 1:5 to 1:6, similar to staffing levels in general nursing home units. The ratio of specially trained RNs to residents on SCUs should be no less than 1:15 so that residents receive assessments and interventions by RNs who can also provide appropriate oversight, training, and role modeling for other staff members (Morgan, Stewart, D'Arcy, & Cammer, 2005). Ideally, social worker, physician, activities/recreation therapist, dietician, and physical therapist should also be members of the care team.

Individualized physical care should follow a consistent routine, as well as emphasize flexibility, unconditional positive regard, and sensitivity when a resident is hesitant to participate in an activity. Catastrophic reactions—responses that are out of proportion to stimuli—can be managed by altering environmental stressors to accommodate an individuals' needs and abilities. Examples include reducing the number of people in the environment, decreasing noise, dimming lights, and using distraction to lessen fear, confusion, and agitation. It is also important to assess for physical discomfort (i.e., pain) that may manifest in undesirable behavioral symptoms. Staff must vigilantly monitor residents' health status and identify adverse effects from medications or treatments. Because people with dementia often cannot interpret or effectively communicate pain and discomfort, monitoring of behavioral clues is especially important. Awareness of conditions that are likely to cause discomfort or pain should guide assessment and intervention.

The physical environment should be modified to reduce overwhelming and disturbing stimuli and provide safe wandering, environmental cues to support memory, and visual, auditory, and other sensory stimulation. The environment should promote resident function and safety, encourage family visitation and involvement, and provide a pleasant, functional workplace for staff. Each environmental component should be evaluated to consider the message it sends to residents and their families. Warm, inviting, homelike environments can be influenced by both the built environment and the staff's sensitivity to their role in shaping the psychosocial climate within dementia SCUs (Edvardsson et al., 2012; Fleming, Goodenough, Low, Chenoweth, & Brodaty, 2014). Finally, care must be taken to avoid residents' sensory deprivation and boredom. Too little stimulation can be as bad as too much, causing feelings and behaviors that are uncomfortable for residents and difficult for staff to manage.

SCUs should provide preadmission support programs for families highlighting policies that govern resident care. Family participation and decision making should be encouraged, with institutional barriers prohibiting their participation removed. Recommended strategies for family involvement include a "buddy system," a family–nurse liaison, and peer support groups.

Systematic evaluations show that the effects of SCUs on resident, family, and staff outcomes are mixed. Consistently reported positive outcomes for SCU residents are reduced agitation, less catastrophic and disruptive behavior, decreased use of physical and chemical restraints, increased participation in activities, and improved quality of life (Reimer, Slaughter, Donalson, Currie, & Eliasziw, 2004). Although SCU staff may also be more knowledgeable about dementia care, the relationship between working on a dementia SCU and staff morale is limited. Dementia SCU staff may experience greater stress compared with those working in traditional nursing homes or assisted-living environments; however, staff commitments to stay in dementia care can increase significantly when opportunities for ongoing training specific to dementia care and person-centered care are provided (Grant, 2002; Lee, Hui, Kng, & Auyerng, 2013; McCarty & Drebing, 2003; Zimmerman et al., 2005). A small number of studies report that family members' satisfaction with care in SCUs improves when emphasis is placed on effective communication between SCU staff, residents, and family members and when end-of-life care is offered within a dementia SCU (Engel, Kiely, & Mitchell, 2006; Robison et al., 2007).

See also Assisted Living; Behavioral Symptoms of Dementia; Depression in Dementia; Family Care for Elders With Dementia; Nursing Homes.

Karis Pressler, Kathleen Abrahamson, and Heather Davila

Abrahamson, K., Clark, D., Perkins, A., & Arling, G. (2012). Does cognitive impairment influence quality of life among nursing home residents? *The Gerontologist*, 52(5), 632–640.

Alzheimer's Association. (2016). 2016 Alzheimer's disease facts and figures. *Alzheimer's & Dementia*, 12(4).

Beerens, H. C., Zwakhalen, S. M. G., Verbeek, H., Ruwaard, D., & Hamers, J. P. H. (2013). Factors associated with quality of life of people with dementia in long-term care facilities: A systematic review. *International Journal of Nursing Studies*, 50(9), 1259–1270.

Cadigan, R. O., Grabowski, D., Givens, J. L., & Mitchell, S. L. (2012). The quality of advanced dementia care in the nursing home: The role of special care units. *Medical Care*, 50(10), 856–862.

Caffrey, C., Sengupta, M., Park-Lee, E., Moss, A., Rosenoff, E., & Harris-Kojetin, L. (2012). Residents living in residential care facilities: United States, 2010. *NCHS Data Brief*, 2(91), 1–8.

Callahan, C. M., Arling, G., Tu, W., Rosenman, M. B., Counsell, S. R., Stump, T. E., & Hendrie, H. C. (2012). Transitions in care for older adults with and without dementia. *Journal of the American Geriatrics Society*, 60(5), 813–820.

Edvardsson, D., Sandman, P. O., & Rasmussen, B. (2012). Forecasting the ward climate: A study from a dementia care unit. *Journal of Clinical Nursing,* 21(7–8), 1136–1144.

Engel, S. E., Kiely, D. K., & Mitchell, S. L. (2006). Satisfaction with end-of-life care for nursing home residents with advanced dementia. *Journal of the American Geriatrics Society,* 54(10), 1567–1572.

Fleming, R., Goodenough, B., Low, L.-F., Chenoweth, L., & Brodaty, H. (2014). The relationship between the quality of the built environment and the quality of life of people with dementia in residential care. *Dementia,* 15(4), 663–680.

Grant, L. A. (2002). Alzheimer's special care units. *Research in Practice, Center for the Study of Healthcare Management.* Minneapolis: University of Minnesota Press.

Harris-Kojetin, L., Sengupta, M., Park-Lee, E., Valverde, R., Caffrey, C., Rome, V., & Lendon, J. (2016). Long-term care providers and services users in the United States: Data from the National Study of Long-Term Care Providers, 2013–2014. *Vital Health Statistics,* 3(38).

Hyde, J., Perez, R., & Forester, B. (2007). Dementia and assisted living. *Gerontologist,* 47, Spec No 3, 51–67.

Jones, D. S., & Greene, J. A. (2016). Is dementia in decline? Historical trends and future trajectories. *New England Journal of Medicine,* 374(6), 507–509.

Lee, J., Hui, E., Kng, C., & Auyeung, T. W. (2013). Attitudes of long-term care staff toward dementia and their related factors. *International Psychogeriatrics,* 25(1), 140–147.

Luo, H., Fang, X., Liao, Y., Elliott, A., & Zhang, X. (2010). Associations of special care units and outcomes of residents with dementia: 2004 National Nursing Home Survey. *The Gerontologist,* 50(4), 509–518.

Maas, M. L., & Buckwalter, K. C. (2006). Providing quality care in assisted living facilities: Recommendations for enhanced staffing and staff training. *Journal of Gerontological Nursing,* 332(11), 14–22.

Marquardt, G., Bueter, K., & Motzek, T. (2014). Impact of the design of the built environment on people with dementia: An evidence-based review. *Health Environments Research & Design Journal,* 8(1), 127–157.

McCarty, E. F., & Drebing, C. (2003). Exploring professional caregivers' perceptions balancing self-care with care for patients with Alzheimer's disease. *Journal of Gerontological Nursing,* 29(9), 42–48.

Morgan, D. G., Stewart, N. J., D'Arcy, C., & Cammer, A. L. (2005). Creating and sustaining dementia special care units in rural nursing homes: The critical role of nursing leadership. *Canadian Journal of Nursing Leadership,* 18(2), 74–99.

Park-Lee, E., Sengupta, M., & Harris-Kojetin, L. D. (2013). Dementia special care units in residential care communities: United States, 2010. *Dementia,* 22, 216–100.

Parker-Oliver, D., Aud, M., Bostick, J., Schwarz, B., & Tofle, R. B. (2005). Dementia special care units: A policy and family perspective. *Journal of Housing for the Elderly,* 19(1), 113–125.

Reimer, M. A., Slaughter, S., Donalson, C., Currie, G., & Eliasziw, M. (2004). Special care facility compared with traditional environments for dementia care: A longitudinal study of quality of life. *Journal of the American Geriatrics Society,* 52(7), 1085–1092.

Robison, J., Curry, L., Gruman, C., Porter, M., Henderson, C. R., & Pillemer, K. (2007). Partners in caregiving in a special care environment: Cooperative communication between staff and families on dementia units. *The Gerontologist,* 47(4), 504–515.

Teri, J. A., Holmes, D., & Ory, M. G. (2000). The therapeutic design of environments for people with dementia. *The Gerontologist,* 40, 417–421.

Zeisel, J., Silverstein, N. M, Hyde, J., Levkoff, S., Lawton, M. P., & Holmes, W. (2003). Environmental correlates to behavior health outcomes in Alzheimer's special care units. *The Gerontologist,* 43(5), 697–711.

Zimmerman, S., Allen, J., Cohen, L. W., Pinkowitz, J., Reed, D., Coffey, W. O.,…Giorgio, P. (2015). A measure of person-centered practices in assisted living: The PC-PAL. *Journal of the American Medical Directors Association,* 16(2), 132–137.

Zimmerman, S., Sloane, P. D., & Reed, D. (2014). Dementia prevalence and care in assisted living. *Health Affairs,* 33(4), 658–666.

Zimmerman, S., Williams, C. S., Reed, P. S., Boustani, M., Preisser, J. S., Heck, E., & Sloane, P. D. (2005). Attitudes, stress, and satisfaction of staff who care for residents with dementia. *The Gerontologist,* 45(Special Issue 1), 96–105.

Web Resources

Administration for Community Living: https://www.acl.gov

Alzheimer's Association: http://www.alz.org/join_the_cause_special_care_units.asp

Alzheimer's Association: http://www.alz.org/documents_custom/2016-facts-and-figures.pdf

Centers for Disease Control and Prevention: http://www.cdc.gov/nchs/data/series/sr_03/sr03_038.pdf

National Center for Health Statistics: http://www.cdc.gov/nchs/data/databriefs/db91.pdf

National Institute of Health, Alzheimer's Disease Education and Referral (ADEAR) Center: http://www.healthfinder.gov/FindServices/Organizations/Organization.aspx?code=HR2426

DEMOGRAPHY OF AGING

The distribution of research among major themes is changing in important ways within the demography of aging. There has been a reduction in the amount of work done on the theme that was the original source of the influence of the demography of aging on other fields, including those of public policy deliberations. This theme is *the increasing proportion of older people in a population*. Themes that are gaining in prominence include the *aging of cohorts or generations* (collections of neighboring birth cohorts) and the *postponement of mortality and compression of morbidity within the population at advanced ages*, which we might call "delayed mortality and compressed morbidity among the oldest old."

Each field of social science activity has, ideally, a set of core concepts, theories, and methods for estimation and analysis. Around the core is a well-defined periphery where researchers are preoccupied with aspects of the core variables. Around the periphery is a boundary that reliably serves to demarcate what is inside and what is outside that field of social science. As a field of social science, the demography of aging approximates this ideal, with one major exception. This field seems to have few markers that help reliably locate its boundary when the research deals with some aspect of aging.

CORE AND PERIPHERY OF THE DEMOGRAPHY OF AGING

The classic theoretical and empirical works were built around the notion that population aging is an increase in the proportion of older persons in a population. However, the basis for classifying whether a person belongs or does not belong to the older population is an unresolved issue.

For decades, it was widely accepted that it is adequate to define *older* in terms of a chronological age such as 65 years or, less often, 60 years. This view has been challenged. First, a collection of persons at the same chronological age can vary widely on a measure of aging based on the functioning of personal biological systems. Second, the number of additional years that a person can be expected to live (derived from the mean of the probability distribution of death at each future possible age) provides the basis for a more policy-relevant measure of population aging than does the numbers of years already lived (Sanderson & Scherbov, 2008). The alternate measure is the change in the proportion of the population with remaining life expectancy of less than 15 years.

The classic concept of *population aging* implies that we should always deal with the *relative size* of the designated older population segment, however defined, within the larger population of all ages to which it belongs. Hence the demography of aging does not have as a core variable the absolute size of the older population.

A *process* of aging is an essential concept in the demography of aging. The most commonly used associated statistical measurement is an increase in the proportion of older persons in the total population. Thus population aging is a process and is not a variable that has a value at a specific point of time or date.

Based on this approach to measurement, the demography of aging has traditionally had at its core comparisons and analyses of variations in the speed of population aging among countries, among regions within a country, and among other defined population segments such as racial/ethnic groups (Rowland, 2012). Some studies have also portrayed variations over time in the speed of population aging in the world and in specific regions (Rowland, 2012). For example, much has been written in the popular media about the higher-than-average speed of aging of the population of European stock across the northern hemisphere during the 20th century (Rowland, 2012).

In the immediate periphery around the core are the analyses that provide explanatory theory and related empirical work designed to achieve advances in the understanding of *why* some populations are aging more rapidly than

D

others (Rowland, 2012). Based on these analyses, models for predicting future population aging for countries, and selected population segments within them, have been developed and applied. The outputs of these models have supported public policy deliberations (Rowland, 2012; Siegel & Olshansky, 2011).

Beyond the core and the immediate periphery off the classic demography of aging is a large and highly influential literature concerning the implications of population aging (Lee & Mason, 2011; Rowland, 2012). However, as one moves from one example to another among relevant research outputs, it can become difficult to decide whether a particular work is an exhibit of the demography of aging.

The decision turns partly on how *demography* is defined. It is beyond the scope of this article to provide an adequate definition. For our purposes, it is sufficient to point to a relevant essential component of demographic work. The units of analysis of demographic work are always collections of persons, often seen as population segments or as whole populations (the latter being an exhaustive collection of designated segments). Demography deals with attributes of these collections. The attributes could be states at a particular point of time or date, changes of states, or behaviors associated with these changes (provided that the units of analysis remain the said collections).

The demography of aging therefore deals with either (a) the measurement and analysis of variations in population aging or (b) the use of variables that measure population attributes in the process of developing and evaluating hypotheses concerning the causation or future evolution of population aging.

It is easy to prepare a profound work about the implications of population aging without making significant research efforts of either type. Some research publications exemplify this property, and others include some aspects of either type. Thus it is inappropriate to take the view that all studies on *the implications* of population aging are instances of the demography of aging. Each case needs to be examined to determine how much the researcher has carried on work in either type of study. Hence, no

simple principle can be used to set the boundary around the demography of aging.

BROADENING THE CORE OF THE DEMOGRAPHY OF AGING

The classic concept of population aging has been joined by two additional concepts that have become the bases for major extensions of theoretical and empirical work in the demography of aging. In the classic concept, a population segment called "the older population" is related to a larger collectivity to which it belongs. The first of the additional concepts abandons this relation and focuses instead on a cohort or a meaningful collection of adjacent cohorts such as a generation (e.g., the Baby Boomers) (Rowland, 2012; Stone, 1999). The aging process for such a cohort, or a collection of cohorts, comprises both increasing chronological age (which would be an average chronological age for a collection of adjacent cohorts) and what is deemed to be a progressive deterioration of functional and cognitive capacities generally called *biological aging*. A way to summarize these ideas is to say that one is speaking about "cohort aging," provided that the unit of analysis remains a collection of persons. A large and growing body of literature analyzes certain implications of the aging of prominent generations and points to related public policy challenges (Universite de Montreal, 2015)

The second "new" concept of population aging involves a special focus within the study of longevity, combined with related research on morbidity rates at the advanced ages. To imagine this focus, one should consider the following questions: For the population that has already passed the life expectancy age (measured in terms of chronological age), what will be the distribution of the ages at death and what will be the age distribution of highly consequential morbidity among the survivors? An important subsidiary question is "How far out in time can the distribution of ages at death reach?" That is, what are the expected extremes of old age, and within each national population or major segment thereof, how many people might survive to such extreme ages? Furthermore, what proportion of the survivors will exhibit extreme levels of dependency? Analyses surrounding these questions are demographic analyses, and they form part of the demography of aging (Christensen, Doblhammer, Rau, & Vaupel, 2009; Ouellette & Bourbeau, 2011).

Another aspect of this third major theme is the increasing proportion of very old people in the total population (Suzman, Willis, & Manton, 1992; Universite de Montreal, 2015). Important issues in elder care policies, as well as long-term care financing, are linked to this increase.

A phrase that can be used to refer to this third *new* concept of population aging is "postponement of mortality and compression of morbidity beyond the age of life expectancy" and perhaps even more pointedly "delayed mortality and compressed morbidity among the oldest old."

It is very important to incorporate this third concept into the demography of aging. Its dimensions and implications go far beyond academic debates about the absolute limit to the length of a human life. It touches on what is perhaps inevitable institutional residence for a high percentage of those who have major declines in functional and cognitive capacities and consequently the unusually burdensome demands on supports exerted by these residents. Directly linked to this question of institutional residence are the probability profiles of major declines in the said capacities as cohorts move into extreme ages. In addition, there are euthanasia-related issues. The analysis and projection of the numbers and the distribution of affected persons are intrinsically instances of demographic analysis, and thus they belong to the field of the demography of aging.

For more than 50 years, starting perhaps with the United Nations Population Division publication cited earlier, the demography of aging has had at its core a focus on aspects of increases in the proportion of the *older segment* within the larger population to which it belongs. To this core has been added two *newer* concepts: *cohort aging* and *postponement of mortality among the oldest old.*

These additions have helped the demography of aging to continue to be influential in other fields, including those of public policy debates. However, statistical measurement of aging across all three concepts has been weakened by almost exclusive reliance on chronological age.

See also African Americans and Health are Disparities; American Indian Elders; Immigrant Elders; Rural Elders.

Leroy O. Stone

Christensen, K., Doblhammer, G., Rau, R., & Vaupel, J. W. (2009). Aging populations: The challenges ahead. *Lancet*, *374*, 1196–1208. Retrieved from http://www.demogr.mpg.de/publications%5Cfiles%5C3444_1264435180_1_Christensen%20et%20al%20Lancet%20374%209696%202009.pdf

Lee, R. D., & Mason, A. (Eds.). (2011). *Population aging and the generational economy: A global perspective.* Edward Elgar.

Ouellette, N., & Bourbeau, R. (2011). Changes in the age-at-death distribution in four low mortality countries: A nonparametric approach. *Demographic Research*, *25*, Article 19, pp. 595–628. Retrieved from http://www.demographic-research.org/volumes/vol25/19/default.htm

Rowland, D. T. (2012). *Population aging. The transformation of societies.* Dordrecht, Netherlands: Springer Science+Business Media.

Sanderson, W., & Scherbov, S. (2008). Rethinking age and aging. *Population Bulletin*, *63*(4). Retrieved from http://www.prb.org/pdf08/63.4aging.pdf

Siegel, J. S., & Olshansky, S. J. (2011) *The demography and epidemiology of human health and aging.* Dordrecht, Netherlands: SpringerScience+BusinessMedia.

Stone, L. O. (Ed.). (1999). *Cohort flow and the consequences of population aging, an international analysis and review.* Ottawa, Canada: Minister of Industry.

Suzman, R. M., Willis, D. P., & Manton, K. G. (1992). *The oldest old.* Oxford, UK: Oxford University Press.

Universite de Montreal. (2015, March 20). The oldest old are changing Canada. *ScienceDaily.* Retrieved from https://www.sciencedaily.com/releases/2015/03/150320101503.htm

Web Resources
NIA Demography of Aging Centers: https://agingcenters.org
UN World Population Aging: http://www.un.org/esa/population/publications/worldageing19502050

D

Dentures

In Western societies, teeth symbolize youth, potency, strength, and virility. Aging is associated with tooth loss. Approximately 70% of people who have lost their teeth express regret, and 60% consider dentures a handicap. Many studies report that 25% to 30% of wearers of complete denture have problems with them, especially the mandibular (i.e., lower) denture. In fact, a person may have a technically perfect denture but be unable to tolerate it (Ettinger & Jakobsen, 1997; Moltzer, Van der Meulen, & Verheij, 1996; van Waas, 1990).

Most natural teeth are lost due to two chronic, infective diseases: caries (decay) and periodontal (gum) disease. In general, both diseases are preventable if the oral cavity is kept clean by the regular removal of plaque. Total loss of all teeth (edentulousness) is declining at a rate of about 1% per year in most industrialized countries (Cooper, 2009). In the United States, the prevalence of edentulism in each age cohort is declining; however, the real increase in the number of older adults means that the number of edentulous adults is not declining. (Douglass Shih, & Ostry, 2002).

TYPES OF DENTURES

Dentures are prosthetic replacements for natural teeth and can be divided into four groups:

1. Complete-removable dentures
2. Removable-partial dentures
3. Fixed-partial dentures
4. Fixed-detachable dentures

A complete denture replaces the chewing surface of all the teeth in an arch. It sits on the mucosa or may have some support from the remaining natural teeth, which have been cut down to 1.5 to 2 mm above the gingival margin. These tooth-supported prostheses are called *overdentures*. Dentures can also be supported by implants.

A removable-partial denture replaces some missing teeth in an arch and is held in place by metal clasps or by special attachments that fit into or onto some of the remaining teeth.

A fixed-partial denture, or bridge, replaces some missing teeth and is supported with a crown or cap on either side of the missing teeth. Bridges are usually cemented in place and are not removable.

A fixed-detachable denture is held in place by screws that go into either implants or natural teeth.

WEARING AND REMOVING DENTURES

Every removable prosthesis moves while it is in use and is potentially traumatic. The mouth needs 6 to 8 hours of rest from a denture each day. The best time to remove a denture is during sleep, when the production of saliva required for lubrication and retention is at its lowest and parafunctional movements such as clenching and grinding are at their highest. A patient being treated for a temporomandibular joint problem may be advised by the dentist not to remove the prosthesis during sleep.

DENTURE HYGIENE AND CARE

A denture, like teeth, becomes covered with plaque and needs to be cleaned regularly—ideally after meals. If a denture is maintained in the mouth continuously, commensal organisms can colonize the plaque. If the denture is not removed and adequately cleaned, organisms such as *Candida albicans* (a fungus) can proliferate and release toxins, resulting in a hypersensitivity reaction of the oral mucosa that looks like contact dermatitis (Berge, Silness, & Sorheim, 1987). Persons who are frail, have xerostomia (i.e., dry mouth), are immunocompromised, or have had radiation therapy of the head and neck are at greater risk for candidiasis. Stafford, Arendorf, and Huggett (1986) showed that if dentures are removed at night and allowed to air dry, the organisms on the denture surface do not proliferate as quickly. However, the dentures need to be rehydrated by soaking them in water for several minutes before they are put back in the mouth.

When teeth are extracted, the bone that was produced during eruption of the teeth—the residual bone—begins to resorb. The rate of resorption for the anterior maxilla has been measured at about 0.1 mm/year; for the mandible, the rate is 4 times greater (0.4 mm) (Tallgren, 1999). This resorption, plus normal wear, results in dentures having a finite life span. The average complete denture needs to be relined or replaced every 5 to 7 years. The life span of a partial denture varies, depending on the amount of tooth support it has. Fixed-partial dentures should last at least 10 years because they are usually made of metal, porcelain, or a combination of the two.

The abutment teeth (i.e., the teeth supporting the denture) for removable or fixed-partial dentures are at higher risk of plaque accumulation, which can result in root surface caries or periodontal disease. Therefore, both dentures and the natural teeth must be cleaned. Fluoride rinses may be helpful for at-risk patients. For fixed-partial dentures and implants, special interproximal brushes and superfloss must be used to clean under and around the bridge (pontic) portion of the prosthesis or the tissues will become inflamed. A daily mouth rinse with 0.12% chlorhexidine gluconate may be helpful for patients who have difficulty cleaning. Because many of these older adults have a dry mouth, an alcohol-free chorhexidine rinse is less irritating (see Sunstar Butler, www.sunstar butler.com/splash.asp).

The best way to clean dentures is to use a denture brush and, if the patient can afford it, a small ultrasonic cleaner. Toothpaste should not be used to clean dentures because it is too abrasive and will damage the surface. A mild dishwashing detergent works well; commercial soaks are also helpful.

DENTURE-INDUCED ORAL DISEASE

Oral lesions associated with the wearing of removable prostheses can be due to microbial colonization of dental plaque, traumatic irritation by the denture, or an allergic response to denture materials.

Microbial Colonization of Dental Plaque

Plaque that is not removed can become colonized by *Streptococcus mutans* and lactobacilli, causing caries on the surface of the remaining teeth. The plaque can also be colonized by a wide variety of aerobic and anaerobic organisms, which can result in bone loss around the teeth, called *periodontal disease*. If *Candida albicans* colonizes the plaque, especially the palatal tissue surface, a denture stomatitis may result. Plaque accumulation is exacerbated by an older person's progressive loss of normal dexterity, poor eyesight, decrease in salivary flow associated with the use of drugs (e.g., anticholinergics), and diseases (e.g., diabetes, depression, Parkinson's disease; Ettinger, 1999; Turner, Jahangiri, & Ship, 2008).

Traumatic Irritation

Traumatic irritation can result in an ulcer due to the changing fit of a denture caused by tissue resorption over time. Also, lack of sufficient saliva for lubrication of the dentures can result in traumatic ulcers (Turner et al., 2008). The ability of oral mucosa to resist this mechanical irritation can be diminished by diabetes, nutritional deficiencies, or xerostomia (dry mouth). Denture wearing can also result in irritation hyperplasia, a chronic inflammatory tissue reaction that leads to edema and tissue overgrowth.

If the residual bone is overloaded or if the tissues over it are chronically inflamed, the bone will resorb and be replaced with fibrous tissue. This commonly occurs in edentulous areas in the anterior maxilla and in tuberosity regions, resulting in so-called flabby tissue, which decreases support for the denture.

Although the main risk factors for oral cancer are tobacco products and alcoholic beverages, there is epidemiological evidence that age, inadequate diet, poor oral hygiene, fractured teeth, and wearing of dentures may be contributing risk factors to the 30,000 new cases diagnosed each year. Therefore, all persons older than 45 years should have their oral cavities evaluated at least yearly for any changes, such as white, red, or mixed lesions, which may be a sign of oral cancer.

Allergic Responses

A small percentage of the population is allergic to the acrylic resins used in complete and partial dentures. A much larger population is allergic

D

to the nickel used in some temporary crowns and in the cast framework of some removable-partial dentures.

PATIENT ACCEPTANCE OF DENTURES

Many persons who wear complete dentures may experience social and psychological problems with their ability to speak, to chew, and to feel comfortable in social situations (Huumonen et al., 2012; Papadaki & Anastassiadou, 2012). The older the patient, the more likely the difficulty wearing complete dentures (Allen & McMillan, 2012). Most problems are associated with the mandibular (lower) arch (Ettinger, 1993). Laird and McLaughlin (1989) stated that although the technical aspects of denture fabrication are important, it is critical to evaluate the patient's motivation and adaptive ability to wear dentures. In other words, a dentist can make a technically correct denture, but the patient may not be able to wear it if the tissues are unable to tolerate it or the patient does not have the necessary neurological skills. Another significant factor in the patient's adaptive ability is effective verbal and nonverbal communication between the dentist and the patient.

Several studies have shown that systemic disease and multidrug regimens increase the number of visits required to fit dentures. However, some patients cannot accept complete dentures either physically or emotionally; for them, implant-supported dentures may be a solution.

See also Geriatric Dentistry: Clinical Aspects; Oral Health Assessment; Xerostomia.

Ronald L. Ettinger

Allen, P. F., & McMillan A. S. (2003). Review of the functional and psychosocial outcomes of edentulousness treated with complete replacement. *Journal of the Canadian Dental Association, 69*, 662.

Berge, M., Silness, J., & Sorheim, E. (1987). Professional plaque control in the treatment of stomatitis prosthetica. *Gerodontics, 3*, 113–116.

Cooper, L. F. (2009). The current and future treatment of edentulism. *Journal of Prosthodontics, 18*, 116–122.

Douglass, C. W., Shih, A., & Ostry, L. (2002). Will there be a need for complete dentures in the United States in 2020? *Journal of Prosthetic Dentistry, 87*(1), 5–8.

Ettinger, R. L. (1993). Managing and treating the atrophic mandible. *Journal of the American Dental Association, 124*, 234–241.

Ettinger, R. L. (1999). Epidemiology of dental caries: A broad view. *Dental Clinics of North America, 43*, 679–694.

Ettinger, R. L., & Jakobsen, J. R. (1997). A comparison of patient satisfaction with dentist's evaluation of overdenture therapy. *Community Dentistry & Oral Epidemiology, 25*, 223–227.

Huumonen, S., Haikola, B., Oikarinen, K., Söderholm, A. L., Remes-Lyly, T., & Sipilä K. (2012). Residual ridge resorption, lower denture stability and subjective complaints among edentulous individuals. *Journal of Oral Rehabilitation, 39*, 384–390.

Laird, W. R., & McLaughlin, E. A. (1989). Management and treatment planning for the elderly edentulous patient. *International Journal of Prosthodontics, 2*, 347–351.

Moltzer, G., Van der Meulen, M. J., & Verheij, H. (1996). Psychological characteristics of dissatisfied denture patients. *Community Dentistry & Oral Epidemiology, 24*, 52–55.

Papadaki, E. & Anastassiadou, V. (2012). Elderly complete denture wearers: A social approach to tooth loss. *Gerodontology, 29*, e721–e727.

Stafford, G. D., Arendorf, T., & Huggett, K. (1986). The effect of overnight drying and water immersion on candidal colonization and properties of complete dentures. *Journal of Dentistry, 14*, 52–56.

Tallgren, A. (1999). The continuing reduction of the residual alveolar ridges in complete denture wearers: A mixed longitudinal study covering 25 years. *Journal of Prosthetic Dentistry, 27*, 120–132.

Turner, M., Jahangiri, L., & Ship, J. A. (2008). Hyposalivation, xerostomia and the complete denture. A systematic review. *Journal of the American Dental Association, 139*, 146–150.

van Waas, M. A. J. (1990). Determinants of dissatisfaction with dentures: A multiple regression analysis. *Journal of Prosthetic Dentistry, 64*, 569–572.

Web Resources

American Academy of Periodontology: http://www.perio.org/consumer/2m.htm

American Dental Association: http://www.ada.org/public/topics/implants.asp

Sunstar Butler: http://www.sunstarbutler.com/splash.asp

DEPRESSION IN DEMENTIA

Prevalence estimates of depression in the general elderly population are between 10% and 15% (Diniz & Reynolds, 2014), with reported prevalence estimates ranging from 19% for concurrent depression and dementia (Verkaik, Francke, van Meijel, Ribbe, & Bensing, 2009) to 30% in vascular dementia and Alzheimer's disease (Enache, Winblad, & Aarsland, 2011) to as high as 40% in Parkinson's and Huntington's diseases (Diniz, Butters, Albert, Dew, & Reynolds, 2013; Reijnders, Ehrt, Weber, Aarsland, & Leentjens, 2008). Despite high rates of depression in dementia, recognition rates by psychiatrists, social workers and nursing home physicians are low across all of these professional disciplines (Engedal, Barca, Laks, & Selbaek, 2011). Clinically significant depression in the elderly—those with and without dementia—is an eminently treatable condition but, if unrecognized and untreated, it is associated with diminished quality of life (Diniz & Reynolds, 2014), may become refractory and chronic (Sherrod, Collins, Wynn, & Gragg, 2010), resulting in a shortened life expectancy due to suicide and other mechanisms (MacQueen et al., 2017); it may cause social dysfunction and disturbing behaviors (Nathanson, 2010).

Recognition of depression in concurrent dementia is hampered not only by the communication problems of the patients, but also by the overlapping symptoms of each disorder (Starkstein & Brockman, 2014). Further complicating the recognition and treatment of depression in dementia are two competing stereotypes held by professional caregivers. The first is that the advent of any mental disorder in advanced age is an indication of an underlying dementing process; the second, that old age is characteristically a time of losses and reactive depression. The former stereotype suggests that depression in old age is inconsequential; the latter that depression is normal. There is no evidence that depression treatment decreases the risk of Alzheimer's disease, although investigators have found that depression improvement results in improved cognition (Bennett & Thomas, 2014; Starkstein & Brockman, 2014).

CLINICAL FEATURES

The overlapping symptoms of Alzheimer's disease and depression make it difficult for diagnosticians to arrive at a differential diagnosis. This is further complicated by the simple fact that many people with Alzheimer's disease are concurrently depressed. Rushing, Sachs-Ericsson, and Steffens (2014) describe, depressive disorders and their symptomatology in old age. The sufferer may report or evince sadness, emptiness, and detachment; anxiety and panic states may occur with or without euphoria and excitement as an associated cyclic aspect of the affective state. Speech is slowed and diminished or repetitive and importuning if anxiety is a dominant symptom. Self-esteem decreases and the patient loses interest in usual activities. Patients may be convinced that they are wicked and have sinned or that their bodily contents are impaired and objectionable. In all but the mildest episodes, sleep, appetite, body weight, and other vital functions may be disordered. In the most severely psychotic depressives, delusions of ill health, poverty, guilt, and self-deprecation may be expressed. Bizarre hypochondriacal and nihilistic delusions and pseudohallucinations may occur. Some patients are mute. In some cases, paranoid symptoms may be conjoined with an empty or hostile affect superficially resembling paraphrenia. Neurotic depressives retain insight into their depressive symptoms and frequently exhibit phobias; anxiety is often more obvious than the underlying depression. The anxiety may be communicated as a feeling of restlessness or fluttering in the abdomen. Depression in dementia is similar to descriptions of depressive disorder, although symptoms may be less severe. In general, significant cognitive decline may be a consequence of the depression alone. Often, a reliable differential diagnosis designed to attribute the cognitive decline to the dementia or the depression can be obtained only after an adequate trial of treatment for depression (Royall, Palmer, Chiodo, & Polk, 2012). However, social isolation, fatigue/loss of energy, and irritability are more frequently reported symptoms in cases of depression in dementia (Zahodne, Stern, & Manly, 2014).

D

The clinical diagnosis of depression is made using diagnostic criteria that are set forth in the *Diagnostic and Statistical Manual for Mental Disorders* (5th ed., *DSM-5*; American Psychiatric Association, 2013). Although the criteria for major depression and its subtypes are clearly described in the *DSM-5*, the tool does not adequately describe the unique manifestation of depression that occurs within the course of dementia in older persons. Olin et al. (2002) have delineated provisional diagnostic criteria for depressive features that occur within the course of dementia. Starkstein and Brockman (2014) elaborate on several significant differences between these diagnostic criteria and those for Major Depressive Disorder found in the *DSM-5*. The provisional diagnostic criteria for depression of Alzheimer disease (PDC-dAD) are distinct from *DSM-5* criteria for Major Depressive Disorder in their focus on the nature and intensity of the symptoms and the inclusion of symptoms of irritability and social isolation and withdrawal. For example, the PDC-dAD require three or more symptoms (vs. five or more for the *DSM-5* classification of Major Depressive Disorder) and do not require the daily presence of symptoms (Starkstein & Brockman, 2014).

Currently, the diagnosis of Major Depressive Disorder using *DSM-5* is made only if it can be established that an underlying organic disorder is not present and that the symptoms are not a normal reaction to the loss of a loved one (i.e., uncomplicated bereavement). In addition, the diagnosis is not made if the disturbance is superimposed on schizophrenia. These criteria relate to the importance of ruling out other psychiatric and organic illnesses that may produce depressive symptoms. Nonetheless, coexisting organic and affective disorders, such as depression and dementia, are common, and the presence of an organic illness does not rule out depression.

The psychiatric disorders that are generally referred to as *the dementias*, are multisymptomatic disorders often accompanied by a variety of noncognitive behavioral symptoms, such as depression, delusions, hallucinations, agitation, and aggressive behaviors. Verkaik et al. (2011) indicate that because people with dementia fall within different and changing levels of awareness (e.g., nearly comatose, confused on an intermittent basis, relatively oriented), different assessment techniques should be used at different points in the disease process. Four major obstacles interfere with the assessment of depression in dementia: the overlap in clinical manifestations of depression and dementia, the inability of patients with dementia to provide accurate information about their moods and inner lives, the narrow range of depressive symptoms addressed by instruments designed for patients with severe dementia, and the transient nature of depressive symptoms in cognitively impaired individuals.

High rates of concurrent depression and dementia have led to attempts to develop tools to measure depression in older people with reversible or irreversible dementia (Alexopoulos, Abrams, Young, & Shamoian, 1988; Brown, Raue, Halpert, Adams, & Titler, 2009; Toner, 2003; Toner, Teresi, Gurland, & Tirumalasetti, 1999). Most of these measures are useful primarily among patients with mild to moderate dementia who can communicate their basic needs. Some measures include informant reports of the presence of depressive symptoms, although studies have found this method to be less valid than direct assessment. Self-report scales of depression have been used with both patients with and without dementia but have a number of limitations that contraindicate their use with physically or mentally frail elderly, particularly those with dementia. Observation scales are limited because adequate validity and reliability estimates are not yet available, the instruments focus on a narrow range of observable depressive symptoms, and they often exclude items that can be assessed only through direct interaction with the patient.

In comparing various assessment instruments and measures of depression in patients with dementia, Toner (2003) suggests that instruments are needed to augment existing observational and informant methods for detecting depressive symptoms among those with severe, moderate, and mild dementia with impaired communication. A measure that uses direct-interview techniques and observation is needed for all levels of dementia. The combination of direct-interview techniques using standard questions about symptoms of depression and observations of affect, or "feeling tone," has been shown to be a reliable and valid measure of depression at all levels of dementia (Toner, 2014; Toner et al., 1999).

Difficult-to-assess populations such as the cognitively impaired need a multisource approach for valid assessment. A methodology of observational, informant, and direct assessment measures is recommended. The Cornell Scale for Depression in Dementia (Alexopoulos et al., 1988) is a useful clinical instrument with an informant focus. The Feeling-Tone Questionnaire (FTQ; Toner, 2003; Toner et al., 1999) augments existing tools by combining a direct-interview focus with informant and clinical observation methods and by adding behaviorally anchored ratings of affect. It was specifically designed for use with communication-impaired patients with dementia, uses standardized questions with simple wording, and can be used by non-clinically trained staff. Finally, because the FTQ requires only 5 to 10 minutes to administer, it can be repeated on several occasions over a prescribed period to capture fluctuating aspects of mood disorder or to obtain an average estimate of depressive symptoms. Toner, Teresi, Ocepek-Welikson, Gurland, and Siu (2016) report that a shortened 13-item version demonstrates good reliability and validity across ethnically, educationally, and cognitively diverse groups of individuals (*N* = 6,621) from a range of living situations, including community, assisted living, and nursing homes.

The FTQ also has been used to facilitate evidence-based team interdisciplinary problem-solving (TIPS) regarding, generally, the recognition of depression and, more specifically, the recognition and treatment of depression in dementia. Evidence-based TIPS expands the six steps of problem solving (Toner, Miller, & Gurland, 1994) and incorporates two additional steps related to evidence-based practices in the treatment of depression. The eight steps of evidence-based TIPS are defining the problem, brainstorming solutions, reviewing the evidence base for solutions, choosing a solution, planning ways to implement the solution(s), carrying out the plan, evaluating the solution, and documenting the evidence for successful and unsuccessful solutions. This program has been used with a training program to enhance the recognition of depression in nursing homes (Abrams et al., 2016).

Brown et al. (2009) have developed a very useful algorithm for detecting depression in older adults with dementia. The authors suggest that the algorithm is most useful for physicians, advance practice nurses, RNs, licensed practical nurses, and social workers practicing in a variety of short- and long-term settings.

See also American Psychiatric Publishing Depression Measurement Instruments.

John A. Toner

Abrams, R., Nathanson, M., Silver, S., Ramirez, M., Toner, J., & Teresi, J. (2016). Performance intervention evaluation: A training program to enhance recognition of depression in nursing homes, assisted living, and other long-term care settings. *Gerontology and Geriatrics Education, 36,* 22–38.

Alexopoulos, G. S., Abrams, R. C., Young, R. C., & Shamoian, C. A. (1988). Use of the Cornell Scale in non-demented patients. *Journal of the American Geriatrics Society, 36,* 230–235.

American Psychiatric Association. (2013). *Diagnostic and statistical manual of mental disorders* (5th ed.). Arlington, VA: American Psychiatric Publishing.

Bennett, S., & Thomas, A. (2014). Depression and dementia: Cause, consequence or coincidence? *Maturitas, 79,* 184–190.

Brown, E., Raue, P., Halpert, K., Adams, S., & Titler, M. (2009). Evidence-based guideline detection of depression in older adults with dementia. *Journal of Gerontological Nursing, 35,* 11–15.

Diniz, B., Butters, M., Albert, S., Dew, A., & Reynolds, C. (2013). Late-life depression and risk of vascular dementia and Alzheimer's disease: Systematic review and meta-analysis of community-based cohort studies. *The British Journal of Psychiatry, 202,* 329–335.

Diniz, B., & Reynolds, C. (2014). Major depressive disorder in older adults: Benefits and hazards of prolonged treatment. *Drugs & Aging, 31,* 661–669.

Enache, D., Winblad, B., & Aarsland, D. (2011). Depression in dementia: Epidemiology, mechanisms, and treatment. *Current Opinions in Psychiatry, 24,* 461–472.

Engedal, K., Barca, M., Laks, J., & Selbaek, G. (2011). Depression in Alzheimer's disease: Specificity of depressive symptoms using three different clinical criteria. *International Journal of Geriatric Psychiatry, 26,* 944–951.

MacQueen, G., Santaguida, P, Keshavarz, H., Jaworska, N., Levine, M., Beyene, J., & Raina, P. (2017). Systematic review of clinical practice guidelines for failed antidepressant treatment response in major depressive disorder, dysthymia, and subthreshold depression in adults. *The Canadian Journal of Psychiatry, 62*, 11–23.

Nathanson, M. (2010). Geriatric assessment for differential diagnosis. In J. Toner (Ed.), *Geriatric mental health disaster and emergency preparedness* (pp. 273–296). New York, NY: Springer Publishing.

Olin, J., Schneider, L., Katz, I., Meyers, B., Alexopoulos, G., Breitner, J.,...Lebowitz, B. (2002). Provisional diagnostic criteria for depression of Alzheimer disease. *American Journal of Geriatric Psychiatry, 10*, 125–128.

Reijnders, J., Ehrt, U., Weber, W., Aarsland, D., & Leentjens, A. (2008). A systematic review of prevalence studies of depression in Parkinson's disease. *Movement Disorders, 23*, 183–189.

Royall, D., Palmer, R., Chiodo, L., & Polk, M. (2012). Depressive symptoms predict longitudinal change in executive control but not memory. *International Journal of Geriatric Psychiatry, 27*, 89–96.

Rushing, N., Sachs-Ericsson, N., & Steffens, D. (2014). Neuropsychological indicators of preclinical Alzheimer's disease among depressed older adults. *Neuropsychology, Development, and Cognition. Section B, Aging, Neuropsychology and Cognition, 21*, 99–128.

Sherrod, R., Collins, A., Wynn, S., & Gragg, M. (2010). Dissecting dementia, depression, and drug effects in older adults. *Journal of Psychosocial Nursing Mental Health Services, 48*, 39–47.

Starkstein, S., & Brockman, S. (2014). Neuropsychiatric approaches to working with depressed older people. In N. Pachana & K. Laidlaw (Eds.), *The Oxford handbook of clinical geropsychology* (pp. 395–413). New York, NY: Oxford University Press.

Toner, J. (2003). *The Feeling-Tone Questionnaire (FTQ): Psychometric properties of a screening instrument for depressive symptoms in cases of dementia in institutional settings.* Ann Arbor, MI: ProQuest.

Toner, J. (2014). Depression in dementia. In E. Capezuti, P. Katz, M. Malone, & M. Mezey (Eds.), *The encyclopedia of elder care* (3rd ed.). New York, NY: Springer Publishing.

Toner, J. A., Miller, P., & Gurland, B. J. (1994). Conceptual, theoretical, and practical approaches to the development of interdisciplinary teams: A transactional model. *Educational Gerontology, 20*(1), 53–69.

Toner, J. A., Teresi, J. A., Gurland, B. J., & Tirumalasetti, F. (1999). The Feeling Tone Questionnaire: Reliability and validity of a direct patient assessment screening instrument for the detection of depressive symptoms in cases of dementia. *Journal of Clinical Geropsychology, 5*, 63–78.

Toner, J., Teresi, J., Ocepek-Welikson, K., Gurland, B., & Siu, A. (2016, November). *Assessing depressive symptoms in communication-impaired elders: The Feeling-Tone Questionnaire (FTQ).* Poster presented at the 69th Annual Scientific Meeting of the Gerontological Society of America, New Orleans, Louisiana.

Verkaik, R., Francke, A., van Meijel, A., Ribbe, M., & Bensing, J. (2009). Comorbid depression in dementia on psychogeriatric nursing home wards: Which symptoms are prominent? *American Journal of Geriatric Psychiatry, 17*, 565–573.

Verkaik, R., Francke, A., van Meijel, A., Spreeuwenberg, P., Ribbe, M., & Bensing, J. (2011). The effects of a nursing guideline on depression in psychogeriatric nursing home residents with dementia. *International Journal of Geriatric Psychiatry, 26*, 723–732.

Zahodne, L., Stern, Y., Manly, J. (2014). Depressive symptoms precede memory decline, but not vice versa, in non-demented older adults. *Journal of the American Geriatrics Society, 62*, 130–134.

Web Resources

American Journal of Geriatric Psychiatry: http://ajgponline.org

American Psychiatric Association Practice Guidelines: http://www.psychiatryonline.org

National Quality Measures Clearinghouse for Evidence-based Quality Measures: http://www.qualitymeasures.ahrq.gov

---

DEPRESSION MEASUREMENT INSTRUMENTS

Depression in the elderly often remains unrecognized and untreated. Frequently, depression is seen as a natural consequence of aging by patients and professionals. Therefore it is not diagnosed or treated. In addition, because depression continues to be seen by many as a personal weakness, they are reluctant to discuss it. Older adults often consider physical illness to be more socially acceptable than psychiatric illness. As a result, they are more likely to report physical or somatic symptoms than emotional ones. Late-life depression increases the risk of medical illness and cognitive decline. Unrecognized and untreated depression has fatal consequences: both suicide and nonsuicide mortality. Suicide is a leading cause of death in the United States, particularly for older adult men.

Depression screening is a recommended part of routine care. The U.S. Preventive Services Task Force (USPSTF) reports that screening improves the accurate identification of depressed patients in primary care settings. In a 2016 update, the USPSTF said that the net benefit of screening for depression in the general adult population is moderate (Siu et al., 2016). They recommend screening all adults regardless of age. Effective screening also requires staff-assisted depression care supports to improve clinical outcomes in both home and clinic-based care of adults and older adults. The treatment of depression with antidepressants and psychotherapy is effective in older adults, and the odds of remission are twice that seen in untreated groups. The optimal timing and frequency of screening remain unclear. The USPSTF suggests screening those who have not been screened before and considering additional screening of high-risk people, taking into account risk factors such as comorbid conditions and life events. Older adults have several risk factors for depression, including disability, poor health status related to medical illness, complicated grief, chronic sleep disturbance, loneliness, and history of depression.

Screening tools for depression are most effective when they are brief, easy to administer and easy to interpret by a variety of providers in a variety of settings, as well as when they have good predictive properties (Richardson, He, Podgorski, Tu, & Conwell, 2010). They are also useful in tracking response to treatment over time. The following scales are used to screen for depressive illness in the community or general medical populations. A positive score on these screening tools can increase or confirm a clinical suspicion of depression. However, a clinical interview is needed to determine the presence or absence of specific depressive disorders.

SELF-REPORT INSTRUMENTS

Beck Depression Inventory

The Beck Depression Inventory (BDI; Beck, Ward, Mendelson, Mock, & Erbaugh, 1961) was developed to measure behavioral manifestations of depression in adolescents and adults. It can monitor change over time or simply identify the illness. In 1996, the BDI (BDI-II) was revised to reflect better the *DSM-IV* criteria (4th ed.; *DSM-IV*; American Psychiatric Association, 1994), which improved its usefulness and use (Rush, First, & Blacker, 2008). The scale is used primarily as a self-report questionnaire and has 21 items that rate symptom severity from absent or mild (a score of 0) to severe (a score of 3). Interpretation of severity scores are as follows: 0 to 13, minimal; 14 to 19, mild; 20 to 28, moderate; and 29 to 63, severe. It takes 5 to 10 minutes to complete, but the oral administration may take 15 minutes. The BDI-II has a sensitivity of 94% and a specificity of 92% in diagnosing major depressive disorder when a cutoff of 18 is used. It is primarily used to assess the severity of depressive symptoms in patients who already have been diagnosed with depression. The BDI is also used to screen patients for depressive illness who may require intervention. Because of its ease of use, simple language, and easy scoring, the BDI is a good tool. The BDI-II, studied in older adults in community-living environments, has been shown to be a good screening measure for depression (Segal, Coolidge, Cahill, & O'Riley, 2008).

Center for Epidemiologic Studies Depression Scale

The Center for Epidemiologic Studies Depression Scale (CES-D; Radloff, 1977) measures symptoms of depression in community populations. This is the most widely used instrument among those in community studies. It has also been validated for use in geriatric populations. Studies have shown that the measurement properties of the CES-D in older adults appear to be comparable to results generated in young and middle-aged adults (Irwin, Artin, & Oxman, 1999). The goals of the scale are to identify health correlates of depressive symptoms and track changes in symptom severity over time. The scale has also been used as a screen for the presence of depressive illness. It is composed of 20 items rated on a scale from 0 (not at all) to 3 (nearly every day). The CES-D scores range from 0 to 60, with a score of 16 or higher indicating illness. The completion time is 5 minutes. The CES-D is in the public domain, so it is free to use (Radloff, 1977; cesd-r.com). Shorter versions, the CES-D-10 and CES-D-8, are also available. The CES-D-10 has been found to be as accurate as the 20-item CES-D version when used with older adults (Boey, 1999), and the validity is similar to that of the BDI when used as first-stage screening devices. It has a sensitivity of 60% to 100% and a specificity of 80% to 85% with a cutoff point of 4. It was also found to have acceptable reliability in a large sample of community-dwelling seniors (Gomez, & McLaren, 2015). One study using the CES-D-8 found it to be a valid instrument for use in older adults. It was easy to understand and administer. However, further research is needed to determine the sensitivity and specificity of this version (Karim, Weisz, Bibi, & Rehmanet, 2015).

Patient Health Questionnaire-9

The Patient Health Questionnaire (PHQ) is a self-administered tool that was designed to screen for several common mental disorders in primary care settings (Spitzer, Kroenke, & Williams, 1999). The PHQ-9 is a derivative of the PHQ specifically for depression. It is one of the most widely used depression screens in primary care settings. It covers nine symptoms of Major Depressive Disorder from the *DSM-5*. The maximum score is 27, with lower scores being better. The authors of the instrument recommend a single screening cutoff point score of 10, which has a sensitivity of 88% for major depression and a specificity of 88% (Kroenke & Spitzer, 2002). A study in elderly primary care patients found that the PHQ-9 performed comparably to the PHQ-2 and Geriatric Depression Scale-15 (GDS; Phelan et al., 2010). In that study, the PHQ-9 performed somewhat better for younger elders and those with less chronic illness. Another study looked at using the PHQ-9 to screen for depression in chronically ill elderly people (Lamers et al., 2008). They found that the summed PHQ-9 score was a valid and reliable screening method for depression in elderly patients with diabetes mellitus and COPD. The PHQ-9 is now incorporated into the minimum data set (MDS) 3.0 in nursing homes. The PHQ is in the public domain and is freely available at www.phqscreeners.com (Saliba et al., 2012).

The USPSTF has suggested that asking two simple questions about "depressed mood" and "diminished interest or pleasure in most activities" may be as effective as using longer instruments. Thus the (PHQ-2 uses the first two items from the PHQ-9: "Over the past 2 weeks, have you felt down, depressed, or hopeless?" and "Over the past 2 weeks, have you felt little interest or pleasure in doing things?" A PHQ-2 score ranges from 0 to 6, and a score of more than 3 is considered positive (Kroenke, Spitzer, & Williams, 2003). The PHQ-2 can be used as a first-step approach to screening for depression. If the patient screens positive on the PHQ-2, they need to be evaluated further with the PHQ-9 or another valid and reliable measure of depression. One study found the PHQ-2 to be a valid screening tool for major depression in older people but should be followed by a more comprehensive diagnostic process (Li, Friedman, Conwell, & Fiscella, 2007). Another study using a sample of older community-dwelling adults used the two-step approach in which only patients who screened positive on the PHQ-2 (cutoff point of 2 or greater) were administered the PHQ-9 (Richardson et al., 2010). The two-step approach (PHQ-2/PHQ-9) performed as well as the PHQ-9 and at least as well as, if not better than, the PHQ-2 alone. It was also found to be more efficient, achieving results with fewer questions, saving time and reducing respondent burden.

Geriatric Depression Scale

The GDS (Yesavage et al., 1983) was developed specifically for the geriatric population. It is the most popular and widely used of the depression scales for seniors. The GDS is easy to score and simple to administer. It can be self-administered, or a clinician can administer it. It has been shortened to 15 items. Others have shortened it even further, so there are 10-item,

5-item, 4-item, and 1-item versions too (Rush, et al. 2008). The 15-item GDS takes 5 to 7 minutes to complete. A recent meta-analysis for the GDS-15 revealed a sensitivity of 0.89% and a specificity of 0.77% at the recommended cutoff score of 5 (Pocklington, Gilbody, Manea, & McMillan, 2016). With a cutoff score of 4, the sensitivity and specificity improved to 0.88% and 0.86%, respectively. Because of a low number of studies, systematic review of the shorter versions has not been done. The GDS has been shown to differentiate older adults with and without depression in studies of patients with various chronic illnesses. The scale has been used in community and nursing-home populations with good results. Both the 30- and 15-item GDS are available at the author's website: www.stanford .edu/~yesavage/GDS.html.

Some elderly patients may find it distressing to be asked about depression. One suggestion is to refer to the GDS as the Geriatric Mood Scale as older adults may react negatively to the word *depression* and may refuse to respond to the items. The word *mood* does not seem to elicit a similar response (Carson & Vanderhorst, 2010).

The GDS is an acceptable instrument for assessing changes in the severity of depression. Cognitive impairment needs to be taken into account with the depression screening of older adults. The validity of self-report depression screening instruments is significantly decreased in patients with a Mini-Mental State Examination score of 15 or less (Sharp & Lipsky, 2002).

INTERVIEWER-ADMINISTERED INSTRUMENTS

Approximately 30% to 40% of elderly patients with dementia experience depression during the course of their disease (Tsai, Levine, & Roemheld-Hamm, 2009). In the setting of dementia, depressive symptoms are less obvious; therefore diagnosing depression is more difficult. This is especially true as the level of cognitive impairment worsens.

Cornell Scale for Depression in Dementia

The Cornell Scale for Depression in Dementia (CSDD; Alexopoulos, Abrams, Young, &

Shamoian, 1988) is a depression scale completed by a clinician by interviewing the patient and a caregiver. Its 19 items are scored on a 3-point scale, absent to severe. Because it is not a self-administered tool and requires caregiver interviews, it does take longer to complete. It typically takes 30 minutes to administer, 20 minutes for the caregiver interview and 10 minutes for the patient interview. It has a sensitivity of 72% and a specificity of 90% with a cutoff score of more than 8. It can be used to assess response to treatment over time. One review of studies using the CSDD found it to be a relatively accurate and well-studied tool for depression with dementia (Tsai et al., 2009). Another study of 242 patients in a memory clinic found CSDD performance to be good for the identification of depression (Hancock & Larner, 2015).

RECOMMENDATIONS

In one study, the CES-D and the GDS had excellent properties for use as screening instruments for major depression in older primary care patients. The researchers felt that the GDS's yes-and-no format makes it easier to administer and that it therefore can be used routinely in primary care practices (Lyness et al., 1997). An expert panel reviewed depression screening instruments from articles published from 1981 to 2005 and made recommendations for screening older adults (Snowden, Steinman, Frederick, & Wilson, 2009). They strongly recommended the use of CES-D 10 and GDS-15 to screen for depression in community-based older adults.

The American Geriatrics Society recommends considering the PHQ-2 as an initial screening test for depression in older adults. If the PHQ-2 is positive, the GDS-15 or the PHQ-9 is recommended as a follow-up (Siu & USPSTF, 2016). Scales with multiple-choice answers can be difficult for some older adults. The GDS with its simple yes-and-no answers and lack of somatic factors appears to be the best choice for this population. Starting with the PHQ-2 is a good first-step screener that would ease the burden on clinicians, as well as patients, by minimizing questions for those who test negative on the PHQ-2. The GDS is the most studied depression scale in senior-specific populations, including community-dwelling and nursing home populations. Studies have now been done on the PHQ-9 in older adults. Therefore it is a good choice as well. The earlier depression screens are well validated, and it may be a matter of finding which one works best in a particular setting. Having the appropriate mechanisms in place to treat and manage patients with positive depression screens is paramount.

Anita Steliga

Alexopoulos, G. S., Abrams, R. C., Young R. C., & Shamoian, C. A. (1988). Cornell Scale for Depression in Dementia. *Biological Psychiatry, 23*, 271–284.

American Psychiatric Association. (2000). *Diagnostic and statistical manual of mental disorders* (4th ed., text rev.). Washington, DC: Author.

Beck, A. T., Ward, C. H., Mendelson, M., Mock, J., & Erbaugh, J. (1961). An inventory for measuring depression. *Archives of General Psychiatry, 4*, 561–571.

Boey, K. W. (1999). Cross-validation of a short form of CES-D in Chinese elderly. *International Journal of Geriatric Psychiatry, 14*(8), 608–617.

Carson, V. B., & Vanderhorst, K. J. (2010). OASIS-C, depression screening, and M1730: Additional screening is necessary, the value of using standardized assessment. *Home Healthcare Nurse, 28*(3), 183–190.

Gomez, R., & McLaren, S. (2015). The Center for Epidemiological Studies Depression Scale: Measurement and structural invariance across ratings of older adult men and women. *Personality and Individual Differences, 75*, 130–134.

Hancock, P., & Larner, A. J. (2015). Cornell Scale for Depression in Dementia: Clinical utility in a memory clinic. *International Journal of Psychiatry in Clinical Practice, 19*(1), 71–74.

Irwin, M., Artin, K. H., & Oxman, M. N. (1999). Screening for depression in the older adult: Criterion validity of the 10-item Center for Epidemiological Studies Depression Scale (CES-D). *Archives of Internal Medicine, 159*, 1701–1704.

Karim, J., Weisz, R., Bibi, Z., & Rehmanet, S. (2015). Validation of the eight-item Center for Epidemiologic Studies Depression Scale (CES-D) among older adults. *Current Psychology: A Journal for Diverse Perspectives on Diverse Psychological Issues, 34*(4), 681–692.

Kroenke, K., & Spitzer, R. (2002). The PHQ-9: A new depression diagnostic and severity measure. *Psychiatric Annals, 32*, 1–7.

Kroenke, K., Spitzer, R., & Williams, J. B. (2003). The Patient Health Questionnaire-2 validity of a two-item depression screener. *Medical Care, 41*(11), 1284–1292.

Lamers, F., Jonkers, C. C., Bosma, H., Penninx, B. W., Knottnerus, J. A., & van Eijk, J. T. (2008). Summed score of the Patient Health Questionnaire-9 was a reliable and valid method for depression screening in chronically ill elderly patients. *Journal of Clinical Epidemiology, 61*, 679–687.

Li, C., Friedman, B., Conwell, Y., & Fiscella, K. (2007). Validity of the Patient Health Questionnaire 2 (PHQ-2) in identifying major depression in older people. *Journal of the American Geriatrics Society, 55*(4), 596–602.

Lyness, J. M., Noel, T. K., Cox, C., King, D. A., Conwell, Y., & Caine, E. D. (1997). Screening for depression in elderly primary care patients: A comparison of the Center for Epidemiologic Studies Depression Scale and the Geriatric Depression Scale. *Archives of Internal Medicine, 157*(4), 449–454.

Phelan, E., Williams, B., Meeker, K., Bonn, K., Frederick, J., LoGerfo, J., & Snowden, M. (2010). A study of the diagnostic accuracy of the PHQ-9 in primary care elderly. *BMC Family Practice, 11*, 63.

Pocklington, C., Gilbody, S., Manea, L., & McMillan, D. (2016). The diagnostic accuracy of brief versions of the Geriatric Depression Scale: A systematic review and meta-analysis. *International Journal of Geriatric Psychiatry, 31*(8), 837–857.

Radloff, L. S. (1977). The CES-D scale: A self-report depression scale for research in the general population. *Applied Psychological Measurement, 1*, 385–401.

Richardson, T. M., He, H., Podgorski, C., Tu, X., & Conwell, Y. (2010). Screening depression aging services clients. *American Journal of Geriatric Psychiatry, 18*(12), 1116–1123.

Rush, A. J., First, M. B., & Blacker, D. (Eds.). (2008). *Handbook of psychiatric measures.* Washington, DC: American Psychiatric Publishing.

Saliba, D., DiFilippo, S., Edelen, M. O., Kroenke, K., Buchanan, J., & Streim, J. (2012). Testing the PHQ-9 interview and observational versions (PHQ-9 OV) for MDS 3.0. *Journal of the American Medical Directors Association, 13*(7), 618–625.

Segal, D. L., Coolidge, F. L., Cahill, B. S., & O'Riley, A. A. (2008). Psychometric properties of the Beck Depression Inventory–II (BDI-II) among community-dwelling older adults. *Behavior Modification, 32*(1), 3–20.

Sharp, L. K., & Lipsky, M. S. (2002). Screening for depression across the lifespan: A review of measures for use in primary care settings. *American Family Physician, 66*(6), 1001–1008.

Siu, A., & U.S. Preventive Services Task Force. (2016). Screening for depression in adults: U.S. Preventive

Services Task Force recommendation statement. *Journal of the American Medical Association, 315*(4), 380–387.

Snowden, M., Steinman, L., Frederick, J., & Wilson, N. (2009). Screening for depression in older adults: Recommended instruments and considerations for community-based practice. *Clinical Geriatrics, 17*(9), 26–32.

Spitzer R. L., Kroenke, K., & Williams, J. B. W. (1999). Validation and utility of a self-report version of PRIME-MD: The PHQ primary care study. Primary Care Evaluation of Mental Disorders, Patient Health Questionnaire. *Journal of the American Medical Association, 282,* 1737–1744.

Tsai, E. H., Levine, J., & Roemheld-Hamm, B. (2009). What is the best way to screen for major depressive disorder in patients with dementia? *Evidence-Based Practice, 12*(12), 4–5.

Yesavage, J. A., Brink, T. L., Rose, T. L., Lum, O., Huang, V., Adey, M., & Leirer, V. O. (1983). Development and validation of a geriatric depression screening scale: A preliminary report. *Journal of Psychiatric Research, 17,* 37–49.

Web Resources
Geriatric Mental Health Foundation: http://www .gmhfonline.org
National Institute of Mental Health: https://www .nimh.nih.gov

DIABETES: MANAGEMENT

The clinical presentation and acute complications of diabetes include a variety of symptoms, most commonly polyuria, polydipsia, polyphagia, weight loss, and fatigue. In the elderly, however, these symptoms may be confused with normal age-related changes or symptoms of other medical disorders. Polyuria may be attributed to the use of diuretics or urinary incontinence. Weight loss may be associated with changes in appetite caused by medications and gastrointestinal disturbances. Whereas some individuals are asymptomatic and are diagnosed during routine medical examinations, others may have fully developed acute or chronic complications at the time of diagnosis (e.g., when a patient comes to the emergency department with severe hyperglycemia or has a diagnostic workup for

pain and burning in the extremities). Thus in older adults, the diagnosis of diabetes must be considered in the workup for a variety of specific and nonspecific symptoms.

MANAGEMENT GOALS

The primary goals in the management of diabetes in the elderly are the prevention of the acute metabolic derangements of diabetes and the prevention of chronic complications. These goals are best achieved through a combination of therapies, such as diet, exercise, and medications.

Glycemic Goals

The glycemic goals in elderly patients with diabetes are highly individualized and generally are based on duration of diabetes and comorbidites. Long-term glucose control is measured by the hemoglobin A1c (A1c), which reflects average glucose readings over the previous 3 months. In recognition in the heterogeneity of physical functioning, comorbidities, and life-expectancy among older adults with diabetes, the American Diabetes Association (ADA) has provided a framework for glycemic goals among the elderly. In this framework, elderly patients are broadly classified into three different categories, healthy, complex and very complex with corresponding glycemic goals of less than 7.5%, less than 8.0%, and less than 8.5% (ADA, 2017c) The ADA discourages maintaining glycemic goals greater than 8.5% as this increases the risk of glycosuria, dehydration, hyperglycemic hyperosmolar syndrome and poor wound healing (ADA, 2017c).

Treatment

Diet

Medical nutrition therapy (MNT)—an essential element in the management of any patient with diabetes, regardless of age—includes maintenance of target blood glucose levels, normalization of serum lipids, attainment and maintenance of a reasonable body weight, and promotion of overall health. The nutritional guidelines of the ADA stress individualization of diet in accordance with blood glucose, lipid, and weight goals (ADA, 2017a). Many older adults, however, may be undernourished due to a variety of physiological, psychological, social, and economic factors such as anorexia and changes in smell, taste, and thirst; dental problems; side effects of medications; inability to shop for food or prepare meals; cognitive impairment, depression, isolation (Kirkman et al., 2012), and loneliness; and inadequate income to purchase food. For older adults unable to meet nutritional needs through a regular meal plan, it may be necessary to modify usual food intake by changing the nutrient content or density, modifying food consistency, providing more frequent meals, using medical nutritional supplements, and considering enteral and parenteral nutritional support (Kirkman et al., 2012). Malnourished elders may require increased calories with an increased adjustment of oral medications or insulin, if indicated, to achieve target blood glucose levels. Older adults residing in long-term care (LTC) facilities many need frequent assessment of nutritional intake to ensure appropriate micronutrient, macronutrient, and caloric intake.

Exercise

Routine exercise is an essential component of the treatment plan. Age-associated loss of muscle mass and strength may be exacerbated by diabetes. Adding an exercise program to the treatment plan improves functional status and decreases the need for insulin or oral medications, but the benefits of exercise must be weighed against the risks and presence of complications in elderly adults with type 2 diabetes mellitus. Many older adults can undertake walking programs and should be encouraged to contact local senior citizen centers for physical activity programs. Adults with limited mobility or those confined to chairs can participate in arm or chair exercises. Older adults without significant complications can participate in activities recommended for all adults with type 2 diabetes as tolerated (ADA, 2017a).

Pharmacological Therapy

Several classes of medications are available in the United States for treating type 2 diabetes: *biguanides* (metformin), *insulin secretagogues, thiazolidinediones, incretin-based therapies,* *alpha-glucosidase inhibitors, sodium-glucose cotransporter 2 inhibitors, pramlintide,* and *insulin.*

Biguanides decrease hepatic glucose production (ADA, 2017b) through reductions in gluconeogenesis and glycogenolysis. Metformin, the only biguanide available in the United States, is often the first line of treatment of type 2 diabetes (ADA, 2017c). Gastrointestinal problems, including abdominal discomfort, are the most common side effects. In addition, metformin is associated with vitamin B_{12} deficiency. An infrequent side effect is lactic acidosis (ADA, 2017b). Metformin is contraindicated in any condition that causes hypoperfusion, such as severe hepatic, renal, and cardiopulmonary disease. More specifically, metformin is contraindicated in patients with an estimated glomerular filtration rate (eGFR) less than 30 mL/min/1.73 m² (U.S. Food and Drug Administration, 2016).

Insulin secretagogues include sulfonylureas and meglitinides. *Sulfonylureas* stimulate insulin secretion from the pancreatic beta-cell (ADA, 2017b). *Meglitinides* stimulate insulin secretion from the pancreatic beta-cell more rapidly than sulfonylureas. Meglitinides are taken before meals to reduce postprandial hyperglycemia. These medications are associated with hypoglycemia and should be used cautiously in the older patient with type 2 diabetes (ADA, 2017c).

Thiazolidinediones increase insulin sensitivity (ADA, 2017b) and have been associated with the risk of weight gain, edema, heart failure, and bone fractures, limiting their usefulness in the elderly (Kirkman et al., 2012).

Alpha-glucosidase inhibitors interfere with the ability of enzymes in the small intestinal brush border to break down oligosaccharides and disaccharides into monosaccharides, thus retarding glucose entry into the systemic circulation. Alpha-glucosidase enzyme inhibitors are associated with a number of gastrointestinal side effects, including bloating, abdominal discomfort, diarrhea, and flatulence; however, they are associated with a low risk of hypoglycemia (ADA, 2017b).

Incretin-based therapies include dipeptidyl peptidase-4 (DPP-4) inhibitors and glucagon-like peptide-1 (GLP-1) agonists. *DPP-4 inhibitors* inhibit the degradation of the incretins, GLP-1 and glucose-dependent insulinotropic peptide (GIP). The net effect of these medications is to reduce postprandial hyperglycemia. These medications are associated with a low risk of hypoglycemia. *GLP-1 agonists* (e.g., exenatide injection [Byetta]) are injectable medications used to reduce postprandial hyperglycemia; however, the risk of nausea and weight loss may limit their use in frail elderly (Kirkman et al., 2012).

Sodium-glucose cotransporter 2 (SGLT2) inhibitors inhibit SGLT2 in the proximal nephron and block glucose reabsorption by the kidney, increasing glucosuria and reducing blood glucose levels. These agents cause modest weight loss and reduce blood pressure. These medications have been associated with the development of ketoacidosis in the absence of severe hyperglycemia (ADA, 2017b). There is limited experience in the use of these medications among the elderly (ADA, 2017c).

Pramlintide is an injectable synthetic analog of human amylin, a hormone secreted by the pancreatic beta-cell. Pramlintide is injected at mealtimes and is indicated for improving glycemic control in type 2 diabetes. Symlin can also be used as adjuvant mealtime therapy for the treatment of type 1 diabetes. Pramlintide is associated with hypoglycemia, so reductions in prandial insulin dosing may be needed to prevent severe hypoglycemia (ADA, 2017b). The risk of hypoglycemia limits the use of these medications in the elderly.

When oral medications cannot reduce blood glucose appropriately, *insulin* may be prescribed for older adults with type 2 diabetes. Extensive algorithms are available for initiating insulin therapy (ADA, 2017b). These regimens range from noncomplex to highly complex. The overall goal of insulin therapy in older patients is to provide the least-complex regimen that provides optimal glycemic control with minimal hypoglycemia. For example, once-daily insulin injections may be appropriate for many older patients with type 2 diabetes. Premixed insulin preparations such as 70/30 (i.e., 70% intermediate insulin/ 30% regular insulin) may provide appropriate coverage and reduce the complexity of mixing and drawing up insulin. Insulin therapy is individualized and relies on the ability of the patient and/or caregiver to draw up and correctly administer the medication. The loss of fine motor skills and visual impairments associated with both diabetes and aging may necessitate the use of adaptive devices, such as magnifiers, insulin dose counters, and prefilled pen devices. A list of such devices is available from the National Federation of the Blind. Elderly patients may need the assistance of home health nurses and family members to draw and administer insulin.

Hypoglycemia

Medications such as biguanides, thiazolidinediones, alpha-glucosidase enzyme inhibitors, and DPP-4 inhibitors generally do not cause hypoglycemia when used alone. However, the medications may cause hypoglycemia when combined with sulfonylureas or insulin. The intensity of the insulin regimen must be balanced between glycemic control and the risk posed by hypoglycemia for a particular patient. For example, the risk of hip fracture from falling in an 80-year-old woman with severe osteoporosis may outweigh the benefits of excellent glucose control. In this case, blood glucose may be maintained at a slightly higher level. Elderly patients with diabetes are more vulnerable to hypoglycemia if they reduce overall caloric intake, skip meals, increase physical activity, or exercise more intensely than usual. Hypoglycemia may be potentiated when gastrointestinal symptoms, such as those associated with alpha-glucosidase inhibitors and biguanides, are present. If hypoglycemia occurs when alpha-glucosidase inhibitors and sulfonylureas or insulin are given simultaneously, glucose tablets or gels provide the fastest recovery from hypoglycemia. In elderly people, the symptoms of hypoglycemia can be confused with cognitive dysfunction. Therefore, patients and their families must understand how to prevent, recognize, and treat hypoglycemia.

BLOOD GLUCOSE MONITORING

Self-monitoring meters that measure capillary blood glucose levels provide immediate feedback, allow individuals to determine patterns of hyperglycemia and hypoglycemia and to make appropriate decisions about insulin doses. Using self-monitoring meters may be a problem for elders with diminished visual acuity and fine motor skills. For these individuals, a meter that has easily read results and requires the least technical skill is recommended. The most appropriate times to monitor blood glucose levels are before breakfast, lunch, dinner, and bedtime snack. These times should be modified, based on each individual's medication regimen.

Medicare coverage for home glucose monitoring is detailed at www.medicare.gov. The blood glucose test strips are considered durable medical equipment, and thus Medicare's Competitive Bidding Program may affect the supplier. Mail-order access to diabetic testing supplies is available nationally. Clinicians should try to reiterate the importance of glucose control and work with patients with limited financial resources. Financial support for equipment and materials may be available from community programs or other resources.

See also Diabetes: Overview.

Lauretta Quinn

American Diabetes Association. (2017a). 4. Lifestyle management. *Diabetes Care, 40*(Suppl. 1), S33–S43. doi:10.2337/dc17-S007

American Diabetes Association. (2017b). 8. Pharmacologic approaches to glycemic treatment. *Diabetes Care, 40*(Suppl. 1), S64–S74. doi:10.2337/dc17-S011

American Diabetes Association. (2017c). 11. Older adults. *Diabetes Care, 40*(Suppl. 1), S99–S104. doi:10.2337/dc17-S014

Kirkman, M. S., Briscoe, V. J., Clark, N., Florez, H., Haas, L. B., Halter, J. B.,…Swift, C. S. (2012). Diabetes in older adults. *Diabetes Care, 35*(12), 2650–2664. doi:10.2337/dc12-1801

U.S. Food and Drug Administration. (2016). Metformin-containing drugs: Drug safety communication—Revised warnings for certain patients with reduced kidney function. Retrieved from https://www.fda.gov/Safety/MedWatch/SafetyInformation/SafetyAlertsforHumanMedicalProducts/ucm494829.htm

Web Resources
American Association of Diabetes Educators: http://www.aadenet.org
American Diabetes Association: http://www.diabetes.org
American Dietetic Association: http://www.eatright.org
Medicare: https://www.medicare.gov
National Federation of the Blind: http://nfb.org

DIABETES: OVERVIEW

Diabetes is a major public health problem affecting approximately 25.8 million people, or 8.3% of the U.S. population (Centers for Disease Control and Prevention, 2014). This epidemic is not limited to the United States; the global prevalence of diabetes has increased dramatically over the past few decades. The number of people living with diabetes has increased from 108 million in 1980 to 422 million in 2014 (WHO, 2016). The incidence of diabetes has increased dramatically in all age groups in the past three decades; however, diabetes remains a disease of aging. Whereas 16.2% of the U.S. population between 45 and 64 years of age have diabetes, this number increases to 25.9% among those 65 years of age or older (Centers for Disease Control and Prevention, 2014). The prevalence of diabetes is expected to increase with the aging of the U.S. population, the number of people from minority populations at high risk for diabetes, and the number of people living longer with diabetes (Boyle, Thompson, Gregg, Barker, & Williamson, 2010).

DIABETES-RELATED COMPLICATIONS IN OLDER INDIVIDUALS

The acute complications of diabetes include diabetic ketoacidosis (DKA), hyperosmolar hyperglycemic syndrome (HHS), and hypoglycemia. Chronic complications include retinopathy, neuropathy, nephropathy, cardiovascular disease, cerebrovascular disease (CVD), and peripheral vascular disease. Older adults with diabetes are at risk for both acute and chronic complications, particularly CVD. The interplay between these complications and age-related comorbidities contributes to increased mortality in older patients with diabetes. The Diabetes Control and Complications Trial (DCCT; Diabetes Control and Complications Trial Research Group, 1993) and the United Kingdom Prospective Diabetes Study (UKPDS; Turner, Cull, Frighi, & Holman, 1999) demonstrated that sustained hyperglycemia is associated with the development of chronic complications, in those with type 1 diabetes mellitus (T1DM) and type 2 diabetes mellitus (T2DM), respectively. In addition, the UKPDS demonstrated that the severity of T2DM increases with longer duration of disease. Clinical trials, such as the Action to Control Cardiovascular Risk in Diabetes (ACCORD; Action to Control Cardiovascular Risk in Diabetes Study Group et al., 2008), the Action in Diabetes and Vascular Disease: Preterax and Diamicron MR Controlled Evaluation (ADVANCE; Advance Collaborative Group et al., 2008) and the Veterans Affairs Diabetes Trial (VADT) (Duckworth et al., 2009) have attempted to delineate the benefits and risks of strict glycemic control on CVD events in T2DM. Subset analyses of ACCORD, ADVANCE, and VADT suggest that patients with shorter durations of T2DM and without established atherosclerosis might receive CVD benefits from intensive glycemic control. The glucose lowering arm of the ACCORD trial was stopped early, however, because of excessive deaths among participants in the intensive glucose-lowering group. In addition, it is possible that potential risks of intensive glycemic control may outweigh its benefits in other patients, such as those with a very long duration of diabetes, a known history of severe hypoglycemia, advanced atherosclerosis, and advanced age/frailty (Skyler et al., 2009).

CLASSIFICATION OF DIABETES AND PREDIABETES

The four primary classifications of diabetes include T1DM, T2DM, gestational diabetes mellitus (GDM), and other types of diabetes (Chamberlain, Rhinehart, Shaefer, & Neuman, 2016). Prediabetes is a category of increased risk for diabetes and is diagnosed as impaired fasting glucose (IFG), impaired glucose tolerance (IGT) or glycosylated hemoglobin (A1c).

Type 1 Diabetes

T1DM affects approximately 5% to 10% of the U.S. diabetes population. Approximately 1.25 million people in the United States live with T1DM, including more than 1 million adults (Juvenile Diabetes Research Foundation, 2017). The number of older patients with T1DM is growing (Schutt et al., 2012) because of a global increase in the incidence of diabetes (Dahlquist, Nystrom, Patterson, Swedish Childhood Diabetes Study Group, & Diabetes Incidence in Sweden Study Group, 2011) and longer survival of those with T1DM (Secrest, Becker, Kelsey, LaPorte, & Orchard, 2010). Clearly, the population of adults and older adults with T1DM is growing along with their associated medical, social, psychological, and social issues. In addition, an increasing number of adults older than 35 years are developing slowly evolving T1DM, known as latent autoimmune diabetes in adults (LADA).

The primary physiological defect in the development of T1DM is the destruction of the pancreatic beta-cell, resulting in an absolute deficiency of insulin secretion. In most individuals with T1DM, this insulin deficiency results from an autoimmune destruction of the pancreatic beta-cell. At the time of diagnosis, 90% to 95% of individuals with T1DM have circulating antibodies directed against the pancreatic beta-cell. In a small number of patients, however, the cause of this pancreatic beta-cell dysfunction is unknown. The inability of the pancreas to secrete insulin, regardless of the cause, results in classic symptoms of T1DM, including polyuria, polydipsia, weight loss, electrolyte imbalances, and DKA.

Type 2 Diabetes

T2DM affects more than 90% of the older diabetic population and increases in the prevalence with age-related alterations in insulin sensitivity and secretion, altered glucose metabolism, dietary changes, obesity, and decreased physical activity. T2DM is characterized by decreased liver, muscle, and adipose sensitivity to insulin and a defect in pancreatic beta-cell insulin secretion. The development of T2DM follows a typical course. There is an initial period of hyperinsulinemia in which the pancreatic beta-cell is able to overcome resistance and maintain normal glucose tolerance. This is followed by a period of postprandial hyperglycemia and increased insulin resistance because hyperinsulinemia is insufficient for maintaining normal postprandial glucose tolerance. In the final stage, fasting hyperglycemia is present as a result of increased insulin resistance, unrestrained hepatic glucose production, and the toxic effects of hyperglycemia on the beta-cell. At this time, the patient usually develops clinical symptoms of T2DM, ranging from polyuria to HHS, a life-threatening state characterized by severe dehydration, increased serum osmolality, and hyperglycemia.

Gestational Diabetes Mellitus

GDM, a type of diabetes that occurs during pregnancy, develops in 2% to 10% of all pregnancies (Centers for Disease Control and Prevention, 2015).

Other Specific Types of Diabetes

Other specific types of diabetes affect approximately 1% to 5% of people with diabetes. (Centers for Disease Control and Prevention, 2015) and result from a variety of causes, such as specific genetic syndromes, surgery, drugs, malnutrition, infections, and other comorbid illnesses. Some of these conditions are more likely to occur in aging populations, such as pancreatic disease, hormonal disease, and medications that cause insulin resistance or decreased insulin secretion (e.g., glucocorticoids).

Prediabetes

Prediabetes is a term used to describe individuals whose plasma glucose levels are higher than normal but are not diagnostic for diabetes. This classification is a major risk factor for the development of both diabetes and CVD. Impaired fasting glucose is diagnosed by a fasting plasma glucose of 100 to 125 mg/dL (Chamberlain et al., 2016). IGT is diagnosed as a 2-hour plasma glucose of 140 to 199 mg/dL during a 75-g oral glucose tolerance test (OGTT) (Chamberlain et al., 2016). Prediabetes is diagnosed through an A1c of 5.7% to 6.4% (Chamberlain et al., 2016).

RISK FACTORS FOR THE DEVELOPMENT OF DIABETES

Risk factors in the development of diabetes include ethnicity (i.e., Native Americans, Hispanics, African Americans, and Asian Americans), age greater than 45 years, first-degree relative with diabetes, obesity, other medical disorders (e.g., hypertension, dyslipidemias), and history of glucose intolerance.

COMPLICATIONS

Diabetic Ketoacidosis

DKA is a life-threatening condition in which severe abnormalities in protein, fat, and lipid metabolism occur as a result of an absolute or relative deficiency in insulin secretion. DKA usually occurs in patients with T1DM but may occur in patients with T2DM during times of severe stress, such as trauma, infection, myocardial infarction, or surgery. Mortality from DKA increases with advancing age. DKA is characterized by hyperglycemia resulting from increased glucose production and decreased glucose utilization, dehydration related to an osmotic diuresis, and metabolic acidosis related to increased production and decreased utilization of acetoacetic acid and beta-hydroxybutyric acid.

Hyperosmolar Hyperglycemic Syndrome

HHS is usually seen initially in middle-aged to older individuals with T2DM or IGT in whom physiological stress results in increased hyperglycemia, severe dehydration, and increased serum osmolality. Older patients who cannot compensate for fluid losses induced by hyperosmolar hyperglycemia (e.g., a patient after a stroke who cannot swallow or articulate their need for fluid) are particularly vulnerable to HHS. Often the patient is unaware of any impairment in glucose tolerance. HHS differs from DKA in that there is no metabolic acidosis caused by an accumulation of serum ketone bodies. Precipitating factors include medications that cause glucose intolerance, such as glucocorticoids; therapeutic procedures, such as peritoneal dialysis; chronic disease, such as renal failure; and acute conditions, such as infection. HHS is characterized by severe dehydration and serum hyperosmolality. Patients may exhibit neurological manifestations from intracerebral dehydration and renal insufficiency or failure from profound dehydration and hyperosmolality. Mortality rates for HHS range from 5% to 20% and are usually attributed to underlying comorbidities (Steenkamp, Alexanian, & McDonnell, 2013).

Hypoglycemia

Hypoglycemia occurs when glucose utilization exceeds glucose production. The low blood glucose level (usually less than 60mg/dL) can cause a variety of adrenergic and neuroglycopenic symptoms, which may be difficult to recognize in vulnerable older patients. Precipitating factors in the development of hypoglycemia include excess exogenous insulin, excess oral hypoglycemic medications, and decreased food intake and increased physical activity in patients using oral hypoglycemic medications. Several abnormalities in the counterregulatory feedback symptoms of T1DM can result in frequent hypoglycemia. Glucagon secretion becomes deficient 2 to 5 years after diagnosis. With prolonged duration of the disease, the epinephrine response is also impaired because of subclinical autonomic neuropathy. Thus some older patients with long-standing T1DM have difficulty both recognizing hypoglycemic symptoms and recovering from hypoglycemia. In other older patients, the symptoms can be mistaken for changes in cognitive function or coexisting diseases. Therefore older patients with diabetes treated with pharmacological therapy (particularly insulin and sulfonylureas) are at increased morbidity and mortality from hypoglycemic episodes.

Chronic Complications

The DCCT and UKPDS demonstrated that chronic hyperglycemia mediates the occurrence and progression of microvascular complications (retinopathy, neuropathy, and nephropathy) and is also a major contributor to the development of macrovascular complications (cardiovascular, cerebrovascular, and peripheral vascular disease). Although the exact physiological mechanisms by which hyperglycemia mediates these complications are unclear, there are several general theories regarding their pathogenesis: increased formation of advanced glycation end products (AGEs), polyol pathway flux, activation of the protein kinase C isoforms, increased expression of the receptor for AGEs, overactivity of the hexosamine and free-radical pathways (Giacco & Brownlee, 2010). Regardless of the physiological cause, hyperglycemia is the primary contributor to the development of diabetes-related complications, but hypertension and lipid abnormalities are major contributors to the development of macrovascular disease.

See also Diabetes: Management.

Lauretta Quinn

Action to Control Cardiovascular Risk in Diabetes Study Group, Gerstein, H. C., Miller, M. E., Byington, R. P., Goff, D. C., Jr., Bigger, J. T.,…Friedewald, W. T. (2008). Effects of intensive glucose lowering in type 2 diabetes. *New England Journal of Medicine, 358*(24), 2545–2559. doi:10.1056/NEJMoa0802743

Advance Collaborative Group, Patel, A., MacMahon, S., Chalmers, J., Neal, B., Billot, L.,…Travert, F. (2008). Intensive blood glucose control and vascular outcomes in patients with type 2 diabetes. *New England Journal of Medicine, 358*(24), 2560–2572. doi:10.1056/NEJMoa0802987

Boyle, J. P., Thompson, T. J., Gregg, E. W., Barker, L. E., & Williamson, D. F. (2010). Projection of the year 2050 burden of diabetes in the US adult population: Dynamic modeling of incidence, mortality, and prediabetes prevalence. *Population Health Metrics, 8*, 29. doi:10.1186/1478-7954-8-29

Centers for Disease Control and Prevention. (2014). *National diabetes fact sheet: National estimates and general information on diabetes and prediabetes in the United States, 2014.* Atlanta, GA: U.S. Department of Health and Human Services.

Centers for Disease Control and Prevention. (2015, March 31). Basics about diabetes. Retrieved from https://www.cdc.gov/diabetes/basics/diabetes.html

Chamberlain, J. J., Rhinehart, A. S., Shaefer, C. F., & Neuman, A. (2016). Diagnosis and management of diabetes: Synopsis of the 2016 American Diabetes

Association standards of medical care in diabetes. *Annals of Internal Medicine, 164*(8), 542–552.

Dahlquist, G. G., Nystrom, L., Patterson, C. C., Swedish Childhood Diabetes Study Group, & Diabetes Incidence in Sweden Study Group. (2011). Incidence of type 1 diabetes in Sweden among individuals aged 0–34 years, 1983–2007: An analysis of time trends. *Diabetes Care, 34*(8), 1754–1759. doi:10.2337/dc11-0056

Diabetes Control and Complications Trial Research Group. (1993). The effect of intensive treatment of diabetes on the development and progression of long-term complications in insulin-dependent diabetes mellitus. *New England Journal of Medicine, 329*(14), 977–986. doi:10.1056/NEJM199309303291401

Duckworth, W., Abraira, C., Moritz, T., Reda, D., Emanuele, N., Reaven, P. D.,…Huang, G. D., for the VADT Investigators (2009). Glucose control and vascular complications in veterans with type 2 diabetes. *New England Journal of Medicine, 360*(2), 129–139. doi:10.1056/NEJMoa0808431

Giacco, F., & Brownlee, M. (2010). Oxidative stress and diabetic complications. *Circulation Research, 107*(9), 1058–1070. doi:10.1161/CIRCRESAHA.110.223545

Juvenile Diabetes Research Foundation. (2017). Type 1 diabetes facts. Retrieved from http://www.jdrf.org/about/fact-sheets/facts-about-jdrf

Schutt, M., Fach, E. M., Seufert, J., Kerner, W., Lang, W., Zeyfang, A.,…German BMBF Competence Network Diabetes Network. (2012). Multiple complications and frequent severe hypoglycaemia in "elderly" and "old" patients with type 1 diabetes. *Diabetes Medicine, 29*(8), e176–e179. doi:10.1111/j.1464-5491.2012.03681.x

Secrest, A. M., Becker, D. J., Kelsey, S. F., LaPorte, R. E., & Orchard, T. J. (2010). All-cause mortality trends in a large population-based cohort with long-standing childhood-onset type 1 diabetes: The Allegheny County type 1 diabetes registry. *Diabetes Care, 33*(12), 2573–2579. doi:10.2337/dc10-1170

Skyler, J. S., Bergenstal, R., Bonow, R. O., Buse, J., Deedwania, P., Gale, E. A.,…Sherwin, R. S. (2009). Intensive glycemic control and the prevention of cardiovascular events: implications of the ACCORD, ADVANCE, and VA diabetes trials: A position statement of the American Diabetes Association and a scientific statement of the American College of Cardiology Foundation and the American Heart Association. *Diabetes Care, 32*(1), 187–192. doi:10.2337/dc08-9026

Steenkamp, D. W., Alexanian, S. M., & McDonnell, M. E. (2013). Adult hyperglycemic crisis: A review

and perspective. *Current Diabetes Reports, 13*(1), 130–137. doi:10.1007/s11892-012-0342-z

Turner, R. C., Cull, C. A., Frighi, V., & Holman, R. R. (1999). Glycemic control with diet, sulfonylurea, metformin, or insulin in patients with type 2 diabetes mellitus: progressive requirement for multiple therapies (UKPDS 49). UK Prospective Diabetes Study (UKPDS) Group. *Journal of the American Medical Association, 281*(21), 2005–2012.

World Health Organization. (2016). *Global report on diabetes.* Geneva, Switzerland: Author.

Web Resources

American Association of Diabetes Educators: http://www.aadenet.org

American Diabetes Association: http://www.diabetes.org

DISCHARGE PLANNING

Discharge planning is defined as the development of a personalized plan for each patient who is leaving the hospital, with the aim of containing costs and improving patient outcomes (Gonçalves-Bradley, Lannin, Clemson, Cameron, & Shepperd, 2016). In 2010, there were 35 million hospital discharges in the United States (excluding newborns; Centers for Disease Control and Prevention [CDC], 2010). The safety and quality issues associated with discharge from acute care settings have been highlighted in multiple studies and consensus reports (Bradway et al., 2012; Coleman et al., 2013; Institute of Medicine [IOM], 2001). The role of high-quality discharge planning is essential in the overall aim of patient safety, particularly for vulnerable elders. In general, the process involves (Centers for Medicare & Medicaid Services [CMS], 2014):

- Determining the appropriate post–hospital discharge destination for a patient.
- Identifying what the patient requires for a smooth and safe transition from the acute care hospital/post-acute care (PCA) facility to the discharge destination.
- Beginning the process of meeting the patient's identified predischarge and postdischarge needs.

Persons older than 65 years who are discharged from acute care hospitals are at risk of 30-day hospital readmission (approximately every fifth hospitalization) and death (Gorina, Pratt, Kramarow, & Elgaddal, 2015). In 2010, adults aged 85 years and older accounted for only 2% of the U.S. population but 9% of hospital discharges (Levant, Chari, & DeFrances, 2015). The financial penalties for avoidable readmissions provide further impetus for health care institutions to meet regulatory mandates in discharge planning. Researchers have estimated that inadequate care coordination, including discharge planning, was responsible for $25 to $45 billion in wasteful spending to pay for avoidable complications and unnecessary readmissions (Health Affairs, 2012). Patients or residents may be discharged from or to acute care hospitals, in-patient rehabilitation facilities, long-term care hospitals, home health agencies, hospice, in-patient psychiatric facilities, long-term care facilities, and swing beds (CMS, 2014). In 2013, 7.96 million in-patient stays were discharged to PCA after hospitalizations; of this, approximately 42% were Medicare fee-for-service patients. Between 2001 and 2013, Medicare spending on PAC doubled from $29 billion to $59 billion annually (Tian, 2016). A systematic review of discharge planning among surgical patients reported that discharge planning programs reduced readmissions by 11.5%, patient education interventions reduced readmissions by 14%, primary care follow-up reduced readmissions by 8.3% for patients after high-risk surgeries, and home visits reduced readmissions by 7.69% respectively (Jones et al., 2016).

The period after discharge from acute care settings is a vulnerable time because of "higher clinical acuity and shorter lengths of stay (that) has contributed to an increased complexity of hospital discharge instructions and higher expectations for patients to perform challenging self-care activities" (Coleman et al., 2013, p. 1). Increased age is associated with a higher illness-related hospital admission rate; consequently, older adults account for one third of hospitalizations (Stranges & Friedman, 2008). The concepts of discharge planning have been used interchangeably or in conjunction with more recent models currently referred to as *transitional care.* Among others, the goal of high-quality and well-organized discharge planning is the safe transition of patients from acute care settings to the next level of care, preventing unplanned readmissions, improving patient care experience satisfaction, and minimizing cost (Li et al., 2016).

COMPREHENSIVE GERIATRIC ASSESSMENT AND DISCHARGE PLANNING

Discharge planning is traditionally thought of as commencing on admission. However, for elective admissions such as a planned hip replacement and other high-risk surgeries, planning for discharge must be integral to the care decisions made even before the patient is admitted. Quality indicators outlined in the Assessing Care of Vulnerable Elders (ACOVE) by the American Geriatrics Society under the Continuity and Coordination of Care heading can be used as a guide in discharge planning (Lim, Foust, & Van Cleave, 2016).

A meta-analysis demonstrated that comprehensive geriatric assessment (CGA) increases patients' survival and discharge to home after an emergency hospital admission (Ellis, Whitehead, Robinson, O'Neill, & Langhorn, 2011). The screening of older hospitalized patients leads to early geriatric-specific interventions and thus shortened hospital stay. In addition, older patients receiving CGA had a greater degree of physical function compared with those receiving usual care. As a result, patients who had CGA were more likely to live in their own homes following discharge (Ellis et al., 2011).

INTERDISCIPLINARY AND COLLABORATIVE DISCHARGE PLANNING: CORE MEASURES

A review involving 36 randomized controlled trials (RCTs) reported that the core measures correlating with positive outcomes in discharge planning are those that are geared toward improving hand-off communication, coordination of care, and communication (Schectman,

2013). Successful discharge planning includes enhancement of patient empowerment, financial systems to support discharge plans, and interdisciplinary collaboration between hospitals and home care (Braet, Weltens, & Sermeus, 2016). Future research is needed to appraise the long-term effects of discharge interventions.

Medication Reconciliation

Medication-related problems were the most common patient safety issue following hospital discharge to home. Older adults are particularly at risk. Nearly one in five older home care patients had at least one adverse drug event within 30 days following hospital discharge. The average number of medication discrepancies during discharge from hospital to home is 3.3 per patient (Corbett, Setter, Daratha, Neumiller, & Wood, 2010). Medication reconciliation is an effective process for avoiding medication errors during care transitions and is recommended by many patient safety organizations (Institute for Healthcare Improvement [IHI], 2008; The Joint Commission [TJC], 2015). The 2016 National Patient Safety Goals require that hospitals maintain and communicate accurate medication information and compare it with the medication information the patient brought to the hospital (TJC, 2016). Because of the complexity of the geriatric medication regimen, study findings have suggested that clinicians review the medications not only for their consistency and accuracy, but also for their appropriateness during medication reconciliation (Hu, Capezuti, Foust, Boltz, & Kim, 2012). The IHI (2008) recommends an interdisciplinary approach in reconciling medications at admission, transfer, and discharge.

Hand-Off Communication

TJC's Center for Transforming Healthcare offers a Targeted Solutions Tool (TST) that promotes high-quality hand-off and successful transfer of patients and residents (TJC, 2009). Its major recommendations are summed up by the mnemonic *SHARE*:

- Standardize critical content
- Hardwire within your system
- Allow opportunity to ask questions
- Reinforce quality and measurement
- Educate and coach

The TST emphasizes well-known strategies such as using standardized checklists and technology to access medical records, as well as novel approaches such as having the patient be present during hand-off between providers (TJC, 2009). For specific guidelines on best practices in discharge planning, the National Guideline Clearinghouse offers evidence-based core measures in conditions such as stroke and congestive heart failure (CHF; U.S. Department of Health and Human Services [n.d.]).

Patient Participation and Caregiver Involvement

Now more than ever, the value of patient participation and the meaningful involvement of caregivers are pivotal in all health care interfaces, particularly in discharge planning. Guiding principles include (a) treating patients with respect and as equal partners; (b) sharing information between providers, patients, and caregivers; (c) developing community-based primary care teams; (d) supporting holistic and individualized discharge care plans for frail older adults; and (e) facilitating a proactive approach to self-care and engaging with caregivers (Winfield & Burns, 2016). The last principle is notable because patients who are discharged from hospitals often feel overwhelmed and unprepared to learn and execute self-care skills on discharge (Graham, Ivey, & Neuhauser, 2009). Patient education and empowerment are vital to this process. To enhance and sustain health literacy and self-advocacy, TJC's *Speak Up* initiative offers patients and their representatives a script for interacting with providers and for medication administration (TJC, n.d.).

Discharge Instructions and Minority Older Adults

Because of increasing ethnic diversity in the United States, addressing specific needs of older ethnic minorities is critical. Older adults from minority populations may have different preferences and disadvantages in post-hospital health service use compared with the general population (Graham et al., 2009). Limited English proficiency is the most common barrier identified in older ethnic minorities (Hu et al., 2012). Graham et al. (2009) found that older ethnic minorities, immigrants, patients with low English proficiency, and low- and middle-income elders experience more barriers to accessing post-hospital services and information than White, English-speaking, and higher-income groups. Discharge planning for older minorities should include specific cultural and financial considerations with sufficient linguistic support. Because of varied literacy levels, the complexity of health information, and the natural process of aging, older patients' capacity to understand and use health information may be compromised (CDC, 2011). Clinicians should consider the older adults' literacy levels when designing effective discharge instructions.

SUMMARY

The interdisciplinary discharge planning team is viewed as a steward of high-quality transitions. High-risk conditions requiring particular attention in health care transitions are admitting-discharge diagnoses such as hip fracture, pneumonia, stroke, chronic obstructive pulmonary disease, and CHF (Gonçalves-Bradley et al., 2016). A Cochrane summary of 24 RCTs suggests that a patient-centered discharge plan leads to reduced hospital length of stay, reduced readmission rates, and increased care satisfaction for older people admitted to a hospital with a medical condition (Shepperd et al., 2013). Hospital strategic planning must implement best practices in discharge planning to stay competitive in an era of value-based purchasing of health care.

Fidelindo Lim and Richard Hsu

Bradway, C., Trotta, R., Bixby, M., McPartland, E., Wollman, M., Kapustka, H., & Naylor, M. D. (2012). A Qualitative analysis of an advanced practice nurse–directed transitional care model intervention. *The Gerontologist, 52*(3), 394–407.

Braet, A., Weltens, C., & Sermeus, W. (2016). Effectiveness of discharge interventions from hospital to home on hospital readmissions: A systematic review. *JBI Database of Systematic Reviews and Implementation Reports, 14*(2), 106–173. doi:10.11124/jbisrir-2016-2381

Centers for Disease Control and Prevention. (2010). National Hospital Discharge Survey: 2010 table, number and rate of hospital discharges. Retrieved from http://www.cdc.gov/nchs/data/nhds/1general/2010gen1_agesexalos.pdf

Centers for Disease Control and Prevention. (2011). Older adults: Why is health literacy important? Retrieved from http://www.cdc.gov/health literacy/developmaterials/audiences/older adults/importance.html

Centers for Medicare & Medicaid Services. (2014). *Discharge planning.* Retrieved from https://www.cms.gov/Outreach-and-Education/Medicare-Learning-Network-MLN/MLNProducts/Downloads/Discharge-Planning-Booklet-ICN908184.pdf

Coleman, E., Chugh, A., Williams, M. V., Grigsby, J., Glasheen, J. J., McKenzie, M., & Min, S. J. (2013). Understanding and execution of discharge instructions. *American Journal of Medical Quality 28*(5), 383–391. doi:10.1177/1062860612472931

Corbett, C. L., Setter, S. M., Daratha, K. B., Neumiller, J. J., & Wood, L. D. (2010). Nurse identified hospital to home medication discrepancies: Implications for improving transitional care. *Geriatric Nursing, 31*(3), 188–196.

Ellis, G., Whitehead, M. A., Robinson, D., O'Neill, D., & Langhorne, P. (2011). Comprehensive geriatric assessment for older adults admitted to hospital: Meta-analysis of randomised controlled trials. *British Medical Journal, 343,* d6553. doi:10.1136/bmj.d6553

Gonçalves-Bradley, D. C., Lannin, N. A., Clemson, L.M., Cameron, I. D., & Shepperd, S. (2016). Discharge planning from hospital. *Cochrane Database of Systematic Reviews, 2016*(1). doi:10.1002/14651858.CD000313.pub5

Gorina, Y., Pratt, L. A., Kramarow, E. A., & Elgaddal, N. (2015). Hospitalization, readmission, and death experience of noninstitutionalized Medicare fee-for-service beneficiaries aged 65 and over. Retrieved from https://www.cdc.gov/nchs/data/nhsr/nhsr084.pdf

Graham, C. L., Ivey, S. L., & Neuhauser, L. (2009). From hospital to home: Assessing the transitional care needs of vulnerable seniors. *The Gerontologist, 49*(1), 23–33.

Health Affairs. (2012). *Improving care transitions.* Retrieved from http://www.healthaffairs.org/healthpolicybriefs/brief.php?brief_id=76

Hu, S. H., Capezuti, E., Foust, J. B., Boltz, M. P., & Kim, H. (2012). Medication discrepancy and potentially inappropriate medication in older Chinese-American home-care patients after hospital discharge. *American Journal of Geriatric Pharmacotherapy, 10*(5), 284–295.

Institute for Healthcare Improvement. (2008). 5 million lives campaign. Getting started kit: Prevent adverse drug events (medication reconciliation) how-to guide. Retrieved from http://www.ihi.org/knowledge/Pages/Tools/HowtoGuidePreventAdverseDrugEvents.aspx

Institute of Medicine. (2001). *Crossing the quality chasm: A new health system for the 21st century.* Washington, DC: National Academies Press.

The Joint Commission. (n.d.). *Speak up: Planning your follow-up care.* Retrieved from http://www.jointcommission.org/assets/1/18/speakup_recovery.pdf

The Joint Commission. (2009). *Improving transitions of care: Hand-off communications.* Retrieved from http://www.centerfortrans-forminghealthcare.org/assets/4/6/CTH_Hand-off_commun_set_final_2010.pdf

The Joint Commission. (2015). National patient safety goals effective January 1, 2015. Retrieved from http://www.jointcommission.org/assets/1/6/2015_NPSG_HAP.pdf

The Joint Commission. (2016). *2016 hospital national patient safety goals.* Retrieved from https://www.jointcommission.org/assets/1/6/2016_NPSG_HAP_ER.pdf

Jones, C. E., Hollis, R. H., Wahl, T. S., Oriel, B. S., Itani, K. M., Morris, M. S., & Hawn, M. T. (2016). Transitional care interventions and hospital readmissions in surgical populations: A systematic review. *American Journal of Surgery, 212*(2), 327–335. doi:10.1016/j.amjsurg.2016.04.004

Levant, S., Chari, K., & DeFrances, C. J. (2015). Hospitalizations for patients aged 85 and over in the United States, 2000–2010. Retrieved from http://www.cdc.gov/nchs/data/databriefs/db182.pdf

Li, J., Brock, J., Jack, B., Mittman, B., Naylor, M., Sorra, J.,…Williams, M. V. (2016). Project ACHIEVE—Using implementation research to guide the evaluation of transitional care effectiveness. *BMC Health Services Research, 16*(70). doi:10.1186/s12913-016-1312-y

Lim, F. A., Foust, J., & Van Cleave, J. (2016). Transitional care models. In M. Boltz, E. Capezuti, T. Fulmer, & D. Zwicker (Eds.), *Evidence-based geriatric nursing protocols for best practice* (5th ed., pp. 633–650). New York, NY: Springer Publishing.

Schectman, J. M. (2013). Review: Interventions for patient transition from hospital to primary care may improve outcomes. *Annals of Internal Medicine, 158*(2), 1539–3704. doi:10.7326/0003-4819-158-2-201301150-02012

Shepperd, S., Lannin, N. A., Clemson, L. M., McCluskey, A., Cameron, I. D., & Barras, S. L. (2013). Discharge planning from hospital to home. *Cochrane Database of Systematic Reviews, 2013*(1), CD000313. doi:10.1002/14651858.CD000313.pub4

Stranges, E., & Friedman, B. (2008). Potentially preventable hospitalization rates declined for older adults, 2003–2007. HCUP: Statistical Brief #83. Retrieved from http://www.hcup-us.ahrq.gov/reports/statbriefs/sb83.jsp

Tian, W. (2016). An all-payer view of hospital discharge to postacute care, 2013: Statistical Brief #205. Retrieved from http://www.hcup-us.ahrq.gov/reports/statbriefs/sb205-Hospital-Discharge-Postacute-Care.pdf

U.S. Department of Health and Human Services. (n.d.). National Guidelines Clearinghouse. Retrieved from http://www.guideline.gov/search/search.aspx?term=discharge+planning

Winfield, A., & Burns, E. (2016). Let's all get home safely: A commentary on NICE and SCIE guidelines (NG27) transition between inpatient hospital settings and community or care home settings. *Age and Ageing, 45*(6), 1–4. doi:10.1093/ageing/afw151 [Epub ahead of print].

Web Resources

Centers for Medicare & Medicaid Services—Your Discharge Planning Checklist: https://www.medicare.gov/Pubs/pdf/11376.pdf

Cochrane Summaries: http://summaries.cochrane.org/CD000313/discharge-planning-from-hospital-to-home

The Joint Commission Center for Transforming Healthcare—Targeted Solutions Tool for Hand-off Communications: http://www.centerfortransforminghealthcare.org/tst_hoc.aspx

The Joint Commission Speak up: Planning Your Follow-up Care, http://www.jointcommission.org/assets/1/18/speakup_recovery.pdf

National Guidelines Clearinghouse: http://guideline.gov/search/search.aspx?term=discharge+planning

National Patient Safety Foundation—Ask Me 3: http://c.ymcdn.com/sites/www.npsf.org/resource/resmgr/AskMe3/AskMe3_HealthLiteracyTrainin.pdf?hhSearchTerms=%22ask+and+3%22

DIZZINESS

Dizziness or vertigo accounts for approximately 3.9 million of all emergency department visits in the United States, with a total extrapolated 2011 national cost of $3.9 billion (Saber Tehrani et al., 2013). In the community and in primary care settings, dizziness is more common in women than in men and increases with age, with an estimated prevalence of dizziness among elderly to be between 20% and 35% (Sloane, Coeytaux, Beck, & Dallara, 2001). Dizziness increases the risk of accidental falls, which leads to hospital admissions, loss of independence, and subsequently, reduced perceptions of quality of life in older adults.

The term *dizziness* applies to various subjective sensory experiences. Patients use this term to refer to lightheadedness, faintness, disequilibrium, vertigo, blurred vision, and giddiness. *The most useful part of the evaluation is the history.* Therefore the clinician must first determine what the patient means by the word. The clinician should elicit the patient's own description of the event *without* prompting, determine character of symptoms (e.g., spinning, fainting, or falling) and any positional effects, and ask about associated complaints. In addition, the most up-to-date medication list should be obtained. Physical examination should include orthostatic blood pressures and pulse, a cardiac examination, a check for nystagmus, and a thorough cerebellar and gait evaluation. For all older patients, the Dix–Hallpike and head-thrust maneuvers are also important to perform. Laboratory assessment helps rule out other metabolic, infectious, and cardiac etiologies of dizziness and should be interpreted in the context of any prior results.

TYPES OF DIZZINESS

Dizziness is classically divided into four types: (a) vertigo—a false sense of movement or spinning of the body or environment, usually caused by problems in the vestibular system; (b) presyncope—a lightheadedness described as a feeling of being about to faint, caused by reduced blood flow to the brain; (c) disequilibrium—a sense of imbalance or postural instability that occurs primarily when walking, which is described as a sensation of unsteadiness in the lower extremities, usually caused by neurological disease; and (d) other—vague sensations not covered by the other three types of dizziness and often associated with anxiety or depression. Of note is a physiological form of dizziness, motion sickness, which is induced by movement (e.g., amusement rides, automobiles, and airplanes), visual stimuli, or odor (e.g., industrial pollutants) that can be induced in almost all humans and is not necessarily indicative of a disease process.

Determining whether dizziness is due to a central (e.g., brain tumor, cerebrovascular disease, multiple sclerosis) or a peripheral (e.g., benign paroxysmal positional vertigo, labyrinthitis, Méniére's disease) cause is key. The sudden onset of dizziness in older persons generally has a single cause, such as an acute illness, new medication, or stroke. Chronic dizziness generally has multiple causes, although one factor is usually most important. Health care providers should search for treatable causes and contributing factors, including anxiety or depression, decreased vision, and medication side effects.

Vertigo

Benign paroxysmal positional vertigo (BPPV) is one of the most common causes of dizziness in older persons (Fife et al., 2008). A spinning sensation usually accompanies changing the position of the head. The sensation is caused when calcium carbonate crystals (otoliths) break loose from the saccule or utricle of the inner ear and move into the posterior semicircular canal. Once positioned in the canal or in its receptor, the particles amplify rotational movements in the plane of the canal. Thus when the patient moves in the plane of the posterior semicircular canal, a short burst of intense vertigo occurs.

Clinically, BPPV is characterized by recurrent episodes of intense vertigo lasting 1 minute or less (usually 5–15 seconds). These episodes are triggered by different head movements such as rolling over in bed, getting in and out of bed, bending over, and straightening up. Typically, patients have vertigo attacks with slight rotatory movement. After intense vertigo, a sensation of lightheadedness or mild vertigo can wax and wane for hours to days. Symptoms improve rapidly and typically resolve in days to weeks.

A simple clinical test, named the Dix–Hallpike or Barany maneuver, can help diagnose this condition. With the patient sitting on an examination table, the head is turned 45 degrees with the neck extended. Then, the patient placed supine so that the head hangs over the table; the clinician observes for nystagmus (e.g., to-and-fro movement of the eyeballs) for 30 seconds and asks about subjective symptoms of vertigo. Return the patient to the sitting position and observe for nystagmus for another 30 seconds. The maneuver is repeated with the patient's head rotated to the opposite side. With older patients, slow or gentle movements should be used, and caution should be exercised when extending the neck of a patient with a prior history of vertebrobasilar compromise or prior stroke. A positive response produces vertigo, rotatory nystagmus, and latency (i.e., dizziness and nystagmus after few seconds), and the symptoms often diminish with repeated testing. Evidence-based review shows repositioning maneuvers such as the Epley and Semont are safe and effective and should be recommended to all patients with BPPV (Fife et al., 2008). On the contrary, medication is generally not helpful for BPPV because symptoms occur only for a short duration.

Labyrinthitis (i.e., inflammation of the inner ear, also known as vestibular neuronitis and vestibular neuritis) is characterized by abrupt onset of severe vertigo and sparing of other neurological functions. The most common cause is viral. Symptomatic treatment using antiemetics, anticholinergics, and antihistamines may be helpful. Vestibular exercises and a short course of high-dose oral corticosteroids may also aid in recovery (Kerber & Baloh, 2011). The condition usually occurs acutely, is self-limited, and typically begins to resolve in 24 to 36 hours.

Ménière's disease is a triad of recurrent vertigo, tinnitus, and hearing loss. Initially, hearing loss is noted only during vertigo attacks; later, a fixed, low-frequency loss can be demonstrated. Attacks of dizziness typically last between 2 and 12 hours. Often, patients complain of "fullness" or "pressure" within the ear but no pain. The frequency and severity of vertigo may improve as hearing impairment progressively worsens. Vestibular rehabilitation (physical therapy) uses exercises to maximize balance and may reduce symptoms of dizziness (Cabrera Kang & Tusa, 2013). Although medical management such as a low-salt diet and diuretics are commonly prescribed, there is insufficient evidence to support any treatment (Kerber & Baloh, 2011). Surgical treatment is reserved for patients with severe symptoms who do not respond to medical management.

Presyncope

Presyncopal dizziness is distinctive and caused by diminished cerebral oxygenation. It leads to a feeling that one is about to pass out. Patients describe a need to sit or lie down, with darkening of the vision (both eyes) or simply as intense lightheadedness. Episodes typically lasts seconds to hours and usually occurs when the patient is upright or in a sitting position. Nausea and weakness often accompany the dizziness. Patients who lose consciousness are said to experience syncope. Some causes of presyncope and syncope are transient conditions that affect systems involved with postural control (e.g., cerebral cortex, brainstem/cerebellum, vestibular portion of the inner ear/eighth cranial nerve, proprioceptive pathways in the neck or lower extremities, peripheral nerves, skeletal muscle, and autonomic nervous system). Also, abnormalities of the cardiovascular system (e.g., arrhythmias, myocardial infarction, and aortic stenosis) and medical conditions (e.g., anemia, excessive diuresis, diabetes, and adrenal insufficiency) are other causes.

Disequilibrium

Chronic disequilibrium in older persons, especially in those aged 85 years and older, is commonly associated with either cervical spondylosis (i.e., neck arthritis) or cerebral ischemia/infarction, often involving small vessels. Persons with ischemic disease generally report a sudden or stepwise onset, have gait abnormalities on physical examination, and demonstrate subcortical white-matter lesions on MRI of the brain. Other factors that may contribute to imbalance include chronic vestibulopathies, visual problems, musculoskeletal disorders, and somatosensory or gait deficits.

Anxiety and Depression

Anxiety and depression are the most common causes of chronic, continual dizziness in younger populations. In older persons with chronic dizziness, psychiatric dysfunction is common, as well, but is rarely the primary cause. Treatment of these secondary psychiatric conditions, however, can reduce disability and improve function.

Many other conditions may cause chronic dizziness. Cerebellar atrophy, which may be idiopathic or secondary to degenerative conditions such as alcoholism, leads to a continuous feeling of disequilibrium. Middle-ear disease or sinusitis can produce vertigo or more vague sensations of continuous dizziness. Bilateral vestibular hypofunction is another cause (e.g., aminoglycoside toxicity). Other causes include sarcoidosis, carcinomatous meningitis, and syphilis. Brain tumors account for less than 1% of cases, the most common being an acoustic neuroma (i.e., tinnitus and hearing loss). In older adults, prescription-drug toxicity is an important contributing factor, especially when five or more medications are taken. High-risk drugs include any that cause orthostatic hypotension (e.g., cardiovascular, antihypertensive, psychotropic, and diuretic medications).

DIAGNOSTIC TESTING

Neuroimaging (i.e., CT scan, MRI) is occasionally needed, especially if there are focal findings on neurologic examination or if stroke is suspected. MRI is more sensitive than CT scan for the evaluation of posterior fossa structures (e.g., brain stem, cerebellum). MRI is also recommended if there is hearing loss associated with vertigo resulting from acoustic neuroma and if the duration of vertigo is prolonged (i.e., several months) for evaluation of multiple sclerosis and cerebellar degeneration. Magnetic resonance angiography of the posterior circulation helps assess for vascular disease in elderly patients with risk factors.

Diagnostic testing with audiometry may help if cochlear symptoms (e.g., tinnitus, asymmetric hearing loss) are present, and abnormal results may indicate Ménière's disease or acoustic neuroma. Vestibular testing (e.g., electronystagmography, brain-stem auditory evoked responses, rotatory chair test, and dynamic posturography) may be helpful. EEG is typically not useful and ECG is low yield with normal cardiac examination and no syncope. Studies that are not useful for isolated dizziness include Holter and event monitors, echocardiography, stress testing, tilt-table, and electrophysiological studies. However, among nonvertigo causes, it is imperative to rule out cardiac causes of dizziness, especially if the patient experiences palpitations, irregular heart rhythm, or tachycardia. If a cardiac cause of dizziness is suspected, then evaluation with ECG, Holter and/or event monitoring, and echocardiography would be indicated.

See also Falls Prevention; Hearing Impairment.

Chin Hwa (Gina) Dahlem and Chin Suk Yi

Cabrera Kang, C. M., & Tusa, R. J. (2013). Vestibular rehabilitation: Rationale and indications. *Seminars in Neurology, 33*(3), 276–285. doi:10.1055/s-0033-1354593

Fife, T. D, Iverson, D. J., Lempert, T., Furman, J. M., Baloh, R. W., Tusa, R. J.,…Gronseth, G. S. (2008). Practice parameter: Therapies for benign paroxysmal positional vertigo (an evidence-based review): Report of the Quality Standards Subcommittee of the American Academy of Neurology. *Neurology, 70,* 2067–2074.

Kerber, K. A., & Baloh, R. W. (2011). The evaluation of a patient with dizziness. *Neurology Clinical Practice, 1*(1), 24–33.

Saber Tehrani, A. S., Coughlan, D., Hsieh, Y. H., Mantokoudis, G., Korley, F. K., Kerber, K. A.,…Newman-Toker, D. E. (2013). Rising annual costs of dizziness presentations to U.S. emergency departments. *Academic Emergency Medicine, 20*(7), 689–696. doi:10.1111/acem.12168

Sloane, P. D., Coeytaux, R. R., Beck, R. S., & Dallara, J. (2001). Dizziness: State of the science. *Annals of Internal Medicine, 134*(9, Pt. 2), 823–32.

D

Web Resources

American Family Physician Dizziness: A Diagnostic Approach: http://www.aafp.org/afp/2010/0815/p361.html

Chicago Dizziness and Hearing: http://www.dizziness-and-balance.com/disorders

Medline Plus: http://www.nlm.nih.gov/medlineplus/dizzinessandvertigo.html

NIH Senior Health: http://nihseniorhealth.gov/balanceproblems/causesriskfactorsandprevention/01.html

Vestibular Disorders Association: http://www.vestibular.org

DRIVING

As the population in the United States ages and continues to be active, there is an increasing number of drivers older than 70 years (Insurance Institute for Highway Safety [IIHS], 2016). Because the majority of older adults prefer the use of a private automobile for mobility, they are driving longer distances and for a greater number of years and, for the first time in history, are outliving their ability to drive safely (American Automobile Association [AAA] Exchange, 2016a). Although research has shown that older drivers are involved in fewer accidents than they were a decade ago and are less likely to be injured, accident and fatality rates start to increase for those drivers aged 70 years and older (IIHS, 2016).

Age alone is a poor predictor of motor vehicle accidents (National Highway Traffic Safety Administration [NHTSA], 2016) because older adults are living longer, healthier, and more active lives. However, driving safety can, in part, be related to physical, visual and/or mental changes associated with aging and/or disease (American Geriatrics Society [AGS] & Pomidor, 2016). If there are any concerns about driving safety, the health professional should assess the older driver, using the Clinical Assessment of Driving-Related Skills (CADReS) Older-Driver Screening Tool, which assesses vision, cognition, motor, and somatosensory skills (AGS & Pomidor, 2016). Computer simulation or an on-road driving assessment can be important pieces in the decision regarding driver safety (Wiese & Wolff, 2016). Depending on the condition affecting driving, a change in medical treatment, including medications, may be necessary, or a referral to physical or occupational therapy may be useful in treating joint dysfunction and muscle atrophy, thereby increasing driving safety. An occupational therapist may recommend changes to the vehicle that will further enhance driving ability and safety.

Health professionals and family members need to recognize that, although many older adults believe that they are safe drivers, they alter their driving habits when their functional abilities decline. Older drivers with reported visual, memory, physical functioning, and/or medical conditions reported self-limited driving, especially reducing driving at night, driving less often, and driving shorter distances (IIHS, 2016). Those who have no reason to drive may live with a family member, have easy access to public transportation, or be within walking distance of needed services.

Older adults may self-screen for driver safety using tools such as the AAA Drivers 65 Plus brochure or the interactive Roadwise Review (AAA, 2016a). AAA also offers a comprehensive website: www.seniordrivers.org, for older drivers and family members to learn about the impact of age-related changes, medical conditions, and medications on driving skills (AAA, 2016b). Self-assessment results should not be the sole assessment of driving safety but can be a starting point in a conversation with the older driver and family regarding safety concerns and risk of accidents.

Health professionals should know whether state laws require them to report unsafe drivers to licensing authorities (AGS & Pomidor, 2016). In states where reporting is not mandated, professional responsibility for the safety of older adults, other drivers, and pedestrians suggests the importance of voluntary reporting. Familiarity with driver's license renewal policies, which vary by state, is also essential. *The Clinicians Guide to Assessing and Counseling Older Drivers*, 3rd edition (AGS & Pomidor, 2016) can assist health professionals in evaluating the ability of older patients to drive safely.

Assessment and discussion regarding the safety of an older driver is an essential but often difficult task for health professionals and should occur annually and prior to restricting driving privileges (AGS & Pomidor, 2016). It may be complicated by well-intentioned family members who have made subtle attempts to convince the older adult to stop driving. The health professional should acknowledge the role that driving has played in the individual's independence and self-esteem. Older adults need to be given the opportunity to discuss the impact that restricted or lost driving privileges may have on their lives. These include lack of access to essential services, such as shopping and health care; social isolation and loneliness; limited recreational opportunities; increased risk of falls due to the need to walk under potentially dangerous conditions, such as ice and snow; loss of income if still employed; and diminished quality of life. The possibility of early or forced entry into assisted-living or nursing home facilities is also a reality that warrants discussion.

The availability of alternate forms of public transportation should be discussed as an option, although they may be inconvenient, expensive, inaccessible, unreliable, or unavailable. Efforts should be made to reduce isolation and help nondriving elders remain engaged in social activities. Friends, family members, and church groups can be queried about their willingness to assist with transportation, particularly when public transportation is unavailable. Although family and friends may promise assistance, such commitments are not always honored, however. Broken promises add to the frustration and isolation already experienced by non-driving elders.

The events leading to a reduction in driving or the loss of a license occur over time. They are not necessarily sequential, and not all older adults experience them. Because many individuals drive safely well into old age, health care providers should not assume that all elders are unsafe drivers.

See also Occupational Therapists; Physical Therapists.

Michelle Pardee

American Automobile Association. (2016a). Senior driver safety. Retrieved from http://exchange .aaa.com/safety/senior-driver-safety

American Automobile Association. (2016b). SeniorDrivingAAA.com. Retrieved from http://www.seniordrivers.org

American Geriatrics Society & Pomidor, A. (Ed.). (2016, January). *Clinician's guide to assessing and counseling older drivers, 3rd edition.* (Report No. DOT HS 812 228). Washington, DC: National Highway Traffic Safety Administration.

Insurance Institute for Highway Safety. (2016). Overview older drivers. Retrieved from http://www.iihs.org/iihs/topics/t/older-drivers/topicoverview

National Highway Traffic Safety Administration, Department of Transportation. (2016). Driving safety—Older drivers. Retrieved from http://www.nhtsa.gov/Driving+Safety/Older+Drivers

Wiese, L., & Wolff, L. (2016, June 6). Supporting safety in the older adult driver: A public health nursing opportunity. *Public Health Nursing,* 1–12. doi:10.1111/phn.12274

Web Resources
Administration for Community Living: https://www.acl.gov

American Automobile Association (AAA): http://seniordriving.aaa.com

American Geriatrics Society (AGS): http://www.americangeriatrics.org

Centers for Disease Control and Prevention: http://www.cdc.gov/features/olderdrivers

National Highway Traffic Safety Administration (driving safety—older driver): http://www.nhtsa.gov

DYSPNEA (SHORTNESS OF BREATH)

Dyspnea, widely defined in the past as an *objective* description of shortness of breath, is now considered by the American Thoracic Society (ATS) to be an umbrella term that encompasses *subjective* experiences of breathing discomfort associated with different sensory qualities. Furthermore, the ATS emphasizes that these distinct sensations often do occur not in isolation, but from "the interactions among multiple physiological, psychological, social and environmental factors and may include secondary physiological and behavioral responses" (pp. 436–437). The most significant finding by the ATS regarding dyspnea is its updated statement of 2012 that declares "as is the case with pain, adequate assessment of dyspnea depends on self report" (Parshall et al., 2012, p. 437).

PREVALENCE IN ELDERLY POPULATIONS

The work of breathing can increase by as much as 20% between the ages of 20 and 60 (Karnani, Reisfield, & Wilson, 2005). Dyspnea is common in the older population, with a pooled prevalence of 36.3% in individuals older than 65 years (Van Mourik et al., 2014), leading to the conclusion that dyspnea may be considered a "normal phenomenon" in the geriatric population. Increasing age affects the prevalence of dyspnea more than gender, although women experience dyspnea more commonly than men (Mahler & Baird, 2005). In the general population, labored breathing or shortness of breath is a frequent problem reported by up to 50% of patients admitted to acute, tertiary care hospitals and by 25% of patients in ambulatory settings; it causes 3 to 4 million emergency department visits each year (Parshall et al., 2012).

MECHANISMS OF DYSPNEA

Three categories are commonly identified as mechanisms of dyspnea: increased work or effort, chest tightness, and air hunger/unsatisfied inspiration. The mechanism behind each helps health care professionals understand and treat the elderly, but these sensations of dyspnea rarely occur in a pure or isolated fashion (Parshall et al., 2012).

Work of breathing: An uncomfortable sense of "work" or "effort" occurs when the capacity to match ventilation to metabolic demand becomes insufficient. Normally, when metabolic demands occur in health individuals, physiological adaptations occur that increase alveolar ventilation so that breathing distress is minimal. Chronic obstructive pulmonary disease (COPD) and asthma, which cause air trapping, impair those physiological adaptations. When the diaphragm, the major muscle of breathing, becomes flattened and weak in cases of COPD, the use of accessory muscles becomes apparent. Similarly, the resistance to bronchial airflow and air trapping seen in asthma increases the work of breathing. Any impairment of respiratory function can cause a heightened awareness of the work of breathing. Motor command to the respiratory muscles is increased, causing the perception of inspiratory effort and work to be substantially magnified in these patients, even if the actual ventilation has not significantly increased.

Chest tightness: Complaints of "pressure or constriction," are frequently related to bronchoconstriction, and this condition is a dominant experience in the early stages of an asthma attack. During asthma exacerbations, patients also report increased work of breathing and air hunger. The mechanism of this tightness or pressure is more specifically related to stimulation of airway afferent receptors rather than to increased respiratory muscle work/effort.

Air hunger/unsatisfied inspiration is the perception of insufficient pulmonary ventilation. Air hunger is not specific to a particular disease but has been reported in patients with asthma, COPD, interstitial lung disease, and neuromuscular disease when there is an increase in spontaneous ventilatory drive such as exercise (hypoxia, hypercapnia, acidosis) or emotions (limbic system). The use of the accessory muscles of breathing and the inability to finish a sentence without pausing to breathe are frequent signs of dyspnea from air hunger. The sensation, described as smothering, suffocating, not enough air, or inability to breathe, is sufficiently distressing to provoke an emergency department visit.

Dyspnea also may be caused by vascular problems such as congestive heart failure (CHF) and pulmonary hypertension in response to vascular J receptors. Paroxysmal nocturnal dyspnea (PND), usually associated with CHF, is the sudden onset, during the night, of difficulty breathing and coughing after sleeping in the recumbent position. It occurs 1 to 2 hours after lying down and is relieved after assuming an upright position. Orthopnea is the inability to breathe when attempting to lie down; to obtain relief, several pillows are usually needed to elevate the upper body. Orthopnea is very common in end-stage COPD but also occurs in other pulmonary diseases and left-sided heart failure. Dyspnea on exertion (DOE) is also very common in obstructive diseases, especially emphysema with its associated hypoxemia, and in restrictive diseases (specifically, interstitial lung disease), because of decreased lung compliance. Painful dyspnea suggests pleural, intercostal, thoracic, or even subdiaphragmatic inflammation. Finally, signs of difficulty inspiring should always be assessed for upper airway obstruction, such as aspiration.

ASSESSMENT

Measurement of dyspnea can be achieved through numerous validated instruments. Several widely used instruments are available to provide assessment of patient experiences and perceptions such as "description of breathlessness" or "severity of breathlessness" (Dorman, Byrne, & Edwards, 2007), categorization of intensity or severity (Mularski et al., 2010), and effects on health-related quality of life (Chhabra, Gupta, & Khuma, 2009; Nishimura, Izumi, Tsukino, & Oga, 2002). Yannacone, Carrieri-Kohlman, and Barbour (2016) found that consistent use of validated scales increases nurses' confidence and assessment in recognizing and treating dyspnea in palliative care patients. Common scales for dyspnea are the Borg Rating of Perceived Exertion (RPE), Respiratory Distress Observation Scale (RDOS), Modified Medical Research Council (MMRC) scale, Baseline Dyspnea Index (BDI), and Oxygen Cost Diagram (OCD). It is worth noting that some people adjust their physical activities to not experience dyspnea, so several instruments may need to be used before an appropriate evaluation can be made. The severity of DOE can be gauged more objectively by distance covered and the pulse oximetry results during a 6-minute walk test (6MWT) or the number of stairs completed in 2 minutes (2MST). Evidence supports the need to include both objective and subjective assessment of dyspnea (Parshall et al., 2012).

Pulmonary function tests (PFTs), arterial blood gas (ABG) sampling or pulse oximetry, and auscultation also provide information for the differential diagnosis. Spirometry is useful in evaluating dyspnea because self-reporting of dyspnea does not always correlate with objective PFTs. ABG results aid in differentiating a respiratory versus a metabolic etiology. Pulse oximetry results are lower in pulmonary patients, due to the decrease in the diffusion of oxygen. Wheezing, heard on auscultation, usually indicates narrowing of the bronchi, as in asthma, but cardiac wheezes also may be heard with CHF. Physical examination of patients with CHF may be remarkable for increased work of breathing associated with dyspnea and fluid overload. Early left-sided heart failure often presents clinically as cough and dyspnea with exertion. With further disease progression, dyspnea at rest may occur.

A chest x-ray is not directly a diagnostic tool for dyspnea but can provide information about heart size, lung parenchyma, pulmonary vasculature, pleural space, and diaphragm position, which may influence breathing patterns or perceptions.

TREATMENT

The treatment of dyspnea may best be correlated to several main categories of shortness of breath: cardiac, pulmonary, central nervous system (CNS), and neuromuscular disorders (Brywczynski, 2010).

One approach to the treatment of dyspnea is to help elderly individuals self-regulate their breathing through biofeedback mechanisms. Pulmonary rehabilitation improves functional capacity in chronically dyspneic lung patients aged 80 years of age or older (Baltzan, Kamel, Alter, Rotaple, & Wolkove, 2004) and has been shown to improve outcomes in quality of life and dyspnea (Schroff et al., 2017). One example of a breathing-retraining strategy is pursed-lip breathing. The external resistance to expiration through pursed lips increases airway pressure and prevents airway collapse. Other techniques

D

include moving at a slower pace with paced breathing, diaphragmatic breathing, use of an inspiratory muscle training device, and relaxation to decrease anxiety. Upper body movements such as hair combing are especially demanding, but elders can learn energy-conservation techniques through evidence-based pulmonary rehabilitation programs.

Symptomatic relief has been reported by directing a fan at the face or sitting before an open window. The air movement is thought to stimulate facial receptors that alter the perception of breathlessness (Mahler, Fierro-Carrion, & Baird, 2003). It is also important to be aware of indoor pollutants that can trigger dyspnea, such as cooking fumes, wood fires, perfume, cleaning agents, dust mites, and dry air.

Obesity and the resulting increased intra-abdominal pressure on the diaphragm and lung can make a dyspneic episode worse. Added pounds increase the workload of the cardio-pulmonary system. Diet modifications and graduated exercise are encouraged and are an important component of pulmonary rehabilitation programs. Exercise benefits dyspneic individuals, especially those with chronic respiratory diseases, by increasing endurance and reducing the subjective sensation of breathlessness.

Fatigue is often a major accompaniment of dyspnea. Elders and their caregivers need to pace periods of activity and rest. Paying attention to the location of elevators and rest rooms and obtaining a handicapped parking permit are helpful ways of decreasing fatigue as well as dyspnea.

Appropriate management of underlying cardiac, pulmonary, infectious, or neurological conditions can offer patients significant relief. When dyspnea occurs or is exacerbated, it may be a sign of pulmonary infection with associated bronchial inflammation and secretions. Teaching a person to cough productively can improve pulmonary reserve. Adherence to prescribed medication schedules is vital. In addition to oral and inhaled medications, low-flow oxygen can help maintain acceptable arterial oxygen saturation, especially for those with DOE. Some elders are reluctant to go out in public with portable oxygen and need encouragement to do so because research has

shown that continuous oxygen therapy (i.e., 24 hours/day and not prn) successfully decreases the progression of right-sided heart failure. Adequate treatment and reasonable control of dyspnea can improve the quality of life for elders who must deal with it as part of their everyday lives.

Joan Kreiger, Christine G. Fitzgerald, and Christine E. Niekrash

Baltzan, M. A., Kamel, H., Alter, A., Rotaple, M., & Wolkove, N. (2004). Pulmonary rehabilitation improves functional capacity in patients 80 years of age or older. *Canadian Respiratory Journal, 11*(6), 407–413.

Brywczynski, J. (2010). Shortness of breath: Prehospital treatment of respiratory distress. *Journal of Emergency Medical Services, 35*(5), 56–63. doi:10.1016/S0197-2510(10)70122-4

Chhabra, S. K., Gupta, A. K., & Khuma, M. Z. (2009). Evaluation of three scales of dyspnea in chronic obstructive pulmonary disease. *Annals of Thoracic Medicine, 4*(3), 128–132.

Dorman, S., Byrne, A., & Edwards, A. (2007). Which measurement scales should we use to measure breathlessness in palliative care? A systematic review. *Palliative Medicine, 21*(3), 177–191.

Karnani, N. G., Reisfield, G. M., & Wilson, G. R. (2005). Evaluation of chronic dyspnea. *American Family Physician, 71*(8), 1529–1537.

Mahler, D. A., & Baird, J. C. (2005). *Dyspnea: Mechanisms, measurement, and management* (2nd ed.). New York, NY: Taylor & Francis.

Mahler, D. A., Fierro-Carrion, G., & Baird, J. C. (2003). Evaluation of dyspnea in the elderly. *Clinics in Geriatric Medicine, 19*(1), 19–33, v.

Mularski, R. A., Campbell, M. L., Asch, S. M., Reeve, B. B., Basch, E., Maxwell, T. L.,...Dy, S. (2010). A review of quality of care evaluation for the palliation of dyspnea. *American Journal of Respiratory and Critical Care Medicine, 181*(6), 534–538.

Nishimura, K., Izumi, T., Tsukino, M., & Oga, T. (2002). Dyspnea is a better predictor of 5-year survival than airway obstruction in patients with COPD. *Chest, 121*(5), 1434–1440.

Parshall, M. B., Schwartzstein, R. M., Adams, L., Banzett, R. B., Manning, H. L., Bourbeau, J.,... American Thoracic Society Committee on Dyspnea. (2012). An official American Thoracic Society statement: Update on the mechanisms, assessment, and management of dyspnea. *American Journal of Respiratory and Critical Care*

Medicine, 185(4), 435–452. doi:10.1164/rccm.201111 -2042ST

Schroff, P., Hitchcock, J., Schumann, C., Wells, J. M., Dransfield, M. T., & Bhatt, S. P. (2017). Pulmonary rehabilitation improves outcomes in chronic obstructive pulmonary disease independent of disease burden. *Annals of the American Thoracic Society, 14*(1), 26–32.

van Mourik, Y., Rutten, F. H., Moons, K. G., Bertens, L. C., Hoes, A. W., & Reitsma, J. B. (2014). Prevalence and underlying causes of dyspnoea in older people: A systematic review. *Age and Ageing, 43*(3), 319–326.

Yannacone, M., Carrieri-Kohlman, V., & Barbour, S. (2016). Use of validated dyspnea scales increase nurses' confidence in their assessment and treatment of dyspnea in palliative care patients. *American Journal of Respiratory and Critical Care Medicine, 193*, A2894.

Web Resources

American Association for Respiratory Care: http:// www.aarc.org

American Heart Association: http://americanheart.gov

American Lung Association: http://www.lungusa .org

American Thoracic Society: http://www.thoracic .org

D

E

ELDER MISTREATMENT: OVERVIEW

Elder mistreatment (EM) is an umbrella term for a variety of behaviors that can cause potential or actual harm to older adults. Actions usually included in this category are abuse, neglect, and financial exploitation of those who are in a trusting relationship to an older adult (Bonnie & Wallace, 2003). Many professionals also include self-neglect, whether intentional or unintentional, as a type of EM. The National Research Council defines *EM* as either: "intentional actions that cause harm or create serious risk of harm (whether or not harm is intended) to a vulnerable elder by a caregiver or other person who is in a trust relationship to the elder" or "failure by a caregiver to satisfy the elder's basic needs or to protect himself or herself from harm" (Bonnie & Wallace, 2003, p. 1). It is important to note that this definition intentionally excludes cases of self-neglect and victimization of older adults by strangers. EM can take place in a variety of settings from the home to institutional settings such as nursing homes, hospitals, and assisted-living facilities.

Data suggest that in the United States, as many as 1 in 10 older adults experience some form of EM. Among community-dwelling older adults with dementia, EM rates appear to be much higher, at approximately 47% (Institute of Medicine and National Research Council, 2014). Although data from recent studies indicate that EM may be twice as common as previously thought (Anetzberger, 2012), it is difficult to estimate the exact number of mistreated elders because EM is widely underreported, with only approximately 16% of cases reported (National Center on Elder Abuse, 1998). For every case of EM reported, it is believed that as many as 5 to 14 cases are unreported (Cohen, Levin, Gagin, & Friedman, 2007; Schecter & Dougherty, 2009).

Cases of EM are expected to increase as the percentage of older adults composing the world's population continues to grow.

Definitions of the types of EM vary from state to state and across countries, which makes measuring its prevalence challenging, but general concepts apply (Institute of Medicine, 2014). All forms of EM may occur in either the community or the institutional setting. *Physical abuse*, for example, is usually defined as deliberate behavior meant to cause physical pain and harm and usually includes actions such as hitting, punching, kicking, biting, and threatening a person with a weapon or using a weapon. Sexual abuse of older adults involves unwanted sexual conduct. *Elder neglect*, which represents approximately 50% of reported cases (National Center on Elder Abuse, 1998), is generally defined as failure to provide for the adequate care of an older adult in terms of housing, food, clothing, personal hygiene, medical care, and medications needed to maintain health and well-being. Neglect can be divided into self-neglect, which occurs when older adults fail to provide these essentials for themselves; active neglect, when caregivers deliberately withhold food, clothing, money, and so forth; and passive neglect, when caregivers do not deliberately withhold necessities but may be unaware of the need because of a lack of knowledge or resources to provide adequate care. Emotional abuse is generally described as any action with the deliberate intent of causing emotional, psychological, or mental pain or distress and includes harassment, verbal assaults, social isolation, insults, threats, and intimidation. Financial exploitation is the intentional obtaining of an older person's money or assets by someone with no legal right to that money for personal use or benefit. This can include fraud, embezzlement, or undue influence (Institute of Medicine, 2014; Bonnie & Wallace, 2003).

The reporting of EM is an important aspect of elder care in the United States. As of 2012, all 50 states have laws addressing this issue; however, three states did not specify mandatory reporting requirements (Jirik & Sanders, 2014). In many states, certain professionals (including doctors, nurses, social workers, other types of health care and home care workers, and law-enforcement officers) must report all suspected cases of EM to the appropriate state agency. For these persons, 42 states have instituted penalties for failing to report suspected abuse (Jirik & Sanders, 2014). In 17 states, mandated reporting has been extended to all adults, meaning that any adult who suspects EM is expected to report it to the responsible agency (Jirik & Sanders, 2014). Definitions for what constitutes EM differ across the United States, with all 50 states offering some protections against physical abuse, 44 against emotional or psychological abuse, 37 against sexual abuse, 13 against abandonment, and 40 against self-neglect, but only 10 states protecting older adults from all types of abuse (Jirik & Sanders, 2014). In many, but not all, states, the name of the person reporting the suspected EM is confidential. In addition, all states have included a Good Samaritan clause in their legislation. This protects the person reporting the suspected mistreatment from a civil lawsuit if the investigating agency decides that no mistreatment has occurred, as long as the reporting person can show that there was no malicious intent. It appears that some are deterred from reporting suspected mistreatment for fear that it may worsen or escalate it; these fears are unsubstantiated.

The individuals protected by EM legislation vary across the country, which further complicates estimating prevalence (Jirik & Sanders, 2014). In some states, the only requirement for protection under the law is the achievement of a certain age, often 60 or 65 (Jirik & Sanders, 2014). In other states, the person must be a certain age and must be considered "vulnerable," meaning that the person has some physical, cognitive, or mental impairment. Other states use a combination of these two concepts. The legal restrictions can sometimes impede attempts to report suspected EM because, in the judgment of the investigator, the alleged victim may not meet the requirements for being a vulnerable adult.

The locations where EM occurs are as varied as the places where older adults live. Much of the early work on EM focused on those living in the community who live independently or with family. This focus is appropriate, because of the majority of older adults, healthy or frail, live in the community. Interest in EM in institutional settings has increased with the realization that older adults residing in these facilities are among the most vulnerable and thus highly dependent on others (Castle, Ferguson-Rome, & Teresi, 2015). For those in caring roles, it is important to recognize that statements of fear or concern about being taken advantage of may be more than a paranoid or delusional response; they may be indications that the older adult is being mistreated.

Providing a general profile of perpetrators of EM is difficult and somewhat less accurate than previously thought because it may vary depending on the type of mistreatment. Therefore the profile of perpetrators has minimal use in identifying at-risk older adults. First, the age of the person who commits EM varies, depending on the relationship between the person who is mistreated and the perpetrator. Perpetrators can be spouses, adult children, parents, grandchildren, other relatives, friends, or complete strangers. In the case of spouses, the age difference may be a few years but with other family members, friends, or strangers, the age span may be greater. Nevertheless, it is still possible to make some general comments about persons who are likely to mistreat older adults. Some research indicates that perpetrators often have problems with substance abuse or other emotional or psychological problems that contribute to their propensity to mistreat older adults (Johannesen & LoGiudice, 2013; Labrum, Solomon, & Bressi, 2015).

Similarly, a profile of the mistreated older adult is difficult to establish and varies with the type of EM; however, some general trends do emerge. Women are more likely to be mistreated than men, and the age of mistreated persons may range from the early 60s to well into the 80s, although the age range is somewhat higher for institutional abuse (Fulmer et al., 2005; National Center on Elder Abuse, 1998). Much of the research suggests that physical frailty or cognitive impairment, such as dementia, may make an older adult more vulnerable to EM (Institute of Medicine, 2014). Finally, social isolation of both the mistreated older adults and perpetrators has also been identified as a factor supported by studies (Anetzberger, 2012).

Recently, EM experts have encouraged a shift away from profiling victims and perpetrators in favor of the development of new theories. One theoretical explanation cannot account for all types of mistreatment or commonalities that may exist between victims of each kind. McDonald and Thomas (2013) utilized the life course perspective as a framework that can be incorporated into other theories of EM and at varying levels of analysis. Four factors were predictive of mistreatment in elders using this approach, including depression, functional deficits, non-White ethnicity, and history of child abuse (McDonald & Thomas, 2013). However, it is important to underscore this does not imply a causal relationship between experiencing abuse as a child and later EM in life. Expanding theory development is a challenging yet important area to guide future EM research.

Although an understanding of the victims and perpetrators of EM is useful, it is most important to examine how we can address and respond to EM. Recent data indicate that older adults suspected of being victims of EM are willing to accept services (Clancy, McDaid, O'Neill, & O'Brien, 2011); however, there is a dearth of intervention research examining the best strategies for addressing EM (Dong, 2015; Ploeg, Fear, Hutchison, MacMillan, & Bolan, 2009). Intervention programs generally focus on providing both the victims and perpetrators with medical and social services. These strategies have shown mixed results (Ploeg et al., 2009). The use of interdisciplinary teams that include experts from the field of law enforcement and criminal prosecution has been recommended, suggesting that this may be the preferred method of protecting vulnerable older adults (Rizzo, Burns, & Chalfy, 2015). The most critical intervention in which individual caregivers or older adults can engage is making that initial report of suspected mistreatment.

See also Adult Protective Services; Crime Victimization; Elder Neglect; Financial Abuse; Institutional Mistreatment: Abuse and Neglect; Money Management.

Billy A. Caceres and Terry T. Fulmer

Anetzberger, G. J. (2012). An update on the nature and scope of elder abuse. *Generations, 36*(3), 12–20.

Bonnie, R. J., & Wallace, R. B. (Eds.). (2003). *Elder mistreatment: Abuse, neglect and exploitation in an aging America.* Washington, DC: National Academies Press.

Castle, N., Ferguson-Rome, J. C., & Teresi, J. A. (2015). Elder abuse in residential long-term care: An update to the 2003 national research council report. *Journal of Applied Gerontology, 34*(4), 407–443. doi:10.1177/0733464813492583

Clancy, M., McDaid, B., O'Neill, D., & O'Brien, J. G. (2011). National profiling of elder abuse referrals. *Age and Ageing, 40*(3), 346–352. doi:10.1093/ageing/afr023

Cohen, M., Levin, S. H., Gagin, R., & Friedman, G. (2007). Elder abuse: Disparities between older people's disclosure of abuse, evident signs of abuse, and high risk of abuse. *Journal of the American Geriatrics Society, 55,* 1224–1230.

Dong, X. Q. (2015). Elder abuse: Systematic review and implications for practice. *Journal of the American Geriatrics Society, 63*(6), 1214–1238. doi:10.1111/jgs.13454

Fulmer, T., Paveza, G., VandeWeerd, C., Guadagno, L., Fairchild, S., Norman, R.,.... Boltan-Blatt, M. (2005). Neglect assessment in urban emergency departments and confirmation by an expert clinical team. *Journals of Gerontology: Medical Sciences, 60A*(8), 1002–1006.

Institute of Medicine and National Research Council. (2014). *Elder abuse and its prevention: Workshop summary.* Washington, DC: National Academies Press.

Jirik, S., & Sanders, S. (2014, November). Analysis of elder abuse statutes across the United States, 2011–2012. *Journal of Gerontological Social Work, 4372,* 37–41. doi:10.1080/01634372.2014.884514

Johannesen, M., & LoGiudice, D. (2013). Elder abuse: A systematic review of risk factors in community-dwelling elders. *Age and Ageing, 42*(3), 292–298. doi:10.1093/ageing/afs195

Labrum, T., Solomon, P. L., & Bressi, S. K. (2015). Physical, financial, and psychological abuse committed against older women by relatives with psychiatric disorders: Extent of the problem. *Journal of Elder Abuse & Neglect, 27*(4–5), 377–391. doi: 10.1080/08946566.2015.1092902

McDonald, L., & Thomas, C. (2013). Elder abuse through a life course lens. *International Psychogeriatrics, 25*(8), 1–9. doi:10.1017/S104161021300015X

National Center on Elder Abuse. (1998). *The national elder abuse incidence study (final report).* Washington, DC: The Administration on Aging (U.S. Department of Health and Human Services).

Ploeg, J., Fear, J., Hutchison, B., MacMillan, H., & Bolan, G. (2009). A systematic review of interventions for elder abuse. *Journal of Elder Abuse & Neglect, 21*(3), 187–210.

Rizzo, V. M., Burnes, D., & Chalfy, A. (2015). A systematic evaluation of a multidisciplinary social work–lawyer elder mistreatment intervention model. *Journal of Elder Abuse & Neglect, 27*(1), 1–18. doi:10.1080/08946566.2013.792104

Schecter, M., & Dougherty, D. (2009). Combating elder abuse through a lawyer/social worker collaborative team approach: JASA legal/social work elder abuse prevention program (LEAP). *Care Management Journals, 10*(2), 71–76.

Web Resources

Center for Elders & the Courts (CEC): http://www.eldersandcourts.org/

Elder Justice Roadmap: https://www.justice.gov/file/852856/download

National Adult Protective Services Association (NAPSA): http://www.napsa-now.org

National Center on Elder Abuse: https://ncea.acl.gov

National Committee for the Prevention of Elder Abuse: http://www.preventelderabuse.org

ELDER NEGLECT

Neglect in older adults causes serious physical and emotional sequelae and is estimated to affect more than 2 million people annually (Acierno et al., 2010). In 2003, the National Research Council published the seminal report, *Elder Mistreatment: Abuse, Neglect, and Exploitation in an Aging America,* in which it defined neglect as "an omission by responsible caregivers that constitutes 'neglect' under applicable federal law" (Bonnie & Wallace, 2003, p. 39). Several studies have documented that elder neglect is a potentially fatal syndrome and that of all elder mistreatment victims, those in the neglect category have significant risk for morbidity and mortality. However, it is clear from current research that cases are severely underreported (Cannell, Jetelina, Zavadsky, & Gonzalez, 2016). All 50 states have procedures for receiving elder neglect reports. In one statewide analysis of California's protective service database, 58 counties were studied to determine variability in adult protective service (APS) investigations (Mosqueda et al., 2016). Large variability was noted county to county, and there were significant differences in the way that APS workers interpreted definitions and provided case management. This deserves further exploration. Another study of neglect based on autopsy cases found that eight cases of suspected neglect resulted in death from sepsis, extreme dehydration, and severe pressure injuries (Collins & Presnell, 2007).

Victims of neglect frequently have the following attributes: having fewer people living in the home, having health problems that limit their activities, and being extremely vulnerable by virtue of advanced age, cognitive impairment, and/or increased functional needs (Fulmer et al., 2005, 2012). The risk of neglect has been associated with minority racial status, low income, poor health, and low social support (Acierno et al., 2010). With increasing age, there is an increase in the prevalence of neglect. This may indicate that the increased care demands present in many older adults may outstrip the capacity of the caregiver to provide for said care. Social isolation is a consistent risk factor for neglect in older adults (Durso & Sullivan, 2016).

Although neglect is the most common form of elder mistreatment, it is the most underreported and least understood. State reporting laws, as well as procedures for investigation and substantiation, vary, leading to challenges in analyzing regional variability in neglect cases. Neglect can be emotional or physical and may be intentional or unintentional. Emotional neglect is the failure to provide dependent older adults with social stimulation or appropriate interpersonal interaction. Physical neglect is the failure to provide assistance with activities of daily living and services necessary for usual functioning. This may include a lack of assistance with bathing, grooming, toileting, and feeding. Forms of physical neglect include withholding

E

food, water, appropriate amenities for weather extremes, or health care; failing to provide eyeglasses, hearing aids, dentures, or other physical aids; and failing to provide safety precautions.

APS workers are the front-line personnel who investigate suspected cases of elder neglect. Other community service providers include police, fire safety inspectors, and others often called to investigate cases of hoarding behavior in older adults; these providers also need to be cognizant of the potential of identifying either neglect or self-neglect. All of these groups consistently describe home environments that are extremely deranged and in many cases unsafe for habitation (Fulmer, 2015). There can be excessive litter, rotting food, and other debris that is inappropriate in the home setting. Poor personal hygiene, contractures, pressure injuries, and malnutrition are other indicators of neglect.

Self-neglect is another serious malady that can be caused by a multitude of factors, including, but not limited to, depression, cognitive impairment, substance abuse, and comorbid health conditions (Dyer, Goodwin, Pickens-Pace, Burnett, & Kelly, 2007). Self-neglect can cause an acceleration of chronic disease manifestations, the creation of new and possibly life-threatening conditions (e.g., hip fracture), and even hazards for others (e.g., hoarding and cluttering behaviors; Dong, Simon, & Evans, 2010).

When conducting a physical examination, health care professionals should be knowledgeable about and assess for neglect. Table E.1 presents signs and symptoms of neglect that should be especially noted during the history and physical examination. The use of standardized clinical assessment instruments that focus on elder neglect is important in the diagnosis and reporting of such cases (Russell et al., 2012). Ageism on the part of clinicians may evoke stereotypical prejudices that preclude appropriate detection of neglect. For example, poor oral hygiene is often accepted as typical in frail older adults and in fact is an indicator of neglect. Cognitive impairment in older adults may interfere with self-report and further contribute to underreporting and missed diagnoses. A careful health history and physical examination that is conducted away from the caregiver/source

Table E.1
INDICATORS OF ELDER NEGLECT

Inadequate/inappropriate clothing

Poor hygiene

Poor nutrition

Poor skin integrity

Contractures

Pressure ulcers

Dehydration

Impaction

Malnutrition

Urine burns/excoriation

Duplication of similar medications

Unusual doses of medications

Dehydration >15%

Failure of caregiver to respond to warning of obvious disease

Repetition of admissions because of probable failure of health care surveillance

Self-report of neglect

of neglect is important. The older adult may be reticent to discuss inadequate care because of fears that caregiving, even if limited, will be withdrawn. If neglect is suspected or substantiated, the state APS department or appropriate unit should be notified. Elder neglect can take place in any setting, and it is important to follow older individuals as they transition across care settings to avoid high-risk situations for neglect.

Intervention in neglect cases can be lifesaving and requires a judicious team approach to ensure that a thoughtful analysis does not disrupt the current caregiving system. Interdisciplinary teams should be constructed to ensure that the relevant clinicians are engaged to address any neglect under review. The police, lawyers, and clergy may be needed for consultation in complex cases. Nurses, social workers, and other allied health care professionals are likely to be in a more optimal position to assess and detect neglect, given their more frequent interaction with older adults across care settings, including the home. Curricula in nursing and other allied health fields should be reviewed to ensure there is adequate instruction related to neglect assessment and intervention. The cost of overlooking neglect cases is not only expensive financially, but also emotionally and personally. Strategies that help older adults express concerns related to neglect need to be studied to determine the most effective interventions for the eradication of elder neglect.

See also Adult Protective Services; Elder Mistreatment: Overview; Financial Abuse; Institutional Mistreatment: Abuse and Neglect.

Terry T. Fulmer

Acierno, R., Hernandez, M. A., Amstadter, A. B., Resnick, H. S., Steve, K., Muzzy, W., & Kilpatrick, D. G. (2010). Prevalence and correlates of emotional, physical, sexual, and financial abuse and potential neglect in the United States: The National Elder Mistreatment Study. *American Journal of Public Health, 100*(2), 292–297. doi:10.2105/AJPH.2009.163089

Bonnie, R. J., & Wallace, R. B. (Eds.) (2003). *Elder mistreatment: Abuse, neglect and exploitation in an aging America.* Washington, DC: National Academies Press.

Cannell, M. B., Jetelina, K. K., Zavadsky, M., & Gonzalez, J. M. R. (2016). Towards the development of a screening tool to enhance the detection of elder abuse and neglect by emergency medical technicians (EMTs): A qualitative study. *BMC Emergency Medicine, 16*(1), 1–10. doi:10.1186/s12873-016-0084-3

Collins, K. A., & Presnell, S. E. (2007). Elder neglect and the pathophysiology of aging. *American Journal of Forensic Medicine and Pathology, 28*(2), 157–162. doi:10.1097/PAF.0b013e31805c93eb

Dong, X. Q., Simon, M., & Evans, D. (2010). Cross-sectional study of the characteristics of reported elder self-neglect in a community-dwelling population: Findings from a population-based cohort. *Gerontology, 56*(3), 325–334. doi:10.1159/000243164

Durso, S. C., & Sullivan, G. M. (2016). *Geriatrics review syllabus* (9th ed.). New York, NY: American Geriatrics Society.

Dyer, C. B., Goodwin, J. S., Pickens-Pace, S., Burnett, J., & Kelly, P. A. (2007). Self-neglect among the elderly: A model based on more than 500 patients seen by a geriatric medicine team. *American Journal of Public Health, 97*(9), 1671–1676. doi:10.2105/AJPH.2006.097113

Fulmer, T. (2015). Nurses and the Elder Justice Act. *American Journal of Nursing, 115*(11), 11.

Fulmer, T., Paveza, G., Vandeweerd, C., Fairchild, S., Guadagno, L., Bolton-Blatt, M., & Norman, R. (2005). Dyadic vulnerability and risk profiling for elder neglect. *The Gerontologist, 45*(4), 525–535.

Fulmer, T., Strauss, S., Russell, S. L., Singh, G., Blankenship, J., Vemula, R., … Sutin, D. (2012). Screening for elder mistreatment in dental and medical clinics. *Geroontology, 29*(2), 96–105.

Mosqueda, L., Wiglesworth, A., Moore, A. A., Nguyen, A., Gironda, M., & Gibbs, L. (2016). Variability in findings from adult protective services investigations of elder abuse in California. *Journal of Evidence-Informed Social Work, 13*(1), 34–44. doi:10.1080/15433714.2014.939383

Russell, S. L., Fulmer, T., Singh, G., Valenti, M., Vermula, R., & Strauss, S. M. (2012). Screening for elder mistreatment in a dental clinic population. *Journal of Elder Abuse & Neglect, 24*(4), 326–339. doi:10.1080/08946566.2012.661683

Web Resources
International Network for the Prevention of Elder Abuse: http://www.inpea.net
National Adult Protective Services Association: http://www.apsnetwork.org
National Center on Elder Abuse: http://www.ncea.aoa.gov

ELDERSPEAK

Caring for older adults can be challenging because of the numerous deficits that they experience as a result of aging, such as impaired communication abilities because of hearing loss. Although their caregivers strive to meet their unique needs and promote overall health, many institutional and noninstitutional settings inadvertently use elderspeak, which fails to support these goals and may produce undesirable effects.

Elderspeak is based on stereotypes that older adults are less able. Consequently, younger adults often simplify their speech, use repetition, and adjust their emotional tones in their attempt to promote clear, effective communication and demonstrate care (Ryan, Hummert, & Boich, 1995). However, research testing the framework of the Communication Predicament of Aging (CPA) Model reveals the failures of elderspeak in accomplishing these goals (Ryan et al., 1995). The CPA model proposes that characteristics of older persons can cue age stereotypes, often leading to the production of patronizing speech. The model is cyclical: Reinforcement of age-stereotyped behaviors and reduced opportunities for meaningful communication lead to negative changes in the older adult recipient (Hummert, Shaner, Garstka, & Henry, 1998).

In addition, research demonstrates that negative stereotypes about older people are both grounded in society and influence intergenerational communication (Hummert et al., 1998) in everyday settings such as department stores, medical waiting rooms, and parks. It also attests that older adults with discernible physical or mental disabilities are more likely to be spoken down to and that those in environments suggesting dependency (e.g., nursing homes), elicit more speech modifications than those in community settings (Hummert et al., 1998).

Exercising high pitch, speaking loudly, and using overstressed intonation are some of the feature components of elderspeak, the often-assumed preference of the elderly. Conversely, older persons receiving home-care or nursing home services report that up to 40% of their caregivers use speech they perceive as demeaning (patronizing and implying incompetence; Caporael & Culbertson, 1986). This may contribute to older adults experiencing a range of psychological ailments associated with dependent behavior. Hence, elderspeak may unintentionally reinforce dependency and generate isolation, adding to the spiral of decline in physical, cognitive, and functional health that often manifests in older people (Ryan et al., 1995). For example, those with negative images of aging have worse functional health over time, including lower rates of survival, than those whose perspective is more positive (Levy, Slade, Kunkel, & Kasl, 2002). In contrast, after controlling participants' health conditions in a study of 660 persons aged 50 and older in a small Ohio town, Levy et al. (2002) found that those who had positive perceptions of aging lived an average of 7.5 years longer, which is more than the benefits of exercising or not smoking.

Other components of elderspeak include less respectful forms of address (e.g., *sweetie, honey,*

darling), the use of the restrictive "we" (e.g., *We'll get you going again.*), belittling nonverbal behavior (e.g., patting the older person's head), and using words and expressions that are commonly used with infants (e.g., *Let's get you cleaned up*). The following nursing home scenario, which depicts an afternoon caregiving interaction between a certified nursing assistant (CNA) and an older man who appears to have fallen asleep in his chair while watching a movie, illustrates some features of elderspeak that frequently occur in nursing homes:

CNA: Hi, George! [long pause] George. [long pause] My goodness. You're missing the movie [accompanied by a sigh]. Are we ready to eat lunch? Are we? We're dazed this afternoon. Aren't we, my boy? Sound asleep.

Communications between caregivers and the elderly habitually include elderspeak, revealing an imbalance of care and control (Hummert et al., 1998). This imbalance, which in trained health care providers could be the consequence of pressure to complete several jobs simultaneously, may incorporate overly directive or bossy talk intended to assert a high degree of authority, yet diminishes the autonomy of older persons. Use of overly nurturing communication reflects improper intimacy, excessive care, and reduced control for older people, which may be an attempt to moderate the directedness in their communication. Most older adults, however, prefer affirming emotional tones that appropriately balance care and control, demonstrating their ability to comprehend the information and act autonomously (Ryan et al., 1995).

Older adults are often aware of when they are being talked down to, and many find it degrading. As a result, caregivers who care disrespectfully, particularly during activities of daily living (ADL), can severely diminish older adults' sense of accomplishment. The combination of these perceptions and the interactions between caregivers and elders are likely to exacerbate any imbalance of power that may already exist.

In addition, trained health care providers who interact with older persons are seldom prepared to communicate with them and may be socialized to use elderspeak. Caregivers are often unaware of their condescension or aware of its negative effects on the elderly. Fortunately, trained health care providers who recognize elderspeak can reduce their use of it, enhance their communication skills, and improve their working relationships with older persons (Williams, Kemper, & Hummert, 2003). Although long-standing behaviors can be difficult to change, interventions, such as communication training based on the Communication Enhancement Model, are available for trained health care providers. This model, which provides a framework for effective communication with older adults, trains professionals to perform individual evaluations of clients' needs by using simplification and clarification strategies only when requested by them (Williams et al., 2003).

Explicit indicators of elderspeak are both recognizable and manageable in one's own communication. Caregivers are expected to significantly improve their discourse with older adults by limiting their use of select features of elderspeak such as diminutives, improper use of collective pronouns, tag questions, and dawdling loud speech.

Sweetie, *buddy*, and *good girl* are among the unsuitably intimate and juvenile names of diminutives, which may suggest a parent–child nature to the relationship. Use of collective pronouns (e.g., *Are we ready to eat our dinner?*) also falls into the unsuitable category and implies that the older person is not capable of acting alone or making autonomous decisions. However, tag questions (e.g., *You want to get out of bed now, don't you?*) appear to offer a choice, yet imply that the older adult needs guidance to select the proper response. Combined, these qualities of elderspeak suggest that the older adult is inept and reliant on others.

Speaking too loudly is another common, yet inappropriate technique for communicating with older people. For some older adults with hearing loss, this technique can be fitting. For others, raising one's voice may further damage their hearing, whereas the use of high-pitched intonation, similar to the pitch commonly used when talking to babies, may provide more difficulties.

Slowed speech and use of short, simple sentences are other features of elderspeak that, when used, may be perceived as condescending by those who are cognitively intact. These do not increase comprehension for older persons experiencing typical age-related difficulties such as reductions in working memory. Using childlike language erroneously implies that older people are retrogressing in terms of communication and that oversimplification is necessary.

Moreover, caregivers may fail to recognize the significance of nonverbal communication, which can deliver a stronger message than spoken words and play a fundamental role in communicating effectively. By overcoming elderspeak, caregivers can promote successful aging, a multidimensional concept that embraces physical health, psychological well-being, functional activity, and social support (Ferri, James, & Pruchno, 2009). With diminished elderspeak, stereotype-based messages that older adults are inept and dependent can be eliminated, which allows for greater fostering of the cognitive and functional abilities of the aging population.

Angel L. Venegas

Caporael, L. R., & Culbertson, G. H. (1986). Verbal response modes of baby talk and other speech at institutions for the aged. *Language & Communication*, 6, 99–112.

Ferri, C., James, I., & Pruchno, R. (2009). Successful aging: Definitions and subjective assessment according to older adults. *Clinical Gerontologist*, 32(4), 379–388.

Hummert, M. L., Shaner, J. L., Garstka, T. A., & Henry, C. (1998). Communication with older adults: The influence of age stereotypes, context, and communicator age. *Human Communication Research*, 25(1), 124–151.

Levy, B. R., Slade, M., Kunkel, S., & Kasl, S. (2002). Longevity increased by positive self-perceptions of aging. *Journal of Personality and Social Psychology*, 83, 261–270.

Ryan, E. B., Hummert, M. L., & Boich, L. H. (1995). Communication predicaments of aging: Patronizing behavior toward older adults. *Journal of Language and Social Psychology*, 14(1–2), 144–166.

Williams, K. N., Kemper, S., & Hummert, M. L. (2003). Improving nursing home communication: An intervention to reduce elderspeak. *The Gerontologist*, 43(2), 242–247.

E

Web Resources
Aging Resources of Central Iowa: http://www.aging
    resources.com
American Society on Aging: http://www.asaging.org/
Nursing   Standard: http://nursingstandard.rcn
    publishing.co.uk
Pioneer Network: http://www.pioneernetwork.net
Right at Home, Inc.: http://www.caringnews.com

EMERGENCY DEPARTMENT CARE

The population of the United States has increased approximately 20% from 2000 to 2010 (U.S. Department of Health and Human Services Administration on Aging, 2016). It is projected that one in five Americans will be more than the age of 65 years by 2030 (Welch, 2014). As the population increases, so do the number of emergency department (ED) visits. Overall, ED visits have increased 43% from 1997 to 2009. As the age of the patient increases, so does the length of stay in the ED. The mean length of stay for children is 1.6 hours compared with the older adult who has a mean stay of 3.5 hours. In addition to the length of stay, the percentage of patients admitted significantly increased, with approximately 50% of older adults being admitted from the ED (Lesney, 2013). Of concern is the frequency of elder visits to the ED. People age 65 years and older are the highest utilizers of health care services, with an estimated six to seven encounters compared with those younger than 65 years, who have only two encounters (Welch, 2014).

Older patients can present to the emergency department atypically. The common signs and symptoms that are seen in younger patients are not typically those of an older patient. Multiple comorbidities, cognitive impairments, depression, polypharmacy, and a decline in functional status are all factors that can complicate the presentation and care of the older adult patient. Financial status and a desire to be independent may also complicate initial care and its continuity for this population.

Older adults may be at risk for suboptimal care in the ED. They may have difficulty expressing their complaints because of underlying cognitive impairment. They likewise may be at risk of adverse drug events because of their concurrent illnesses. Some older patients are cared for in the ED as a culmination of a stressful period of the caregiver's attempt to help the patient at home. Similar to other settings, care of the older adult in the ED requires a multidisciplinary team approach.

Numerous studies have reported the importance of early identification, evaluation, and management of older adults in the ED (Samaras, Chevalley, Samaras, & Gold, 2010; Schnitker, Martin-Khan, Beattie, & Gray, 2013; Shapiro, Clevenger, & Dowling Evans, 2012). Early identification of a potentially life-threatening event is an imperative of nurses and providers in this setting. As stated previously, older patients may not present typically. A patient may present with the confusion that is actually the symptom of an infection. The patient may downplay symptoms for fear of admission to the hospital or loss of independence. Evidence also supports the enhancement of basic nursing care and interventions, as well as the need for atypical diagnostic workups for atypical presentations. It is imperative for providers to obtain a comprehensive history and physical examination inclusive of baseline mental and physical/functional status, cognition, and medications (prescribed, over the counter, and herbal).

Older adults require specialized care to meet the complexity of their needs. The ED can be foreign and intimidating to them. It is important to consider the special needs of this population throughout the entire stay in the ED. Numerous programs have been developed to increase awareness and enhance care to older adults.

The Emergency Nurses Association (ENA) offers an educational program entitled, "Geriatric Emergency Nursing Education," on their website (www.ena.org). This program covers the topics of triage and assessment, abuse and neglect, attitudes and ageism, polypharmacy, physical and psychological changes, palliative care, pain management, and discharge planning. Its intention is to educate emergency nurses in the identification, triage, and care of the older adult.

These various programs have led to innovative changes in EDs across the country. When patients enter the ED, they are triaged by a nurse. The term *triage* is of French origin and was initiated during the Korean War. Triage is based on a severity index that was originally a three-tiered system but has now expanded to a five-tiered system. Once triaged, the patient is placed in a room for evaluation by additional nursing staff and health care providers. There, the patient receives continued assessment, interventions, procedures, medications, and then finally disposition. Disposition may be home, a family member's home, another facility, an observational stay, or an admission to the inpatient setting.

Some EDs have initiated additional screening of the older patient, including cognitive function, depression, delirium, mobility, caregiver strain, and current use of community resources. Successful programs have screening tools, as well as protocols and resources, to assist those who have abnormal findings. In addition, some EDs have designated areas that care specifically for older adults. These areas may have soft lighting, earth-toned walls, nonglare and nonskid floors, large-print signs, pressure-reducing mattresses, warmed blankets, and reclining chairs in place of stretchers to help reduce and prevent pain (Jaworski, 2013; Shapiro et al., 2012).

During the stay in the ED, the patient may encounter not only nurses and providers, but also social workers, case managers, respiratory therapists, radiology technicians, and clergy. To have a successful program of care for the older adult, it is important to educate all members of the health care team, initiate evidence-based practice protocols, and encourage a culture of care inclusive of physical, psychosocial, and spiritual care for the patient and family.

There is a trend for EDs or areas of them to be devoted to the elder patient. These areas or departments specialize in the care of the elderly and identify and treat their complex and simple problems. These areas take into consideration the environmental factors that can comfort older patients, as well as enhance their time in the ED with beds instead of stretchers or recliners in place of stretchers (Welch, 2014). EDs that specialize in the older population can have cost and staff issues that must be considered. Specialized ED cost, staffing, and most of all, outcomes are areas in need of further scientific evaluation.

Caring for the older adult in the emergency care setting can be complex and challenging but also very rewarding. Having a good foundation of knowledge in the physiological and psychosocial changes that occur with aging and consideration of emotional and spiritual well-being help make the older patient's stay in this setting beneficial and lifesaving.

Theresa M. Campo

Jaworski, M. (2013). Senior emergency departments deliver the best care for older adults. *Parentgiving: The Ultimate Senior Resource*. Retrieved from http://www.parentgiving.com/elder-care/senior-emergency-departments-deliver-best-care

Lesney, M. S. (2013). Aging population will need more ED capacity. *ACEP News*. Retrieved from http://www.acepnews.com/specialty-focus/practice-trends/single-article-page/aging-population-will-need-more-ed-capacity-admissions/cf6c29862e54ba2bc3478651462497dd.html

Samaras, N., Chevalley, T., Samaras, D., & Gold, G. (2010). Older patients in the emergency department: A review. *Annals of Emergency Medicine, 56*(3), 261–269.

Schnitker, L., Martin-Khan, M., Beattie, E., & Gray, L. (2013). What is the evidence to guide best practice for the management of older people with cognitive impairment presenting to emergency departments? *Advanced Emergency Nursing Journal, 35*(2), 154–169.

Shapiro, S. E., Clevenger, C. K., & Dowling Evans, D. (2012). Enhancing care of older adults in the emergency department. *Advanced Emergency Nursing Journal, 34*(3), 197–203.

Total number of Medicare beneficiaries accessed. Retrieved from http://kff.org/medicare/state-indicator/total-medicare-beneficiaries

U.S. Department of Health and Human Services Administration on Aging. (2016). A profile of older Americans: 2016. Retrieved from https://www.acl.gov/sites/default/files/Aging%20and%20Disability%20in%20America/2016-Profile.pdf

Welch, S. (2014). *13*—The geriatric emergency department. *The American College of Emergency Physicians*. Retrieved from https://www.acep.org/content.aspx?id=87577

Web Resources
AARP: http://www.aarp.org
American Academy of Emergency Nurse Practitioners: http://www.aaenp-natl.org

American College of Emergency Physicians: http://www.acep.org

American Nurses Association: http://www.nursingworld.org

Centers for Medicare & Medicaid Services—CMS Program Statistics: https://www.cms.gov/Research-Statistics-Data-and-Systems/Statistics-Trends-and-Reports/CMSProgramStatistics

Emergency Nurses Association: http://www.ena.org

EMPLOYMENT

The face of America's workforce has changed dramatically since the end of World War II, when almost all "prime-age" men (ages 25–54 years) and more than two thirds of "older" men (aged 55 and older) were in the labor force; that is, they were either working or jobless but looking for work. Only a minority of women in either age group was in the labor force. However, men's growing propensity to retire at fairly early ages over the following four-plus decades led to a steep decline in participation on the part of older men, one of the more significant labor force developments of the 20th century. At the same time, women began entering, reentering, or remaining longer in the labor force in growing numbers.

Older men's behavior changed in the mid-1990s, when their declining participation came to a halt and eventually started to rise. Over the past 30 years, older men and women have increased their labor force participation rates, women more so than men. Among some older age subgroups, the increases have been especially noteworthy. For example, in 1985, only 18.4% of people aged 65 to 69 were working or looking for work; by 2015, that figure had reached 32.1% (U.S. Department of Labor, 2016), a sharp rise for a group commonly considered "retirement age." Rates are rising among even older age groups as well.

More than 8 in 10 prime-age Americans were in the labor force as of 2015. Those aged 55 and older are far less likely to be working or looking for work than are their prime-age counterparts—only about four in 10 in 2015.

As they have in the total workforce, women have become a more prominent part of the older workforce: less than one fourth in 1950 compared to close to half in 2015. In fact, in 1950, men were more than three and a half times as likely as their female counterparts to be in the labor force. They are now only somewhat more than 30% more likely. At the same time, the total labor force has been aging: Its median age has risen by more than 4 years over the past quarter century (Toossi, 2015).

A LOOK TO THE FUTURE

The Bureau of Labor Statistics (BLS) projects that by 2024, participation rates will rise somewhat for prime-age workers but dip slightly for those aged 55 years as Baby Boomers move into older age groups, with their lower labor force participation rates (Toossi, 2015). Nonetheless, specific older age subgroups (e.g., 60–64 or 65–69) may see participation rates rise by up to 4.6 percentage points. Increases will be substantially greater for women. Americans work at older ages for a variety of reasons. They enjoy their jobs; work makes them feel useful; and employment is a way to remain active (AARP, 2014). However, they also work because they need the money and/or the health insurance that employers provide to a large portion of the workforce.

Greater interest in retirement-age employment is the result of a number of factors. Rising life expectancy means more years of retirement to plan and save for. Defined benefit pension plans have been replaced by defined contribution or 401(k) plans, which shift the burden investment decisions and risk to workers and away from employers. Retiree health benefits have been cut back. Although workers need more of their own resources to finance a secure retirement today, too many older households have not saved enough to supplement Social Security, as evidenced by the size of the 401(k) balances of near-retirees (Miller, Madland, & Weller, 2015).

Working longer can help compensate for inadequate retirement savings. The decline in physically demanding jobs and improved health status, along with enhanced medical care for many chronic health conditions, should be making longer work lives more feasible. However, these developments do not account for all of the increased activity near or in the retirement years. Public policies such as increases in the full benefit age of Social Security and the delayed retirement credit (DRC) paid for postponing Social Security benefit receipt beyond the full retirement age may, respectively, discourage early retirement and encourage more work.

It appears, however, that rising educational attainment on the part of older workers may have had a more substantial impact on work behavior than any specific policy. Burtless (2013) concludes that it may account for more than half of the rise in older men's labor force participation. At all ages, labor force participation rates are higher for the better educated, whose jobs are typically less arduous and less likely to have an adverse impact on health, than those held by workers with fewer years of schooling. Also, the better educated tend to be more attractive to employers and thus have employment opportunities that are more conducive to prolonged employment. Nonetheless, gains in educational attainment at older ages are expected to slow, so Burtless also foresees a slowdown in the trend toward later retirement.

CONTINUING TO WORK AT OLDER AGES

Continuing to work at older ages is not always as simple as opting to remain longer with one's current employer. Employee Benefit Research Institute (EBRI) Retirement Confidence Surveys have found that workers are far more likely to say that they expect to work in retirement than to end up doing that. Although two thirds of workers, aged 25 and older when interviewed, said that they planned to work for pay in retirement, but only 27% of them reported having worked at that time (EBRI, 2016). Older workers lose their jobs, develop health problems or disabilities, or fail to find the type of job or work arrangements that might make continued employment more appealing.

Older job seekers typically find it more difficult than younger ones to find work as a result of age discrimination, skills obsolescence, and employer misconceptions about their ability to learn new technology. Employers may also have

concerns about the health care costs of older workers, as well as the likelihood of recouping training expenditures for workers nearing retirement. The consequences of job displacement can be more severe in the case of older workers, who tend to be unemployed longer than their younger counterparts, less likely to find work, and more apt to experience earnings and benefit losses when they are successful in the job search (Johnson & Butrica, 2012). Moreover, they have less time to recover lost earnings and neglected savings.

The majority of employed older workers are employed full time, although part-time employment increases with age. Older workers of both sexes are more likely to work part time than prime-age workers, and in both groups, women are much more likely than men to work part time. Self-employment rates are also higher at older ages. Both work arrangements may make it easier to combine paid work and caregiving responsibilities.

EMPLOYMENT AND CAREGIVING

Workers of all ages have caregiving responsibilities, with the typical family caregiver for an adult well into middle age (age 49 on average); some are aged 75 or older (National Alliance for Caregiving & AARP 2015). Much of the care provided by prime-age and especially older workers is elder care: Nearly 6 in 10 workers aged 45 to 74 reported caring for a spouse, parent, or other relative in 2013 (AARP, 2014). Workers' elder caregiver responsibilities are likely to grow as life expectancy increases, more workers push back the date of retirement, and the workforce ages. Employers should be preparing for this development.

Many employers offer a variety of flexible work options that could facilitate caregiving to some, but generally not all, of their workers (Matos & Galinsky, 2014). Although three fourths of employers with at least 50 employees report that their employees can take time off for elder care without jeopardizing their jobs (Matos & Galinsky, 2014), there may be limits to how easily that leave can be accessed and how much time away from work is acceptable. Some employed caregivers report having been

E

warned about their performance or work attendance (Feinberg, 2016).

Combining work and family responsibilities can prove daunting. One survey of older caregivers found that one in six had taken leave in the previous 5 years because of elder caregiving and one in five anticipated that they might need to do so in the future (AARP, 2014). Other work impacts because of family caregiving include going in to work late, leaving early, or taking time off and reducing work hours or shifting to less-demanding jobs (Feinberg, 2016)

Relatively few working caregivers report having quit work entirely as a result of caregiving, but others retired (Feinberg, 2016). Older caregivers might find it particularly difficult to reenter the workforce at a later date, with potentially significant consequences for future retirement-income security.

In fact, lost work time for caregiving can take a heavy toll on current financial well-being as well. The Family and Medical Leave Act (FMLA) requires employers with 50 or more employees to provide up to 12 weeks of leave in a 12-month period for caregiving or to deal with a serious health condition, but the leave is unpaid. Workers in the few states that offer paid family leave, as well as the more than four in 10 civilian workers with access to paid personal leave, may find elder care easier when they can take time to deal with care responsibilities. Lack of access to paid leave, however, makes it difficult for many workers, particularly low earners, to take advantage of the FMLA. Workers in small firms cannot even count on the unpaid benefit.

RESPONSES TO AN AGING WORKFORCE

Employers, for the most part, have been slow to respond to a workforce that is getting older. Out of business necessity, employers in some industries, such as health care, have reached out with innovative programs and policies designed to attract and retain older workers, but they are not yet the majority of employers. Nor has the government placed issues associated with an aging workforce, including elder care or the economic advantages of prolonging working life, high on the legislative agenda. This may change if more employers

find themselves facing significant labor and skills shortages or when attention turns to Social Security reform, which will likely include proposals to further increase the retirement age. More widely implemented flexible work options, along with opportunities to shift to new, less demanding work, could facilitate the continued employment of more older workers, with health problems, caregiving responsibilities, and/or interest in a new balance between paid work and other activities.

See also Active Life Expectancy; Ageism; Caregiving Relationships; Retirement; Social Security.

Sara E. Rix

AARP. (2014). *Staying ahead of the curve 2013: The AARP work and career study*. Washington, DC: Author. Retrieved from http://www.aarp .org/content/dam/aarp/research/surveys_ statistics/general/2014/Staying-Ahead-of-the -Curve-2013-The-Work-and-Career-Study-AARP -res-gen.pdf

Burtless, G. (2013). *Can educational attainment explain the rise in labor force participation at older ages? IB No. 13-13.* Chestnut Hill, MA: Center for Retirement Research at Boston College. Retrieved from http://crr.bc.edu/wp-content/uploads/2013/ 09/IB_13-13-508x.pdf

Employee Benefit Research Institute. (2016). *Expectations about retirement: 2016 RCS fact sheet #2.* Washington, DC: Author. Retrieved from https:// www.ebri.org/pdf/surveys/rcs/2016/RCS _16.FS-2_Expects.pdf

Feinberg, L. F. (2016). *The dual pressures of family caregiving and employment.* Washington, DC: AARP. Retrieved from http://www .aarp.org/content/dam/aarp/ppi/2016-03/ The-Dual-Pressures-off-Family-Caregiving-and -Employment.pdf

Johnson, R. W., & Butrica, B. A. (2012). *Age disparities in unemployment and reemployment during the Great Recession and recovery: Brief #03.* Washington, DC: Urban Institute. Retrieved from http:// www.urban.org/sites/default/files/alfresco/ publication-pdfs/412574-Age-Disparities-in -Unemployment-and-Reemployment-During-the -Great-Recession-and-Recovery.PDF

Matos, K., & Galinsky, E. (2014). *2014 national study of employers.* New York, NY: Families and Work Institute. Retrieved from http://familiesandwork .org/downloads/2014NationalStudyOfEmploy ers.pdf

Miller, K., Madland, D., & Weller, C. E. (2015). *The reality of the retirement crisis.* Washington, DC: Center for American Progress. Retrieved from https://www.americanprogress.org/issues/economy/reports/2015/01/26/105394/the-reality-of-the-retirement-crisis/

National Alliance for Caregiving & AARP. (2015). *Caregiving in the U.S. 2015.* Bethesda, MD: NAC, and Washington, DC: AARP. Retrieved from http://www.caregiving.org/wp-content/uploads/2015/05/2015_CaregivingintheUS_Final-Report-June-4_WEB.pdf

Toossi, M. (2015). Labor force projections to 2024: The labor force is growing, but slowly. *Monthly Labor Review.* Retrieved from http://www.bls.gov/opub/mlr/2015/article/pdf/labor-force-projections-to-2024.pdf

U.S. Department of Labor, Bureau of Labor Statistics. (2016). Labor force statistics from the current population survey. Retrieved from http://data.bls.gov/pdq/querytool.jsp?survey=ln

Web Resources

AARP: Job and career information: http://www.aarp.org/work

Age discrimination in employment legislation, regulations, guidance, and statistics: http://www.eeoc.gov

American Job Center Network/CareerOneStop: https://www.careeronestop.org

Families and Work Institute: http://www.whenworkworks.org/about-us/our-partners/families-and-work-institute-fwi

Labor force statistics: http://data.bls.gov/pdq/querytool.jsp?survey=ln

Labor force statistics: http://www.bls.gov

National Alliance for Caregiving: http://www.caregiving.org

Unemployment information: http://www.dol.gov/dol/topic/unemployment-insurance

ENVIRONMENTAL MODIFICATIONS: HOME

Most older persons desire to live at home for as long as possible. Familiar surroundings, control over one's daily activities, and established community bonds are among the many benefits. With the rapid growth of home health services and "smart" technologies that monitor health status, living at home can be a viable long-term-care option. However, the very home that offers comfort and control can itself be a barrier to independent living. Most dwellings have not been designed to accommodate the sensory, physical, and cognitive disabilities that often accompany aging, a time when a supportive environment is *most* needed (Lawton, 1980). A ramp, walk-in shower, and other modifications can make the difference between living at home or in a facility. In the last decade, the focus on healthy aging has been on diet, exercise, and access to health care. With the coming age wave and the rapid growth of the older population, the home environment needs to be included in healthy aging *and* chronic disease management.

BENEFITS OF HOME MODIFICATIONS

Research on home modification (HM), defined as environmental modifications and assistive devices, has taken a back seat to design research in institutional settings, where, until recently, long-term care services were primarily offered and reimbursed. In addition, HM research presents several challenges, including the variability of subjects and housing structures. However, in the last couple of decades, HM research has emerged to examine its role in (a) providing cost-effective care in the home as opposed to an institution, (b) preventing fall injuries, (c) increasing the ability to perform activities of daily living (ADL), and (d) decreasing caregiving help and burden. The research findings show that HM can:

- Improve ADL performance, including bathing, toileting, and transferring (Stark, Keglovits, & Somerville, 2016)
- Reduce home care costs for frail elders and help to delay institutionalization when combined with home health services (Jutkowitz, Gitlin, Pizzi, Lee, & Dennis, 2012; Mann, Ottenbacher, Fraas, Tomita, & Granger, 1999)
- As part of a fall-reduction program, reduce falls among older adults (Chase, Mann, Wasek, & Arbesman, 2012; Panel on Prevention of Falls in Older Persons, American Geriatrics Society and British Geriatrics Society, 2011)

E

- Enhance caregiver ability to provide assistance and with reduced burden (Gitlin, Corcoran, Winter, Boyce, & Hauck, 2001; Unwin, Andrews, Andrews, & Hanson, 2009)

KEY STRATEGIES FOR ADDRESSING CHALLENGES OF HMs

Even though HMs are increasingly recognized as a key element in successful aging-in-place, problems for intervention abound. Individuals have insufficient knowledge about how the environment can reduce an avoidable disability or how to properly assess for and carry out needed modifications. Understanding the major obstacles can assist stakeholders in developing creative strategies for successful interventions.

Increasing Awareness of Person/ Environmental Fit

Many people inaccurately blame decreased functioning on the individual's age-related decline, as opposed to the dynamic interface between a user's capabilities and the designed environment. For example, a person with age-related arthritis may engage in unsafe bathing transfers, blaming difficulties on "getting old" and a "bad knee" instead of the tub's design. Consequently, safer alternatives are not explored. That same individual, however, may be able to bathe/shower in a safe, independent manner using a transfer bench or walk-in shower. Enlightening seniors that difficulties in ADL are often because of the youth-oriented design of their homes, not their impairment, can promote constructive interventions.

Engaging in Prevention and Planning

Obvious environmental hazards are often overlooked until injuries or health crises occur. For example, often it is only after a hip fracture that a senior with a shuffling gait will remove slippery area rugs or install stair handrails. Encouraging seniors to engage in preventive strategies can help them focus on the benefits of HM *before the crisis*. Healthy seniors can be counseled to consider HM that increase comfort while reducing fall risk (e.g., grab bars, supportive seating, and

bedding, nonslip finishes on floors, increased lighting) and to develop contingency plans (e.g., first-floor living) if their needs change. Newly diagnosed individuals with impairments that will severely limit mobility over time can be advised to plan for future needs (e.g., ramps, widened doorways, and roll-in showers).

Conducting Assessments and Solving Problems

Some providers encourage patients to have their home environment assessed, but confusion arises over who conducts the assessment: a nurse, occupational or physical therapist, social worker, interior designer, or family member? To contain health care costs and raise awareness of the value of HM, cross-training of health care and design professionals, as well as consumers, is warranted. Another confusing issue is assessment of the need for HM. Many checklists assess for problems but do not offer potential solutions. In considering interventions, no one size fits all, especially in the older population, where there is a greater range of physical and psychological differences than in any other age group. Solutions should be tailored to the functional and personal needs of the individual, the characteristics of the housing structure, and the available funding streams. Web-based resources offer practical guidance in conducting assessments and choosing appropriate interventions for general safety and disability-specific interventions. Taking into account personal preferences and offering choices greatly increase chances for success. In the last decade, there has been an explosive growth in senior-friendly products and furnishings that are also aesthetically pleasing. For example, well-designed grab bars can take the stigma out of using a "disability" product and increase usage.

Implementation and Service Delivery

Locating, purchasing, and installing equipment and furnishings and hiring and supervising contractors can require more stamina than many seniors have. Often it is difficult to locate reliable contractors with the necessary skills and understanding of the older population's needs.

Providers can assist caregivers and seniors by creating a list of (a) national organizations with members in local communities, including universal-design homebuilders or aging-in-place contractors, and (b) local resources such as home health and home remodeling stores, senior centers (a good source for word-of-mouth renovator referrals), area agencies on aging, and centers for independent living. The National Association of Home Builders (NAHB) also maintains a national listing of contractors certified in aging-in-place (CAPS).

Funding

Lack of government reimbursement has made access to HM beyond the reach of many low-income individuals with disabilities. Until recently, states primarily funded long-term care within the nursing home setting. Due to cost containment, consumer demands, and new legislation, state funding is being channeled into HM to provide long-term care "in the most integrated setting appropriate to the needs of qualified individuals with disabilities" (*Olmstead v. L. C.* 1999). For example, the *Access to Home* Program (2017) funds organizations to assess, coordinate, and implement HM for income-eligible New Yorkers with disabilities so that they can remain at home. Funding includes accessibility features (e.g., lifts, widened doorways, remodeled bathrooms) and assistive devices (e.g., raised toilet seats, listening devices) up to $25,000, for both home owners and renters.

Increasing Access to Education and Resources

Universities and nonprofit organizations are actively promoting living environments that promote healthy aging and lifetime use (i.e., universal design). For example, no-step entrances and wider doorways are beneficial for families with baby carriages, teenagers on crutches, and seniors using walkers or wheelchairs. A wide variety of resources on HM are available to educate consumers and providers and include online courses and tours of homes that have accessibility features as an integral part of the design

THE FUTURE IS NOW—THE "SMART" HOUSE

"Smart" monitoring technologies can further extend independent living for seniors who are frail, have chronic health conditions, or have memory disorders. These systems can monitor health status (e.g., glucose or blood pressure changes), ADL, and environmental conditions, sending data to caregivers via computers (i.e., broadband wiring) or regular telephone lines. These passive systems allow distant caregivers to assess whether a person is able to live alone or needs additional support or if emergency attention is required. Most systems use wireless sensors to record activity within the home, sending alerts when there are deviations from the norm (e.g., a person's getting-up time, medication usage, or meal preparation). Caregivers can then determine whether the person is sick, has fallen, or needs an activity reminder. Environmental hazards (e.g., extreme indoor temperature) are also recorded. Although passive monitoring can present ethical issues (e.g., if an adult child uses the system without consent in the home of a parent with dementia), these new technologies have tremendous potential to reduce health care costs and extend independent living.

Other smart home systems anticipate a person's routines and accordingly control environmental features, such as lighting, heating, and cooling systems. There are new technologies to help persons with dementia live at home with greater efficiency and safety, including automatic stove turnoffs and caregiver alerts during nighttime wandering.

PREPARING FOR THE FUTURE

The home environment, along with diet, exercise, and health care, is a key factor in quality of life and ability to age in place. Along with addressing the housing needs of the existing senior cohort, baby boomers should be encouraged to plan for their retirement. This techno-savvy cohort will more readily accept and demand accessible, attractive, and smart features that promote independence and well-being. With the coming increase in the aging population comes an exciting opportunity to

E

transform the existing youth-oriented housing model into user-friendly residences that encourage health and independence at all ages.

See also Environmental Modifications: Shared Residential Settings; Ergonomics; Technology.

Rosemary Bakker

Chase, C. A., Mann, K., Wasek, S., & Arbesman, M. (2012). Systematic review of the effect of home modification and fall prevention programs on falls and the performance of community-dwelling older adults. *American Journal of Occupational Therapy, 66*(3), 284–291.

Gitlin, L. M., Corcoran, M., Winter, L., Boyce, A., & Hauck, W. W. (2001). A randomized, controlled trial of a home environmental intervention: Effect on efficacy and upset in caregivers and on daily function of persons with dementia. *The Gerontologist, 41*(1), 4–14.

Jutkowitz, E., Gitlin, L., Pizzi, T., Lee, E., & Dennis, M. (2012). Cost effectiveness of a home-based intervention that helps functionally vulnerable older adults age in place at home. *Journal of Aging Research*. doi:10.1155/2012/680265

Lawton, M. P., (1980). Housing the elderly, residential quality and residential satisfaction. *Research on Aging, 2*, 309–328.

Mann, W. C., Ottenbacher, K. J., Fraas, L., Tomita, M., & Granger, C. V. (1999). Effectiveness of assistive technology and environmental interventions in maintaining independence and reducing home care costs for the frail elderly. *Archives of Family Medicine, 8*, 210–217.

Olmstead v. L. C. 527 U.S. 581 (1999).

Panel on Prevention of Falls in Older Persons, American Geriatrics Society & British Geriatrics Society. (2011). Summary of the updated American Geriatrics Society/British Geriatrics Society clinical practice guideline for prevention of falls in older persons. *Journal of the American Geriatrics Society, 59*(1), 148–157.

Stark, S., Keglovits, M., & Somerville, E. (2016). A randomized controlled feasibility trial of tailored home modifications to improve activities of daily living. *American Journal of Occupational Therapy, 70*(4, Suppl. 1), 7011520290p1. doi:10.5014/ajot.2016.70S1-RP103E

Unwin, B., Andrews, C., Andrews, P., & Hanson, L. (2009). Therapeutic home adaptations for older adults with disabilities. *American Family Physician, 80*(9), 963–968.

Web Resources

AARP: Livable Communities: http://www.aarp.org/livable-communities

Center for Inclusive Design and Environmental Access, University of Buffalo: http://www.ap.buffalo.edu/idea

Center for Universal Design, North Carolina State University: http://www.design.ncsu.edu

National Association of Home Builders: http://www.Nahb.org

National Clearing House for Long Term Care Information: Home Modifications, U.S. Department of Health and Human Services: http://www.longtermcare.gov/LTC/Main_Site/Resources/Home_Mod.aspx

National Resource Center on Supportive Housing and Home Modification, University of Southern California: http://homemods.org

This Caring Home, A project of Weill Cornell Medical College: http://thiscaringhome.org

ENVIRONMENTAL MODIFICATIONS: SHARED RESIDENTIAL SETTINGS

Shared residential settings for seniors are defined as sponsor-supported housing and services that range from independent living to assisted-living facilities (which go by many names in different states) to short-stay/post-acute rehabilitation to nursing homes. Independent-living settings are essentially apartment buildings or campus-type housing, typically age-limited to adults aged 65 years and over (although some active living communities include individuals 50 and older), in which maintenance, a variety of dining options, and scheduled activities are provided. A variety of other services is often available, sometimes for additional fees. Assisted living was initially conceptualized as independent living with services so that individuals who needed some support with independent activities of daily living (IADL) or activates of daily living (ADL) could get personal care. Since their emergence with the Hill–Burton Act (1946), nursing homes (or skilled nursing facilities) have primarily been considered long-term care settings where people live for months or years. Excluded, for the purposes of this chapter, are short-stay/post-acute rehabilitation centers, day care, respite programs, and residential hospices, settings where individuals stay for short periods of time but generally do not consider their residence.

Over the past few decades, there has been increasing pressure from advocacy organizations, residents, and families to move to a model that views the nursing home as a residence with supportive services, more consistent with the underlying principles of assisted living. At the same time, many assisted-living communities are now providing significant care—personal and medical—to residents who prefer not to live in a nursing home. There are also more home-care options for individuals in independent living, thus blurring the lines between these different regulatorily-defined settings.

Although all residential settings need to be designed for elders and their care partners, the most significant physical environmental changes are occurring in nursing homes, which are moving—either through renovation or reconstruction—away from hospital-style (i.e., institutional) architecture to settings that feel more like home. These modifications can occur at multiple levels of the setting, including overarching spatial layout and adjacencies, elimination of institutional "icons" such as prominent nursing stations and day rooms, development of residential spaces such as kitchens and living rooms, and redecoration to include more familiar patterns and décor.

SCALE AND UNIT CONFIGURATION

One of the largest, and perhaps most difficult, changes to achieve within existing long-term care communities is the breakdown of the scale of spaces in which residents spend their time. Traditionally, nursing units were based on groups of 40 to 60 beds arranged along long, double-loaded corridors, with a single large multipurpose room across from the nursing station that served for group activities and meals. Care communities dedicated to residential-style care generally group residents in households of 12 to 24 residents, containing all the spaces of a typical house. Positive outcomes associated with smaller groups of residents and staff interacting together include decreased anxiety and depression; less use of antibiotics and psychotropic drugs; higher motor functions; increased mobility, social interaction, and friendship formation; and increased rates of supervision and interaction between staff and residents (Bicket et al., 2010; Calkins 2009; McAllister & Silverman, 1999; Milke, Beck, Danes, & Lesak 2009; Pekkarinen, Sinervo, Perala, & Elovainio 2004). There is also evidence that such modifications benefit staff working in residential settings (Adams, Verbeek, & Zwakhalen, 2017; Parker et al., 2004).

Traditional institutional-care settings were laid out along long, straight corridors to maximize staff's ability to monitor residents while sitting behind the centrally located nursing station. With the reduction of the scale of spaces, there is an emphasis on both spatial organization and design of specific rooms. Increasingly common, household models place a value on a front door that opens to the social areas of the house (kitchen, dining, and living rooms), with the bedrooms and personal care areas more privately located. This configuration reflects the public-to-private transitions common in most homes in the community and appears to have a positive impact on orientation, quality of life, and agitation; households are associated with higher levels of orientation, higher quality of life, and less agitation than traditional units (Day & Calkins, 2002; Kane, Lum, Cutler, Degenholtz, & Yu, 2007; Milke et al., 2009; Parker et al., 2004).

PRIVACY

Traditional long-term care settings provide little in the way of privacy protections; bedrooms are shared with one to three other people, separation between personal space is limited to a curtain, staff routinely enter bedrooms without knocking and waiting to be invited in, and there are few or no designated spaces where one can be alone or share a private visit with family and friends. There is strong evidence linking lack of privacy to myriad negative outcomes (Mazer, 2012; Nordin, McKee, Wijk, & Elf, 2017). There is also clear evidence of positive outcomes

E

associated with private rooms, including fewer nosocomial infections and hospitalizations, decreased staff time spent managing roommate conflicts, higher quality of life, and reduced housekeeping and maintenance costs (Bicket et al., 2010; Calkins & Cassella, 2006).

The Centers for Medicare & Medicaid (CMS) published new guidelines in 2016 that limit the number of residents per bedroom to two individuals, and each bedroom must have its own bathroom with toilet and sink (at a minimum), for renovation or new construction (CMS, 2016). These guidelines do not address room configuration, but architects have developed ingenious privacy-enhanced shared room designs, wherein each individual has an equally accessible, spatially defined territory that includes a personal window and equal access to a shared bathroom. Anecdotal reports suggest that residents find these rooms more acceptable, even considering them "private" rooms (Calkins & Cassella, 2006). The 2018 edition of the Facility Guidelines Institute (FGI), *Guidelines for the Design and Construction of Residential Health, Care and Support Facilities,* recommends these enhanced shared rooms in all facilities.

PERSONAL POSSESSIONS

One of the traumatic aspects of leaving one's home and relocating into a shared residential setting is the loss of personal possessions, which reflect both personality and a life-time of memories, accomplishments, and activities (Rowles & Bernard, 2013). Lack of personal possessions also makes it harder for staff to get to know residents as people, not just diagnoses or bodies that need care and assistance. This is especially true for those with communication difficulties such as persons with dementia or expressive aphasia. Increasingly, policies are changing to accommodate and actively encourage bringing more personal possessions, including furniture (including larger beds, when state codes allow for it) art, and memorabilia. Placement of personal items is not always limited to the individual's bedroom. China cupboards or other large pieces are sometimes placed in shared spaces, which helps people to feel like the whole household is their home.

LIGHTING AND ACOUSTICS

Although there has been solid research for decades documenting age-related changes to vision and hearing, there has been relatively little design guidance until recently that reflect these difficulties in long-term care settings. The *Design Guidelines for the Visual Environment* (National Institute of Building Sciences [NIBS], 2015) provides detailed visual and lighting recommendations for interior and exterior spaces, including information about the health effects of natural and artificial lighting. Unfortunately, there is evidence that nursing homes, in particular, are woefully underlit. Several studies have suggested that higher ambient lighting is associated with less agitation and distress (Brush, Threats, & Calkins, 2003) and that increasing light and contrast at the place setting can promote independence in eating and increase caloric intake by an average of 1,000 calories per day (Sloane et al., 2005). Not only are dining rooms underlit, but also they are often places of excessive noise levels, which makes eating less pleasurable for some and positively overwhelming for others. New acoustic standards can be found in the 2018 Edition of the FGI's guidelines, which address acoustic in bedrooms, apartments, and shared living spaces.

The movement away from staff-centric, institutional settings—reflecting Goffman's *Total Institutions* that reward passive acceptance of staff-determined routines—to settings that promote person- or self-directed, relationship-based models of care honoring the individual and respecting individuality and right to self-determination—can no longer be considered a passing fad. Person-centered care (PCC) is now codified in federal codes, such as the *Conditions of Participation for Long Term Care: Client Protections* (CMS, 2016) and numerous other codes and guidelines (e.g., National Fire Protection Agency's *Life Safety Code*, International Code Council *Building Codes*, and the FGI's guidelines). PCC, as it is most commonly referred to, represents a fundamental shift by valuing the quality of life as equally important as the quality of care. It is more than "a program" or set of activities and requires philosophical, organizational, operational, and behavioral changes. Although some experts argue that radical environmental changes may be difficult to implement (Koren, 2010), most agree that without at least some level of de-institutionalization of the environment, it is impossible to create a place where residents can feel that they are living at home.

Margaret P. Calkins

Adams, J., Verbeek, H., & Zwakhalen, S. M. (2017). The impact of organizational innovations in nursing homes on staff perceptions: A secondary data analysis. *Journal of Nursing Scholarship, 49*(1), 54–62.

Bicket, M. C., Samus, Q. M., McNabney, M., Onyike, C. U., Mayer, L. S., Brandt, J., … Rosenblatt, A. (2010). The physical environment influences neuropsychiatric symptoms and other outcomes in assisted living residents. *International Journal of Geriatric Psychiatry, 25*(10), 1044–1054.

Brush, J. A., Threats, T. T., & Calkins, M. P. (2003). Influences on perceived function of a nursing home resident. *Journal of Communication Disorders, 36*(5), 379–393.

Calkins, M. (2009). Evidence-based long term care design. *NeuroRehabilitation, 25*(3), 145–154.

Calkins, M., & Cassella, C. (2006). *Exploring the cost and value of private versus shared bedrooms in nursing homes.* Kirtland, OH: IDEAS Institute.

Centers for Medicare & Medicaid Services. (2016). Conditions of participation for long term care: Client protections (42 CFR § 483.420). *U.S. Dept. of Health and Human Services.* Retrieved from https://www.gpo.gov/fdsys/pkg/CFR-2016-title42-vol5/pdf/CFR-2016-title42-vol5-sec483-420.pdf

Day, K., & Calkins, M. P. (2002). Design and dementia. In R. B. Bechtel & A. Churchman (Eds.), *Handbook of environmental psychology* (pp. 374–393). New York, NY: Wiley.

Goffman, E. (1968). *Asylums: Essays on the social situation of mental patients and other inmates.* Chicago, IL: Aldine Transaction.

Kane, R., Lum, T., Cutler, L., Degenholtz, H., & Yu, T. (2007). Resident outcomes in small-house nursing homes: A longitudinal evaluation of the initial Green House program. *Journal of the American Geriatrics Society, 55*, 832–839.

Koren, M. J. (2010). Person-centered care for nursing home residents: The culture-change movement. *Health Affairs, 29*(2), 312–317.

Mazer, S. (2012). *The role and perception of privacy and its influence on the patient experience.* Chicago IL: The Beryl Institute.

McAllister, C. L., & Silverman, M. A. (1999). Community formation and community roles among persons with Alzheimer's disease: A comparative study of experiences in a residential Alzheimer's facility and a traditional nursing home. *Qualitative Health Research, 9*(1), 65–85.

Milke, D., Beck, C., Danes, S., & Lesak, J. (2009). Behavioral mapping of residents' activity in five residential style care centers for elderly persons diagnosed with dementia: Small differences in sites can affect behaviors. *Journal of Housing for the Elderly, 23*(4), 335–367. doi:10.1080/02763890903327135

National Institute of Building Sciences. (2015). *Design guidelines for the visual environment.* Washington DC: Author. Retrieved from http://www.nibs.org/?page=lvdc_guidelines&hhSearchTerms=%22visual+and+environment%22

Nordin, S., McKee, K., Wijk, H., & Elf, M. (2017). Exploring environmental variation in residential care facilities for older people. *Health Environments Research & Design Journal, 10*(2), 49–65.

Parker, C., Barnes, S., McKee, K., Morgan, K., Torrington, J., & Tregenza, P. (2004). Quality of life and building design in residential and nursing homes for older people. *Ageing & Society, 24*, 941–962.

Pekkarinen, L., Sinervo, T., Perala, M., & Elovainio, M. (2004). Work stressors and the quality of life in long-term care units. *The Gerontologist, 44*, 633–643.

Rowles, G. D., & Bernard, M. (2013). *Environmental gerontology: Making meaningful places in old age.* New York, NY: Springer Publishing.

Sloane, P. D., Noell-Waggoner, E., Hickman, S., Mitchell, C. M., Williams, C. S., Preisser, J. S., … Brawley, E. (2005). Implementing a lighting intervention in public areas of long-term care facilities: Lessons learned. *Alzheimer's Care Today, 6*(4), 280–293.

Web Resources

American Institute of Architects: Design for Aging Knowledge Network: https://network.aia.org/designforaging/home

Facilities Guidelines Institute: https://www.fgiguidelines.org

Society for the Advancement of Gerontological Environments: http://www.SAGEFederation.org

The Mayer-Rothschild Foundation: https://www.TheMayer-RothschildFoundation.org

ERGONOMICS

Ergonomics is a multidisciplinary field of study that has its origins in the late 1930s and early 1940s. The early foundations of ergonomics (or

E

human factors) were drawn from the areas of anatomy, physiology, psychology, medicine, and engineering. The evolution of ergonomics into a discipline, in its own right, required a formal definition of what ergonomics entails. The International Ergonomics Association (IEA, 2016) defines ergonomics as the scientific discipline concerned with the understanding of interactions among humans and other elements of a system, and the profession that applies theory, principles, data, and methods to design in order to optimize human well-being and overall system performance. More simply put, ergonomics helps optimize the interaction between humans and products, tasks, jobs, organizations, and environments based on their needs, abilities, and limitations. The discipline of ergonomics is now involved in all aspects of human activity and has areas of specialization in physical, cognitive, and organization ergonomics (IEA, 2016).

According to the United Nations (2015), the world's population is aging at a rate unprecedented in history. The percentage of persons older than 60 is projected to double from 10% in 2000 to 21% in 2050. This demographic shift requires greater attention on ergonomic designs to improve performance, safety, comfort, and user satisfaction and to minimize the likelihood of errors, injury, fatigue, and user dissatisfaction of older adults. As early as the 1990s, researchers recognized that ergonomic designs should take into consideration the heterogeneous changes in sensation, cognition, movement control, and perception that are associated with aging because they may all affect how older adults interact with products, tasks, jobs, organizations, and the environment.

Two main philosophies guide ergonomic design for older adults; these are the systems approach and "user-centered design/human-centered design" (UCD/HCD) practices. The systems-based approach, initially described by L. E. Morehouse in 1958, aims to achieve the optimal use of both human and machine capabilities for optimal performance of the total system. UCD/HCD design, initially described by Donald Norman in the 1980s, requires that users (older adults) be involved in the design of the final product. UCD practices are critical to improving a product's usefulness and usability, which are inadequately addressed by the systems approach alone (Mao, Vredenburg, Smith, & Carey, 2005).

Systems theory suggests that when interactions between older adults and the things they interact with are not optimal, the lack of person–environment fit can negatively affect health. Interactions between older adults and their environment occur in a wide range of areas; this chapter focuses on ergonomic considerations in the healthcare system, home, and work, because of their potential impact on the overall health of older adults.

HEALTH CARE SYSTEM

Within the health care field, "connected health technologies," or technologies for delivering healthcare remotely, is a burgeoning field that could transform the health management of older adults (Harte et al., 2014). The benefits of such technologies on the health of older adults are numerous and include, but are not limited to, improved quality of life and independence. By improving how well the user can access the functionality of technology (i.e., its usability), ergonomics can have an immense impact on connected health technologies by reducing the incidence of errors.

Czaja (2015) classified connected health technologies into the three categories: monitoring and sensing technologies, e-health applications, and robotic-coaching technologies:

- *Monitoring and sensing technologies* include in-home fall-detection and vision-sensing systems, smart home technology, and wearable monitoring technology. This technology allows for the management of chronic illnesses, health promotion and maintenance, and activity monitoring.
- *E-health applications* include websites, telemedicine, mobile health applications, electronic health records (EHRs), and personal health records (PHRs). This technology allows the older adult to access health information or support.

- *Robotic-coaching technologies* include robotic devices and virtual coaches. This technology allows for support in the form of instructions on device use, medication adherence, appointment reminders, as well as provision of companionship and supplementation of physical ability (Czaja, 2015).

HOME

The U.S. Department of Health and Human Serivces Administration for Community Living (2016) estimates that in 2014, more than 96% of adults aged 65 and older live in noninstitutionalized settings. This section focuses on ergonomic considerations that let older adults maintain independence in their home, allowing them to "age-in-place." Some of the major factors to consider when evaluating or implementing ergonomic designs to help older adults age-in-place are falls and performance of activities of daily living (ADL).

The Centers for Disease Control and Prevention (2016) estimates that one in every three older adults fall annually. The consequences of falls include soft tissue injuries, fear of falling, fractures, traumatic brain injury, and death. Because falling is a multifaceted problem, home evaluation for falls involves multiple considerations. Home evaluations include assessments of whether home lighting is adequate; high-contrast visual cues at stair edges or rises are present, particularly in bathrooms and kitchens; handrails are installed; cues to improve handrail use are present; furnishings that increase the risk of tripping are present; and grab bars are installed in bathrooms (Cisneros, Dyer-Chamberlain, & Hickie, 2012; Fisk, Rogers, Charness, Czaja, & Sharit, 2009; Jacobs, 2016).

An estimated 30% of community-dwelling Medicare beneficiaries aged 65 years or older report having difficulty in one or more ADL (U.S. Department of Health and Human Services, Administration for Community Living, 2016). The ability to perform ADL may be affected by cognitive, perceptual, or motor control changes that occur with normal aging. Devices can be provided to older adults to assist in performing ADL, including hip-high chairs, transfer benches, walk-in tubs, nonslip mats, hand-grip adaptations, bed rails, grabbers/reachers, sock-pull aids, and button and zipper pullers.

WORK

Since 2002, the Bureau of Labor Statistics has reported a steady increase in the number of older adults in the labor force (working or actively seeking work), and in 2015 persons 65 and older constituted 5.6% of the workforce. This increase in older adult workers is because of financial issues, job enjoyment, an aging population, and extended life expectancy. With an increasing older adult workforce, occupational ergonomic designs should consider the older adult worker to ensure their safety and efficacy.

As noted previously, older adults experience several changes; however, the relationship between the changes and ability to perform the physical and mental tasks associated with work is complex (Fox, Brogmus, & Maynard, 2015). For instance, declines in strength with aging are generally based on tests of maximal strength (e.g., isometric, isokinetic). However, in industrial working environments, task demands are submaximal; therefore, the ability to perform a task may involve more factors than strength. In addition, the effects of aging on an individual worker's ability are not uniform. Because all areas of age-related declines may not be relevant in an ergonomic assessment, Fox et al. (2015) propose a more targeted approach to ergonomic workplace evaluations for older adults; these evaluations focus on identifying injury hazards that are relevant to the specific work environment. Furthermore, the authors provide general guidelines for ergonomic assessments. To reduce the incidence of same-level falls, which are prevalent in those aged 65 and older, they recommend that workplaces use appropriate mats, eliminate tripping and slipping hazards, and use proper stairway designs. In addition, there should be proper lighting and appropriate use of colors and contrast for transitions (e.g., steps); the use of wellness programs and training methods should be encouraged to reduce risks or errors.

Sylvester Carter

E

Centers for Disease Control and Prevention. (2016, January 20). Home and recreational safety: Important facts about falls. Retrieved from http://www.cdc.gov/homeandrecreationalsafety/falls/adultfalls.html

Cisneros, H., Dyer-Chamberlain, M., & Hickie, J. (2012). *Independent for life: Homes and neighborhoods for an aging America:* Austin: University of Texas Press.

Czaja, S. J. (2015). Can technology empower older adults to manage their health? *Generations, 39*(1), 46–51.

Fisk, A. D., Rogers, W. A., Charness, N., Czaja, S. J., & Sharit, J. (2009). *Designing for older adults: Principles and creative human factors approaches.* Boca Raton, FL: CRC Press.

Fox, R. R., Brogmus, G. E., & Maynard, W. S. (2015). Aging workers & ergonomics: A fresh perspective. *Professional Safety, 60*(1), 33–41. doi:10.5888/pcdlO.120203

Harte, R. P., Glynn, L. G., Broderick, B. J., Rodriguez-Molinero, A., Baker, P. M., McGuiness, B., …ÓLaighin, G. (2014). Human centred design considerations for connected health devices for the older adult. *Journal of Personalized Medicine, 4*(2), 245–281. doi:10.3390/jpm4020245

International Ergonomics Association. (2016). Definition and domains of ergonomics. Retrieved from http://www.iea.cc/whats/index.html

Jacobs, J. V. (2016). A review of stairway falls and stair negotiation: Lessons learned and future needs to reduce injury. *Gait Posture, 49*, 159–167. doi:10.1016/j.gaitpost.2016.06.030

Mao, J.-Y., Vredenburg, K., Smith, P. W., & Carey, T. (2005). The state of user-centered design practice. *Communications of the ACM, 48*(3), 105–109.

United Nations Department of Economic and Social Affairs, Population Division. (2015, October). Population fact-sheets. Retrieved from http://www.un.org/en/development/desa/population/publications/factsheets/index.shtml

U.S. Department of Health and Human Services, Administration for Community Living. (2016). Profile of older Americans. Retrieved from https://www.acl.gov/node/537

ETHICS CONSULTATION

Clinical ethics consultation is a service that an individual or group provides to help health care professionals, patients, and families identify and resolve ethical conflicts and problems that arise in the care of patients. The practice of offering clinical ethics consultations began informally in the 1970s and during the past 45 years, has become an established part of the clinical services of many health care institutions. The increased importance of ethics consultations can be traced to at least two sources: (a) the rapid growth of medical technology, which has presented patients, families, and health care providers with new and difficult ethical choices, and (b) the rise of the patient's rights movement and the correlative attack on medical paternalism. Clinical ethics consultation was also given a major impetus by The Joint Commission, which in 1992, mandated that all accredited health care institutions have a "mechanism" for dealing with disputes concerning end-of-life care.

MODES

Clinical ethics consultations can be conducted in various ways: by an ethics committee, by a small team (possibly a subgroup of the ethics committee), or by individual consultants. Consultations by committee are often difficult to organize in a timely fashion and may become bureaucratic and depersonalized, but they can provide multiple perspectives and reveal relevant aspects of a case that might otherwise be overlooked. Consultations by individuals—typically clinicians, lawyers, or philosophers specializing in bioethics—are generally more flexible and personal and can be arranged more expeditiously. Many ethics consultative services require that individual consultants report to an ethics committee or consultation group, either for retrospective review of cases or for help with ongoing cases. This supervision provides peer review and quality assurance and is a way of holding consultants accountable for their activities. Consultations by small teams occupy a middle ground between these two approaches.

GOALS

The main goal of clinical ethics consultation is to improve the quality of care by providing a mechanism for the identification, analysis, and resolution of ethical problems and conflicts that arise in the clinical setting. Other important goals include facilitating institutional efforts at quality improvement by identifying common sources of ethical problems and helping health care providers handle ethical problems by providing education in clinical bioethics (Wasson et al., 2016).

ROLE OF THE CLINICAL ETHICS CONSULTANT

The role of the clinical ethics consultant has been described variously as a professional colleague, educator, facilitator of moral reflection, mediatory of moral conflict, and patient advocate. Associated with each description is a particular set of skills and competencies (American Society for Bioethics and Humanities, 2011). Some view the consultant primarily as a patient advocate responsible for protecting the patient's rights and interests; others perceive the consultant as a neutral mediator whose goal is to forge consensus among the involved parties, all of whose rights, interests, and responsibilities are acknowledged. Even though complete neutrality is not possible, since consultants are part of the health system, an ethics consultant must strive not just for a mutually agreeable solution, but also for a morally principled consensus (Dubler, 2011). At the same time, ethics consultants should not be considered moral police; their authority is qualitatively different.

A model that has attracted considerable interest in the field of ethics consultation is mediation (Dubler & Leibman, 2011). Ethics consultants, as mediators, use many of the techniques of classical mediation, including active listening, reframing, acknowledging the feelings and concerns of the involved parties, and developing options. However, these techniques must be modified to fit the peculiar features of the medical setting.

As facilitators or moral reflection, consultants are regarded as having particular skills and knowledge that their professional colleagues lack. What they bring to the clinical encounter is not "the right answer," but rather the ability to uncover value conflicts, articulate different moral positions on issues, and apply moral reasoning and ethical theory to the issue at hand.

There is considerable literature on whether there is such a thing as *ethical expertise* and whether the ethics consultant has or is supposed to have it (Steinkamp, Gordijn, & ten Have, 2008). The notion of ethical expertise, however, has a number of unfortunate connotations. Properly understood, the role of the ethics consultant is to offer reasoned ethical advice and guidance to patients, families, and health professionals, not to make decisions or to override the views of others. A criticism related to concerns about ethical expertise is that ethics consultation promotes the segregation of ethical decision making from the clinical practice of medicine. However, this danger can be avoided if ethics consultants work collaboratively with clinicians and regard the education of staff as one of their main responsibilities.

ISSUES ADDRESSED BY CLINICAL ETHICS CONSULTANTS

Patients, families, and health care professionals may call on clinical ethics consultants to address a wide range of issues, including the following:

- Confidentiality and privacy
- Decisional capacity
- Informed consent and truth telling
- Surrogate decision making
- Withdrawal or withholding of life-sustaining treatment
- Shift from curative to palliative care
- Allocation of scarce medical resources
- Conflicts among health care providers
- Role of economic considerations in clinical care.

The patient's attending physician retains decision-making responsibility and authority. As such, the physician should be informed of the request for an ethics consultation and the source of the request (i.e., patient, family member, or other member of the health care team). Many institutions allow anyone to initiate an ethics consult anonymously.

COMPETENCIES OF THE CLINICAL ETHICS CONSULTANT

The core competencies of ethics consultants can be divided into two categories: skills and knowledge. Core skills include the ability to:

- Identify the value conflict or problem in the clinical situation
- Listen attentively, respectfully, and supportively to the involved parties
- Elicit the interests and moral concerns of all involved parties
- Promote effective communication among the involved parties
- Articulate care options and their consequences
- Work toward a moral consensus

Core knowledge includes competency in the following:

- Terms used in the diagnosis, treatment, and prognosis of common medical problems
- Key bioethical concepts, principles, and theories
- Techniques of moral reasoning
- Main ethical positions on important clinical issues
- Applicable health law
- Ways that cultural beliefs may influence decision making in the population served
- Organization, corporate structure, and culture of the institution

METHODS OF CLINICAL ETHICS CONSULTATION

At a minimum, these four elements must be performed and documented for each ethics consultation: ethics question; consultation-specific information; ethical analysis; conclusions and/or recommendations. The *CASES approach* incorporates all of these elements. It is a systematic approach to clinical ethics consultation whereby the consultant follows these five steps: clarify the consultation request, assemble the relevant information, synthesize the information, explain the synthesis, and support the consultation process. Decision-making tools such as the *four box method* are useful in the analysis of each case. This approach requires the consultant to consider and balance these four intrinsic elements of each clinical encounter: medical indications, patient preferences, quality of life, and contextual features.

EVALUATION OF CLINICAL ETHICS CONSULTATION

Evaluation of clinical ethics consultation is a matter of considerable interest and debate among those in the field (Magnus, 2015). Meaningful evaluation of the ethics consultation is particularly important in light of efforts to control health care costs by eliminating unnecessary and unprofitable services. Such an evaluation must keep in mind the goals of that consultation. Both the process of consultation and its outcomes need to be evaluated (Batten, 2013). The process is evaluated by asking whether the consultation was conducted in a timely fashion, whether all interested parties were included in the consultation, and whether participants were satisfied with the quality of communication. Outcomes are evaluated by asking such questions as whether a principled ethical resolution of the problem was achieved, whether the participants were satisfied with the outcome, whether the consultation altered the plan of care, and whether the consultant's services were frequently used. Chart reviews, questionnaires, and interviews are some useful evaluation techniques. The American Society for Bioethics and Humanities has created a Quality Attestation Presidential Task Force to ensure that individual ethics consultants are qualified (Fiester, 2014). Sound methods of evaluation should be implemented (Wasson, Parsi, McCarthy, Siddall & Kuczewski, 2016).

See also Advance Directives; Hospice; Palliative Care; Physician Aid in Dying, Physician-Assisted Suicide, and Euthanasia.

Lara Wahlberg and
Anne Steinfeld Rugova

American Society for Bioethics and Humanities. (2011). *Core competencies for health care ethics consultants* (2nd ed.). Glenview, IL: Author.
Batten, J. (2013). Assessing clinical ethics consultation: Process and outcomes. *Medicine and Law, 32*, 141–152.

Dubler, N. N. (2011). A "principled resolution": The fulcrum for bioethics mediation. *Law and Contemporary Problems, 74*(3), 177–200.

Dubler, N. N., & Liebman, C. B. (2011). *Bioethics mediation: A guide to shaping shared solutions, revised and expanded edition.* Nashville, TN: Vanderbilt University Press.

Fiester, A. (2014). The "quality attestation" process and the risk of the false positive. *Hastings Center Report, 44*(3), 19–22. doi:10.1002/hast.311

Magnus, D. (2015). Clinical ethics consultation: A need for evidence. *The American Journal of Bioethics, 15*(1), 1–2. doi:10.1080/15265161.2015.987577

Steinkamp, N. L., Gordijn, B., & ten Have, H. A. M. J. (2008). Debating ethical expertise. *Kennedy Institute of Ethics Journal, 18*(2), 173–192.

Wasson, K., Anderson, E., Hagstrom, E., McCarthy, M., Parsi, K., & Kuczewski, M., (2016). What ethical issues really arise in practice at an academic medical center? A quantitative and qualitative analysis of clinical ethics consultations from 2008 to 2013. *HEC Forum, 28*(3), 217–228. doi:10.1007/s10730-015-9293-5

Wasson, K., Parsi, K., McCarthy, M., Siddall, J., & Kuczewski, M. (2016). Developing an evaluation tool for assessing clinical ethics consultation skills in simulation based education: The ACES project. *HEC Forum, 28*(2), 103–113. doi:10.1007/s10730-015-9276-6

Web Resources

American Bar Association: Surrogate Decision Making and Advance Directives: http://www.americanbar.org/content/dam/aba/migrated/aging/pdfs/nalc_sur_d_m.authcheckdam.pdf

American Medical Association Code of Medical Ethics: http://www.ama-assn.org/ama/pub/physician-resources/medical-ethics/code-medical-ethics.page

American Society for Bioethics and Humanities: http://asbh.org

Ethics in Medicine: http://depts.washington.edu/bioethx/tools/cesumm.html

Hastings Center: http://www.thehastingscenter.org

National Center for Ethics in Healthcare: http://www.ethics.va.gov/integratedethics/ecc.asp

EUTHANASIA

Euthanasia comes from Greek words meaning "a gentle and easy death" and "the means of bringing about a gentle and easy death." Most ancient Greek and Roman practitioners, Socrates, Plato, and Stoic philosophers from Zeno to Seneca, supported physician-induced death of the sick and suffering to bring about a gentle and easy death (Vanderpool, 1995). In contrast to these dominant Graco-Roman traditions, the *Hippocratic oath* required physicians to swear "neither to give a deadly drug to anybody if asked for it, nor … [to] make a suggestion to this effect" (Edelstein, 1989, p. 6). The oath, which continues to exert a towering influence in Western medicine, reflects the Pythagorean conviction that human beings are owned by God or gods and should abide by a divine determination of life's completion (Carrick, 1985).

In contemporary usage, discussion of euthanasia has increasingly dealt with "the action of inducing a gentle and easy death." Thus ethical debates about the permissibility of physician involvement in euthanasia concern the question: Are physicians ethically permitted to act to end a patient's life? This question should be distinguished from other ethical questions that may arise at the end of life. For example, as the term *euthanasia* is commonly used today, it does not concern questions related to refraining from using or continuing life-sustaining treatments (i.e., passive euthanasia), nor does it concern questions related to providing patients with the means necessary to end their own lives (i.e., assisted suicide). Many who defend the permissibility of physician-assisted suicide do not support physician-assisted euthanasia. Advocates of physician-assisted suicide approve of letting physicians prescribe medications that patients may use to end their own life; they do not necessarily approve of letting physicians administer, for example, lethal injections for the purpose of terminating a patient's life. Other means of achieving the goal of a "gentle and easy death" include accelerating opioids for the purpose of relieving pain or dyspnea, with death as a foreseeable yet unintended consequence (Quill, Dresser, Brock, 1997); administering continuous deep sedation to reduce or take away consciousness at the end of life until death follows (Raus, Sterckx, & Mortier, 2011); and voluntarily withholding fluids and nutrition until death occurs (Quill, 2012).

ETHICAL PERSPECTIVES

E Contemporary ethical arguments supporting euthanasia often appeal to compassion for the suffering of a terminally ill and imminently dying patient. These arguments purport to show that physician aid in dying is ethically permissible under circumstances in which the patient's condition is associated with severe and unrelenting suffering that is not the result of inadequate pain control or comfort care.

Alternatively, arguments defending the permissibility of euthanasia reference the ethical principle of autonomy. The principle of autonomy requires respecting the informed choices of competent patients. Under this approach, physician involvement in euthanasia is ethically limited to situations in which competent patients make informed repeated requests for aid in dying.

Critics of euthanasia charge that both compassion and autonomy-based ethical arguments are unpersuasive. Arguments invoking compassion are faulted on the grounds that there is no principled basis for limiting euthanasia to competent patients who choose it. After all, many suffering patients are not competent. Therefore, if the ethical basis for providing aid in dying is compassion, then aid in dying should logically be extended to incompetent persons.

Arguments relying on the ethical principle of autonomy are also criticized for failing to offer a principled basis for appropriately limiting euthanasia. Thus autonomy-based arguments do not require limiting euthanasia to patients who experience severe and unrelenting suffering but would presumably allow applying euthanasia to healthy people who wish to die. Critics of autonomy-based arguments also doubt that patients' requests to die reflect patients' autonomous choices. Instead, such requests may occur because of inadequate palliative and comfort care, continued use of invasive and futile interventions, or failure to diagnose and treat other underlying causes of the request, such as depression. In such cases, meeting a patient's request for assistance in dying is not supported by a principle of respect for patient autonomy.

Both autonomy and compassion-based arguments are vulnerable to the further objection that there is no principled basis for restricting euthanasia to persons who are imminently dying. After all, the prospect of suffering for a long period is arguably worse than the prospect of suffering briefly. Likewise, the principle of respect for autonomy presumably applies to all competent individuals, irrespective of whether they are about to die.

LEGAL PERSPECTIVES

Just as the ethical status of euthanasia is controversial, the legal status of both euthanasia and assisted suicide is the subject of intense debate in the United States. Historically, legislative statutes made assisted suicide a criminal act in many states; however, the constitutionality of these statutes has been challenged. Defenders of physician-assisted death have placed citizen initiatives on the ballots of several Western states to decriminalize euthanasia and/or assisted suicide. In 1997, Oregon became the first state to allow physician-assisted suicide. In 2008, Washington became the second. In 2013, Vermont became the first state to approve physician-assisted suicide through legislation (rather than through citizen initiatives). Montana and California subsequently became the fourth and fifth states to allow physician-assisted suicide for the terminally ill. No state currently allows euthanasia, which would involve physicians (or others) directly administering a medication to end a patient's life (Lindsay, 2009).

Although euthanasia is illegal in the United States and in most other nations, it is no longer against the law in The Netherlands. In 2002, the Dutch Parliament passed an act formally exempting physicians from criminal liability for euthanasia and assisted suicide, provided that certain conditions are met. These conditions include that (a) the patient's request is voluntary and well considered, (b) the patient experiences lasting and unbearable suffering, (c) the physician has informed the patient about the situation and prospects, (d) the physician and patient believe there is no other reasonable solution, (e) the physician consults with one other independent physician regarding the first four conditions, and (f) the physician exercises due care in terminating life or assisting with suicide.

EUTHANASIA AND THE ELDERLY

Although debates about euthanasia apply to persons of all ages, they may bear special relevance to elderly persons (Jecker, 2014). Because death is generally nearer in old age, aging individuals may be more likely than younger persons to think about death and the dying process. Perhaps the rapid aging of populations occurring in developed nations will lead societies to focus greater attention on how to assure humane care at the end of life. The question of whether euthanasia represents humane medical care for dying patients is an ongoing ethical debate.

See also Physician Aid in Dying; Physician-Assisted Suicide; and Euthanasia.

Nancy S. Jecker

Carrick, P. (1985). *Medical ethics in antiquity: Philosophical perspectives on abortion and euthanasia.* Dordrecht, Netherlands: D. Reidel.

Edelstein, L. (1989). The Hippocratic oath: Text, translation and interpretation. In O. Temkin & C. L. Temkin (Eds.), *Ancient medicine: Selected papers of Ludwig Edelstein* (pp. 6–8). Baltimore, MD: John Hopkins University Press.

Jecker, N. S. (2014). Against a duty to die. *Virtual Mentor: AMA Journal of Ethics, 16*(5), 390–394.

Lindsay, R. A. (2009). Oregon's experience: Evaluating the record. *American Journal of Bioethics, 9*(3), 19–27.

Raus, K., Sterckx, S., & Mortier, F. (2011). Is continuous sedation at the end of life an ethically preferable alternative to physician-assisted suicide? *American Journal of Bioethics, 11*(6), 32–40.

Quill, T. E. (2012). Physicians should "assist in suicide" when it is appropriate. *Journal of Law, Medicine & Ethics, 40*(1), 57–65.

Quill, T. E., Dresser, R., & Brock, D. W. (1997). Rule of double effect: A critique of its role in end-of-life decision making. *New England Journal of Medicine, 337*, 1768–1771.

Vanderpool, H. Y. (1995). Death and dying: Euthanasia and sustaining life. In T. R. Warren & T. Reich (Eds.), *Encyclopedia of bioethics* (Rev. ed., pp. 554–561). New York, NY: Simon & Schuster, MacMillan.

Web Resources

Bioethics.net: http://www.bioethics.net
Hastings Center: http://www.thehastingscenter.org
Stanford Encyclopedia of Philosophy: http://www.science.uva.nl/~seop

EVIDENCE-BASED HEALTH CARE

E

The U.S. Department of Health and Human Services, Administration for Community Living (2016) estimates that 14% of Americans are elderly and this number is expected to double by the year 2030, to almost 78 million. With such an unprecedented surge in this segment of the population, health care clinicians are challenged with providing high-quality, evidence-based health care for a growing population of older Americans who are interested in staying healthy, preventing physical and cognitive decline, and coping with cognitive and functional decline. *Evidence-based practice (EBP)* is defined as the "conscientious and judicious use of the current best evidence from clinical care research in the management of individual patients" (Sackett, Rosenberg, Gray, Haynes, & Richardson, 1996, p. 71). Recently, experts suggest that the better term is *evidence-based decision making*, described as the formulation of clinical decisions based on the best available research evidence while considering the patient's preferences and acknowledging a central role for the clinician's expertise to coordinate these components. Decisions regarding the best nutritional approaches, exercise regimens, and screening approaches represent just a few of the many decisions clinicians encounter when providing treatments for a healthy and long life span.

The Institute of Medicine ([IOM], 2008) has designated 2020 as the target year when 90% of all clinical decisions should be based on the best available evidence. Yet health care clinicians encounter considerable constraints when using evidence-based approaches, including inefficient information systems, inadequate knowledge of EBP, and a lack of evidence-based critical appraisal skills. Compounding these barriers is the preponderance of existing research studies in electronic databases, with the number of English-language citations in PubMed surpassing 20 million in 2012 (U.S. National Library of Medicine, 2013). Reviewing all of the research studies is not possible, therefore efficient methods of searching databases to attain the best

E

available evidence are needed to support clinical decision making.

In everyday practice, clinicians ask multiple questions concerning the validity of diagnostic tests, the effectiveness of pharmacological interventions, and the accuracy of prognostic data. The EBP framework provides a step-by-step approach for generating different types of evidence-based clinical decisions (Strauss, Richardson, Glasziou, & Haynes, 2011). The first step begins by structuring a searchable question that encompasses the patient/population (P), the intervention (I), the comparison or control intervention (C), and the outcome (O), known by the acronym PICO. The second step involves searching electronic databases for high-quality evidence using the PICO components as the key search terms. Once the evidence is located, the next step involves a critical appraisal of the evidence for validity, evaluation of bias, and clinical usefulness. Once the evidence is assessed as high quality and relevant for the patient, the fourth step involves aligning the preferences of patients with the recommended evidence-based approach. A fifth step requires an evaluation of the patient's response to the intervention.

Information resources are being developed to facilitate efficient evidence-based decision making. The "6S Organization of Evidence" describes the ideal, hierarchical systems approach for accessing the best available evidence and encourages the use of "preprocessed," or previously appraised, evidence (Strauss et al., 2011). In this model, the search for the best evidence begins with a computerized information-support system, where evidence has been integrated into an electronic medical records system and, on request, connects to the patient's problem or diagnosis. Because many of these sophisticated, computerized systems have not yet been developed or implemented, the next step involves a search for summaries, evidence-based guidelines, or textbooks that succinctly summarize the best available evidence for a given problem. Synopses or syntheses of systematic reviews represent the next level of "preprocessed" evidence and may be accessed at the American College of Physicians Journal Club (www.acpjc.org) or Evidence-Based Nursing (www.ebn.bmjjournals.com). In the absence of

synopses, the next step involves searching for a single systematic review, a systematic synthesis of the best available evidence related to a clinical question. The Cochrane Collaboration is an example of an electronic database that contains a large repository of systematic reviews (www.cochranecollaboration.org). If a systematic review does not exist for a particular problem, the next step involves searching for a synopsis of a single, high-quality study. If a synopsis of a single study is not located, the search for single studies begins.

Professional organizations publish evidence-based guidelines based on the most recent research studies and provide recommendations regarding the screening, diagnosis, and treatment of a medical problem such as coronary artery disease, heart failure, and hypertension, medical conditions that disproportionately afflict older individuals. However, not all guidelines are alike. To help guide clinicians in selecting the best evidence, Grades of Recommendation, Assessment, Development, and Evaluation (GRADE) Working Group developed the GRADE rating scale in 2004. In this rating scale, the quality of the evidence is evaluated. For example, a Grade A recommendation indicates considerable confidence in the treatment benefit over harm. Grade B recommendations indicate moderate certainty the treatment will have a moderate benefit. Grade C recommendations are weaker recommendations and indicate that the purported benefits are small. Clinicians should assess the individual patient to determine whether these treatments may be beneficial for an individual and not outweigh the potential harm. Grade D recommendations advise against the treatment indicating no benefit of this approach. The United States Preventive (USPSTF, 2016) uses this grading approach to generate recommendations for or against treatments. For example, the USPSTF provides a Grade B recommendation for both physical therapy and vitamin D supplements in the prevention of falls in adults who are 65 years of age or older and at risk of falling, indicating moderate certainty that these treatments will have a moderate effect.

When preprocessed evidence, guidelines, or systematic reviews are not available, clinicians need to search for a single study that represents the highest level of evidence to address the clinical question. Numerous hierarchies of evidence rank the strength of research according to the most appropriate design/methodology for the question. McMaster's University has suggested the "Hierarchy of Strength of Evidence for Treatment Decisions" (DiCenso, Ciliska, & Guyatt, 2005, p. 12). For therapy questions, systematic reviews, syntheses of randomized controlled trials, are the highest level of evidence. The next level includes the single randomized controlled trial. Systematic reviews of observational studies represent the next level, followed by a single observational study, including both cohort and case-control studies. Physiological studies that use surrogate outcomes, such as blood pressure, total cholesterol, and hemoglobin A1c, as substitute measures of clinical outcomes, are included in the next level, followed by unsystematic expert opinions (DiCenso et al., 2005). Similarly, if the question pertains to the validity of a diagnostic study, the highest level of evidence would include a systematic review of diagnostic studies using cross-sectional designs; if the question pertains to the accuracy of a prognostic sign, the highest level of evidence would be a cohort study.

The search for evidence reveals substantial discrepancies in the quality of individual studies. Multiple critical appraisal tools (CATs) are designed to help clinicians evaluate the quality of different types of studies, including systematic reviews, randomized controlled trials, and diagnostic and prognostic studies. The selection of a CAT linked to the study design allows clinicians to evaluate the critical aspects of the design. For example, a CAT for a randomized controlled trial asks key questions pertaining to the type of sample, the randomization process, and the results. Of the existing tools, few have demonstrated psychometric reliability and validity, highlighting one of the limitations of the critical appraisal process (Crowe & Sheppard, 2011).

Evidence-based statistics help translate statistical data into understandable and clinically useful data. To illustrate, if a study evaluated the effectiveness of Drug A compared with Drug B on mortality, and if the outcomes revealed a statistically significant reduction in mortality with Drug A, the clinician may want to know the extent of the difference for the individual patient and/or patient population. The absolute risk reduction (ARR) or risk difference may be calculated by subtracting the experimental event rate (EER) from the control event rate (CER), as seen in the following equation (CER − EER = ARR). To calculate the number of individuals needed to treat to reduce one death, the number needed to treat (NNT) is determined using the inverse of the ARR (1/ARR = NNT). The risk in the control group (CER) relative to the risk in the experimental group (EER), known as the *relative risk ratio*, is derived by the following equation: (CER/EER). The relative risk reduction is determined by the difference between the CER and the EER relative to the CER (CER − EER/CER). Similarly, the clinician may calculate the probability of an increase in a beneficial outcome and/or an increase in a deleterious outcome by examining the relative benefit increase (RBI = EER − CER/CER) or the relative risk increase (RRI = EER − CER/CER), respectively, depending on the designated outcome of the study (Strauss et al., 2011).

Older adults are likely to have more comorbidities, take more medications, and experience more impairments in cognition, function, and/or mood. By applying the principles of EBP, health care providers will ensure that all older adults have access to the most effective evidence-based approaches associated with health promotion, injury prevention, comorbidity management, and end-of-life issues. To recognize the IOM's vision for evidence-based decision making, educators, health care administrators, researchers, and clinicians need to collaborate to teach EBP, implement evidence-based systems, produce more clinical evidence and research, and finally, support shared decision making for both patients and populations with the best evidence.

See also Clinical Pathways; Telehealth.

Mary M. Brennan

Crowe, M., & Sheppard, L. (2011). A review of critical appraisal tools show they lack rigor: Alternative tool structure is proposed. *Journal of Clinical*

Epidemiology, 64(1), 79–89. doi:10.1016/j.jclinepi.2010.02.008

DiCenso, A., Ciliska, D., & Guyatt, G. (2005). Introduction to evidence-based nursing. In A. DiCenso, G. Guyatt, & D. Ciliska (Eds.), *Evidence-based nursing: A guide to clinical practice* (pp. 3–19). St. Louis, MO: Elsevier Mosby.

GRADE Working Group. (2004). Grading quality of evidence and strength of recommendations. *British Medical Journal, 328,* 1490–1494.

Institute of Medicine. (2008). *Evidence-based medicine and the changing nature of health care: 2007 Institute of Medicine annual meeting summary.* Washington, DC: National Academies Press. Retrieved from http://www.ncbi.nlm.nih.gov/books/NBK52819/#summary.r3

Sackett, D. L., Rosenberg, W. M., Gray, J. A., Haynes, R. B., & Richardson, W. S. (1996). Evidence-based medicine: What it is and what it isn't. *British Medical Journal, 312*(702), 71–72.

Strauss, S. E., Richardson, W. S., Glasziou, P., & Haynes, R. B. (2011). *Evidence-based medicine: How to practice and teach EBM* (4th ed.). Edinburgh, UK: Churchill Livingstone Elsevier.

U.S. Department of Health and Human Services, Administration for Community Living, Administration on Aging. (2016). Retrieved from https://www.acl.gov/node/537

U.S. National Library of Medicine. (2013). MEDLINE: Number of citations to English language articles; number of citations containing abstracts. Retrieved from http://www.nlm.nih.gov/bsd/medline_lang_distr.html

U.S. Preventive Services Task Force. (2016). Grade A and grade B recommendations. Retrieved from www.uspreventiveservicestaskforce.org/Page/Name/uspstf-a-and-b-recommendations

Web Resources

Agency for Healthcare Quality Research (AHRQ), Evidence Reports: https://www.ahrq.gov/research/findings/evidence-based-reports/index.html

American College of Physicians (ACP) Journal Club: http://www.acponline.org

Centre for Evidence-Based Medicine: http://cebm.jr2.ox.ac.uk

Clinical Evidence: http://www.clinicalevidence.org

Cochrane Collaboration: http://www.cochrane.org

Complementary and Alternative Medicine: http://www.jr2.ox.ac.uk/bandolier

Cumulative Index to Nursing and Allied Health Literature (CINAHL): http://www.ebscohost.com/academic/cinahl-plus-with-full-text

Evidence-Based Nursing: http://ebn.bmjjournals.com

National Guideline Clearing House: http://www.guidelines.gov/index.asp

U.S. Department of Health and Human Services, Administration for Community Living: https://aoa.acl.gov/Aging_Statistics/Index.aspx

U.S. National Library of Medicine and National Institutes of Health/PubMed.gov: http://www.ncbi.nlm.nih.gov/pubmed

U.S. Preventive Services Task Force: https://www.uspreventiveservicestaskforce.org

EXERCISE

Physical activity consists of movements that involve energy expenditure. Exercise is a specific type of physical activity that is planned and structured. The benefits of physical activity and exercise in the overall health and well-being of persons of all ages are well known, yet older adults are the least active of all age groups (Elsawy & Higgins, 2010). Older adults who begin physical activity after 50 years old have been found to have a 50% decreased risk of mortality, which has equal benefits as smoking cessation (Batt, Tanji, & Borjesson, 2013). In addition, older adults who engage in regular physical activity may have lower medical expenditures than sedentary adults (Snell, 2016). Conversely, physical inactivity increases the cost of health care expenses and contributes to many chronic diseases that affect older adults such as heart disease, stroke, diabetes, lung disease, Alzheimer's disease, hypertension (HTN), obesity, osteoporosis, and certain cancers. In fact, physical inactivity is one of the leading risk factors for death worldwide, accounting for about 3.2 million deaths yearly per the WHO (2017). Three of the other leading risk factors (high blood pressure, high blood glucose, and obesity) are also connected with physical inactivity (Taylor, 2014).

Health care providers have a unique role in helping older adults become more physically active. Those who received advice from their physician performed more moderate-to-vigorous intensity activity than those who did not (Taylor, 2014). Therefore it is imperative that those involved in the care of older adults understand the benefits of, barriers to, and guidelines for physical activity to improve both the quantity and quality of life.

PHYSIOLOGIC CHANGES IN STRUCTURE AND FUNCTION IN NORMAL AGING

Body composition changes with aging. Older adults gradually accumulate more body fat centrally and viscerally and lose muscle mass and strength, also known as sarcopenia. Bone mineral density also starts to decline after age 40 (0.5% per year) and declines more rapidly in postmenopausal females (2%–3% per year). Cardiovascular changes include decreased cardiac output, a major determinant of reduced exercise capacity in aging, and increased systolic blood pressure at rest. Thirst sensation also decreases, and the kidneys have a decreased ability to conserve sodium and water, both of which can increase the risk of dehydration. Even in healthy older adults, skeletal muscle performance declines. This leads to decreased exercise tolerance and increased risk of losing the ability to do basic and instrumental activities of daily living and therefore physical independence.

BENEFITS OF EXERCISE

The benefits of regular physical are seen in all areas of well-being: physical, emotional, and cognitive. Age-related functional decline, falls, and unhealthy weight gain can be averted or prevented with regular physical activity (Snell, 2016). Low physical activity is a key component of frailty, and systematic reviews have shown that frailty is amenable to exercise interventions, although further studies need to be done regarding which exercises are most beneficial (De Labra, Guimaraes-Pinheiro, Maseda, Lorenzo, & Millán-Calenti, 2015). All-cause mortality and morbidity may decrease with regular exercise. Even a sedentary smoker or obese older adult who becomes physically active can experience health benefits, even if they continue to smoke or do not lose weight. Progressive weight training

can increase muscle strength, size and power, which helps with sarcopenia (American College of Sports Medicine [ACSM], 2009). Recent literature shows that the volume of the hippocampus, the area of the brain involved in memory, increases with exercise. Improved cognition and attention and decreased risk of dementia have also been demonstrated (Batt et al., 2013). In addition, clinical guidelines include physical activity as an important component in the treatment of many chronic conditions such as coronary artery disease (CAD), peripheral vascular disease, HTN, type 2 diabetes, osteoarthritis, osteoporosis, some lipid disorders, obesity, claudication, and chronic obstructive pulmonary disease (COPD). Physical activity also aids in the management of depression, anxiety disorders, pain, heart failure, syncope, sleep disorders, stroke, dementia, back pain, and constipation and in the prevention of venous thromboembolism (Snell, 2016). The Lifestyle Interventions and Independence for Elders (LIFE) study of a structured, moderate-intensity physical activity program for a sample of sedentary community-dwelling older persons found that those who participated in the exercise program over 2.6 years were less likely to develop major mobility disability (Pahor, 2014).

BARRIERS TO EXERCISE

Despite the many benefits of exercise, older adults often have numerous reasons, real or perceived, for not engaging in it. The most common reason for not exercising is poor health (Schutzer & Graves, 2004). Older adults often perceive themselves as being too old or frail to exercise. Pain is reported as another common barrier (Schutzer, 2004). The physical environment can also be a barrier; high crime rates and no access to sidewalks, parks, recreation centers, and fitness facilities have been linked to decreased adherence to exercise.

TYPES OF EXERCISE

Aerobic exercise includes aerobic exercise classes, bicycle riding, dancing, golfing (without a golf cart), raking, lawn mowing (push mower), vacuuming, swimming, water aerobics, tennis, walking, and jogging. Examples of muscle-strengthening options are performing calisthenics, carrying groceries, and using exercise bands, weight machines or hand-held weights, Pilates, and washing windows or floors.

The self-perceived rate of exertion is a simple scale for measuring intensity, with 0 as no effort and 10 being greatest effort possible (ACSM, 2009). Moderate-intensity aerobic activity is a 5 or 6, or 3 to 6 metabolic equivalents (METS), roughly equating to walking briskly at 3 to 4 miles per hour. One is often able to talk, but not sing, the words to a song while exercising. Vigorous-intensity activity is 7 or 8, or greater than 6 METS; heart rate is significantly increased and breathing can be difficult, so only a few words can be said before needing to catch one's breath. General physical activity guidelines are available through the Centers for Disease Control and Prevention (n.d.).

HOW TO RECOMMEND EXERCISE IN OLDER ADULTS

Before an older person starts an exercise program, a medical evaluation to look for any cardiac issues that can preclude exercising independently in an unmonitored environment should be performed. Those who develop shortness of breath or chest pain climbing a flight of stairs are not considered good candidates to start an exercise program without being monitored. Older adults who do not have a diagnosed chronic condition, such as diabetes mellitus, heart disease, or osteoarthritis, and who do not have symptoms (e.g., chest pain or pressure, dizziness, joint pain) *do not* need to consult a physician before starting physical activity (U.S. Department of Health and Human Services [USDHHS], 2008). Absolute contraindications to aerobic and resistance exercise include recent myocardial infarction within the last 6 months, changes in electrocardiogram, complete heart block, acute congestive heart failure (CHF), unstable angina, and uncontrolled HTN (systolic greater than or equal to 200 or diastolic greater than or equal to 110; Elsawy & Higgins, 2010). These individuals may benefit from cardiac rehabilitation programs supervised by health professionals.

Some sedentary older adults who begin exercise programs may be at an increased risk of hospitalization because symptoms of underlying medical conditions be unmasked. Further research must study the effects of exercise on the hospitalization and mortality rates of previously sedentary older adults.

EXERCISE PRESCRIPTION

Exercise prescriptions for most older adults should include aerobic, muscle-strengthening, and flexibility exercises. Individuals who are at risk for falling or mobility impairment should also perform specific exercises to improve balance, in addition to the other components of health-related physical fitness (ACSM, 2009).

Key recommendations adapted from the WHO in 2017 and ACSM in 2011 include (a) at least 150 minutes per week of moderate-intensity aerobic activity, at least 75 minutes of vigorous-intensity activity, or at least 20 minutes of vigorous-intensity physical activity at least three times per week; (b) aerobic activity in bouts of at least 10 minutes duration; (c) muscle-strengthening activities that work all major muscle groups at least two or more days; and (d) balance exercises to prevent falls in those with poor mobility on three or more days. Additional benefits occur with up to 300 minutes of moderate-intensity or 150 minutes of vigorous-intensity aerobic activity (Taylor, 2014). If 150 minutes of moderate-intensity aerobic activity per week cannot be done because of chronic medical conditions, the older adult should be as physically active as individual abilities and conditions allow. Flexibility exercises are also recommended at least 2 days a week, consisting of a moderate-intensity static (not ballistic) stretching program. Further detailed recommendations can be found in the ACSM 2011 Position Stand on Quality and Quality of Exercise.

Pedometers are being studied to determine an ideal number of steps per day that can be used as another means of tracking and improving physical activity in older adults (Tudor-Locke, Hatano, Pangrazi, & Kang, 2011). Common exercise monitors such as Fitbit wristbands are available at retail stores.

ADDITIONAL CONSIDERATIONS IN SEDENTARY OLDER ADULTS

Those with previously sedentary lifestyles can and should start on a low-intensity program. These individuals start with light activities lasting no more than 10 minutes, and gradually increase the duration and the number of days exercise is performed. Warm-ups and cooldowns are advised, and at least one session should be monitored to make sure that it is safely and successfully done. If older adults develop chest pain, shortness of breath, or dizziness, they should be advised to stop the exercise immediately and see their physician as soon as possible before they resume the exercise program. Exercise stress testing is recommended for *all* sedentary older adults, even without known or suspected CAD, as well as persons with known CAD, cardiac symptoms, or two or more CAD risk factors, who want to start a *vigorous* exercise program (Elsawy & Higgins, 2010). Muscle strengthening and/or balance training may be the first step before starting aerobic exercise among very frail individuals. Aerobic and strengthening programs are absolutely contraindicated for patients who have had a recent myocardial infarction or have EKG changes, third-degree heart block, CHF, unstable angina, and uncontrolled HTN (Elsawy & Higgins, 2010).

Karen Padua

American College of Sports Medicine position stand. (2009). Exercise and physical activity for older adults: 2009 update. *Medicine and Science in Sports and Exercise, 41*(7), 1510–1530.

American College of Sports Medicine position stand. (2011). Quantity and quality of exercise for developing and maintaining cardiorespiratory, musculoskeletal, and neuromotor fitness in apparently healthy adults: Guidance for prescribing exercise. *Medicine and Science in Sports and Exercise, 43*(7), 1334–1359.

Batt, M. E., Tanji, J., & Borjesson, M. (2013). Exercise at 65 and beyond. *Sports Medicine, 43*, 525–530. doi:10.1007/s40279-013-0033-1

Centers for Disease Control and Prevention. (n.d.). General physical activities defined by level of intensity. Retrieved from https://www.cdc.gov/nccdphp/dnpa/physical/pdf/PA_Intensity_table_2_1.pdf

De Labra, C., Guimaraes-Pinheiro, C., Maseda, A., Lorenzo, T., & Millán-Calenti, J. C. (2015). Effects of physical exercise interventions in frail older adults: A systematic review of randomized controlled trials. *BMC Geriatrics, 15*, 154–170. doi:10.1186/s12877-015-0155-4

Elsawy, B., & Higgins, K. E. (2010). Physical activity guidelines for older adults. *American Family Physician, 81*(1), 55–59, 60–62.

Pahor, M., Guralnik, J. M., Ambrosius, W. T., Blair, S., Bonds, D. E., Church, T. S., & LIFE Study Investigators. (2014). Effect of structured physical activity on prevention of major mobility disability in older adults—The LIFE study randomized clinical trial. *Journal of the American Medical Association, 311*(23), 2387–2396.

Schutzer, K. A., & Graves, B. S. (2004). Barriers and motivations to exercise in older adults. *Preventative Medicine, 39*, 1056–1061.

Snell, P. G. (2016). Physical activity. In A. Medina-Walpole & J. T. Pacala (Eds.), *Geriatrics review syllabus* (9th ed.). [Online]. New York, NY: American Geriatrics Society.

Taylor, D. (2014). Physical activity is medicine for older adults. *Postgraduate Medical Journal, 90*, 26–32. doi:10.1136/postgradmedj-2012-131366

Tudor-Locke, C., Hatano, Y., Pangrazi, R. P., & Kang, M. (2011). How many steps/day are enough? For older adults and special populations. *International Journal of Behavioral Nutrition and Physical Activity, 8*, 80–99.

U.S. Department of Health and Human Services. (2008). Physical activity guidelines for Americans. Retrieved from https://health.gov/paguidelines/guidelines/chapter5.aspx

World Health Organization. (2017). Physical activity: Fact sheet. Retrieved from http://www.who.int/mediacentre/factsheets/fs385/en

EYE CARE PROVIDERS

The need for eye care services increases significantly with aging. The majority of persons older than 65 years of age require some type of corrective lenses to improve distance or near visual performance, or both, and the prevalence of ocular disease rises substantially with age. Over half of all seniors older than 74 have cataracts. In this age group, age-related macular degeneration (8.3%) and glaucoma (6.3%)

follow in the prevalence of eye diseases in the United States (Prevent Blindness America, 2012). There have been significant increases in the number of people with eye disease, particularly diabetic retinopathy. Blindness and visual impairment are prevalent among the elderly, especially among nursing home residents and those living in assisted-living facilities (Elliott, McGwin, & Owsley, 2013). A significant proportion of visual impairment can be remedied by refractive correction, medical eye treatment, and cataract surgery. Much of the loss can be treated or prevented with appropriate eye care (Prevent Blindness America, 2012). Eye care services in the United States are provided largely by two groups: ophthalmologists and optometrists. Although both professions are trained to provide eye care, these two groups have specific education, training, licensure, and reimbursement for eye care services.

OPHTHALMOLOGISTS

Ophthalmologists are medical doctors who specialize in the medical and surgical care of the eyes. Ophthalmology is 1 of 24 medical specialties certified by the American Board of Medical Specialties. All ophthalmologists complete 4 years of education in a medical school or college of osteopathic medicine, a 1-year internship, and 3 years of postgraduate medical and clinical training in ophthalmology, and they must pass written and oral examinations to practice as licensed ophthalmologists. Many ophthalmologists take a postresidency fellowship in a subspecialty area such as retina, cornea, and glaucoma. Since 1992, board certification is limited to 10 years and must be renewed.

In 2016, there were 468 positions in 116 ophthalmology residency training programs accredited by the Accreditation Council for Graduate Medical Education (ACGME) (Ophthalmology Residency, 2016). According to the American Academy of Ophthalmology (AAO), in 2014, there were 19,216 active ophthalmologists in the United States (AAO, 2014). This amounts to approximately 1 ophthalmologist per 17,000 people in the United States (Association of American Medical Colleges

[AAMC], 2014). Ophthalmology has long been a male-dominated specialty; almost 78% of practicing ophthalmologists are men. However, this is shifting, and more than 40% of ACGME ophthalmology trainees were female in 2013 (AAMC, 2014). Ophthalmology has become more specialized. In 2016, the most popular fellowships included retina, cornea, and glaucoma, which matched 124, 78, and 76 trainees, respectively (Ophthalmology Fellowship, 2016). Ophthalmologists are the only practitioners trained to perform major ocular surgery. Ophthalmologists also treat ocular diseases and conduct basic vision examinations, including refractions.

OPTOMETRISTS

Optometrists, or doctors of optometry (OD), are independent health care professionals and are the major providers of primary eye care in America. Optometry practice is specifically defined by each state; thus the scope of practice and licensure requirements vary from state to state. All states now authorize optometrists to use prescribed drugs to treat eye infections, allergies, inflammation, and glaucoma. Licensed optometrists must take specified courses, pass written examinations, and demonstrate clinical aptitude to have their licenses extended to use and prescribe pharmaceutical agents. These educational requirements are included in the current optometric curricula and licensing examinations, so new licensees automatically meet state requirements.

Optometric education consists of a minimum of 3 years of undergraduate study, followed by 4 years of professional training. There are 23 accredited DO programs in the United States and one located in Puerto Rico. All states require optometric graduates to pass the National Board of Examiners in Optometry test, and many states require graduates to pass an additional state-administered practical examination. Optometric postgraduate clinical residency programs are available in ocular disease, geriatric care, vision rehabilitation, contact-lens fitting, and pediatric care. All states have continuing education requirements for relicensure. In

2014, the Bureau of Labor Statistics estimated that there were 40,600 practicing optometrists in the United States, which is more than double the number of practicing ophthalmologists. About half of optometrists worked in stand-alone offices of optometry. Others may work in optical good stores, doctors' offices, hospitals, the military, or ophthalmological practices (Bureau of Labor Statistics, 2016).

COVERAGE AND REIMBURSEMENT FOR VISION SERVICES

Despite the large need for vision care among older adults, Medicare coverage for eye examinations and eyeglasses is limited. This limitation in insurance coverage can lead to underutilization of needed eye services among those in lower socioeconomic groups (Caban-Martinez et al., 2012). Routine eye examinations and refraction are not covered by Medicare, whether provided by an optometrist or an ophthalmologist. Medicare does not cover eye examinations for prescribing, fitting, or changing eyeglasses or contact lenses for refractive errors. Eye examinations are reimbursable only for patients with complaints or symptoms of an eye disease or injury. Medicare Part B does cover yearly eye examinations for diabetic retinopathy. Medicare Part B also covers a glaucoma test once every 12 months for people at high risk, which includes those with diabetes mellitus, those with a family history of glaucoma, African Americans aged 50 or older, or Hispanic Americans aged 65 or older. Medical eye care for ocular diseases rendered by optometrists and ophthalmologists is a covered benefit under Medicare. Similarly, surgical eye care is covered. A major gap in coverage exists in rehabilitative services.

Generally, Medicare does not cover eyeglasses or contact lenses. However, following cataract surgery with implantation of intraocular lens, Medicare Part B does pay for one pair of corrective lenses per surgery per lifetime (Medicare, 2016). Medicare Part D helps pay the cost of prescription drugs such as those required or glaucoma, although often, those with glaucoma have multiple prescriptions that can become expensive, which is a significant barrier to adherence (Blumberg, Prager, Liebmann, Cioffi, & De Moraes, 2015).

Many Medicaid programs cover routine eye examinations and eyeglasses annually or biennially, even though it is considered an optional benefit, and coverage varies widely. HMOs frequently offer additional benefits to Medicare patients at little or no extra cost, and eye care coverage is one of the more popular additions. Although few HMOs offer eyeglasses as a cost-free benefit, a number do offer ophthalmic materials with moderate co-payments or discounts. Unlike most other care, which requires patients to visit a gatekeeper or primary care provider initially, most managed-care plans waive the referral requirement and allow direct access to an eye care provider (i.e., optometrist or ophthalmologist). Some plans, however, may require patients to consult an optometrist before seeking ophthalmological care.

See also Cataracts and Glaucoma.

Angela Beckert and Duthie Edmund

Association of American Medical Colleges. (2012). Physician specialty data book: Center for Work force Studies. Retrieved from https://www.aamc.org/ownload/313228/data/2012phyiscian specialtydatabook.pdf

Blumberg, D. M., Prager, A. J., Liebmann, J. M., Cioffi, G. A., & De Moraes, C. G. (2015). Cost-related medication nonadherence and cost saving behaviors among patients with glaucoma before and after the implementation of Medicare Part D. *JAMA Ophthalmology, 133,* 985–996.

Bureau of Labor Statistics. (2016). Occupational outlook handbook, 2016–17 edition, Optometrists. Retrieved from https://www.bls.gov/ooh/healthcare/optometrists.htm

Caban-Martinez, A. J., Davila, E. P., Lam, B. L., Arheart, K. L., McCollister, K. E., Fernandez, C. A., … Lee, D. J. (2012). Sociodemographic correlates of eye care provider visits in the 2006–2009 Behavioral Risk Factor Surveillance Survey. *BMC Research Notes, 5,* 253.

Elliott, A. F., McGwin, G., & Owsley, C. (2013). Vision impairment among older adults residing in assisted living. *Journal of Aging Health, 25,* 364–378.

Medicare. (2016). Eye exams and eyeglasses. Retrieved from http://www.medicare.gov/coverage

E

Ophthalmology Fellowship Match. (2017). Retrieved from https://sfmatch.org/SpecialtyInsideAll.aspx?id=2&typ=1&name=Ophthalmology

Ophthalmology Residency Matching Program. (2016). Retrieved from https://sfmatch.org/SpecialtyInsideAll.aspx?id=6&typ=2&name=Ophthalmology

Prevent Blindness America. (2012). Vision problems in the U.S. Retrieved from http://www.visionproblemsus.org

Web Resources

American Academy of Ophthalmology: http://www.eyenet.org

American Optometric Association: http://www.aoa.org

Medicare coverage: http://www.medicare.gov/Coverage/Home.asp

National Eye Institute: http://www.nei.nih.gov

F

Falls Prevention

WHAT IS A FALL?

A fall is a sudden unexplained change in position to a next lower surface (e.g., chair to floor, bed to mat). A fall is a common geriatric syndrome that may threaten seniors' independence. Most of the literature about falls among seniors does not usually include falls related to syncope, seizure, or loss of consciousness.

WHY FALLS MATTER

Falls are problematic for individuals, families, caregivers, and the entire health economy. Approximately 30% to 40% of people older than age 65 fall at least once a year. Of those who fall, 5% to 10% sustain a head injury, a fracture, or laceration (Moyer, 2012). Falls also may lead to hospitalization, admissions to extended-care facilities, and even death (Huang et al., 2012). Rates of falls in hospitals and extended-care settings are as high as 13 falls per 1,000 bed days. In hospitals and nursing homes, falls constitute the most common adverse incident and often lead to concerns, complaints, or litigation from patients and families (Oliver et al., 2006).

Fracture of the femur alone is pandemic in developing countries, with WHO estimates of more than 6 million fractures worldwide by 2030 (WHO, 2008). Even with modern treatment, fractures of the proximal femur still carry a 30% 12-month mortality rate and very high physical and functional morbidity. Falls may also result in head injury and subdural hematoma. In frail older people with limited functional ability, even "trivial" soft tissue injuries may be disabling. A "long lie" following a fall can lead to pressure damage, hypothermia, and fear. Falls also result in anxiety, loss of confidence, limitation of activities, caregiver stress, and institutionalization. Many seniors develop delirium after injurious fall, which adds to their short- and long-term mortality.

WHY FALLS HAPPEN

Although falls may occur in ambulatory older people with no comorbidities, they most commonly happen at home, increasingly with age. They are usually the result of synergistic interaction between several physiological risk factors and causative pathologies: the physical environment and the older person's own behavior and beliefs. Several reports have summarized risk factors for falling (American Geriatrics Society, 2009; Oliver et al., 2006), but clinicians need a framework to ensure that they consider all common reversible risk factors. One such framework is the Drugs and Alcohol, Age-Related Physiological Changes, Medical Causes, and Environmental Causes (DAME) classification.

- *Drugs and alcohol:* Older people are more sensitive to the effects of drugs and are often prescribed multiple medications for long-term conditions. The key "culprit drugs" are either centrally sedating agents (i.e., sedative/hypnotics, opiates, anticonvulsants) or those that can precipitate postural hypotension, arrhythmia, or presyncope (e.g., antihypertensives, diuretics, antiarrhythmics, antiparkinsons). The risk from several co-prescribed agents is cumulative. Alcohol use may contribute to falls as well.
- *Age-related changes:* Although it can be improved by resistance exercise, muscle strength declines by 30% to 40% between ages 30 and 80. Sway increases, reaction times and reflexes decrease, visual problems

accumulate (including field defects, worsening acuity, contrast, and depth perception), gait patterns change, and cognitive impairment increases. Baroreceptor reflex and cerebral autoregulation, which maintain upright posture, detection, computation, and correction, may be easily affected by acute illness, dehydration, and drugs. Lifestyle factors such as insufficient exercise, calcium intake, and vitamin D levels may also play a part, as may the person's own beliefs and attitudes about risk, acceptance of falls-prevention advice, and activity level. Cardiovascular changes with aging put seniors at greater risk of falling from orthostatic hypotension (Huang et al., 2012).

- *Medical causes:* Medical causes include any cause of gait instability or muscle weakness (e.g., cerebrovascular disease, parkinsonism, cerebellar disease, neuropathy, myopathy, osteoarthritis, foot disorders) and any cause of presyncope or syncope (e.g., aortic outflow obstruction, arrhythmia, postural hypotension, vasovagal syncope, carotid sinus hypersensitivity). Any acute or subacute medical illness (e.g., acute infection, metabolic disturbance, acute gouty arthritis) may present with falls or immobility. Falls are especially common in persons with dementia or delirium (especially if there is concurrent impulsiveness).
- *Environmental causes:* Environmental causes include inadequate footwear, unsuitable walking aids, poor ambient lighting levels or contrast between surfaces, loose mats, slippery surfaces, trailing cables, and difficult stairs or access. Bifocal glasses can contribute to falls especially with an uneven surface.

HOW WE SHOULD APPROACH PATIENTS WHO HAVE FALLEN

The American Geriatrics Society recommends that primary care physicians ask their older patients if they have fallen in the last year, and it has developed a pathway for assessing patients for falls and ways to prevent them (American Geriatrics Society [AGS] & British Geriatrics Society [BGS], 2009). A thorough history is especially important for determining frequency, circumstances, precipitants, and consequences of falls, as well as associated syncope or dizziness. The medication history is crucial for identifying medications that are associated with an increased risk of falls. The physical examination should focus on risk factors, including gait assessment, assessment of integrated musculoskeletal function using the functional reach test or other similar tests. Another test is the Timed Up and Go test, which can be easily performed in any clinical setting (e.g., clinic, emergency department, hospital, nursing home). Laboratory tests for anemia, electrolyte abnormalities, dehydration, and vitamin D deficiency as causes or contributing factors for falls are important to review. If cardiac rhythm disturbances exist, a Holter monitor and other cardiac evaluations may be considered, but it is important to emphasize that this test is not routinely done for older patients with falls. Radiologic studies should be driven only by history and physical examination findings; for example, MRI of the spine can be useful in patients with gait disorders.

A balance must be struck between maximizing safety and respecting the autonomy of cognitively intact individuals. This is especially important in the hospital setting, where falls risk is an inevitable part of recovery from acute illness, or in extended care, where autonomy should not be compromised by an excessively risk-averse or custodial approach (Oliver et al., 2006).

EVIDENCE FOR INTERVENTIONS

Interventions to prevent falls and fractures may be multifaceted or single and may be targeted at general at-risk groups or specific groups (Chang et al., 2004). The evidence is much stronger for secondary prevention in people who have already fallen (AGS & BGS, 2009). Interventions usually have high internal validity for specific target populations, which does not necessarily confer external validity or effectiveness outside of closely supervised research trials. There is good evidence that interventions should be group specific, just as individual treatments are person specific. Key risk factors targeted in successful interventions have been (a) lower-limb muscle strength, (b) balance, (c) medication withdrawal (especially psychotropic medications), (d) postural hypotension and syncope, (e) vision and hearing, (f) vitamin D deficiency, (g) physical environment, (h) injury prevention (e.g., appropriate footwear, bone-strengthening medications), (i) home safety evaluation, and (j) treatment of other geriatrics syndromes (e.g., dementia, delirium, depression). Multifaceted interventions often include assessment and treatment for some or all of these factors, sometimes combined with other approaches such as patient and caregiver education, assistive technology, comprehensive geriatric assessment, and nursing or medical review.

The best evidence is for progressive strength balance training in older women who are at risk for falls but who are able to adhere to an exercise regimen (in one case, coupled with the withdrawal of psychotropic medication). There has been at least one positive trial of tai chi. Structured medical and occupational therapy assessment/intervention for patients brought to the emergency room following a fall has been effective in fall prevention, as has structured multidisciplinary review and intervention for patients with falls living in their own homes. High-dose oral calcium and vitamin D, together with environmental assessment for home hazards, may decrease the risk of falling in institutionalized populations. There is some evidence on the effectiveness of investigation and treatment of syncope in fall prevention. Hip protectors do not show the benefit once assumed to protect older persons from injury in the long-term care setting.

Several trials of multifaceted interventions in hospitals have shown moderate effects in reducing falls (although not fractures). Only a few have been designed using a randomized controlled trial (RCT). In nursing homes, more high-quality RCTs have been performed, some demonstrating significant reductions in falls (not fracture) rates from multifaceted interventions (Oliver et al., 2006). There is no evidence that the use of physical restraints or bedrails prevents injurious falls.

There are many gaps in the evidence base, including tests of single interventions (e.g., medication review, footwear, use of alarm devices), the effectiveness of fall prevention in older persons who have dementia, the role of assistive technology and environment, and community or public health approaches to fall prevention.

CAN THE EVIDENCE BE IMPLEMENTED IN REAL LIFE TO HELP WHOLE POPULATIONS?

Specialist assessment services would not meet the demand if all patients with recurrent or injurious falls were referred for assessment. Therefore all professionals working in hospitals, primary care, and skilled nursing facilities should be able to assess fall risk factors and take appropriate actions. Referral for specialist assessment and investigation services should be reserved for patients with more complex histories. In the short term, investment is required in exercise programs, screening, medication review, and specialist assessment services.

Soryal A. Soryal and Laila M. Hasan

American Geriatrics Society & British Geriatrics Society. (2009). *Clinical practice guideline for the prevention of falls in older persons*. New York, NY: Author. Retrieved from http://www.american geriatrics.org

Chang, J., Morton, S., Rubenstein, L., Mojica, W., Maglione, M., Suttorp, M., ... Shekelle, P. G. (2004). Interventions for the prevention of falls in older adults: Systematic review and meta-analysis of randomised clinical trials. *British Medical Journal, 328,* 680.

Huang, A., Mallet, L., Rochefort, C., Equale, T., Buckeridge, D. L., & Tamblyn, R. (2012). Medication-related falls in the elderly: Causative factors and preventive strategies. *Drugs Aging, 29*(5), 360–371.

Moyer, V. (2012). Prevention of falls in community-dwelling older adults: U.S. Preventive Services Task Force recommendation statement. *Annals of Internal Medicine, 157,* 197–204.

Oliver, D., Connelly, J. B., Victor, C. R., Shaw, F. E., Whitehead, P. A. Genc, Y., ... Gosney, M. A. (2006). Strategies to prevent falls and fractures in hospitals and care homes and effect of cognitive impairment: Systematic review and meta-analyses. *British Medical Journal, 334*(7584), 82. Retrieved from http://www.bmj.com/cgi/content/abstract/bmj .39049.706493.55v1

World Health Organization. (2008). *WHO global report on falls prevention in older age*. Geneva, Switzerland: Author.

Web Resources
Cochrane Review: Hip protectors, The Cochrane Library, Issue 4, Oxford, UK: http://www.the cochranelibrary.com
Queensland Falls Prevention Best Practice Guidelines: http://www.health.qld.gov.au/fallsprevention/best practice/default.asp
Registered Nurses Association of Ontario: Prevention of falls and fall injuries in the older adult: Best practice guidelines: http://rnao.ca/fr/bpg/guidelines/prevention-falls-and-fall-injuries
UK National Institute for Health and Care Excellence (NICE): http://www.nice.org.uk
Welsh Assembly Bulletin: accidents and injuries, Issue 1—Falls; March 2005: http://www.cmo.wales.gov.uk/content/publications/research/bulletin-accidents-mar05-e.PDF

FAMILY CARE FOR ELDERS WITH DEMENTIA

Although many issues are important in understanding the needs of family caregivers of patients with dementia, three are key: (a) the importance of early diagnosis and prognosis, (b) common problems associated with memory loss that families find difficult to cope with, and (c) the family's emotional needs throughout the caregiving experience.

EARLY DIAGNOSIS AND PROGNOSIS

With early diagnosis, it may be possible to begin treatment that can slow cognitive decline while there is still minimal impairment. Most important for family members is that early diagnosis allows the patient and family time to plan for future needs, such as executing a power of attorney and appointing a health care representative. Patient and family members often fear that after the diagnosis, the physician will abandon them because of the stigma associated with cognitive decline (Boustani et al., 2011; Fowler et al., 2012). It is essential that physicians convey to the family that they will continue to be involved with the patient and family

and that management issues will be reviewed as they arise (Austrom & Lu, 2009; Callahan et al., 2011; McKhann et al., 2011). Health care providers should also educate the patient and the family regarding disease progression and prognosis, provide support, and monitor judgment and safety issues so that the patient can remain independent or live in a community dwelling as long as possible (Boustani et al., 2011; Callahan et al., 2012).

COMMON PROBLEMS ASSOCIATED WITH MEMORY LOSS

Unlike other illnesses, dementia has the additional problem of memory loss. Most family caregivers have difficulty providing care simply because they do not understand what is happening to the patient in the early stages of the disease and do not know how to respond appropriately to changes in the patient's behavior. Table F.1 describes some of the most common problems associated with memory loss and the ways that caregivers should respond (Austrom & Lu, 2009; Boustani et al., 2006).

One of the most important things for family caregivers to remember is that a patient diagnosed with dementia does not behave in these ways intentionally. These behaviors are manifestations of a brain disorder, and caregivers should not take personally anything the patient says or does. This can help avoid conflicts, anger, and subsequent feelings of guilt. Patients cannot be held responsible for their behaviors, but all behavior has a purpose. It is up to the caregiver to look for that underlying purpose. For example, patients may be agitated and wander around the house because they have forgotten where the bathroom is and need to use it. Or constant disrobing may occur because the patient is too hot. The caregiver should not blame the patient for these behaviors but should remain calm, try to figure out what is causing the behavior, and redirect the patient while protecting dignity (Whitlatch, Judge, Zarit, & Femia, 2006).

FAMILY'S EMOTIONAL RESPONSE TO DEMENTIA

A person with dementia may need care for many years. Successful caregiving is based on

Table F.1
Common Problems Associated With Memory Loss

Problem	Common Response	More Appropriate Response
Is unaware of memory loss or denies it.	Patients should remember. Why will they not face it?	Patients cannot remember that they cannot remember. They are not doing this intentionally.
Memory fluctuates from day to day.	Patients are not trying. They remember only what they want to remember.	Some fluctuation in memory is normal. Take advantage of the "good" days.
Asks repetitive questions.	Patients are doing this to annoy me. I have answered them 10 times already. They can control this.	Patients cannot remember asking. They no longer know how to ask for attention.
Makes accusations (e.g., stealing).	Patients are crazy. No one is stealing their possessions.	This may be a way for patients to deal with the insecurity caused by not being able to remember. They can no longer interpret the situation correctly.
Will not bathe; becomes agitated and violent about it.	Patients know that it is important to shower every day.	Patients cannot remember all the steps necessary to shower or get confused in the bathroom. It is embarrassing for them to ask for help. It is not critical to shower every day.
Insists on driving, although it is obvious that patient has trouble behind the wheel.	Ignore it and hope that nothing bad happens. Rationally try to explain that driving is dangerous.	Enlist professional help (e.g., a physician, lawyer, or insurance agent). Driving cessation is a complicated decision.
Lowered inhibitions.	Patients should be able to control themselves. They know that they should be dressed to go outside.	This is a symptom of the disease. Patients cannot help it. They are not doing it to embarrass anyone.

understanding the caregiver's emotional response to the disease, to the patient, and to the patient's behaviors, which change over time. Families must endure an ongoing grief process as they strive to cope with the demands of caregiving while watching the psychological death of their loved one and the death of that individual's personality—that quality or assemblage of qualities that makes a person who he or she is. Unfortunately, many caregiving families fail to realize that *grief* is an appropriate response when caring for a person with dementia (Austrom & Lu, 2009; Schulz et al., 2012).

Denial is a common response when confronted with emotionally difficult information, such as the diagnosis of dementia. Although early denial may lessen the emotional impact of the diagnosis, continued denial is counterproductive (Austrom & Lu, 2009; Fowler et al., 2012). It may foster unrealistic expectations about the patient's capabilities and interferes with appropriate planning for the future. Clinicians should recognize that denial and disbelief are common

when caregivers first learn about the diagnosis. Families need a second opportunity to review the information with the clinician.

Anger is commonly experienced by caregiving families who must provide long-term care. Sometimes this anger is directed at the patient. Often, families are angry with the government or the health care system. The cost of long-term care can be devastating to middle-income families, shattering their plans for retirement. Anger may also be directed at other family members for not understanding the toll that caregiving takes and for criticizing their efforts. Family members who do not live with the patient and have not had to provide constant care may not appreciate the extent of the demands placed on the caregiver and may offer suggestions about how to provide better care. Conflicts among family members are not unusual, and relationships are further strained when they cannot agree on the patient's care. Old resentments may resurface and interfere with sensible problem solving. The decision whether to institutionalize the patient

F

often exacerbates these family conflicts and associated guilt (Austrom & Lu, 2009; MacNeil et al., 2010).

The emotions of *anger* and *guilt* are often intertwined. Family members may experience guilt for many reasons: not being attentive enough to the patient before the illness, remembering unresolved past conflicts, or making decisions to which the patient objects. Some feelings of guilt may be a normal reaction to feelings of anger or wishes that the demented patient would die. When the patient finally dies, bereavement reactions are often mixed with relief that it is finally over and guilt for having wished that it would end (Austrom & Lu, 2009; Schulz, Boerner, Shear, Zhang, & Gitlin, 2006). It is important that caregivers know that such mixed emotions are both understandable and common.

Several recent studies have demonstrated benefits from dyadic interventions for both family caregivers and persons with subjective cognitive complaints (SSCs) or early stage dementia. Counseling, emotional support, education, and skills training provided to the family caregiver–patient dyads improved dyadic relationships, and overall quality of life, increased knowledge about disease and coping skills, reduced caregiver depression and/or anxiety, maintained patient engagement in activities, and helped caregivers keep patients at home longer (Lu et al., 2016; Moon & Adams, 2013).

A number of online technologies and interventions have been designed to support caregivers of patients with dementia. With the advent and ever-increasing availability of mobile technology and access to the Internet, more support options are available to caregivers without having to leave home or find someone to spend time with the person with dementia (even though some respite for the caregiver is highly recommended). Online forums are one area where dementia caregivers can receive informational and emotional support. Although these forums offer a lot of benefits, there can be cause for concern for unmoderated online caregiver forums, where caregivers might receive inaccurate information or inappropriate medical advice. One observational study of 61 participants who used a reputable online dementia forum in the United Kingdom, showed that after 12 weeks,

caregivers who used the forum rated their relationship with the person with dementia as improved (McKechnie, Barker, & Stott, 2014). A recent systematic review of Internet-based supportive interventions for caregivers of patients with dementia found that 6 of the 12 studies reported significant improvements in caregiver well-being. These areas included depression, sense of competence, decision-making confidence, self-efficacy, and caregiver burden (Boots, de Vugt, van Knippenberg, Kempen, & Verhey, 2014). More recent online caregiver interventions have demonstrated improvements in empathy and distress (Hattink et al., 2015) and caregiver depression and anxiety (Blom, Zarit, Groot Zwaaftink, Cuijpers, & Pot, 2015). Similarly, one research group's web-based videoconference caregiver support group improved caregiver anxiety and depression while reducing barriers to attendance (Austrom et al., 2015). In summary, these new online interventions offer a lot of promise, but much still needs to be learned about their potential risk and benefits.

When dealing with patients with dementia, family caregivers face the progressive deterioration of the patient's higher mental functions, behavioral problems associated with the disease, the financial burden, the eventual institutionalization of the patient, and the grief associated with the loss of the patient as previously known. Caregivers must take the necessary time to deal with their own emotions so that they can continue to function effectively as caregivers. Health care professionals, who should provide appropriate long-term support to these families, rarely recognize this massive burden. In a recent major study, however, it was demonstrated that the key principles of management can indeed be implemented in a primary care setting and are associated with a highly significant reduction in behavioral and psychological symptoms of Alzheimer's disease (AD) with minimal use of psychotropic drugs, effectively reducing caregiver stress and increasing caregiver skills. This type of interdisciplinary team-based approach, which includes comprehensive biopsychosocial care management, may serve as a model for effective AD patient and caregiver management in primary care (Boustani et al., 2011; Callahan et al., 2012).

AUTHORS' NOTE

This work was supported in part by NIA Grant No. P30AG10133a and in part by NINR Grant No. 1R21NR013755–01b

See also Caregiver Burnout; Family Care for Frail Elders; Social Supports: Formal and Informal.

Mary Guerriero Austrom, Yvonne Lu, Daniel R. Bateman, and Hugh C. Hendrie

Austrom, M. G., Geros, K. N., Hemmerlein, K., McGuire, S. M., Gao, S., Brown, S. A., ... Clark, D. O. (2015). Use of a multiparty web based videoconference support group for family caregivers. *Dementia, 14*(5), 682–690. doi:10.1177/1471301214544338

Austrom, M. G., & Lu, Y. Y. F. (2009). Long term caregiving: Helping families of persons with mild cognitive impairment cope. *Current Alzheimer Research, 6,* 392–398.

Blom, M. M., Zarit, S. H., Groot Zwaaftink, R. B. M., Cuijpers, P., & Pot, A.M. (2015). Effectiveness of an internet intervention for family caregivers of people with dementia: Results of a randomized controlled trial. *PLOS ONE, 10*(2), e0116622. doi:10.1371/journal.pone.0116622

Boots, L. M. M., de Vugt, M. E., van Knippenberg, R. J. M., Kempen, G. I. J. M., & Verhey, F. R. J. (2014). A systematic review of Internet-based supportive interventions for caregivers of patients with dementia. *International Journal of Geriatric Psychiatry, 29*(4), 331–344. doi:10.1002/gps.4016

Boustani, M. A., Justiss, M. D., Frame, A., Austrom, M. G., Perkins, A. J., Cai, X., ... Hendrie, H. C. (2011). Caregiver and noncaregiver attitudes toward dementia screening. *Journal of the American Geriatrics Society, 59,* 681–686. doi:10.1111/j.1532–5415.2011.03327.x

Boustani, M. A., Perkins, A. J., Fox, C., Unverzagt, F., Austrom, M. G., Fultz, B., ... Hendrie, H. C. (2006). Who refuses the diagnostic assessment for dementia in primary care? *International Journal of Geriatric Psychiatry, 21,* 556–563.

Boustani, M. A., Sachs, G. A., Alder, C. A., Munger, S., Schubert, C. C., Austrom, M. G., ... Callahan, C. M. (2011). Implementing innovative models of dementia care: The Healthy Aging Brain Center. *Aging and Mental Health, 15*(1), 13–22. doi:10.1080/13607863.2010.496445

Callahan, C. M., Boustani, M. A., Schmid, A. A., Austrom, M. G., Miller, D. K., Gao, S., ... Hendrie, H. C. (2012). Alzheimer's disease multiple intervention trial (ADMIT): Study protocol for a randomized controlled clinical trial. *Trials, 13,* 90. doi:10.1186/1745-6215-13-92

Callahan, C. M., Boustani, M. A., Weiner, M., Beck, R., Livin, L. R., Kellams, J. J., ... Hendrie, H. C. (2011). Implementing dementia care models in primary care settings: The Aging Brain Care Medical Home [Special supplement]. *Aging Mental Health, 15*(1), 5–12. doi:10.1080/13607861003801052

Fowler, N. R., Boustani, M. A., Frame, A., Perkins, A. J., Monahan, P., Gao, S., ... Hendrie, H. C. (2012). Effect of patient perceptions on dementia screening in primary care. *Journal of American Geriatric Society, 60,* 1037–1043. doi:10.1111/j.1532–5415.2012.03991.x

Hattink, B., Meiland, F., van der Roest, H., Kevern, P., Abiuso, F., Bengtsson, J., ... Dröes, R.-M. (2015). Web-based STAR E-learning course increases empathy and understanding in dementia caregivers: Results from a randomized controlled trial in the Netherlands and the United Kingdom. *Journal of Medical Internet Research, 17*(10), e241. doi:10.2196/jmir.4025

Lu, Y. Y. Bakas, T., Yang, Z., Stump, T., Weaver, M. T., Austrom, G. M., & Haase, J. E. (2016). Feasibility and effect sizes of the revised daily engagement of meaningful activities intervention for persons with mild cognitive impairment and their caregivers. *Journal of Gerontological Nursing, 42*(3), 45–58. doi:10.3928/00989134-20160212-08

MacNeil, G., Kosberg, J. I., Durkin, D., Dooley, W. K., DeCoster, J., & Williamson, G. M. (2010). Caregiver mental health and potentially harmful caregiving behavior: The central role of caregiver anger. *The Gerontologist, 50*(1), 76–86. doi:10.1093/geront/gnp099

McKechnie, V., Barker, C., & Stott, J. (2014). The effectiveness of an internet support forum for carers of people with dementia: A pre-post cohort study. *Journal of Medical Internet Research, 16*(2), e68. doi: 10.2196/jmir.3166

McKhann, G. M., Knopman, D. S., Chertkow, H., Hyman, B. T., Jack, C. R. J., Kawas, C. H., ... Phelps, C. H. (2011). The diagnosis of dementia due to Alzheimer's disease: Recommendations from the National Institute on Aging-Alzheimer's Association workgroups on diagnostic guidelines for Alzheimer's disease. *Alzheimer's & Dementia: Journal of Alzheimer Association, 7,* 263–269. doi:10.1016/j.jalz.2011.03.005

Moon, H., & Adams, K. B. (2013). The effectiveness of dyadic interventions for people with dementia and their caregivers. *Dementia, 12*(6), 821–839. doi:10.1177/1471301212447026

Schulz, R., Beach, S. R., Cook, T. B., Martire, L. M., Tomlinson, J. M., & Monin, J. K. (2012). Predictors and consequences of perceived lack of choice in becoming an informal caregiver. *Aging Mental Health, 16*, 712–721.

Schulz, R., Boerner, K., Shear, K., Zhang, S., & Gitlin, L. (2006). Predictors of complicated grief among dementia caregivers: A prospective study of bereavement. *American Journal of Geriatric Psychiatry, 14,* 650–658. doi:10.1097/ 01.JGP.0000203178.44894.db

Whitlatch, C. J., Judge, K., Zarit, S. H., & Femia, E. (2006). Dyadic intervention for family caregivers and care receivers in early-stage dementia. *The Gerontologist, 45,* 688–694.

Web Resources

Alzheimer's and Dementia Caregiver Center: http:// www.alz.org/care/2016

Alzheimer's Association: http://www.alz.org/alzhei mers_disease_what_is_alzheimers.asp

ClinicalTrials.gov: http://clinicaltrials.gov

Family Caregiver Alliance—National Center on Caregiving: http://www.caregiver.org

National Institute on Aging: Alzheimer's Disease Education and Referral Center (ADEAR): http:// www.nia.nih.gov/Alzheimers

National Institutes of Health, Senior Health— Alzheimer's Disease: http://nihseniorhealth.gov/ index.html

National Library of Medicine—MedlinePlus: http:// www.nlm.nih.gov/medlineplus

National Task Group on Intellectual Disabilities and Dementia Practices 'My Thinker's Not Working': http://www.aadmd.org/ntg; http://www.rrtcadd .org

FAMILY CARE FOR FRAIL ELDERS

Frailty is a geriatric syndrome characterized by accumulated age-related vulnerability and declines in physiological reserve that are associated with increased disability, vulnerability to falls and hospitalization, and mortality (Clegg, Young, Iliffe, Rikkert, & Rockwood, 2013). Frail older adults commonly experience weight loss, muscle weakness, reduced physical activity and slowness, fatigue and exhaustion, and increased impairment in mobility. Additional signs of frailty include gait and balance disorders, falls, cognitive decline, depressive affect, multiple comorbidities, and increasing dependence in physical and instrumental activities of daily living (Romero-Ortuno, Walsh, Lawlor, & Kenny, 2010).

Aging, chronic disease, and functional decline, woven together, create frail elders, which is estimated to affect at 25% to 50% of people aged 85 years or older (Clegg et al., 2013). Caring for frail, community-dwelling older adults may amplify burden among informal caregivers. As people grow more vulnerable to multiple chronic illnesses during the coming century, a growing number of frail older adults who wish to remain in the community will require informal support and care from loved ones, friends, and neighbors

HELPING FAMILIES MANAGE PHYSICAL FRAILTY

An estimated 34.2 million Americans provide at least one older adult aged 50 years or older with unpaid care each year, including help with medications, bathing, dressing, eating, transferring, and even toileting (National Alliance for Caregiving [NAC] & AARP, 2015). Approximately 45% (15.7 million) of these provide care for older adults with Alzheimer's disease (Alzheimer's Association, 2017), a role particularly associated with caregiving burden. Research demonstrates that informal caregivers are responsible for complex physical care tasks associated with medical needs (e.g., wound care, infusions) and managing problems such as poor nutrition, incontinence, depression, and dementia-related behavioral changes (Gaugler, Roth, Haley, & Mittelman, 2011). Family caregivers thus need illness-specific information, direct-care skill training, counseling and support, and periodic respite (Martín-Carrasco et al., 2009; Pinquart & Sörensen, 2005).

Under the auspices of the Older Americans Act, the National Family Caregiver Support Program (NFCSP) distributes funds to states for programs that offer family caregivers counseling, training, support groups, respite care, and informational programs on home care for frail older adults. As of 2012, there were more than 600 area agencies on aging around the country. Eldercare Locator, a public service of the U.S. Administration on Aging provides information on services and resources for older adults and their families (see Table F.2).

HELPING FAMILIES MANAGE PSYCHOLOGICAL FRAILTY

Another challenging issue for family caregivers is managing the emotional and behavioral reactions associated with negative moods and depressive affect. Frail elders are at high risk for depression because of cascading personal losses, including the loss of energy, mobility, autonomy, and family members and friends. Four factors are associated with depression in the aged: bereavement, sleep disturbance, disability, and prior depression. Depressive symptoms often are mistakenly diagnosed as the early onset of dementing illness.

Increased pleasant life events and social engagement can reduce depressive symptoms

and enhance cognitive well-being in frail elders, and helping family caregivers increase the number of simple pleasures (e.g., listening to music, getting out of the house, visiting with friends and family, participating in familiar social activities) can enhance mood and improve positive affect (Teri, McCurry, Logsdon, & Gibbons, 2005).

HELPING FAMILIES MANAGE END-OF-LIFE CARE

Frailty in later life is highly associated with mortality (Buchman, Wilson, Bienias, & Bennett, 2009; Kulmala, Nykänen, & Hartikainen, 2014). Providing end-of-life care for older loved ones presents another challenge for families. Although policies enacted in the past 20 years have increased the likelihood that hospitalized patients have the opportunity to participate in their treatment decisions, this legislation did not extend beyond hospital walls, and families of older adults are often faced with making advance directive decisions about when the care recipient becomes incapacitated and unable to voice care wishes. Education and support about

Table F.2
INTERNET RESOURCES FOR FAMILY CAREGIVERS

Resource	Contents
www.caregiver.va.gov	Provides a toolbox for caregivers of veterans; includes "Help near Home" a resource connecting caregivers to closest VA Caregiver Support Coordinator
www.ltcombudsman.org/ombudsman	National Consumer Voice for Quality Long-Term Care: Ombudsman Resource Center; ombudsmen advocate for the rights of residents of nursing homes
www.benefitscheckup.org/cf/index.cfm?partner_id=58	National Center for Benefits and Outreach and Enrollment (supported by the U.S. Administration on Aging, U.S. Department of Health and Human Services)
www.usa.gov/Topics/Seniors.shtml	Senior Citizen Resources; includes link to caregiver resources
www.usa.gov/Citizen/Topics/Health/caregivers.shtml	For help locating nursing home, assisted living, or hospice; checking eligibility for benefits; obtaining resources for long-distance caregiving; addressing legal considerations; and supporting caregivers
www.caregiver.org/caregiver/jsp/fcn_content_ node.jsp?nodeid=2083	Supported by Family Caregiver Alliance: National Center on Caregiving
www.eldercare.gov/Eldercare.NET	Sponsored by the Administration on Aging
Public/Index.aspx	U.S. Department of Health and Human Services; provides information on aging services in communities

F

advance care planning should be a standard part of family home care preparation.

HELPING FAMILIES MANAGE CONFLICT

Although caring for parents and spouses is an expected norm in most cultures, caregiving often generates intrafamilial stress as older adults' health and independent function decline or they experience unexpected health crises such as falls, broken bones, or cardiac episodes; such changes often require family caregivers to take on new roles and responsibilities, often for an uncertain and extended time. Caregiving conflicts within families and between families and health care providers are common (Kramer, Boelk, & Auer, 2006; Levine, Murray, & Cassell, 2007). When this happens, it can be helpful to facilitate family communication and attempt to normalize the conflicts that families encounter in home care such as competing time demands, role confusion, uncertainty, communication difficulties, and dealing with providers and medical emergencies. Family conferences have been found to be helpful in increasing family communication, problem solving, and confidence in collaborating with providers and in solving care conflicts (Fineberg, 2005). Because frail elders and their families often need protection from abuse and financial loss, another vital resource is the elder law attorney. Elder law attorneys can advise elders and their families on benefits rights and how best to ensure that health choices care are fulfilled.

Recent Home Care Innovations

Technology has transformed how families find and use health care information. Today's home care technologies include:

- Internet-based information on caregiving resources, webinars on how to provide care, and web-cameras caregiving assessments
- "Smart" technology sensors to gather data on normal patterns of daily living, provide medication reminders, and alert caregivers about unsafe wandering
- Telecare services to monitor vital signs such as blood pressure and blood glucose

- Assistive devices such as medicine dispensers, intelligent walkers for the visually impaired, safety alarms for alerting providers of the need for assistance, and alarms that show a fall has just occurred (Smith, 2008, p. 64)

These new technologies are promising resources for caregiving families. Medline Plus (2012), a National Library of Medicine and National Institutes of Health (NIH) service provides information for evaluating web-based health information such as looking for the health evaluation logos or information located under "about this site."

Increasingly, families and health care providers are opting to treat frail older adults at home when feasible, supported by patient care preferences and payment systems such as Medicare Advantage and Medicaid (Cryer, Shannon, Van Amsterdam, & Leff, 2012). Although research on interventions for frail adults and their family caregivers is still in its infancy, several models have demonstrated promising results (Cameron et al., 2015; Janse, Huijsman, de Kuyper, & Fabbricotti, 2014). In the United States, the Johns Hopkins "Hospital at Home" model, for example, shows that frail older adults have comparable or better outcomes compared with inpatients (Boult et al., 2009).

HELPING FAMILIES VIEW HOME CARE AS A SERIES OF TRANSITIONS

Helping families view elder care needs as evolving over time enables them to accept the idea that they will likely need to make decisions during periods of uncertainty. For these families, managing those periods of uncertainty is aided by health and social care professionals (i.e., social workers, nurses, physicians, clergy) who can offer education, professional support, and assistance.

Daniel S. Gardner

Alzheimer's Association. (2017). Alzheimer's Association: Facts & figures, 2017. *Alzheimer's & Dementia, 13,* 325–373.

Boult, C., Green, A. F., Boult, L. B., Pacala, J. T., Synder, C., & Leff, B. (2009). Successful models of comprehensive care for older adults with chronic conditions: Evidence for the Institute of Medicine's "retooling for an aging America" report. *Journal of the American Geriatrics Society, 57*(12), 2328–2337.

Buchman, A. S., Wilson, R. S., Bienias, J. L., & Bennett, D. A. (2009). Change in frailty and risk of death in older persons. *Experimental Aging Research, 35*(1), 61–82.

Cameron, I. D., Fairhall, N., Gill, L., Lockwood, K., Langron, C., Aggar, C., … Kurrle, S. (2015). Developing interventions for frailty. *Advances in Geriatrics, 2015*, Article ID 845356. doi:10.1155/2015/845356

Clegg, A., Young, J., Iliffe, S., Rikkert, M. O., & Rockwood, K. (2013). Frailty in elderly people. *The Lancet, 381*(9868), 752–762.

Cryer, L., Shannon, S. B., Van Amsterdam, M., & Leff, B. (2012). Costs for 'hospital at home' patients were 19 percent lower, with equal or better outcomes compared to similar inpatients. *Health Affairs, 31*(6), 1237–1243.

Fineberg, I. C. (2005). Preparing professionals for family conferences in palliative care: Evaluation results of an interdisciplinary approach. *Journal of Palliative Medicine, 8*(4), 857–866.

Gaugler, J. E., Roth, D. L., Haley, W. E., & Mittelman, M. S. (2011). Modeling trajectories and transitions: Results from the New York University caregiver intervention. *Nursing Research, 60*(3 Suppl.), S28–S37.

Janse, B., Huijsman, R., de Kuyper, R. D., & Fabbricotti, I. N. (2014). The effects of an integrated care intervention for the frail elderly on informal caregivers: A quasi-experimental study. *BMC Geriatrics, 14*, 58.

Kramer, B. J., Boelk, A. Z., & Auer, C. (2006). Family conflict at the end of life: Lessons learned in a model program for vulnerable older adults. *Journal of Palliative Medicine, 9*(3), 791–801.

Kulmala, J., Nykänen, I., & Hartikainen, S. (2014). Frailty as a predictor of all-cause mortality in older men and women. *Geriatrics & Gerontology International, 14*(4), 899–905.

Levine, C., Murray, T., & Cassell, C. (2007). *The cultures of caregiving: Conflict and common ground among families, health professionals, and policy makers.* Baltimore, MD: Johns Hopkins University Press.

Martín-Carrasco, M., Martín, M. F., Valero, C. P., Millán, P. R., García, C. I., Montalbán, S. R., … Vilanova, M. B. (2009). Effectiveness of a psychoeducational intervention program in the reduction of caregiver burden in Alzheimer's disease patients' caregivers. *International Journal of Geriatric Psychiatry, 24*(5), 489–499.

MedlinePlus. (2012). Evaluating health information. Retrieved from http://www.nlm.nih.gov/medlineplus/evaluatinghealthinformation.html

National Alliance for Caregiving, & AARP. (2015). *Caregiving in the U.S.* Washington, DC: Authors.

Pinquart, M., & Sörensen, S. (2005). Ethnic differences in stressors, resources, and psychological outcomes of family caregiving: A meta-analysis. *The Gerontologist, 45*(1), 90–106.

Romero-Ortuno, R., Walsh, C. D., Lawlor, B. A., & Kenny, R. A. (2010). A frailty instrument for primary care: Findings from the Survey of Health, Ageing and Retirement in Europe (SHARE). *BMC Geriatrics, 10*, 57.

Smith, C. (2008). support. *American Journal of Nursing, 108*(9 Suppl.), 64–68; quiz 68.

Teri, L., McCurry, S. M., Logsdon, R., & Gibbons, L. E. (2005). Training community consultants to help family members improve dementia care: A randomized controlled trial. *The Gerontologist, 45*(6), 802–811.

FEEDING: NON-ORAL

DEFINITION

Non-oral feeding refers to ways in which nutrient needs are met by either parenteral nutrition (intravenous route) or enteral nutrition (tube feeding). The focus of this discussion is to provide an overview of non-oral feeding modalities. For further in-depth information on best practices on parenteral and enteral nutrition, review the American Society for Parenteral and Enteral Nutrition's (www.nutritioncare.org) published standards of practice.

INDICATIONS FOR NON-ORAL FEEDING

The determining factor whether to initiate non-oral feeding in the older person in the form of parenteral or enteral nutrition is based on whether the gastrointestinal tract is functional and can be used. Parenteral nutrition "delivers nutrients that support physiologic needs while targeted medical interventions take place, in situations when oral intake or enteral nutrition is not feasible" (Worthington et al., 2017, p. 8). Enteral is preferred over parenteral nutrition

F

because enteral nutrition is more physiologic, maintains gut integrity, costs less, is associated with reduced infection and decreased length of hospital stay (Seres, Valcarcel, & Guillaume, 2013). Non-oral feedings should be implemented only if such use is in accordance with the individual's advanced directives and if the benefits of improved nutrition outweigh the associated risks of therapy (Barrocas et al., 2010). Providers should exercise clinical judgment when deciding to initiate parenteral or enteral nutrition (Barrocas et al., 2010). A discussion should take place with the patient and/or health care surrogate regarding the treatment goals (curative, rehabilitative, or palliative), as well as the anticipated outcome of providing or withholding parenteral or enteral nutrition (Pioneer Network, 2011). The medical futility of non-oral feeding should be considered prior to starting therapy. For example, a Cochrane Review concluded there was insufficient evidence that enteral nutrition prolonged survival, improved quality of life or nutrition status, or prevented complications in advanced dementia (Sampson, Candy, & Jones, 2009).

PARENTERAL NUTRITION

Parenteral nutrition refers to nutrients administered by the intravenous route, either through a large-diameter vein usually in the superior vena cava (i.e., central parenteral nutrition) or through a peripheral vein usually in the hand or forearm (i.e., peripheral parenteral nutrition). Catheters used for central parenteral nutrition can be placed at the bedside using full barrier precautions (O'Grady et al., 2011). However, if a patient requires prolonged central parenteral nutrition, then a central venous access device is inserted surgically. Peripheral parenteral nutrition is indicated primarily for short-term use (i.e., fewer than 14 days) because it contains a lower concentration of nutrients; therefore, increased nutrient needs cannot be met with this route (Worthington et al., 2017).

A parenteral nutrition formulation contains amino acids, dextrose, fat emulsions, water, electrolytes, trace elements, and vitamins. The compounding of a parenteral nutrition formulation is complex, and care is taken to ensure

the stability of the solution (Boullata et al., 2016). Select medications, such as insulin, may be added to parenteral nutrition formulations, depending on medication stability and compatibility with parenteral nutrition. Each parenteral nutrition solution is individualized based on the patient's nutrient requirements.

Equipment needed for the administration of parenteral nutrition includes an intravenous infusion pump and an in-line filter. The infusion pump ensures consistent delivery of the prescribed rate, and the inline filter reduces infusion particulates, microorganisms, and air (Ayers et al., 2014). Parenteral nutrition delivered via a central vein contains high amounts of dextrose; therefore, to prevent hypoglycemia, the solution should not be abruptly discontinued. Complications of parenteral nutrition include catheter-related complications, infection, refeeding syndrome, fluid and electrolyte abnormalities, and hepatobiliary alterations, as well as metabolic complications associated with long-term parenteral nutrition (Worthington et al., 2017). Parenteral nutrition is administered over a 24-hour period. However, older adults requiring home parenteral nutrition may be started on a compressed, cyclical administration schedule. With a cyclical schedule, a 24-hour supply of parenteral nutrition is administered over 12 to 16 hours, usually at night so that the person can be free from the infusion device during the day. Cyclical schedules help stimulate normal eating and fasting patterns, as well as increase quality of life (Worthington et al., 2017).

ENTERAL NUTRITION

Enteral nutrition is the administration of nutrition through the stomach or small intestine via a tube, catheter, or stoma (American Society for Parenteral and Enteral Nutrition, 2015). Although the stomach is the most commonly used route, enteral nutrition may be infused into the small intestine in patients at risk for aspiration or with impaired gastric functioning.

Patients requiring short-term enteral nutrition (i.e., fewer than 30 days) may have a feeding tube placed nasally or orally (Boullata et al., 2017). Large-bore tubes used for gastric decompression or suction may temporarily be used to provide enteral nutrition because they are uncomfortable and are associated with sinusitis, otitis media, mucosal ulcerations, necrosis, and vocal cord injury (Bankhead et al., 2009). Small-bore tubes are more comfortable for the patient and are the recommended first choice for short-term enteral access (Bankhead et al., 2009). An x-ray must be obtained to confirm placement of nasally or orally placed feeding tubes prior to the initiation of enteral nutrition because these tubes can inadvertently be placed in the lung during insertion (Boullata et al., 2017).

Long-term enteral feeding should be provided through a tube placed in the stomach (i.e., gastrostomy) or jejunum (i.e., jejunostomy). Gastrostomy tubes can be placed surgically, laparoscopically, endoscopically, or radiologically. A gastrostomy tube placed endoscopically is referred to as a percutaneous endoscopic gastrostomy (PEG) tube. Jejunostomy tubes can be placed surgically or endoscopically (PEJ). Combination dual-lumen tubes are used in patients who require gastric decompression while being fed distally into the jejunum.

Selection of the most appropriate commercially prepared formula to deliver enteral nutrition is based on the patient's underlying disease state and clinical characteristics. Standard enteral formulas are lactose free, are available with and without fiber and provide approximately 1,000 calories (1 kcal/mL); concentrated formulas provide 1.5 to 2.0 kcal/mL and are used primarily for fluid-restricted patients or those with increased nutrient needs. formulas (i.e., renal failure, hepatic failure) as well as formulas for those with diabetes mellitus, are available (Dorner, Posthauer, Friedrich, & Robinson, 2011).

Enteral nutrition can be administered by bolus, gravity, or pump-controlled delivery methods. With the bolus method, a large syringe is connected to the feeding tube and formula flows by gravity into the stomach. Similarly, with the gravity-drip method, formula is placed into an administration set and allowed to flow by gravity into the stomach, usually for 30 to 60 minutes. A pump-controlled delivery method provides a continuous slow infusion of formula, usually for 18 to 22 hours (Dorner et al., 2011). Enteral nutrition can be administered via an open or closed administration system. With an open system, formula is poured into a refillable administration set several times per day; with a closed system, the enteral formula in the delivery container is prefilled by the manufacturer. Closed systems reduce nursing time and are associated with decreased contamination (Boullata et al., 2017). Enteral nutrition complications include tube-related complications, aspiration, gastrointestinal disturbances, dehydration, fluid and electrolyte imbalances, and bacterial contamination of formula (Boullata et al., 2017).

MEDICARE REIMBURSEMENT FOR NON-ORAL FEEDING

Home parenteral and enteral nutrition is covered under Medicare Part B's prosthetic-device benefit only if the patient has a permanently inoperative internal body organ or function (Centers for Medicare & Medicaid Services [CMS], n.d.). The test of permanence is met if the medical record includes a judgment by a physician that the impairment will be of long and indefinite duration. Enteral and parenteral therapies are not covered if the therapy is due to a temporary impairment.

Vulnerable older adults can benefit from the appropriate use of these nutritional interventions.

See also Dehydration; Gastrointestinal Bleed.

Rose Ann DiMaria-Ghalili

American Society for Parenteral and Enteral Nutrition. (2015). *Definition of terms, style, and conventions used in A.S.P.E.N. Board of Directors-approved documents.* Retrieved from http://www.nutritioncare.org/uploadedFiles/Home/Guidelines_and_Clinical_Practice/DefinitionsStyleConventions.pdf

Ayers, P., Adams, S., Boullata, J., Gervasio, J., Holcombe, B., Kraft, M. D., . . . American Society for Parenteral and Enteral Nutrition. (2014). A.S.P.E.N. parenteral nutrition safety consensus recommendations. *Journal of Parenteral and Enteral Nutrition, 38,* 296–333.

Bankhead, R., Boullata, J., Brantley, S., Corkins, M., Guenter, P., Krenitsky, J., . . . Wessel, J.; A.S.P.E.N. Board of Directors. (2009). Enteral nutrition practice recommendations. *Journal of Parenteral and Enteral Nutrition, 33,* 122–167.

Barrocas, A., Geppert, C., Durfee, S. M., Maillet, J. O. S., Monturo, C., Mueller, C.,... American Society for Parental and Enteral Nutrition. (2010). ASPEN ethics position paper. *Nutrition in Clinical Practice, 25*(6), 672–679.

Boullata, J. I., Carrera, A. L., Harvey, L., Escuro, A. E., Hudson, L., Mays, A., ... American Society for Parenteral and Enteral Nutrition. (2017). ASPEN safe practices for enteral nutrition therapy. *Journal of Parenteral and Enteral Nutrition, 41,* 15–103.

Boullata, J. I., Holcombe, B., Sacks, G., Gervasio, J., Adams, S. C., Christensen, M., ... American Society for Parenteral and Enteral Nutrition. (2016). Standardized competencies for parenteral nutrition order review and parenteral nutrition preparation, including compounding: The ASPEN model. *Nutrition in Clinical Practice, 31,* 548–555.

Centers for Medicare & Medicaid Services. (n.d.). National coverage determination (NCD) for enteral and parenteral nutritional therapy (180.2). Retrieved from https://www.cms.gov/medicare -coverage-database/details/ncd-details.aspx?NC AId=231&NcaName=Outpatient+Intravenous+In sulin+Treatment+(Therapy)&ExpandComments= n&CommentPeriod=0&NCDId=242&ncdver=1& SearchType=Advanced&CoverageSelection=Both &NCSelection=NCA%257CCAL%257CNCD%257 CMEDCAC%257CTA%257CMCD&ArticleType= Ed%257CKey%257CSAD%257CFAQ&PolicyType =Final&s=5%257C6%257C66%257C67%257C9%2 57C38%257C63%257C41%257C64%257C65%257C 44&KeyWord=enteral+nutrition+therapy&KeyW ordLookUp=Doc&KeyWordSearchType=And&k q=true&bc=IAAAABAAEEAAAA%3D%3D&

Dorner, B., Posthauer, M. E., Friedrich, E. K., & Robinson, G. E. (2011). Enteral nutrition for older adults in nursing facilities. *Nutrition in Clinical Practice, 26*(3), 261–272.

O'Grady, N. P., Alexander, M., Burns, L. A., Dellinger, E. A., Garland, J., Heard, S. O., & the Healthcare Infection Control Practices Advisory Committee. (2011). Guidelines for the prevention of intravascular catheter-related infections. *Clinical Infectious Diseases, 52*(9), e162–e193.

Pioneer Network, Food and Dining Clinical Standards Taskforce. (2011). New dining practice standards. Retrieved from https://www.pioneernetwork .net/resource-library

Sampson, E. L., Candy, B., & Jones, L. (2009). Enteral tube feeding for older people with advanced dementia. *Cochrane Database of Systematic Reviews, 2,* CD007209. doi:10.1002/14651858.CD007209.pub2

Seres, D. S., Valcarcel, M., & Guillaume, A. (2013). Advantages of enteral nutrition over parenteral nutrition. *Therapeutic Advances in Gastroenterology, 6*(2), 157–167.

Worthington, P., Balint, J., Bechtold, M., Bingham, A., Chan, L., Durfee, S., ... Holcombe, B. (2017). When is parenteral nutrition appropriate? *Journal of Parenteral and Enteral Nutrition, 41*(3), 324–377. doi:10.1177/0148607117695251

Web Resources

Academy of Nutrition and Dietetics: http://www .eatright.org

American Gastroenterological Association: http://www .gastro.org

American Society for Parenteral and Enteral Nutrition: http://www.nutritioncare.org

American Society of Health-System Pharmacists: http://www.ashp.org

Centers for Medicare & Medicaid Services: http:// www.cms.hhs.gov/home/medicare.asp

Infusion Nurses Society: http://www.ins1.org

National Institutes of Health: Nutritional support information: http://www.nlm.nih.gov/medline plus/nutri tionalsupport.html

Oley Foundation: http://oley.org

FINANCIAL ABUSE

Financial abuse (also commonly referred to as *financial exploitation*) has been defined as the illegal or improper use of another's' funds, property or assets (National Center on Elder Abuse [NCEA], 1998). Although anyone can experience financial abuse, older adults may be particularly vulnerable; older adults are more likely to have financial resources than younger adults and may also be more trusting (Jackson & Hafemeister, 2011).

Legally, the definition of financial abuse varies among states (Jackson & Hafemesiter, 2011). Nor is abuse a simple phenomenon; it encompasses a range of behaviors, motivations, and relationships between victim and perpetrator (Jackson & Hafemesiter, 2011). Examples of financial abuse include taking money without the victim's knowledge or permission, forging a signature on checks or documents, denying the victim access to assets; improperly using a conservatorship/guardianship or power of attorney, misusing ATM or credit cards, coercing or deceiving the victim into signing a document, being guilty of negligence in handling assets, and overcharging for or not delivering caregiving services.

Data suggest that there are at least 5 million financial abuse victims each year, with approximately 5% of adults 65 and older experiencing financial abuse (Acierno et al., 2010; Lichtenberg, Stickney, & Paulson, 2013; Peterson et al., 2014). Financial abuse occurs in 30% of substantiated adult protective services (APS) elder abuse cases nationwide (NCEA, 1998) and is the third most frequent type of abuse, behind only neglect and emotional or psychological abuse (35%; NCEA, 1998). However, the prevalence is likely underestimated; a New York State study found that for every financial abuse case reported to an agency, 44 are not reported (Lachs & Berman, 2011). Potential reasons for under-reporting include failure to recognize the abuse as such, physical or cognitive impairments that limit ability to report, fear of not being believed, stigma about being labeled a victim, fear of getting the perpetrator into trouble (especially when the perpetrator is a family member or friend), and fear that exposure of abuse will lead to appointment of a guardian or placement in a long-term care facility (Stiegel, 2012). The incidence of financial abuse is likely to increase as opportunities for abuse expand with technological developments.

RISK FACTORS

A number of conditions or factors have been identified as increasing the likelihood for financial abuse in older adults, although systematic research on this topic is limited. A national study of APS reports found that the oldest of older adults are most likely to experience abuse, with 48% involving victims 80 years of age or older, although they composed only 19% of the total older population at the time (NCEA, 1998). Another set of identified risk factors focuses on social factors; older adults who are socially isolated and lonely and who recently lost a loved one are more likely to experience financial abuse (Choi & Mayer, 2000; Jackson

& Hafemeister, 2012). Having family members who are unemployed or who have substance abuse problems also increases the risk (National Committee for the Prevention of Elder Abuse [NCPEA], 2001).

Physical or mental disabilities in the victim also appear to increase risk. This includes medical conditions that limit their ability to understand and comprehend financial issues, as well as conditions that make managing finances difficult, such as the presence of depression (Beach, Schulz, Castle, & Rosen, 2010) and cognitive impairment (Jackson & Hafemeister, 2012).

Data on risk for financial abuse by race/ethnicity are mixed. A review of APS cases found that 83% of the substantiated APS reports involved white victims (NCEA, 1998), yet a recent study of adults aged 60 years and older in Pittsburgh found that financial abuse prevalence rates were significantly higher for African Americans than for non–African Americans (23.0% vs. 8.4%; Beach et al., 2010), and a New York State sample of older adults found that those of African American/Black race had 3.8 higher odds of experiencing financial abuse than other groups (Peterson et al., 2014). Data on risk by economic status are also mixed. Although two national studies found that the likelihood of financial abuse did not increase with higher levels of income (Acierno et al., 2010; NCEA, 1998), a recent New York State sample of community-dwelling older adults found significantly more financial abuse in those who lived below the poverty line (Peterson et al., 2014). Differences may be because of the samples selected (including whether APS cases or community-dwelling older adults are examined) and location.

PERPETRATION OF FINANCIAL ABUSE

Family and friends are the most common perpetrators of financial abuse. Adult children are the most frequent perpetrators; other common perpetrators include friends and neighbors, other relatives, and paid home care aides (Lachs & Berman, 2011; NCEA, 1998; Stiegel, 2012). Cited motivations include the perpetrator's substance abuse, mental health, gambling, or financial problems (NCPEA, 2001). Cultural context is

F

important to consider; within some cultures, there may be expectations that older adults will share their resources with family members in need, even though the elder person might not agree to such sharing (Moon, 2000).

Less frequent, but still extremely harmful are scams by strangers, including Internal Revenue Service and tax scams, sweepstakes and lottery scams, sweetheart (affinity) scams (which often use online dating platforms to trick unsuspecting seniors to send money) and tech support scams (in which scammers pretend to be computer techs to trick people into giving them remote computer access or paying for unneeded software; U.S. Department of Justice, 2016).

Financial abuse is associated with annual losses of at least $530 million, and loss has been estimated to be as high as $2.9 billion (MetLife Mature Market Institute, 2011). Most immediately, the experience of financial abuse can be financially devastating. It is generally not as viable for an older adult to recoup lost assets as a younger adult, particularly if they are retired (Jackson & Hafemeister, 2011). Such depletion of assets may result in a loss of independence and security, create a financial burden on family members now required to support the individual, or lead to dependence on social welfare agencies (Jackson & Hafemeister, 2011).

Financial abuse has been linked to lower 5-year survival rates in victims compared with victims of physical and psychological abuse (Burnett et al., 2016). Emotional and psychological consequences of financial abuse can include loss of trust in others, increased fearfulness of crime, loss of confidence in one's financial abilities, feelings of shame and self-criticism, isolation from family or friends, and increased risk for depression (National Adult Protective Services Association [NAPSA], 2016).

PREVENTING, DETECTING, AND REPORTING FINANCIAL ABUSE

Health care and other clinical professions workings with older adults are well positioned to prevent and detect elder abuse. They may be the first to identify risk factors, such as cognitive decline. Potential indicators of financial abuse

include financial transactions that are uncharacteristic of the older adult (e.g., the older adult was always frugal but suddenly spends large amounts on a new acquaintance). Behavioral indicators include fear, withdrawal, depression, hopelessness, hesitation to talk openly, and confusion or disorientation. Indicators related to the elder's health, such as unmet physical needs, untreated health problems, and declining health, may also be present.

When financial abuse is suspected, the provider should document both the elder's cognitive and functional status and financial knowledge. Four important questions may guide the clinician in determining whether further investigation is needed: (a) Are there risk factors that contribute to the elder's susceptibility? (b) Is there a confidential relationship between the two parties? (c) Is the caregiver active in procuring the legal/financial transactions? (d) Is there monetary loss to the elder's estate and gain to the other party? Because so many older adults are reluctant to report financial abuse, professionals working with older adults should screen for financial abuse; although victims may not disclose without prompting, they may do so if asked. Moreover, screening consistently can both normalize questioning (potentially reducing stigma) and help the professional become more comfortable asking questions about abuse (Stiegel, 2012). A screening tool for financial abuse is the Financial Exploitation Measure (Conrad, Iris, Ridings, Langley, & Wilber, 2010). In addition, specific training programs have been created to help physicians and other providers identify vulnerable patients (NAPSA, 2016). It is not the health care professional's responsibility to confirm that abuse has occurred, but a reasonable suspicion should be reported to the appropriate investigative entity.

ADDRESSING FINANCIAL ABUSE

All states have elder abuse prevention laws and have a system in place for investigating elder abuse; usually, APS is responsible for these activities (NAPSA, 2016). However, although almost all states specifically mention financial abuse in their reporting of elder abuse, only rarely do they establish special procedures for investigating and responding to financial abuse in particular (Jackson & Hafemeister, 2011). When an allegation of elder abuse is made, APS investigates the allegations, assesses the victim's cognitive capacity, and intervenes to stop or reduce the abuse.

Interventions for addressing financial abuse include closing joint bank accounts, arranging for direct-deposit banking, having the victim revoke the power of attorney of the abuser, putting an agency or responsible person in place to assist with managing funds, and restarting utilities that have been turned off. APS also works to reduce the isolation of the victim by putting into place services, such as case management, that reduce the risk of continued abuse. In many cases, APS refers cases to law enforcement for investigation and prosecution (NAPSA, 2016).

The complexity of financial abuse also means that no single agency can fully address the issue. Multiple disciplines often become involved in cases; these include aging and other social service agencies, civil legal services, financial services, forensic and other accountants, guardians/conservators, mental health professionals, and victim services. Multidisciplinary teams made up of attorneys, mental health professionals, law enforcement, banks, and others may be particularly useful, and many such teams exist throughout the United States (NAPSA, 2016). Reducing or eradicating financial abuse requires working closely with banks to recognize, report, and investigate financial abuse (NAPSA, 2016). The least restrictive alternatives should be used to maintain the seniors' autonomy to the fullest extent possible.

FUTURE DIRECTIONS

A number of barriers need to be addressed to prevent and respond effectively to elder abuse, including the reluctance of victims to report; difficulty establishing whether financial transactions were conducted the with the victim's consent; lack of training of professionals working with older adults to identify and address financial abuse; and challenges in the coordinated prompt response to abuse, including a lack of resources to do so (Jackson & Hafemeister, 2011).

As a first step, it important that aging services and other professionals working with older adults understand the types of and risks for financial abuse and ways to address it. Work is also needed to foster greater communication between APS caseworkers and prosecutors to facilitate both investigation of financial abuse and prosecution. Law enforcement officials would likely benefit from engaging in a multidisciplinary team approach. Services for perpetrators should also be part of any intervention; only by understanding the perspectives and characteristics of each participant can financial abuse be truly understood and addressed.

All elder abuse interventions require further, more in-depth evaluation, and interventions should be tailored to meet the needs of at-risk populations, such as those with cognitive decline. More research is also needed to understand the development and course of financial abuse, as well as its prevalence and costs. Existing research on prevalence, although extremely useful for increasing knowledge about the extent of financial abuse, has not included individuals who lacked telephones, did not have the capacity to participate in the survey (e.g., care. Similarly, cost studies have been based on cases covered by media or on substantiated APS cases and have not considered the indirect costs of abuse such as those related to health and medical care and taxes (Stiegel, 2012).

Angela Ghesquiere

Acierno, R., Hernandez, M. A., Amstadter, A. B., Resnick, H. S., Steve, K., Muzzy, W., & Kilpatrick, D. G. (2010). Prevalence and correlates of emotional, physical, sexual, and financial abuse and potential neglect in the United States: The National Elder Mistreatment Study. *American Journal of Public Health, 100*(2), 292–297.

Beach, S. R., Schulz, R., Castle, N. G., & Rosen, J. (2010). Financial exploitation and psychological mistreatment among older adults: Differences between African Americans and non-African Americans in a population-based survey. *Gerontologist, 50*(6), 744–757.

Burnett, J., Jackson, S. L., Sinha, A., Aschenbrenner, A. R., Xia, R., Murphy, K. P., & Diamond, P. M. (2016). Differential mortality across five types of substantiated elder abuse. *Journal of Elder Abuse and Neglect, 28*(2), 59–75.

Choi, N. G., & Mayer, J. (2000). Elder abuse, neglect, and exploitation: Risk factors and prevention strategies. *Journal of Gerontological Social Work, 33*(2), 5–25.

Conrad, K. J., Iris, M., Ridings, J. W., Langley, K., & Wilber, K. H. (2010). Self-report measure of financial exploitation of older adults. *The Gerontologist, 50*(6), 758–773.

Jackson, S. L., & Hafemeister, T. L. (2011). Financial abuse of elderly people vs. other forms of elder abuse: Assessing their dynamics, risk factors, and society's response. *Final Report to the National Institute of Justice.* Retrieved from http://www .dss.virginia.gov/files/about/reports/adults/ adult_services_annual/elder_abuse_financial_ exploitation_nij_exec._summ._11-22-10.pdf

Jackson, S. L., & Hafemeister, T. L. (2012). Pure financial exploitation vs. hybrid financial exploitation co-occurring with physical abuse and/or neglect of elderly persons. *Psychology of Violence, 2*(3), 285–296.

Lichtenberg, P. A., Stickney, L., & Paulson, D. (2013). Is psychological vulnerability related to the experience of fraud in older adults? *Clinical Gerontologist, 36*(2), 132–146.

Lachs, M., & Berman, J. (2011). Under the radar: New York State elder abuse prevalence study. Retrieved from http://www.preventelderabuse.org/ library/documents/UndertheRadar051211.pdf

MetLife Mature Market Institute. (2011). *The MetLife study of elder financial abuse: Crimes of occasion, desperation, and predation against America's elders.* New York, NY: Author.

Moon, A. (2000). Perceptions of elder abuse among various cultural groups: Similarities and differences. *Generations—Journal of the American Society on Aging, 24*(2), 75–80.

National Adult Protective Services Association. (2016). Elder financial exploitation. Retrieved from http://www.napsa-now.org/policy-advo-cacy/exploitation

National Center on Elder Abuse. (1998). *The National Elder Abuse Incidence Study: Final report.* Washington, DC: National Aging Information Center.

National Committee for the Prevention of Elder Abuse. (2001). *Elder abuse: Financial abuse.* Retrieved from http://www.preventelderabuse.org/elderabuse/ fin_abuse.html

Peterson, J. C., Burnes, D. P., Caccamise, P. L., Mason, A., Henderson, C. R., Jr., Wells, M. T., ... Lachs, M. S. (2014). Financial exploitation of older adults: A prevalence study. *Journal of General Internal Medicine, 29*(12), 1615–1623.

Stiegel, L. A. (2012). An overview of elder financial exploitation. *Generations—Journal of the American Society on Aging, 36*(2), 73–80.

U.S. Department of Justice. (2016). *Senior scam alert.* Retrieved from https://www.justice.gov/elder justice/senior-scam-alert

Web Resources

Administration on Aging: https://aoa.acl.gov

American Bar Association Commission on Law and Aging: http://www.americanbar.org/groups/law_ aging.html

BITS Fraud Protection Toolkit: Protecting the elderly and vulnerable from financial fraud and exploitation: http://www.actonalz.org/sites/default/files/ documents/bitstoolfeb06.pdf

Consumer Financial Protection Bureau's Office for Older Americans: http://www.consumerfinance .gov/older-americans

Federal Trade Commission: https://www.ftc.gov

Investor Protection Trust: http://www.investor protection.org

National Center on Elder Abuse: https://ncea.acl .gov

National Committee for the Prevention of Elder Abuse: http://www.preventelderabuse.org

National Institute of Justice: http://www.nij.gov/nij/ topics/crime/elder-abuse/financial-exploitation .htm

FOOT PROBLEMS

Managing foot problems in older patients begin with a comprehensive clinical podogeriatric assessment, continuing surveillance, education, prevention strategies, treatment of specific diseases and disorders, and a team approach. The inclusion of appropriate podiatric services in geriatric care programs often produce dramatic effects. Immobility can be replaced by activity. The quality of care translates into quality of life. Support and encouragement can be directed to independence and a strong sense of personal identity and worth. Isolation can be replaced by interaction. When the quality of life decreases as a result of disease, disability, and age, those precious aspects of dignity must be restored to a maximal level by people who care. Because walking is a catalyst for an active life, podiatric care can help restore some of the lost dignity by keeping patients walking and moving so that they can accept and participate in the social activities of life and live life.

The Helfand Index, developed by the Pennsylvania Department of Health, is a protocol for developing prevention (primary, secondary, and tertiary) management strategies. It reviews information related to demographics; primary medical facilities and management; history of present problems; pertinent past medical history; a systems review; current and past medications; visual evaluation; dermatologic, musculoskeletal, orthopedic (biomechanical and pathomechanical), peripheral vascular, and neurologic evaluation; neurologic risk stratification; peripheral arterial risk stratification; footwear evaluation; primary assessment; an initial management plan; referral direction; Medicare's class findings; risk stratification of onychomycosis, plantar pressure; keratotic patterns; preulcer and ulcer classification; and the classification of mechanical or pressure hyperkeratotic lesions.

The demographics, past medical history, system review, medications and therapeutic programs, and current health conditions should be reviewed and noted. Primary foot problems, as well as their relationship to chronicity and activities, should also be noted and include swelling, pain, hyperkeratosis, joint deformities, onychial diseases and disorders, infections, coldness, and other problems, as well as location, quality, severity, duration, context, modifying factors, and associated signs and symptoms. The primary and secondary "at risk" diseases and disorders include complications associated with diabetes mellitus and metabolic disorders, peripheral vascular disease, lower extremity arterial and venous diseases, sensory and motor impairment, edema, degenerative joint changes and the residuals of arthritis and collagen diseases, ambulatory dysfunction, obesity, and cognitive impairment.

In 1971, Medicare regulations identified, as risk factors related to management, a number of diseases and/or disorders that develop vascular insufficiency and neurological insensitivity and their complications. The primary examples include the following but are not exclusive: amyotrophic lateral sclerosis; arteriosclerosis obliterans (ASO; arteriosclerosis of the extremities, occlusive peripheral arteriosclerosis); arteritis of the feet; Buerger's disease (thromboangiitis obliterans); chronic indurated cellulitis; chronic thrombophlebitis; chronic venous insufficiency; diabetes mellitus; intractable edema secondary to a specific disease (e.g., congestive heart failure, kidney disease, hypothyroidism); lymphedema secondary to a specific disease (e.g., Milroy's disease, malignancy); peripheral neuropathies involving the feet (associated with malnutrition and vitamin deficiency); malnutrition (general, pellagra); alcoholism; malabsorption (celiac disease, tropical sprue); pernicious anemia associated with carcinoma, diabetes mellitus, drugs and toxins, multiple sclerosis, uremia (chronic renal disease), traumatic injury, leprosy or neurosyphilis, and hereditary disorders; hereditary sensory radicular neuropathy; angiokeratoma corporis diffusum (Fabry's syndrome); amyloidosis; peripheral vascular disease; and Raynaud's disease.

In 2009, the Department of Veterans Affairs (VHA Directive 2009–030) expanded the Medicare primary risk categories to appropriately include the following conditions: documented peripheral arterial disease, documented sensory neuropathy, prior history of foot ulcer or amputation (above the knee, below the knee, forefoot, and toes), visual impairment, physical impairment, neuromuscular disease (i.e., Parkinson's disease), severe arthritis and spinal disc disease, cognitive dysfunction, chronic anticoagulation therapy, age greater than 70 years without other risk factors, diabetes without foot complications, and obesity.

The dermatological and onychial section focuses on skin integrity and multiple changes that affect pressure, mechanical keratosis, onychial changes, infections, and pre-ulcerative states. The primary clinical signs and findings include the following: hyperkeratosis, keratotic lesions without hemorrhage or hematoma, tyloma, heloma durum, heloma milliare, heloma, molle, heloma neurofibrosum, heloma vasculare, pigmentation (hemosiderin), onychophosis, intractable plantar keratosis, sub-keratotic hematoma

F

(preulceration), subungual hematoma, maceration, xerosis, onychauxis, tinea pedis, bacterial infection, verruca, ulceration, onychomycosis, rubor, onychodystrophy, onychodysplasia, incurvation, preulcerative conditions, cyanosis, and discoloration.

Onychomycosis evaluation includes documentation of mycosis/dystrophy causing secondary infection and/or pain that results in marked limitation of ambulation and includes discoloration, hypertrophy, subungual debris, onycholysis, secondary infection, and limitation of ambulation and pain.

Hyperkeratosis classification identifies the major functions of the foot as static and dynamic. The foot is an organ of weight bearing, propulsion, and locomotion. The foot is relatively rigid and changes are related to activities of daily living, excessive and repetitive stress, the normal aging process, degeneration, and disease, producing functional disability and ambulatory dysfunction. Factors that do not provide for a compensatory element for weight diffusion and/or weight dispersion include repetitive stress, hard and flat surfaces, increased shock, tissue trauma, past occupational stress, and the environmental factors associated with ambulation. Examples of related complications include atrophy of the intrinsic foot muscles, atrophy and anterior displacement of the plantar fat pad, morphologic changes, digital contractures and deformities, inflammation, pain, and the residuals of biomechanical, pathomechanical, and balance and gait change. Stress factors related to the development of hyperkeratosis include force, compression, tensile stress, shearing, friction, elasticity, and fluid pressure.

The Ulcer Classification, adapted from Sims, Cavanaugh, and Ulbrecht (1988), provides an earlier identification of risk, given it's 10-grade classification. Other classifications include the Wagner Ulcer Classification System (grades 1–5), the Liverpool Classification System for diabetic ulcers (primary and secondary), the University of Texas Foot Ulcer Wound Classification Systems with stages A–D and grades 1–3.

The musculoskeletal–orthopedic section highlights altered biomechanics and pathomechanics and the most common foot, ankle, and joint deformities and syndromes identified in the older patient and patients with chronic diseases. These include arthritis (rheumatoid, degenerative [osteo], gouty, psoriatic), hallux valgus (bunion), anterior imbalance (identifies inappropriate weight bearing and correlates with the plantar keratoma pattern noted later in the examination), digiti flexus (hammer toes, claw toes, mallet toes, and rotational deformities), prominent metatarsal heads, plantar fat pad displacement and/or atrophy), Morton's syndrome, improper weight distribution and pressure areas, and soft tissue inflammation. Other primary findings include diminished joint mobility (flexion, extension, eversion, and inversion); pes planus, pes valgo planus; pes cavus (equinus); hallux limitus or rigidus; bursitis; Charcot joints (neuropathic arthropathy); foot drop; osseous reabsorption; rear and/or forefoot varus; plantar-flexed first ray; digital and or partial foot amputation; toe, partial foot, below-knee and above-knee amputation; and other clinical findings.

Gait evaluation includes mobility, gait speed, and balance as it relates to fall risk that may be associated with a foot deformity and inappropriate footwear. Ambulatory aids such as canes and walkers, as well as physical activities, are also a consideration. Mobility should consider independent activity, independence with assistance, homebound status, nonambulatory status, and wheelchair use. The ranges of motion include dorsiflexion, plantar flexion, inversion, and eversion of the foot and ankle, as well as flexion and extension of the great toe and intrinsic foot muscles.

Vascular evaluation identifies symptoms associated with arterial insufficiency and ischemia. The primary findings include coldness; trophic changes; diminished or absent pedal pulses, such as the dorsalis pedis pulse and posterior tibial pulses; night cramps; edema; claudication; varicosities; atrophy; and amputation, if present (above the knee, below the knee, forefoot, and toes); these findings are particularly important in patients with diabetes and arterial insufficiency. Vascular risk stratification includes the following as part of the initial assessment: no change, mild claudication, moderate claudication, severe claudication, ischemic rest pain, minor tissue loss, and major tissue loss.

Medicare currently may provide payment for therapeutic shoes for patients with diabetes mellitus who meet specific criteria. These criteria include a history of partial or complete amputation of the foot, a history of previous foot ulceration, a history of preulcerative callus, peripheral neuropathy with evidence of callus formation, evidence of foot and/or osseous deformity, and evidence of poor circulation.

The neurological evaluation identifies primary reflex and sensory changes. Those findings include the deep tendon reflexes (DTRs; i.e., patellar and Achilles) and superficial plantar reflex, joint position, vibratory sensation, vibration perception threshold (VPT), sharp and dull reactions, evidence of paresthesia and burning.

Medicare also provides a process for the evaluation and management of a diabetic patient with diabetic sensory neuropathy, resulting in a loss of protective sensation (LOPS) to include a diagnosis of LOPS, a patient history of diabetes mellitus, and a physical examination consisting of the following elements: (a) visual inspection of the forefoot, hind foot, and toe web spaces; (b) evaluation of protective sensation; (c) evaluation of foot structure, pathomechanics, and biomechanics; (d) evaluation of vascular status; (e) evaluation of skin integrity; (f) evaluation and recommendation of footwear; and (g) patient education.

The neurological risk stratification includes the following classification: no sensory loss; sensory loss; sensory loss and foot deformity; and sensory loss, a history of ulceration, and deformity.

Medicare also has a series of class findings that need to be evaluated and documented as qualifiers for primary foot care for patients with noted primary risk diseases. These findings include the following: A–1, nontraumatic amputation of the foot or part of the foot; B–1, absent posterior tibial pulse; B–2, advanced trophic changes; B–2–a, hair growth (decreased or absent); B–2–b, nail changes (thickening); B–2–c, pigmentary changes (discoloration); B–2–d, skin texture (thin, shiny); B–2–e, skin color (rubor or redness); B–3, absent dorsalis pedis pulse; C–1, claudication; C–2, temperature changes (cold); C–3, edema; C–4, paresthesia; and C–5, burning.

Other assessment areas include footwear, hygiene, and type of stocking (nylon, cotton, wool, other) or lack thereof. Stockings or socks should also be inspected for stains and excessive wear (friction). The shoe or footwear evaluation includes the type of shoe, fit, depth, size, last, flare, shoe lining wear, shoe wear pattern (outsole and upper counter distortion), foreign bodies, insoles, and orthoses. When special shoes, such as those defined as "therapeutic" by Medicare, are prescribed, they should generally include a padded collar and tongue, laces; adjustable straps or "Velcro" closures; a wide toe box to accommodate deformities; added depth in the upper section to accommodate deformities, orthotics, and/or padded inserts to evenly distribute plantar pressure; a steel shank for stability; cushioning; and a broad sole base for support and traction.

The plan of care includes the following, as an example: podiatric referral, patient education, medical referral, special footwear, vascular studies, clinical laboratory studies, imaging (including radiographs, sequential bone scans, CT, MRI, and duplex ultrasound), prescriptions, and follow-up assessment and management.

PRIMARY MANAGEMENT OF COMMON PROBLEMS

Onychia is an inflammation of the posterior toe nail wall and bed. It is usually precipitated by local trauma or pressure or is a complication of systemic diseases such as diabetes mellitus and peripheral arterial insufficiency. Onychia is usually an early sign of a developing local infection. Mild erythema, swelling, and pain are common, and tepid saline compresses and pressure reduction help initially. Untreated, it may progress to paronychia, with significant infection and abscess of the posterior nail wall. Infection progresses proximally and deeper structures become involved, possibly leading to necrosis, gangrene, and even amputation. Management includes pressure reduction, drainage, imaging, and antibiotics.

Toenail deformities result from repeated microtrauma, degenerative changes, or disease. Without periodic debridement, the nail structure hypertrophies, thickens (onychauxis), and becomes deformed. Onychogryphosis is usually complicated by fungal infection with disability

F

and pain that can limit ambulation. Exaggerated curvature or onychodysplasia may cause the nail to penetrate the skin, leading to infection and ulceration. Traumatic avulsion of the nail is common, and management consists of local debridement, mild keratolytics, and emollients. Patients with sensory loss may not complain of pain and discomfort.

The most common nonbacterial infection of the toenails is onychomycosis, a chronic and communicable disease. In superficial infections (white onychomycosis), changes appear on the superior surface of the toenail and generally do not invade the deeper structures. In more complicated cases, the nail bed and nail plate are infected from the distal edge (i.e., onycholysis). *Candida* infections are common in patients with mucocutaneous manifestations. Mycotic onychia; auto-avulsion; subungual hemorrhage; a foul, musty odor; and degeneration of the nail plate are common. When the nail matrix becomes involved, hypertrophy and deformity occur. Multiple medications and vascular impairment in older patients complicate systemic treatment. Initial management includes topical fungal solutions, keratolytics, and systemic antifungals. Laser application is also now a part of the management process.

Ingrown toenails in the elderly are usually the result of deformity, onychodysplasia, and improper self-care. When the nail penetrates the skin, abscess and infection result. If not managed early, periungual granulation tissue develops and complicates treatment, which entails removal of the offending nail segment to establish drainage, saline compresses, and antibiotics. Excision, fulguration, desiccation, caustics, and/or astringents reduce granulation tissue. In all cases, removal of the penetrating portion of the nail is essential. Long-standing cases usually require surgical revision.

Many elderly patients develop hyperkeratotic lesions, such as tyloma (i.e., callus) and heloma (i.e., corn), including the hard, soft, vascular, neurofibrous, seed, and subungual types. Intractable keratoma, eccrine poroma, porokeratosis, and verruca must be differentiated from keratotic lesions, although each may present initially as a hyperkeratotic area. Compressive, tensile, or shearing stress creates

these problems. Soft tissue loss and atrophy of the plantar fat pad increase pain and limit ambulation. Contractures, gait changes, deformities, incompatibility between foot type and shoe last, and arthritis are additional factors that need consideration. Many factors, including skin tone and elasticity, predispose patients to keratotic lesions.

Management focuses on functional and activity needs, including debridement, padding, weight dispersion and diffusion, emollients, shoe modifications and shoe last changes, orthoses, and surgical revision. Keratotic lesions can become primary irritants and produce local avascularity, thus precipitating ulceration. Pressure ulcers in the foot usually begin with subkeratotic hemorrhage. If debrided and managed properly, ulcers usually heal. However, the problems may persist because of residual deformity and systemic diseases, such as diabetes mellitus.

Dryness of the skin, or xerosis, due in part to decreased hydration and lubrication, is part of normal aging. Fissures that develop with associated stress are at risk for ulceration. Initial management includes using an emollient and a mild keratolytic. Pruritus is also common and is more severe in cold weather.

Treatment of hyperhidrosis and bromhidrosis depends on the cause. If local, astringents may control excessive perspiration and odor; for example, the short-term use of neomycin powder helps control odor by reducing the bacterial decomposition of perspiration. Topical antifungal foot powders and footwear and stocking modifications should be considered. Dampness and cold can predispose patients to vasospastic effects.

Tinea pedis in elderly patients is often an extension of onychomycosis and common in warm weather. Poor foot hygiene and the inability to see their feet may cause patients to postpone seeking care until the condition becomes clinically significant. Many topical medications can initially manage this condition. Antifungal foot powders provide effective prevention.

Most foot and leg ulcerations in older patients are related to diabetes mellitus, peripheral arterial insufficiency, venous insufficiency, and continuing pressure and trauma. Care involves supportive measures to reduce trauma and pressure to the ulcerated area, orthoses, shoe modifications, and special shoes. Therapeutic shoes are a Medicare entitlement and are appropriate for diabetic patients. Prevention and control of infection are important, and keratosis must be debrided to prevent the ulcer from roofing. Physical modalities and exercises can improve the local vascular supply. Atrophy of soft tissue and arthritis residuals are associated with ulcerations. Management focuses on identifying the cause, instituting local supportive measures, treating related systemic diseases, minimizing osteomyelitis, and maintaining ambulation as long as possible.

Structural deformities or abnormalities of the feet create pain and functional problems in gait and balance and make it difficult to obtain proper footwear. Several conditions involve the hallux (i.e., great toe) such as hallux valgus and hallux rigidus, digitus flexus (i.e., hammertoe), digitus quintus varus, overlapping and underriding toes, prolapsed metatarsals, pes cavus, pes planus, pronation, and splay foot. Treatment can be nonsurgical or surgical and depends on the patient's ability to adapt to structural changes.

These deformities may produce inflammatory changes such as periarthritis, bursitis, myositis, synovitis, neuritis, tendinitis, sesamoiditis, plantar myofasciitis, plantar fasciitis, calcaneal spurs, periostitis, tenosynovitis, atrophy of the plantar fat pad, metatarsal prolapse, metatarsalgia, anterior imbalance, Haglund's deformity, entrapment syndrome, and neuroma. Conservative interventions include shoe modifications, orthoses, braces, physical medicine, exercises, and mild analgesics. Surgical management may be considered when discomfort and pain cannot be managed with conservative measures and when the operative outcome will improve the quality of life. Shoes themselves do not cause pain; rather, pain arises when shoes are improperly used, designed, or incompatible with the foot type and deformities present.

Shoe modifications for the elderly include mild calcaneal wedges to limit motion and alter gait, metatarsal bars to transfer weight, Thomas heels to increase calcaneal support, long shoe counters to increase midfoot support and control

foot direction, heel flares to add stability, shank fillers or wedges to produce a total weight-bearing surface, steel plates to restrict motion, and rocker bars to prevent flexion and extension. Other internal modifications include longitudinal arch pads, wedges, bars, lifts, and tongue or bite pads.

Rheumatoid changes cause early morning stiffness, pain, fibrosis, ankylosis, contracture, deformity, impairment, ambulatory dysfunction, and reduced ambulation. Management includes nonsteroidal anti-inflammatory drugs, local steroid injections, physical medicine, shoe modifications, and orthoses for weight diffusion, dispersion, support, and stabilization. Surgical revision of deformities is also an option. Supportive devices such as a cane may also be indicated with balance concerns and fall prevention.

Foot complaints associated with peripheral arterial, sensory, and diabetic changes include fatigue, resting pain, coldness, burning, color changes, tingling, numbness, diminished hair growth, thickening toenails, ulcerations, phlebitis, cramps, edema, claudication, and repeated foot infections. Primary physical findings include diminished or absent pulses in the foot and throughout the entire extremity, depending on the location and degree of occlusion. Hypertensive patients may demonstrate pulsations that falsely reflect vascular supply. Color changes include rubor and/or cyanosis, and the foot usually feels cool. Vasospastic changes are especially pronounced in colder climates. The skin is usually dry, with pronounced atrophy of the skin and soft tissues. Superficial infections are common and painful when they persist. Neurological assessment of the foot should include Achilles reflex, vibratory sensation, sharp and dull response, superficial plantar response (Babinski), paresthesia, burning, joint position, and testing for LOPS with a monofilament or vibratory threshold meter.

Older diabetic patients have special foot problems. It is estimated that 50% to 75% of all amputations in patients with diabetes could be prevented by early intervention, improved health education, preventive strategies, and periodic evaluation before the onset of significant symptoms and pathology. Elderly patients with diabetes and neuropathy have insensitive feet, with paresthesia, sensory impairment to pain and temperature, motor weakness, diminished or lost Achilles and patellar reflexes, decreased vibratory sense, sensory loss, loss of proprioception, xerotic changes, anhidrosis, neurotrophic arthropathy, atrophy, neurotrophic ulcers, and possibly a marked difference in size between the two feet. There is increased prevalence and incidence of infection, necrosis, and gangrene. Vascular impairment is characterized by pallor, absent or decreased posterior tibial and dorsalis pedis pulses, dependent rubor, decreased venous filling time, skin coolness, trophic changes, numbness, tingling, cramps, and pain. Loss of the plantar metatarsal fat pad predisposes ulceration relative to the existing deformities of the foot.

Hyperkeratotic lesions form as space replacements and are prone to ulceration because of increased pressure on the soft tissues, subcallosal hematoma, and localized avascularity. Tendon contractures and claw toes (i.e., hammertoes) are common. A warm foot with pulsations in an elderly patient with diabetes and neuropathy is common. When ulceration is present, keratosis tends to roof the lesion, retards or prevents closure, and may progress to infection, necrosis, and gangrene. Foot drop, a loss of position sense, and pretibial lesions are indicative of neuropathy and microvascular infarction. Arthropathy gives rise to deformity, altered gait patterns, and increased risk for ulceration and limb loss.

X-rays and other imaging studies of the feet of elderly patients with diabetes usually demonstrate thin trabecular patterns, decalcification, joint position changes, osteophyte formation, osteolysis, deformities, and osteoporosis. Bone scans and MRI studies should be completed.

Management begins by reducing local trauma with orthotics, shoe modifications, and specialized footwear; efforts to maximize weight diffusion and weight dispersion; exercise; local debridement; and appropriate antibiotics. Asymptomatic elderly patients with diabetes mellitus should be assessed at least twice a year to prevent and manage foot problems. Surgical consultation and reconstruction are additional considerations to help reduce pain and increase ambulation.

See also Gait Disturbances.

Arthur E. Helfand and Jeffrey M. Robbins

Sims, D. S., Jr., Cavanagh, P. R., & Ulbrecht, J. S. (1988). Risk factors in the diabetic foot: Recognition and management. *Physical Therapy, 68*(12), 1887–1902.

Web Resources
American Podiatric Medical Association: http://www.apma.org
National Institute on Aging: http://www.niapublications.org/engagepages/footcare.asp
U.S. Department of Veterans Affairs Publications: https://www.va.gov/vhapublications/publications.cfm?Pub=1

FUTURE OF CARE

Caring is fundamental to individual and community flourishing and needs to be seen in the larger global context of human life on the planet and its current and future challenges. Aging is best viewed as a lifelong process and care as a reciprocal activity amongst different generations at a societal level and among individuals interpersonally. Whereas global aging and environmental deterioration may not seem interrelated, how we care for the elderly, as well as children and the environment, in the future will affect not only our ethical legacy, but also the viability of our species. Global aging and environment are linked through the growth of our population, especially the number of elders, and human impact on our planet, particularly global warming and environmental deterioration. We are living in the Anthropocene, the geological scale era on our planet defined by the enormous ecological footprint of our species. As a part of our vision of care into the future, we must recognize elders as an untapped natural resource and source of social capital and ageism as discrimination based on age, not of just advanced age. In this fundamentally important sense, children can be and are victims of ageism. The future of elder care is intimately tied to the future of care generally. In the long-term perspective, children are both our most fundamental current natural resource and the future elders of the world. Thinking through and acting on these challenges creates new opportunities for changing not only how we care, but also how we live.

Arguably, global climate change and associated income inequities and health challenges are the most critical long-term, species–challenging issues we face. Wars, epidemics, famines, and other disasters, such as fires, droughts, and floods, will likely happen with increasing frequency as competition for resources, such as water and energy sources, heat up and ecosystems and human communities are increasingly challenged. Public health will become even more important than in the past. The science of ecology—conceptually superordinate but politically weaker than molecular biology in medicine—should receive more emphasis because it is critical to our health improvement efforts.

New approaches to the economy will be needed to support care systems, including attention to natural resources. In addition, the growing divide between the economic and educational haves and have-nots will create social tension and health consequences. Information systems (e.g., social networking, multimedia narrative, mobile computing) will be important aspects of the world's future in relation to the economy and education. It remains to be seen how the revolution in the creation and distribution of knowledge and the associated shifts in social and economic power will benefit individuals within and among different societies.

A world filled with elders and fewer younger people will create economic challenges with fewer adult workers but also opportunities for positive individual growth and cultural evolution. However, generational inequities and conflicts could grow as a problem. Focusing on the positive aspects of aging, such as the wisdom to appreciate limits, and the reciprocity of caring relationships will be key. Medical models of care focus on "caregiver burden," but giving and receiving care throughout the life course is a part of the basic human condition. We are or should be carers or care partners for each other.

The field of biomedical ethics could become a more important focal point for social discussion of value, particularly if this field broadens its scope beyond the limited philosophical and empirical analysis of medical technologies (such as so-called biomarkers for disease and biological treatments) to explore the relationships between health and other values, such as the quality of our environment and commitment to future generations. Medical models tend to focus on expensive and unrealistic goals such as curing dementia. The often-used aphorism in the Alzheimer's field is "Care today, cure tomorrow," as if a cure can be found for this complex set of age-related conditions and if such imagined cures will replace care. The hype contributed by so-called antiaging medicine movement also contributes to false hopes associated with promised quick-fix solutions to the challenges of aging.

Further research on health care systems is an important aspect of preparing for the future. Emerging information technologies include smart homes, robots, and social media. However, attending to the integration of what we already know and the development of processes for making wise social decisions, often with incomplete information, will be important goals for scholarship and practice.

SOCIAL CARE ISSUES

We will be caring for more older people who have chronic diseases, despite all medical advances. Chronic diseases affect people of all ages. How many resources will society allocate to the future care of the elderly? Questions about how much informal care is, and should be, provided by families and others and how much formal care should be provided by the health care system will continue to be answered in different ways in different cultures. Continued urbanization will disrupt family networks and alter care patterns.

The political will to support formal health care systems for the elderly will be challenged by the need to support other initiatives, such as improvement of the environment and the health and education of children. Intergenerational conflicts over resources could become a political issue at a time of resource scarcity. The resources available for caring for the elderly and the young will depend on the economic well-being of the

F

country. Yet, economic development depends, in part, on the educational level of children. As environmental deterioration continues, the economy will need to adapt. Many of these general social issues, such as the state of the economy and the environment, the political issues around resource allocation, and the development of information systems, will directly and indirectly affect health care systems.

Intergenerational programs offer one hope for avoiding conflict and creating collective wisdom. Planning for the future is relatively well developed evolutionarily in human beings, but our ability to think very long term will need to develop further, enhanced by technologies such as computer modeling and education about systems thinking. Another chapter, Intergenerational Programs, examines how we can both develop intergenerational care programs that meet the needs of vulnerable populations and help society in general.

It is likely that the locus of care in society will also shift. Self-care by being responsible for lifestyle and prevention behaviors will get more emphasis. On the other hand, movements to create age- and dementia-friendly communities need to be expanded and be better integrated with each other and the larger community. In general, "friendly" communities will be better for children, elders, those with cognitive impairment, and in fact all of us and the environment as well. As individuals, communities, and health care systems, we will need to be more adaptable.

HEALTH SYSTEM ISSUES

Major forces driving health care system change will continue to be the aging population and chronic diseases. It is also likely, however, that we will see greater resources being put toward the health consequences of disasters, including emergent infections and trauma.

The evolution of health care systems will need to balance preserving what has worked in the past with developing new concepts and behaviors that will work in the future. The very concept of health and disease will continue to change and influence how we establish both informal and formal systems for providing care.

Encompassing conceptions of health such as ecopsychosocial models and adding the arts, including music, dance, and theater, and the humanities in care will be key. A focus on spiritual, mental, and physical well-being suggests that we should look at broad concepts such as quality of life as desired outcomes of social and health care.

The popularity of alternative and complementary medicine (CAM) suggests that ill persons are seeking nontraditional health concepts and practices. Although not enough CAM is evidence based (much of allopathic medicine is not evidence based either), the concepts of personal centeredness, environmental and community health, and holism are attractive to many. Cultural competence and humility will be increasingly important in a world altered by complex immigration patterns. The philosophies and practices of nursing offer us more integrated approaches than typical biomedicine.

EXAMPLES: CARE FOR PEOPLE WITH DEMENTIA AND END-OF-LIFE CARE

People with dementia often face both a chronic disease process and vulnerabilities to acute health problems such as delirium caused by changes in somatic health or environmental insults. Dementia is not only a prototypical chronic disease, but also one of the most common. It adds to the complexity of providing care in that affected individuals have an impaired decision-making capacity, which means that other people may need to assist in or make health care and other decisions for them. Yet we must challenge our current concepts of age-related cognitive conditions and avoid the over-medicalization of aging. For example, the concept of so-called mild cognitive impairment (i.e., thinking difficulties not yet causing impairments in activities of daily living) illustrates the challenges of separating normal aging from dementia, such as so-called Alzheimer's disease, which is itself closely related to aging and is so heterogeneous as to not likely be a single condition. The pressure from academics and pharmaceutical companies to create more disease categories and overpromise biological fixes must be more strongly addressed. To address the growing number of older individuals with dementia and other chronic diseases, better integration of acute and chronic care systems is needed. Much of the current investment in health care from government and industry focus on bio-medical interventions. The future will require more psychosocial, information systems, educational, and arts innovations. Efforts should continue to ensure that results of outcome studies are incorporated into practice.

End-of-life care is a component of the health care system that needs further development. We must be sure that such care reflects the values of the individuals who are dying. Our desire to prevent death must be balanced by our concern that quality of life is preserved to the end. It is said that the best way to predict the future is to create it. Therefore it is essential that all health care professionals, particularly those working in geriatrics, educate their patients and communities about the challenges ahead. If we continue to focus on biologically dominated efforts to cure the chronic diseases of the elderly, out of proportion to the efforts needed to improve the health care system overall, the quality of life of older individuals may suffer.

Aging is a worldwide phenomenon. We need to create sustainable and resilient health and social care systems that will serve current and future generations of older individuals, as well as the younger people who will care for their elders and who will eventually need such care themselves.

See also Environmental Modifications: Home; Intergenerational Programs; Long-Term Care Policy; Technology.

Peter J. Whitehouse

Web Resources
Family Caregivers: http://www.pewinternet.org/files/old-media//Files/Reports/2013/Pew Research_FamilyCaregivers.pdf
Institute for the Future: Caregiving 2031: http://www.iftf.org/caregiving2031
Mehta, R., & Nafus, D. (2016). *Pilot study report, atlas of caregiving*. Retrieved from http://atlasofcaregiving.com/wp-content/uploads/2016/03/Study_Report.pdf
National Alliance for Caregiving & AARP Public Policy Institute. (2015). Caregiving in the U.S. http://www.caregiving.org/wp-content/uploads/2015/05/2015_CaregivingintheUS_Final-Report-June-4_WEB.pdf
Redfoot, D., Feinberg, L., & Houser, A. (2013). The aging of the baby boom and the growing caregap: A look at future declines in the availability of family caregivers. *AARP Public Policy Institute*. Retrieved from https://www.aarp.org/home-family/caregiving/info-08-2013/theaging-of-the-baby-boom-and-the-growing-care-gap-AARPppi-ltc.html
Reinhard, S. C., Levine, C., & Samis, S. (2012). *Home alone: Family care givers providing complex chronic care*. AARP Public Policy Institute/UHF. Retrieved from https://www.aarp.org/content/dam/aarp/research/public_policy_institute/health/home-alone-family-caregivers-providingcomplex-chronic-care-rev-AARP-ppi-health.pdf

G

GAIT ASSESSMENT INSTRUMENTS

Gait assessment requires a thorough subjective and objective evaluation to determine whether gait changes are related to advancing age or a specific pathology. The clinician must identify and correlate any underlying pathologies with physical impairments of certain body structures or altered body functions. These impairments, in turn, may cause specific functional limitations and decreased participation in a certain task. For example, an elderly man is unable to visit his daughter as he can no longer walk to a bus stop; he has decreased balance in stance caused by diminished strength and initiation of hip and knee flexors because of a stroke 1 year ago.

A pathological gait pattern is different than the gait pattern normally seen in aging adults and is related to a specific medical condition that may be remediable (see Table G.1). As individuals age, muscle size, strength, and power may reduce by greater amounts due to a sedentary lifestyle (Nilwik et al., 2013). As a result, the gait of older adults may present as slower walking speeds, smaller step lengths, and shorter stride lengths (Afiah, Nakashima, Loh, & Muraki, 2016). According to Berryman et al. (2017), the energy cost of walking is negatively correlated with mobility and function in elderly individuals, suggesting that inefficient movement patterns require greater amounts of energy, resulting in poorer functional outcomes. Specifically, strong hip extension and flexion strength is related to decreased energy expenditure during walking, making these muscles important for maintenance of ambulatory status and function (Berryman et al., 2017). Earlier studies show that elderly individuals have decreased knee range of motion and ambulate with lower plantar flexion force, which can

reduce the overall force during push-off (Afiah et al., 2016). Regular strength training can improve strength and muscle fiber size in an elderly population and may help prevent or potentially reverse adverse gait mechanics; therefore it is important to have a thorough understanding of an individual's past and present activity level (Nilwik et al., 2013).

The subjective portion of the examination should include medical history and the patient's report on current ambulation status and restrictions (see Table G.2). Specific to ambulation, important information pertains to the typical distance or time walked daily and conditions under which they walk, requirements for an assistive device and specific footwear (if so, what kind), the progression in use of assistive devices (if applicable), any recent onset of changes in walking habits, any rest required during and after walking, any avoidance of situations (i.e., uneven terrain such as grassy hills, uneven pavement) and any pain while walking. The medical history should focus on use of alcohol, benzodiazepines, neuroleptic agents, antihypertensives, and vasodilators; surgical history; and previous orthopedic injuries.

Objectively, gait can be measured functionally and biomechanically. Functionally, assessments such as the Functional Gait Assessment (FGA), Timed Up and Go Test (TUG), Dynamic Gait Index (DGI), and 6-Minute and 10-Minute Walk Tests (6MWT and 10MWT) can identify limitations in gait speed, endurance, and stability under different conditions (see Table G.3). These tests are ideally performed fatigued, not fatigued, in different lighting, and with different levels of distractions.

Biomechanical evaluation of gait requires observation of the full gait cycle which is divided into stance (60% of the cycle) and swing (40% of the cycle). Stance involves weight acceptance (initial contact and loading

Table G.1
PATHOLOGICAL GAIT ASSESSMENT

Pathology	Typical Presentation
Parkinson's disease (PD)	Flexed-forward, flatfooted, shuffling, and at times festinating gait, coupled with neurological findings of rigidity, bradykinesia, masked facies, and resting tremor, are typical. Findings may begin unilaterally and progress to bilaterally as Parkinson's disease progresses.
Cerebrovascular accident	Hemiplegia (unilateral loss of lower extremity and/or upper extremity movement) leading to gait asymmetry. Possible synergy posturing due to flexor or extensor tone, with positive findings for spasticity, hyperreflexia, and pathological reflexes on the involved side. Foot drop, Trendelenburg, circumduction, lateral, or posterior lean are all possible.
Multiple sclerosis (MS)	Progressive muscle fatigue, limiting gait endurance, is typical. Performance may worsen in heat. Can have any neurologic presentation but most common findings are due to progressive worsening of symptoms with increased activity. Can have spasticity, ataxia, hyperreflexia, pathological reflexes, and sensory loss, as well as cognitive and attention dysfunctions.
Cerebellar dysfunction	Ataxic: Wide-based, uncoordinated movement of legs, abrupt adjustments to trunk position, positive findings for dysmetria, dysdiadochokinesia, and possibly vestibular ocular reflex impairment.
Sensory loss (peripheral neuropathy)	Ataxic: Wide-based, high-stepping, or stamping walk, possible inability to shift full weight onto affected side, diminished light touch, vibration, and position sense. May correlate with lower motor neuron signs: loss of reflexes, muscle wasting. Check for nerve entrapment via bony alignment or hypertonic musculature in body regions more proximal than symptoms.
Sensory loss (central dysfunction)	Ataxic: Wide-based, high-stepping, or stamping walk; possible inability to shift full weight onto affected side; diminished light touch, vibration, and position sense. May be found with acute spinal or cortical shock: loss of reflexes, decreased tone, or, with upper motor neuron signs, spasticity, hyperreflexia, and pathological reflexes. Possible in stroke, spinal cord injury, multiple sclerosis, and traumatic brain injury.
Osteoarthritis (OA)	Antalgic: decreased weight bearing on painful side, possible trunk side-bend away from painful side.

Table G.2
COMPONENTS OF GAIT ASSESSMENT

Assessment Components	Specific Aspects to Include
Patient history	Age, height, weight, diagnosis, prognosis, ambulation limitations, date of onset of the problem, goals, use of an assistive device, medications, usual activity level, past medical problems.
Muscular and neurological evaluation	Motor deficits, strengths/weaknesses, muscle tone, proprioceptive deficits, range of motion limitations, coordination limitations, cognitive limitations, safety awareness.
Static alignment	Patient standing in a relaxed, comfortable position with equal weight on both lower extremities while examiner observes for malalignments
Dynamic alignment	Observation of the patient ambulating through stance and swing phase.

response) and single-limb support (midstance, terminal stance, and preswing). Swing phase consists of limb advancement, including the end of preswing, initial swing, midswing, and terminal swing. At any point within the gait cycle, deviations can reduce efficiency and create a potential mechanism for injury (see Table G.4).

The most efficient means of performing a physical examination is to first observe the patient walking and in quiet standing under different conditions (even vs. uneven ground,

G

Table G.3
GAIT ASSESSMENT TOOLS

Functional Test	Indications	Summary	Normal
Six-Minute Walk Test (6MWT)	Alzheimer's disease Geriatrics Heart failure Multiple sclerosis Osteoarthritis Parkinson's disease Pulmonary disease Spinal cord injury Stroke	Walk for 6 minutes. Documentation should include the speed tested if fastest speed is not used (preferred vs. fast). Assistive device okay to use, using the same each trial. Individual should be able to ambulate without physical assistance.	For community-dwelling, healthy adults: 60–69 years old: M: 572 m F: 538 m 70–79 years old: M: 527 m F: 471 m 80–89 years old: M: 417 m F: 392 m
Dynamic Gait Index (DGI)	Brain injury Geriatrics Multiple sclerosis Parkinson's disease Stroke Vestibular disorders	Performed with a marked distance of 20 feet. 8-item test. Assistive device okay to use, using the same each trial. Scores are based on a 4-point scale: 0 = severe impairment 1 = moderate impairment 2 = mild impairment 3 = normal ambulation Highest possible score is 24 points.	Community-dwelling elderly >65 years old: ≤19/24 indicative of increased fall risk
Functional Gait Assessment (FGA)	Older adults ranging from 40 to 80 years Parkinson's disease Spinal cord injury Stroke Vestibular populations	Modification of the DGI to improve reliability and decrease the ceiling effect. 10-item test, with 7 of the 8 items of the DGI. Scores are based on a 4-point scale: 0 = severe impairment 1 = moderate impairment 2 = mild impairment 3 = normal ambulation Assistive device okay to use, using the same each trial. Highest possible score is 30 points.	≤22/30 = effective in predicting falls ≤20/30 = optimal to predict community-dwelling older adults who would sustain unexplained falls in next 6 months Healthy adults 60–69 years old: Mean: 27.1/30 70–79 years old: Mean: 24.9/30 80–89 years old: Mean: 20.8/30
Timed Up and Go (TUG) Test	Acute medical patients (on wards) Amputations Alzheimer's disease Arthritis (before and/or after joint arthroplasty) Cerebral palsy Community-dwelling older adults Frail elderly Low back pain Lower extremity Multiple sclerosis Osteoarthritis Parkinson's disease Rheumatoid arthritis Spinal cord injury Stroke Vestibular disorders	Rise from a chair, walk 10 feet (3 m), turn, walk back to the chair, and sit down. Timing begins at "go" and stops when the patient is seated completely. It is suggested to use an average of 3 trials. Assistive device okay to use, using the same each trial.	Cut off scores for falls risk: Community-dwelling adults in general >65 years old: >13.5 seconds Frail elderly: >32.6 seconds 60–69 years old: M: 8 seconds F: 8 seconds 70–79 years old: M: 9 seconds F: 9 seconds 80–89 years old: M: 10 seconds F: 11 seconds

(continued)

Table G.3
GAIT ASSESSMENT TOOLS   (*continued*)

Functional Test	Indications	Summary	Normal
Tinetti Performance Oriented Mobility Assessment (POMA)	Older adults	Task-oriented. Assesses gait and balance ability. Composed of a 9-item gait portion (POMA-G) and 7-item balance portion (POMA-B). POMA-G: maximum score of 12 points. POMA-B: maximum score of 16 points.	65–79 years old: M: 26.21/28 F: 25.16/28 >80 years old: M: 23.29/28 F: 17.2/28 Cut off: POMA total: 21/28 POMA B: 11/16 <19/28: high fall risk 19–24/28: med fall risk 25–28/28: low fall risk
10-Minute Walk Test (10MWT)	Alzheimer's disease Brain tumor Community-dwelling older adults General neurological movement disorders Hip fracture Lower limb amputation Multiple sclerosis Parkinson's disease Spinal cord injury Stroke Traumatic brain injury Vestibular disorders	Average 3 trials: Walk 33 feet (10 m) while timed. Divide distance by time. Assistive device okay to use but must be kept consistent each trial. Not appropriate if individual requires physical assistance to ambulate. Perform at preferred walking speed or fastest speed possible (document).	60–69 years old: M: Comfortable speed (CS): 1.36 m/s Fast speed (FS): 1.93 m/s F: CS: 1.3 m/s; FS: 1.77 m/s 70–79 years old: M: CS: 1.33 m/s; FS: 2.08 m/s F: CS: 1.27 m/s; FS: 1.74 m/s

Table G.4
COMMON GAIT IMPAIRMENTS

Phase	Impairments
Initial contact	No heel strike (step on flat foot), foot slap (L4, dorsiflexors), excessive trunk extension, equinus deformity, plantar flexor spacticity
Loading response	Backward trunk lean, anterior trunk lean, plantar flexion contracture/spasticity, knee remains flexed
Midstance	Trendelenburg sign of stance leg, antalgic gait (shortened stance), forward trunk bend (contracture), excessive lordosis (contracture), genu recurvatum (weak quadricepts)
Terminal stance	Trendelenburg sign, excessive lumbar lordosis; forward trunk, trunk moves backward, genu recuvatum, flexed knee
Preswing	Weak plantar flexors, MTP dysfunction/pain, backward trunk lurch
Initial swing	Posterior pelvic tilt/backward trunk lean, vaulting and circumducting, drop foot/steppage gait
Mid and terminal swing	Weak hamstrings/gluteals, quadriceps weakness, vaulting and circumducting, drop foot/steppage

Source: Perry (1992).

G

at different velocities, uphill vs. downhill), and during different tasks. Deviations are recorded by body region (ankle, knee, hip, pelvis, trunk, scapula, arms, and head/neck) or body function (single leg balance). Equally important are static malalignments such as genu valgus/varus, pes planus/cavus, and excessive kyphosis or lordosis. Further tests are performed to determine impairments in cardiopulmonary function (respiratory rate, blood pressure, and heart rate measures), flexibility, strength (manual muscle tests), sensation (light touch, proprioception, kinesthesia), vestibular (vestibular ocular reflex, Dix–Hallpike test), coordination (dysmetria, dysdiadochokinesia), motor control (ability to modify motor behavior in response to internal or external cues), or decreased attention and cognitive awareness. The use of a force plate and video analysis can assist the clinician in identifying specific objective data pertaining to a patient's gait mechanics and assist in finding more subtle deviations. Once identified, deviations, or impairments, can be further broken down: decreased range of motion can be due to lack of muscle flexibility, joint malalignment, ligamentous or capsular restrictions, muscle spasms or hypertonicity, or pain. Manual muscle tests identify directional or muscle-specific weakness, but muscles should be tested with and without external proximal stability (i.e., hip extension may test weak due to poor pelvic core stability). Sensation tests should be correlated with other findings to determine if it is of a peripheral or central nature. Peripheral findings should be further examined for areas of nerve entrapment that can be resolved with soft tissue or joint mobilization.

Cognitive function and mood testing should include levels of anxiety, attention, and safety awareness. Observation of dual tasking can assist with attention testing. There is increasing evidence that there is an interrelationship between gait and cognitive processes such as attention, executive function, and working memory (Montero-Odasso, Verghese, Beauchet, & Hausdorff, 2012).

See also Gait Disturbances.

Laura Isham and Herbert Karpatkin

Afiah, I. N., Nakashima, H., Loh, P. Y., & Muraki, S. (2016). An exploratory investigation of changes in gait parameters with age in elderly Japanese women. *SpringerPlus*, 5(1), 1069. doi:10.1186/s40064-016-2739-7

Berryman, N., Bherer, L., Nadeau, S., Lauzière, S., Lehr, L., Bobeuf, F., … Bosquet, L. (2017). Relationships between lower body strength and the energy cost of treadmill walking in a cohort of healthy older adults: A cross-sectional analysis. *European Journal of Applied Physiology*, 117(1), 53–59. doi:10.1007/s00421-016-3498-4

Montero-Odasso, M., Verghese, J., Beauchet, O., & Hausdorff, J. M. (2012). Gait and cognition: A complementary approach to understanding brain function and the risk of falling. *Journal of the American Geriatrics Society*, 60(11), 2127–2136. doi:10.1111/j.1532-5415.2012.04209.x

Nilwik, R., Snijders, T., Leenders, M., Groen, B. B., van Kranenburg, J., Verdijk, L. B., & van Loon, L. J. (2013). The decline in skeletal muscle mass with aging is mainly attributed to a reduction in type II muscle fiber size. *Experimental Gerontology*, 48(5), 492–498. doi:10.1016/j.exger.2013.02.012

Perry, J. (1992). *Gait analysis: Normal and pathological function slack incorporated*. Thorofare, NJ: Slack.

Web Resources
Functional Balance Assessment of Older Community Dwelling Adults: http://ijahsp.nova.edu/articles/vol5num4/pdf/langley.pdf
Performance-Oriented Mobility Assessment: http://www.hospitalmedicine.org/geriresource/toolbox/pdfs/poma.pdf
Timed Up and Go: http://gsa.buffalo.edu/DPT/tug_0109.pdf

GAIT DISTURBANCES

Despite aging being associated with changes to gait quality, one cannot assume that the aging process causes gait disturbances. Age-related changes are multifactorial, influenced by insults to the musculoskeletal, cardiovascular, pulmonary, and neurological systems. A population-based study has shown a 35% prevalence of gait disorders among persons older than the age of

70 years (Verghese et al., 2006). Approximately, 85% of individuals living in the community, older than 60 years of age, still have a normal gait pattern, but only 20% of those 85 years old or older walk normally (Sudarsky, 2001). Any minor alteration in gait pattern can increase energy expenditure (Waters, 2010), affecting function and decreasing quality of life. This further influences a person's level of independence. Clinicians working with older adults must effectively evaluate older patients for contributors to gait changes, identify potentially treatable conditions, and provide patients and caregivers with appropriate interventions to compensate for changes.

There are no clear definitions of a normal gait according to age, and many changes of an older individual's gait may be because of underlying disease (Alexander & Goldberg, 2005). With aging, there tends to be a decline in gait speed and stride length of about 10% to 20% from age 20 to 70 years (Winter, Patla, Frank, & Walt, 1990). This decline has no distinct mechanism, and it could be caused by pain, changes to the central nervous system (CNS) or peripheral nervous system (PNS), degenerative joint disease, or cardiopulmonary dysfunction. Other gait characteristics that may occur with aging include a decline in ankle range of motion (ROM), decreased spinal rotation, decreased arm swing, increased length of the double-limb stance portion of the gait pattern, and reduced propulsive force generalized at preswing (Salzman, 2010). Although commonly occurring with age, gait disorders are not endemic among all older individuals. Most disorders are pathological in origin. If the examination and evaluation findings discover nothing specific, the disturbance may be idiopathic in nature, requiring further consultation with the medical team.

Abnormal patterns of movement occur because of pain from spasticity, weakness, or deformity. Furthermore, the movement may compensate for other problems, such as visual or vestibular dysfunction. Alterations in gait can also be compromised by cardiovascular, arthritic, and orthopedic disorders. Most gait disorders are influenced by chronic neurological disorders.

NEUROLOGIC

a. Parkinson's disease
  - Festinating gait—progressively small, quick steps with narrower base of support or shuffling, often culminating in a fall
  - Delayed initiation of postural reactions
  - Freezing, especially during a change to environment (i.e., walking through a doorway)
  - Decreased heel strike, arm swing, and trunk rotation
  - Kyphosis
  - Turning as one unit, rather than dissociating head and trunk rotation from the pelvis and legs
  - Marked rigidity throughout the joints

b. Multiple sclerosis
  - No "typical" pattern because of different presentations and progression
  - Gait worsening with fatigue
  - Demyelination and disuse may lead to joint contractures, decreased sensation, and muscle weakness
  - Ataxia with a wider base of support and stiff knees for added stability

c. Cerebrovascular accident
  - Most persons with stroke experience paralysis on one side of the body (hemiparesis), whether affecting the upper and lower extremity similarly or sparing/recovering strength in the lower extremity
  - Compensations based on muscle imbalances and decreased proprioception because of where the infarct occurred in the brain
  - Sequelae may include spasticity and alterations in muscle tone
  - Extensor and flexor synergies, often referred to as *spastic hemiplegia*
  - A lean to the unaffected side and a thrust forward of the affected hip
  - External rotation and circumduction of the affected leg in swing
  - Toe drag because of decreased ability at the affected dorsiflexors and genu recurvatum/extension thrust of the affected leg in stance

- Or crouched/flexed posture because of flexor synergy
- Because of gluteal weakness of the paretic side, a Trendelenburg pattern is possible, with a trunk lean to the affected side and contralateral hip drop

d. Alzheimer's disease
- No "typical" pattern but generalized weakness because of muscle wasting
- Impaired posture because of atrophy of the spinal musculature
- Decreased proprioception
- Decreased safety awareness because of cognitive decline
- Wandering because of inability to recognize familiar landmarks

Sensory Loss

There are numerous mechanisms of sensory loss, including, degenerative joint disease (DJD), radiculopathy, and multiple sclerosis (MS). A common finding is ataxia, a complex disorder caused by a disruption to the nerve pathways in the brain involved in coordination.

Sensory ataxia: absent/impaired proprioception, or knowing where the body is in space
Motor/cerebellar ataxia: impaired motor control and coordination
Vestibular ataxia: impaired balance and body position because of involvement of vestibular nuclei

Presentation may include:

- Short, small strides and wider base of support
- Occasional scissoring of one or both lower extremities
- High steppage pattern
- Foot drop, a slap of the forefoot for greater feedback through the foot

ORTHOPEDIC

Orthopedic changes with age are associated with decreased integrity of the musculoskeletal system. Bone and muscle are affected by decreased osteoblast activity and decreased calcium absorption, with stiffness because of decreased elastin and decreased bone tensile strength and fat or collagen replacing muscle fiber. These systemic changes can lead to sarcopenia or frailty, further affecting gait quality, speed, and level of independence.

a. Foot/ankle: Decreased ROM is possible in all planes of movement but is seen mostly with ankle dorsiflexion and great toe extension. Decreased mobility at presswing changes the force of the swing, causing an overall slower speed and/or shorter step length. Pain is often associated with decreased ROM and weight bearing affecting the stance sequence. Other factors include fractures, deformities such as claw-foot or bunions, plantar fasciitis, effects of rheumatoid arthritis or gout, cellulitis, and gangrene (Naser & Mahdi, 2016). Gait abnormalities are also possible because of cumulative years of weight bearing and improper shoe wear, which can either be cause or effect of overpronation, creating malalignment and issues up the kinetic chain.

b. Knee: Knee osteoarthritis (OA) is a leading cause of disability according to the American Association of Orthopedic Surgeons. Pain, inflammation, decreased strength, and impaired balance affect gait quality. Patellofemoral dysfunction and meniscal tears also contribute to an antalgic pattern; there is noted decreased weight acceptance on the affected leg and/or decreased knee flexion with swing because of pain with active ROM, presenting a limp.

c. Hip: Hip OA is also common, causing pain with active or passive motion and weight bearing, which in turn decreases stance time, step length, and speed. Other common findings are fractures because of falls or osteopenia/osteoporosis, usually requiring surgical intervention. Bursitis also occurs, often at the greater trochanter, affecting gait quality, overall body mechanics, and independence.

d. Trunk: Because of decreased bone formation and change in hormone levels with advanced age, osteoporosis is common. Trunk instability ensues because of decreased vertebral height and decreased integrity of the rib cage to provide support. Breathing difficulties, as well as abdominal pain, follow, impairing balance and mobility. Stiffness throughout the spine inhibits rotation and postural reactions. The common presentation is increased kyphosis with increased risk of vertebral fracture.

e. Arms: Degeneration is noted throughout the spine and shoulders, decreasing arm swing, with rounding of the shoulders, exaggerating forward head posture and kyphosis. Common findings are pain with active or passive movement because of atraumatic rotator cuff dysfunction or adhesive capsulitis. This further decreases the ability to walk while carrying/lifting, limiting ability to perform self-care appropriately.

EVALUATION/EXAMINATION

It is imperative to perform an evaluation that includes history of falls, surgeries, medications, need for assistance, a simple cognitive screen (e.g., Mini-Cog), and the person's health goals. The examiner should pay close attention to vision, coordination, and sensation, including proprioception and balance, as well as muscle strength and joint ROM.

Because gait speed can predict mortality (Studenski et al., 2011), a thorough kinematic/kinetic analysis should be performed during the examination. This can be done with a stopwatch and marks on the floor or with high-tech equipment in a movement/gait analysis laboratory. Other functional analysis should be completed to determine the more difficult aspects of gait and to assess endurance. Tests include the Timed Up and Go Test, Functional Gait Analysis, 6-Minute Walk Test, and Sit to Stand Test. The Tinetti Performance Oriented Mobility Assessment (POMA) or Berg Balance Scale should be included to correlate balance dysfunction with gait disturbance.

INTERVENTIONS

Rehabilitation

In the treatment of gait disturbances in older adults, the clinician must decide whether the intervention should be based on remediation or

compensation. *Remediation* refers to the use of physical or medical interventions to restore the lost function to its premorbid state. *Compensation* refers to using an alternative strategy or assistive device to take over the work of the lost function. For example, a patient with a foot drop because of calf muscle tightness or dorsiflexor weakness could be treated with plantiflexor stretching and dorsiflexor strengthening to remediate the problem or could be given an ankle brace and a cane to compensate for the problem. Giving compensatory interventions before attempting remediation may result in worsening of the deficit because of non-use.

If remediation is unsuccessful, to maintain quality of life and independence, compensations for gait dysfunction in the form of assistive devices and orthoses may be required. One might choose a front-wheeled walker or a rollator with seat for energy conservation. For less support, walking poles or a single-point cane may be appropriate. Orthoses offer support to permanent changes of the musculoskeletal system. A Dorsi-Assist or a plantar-flexion stop provides mechanical advantage during swing, and knee bracing prevents extensive extension thrust or buckling in stance.

As mentioned, it is imperative to request a medication list with dosages to screen for polypharmacy. This geriatric syndrome is associated with decline in functional capacity, nutritional status, and cognition (Jyrkkä, Enlund, Lavikainen, Sulkava, & Hartikainen, 2011). Frequent communication between all members of the health care team is beneficial to prevent polypharmacy and to better coordinate care. Gait disturbances are not guaranteed in the older population and warrant the same care as one would offer to a younger person with the same presentation.

Herbert Karpatkin

Alexander, N. B., & Goldberg, A. (2005). Gait disorders: Search for multiple causes. *Cleveland Clinic Journal of Medicine, 72*(7), 586–600.

Jyrkkä, J., Enlund, H., Lavikainen, P., Sulkava, R., & Hartikainen, S. (2011). Association of polypharmacy with nutritional status, functional ability and cognitive capacity over a three-year period in an elderly population. *Pharmacoepidemiology and Drug Safety, 20*, 514–522. doi:10.1002/pds.2116

Naser, S. S. A., & Mahdi, A. O. (2016). A proposed expert system for foot diseases diagnosis. *American Journal of Innovative Research and Applied Sciences, 2*(4), 155–168.

Salzman, B. (2010). Gait and balance disorders in older adults. *American Family Physician, 82*(1), 61–68.

Studenski, S., Perera, S., Patel, K., Rosano, C., Faulkner, K., Inzitari, M., … Guralnik, J. (2011). Gait speed and survival in older adults. *Journal of the American Medical Association, 305*(1), 50–58. doi:10.1001/jama.2010.1923

Sudarsky, L. (2001). Neurologic disorders of gait. *Current Neurology and Neuroscience Reports, 1*(4), 350–356. doi:10.1007/s11910-001-0089-4

Verghese, J., LeValley, A., Hall, C. B., Katz, M. J., Ambrose, A. F., & Lipton, R. B. (2006). Epidemiology of gait disorders in community-residing older adults. *Journal of the American Geriatrics Society, 54*(2), 255–261. doi:10.1111/j.1532-5415.2005.00580.x

Waters, R. (2010). Energy expenditure. In A. Perry & J. M. Burnfield (Eds.), *Gait analysis: Normal and pathological function* (p. 496). Thorofare, NJ: SLACK.

Winter, D. A., Patla, A. E., Frank, J. S., & Walt, S. E. (1990). Biomechanical walking pattern changes in the fit and healthy elderly. *Physical Therapy, 70*(6), 340–347.

GASTROINTESTINAL BLEED

Gastrointestinal (GI) bleeding emergencies in older adults require rapid diagnosis and aggressive intervention because they are associated with significant morbidity and mortality. More than 1 million patients are hospitalized for acute GI bleeding each year in the United States, with an annual rate of hospitalization of approximately 350 per 100,000 population (J. D. Lewis, Bilker, Brensinger, Farrar, & Strom, 2002). Approximately 50% of these admissions are secondary to bleeding from the upper GI tract (esophagus, stomach, or duodenum), 40% are secondary to lower GI sources (colon, anus, and rectum), and the remainder from the small intestine (Feldman, Friedman, & Brandt, 2010).

Comorbid conditions and decreased physiologic reserve make persons 65 years and older particularly vulnerable to the adverse consequences of acute blood loss. Thus GI bleeding in older individuals is a significant clinical challenge. The etiology of most GI bleeding can be suspected by the presenting clinical symptoms and physical examination. Initial management should focus on resuscitation to achieve and maintain hemodynamic stability. Optimal patient outcomes depend on appropriate diagnosis, pharmacologic therapy, and if needed, therapeutic endoscopy.

Patients with severe GI bleeding may have shock, tachycardia, orthostatic hypotension, decrease in hematocrit of 6% or more, and need for transfusion of at least two units of packed red blood cells (PRBCs). These patients should be admitted to the intensive care unit for careful resuscitation and treatment. Depending on the GI site of the blood loss, a patient may vomit bright red or coffee grounds–like material (upper GI tract bleeding), pass black tarry or mahogany stools (upper GI tract bleeding), or pass bright red blood from the rectum (lower or brisk upper GI tract bleeding). Disorders associated with GI hemorrhage include *Helicobacter pylori* infection (gastritis/ulcers), vascular abnormalities such as arteriovenous malformations or Dieulafoy's lesions, inflammatory bowel disease, GI tract malignancies, aortoenteric fistulas, diverticulosis, hemorrhoids, and cirrhosis. Medications implicated in GI hemorrhage include nonsteroidal anti-inflammatory drugs (NSAIDs), antithrombotic agents, and chemotherapeutic agents. Other medications, including selective serotonin reuptake inhibitors (SSRIs) and steroids, are associated with increased risk of bleeding when used with NSAIDs. Newer antithrombotic medications have complicated the management of GI hemorrhage because of a lack of reversibility. Expert consultation from cardiology or hematology should be considered to assist in management.

ACUTE UPPER GI BLEEDING

Upper GI bleeding (UGIB) is defined as blood loss proximal to the ligament of Treitz. As many as 70% of all episodes of acute UGIB occur in patients aged 60 years and older (Van Leerdam et al., 2003). Older patients have been shown to have a higher mortality from UGIB, likely because of higher prevalence of comorbid illnesses (Farrell & Friedman, 2001). Peptic ulcer disease (PUD), followed by esophagitis, gastropathy, and varices, is the most common cause of UGIB in the elderly. UGIB rates and hospital admissions have increased among older adults with PUD (Thomopoulos et al., 2004). Older patients are more likely to have bleeding lesions because of NSAID use, probably because of age-related gastric mucosa susceptibility to NSAID damage.

In an older patient, emesis of any coffee grounds–like material or bright red blood requires immediate evaluation. Melena, or passage of back, tarry stool, is considered to be a sign of UGIB until proved otherwise. Approximately 10% of patients presenting with hematochezia have brisk UGIB. Concurrent vascular disease with UGIB increases the risk of cardiac ischemia. Initial laboratory studies are vital in guiding intervention because renal failure, thrombocytopenia, or medications may compromise the coagulation system in older patients. GI bleeding in patients taking warfarin or clopidogrel can be more rapidly life-threatening than a thrombotic event. Risk scores, which are based on age, comorbidities, endoscopic findings, blood urea nitrogen, hemoglobin, systolic blood pressure, pulse, and presenting symptoms, have been developed to predict the need of clinical intervention, rebleeding, and mortality (Ohmann et al., 2005).

Treatment

The primary aim is to achieve hemodynamic stability with intravenous fluids, PRBC transfusion, and vasopressor support. Continuous infusion of a proton pump inhibitor (PPI) is usually initiated if upper GI bleed is suspected because it decreases the proportion of patients who have higher-risk stigmata of bleeding at endoscopy (Cappell, 2010). Infusion of a somatostatin analog (i.e., octreotide) to decrease splanchnic circulation inflow may be used in patients with cirrhosis if variceal bleeding is

under consideration. Placement of a nasogastric (NG) tube can confirm or exclude the presence of an upper GI source but has not been shown to affect outcome (Rockey, 2005). In 10% to 15% of cases, NG lavage is clear even in the presence of active bleeding (usually duodenal ulcer bleeding). Early endoscopy, within 24 hours of presentation, allows for discharge of patients at low risk of recurrent bleeding and leads to reduced hospital admission and resource use. Early endoscopy in high-risk patients potentially offers an opportunity to stop the bleeding and improve clinical outcomes (Laine & Jensen, 2012).

Outpatient care of patients after UGIB depends on the cause of bleeding and may include maintenance of PPI therapy and eradication of *H. pylori* infection in patients with PUD. Patients with UGIB may continue low-dose aspirin for secondary prevention of vascular events. The risks and benefits of continuing NSAIDs and other antiplatelet agents should be discussed with the patient and the appropriate specialist (Dworzynski, Pollit, Kelsey, Higgins, & Palmer, 2012). Patients diagnosed with a gastric ulcer should repeat upper endoscopy in 6 to 8 weeks to document healing and exclude malignancy. Future bleeding from esophageal varices may be prevented by the use of portal antihypertensive therapy and repeat endoscopic banding to fully eradicate the varices.

ACUTE LOWER GI BLEEDING

Lower GI bleeding (LGIB) mostly presents as hematochezia although a proximal colonic source of bleeding can cause melena. Compared with acute UGIB, patients with LGIB have a higher presenting hemoglobin level, are less likely to experience shock (19% vs. 35%), and require fewer blood transfusions (36% vs. 64%; Barnert & Messmann, 2008). Acute LGIB stops spontaneously in 80% to 85% of patients, with an overall mortality rate of 2% to 4% (Farrell & Friedman, 2005). Diverticulosis and angiodysplasias are the two most common causes of LGIB, followed by hemorrhoids and colonic neoplasms. Other etiologies include inflammatory bowel disease, ischemic or infectious colitis, and radiation proctitis. Clinical history, such

G

as the absence or presence of abdominal pain, consistency and color of stool, and the timing of bleeding, combined with a digital rectal examination often suggests the etiology. Once hemodynamic stability has been achieved, further investigation via anoscopy, sigmoidoscopy, or colonoscopy can be performed.

Diverticular Bleeding

Most patients with diverticulosis are asymptomatic, but a small percentage can have acute diverticular hemorrhage presenting as painless hematochezia. Although approximately 70% to 90% of diverticula are located in the descending and sigmoid colon, hemorrhage disproportionately occurs from right-sided diverticula (Wilkins, Baird, Pearson, & Schade, 2009). Most often, bleeding from diverticulosis occurs in the elderly and is rare in patients under the age of 50 years (M. Lewis, 2008). Patients with an episode of diverticular hemorrhage are at an increased risk of recurrent episodes (Psarras et al., 2011). Diverticular hemorrhage ceases spontaneously in approximately 80% of cases (Wilkins et al., 2009). Most patients can be managed endoscopically or via angiography, and few patients now require surgery.

Ischemic Colitis

Transient colonic hypoperfusion can cause cramping lower abdominal pain with hematochezia. Incidence of ischemic colitis is associated with advanced age and medical comorbidities (e.g., atherosclerotic vascular disease, end-stage renal disease requiring dialysis). Most patients improve with supportive care alone, and overall mortality is low (Feuerstadt & Brandt, 2010).

Other Causes

Bleeding from colonic angioectasias can present as either brisk hemorrhage or chronic blood loss. Endoscopic therapy can be targeted at sites of active bleeding but is difficult if multiple lesions are present. Rectal bleeding from hemorrhoids may be associated with constipation and can present as stool coated with blood. Colonic malignancy usually presents as occult blood loss (more common), or overt bleeding accompanied

by weight loss change in bowel habits, change in stool caliber, and iron deficiency anemia. Radiation proctitis should be suspected in patients with hematochezia who have undergone previous radiation therapy for GI, genitourinary, prostate, or gynecologic malignancy.

Treatment

Advances in endoscopy and angiography have improved treatment and patient outcomes. However, benefits are sometimes limited by patients' advanced age and multiple comorbidities. Colonoscopic evaluation can be useful in identifying the source of bleeding. However, it may be difficult to localize the single "culprit" diverticulum in a colon that is filled with fresh blood and multiple large diverticula. If a bleeding diverticulum is localized, injection with epinephrine to cause localized tamponade and vasoconstriction may be effective. Placing a hemostatic clip across the mouth of the bleeding diverticulum has also been shown to control the bleeding. Bleeding angioectasias are treated with argon plasma coagulation or electrocautery.

Nuclear scanning using radionuclide-tagged red blood cells can detect sources of colonic bleeding at rates as low as 0.1 mL of blood per minute (Dusold, Burke, Carpentier, & Dyck, 1994). This noninvasive modality can be helpful in detecting the site of bleeding before angiography or surgical resection is pursued. Mesenteric arteriography can detect hemorrhage at a rate of 0.5 to 1 mL/minute and can provide hemostatic therapy via intra-arterial infusion of vasopressin or embolization of the bleeding arterial vessel with gel foam or microscopic coils (Zuckerman, Bocchini, & Birnbaum, 1993). The morbidity of arteriography is considerably less than that of urgent hemicolectomy or subtotal colectomy. However, patients with renal impairment and older patients, because of their lower glomerular filtration rate, are at greater risk of nephrotoxicity from arteriography.

Bleeding lesions in the small intestine (i.e., angioectasias, tumors, and Crohn's disease) may be detected via video capsule endoscopy (VCE), push enteroscopy, or single- or double-balloon enteroscopy. VCE involves the swallowing of a capsule that contains a LED light source, camera, and transmitter, which transmits images to an external recording device. VCE allows rough localization of the lesion in the small bowel using a positioning system, which can direct definitive therapy. Push or balloon-assisted enteroscopy can then be used for the treatment of identified bleeding lesions.

Jonathan Fahler and Aboud Affi

Barnert, J., & Messmann, H. (2008). Management of lower gastrointestinal tract bleeding. *Best Practice & Research Clinical Gastroenterology, 22*(2), 295–312.

Cappell, M. S. (2010). Therapeutic endoscopy for acute upper gastrointestinal bleeding. *Nature Reviews Gastroenterology and Hepatology, 7*(4), 214–229.

Dusold, R., Burke, K., Carpentier, W., & Dyck, W. P. (1994). The accuracy of technetium-99m-labeled red cell scintigraphy in localizing gastrointestinal bleeding. *American Journal of Gastroenterology, 89,* 345–348.

Dworzynski, K., Pollit, V., Kelsey, A., Higgins, B., & Palmer, K. (2012). Management of acute upper gastrointestinal bleeding: Summary of NICE guidance. *British Medical Journal, 13*(344), e3412. doi:10.1136/bmj.e3412

Farrell, J. J., & Friedman, L. S. (2001). Gastrointestinal bleeding in the elderly. *Gastroenterology Clinics of North America, 30*(2), 377–407.

Feldman, M., Friedman, L. S., & Brandt, L. J. (2010). *Sleisenger and Fordtran's gastrointestinal and liver disease: Pathophysiology, diagnosis, management.* Philadelphia, PA: Saunders Elsevier.

Feuerstadt, P., & Brandt, L. J. (2010). Colon ischemia: Recent insights and advances. *Current Gastroenterology Reports, 12*(5), 383–390.

Laine, L., & Jensen, D. M. (2012). Management of patients with ulcer bleeding. *American Journal of Gastroenterology, 107*(3), 345.

Lewis, J. D., Bilker, W. B., Brensinger, C., Farrar, J. T., & Strom, B. L. (2002). Hospitalization and mortality rates from peptic ulcer disease and GI bleeding in the 1990s: Relationship to sales of nonsteroidal anti-inflammatory drugs and acid suppression medications. *American Journal of Gastroenterology, 97,* 2540–2549.

Lewis, M. (2008). Bleeding colonic diverticula. *Journal of Clinical Gastroenterology, 42*(10), 1156–1158.

Ohmann, C., Imhof, M., Ruppert, C., Janzik, U., Vogt, C., Frieling, T., & Reinhold, C. (2005). Time-trends in the epidemiology of peptic ulcer bleeding. *Scandinavian Journal of Gastroenterology, 40,* 914–920.

Psarras, K., Symeonidis, N. G., Pavlidis, E. T., Micha, A., Baltatzis, M. E., Laloutas, M. A., & Sakadamis, A. (2011). Current management of diverticular disease complications. *Techniques in Coloproctology, 15*(Suppl. 1), S9–S12.

Rockey, D. C. (2005). Gastrointestinal bleeding. *Gastroenterology Clinics of North America, 34,* 581–588.

Thomopoulos, K. C., Vagenas, K. A., Vagianos, C. E., Margaritis, V. G., Blikas, A. P., Katsakoulis, E. C., & Nikolopoulou, V. N. (2004). Changes in aetiology and clinical outcome of acute upper gastrointestinal bleeding during the last 15 years. *European Journal of Gastroenterology & Hepatology, 16,* 177–182.

Van Leerdam, M. E., Vreeburg, E. M., Rauws, E. A., Geraedts, A. A., Tijssen, J. G., Reitsma, J. B., & Tytga, G. N. J. (2003). Acute upper GI bleeding: Did anything change? *American Journal of Gastroenterology, 98,* 1494–1499.

Wilkins, T., Baird, C., Pearson, A. N., & Schade, R. R. (2009). Diverticular bleeding. *American Family Physician, 80*(9), 977–983.

Zuckerman, D. A., Bocchini, T. P., & Birnbaum, E. H. (1993). Massive hemorrhage in the lower gastrointestinal tract in adults: Diagnostic imaging and intervention. *American Journal of Roentgenology, 161,* 703–711.

GERIATRIC CONSULTATION

The purpose of a geriatric consultation is to assess a patient from a medical, cognitive, psychological, social, environmental, and functional perspective. Geriatric consultations also clarify the patient's goals of care and make recommendations or comanage with other providers.

Geriatric consultations have developed all over the world under different names, including comprehensive geriatrics assessment (CGA), geriatrics evaluation units (GEUs) geriatric evaluation and management (GEM), geriatric floating interdisciplinary transition team (Geri-FITT), and acute care for elders (ACE) units, and ACE consult programs.

A core interdisciplinary team consisting of a gerontological nurse practitioner, social worker, and geriatrician usually perform the evaluation. The team may also include other professionals

G

such as a physical therapist, occupational therapist, speech therapist, physiatrist, nutritionist, pharmacist, and geriatric psychiatrist. The team usually starts by asking the referring physician the reason for the consult and likewise asking the patient/caregiver for what they are looking for the geriatrician to address.

Geriatric consultations can occur in both the outpatient and the hospital setting. In the outpatient environment, a geriatric evaluation may occur during a house-call visit or in a geriatric outpatient clinic. Patients may be self-referred or referred by other health professionals (i.e., primary care provider, specialist, emergency-department physician, or social worker on discharge from an acute hospitalization/skilled nursing facility).

In the hospital setting, consultations may be initiated in several ways. Some hospitals provide geriatrics consult services starting in the emergency department, whereas others have triggers for the consult service. Some triggers could be multiple recent admissions or delirium. In some hospitals, older patients who receive their care at a geriatric clinic, house-call program, or nursing home are routinely evaluated by the geriatric service once they are admitted to the hospital. Finally, geriatric consultation may be initiated by case finding during daily interdisciplinary team huddles.

In the outpatient setting, consultation is often sought for evaluation of cognitive disorders, falls, polypharmacy, incontinence, and depression. In addition, families often look for assistance with long-term care planning when an older person's ability to perform self-care declines. Some consultations are intended to establish subsequent primary care with a geriatrician. In the hospital, consultation requests may be for general medical management, transitions planning for the next level of care, "failure to thrive," rehabilitation potential, assistance with ethical dilemmas, preoperative screening, delirium, incontinence, gait instability, falls, frailty and social evaluation. A consult team that provides liaison services aims to prevent delirium and iatrogenic complications and provides extra attention to medication orders, skin care, bowel regimen, removal of unnecessary tethers (i.e., urinary catheters and intravenous lines),

and early mobilization. The geriatrics team also is able to communicate with all other interdisciplinary caregivers and families to help coordination of care, delineate goals of care, and be the best advocate for the patient.

Geriatric consultations are comprehensive and require a detailed review of the medical record to appropriately identify geriatric syndromes. Collaboration with an interdisciplinary team is a feature that makes geriatric consultation unique from many other specialties. The geriatrician collects information from family or caregivers, health care providers, and social services. This information is particularly valuable in caring for vulnerable older patients. The geriatric team pays particular attention to issues of functional status, cognition, caregiver stress, advance directives, medication review, gait and balance, behavioral health needs, use of community resources, nutrition, hearing, and vision. It is also important to mention that collaboration with the multidisciplinary team is key for detecting and reporting any form of abuse or neglect.

Research results may differ depending on the setting in which the consultation services are provided (i.e., outpatient vs. inpatient; Veterans Administration hospital vs. academic teaching hospital vs. community hospital), types of patients targeted (i.e., based on age only vs. degree of functional impairment), and the structure of the geriatric consultation program itself. Studies to date show mixed results in mortality, function, hospital-acquired complication rates, rehospitalization rates, and cost savings (Ellis & Langhorne, 2005; Rubenstein, Stuck, Siu, & Wieland, 1991).

Geriatric consultations identify new treatable diagnoses, including sensory impairment, depression, dementia, adverse medication effects, delirium, dysphagia, cardiovascular disorders, malnutrition, anemia, pressure injuries, constipation, urine retention, and orthostatic hypotension. Geriatric consultations help define the patient's goals, discussing advance directives, code status, and transition to palliative or end-of-life care when appropriate.

The combination of the traditional geriatric consult and ACE can improve outcomes when caring for vulnerable seniors in the acute setting. Generally, the ACE model of consultation has been effective in helping vulnerable older patients. Many ACE studies report reduced cost of care. The length of stay was increased and was more often reduced for hospitalized older adults compared with general medical care. Readmission to acute care hospitals was predominantly lower for patients discharged from ACE units. Existing evidence suggests that the ACE model contributes to reductions of polypharmacy. Finally, all studies that report satisfaction survey results noted superior evaluations for the ACE intervention group (Ahmed & Pearce, 2010).

New models of care and initiatives have been created to care for older adults in the acute care setting. The authors of a recent study modified the ACE unit model of care in the inpatient setting to a mobile acute care of the elderly (MACE) service without the limitations of physical unit. The MACE service consists of an interdisciplinary team of geriatricians, social workers, and clinical nurse specialists. In this single-site study of a redesigned ACE program, the authors found that the MACE service was associated with lower rates of adverse events, shorter hospital stays, and improved satisfaction with transitions of care (Hung, Ross, Farber, & Siu, 2013).

For any consultation to be effective, the recommendations suggested should be implemented. In general, several factors determine the likelihood of this happening. The institution must have the resources necessary to carry out suggested recommendations. Having adequate nursing staff is imperative for patient safety and activity. The likelihood of compliance with consultant recommendations is increased if the expectations of the referring team are met by making a few but concise recommendations pertaining to gait instability, falls, and discharge planning (Allen et al., 1986). Many of the best consultants are good communicators. They simply call the referring physician to succinctly explain their assessment and recommendation. Some referring physicians might have a misconception that the geriatric consult service is effective only for discharge planning. To address such misconceptions, geriatric consultation programs can educate staff about common geriatric syndromes through both formal and informal teaching activities. The geriatric consultation

service may have a role in educating specialty physicians who care for older patients.

Multidisciplinary geriatric consultation teams provide comprehensive assessment of physical, emotional, and functional status in older persons and make recommendations regarding the prevention and management of common geriatric syndromes. Through their expertise, geriatric consultations improve the safety of hospitalized elders (or nursing home residents) by reducing hospital-acquired complications such as falls, delirium, and functional decline.

In summary, geriatric consultants bring a global knowledge base that utilizes interdisciplinary expertise to coordinate care that is sensitive to the physiological, functional, cognitive, and social changes that occur with aging. An extensive study of geriatric in-patient consult services done in the United Kingdom concluded that such service may reduce short-term mortality, increase the chances of living at home at 1 year, and improve physical and cognitive function (Ellis & Langhorne, 2005).

See also Geriatric Evaluation and Management Units; Hospital-Based Services.

Jonny A. Macias Tejada, Soryal A. Soryal,
and Michael L. Malone

Ahmed, N. N., & Pearce, S. E. (2010). Acute care for the elderly: A literature review. *Population Health Management, 13,* 219–225.

Allen, C. M., Becker, P. M., McVey, L. J., Saltz, C., Feussner, J. R., & Cohen, H. J. (1986). A randomized, controlled clinical trial of a geriatric consultation team: Compliance with recommendations. *Journal of the American Medical Association, 255*(19), 2617–2621.

Ellis, G., & Langhorne, P. (2005). Comprehensive geriatric assessment for older hospital patients. *British Medical Bulletin, 71,* 45–59.

Hung, W. W., Ross, J. S., Farber, J., & Siu, A. L. (2013). Evaluation of the mobile acute care of the elderly (MACE) service. *JAMA Internal Medicine, 173*(11), 990–996.

Rubenstein, L. Z., Stuck, A. E., Siu, A. L., & Wieland, D. (1991). Impacts of geriatric evaluation and management programs on defined outcomes: Overview of the evidence. *Journal of the American Geriatrics Society, 39*(9, Pt. 2), 8S–16S.

Web Resource

Talking with Your Doctor: A Guide for Older People,
National Institute on Aging: https://www.nia.nih
.gov/health/talking-your-doctor-presentation
-toolkit

GERIATRIC DENTISTRY: CLINICAL ASPECTS

The head, neck, and oral structures undergo changes across a person's life span. Older adults are more susceptible to systemic conditions, predisposing them to develop oral and maxillofacial diseases that can directly or indirectly lead to malnutrition, altered communication, increased susceptibility to infectious diseases, and diminished quality of life (Scully & Ettinger, 2007; Ship, 2003; Tavares, Lindefjeld Calabi, & Martin, 2014). Interestingly, age alone does not seem to play a major role in impaired oral health (de Andrade et al., 2012). Rather, oral diseases (e.g., dental caries, gingivitis and periodontitis, oral mucosal diseases, salivary dysfunction, alveolar bone resorption), systemic conditions (e.g., diabetes mellitus, stroke, Alzheimer's disease), prescription and nonprescription medications, and head and neck radiotherapy predispose older persons to developing oral and pharyngeal (i.e., throat) disorders. The effects of these disorders are not limited to the oral cavity and its functions. Oral diseases give rise to pathogens, which can be blood-borne or aspirated into the lungs, bringing about severe, even life-threatening consequences, such as aspiration pneumonia (Sura, Madhavan, Carnby, & Crary, 2012). Systemic mucosal and skin diseases can manifest initially in the oral cavity, which can predispose older individuals to additional oral and pharyngeal problems.

Today's older adults are more likely to have natural teeth compared with previous aged cohorts (Manski et al., 2014; Ship, Allen, & Lynch, 2004). Thus older persons are at higher risk of developing a serious dentally derived medical problem than earlier cohorts of elders. Older adults are also more likely to use dental health care services and perform regular oral hygiene compared with previous older generations (Manski et al., 2014). Therefore it is imperative that health care professionals become familiar with the common aspects of oral diseases so that early diagnosis can lead to interventions with a high likelihood of preserving oral function (Ship, 2003). The goal is to develop universal oral disease–prevention strategies that will help all older persons maintain a good oral health-related quality of life (Sarment & Antonucci, 2002).

TEETH

The most common age-related changes in teeth include wearing of the enamel (i.e., attrition), recession of the dental pulp, and decreased cellularity of tooth structures (Ship et al., 2004). With increasing age, teeth undergo staining, chipping, and cracking and become more susceptible to fracture. Older people are at risk for developing new and recurrent coronal (i.e., chewing surfaces of teeth) caries, and they are more likely to have root-surface caries compared with younger adults (Gonsalves, Wrightson, & Henry, 2008). Coronal dental caries are the most common cause of tooth loss in the elderly and account for more extractions than periodontal diseases (Gregory & Hyde 2015). Gingival recession, salivary gland hypofunction (i.e., dry mouth), ineffective oral hygiene, removable prostheses (i.e., partial dentures), and diminished oral motor function all contribute to root-surface caries, as does having less than a high school education and two or more chronic health conditions (McNally et al., 2014). Large restorations (i.e., fillings) place coronal surfaces at risk for decay as well.

Caries treatment in older adults does not differ dramatically from that in younger patients. Fluoride-releasing restorative materials (i.e., glass ionomers) are particularly useful for root-surface decay and in patients with a dry mouth. Composite resins are indicated for repairing defective restorations and/or carious tooth surfaces, whereas the new generation of glass ionomer liners provides sustained fluoride release that reduces the incidence of recurrent caries. For frail older adults and residents of nursing

G

homes, conventional dental treatment of caries may not be acceptable; therefore atraumatic restorative treatment (ART), which was developed for restoring teeth in developing countries, has proved useful (da Mata et al., 2015).

An assessment for caries risk is advised for all patients; risk factors found in the geriatric population include use of medications that inhibit salivation, gingival recession, and poor oral hygiene secondary to debilitation. Dental caries and subsequent tooth loss can be prevented in high-risk patients with regular recall; application of topical fluoride rinses, gels, and varnishes; appropriate oral hygiene; and early intervention for dry mouth. Older patients with cognitive and/or motor disturbances (e.g., stroke, Parkinson's disease) usually require daily assistance to maintain the health of their dentition (Coleman 2002).

PERIODONTAL TISSUES

Although age-related changes in the periodontal tissues are not sufficient to lead to tooth loss, gingival recession and loss of periodontal attachment and bony support are almost universal in older persons (Holm-Pedersen, 1996). Multiple oral factors and systemic diseases, and the medications taken to treat them have an adverse influence on periodontal health, and these conditions are more prevalent among older adults; therefore older individuals are at higher risk for experiencing periodontal disease–related morbidity (Tavares et al., 2014). Diabetes mellitus, for example, leads to a higher prevalence and severity of periodontal diseases (Lee et al., 2014). Three types of medications frequently prescribed in older people have been associated with gingival enlargement (e.g., calcium channel blockers used for cardiovascular diseases, the antiseizure drug phenytoin, and the immunosuppressant cyclosporine A) (Kataoka, Kido, Shinohara, & Nagata, 2005).

Periodontal diseases have oral and systemic effects on the health of older persons. They have been associated with halitosis (bad breath), gingivitis (inflamed and bleeding gum tissues), and tooth loss, which can affect mastication (chewing), swallowing, tasting, and nutritional intake (Gonsalves et al., 2008). Periodontal diseases have also been associated with cardiovascular, cerebrovascular, endocrine, pulmonary, and infectious diseases (Tavares et al., 2014).

The treatment of periodontal diseases is the same regardless of age and starts with prevention. Thorough toothbrushing and flossing preferably after each meal, are recommended for patients of all ages. Periodontal infections can be resolved with conservative surgical procedures, although wound healing after soft tissue procedures may take slightly longer in older patients. Patients with bleeding disorders, extensive heart and lung problems, and immunosuppression may be poor candidates for periodontal surgery; local methods (i.e., extensive cleanings, including scaling/root planning) and antimicrobial and anti-inflammatory agents delivered topically or, occasionally, systemically are preferred (Tariq et al., 2012).

ORAL MUCOSA

Both normal aging changes and pathological factors contribute to disorders of oral mucosal tissues (Lamster, Asadourian, Del Carmen, & Friedman, 2016). The mucosa that lines most of the oral cavity (i.e., stratified squamous epithelium) tends to become thinner, loses elasticity, and atrophies with age (Pindborg & Holmstrup, 1996). Simultaneously, there are declines in immunological responsiveness that increase susceptibility to infection and trauma. Increases in the incidence of oral and systemic diseases and the use of multiple medications lead to oral mucosal disorders among older persons (Tavares et al., 2014). The oral mucosa is a common site for a large variety of lesions, ranging from benign and asymptomatic to malignant and potentially life threatening. For example, many older adults are at risk for developing oral fungal infections, which when diagnosed appropriately, usually resolve with topical therapies (Gonsalves et al., 2008). Oral cancer, primarily a disease of adults aged 50 years and older, has a survival rate of approximately 50% at 5 years, due in part to late diagnosis (Neville & Day, 2002). Any mucosal lesion that persists for 3 to 4 weeks despite all attempts to remove suspected causes (e.g., ill-fitting denture flange) must be biopsied to determine a diagnosis. Regularly

G

scheduled head, neck, and oral examinations are required to diagnose oral mucosal diseases at an early stage and to intervene with appropriate therapy. Even edentulous (i.e., missing all teeth) older adults require at least an annual head, neck, and oral examination to evaluate for benign and malignant lesions.

SALIVARY GLANDS

Although studies have demonstrated that in healthy older adults, the volume of saliva does not decrease, many older persons complain of a dry mouth (xerostomia) and have diminished salivary output (salivary hypofunction) (Villa, Connell, & Abati, 2015). Medical diseases, medications, and radiation therapy for head and neck tumors are the most common causes (Ship, Pillemer, & Baum, 2002). More than 400 drugs, especially tricyclic antidepressants, sedatives and tranquilizers, antihistamines, antihypertensives, cytotoxic agents, and anti-Parkinson drugs, have been reported to decrease salivary flow. Diseases such as Sjögren's syndrome, lupus erythematosus, diabetes mellitus, and Alzheimer's can also cause dry mouth.

Insufficient salivary output leads to dry and friable oral mucosa; greater susceptibility to microbial infections (e.g., fungal or yeast infection); diminished lubrication; caries development; pain; difficulty with chewing, tasting, and swallowing; and impaired retention of removable prostheses and therefore quality of life (Singh & Papas 2014). Early diagnosis and intervention are necessary to help preserve oral health in the adult with a dry mouth (Villa et al., 2015).

Effective collaboration with the patient's physicians can promote elimination of causative medications or help change to medications with fewer dry-mouth side effects. Salivary substitutes and oral moisturizers can assist in preventing complaints of dry mouth, and sugar-free candies and mints increase salivary output. Several drugs are available to increase saliva and should be considered for some patients. Teeth in the dry-mouth patient must be protected with daily exposure to high-dose fluorides, and periodontal health can be maintained with thorough toothbrushing and flossing.

ORAL MOTOR AND SENSORY FUNCTION

Age-related changes in chewing, swallowing, and oral muscular posture can affect nutritional health and a person's quality of life (Palmer, 2005). The most often reported oral motor disturbance in older people is altered mastication, and although older persons with all of their natural teeth are less able to prepare food for swallowing as efficiently as younger adults, rarely do these changes have any adverse effects in a healthy older person. Alternatively, systemic diseases (e.g., strokes, Parkinson's disease) and certain drugs (e.g., phenothiazines) can cause significant and even permanent changes in chewing and swallowing, predisposing a person to choking or aspiration. Other age-related diseases such as osteoarthritis may affect the temporomandibular joint (TMJ), yet older persons are less likely to report symptoms of TMJ-related pain.

Diminished food enjoyment, smell, and taste are common complaints in older individuals (Spielman & Ship, 2004). Although taste function is remarkably stable, olfaction (i.e., smell) is dramatically diminished with age. Decreased smell capacity combined with changes in oral motor, salivary, and other sensory modalities most likely account for the loss of flavor perception and interest in food in some older persons. An adult reporting these symptoms requires a comprehensive evaluation to determine the cause of the problem. Nutritional counseling helps prevent malnutrition, dehydration, and a diminished quality of life.

See also Dentures; Oral Health Assessment; Xerostomia.

Ronald L. Ettinger

Coleman, P. (2002). Improving oral health care for the elderly: A review of widespread problems and best practices. *Geriatric Nursing, 23*(4), 189–199.

de Andrade, F. B., Lebrão, M. L., Santos, J. L. F., Teixeira, D. S. D. C., & de Oliveira Duarte, Y. A. (2012). Relationship between oral health–related quality of life, oral health, socioeconomic, and general health factors in elderly Brazilians. *Journal of the American Geriatrics Society, 60*(9), 1755–1760.

da Mata, C., Allen, P. F., McKenna, G., Cronin, M., O'Mahony, D., & Woods, N. (2015). Two-year survival of ART restorations placed in elderly patients: A randomised controlled clinical trial. *Journal of Dentistry, 43*(4), 405–411.

Gonsalves, W. C., Wrightson, A. S., & Henry, R. G. (2008). Common oral conditions in older persons. *American Family Physician, 78*(7), 845–852.

Gregory, D., & Hyde, S. (2015). Root caries in older adults. *Journal of the California Dental Association, 43*(8) 439–445.

Holm-Pedersen, P. (1996). Pathology and treatment of periodontal diseases in the aging individual. In P. Holm-Pedersen & H. Loe (Eds.), *Textbook of geriatric dentistry* (2nd ed., pp. 388–405). Copenhagen, Denmark: Munksgaard.

Kataoka, M., Kido, J., Shinohara, Y., & Nagata, T. (2005). Drug-induced gingival overgrowth—a review. *Biological and Pharmaceutical Bulletin, 28*(10), 1817–1821.

Lamster, I. B., Asadourian, L., Del Carmen, T., & Friedman, P. K. (2016). The aging mouth: Differentiating normal from disease. *Periodontology, 72*, 96–107.

Lee, K.-S., Kim, E.-K., Kim, J.-W., Choi, Y.-H., Mechant, A. T., Song, K.-B., & Lee, H.-K. (2014). The relationship between metabolic conditions and prevalence of periodontal disease in rural Korean elderly. *Archives of Gerontology and Geriatrics, 58*(1), 125–129.

Manski, R. J., Cohen, L. A., Brown, E., Carper, K. V., Vargas, C., & Macek, M. D. (2014). Dental service mix among older adults aged 65 and over, United States, 1999 and 2009. *Journal of public Health Dentistry, 74*(3), 219–226.

McNally, M. E., Matthews, D. C., Clovis, J. B., Brillant, M., & Filiaggi, M. J. (2014). The oral health of ageing baby boomers: A comparison of adults aged 45–64 and those 65 years and older. *Gerodontology, 31*(2), 123–135.

Neville, B. W., & Day, T. A. (2002). Oral cancer and precancerous lesions. *CA: Cancer Journal for Clinicians, 52*(4), 195–215.

Palmer, C. A. (2005). Age-related changes in oral health status: Effects of diet and nutrition. In R. Touger-Decke, D. A. Sirois, & C. C. Mobley (Eds.), *Nutrition and oral medicine* (pp. 31–43). Totawa, NJ: Humana Press.

Pindborg, J. J., & Holmstrup, P. (1996). Pathology and treatment of diseases in oral mucous membranes and salivary glands. In P. Holm-Pedersen & H. Loe (Eds.), *Textbook of geriatric dentistry* (2nd ed., pp. 405–428). Copenhagen, Denmark: Munksgaard.

Sarment, D. P., & Antonucci, T. C. (2002). Oral health-related quality of life and older adults. In M. R. Inglehart & R. A. Bagramian (Eds.), *Oral health-related quality of life* (pp. 99–110). Copenhagen, Denmark: Quintessence.

Scully, C., & Ettinger, R. L. (2007). The influence of systemic diseases on oral health care in older adults. *Journal of the American Dental Association, 138*(Suppl), 7S–14S.

Ship, J. A. (2003). Geriatrics. In M. S. Greenberg & M. Glick (Eds.), *Burket's oral medicine: Diagnosis and treatment* (10th ed., pp. 605–622). Hamilton, Ontario, Canada: BC Decker.

Ship, J. A., Allen, K. L., & Lynch, E. (2004). Dental caries in the elderly. In E. Lynch (Ed.), *Ozone: The revolution in dentistry* (pp. 295–300). Copenhagen, Denmark: Quintessence.

Ship, J. A., Pillemer, S. R., & Baum, B. J. (2002). Xerostomia and the geriatric patient. *Journal of the American Geriatrics Society, 50*(3), 535–543.

Singh, M. L., & Papas, A. (2014). Oral implications of Polypharmacy in the elderly. *Dental, Clinic of North America, 58*(4), 783–796.

Spielman, A. I., & Ship, J. A. (2004). Taste and smell. In T. S. Miles, B. Nauntofte, & P. Svensson (Eds.), *Clinical oral physiology* (pp. 53–70). Copenhagen, Denmark: Quintessence.

Sura, L., Madhavan, A., Carnby, G., & Crary, M. A. (2012). Dysphagia in the elderly: Management and nutritional considerations. *Clinical Interventions in Aging, 7*, 287–298.

Tariq, M., Iqbal, Z., Ali, J., Baboota, S., Talegaonkar, S., Ahmad, Z., & Sahni, J. K. (2012). Treatment modalities and evaluation models for periodontitis. *International Journal of Pharmaceutical Investigation, 2*(3), 106.

Tavares, M., Lindefjeld Calabi, K. A., & Martin, L. S. (2014). Systemic diseases and oral health. *Dental Clinics of North America, 58*, 797–814.

Villa, A., Connell, C. L., & Abati, S. (2015). Diagnosis and management of xerostomia and hyposalivation. *Therapeutics and Clinical Risk Management, 11*, 45–51.

Web Resources

American Academy of Periodontology: http://www.perio.org/consumer/2m.htm

American Dental Association: http://www.ada.org/public/topics/implants.asp

International Association for Dental Research: http://www.iadr.com

National Institute of Dental and Craniofacial Research: http://www.nidcr.nih.gov

Oral Health America: http://oralhealthamerica.org

GERIATRIC EVALUATION AND MANAGEMENT UNITS

Geriatric evaluation and management (GEM) is a specialized program of services provided by an interdisciplinary team of health care professionals for a targeted group of older patients with medical complexity who are likely to benefit from the services. Such services are most often provided in inpatient or outpatient settings, and include evaluation and management components. GEM units are most often found in VA medical centers (Hornick & Rubenstein, 2015). The GEM unit couples comprehensive geriatric assessment with specific treatment plans implemented by an interdisciplinary team, and individualized to the patient's needs. Interdisciplinary teams often include a geriatrician, advanced practice nurse (i.e., clinical nurse specialist or nurse practitioner) or physician assistant with training in geriatrics, social worker, dietician, and physical and occupational therapists. An extended team of health professionals might include a speech therapist, clinical pharmacist, geriatric psychiatrist, psychologist, dentist, and physiatrist.

The team considers the patient's present medical conditions, medical history, social supports, living conditions, and ability to perform activities of daily living (ADL). The physician catalogues the patient's medical diagnoses, orders laboratory studies, and makes referrals to other specialists as warranted (the evaluation), and the interdisciplinary team members generate a plan of care designed to optimize management of the patient's medical and psychosocial issues and level of physical functioning (management). Team meetings provide a regular opportunity to review the patient's functional status and reassess plans of care.

COMPONENTS OF GEM PROGRAMS

In hospital-based GEM units, patients are either directly admitted or transferred to the unit after acute care hospitalization. The specific components of GEM programs differ somewhat, depending on the setting and the goal of the GEM unit. However, there are many similarities across units. Most GEM protocols begin with a specific targeting strategy directed at identifying patients who are most likely to benefit from a comprehensive geriatric assessment (Ellis, Whitehead, O'Neill, Langhorne, & Robinson, 2011). The general goal is to identify patients at high risk for adverse outcomes such as functional deterioration and nursing home placement while conserving health care resources by not targeting patients who are so ill or dependent that they are unlikely to benefit from services. Comprehensive evaluations usually include an assessment of caregiving needs and caregiver stress. Examples of high-risk patients targeted by GEM units include those who are dependent in one or more basic or instrumental activities of daily living (IADL), those with cognitive impairment or depressive symptoms, those recently hospitalized, and those who live alone or with a stressed caregiver.

The results of the evaluation are reviewed in a team conference, often with the patient or family in attendance; team members make specific preventive and restorative recommendations regarding treatment, rehabilitation, health promotion, and social service interventions. The outcome of the comprehensive geriatric assessment is a written care plan that addresses all functional, medical, and psychosocial issues and an action plan for immediate and future care of the patient.

HOSPITAL-BASED GEM UNITS: VETERANS AFFAIRS GEM UNITS

The initial inpatient GEM units, developed and evaluated in the Veterans Affairs (VA) hospitals (Rubenstein et al., 1984), are common in VA Geriatric Research, Education, and Clinical Centers (GRECCs). The VA has established explicit definitions of GEM and team members in the *Veterans Health Benefits Handbook* (U.S. Department of Veterans Affairs, 2017). GEM services can be found in inpatient units, outpatient clinics, and geriatric primary care clinics. The VA operates 34 inpatient GEM programs and 64 GEM clinics. Patients may be admitted to inpatient GEM Units from inpatient acute care units, outpatient clinics, or home. Subacute care, respite care and acute care are often provided on these units. The goal of the VA GEM unit is to improve the process and outcome of clinical care using the following objectives:

- Improving diagnostic accuracy
- Optimizing drug prescribing
- Ensuring the most appropriate discharge location (i.e., most independent and least restrictive level of care)
- Minimizing repeated hospitalizations
- Maximizing physical and psychosocial functional status
- Reducing inappropriate use of resources (e.g., acute hospital or nursing home)
- Providing interdisciplinary patient evaluations
- Establishing and coordinating an interdisciplinary plan for long-term management of care
- Developing clinical indicators and monitoring the quality of care provided

The first controlled trial of the VA GEM unit demonstrated positive effects on important patient outcomes. Reduced mortality, fewer acute-care hospital days, improved functional status, and better morale were reported among patients assigned to the GEM unit compared with control patients who received usual care (Rubenstein et al., 1984). Subsequent controlled clinical trials have shown important, if less impressive, findings. In a multicenter study of inpatient GEM with subsequent outpatient follow-up, functional decline was reduced during inpatient GEM admission, and mental health was improved among veterans receiving outpatient GEM (Cohen et al., 2002). Nursing home admissions were less common among patients on the GEM unit (Phibbs et al., 2006). Quality-of-life measures were significantly better for cancer patients admitted to the unit compared with those receiving usual care (Rao, Hsieh, Feussner, & Cohen, 2005).

COMMUNITY HOSPITAL–BASED GEM UNITS

Community hospital GEM units are typically separate hospital units that have been designed to facilitate care of the geriatric patient. Multidisciplinary team rounds and patient-centered team conferences are hallmarks of care on

these units, which in contrast to geriatric consultation services, have direct control over the implementation of team recommendations.

The inpatient GEM unit overlaps in its goals of care with other acute care models such as the acute care for elders (ACE) unit and the Hospital Elder Life Program (HELP) but differs in several ways. In contrast to inpatient GEM units, the ACE and HELP models of care are based on acute care units where the short length of stay and high acuity of illness predispose patients to functional decline and loss of mobility. The geriatric assessment is brief and targeted at risk factors for functional decline or delirium, and management focuses on acute care issues. The management of chronic diseases occurs following transition of care from hospital to home or to an other site such as a GEM unit. Systematic reviews of inpatient GEM often include both acute care units and subacute (post-acute hospitalization) programs, such as the VA GEM. These reviews identify multidisciplinary team involvement as a key element and suggest the benefits of reduced rates of functional decline at discharge and 1-year institutionalization of patients admitted to GEM units compared with usual care (Van Craen et al., 2010).

OUTPATIENT-BASED GEM UNITS

Similar to inpatient units, outpatient GEM units complete a comprehensive geriatric assessment of complex older adults, including their medical, psychosocial, and functional capabilities and limitations. This assessment is followed by comprehensive, interdisciplinary, and ongoing care that is tailored to the patient's individual needs. Recommendations are typically shared with the patient's primary care physician and the patient in a summary report or by direct communication that reflects recommendations from the team. The implementation of these recommendations varies considerably among outpatient GEM units. In some units, the GEM team assumes overall responsibility for the patient for a finite length of time. The effectiveness of this approach was shown in a population-based sample of community-dwelling Medicare beneficiaries who were at high risk for hospital admission in the future. The GEM intervention included a comprehensive geriatric assessment, followed by primary care provided by the team for up to 6 months. Patients receiving the intervention, compared with patients receiving usual care, were significantly less likely to lose functional ability, experience increased health-related restrictions in their ADL, have possible depression, or use home health care services (Boult et al., 2001).

The Geriatric Resources for Assessment and Care of Elders (GRACE) model of primary care was developed specifically to improve the quality of care for low-income seniors (Counsell, Callahan, & Clark, 2007). Unique features of the GRACE intervention, compared with prior studies of home-based integrated geriatric care, include an in-home assessment and care management provided by a nurse practitioner and social worker team; an individualized care plan reviewed with the primary care physician using GRACE protocols; utilization of an integrated electronic medical record and a web-based care-management tracking tool; and integration with affiliated pharmacy, mental health, home health, and community-based and inpatient geriatric care services (Butler, Frank, & Counsell, 2015). In a randomized controlled trial, high-risk patients who were aged 65 years and older, who had incomes below 200% of the federal poverty level, and who were enrolled in the GRACE intervention had fewer visits to emergency departments, hospitalizations, and readmissions; as well as reduced hospital costs, compared with the control group.

In summary, both inpatient and outpatient GEM units have been effective in improving the functional status of elderly patients at risk for functional decline or hospitalization. Although the process of a comprehensive geriatric assessment linked to chronic care management can be time-consuming for an interdisciplinary care team of health professionals, the GEM model remains an attractive option for accountable care organizations and Medicare Advantage programs as a cost-effective alternative to usual fee-for-service Medicare.

See also Gait Assessment Instruments; Geriatric Resource Nurse; Hospital-Based Services; Nurses Improving Care of Healthsystem Elders (NICHE), Veterans and Veteran Health.

Robert M. Palmer

Boult, C., Boult, L. B., Morishita, L., Dowd, B., Kane, R. L., & Urdangarin, C. F. (2001). A randomized clinical trial of outpatient geriatric evaluation and management. *Journal of the American Geriatrics Society, 49*(4), 351–359.

Butler, D. E., Frank, K. I., & Counsell, S. R. (2015). The GRACE model. In M. L. Malone, E. Capezuti, & R. M. Palmer (Eds.), *Geriatrics models of care: Bringing "best practice" to an aging America* (pp. 125–138). Cham, Switzerland: Springer Publishing.

Cohen, H. J., Feussner, J. R., Weinberger, M., Carnes, M., Hamdy, R. C., Hsieh, F., … Lavori, P. (2002). A controlled trial of inpatient and outpatient geriatric evaluation and management. *New England Journal of Medicine, 346*, 905–912.

Counsell, S. R., Callahan, C. M., & Clark, D. O. (2007). Geriatric care management for low-income seniors: A randomized controlled trial. *Journal of the American Medical Association, 298*, 2623–2633.

Ellis, G., Whitehead, M. A., O'Neill, D., Langhorne, P., & Robinson, D. (2011). Comprehensive geriatric assessment for older adults admitted to hospital. *Cochrane Database of Systematic Reviews, 7*, CD006211. doi:10.1002/14651858.CD006211.pub2

Hornick, T. R., & Rubenstein, L. (2015). Outpatient evaluation and management. In M. L. Malone, E. Capezuti, & R. M. Palmer (Eds.), *Geriatrics models of care: Bringing "best practice" to an Aging America* (pp. 183–191). Cham, Switzerland: Springer Publishing.

Phibbs, C. S., Holty, J. E., Goldstein, M. K., Garber, A. M., Wang, Y., & Cohen, H. J. (2006). The effect of geriatrics evaluation and management on nursing home use and health care costs: Results from a randomized trial. *Medical Care, 44*, 91–95.

Rao, A. V., Hsieh, F., Feussner, J. R., & Cohen, H. J. (2005). Geriatric evaluation and management units in the care of the frail elderly cancer patient. *Journals of Gerontology: Series A, Biological Sciences and Medical Sciences, 60*(6), 798–803.

Rubenstein, L. Z., Josephson, K. R., Wieland, G. D., English, P. A., Sayre, J. A., & Kane, R. L. (1984). Effectiveness of a geriatric evaluation unit. A randomized clinical trial. *New England Journal of Medicine, 311*(26), 1664–1670.

U.S. Department of Veterans Affairs. (2017). Veterans health benefits handbook. Retrieved from https://www.va.gov/healthbenefits/vhbh

Van Craen, K., Braes, T., Wellens, N., Denhaerynck, K., Flamaing, J., Moons, P., & Milisen, K. (2010).

The effectiveness of inpatient geriatric evaluation and management units: A systematic review and meta–analysis. *Journal of the American Geriatrics Society, 58*(1), 83–92.

Web Resource
U.S. Department of Veterans Affairs: Geriatrics and Extended Care Program: http://www.patient care.va.gov/geriatrics.asp

GERIATRIC RESOURCE NURSE

The geriatric resource nurse (GRN) model is an educational and clinical intervention model that prepares staff nurses to be clinical resources on geriatric care to nurses on their unit. The GRN model provides staff nurses, via education and modeling by a geriatric advanced practice nurse, with specific content on geriatric syndromes (e.g., falls, incontinence) to improve the knowledge and manage the care of older adults. GRNs identify and address specific geriatric syndromes such as falls and delirium and implement care strategies that discourage the use of restrictive devices and promote patient mobility. Thus this model facilitates the integration of evidence-based geriatric care at the bedside. It also supports the role of the staff nurse on the interdisciplinary team. GRNs function in all types of units that serve older adults, such as medical–surgical, specialty units, critical care areas, and dementia programs (Boltz et al., 2008; Capezuti et al., 2012).

Within the Nurses Improving Care for Healthsystem Elders (NICHE) program, the GRN model is considered the foundation for improving geriatric care. The GRN is meant to function as a leader who participates in patient family rounds, bedside teaching, quality initiatives, and hospital committees to increase gerontological knowledge and maximize the coordination of care across disciplines (Capezuti et al., 2012). GRNs are also actively engaged in teaching patient/families as well as preparing nursing assistants as geriatric patient care associates.

Dr. Terry Fulmer initiated the GRN model in 1981 at Boston's Beth Israel Hospital to provide consultation to other staff nurses regarding specific geriatric clinical syndromes. As part of the The John A. Hartford Foundation Hospital Outcomes Program for the Elderly multisite initiative, Dr. Fulmer and colleagues adapted the GRN model within a geriatrician-led care team at Yale New Haven Hospital. A randomized controlled trial using matched units found that this model was successful in improving management of delirium, immobility, bladder/bowel problems, and pressure injury treatment and prevention (Inouye et al., 1993). Building on the knowledge gained from the Yale New Haven Hospital efforts, The John A. Hartford Foundation funded the NICHE program in 1994 at New York University.

Most NICHE member sites use the GRN model. Outcome studies from individual NICHE hospitals suggest that the GRN model results in positive outcomes, including reduced use of physical restraints and improvements in functional mobility (Capezuti et al., 2012). The Geriatric Institutional Assessment Profile (GIAP) is an instrument designed to help NICHE member sites to examine self-reported measures of nurses' knowledge and attitudes about care of the hospitalized elderly and perceived institutional support (Capezuti, Boltz, et al., 2013). The GRN model is considered by NICHE sites as a useful system-wide strategy for maximizing the education of nurses and for promoting quality care to hospitalized older adults (Capezuti, Bricoli, & Boltz, 2013; Capezuti et al., 2012). The GRN model has demonstrated a positive influence on the geriatric nursing practice environment (Boltz et al., 2008); the principles of this model are consistent with professional nursing practice models (Boltz, Capezuti, & Shabbat, 2010).

See also Advanced Practice Nursing; Hospital-Based Services; Nurses Improving Care for Healthsystem Elders (NICHE).

Elizabeth A. Capezuti

Boltz, M., Capezuti, E., Bowar-Ferres, S., Norman, R., Secic, M., Kim, H., ... Fulmer, T. (2008). Changes

G

in the geriatric care environment associated with NICHE (Nurses Improving Care for HealthSystem Elders). *Geriatric Nursing, 29*(3), 176–185.

Boltz, M., Capezuti, E., & Shabbat, N. (2010). Building a framework for a geriatric acute care model. *Leadership in Health Services, 23*, 334–360.

Capezuti, E., Boltz, E., Cline, D., Dickson, V., Rosenberg, M., Wagner, L., … Nigolian, C. (2012). Nurses Improving Care for Healthsystem Elders—A model for optimizing the geriatric nursing practice environment. *Journal of Clinical Nursing, 21*, 3117–3125.

Capezuti, E., Boltz, M., Shuluk, J., Denysyk, L., Brouwers, J., Roberts, M.C., … Secic, M. (2013). Utilization of a benchmarking database to inform NICHE implementation. *Research in Gerontological Nursing, 6*(3), 198–208.

Capezuti, E., Bricoli, B., & Boltz, M. (2013). NICHE: Creating a sustainable business model to improve care of hospitalized older adults. *Journal of the American Geriatrics Society, 61*(8), 1387–1393.

Inouye, S. K., Acampora, D., Miller, R. L., Fulmer, T., Hurst, L. D., & Cooney, L. M. (1993). The Yale Geriatric Care Program: A model of care to prevent functional decline in hospitalized elderly patients. *Journal of the American Geriatrics Society, 41*(12), 1345–1352.

Web Resource
Nurses Improving Care for Healthsystem Elders (NICHE) Program: http://nicheprogram.org

GERIATRICIAN

A geriatrician is a physician with expertise in the care of older adults. Unlike gerontologists, who study the science of aging, geriatricians are allopathic or osteopathic physicians whose clinical focus on the older patient parallels that of their colleagues working at the other end of the life span, pediatricians. After graduating medical school, a physician must first complete 3 years of residency in family practice or internal medicine followed by at least 1 year of accredited geriatrics fellowship training to be eligible to take the examination for certification in the subspecialty of geriatric medicine (before July 2006, eligible candidates received a Certificate of Added Qualifications).

Although George Day and J. M. Charcot wrote medical texts in the 19th century about the diseases of late life (Chase, Mitchell, & Morley, 2000), Ignatz Nascher coined the term *geriatrics* in the early 1900s, noting the parallel with pediatrics (Nascher, 1909). As Nascher is often considered as the "father" of geriatrics, Marjory Warren is viewed as its "mother"; she created the first geriatrics unit, calling attention to the role of the environment and the importance of rehabilitation (Warren, 1946).

Patients and physicians may fail to appreciate what geriatricians have to offer. Expertise in geriatric problems (e.g., polypharmacy, cognitive impairment, incontinence, gait disorders) and in a broad range of functional, medical, and psychosocial domains of elder care distinguishes geriatricians from their colleagues. Geriatrics requires specially honed team skills because comprehensive care of older patients necessitates collaboration with experts in fields other than medicine.

Despite the proliferation of geriatric medicine fellowship programs, which increased from 92 in 1991–1992 to 145 in 2017 (Electronic Residency Application Service, n.d.), and the "demographic imperative," the number of practicing geriatricians is not increasing. The Association of Directors of Geriatric Academic Programs (ADGAP) and the American Geriatrics Society estimate that there were 7,000 active certified geriatricians in 2011, a gradual decrease from 1998 (Bragg & Warshaw, 2012). Relatively low pay compared with that of subspecialty colleagues (in large part due to its lack of highly remunerative procedures and its dependence on Medicare reimbursement) limits the number of candidates who enter and remain in the field; burnout may also contribute. Nonetheless, a recent cross-specialty survey found that geriatricians were most likely to be highly satisfied with their careers (Leigh, Kravitz, Schembri, Samuels, & Mobley, 2002).

Because of the anticipated demographic changes and the lack of sufficient geriatricians to provide direct care, our field has had to re-think our primary goals (Kane, 2002; Tinnetti, 2016). A clear direction forward has been provided in separate essays by Robert Kane and Mary Tinetti. First, geriatricians need to provide direct care for the subset of the most complex older patients. This could focus on older adults with chronic conditions or multiple comorbid conditions. Second, geriatricians should teach the principles of geriatrics to all health professionals and to the public. Third, geriatricians should increase the number of health professionals who practice the principles of geriatric medicine as they care for older adults. This means teaching in undergraduate and graduate medical education. Beyond this role, geriatricians should train nurses, therapists, pharmacists, specialist physicians, and surgeons. Next, geriatricians should ensure that health systems are guided by geriatrics principles and goal-directed care. Furthermore, geriatricians should lead research on the science of aging, and likewise they should study strategies to improve the care of vulnerable older adults across multiple settings. Last, geriatricians should engage in health care policy to ensure access to patient-centered care for all older Americans.

Because of the anticipated demographic changes, geriatricians must see themselves as champions for improved care for vulnerable populations. Furthermore, geriatrics providers are role models for future trainees. Geriatricians thrive on the challenges of managing patients with complex medical and psychosocial needs. Team support adds to the sense of satisfaction. Conveying that satisfaction and challenge to trainees is one of our responsibilities. Adding new geriatricians to the ranks is ideal, but we can also teach medical students and house staff destined for subspecialty careers to enjoy caring for older patients (Siegler & Capello, 2005).

Ariba Khan

Bragg, E., & Warshaw, G. (2012). The ADGAP status of the geriatric workforce study—Geriatric medicine in the United States 2012 update. Retrieved from http://dev.americangeriatrics.org/advocacy_public_policy/gwps

Chase, P., Mitchell, K., & Morley, J. E. (2000). In the steps of giants: The early geriatrics texts. *Journal of the American Geriatrics Society, 48*(1), 89–94.

Electronic Residency Application Service. (n.d.). ERAS 2018 participating specialities & programs. Retrieved from https://services.aamc.org/eras/erasstats/par/index.cfm

Kane, R. L. (2002). The future history of geriatrics: Geriatrics at the crossroads. *Journals of Gerontology, 57*(12), M803–M805.

Leigh, J. P., Kravitz, R. L., Schembri, M., Samuels, S. J., & Mobley, S. (2002). Physician career satisfaction across specialties. *Archives of Internal Medicine, 162*(14), 1577–1584.

Nascher, I. L. (1909). Longevity and rejuvenescence. *New York Medical Journal, 89*, 795–800.

Siegler, E. L., & Capello, C. F. (2005). Creating a teaching geriatric service: Ten important lessons. *Journal of the American Geriatrics Society, 53*(2), 327–330. doi:10.1111/j.1532-5415.2005.53122.x

Tinnetti, M. (2016). Mainstream or extinction: Can defining who we are save geriatrics? *Journal of the American Geriatrics Society, 64*, 1400–1404.

Warren, M. W. (1946). Care of the chronic aged sick. *Lancet, 1*(6406), 841–843.

Web Resources
AGS Foundation for Health in Aging (FHA): http://www.healthinaging.org
American Geriatrics Society: http://www.americangeriatrics.org
British Geriatrics Society: http://www.bgs.org.uk
Canadian Geriatrics Society: http://canadiangeriatrics.ca

GERONTOLOGICAL SOCIAL WORKERS

It is widely recognized that social workers play a critical role in health care for older persons. The role and function of geriatric social workers has evolved along with the transformation of community health care. Geriatric social workers increasingly monitor and manage care transitions between community and institutional settings and mobilize an array of both formal and informal community services to address the evolving care needs of the older client. The field of social work more broadly has historically been concerned with underserved and vulnerable populations; thus geriatric social workers are often on the forefront of specialized programming for minority, immigrant, and poor older populations. Although a majority of geriatric social workers provide clinical social work

G

service, many others also function as program planners, administrators, and evaluators. Some geriatric social workers are also found in local, state, and national policy settings.

ROLE AND KNOWLEDGE BASE

Social work is especially concerned with working with the family and other social support systems that are relevant to the older adult's overall functioning. There is first a focus on enhancing older persons' self-care capacity and then on enhancing the web of social supports that might be mobilized on their behalf to buttress what they could do for themselves. Generally, this means helping older persons' families to most effectively back up the their resources (Damron-Rodriguez & Lubben, 2007).

Gerontological social workers are called on to support persons and families dealing with end-of-life issues, for example, by helping plan advance directives and facilitating the grief process. Indeed, advance care planning, in which social workers assess client preferences for care at the end of life, is an area of practice that is increasingly central to gerontological practice (Kass-Bartelmes & Hughes, 2003). In addition, social workers might deal with transitional tasks, such as retirement and widowhood, which may precipitate a crisis and direct their attention to past conflicts, roles, alliances, and communication patterns.

Gerontological social workers base their family interventions on a number of conceptual frameworks (e.g., systems theory, family life cycle, transpersonal theory, social behavioral model, equity theory). Issues of interdependence versus dependence often inform family-centered practice models. In family crisis situations, the practitioner takes into account developmental issues as well as the changing needs of family members. Using an ecological approach focused on person–environment fit (P-EF) and the press-competence model, practitioners emphasize a healthy, realistic adaptation to problems in living. This multisystem approach allows practitioners to understand how clients function within their total environment and permits a range of interventions. In

addition, the ecological perspective underscores the need for social workers to promote everyday competence among older adults (McInnis-Dittrich, 2009).

EDUCATION

Bachelor's degrees in social work (BSW) prepare students for generalist social work practice, whereas master's degree programs (MSW) prepare students for advanced or specialized practice. An increasing number of MSW programs are offering a concentration in older adults and families or certificates in gerontology. Doctoral programs in social work prepare graduates to become social work research scholars and academics (PhD). There is also an increasing number of advanced practice doctorates (DSW). BSWs, MSWs, PhDs, and DSWs in most states need licenses to practice clinical social work (e.g., LICSW, LCSW); however, there are generally no formal licensing or certification for social workers to work with older adults.

It has been widely recognized that the demand for geriatric social workers continues to outpace the number of social workers entering the workforce who are trained to work with older adults, and as the large Baby Boomer generation ages, this demand will only increase. This is particularly the case in the health care arena. Various initiatives have been implemented to increase the training of social workers to work with older adults. For example, from 2009 to 2014, The John A. Hartford Foundation funded the Hartford Partnership Program for Aging Education (HPPAE)—a nationally recognized training model that has proved to be effective in recruiting master's-level social work students who will go on to pursue careers in the aging field. HPPAE offers a new field approach that exposes students to older adults beyond the nursing home setting and blurs the line between classroom learning and internships so that graduates are prepared for the realities of the workplace. The HPPAE program has continued in some schools of social work across the country since the Hartford funding ended. Another program originally supported by the Hartford Foundation is the Council on Social Work Education's National Center for Gerontology

Social Work Education, or Gero-Ed Center. This Center developed curriculum standards for geriatric social work education and a clearinghouse for geriatric teaching tools with the aim of promoting gerontology competencies in baccalaureate and master's-level social work programs nationwide to prepare students to enhance the health and well-being of older adults and their families.

PRACTICE SETTINGS

Clinical/Direct Service Settings

In clinical or direct service settings, gerontological social workers care for and interact with older adults to assist them with everyday life. This can include connecting older adults with community resources, coordinating care for individuals who need a number of services and care at different levels, helping older individuals and their families examine their needs and facilitate family communication, assisting older adults in applying for needed services and programs, and providing support in dealing with end-of-life issues (e.g., preparing advance directives, helping prepare individuals and families). Social workers working in direct practice settings are increasingly in roles in which they serve as the only social worker within a team of other professionals providing care for older adults (e.g., in medical settings). Geriatric social workers are often the ones on the team who recognize and support older adults' desires to age-in-place and remain independent, point out and address the various social determinants of health at play for individuals and groups, and bring unique skills and training with regard to care coordination and transition management. Clinical/direct service settings may include private practice, in-home, neighborhoods, hospitals, senior congregate housing, hospice/end-of-life care, area agencies on aging, senior centers, Programs of All-Inclusive Care for the Elderly (PACE), continuing care communities, and residential long-term care facilities such as nursing facilities.

Management/Administration Settings

Managers or administrators run or have leadership roles within facilities that care for older adults, whereas program planners and evaluators ensure that programs function effectively to address the needs of older adults. Gerontological social workers may use such roles within a wide range of community-based agencies (e.g., mental health clinics, senior centers, housing-related agencies).

Policy and Advocacy Settings

Other gerontological social workers work on macropolicy issues for either government or nonprofit agencies. For example, former Maryland Senator Barbara Mikulski, a social worker, supported stronger pension plans for retirees, helped make quality psychological care available to seniors in nursing homes, and encouraged the Senate to renew and strengthen the Older Americans Act (OAA; Geriatric Social Work Initiative, 2013). Advocates work to inform various audiences about issues of concern, working with older adults to raise awareness about their needs and concerns, and the appropriate responses to those concerns. Gerontological social workers in policy/advocacy settings may work, for example, for state departments of health, state Veterans Affairs offices, adult protective services, Centers for Medicare & Medicaid Services, or the Department of Veterans Affairs.

Research Settings

Some gerontological social workers can be found in roles that involve skills in planning, designing, and implementing social research. For example, some serve in grant writing, policy analyst, and program evaluation within agencies that serve older adults.

ELDER CARE NEEDS ADDRESSED BY SOCIAL WORKERS

Assessment

Almost two of five older persons report some type of disability (i.e., difficulty hearing, vision, cognition, ambulation, self-care, or independent living); these disabilities range from minor to requiring extensive assistance (Administration on Aging, U.S. Department of Health and

G

Human Services, 2011). Thus sound assessment of the functional and social capacities of this population is critical. Older persons' problems are often complex and involve interrelated biological/health, psychological, social, and cultural dimensions.

To determine the need for particular resources, therefore, it is best for an older adult to receive a comprehensive geriatric assessment. An assessment that involves a very frail older adult with multiple, complex needs is ideally conducted by an interdisciplinary team (Damron-Rodriguez & Corley, 2002). Team members from different disciplines collectively set goals and share responsibilities and resources. The client and caregivers may also attend team meetings. The aim of assessment, by examining the status of physical, mental, and social well-being, is to gain an understanding of the older adults' problems, needs, and strengths to develop an intervention plan (McInnis-Dittrich, 2009).

Some particular assessment skills are crucial to gerontological social work practice. The use, for example, of empathic interviewing skills to engage older clients in identifying both their strengths and problems is especially important. Along these lines, it is often necessary to adapt interviewing methods to potential sensory, linguistic, and cognitive limitations of the older adult. Ascertaining the health status and assessing the physical functioning (e.g., activities of daily living [ADL] and instrumental activities of daily living [IADL]) of older clients has long been a part of elder care, as has assessing their cognitive functioning and mental health status (e.g., depression, dementia). Proper assessment depends on administering standardized assessment and diagnostic tools that are appropriate for use with older adults (e.g., Blozik et al., 2009; Kane, 2006).

Care Coordination and Management

Because the care an older person often involves multiple sources, effective coordination and monitoring are essential. The focus of a long-term care system is the persons (and families) whose decreased functional capacity places them in a position to need assistance with ADL,

such as housekeeping, finances, transportation, meal preparations, or administration of medication. The care manager facilitates the client's movement through the service-delivery system and is responsible for ensuring that a client's needs are met. Gerontological social workers who function as care managers are skilled at navigating the Aging Services Network to identify the best options for the older adults with whom they work.

Social Integration

A major focus for geriatric social workers is to assist the older person's social engagement and integration. Sometimes this involves helping the older person stay involved in an array of meaningful activities such as work, volunteering, and general recreational activities, with a focus on promoting activities that support physical, cognitive, and social well-being (Matz-Costa, Besen, James, & Pitt-Catsouphes, 2014; Matz-Costa, Carr, McNamara, & James, 2016). However, geriatric social workers are also concerned with the older persons whose web of social ties has been weakened. Thus screening for social isolation and developing programs for those older persons with extremely limited social networks is also a critical function of geriatric social workers (Lubben et al., 2006).

Advocacy

To facilitate what the WHO (2002) has deemed as crucial for elder care—namely, the joint efforts of public and private domains—advocacy on the part of social workers is indispensable. Advocacy cuts across multiple points of service delivery: On behalf of clients, with agencies and other professionals to help obtain quality services; with service providers, community organizations, policy makers, and the public to promote the needs and issues of a growing aging population; and for the adaption of organizational policies, procedures, and resources to facilitate the provision of services to diverse older adults and their family caregivers. All of these have the goal of formalizing changes within an organization and publicizing the process.

EMERGING ROLES FOR GERONTOLOGICAL SOCIAL WORKERS

The Patient Protection and Affordable Care Act (PPACA) was signed into law in 2010. The PPACA emphasizes health promotion and increased community care alternatives designed to keep older people well rather than focused on picking up the pieces once they have suffered major health events (Fielding, Teutsch, & Koh, 2012). The PPACA has challenged traditional hospital-based social work but has provided new venues for social work practice as well (Reisch, 2012). Indeed, many new opportunities for social work have begun to unfold with the full implementation of this legislation. However, the future of the PPACA is unclear, as the Trump administration promises to repeal and replace the Act (Lee, 2017). Gerontological social workers will likely play a large role in advocating for affordable health care coverage, Medicaid expansion, coverage for pre-existing conditions, access to mental health and substance use disorder services at parity, essential health benefits and preventive care, lack of annual or lifetime dollar limits, and promotion of new, integrated models of care and delivery systems during these times of uncertainty.

In addition to changes in the delivery of health care service, multiple other trends will promote opportunities for gerontological social work practice. Social workers will play an important role in responding to the impending retirement of the Baby Boomer generation, specifically the retirement of the health and human service workforce; reacting to the expanded focus on interdisciplinary/interprofessional service delivery; increasing pressure to implement tested interventions and evidence-based practices; addressing the needs of the military and their families and the many generations of veterans (Social Work Policy Institute, 2011); and addressing the growing demand for quality consumer-centered care and decision making (Mahoney, 2011). There could also be increasing opportunities for gerontological social workers in business and in the for-profit sector given emerging trends in the healthy aging market. These include an increased corporate interest in issues of life planning and supporting alternative retirement options.

Finally, the American Academy of Social Work and Social Welfare (see aaswsw.org) recently announced the Grand Challenges for Social Work. These Grand Challenges establish a social agenda for the next decade (Uehara et al., 2013). Many of the Grand Challenges, such as eradicating social isolation (Lubben, Gironda, Sabbath, Kong & Johnson, 2015) and promoting long and productive lives (Morrow-Howell, Gonzales, Matz-Costa, & Greenfield, 2015), are very relevant to the health and well-being of older populations and will be the focus of increased attention by social workers in the coming years.

See also Advance Directives; Caregiver Burnout; Discharge Planning; Social Supports: Formal and Informal.

Christina Matz-Costa and James Lubben

Administration on Aging, U.S. Department of Health and Human Services. (2011). *A profile of older Americans: 2011*. Retrieved from http://www.aoa.gov/Aging_Statistics/Profile/2011/docs/2011profile.pdf

Blozik, E., Wagner, J. T., Gillman, G., Iliffe, S., von Renteln-Kruse, W., Lubben, J., … Clugh-Gorr, K. M. (2009). Social network assessment in community-dwelling older persons: Results from a study of three European populations. *Aging Clinical and Experimental Research, 21*(2), 150–157.

Damron-Rodriguez, J., & Corley, C. S. (2002). Social work education for interdisciplinary practice with older adults and their families. *Journal of Gerontological Social Work, 39*, 37–55.

Damron-Rodriguez, J. A., & Lubben, J. (2007). Family and community health care for older persons. In S. Carmel, F. Torres-Gil, & C. Morris (Eds.) with J. Damron-Rodriguez, S. Feldman, & T. Seedsman (Co-Eds.), *The art of aging well: Lessons from three nations* (pp. 75–90). New York, NY: Baywood.

Fielding, J. E., Teutsch, S., & Koh, H. (2012). Health reform and Healthy People initiative. *American Journal of Public Health, 102*(1), 30–33. doi:10.2105/AJPH.2011.300312

Geriatric Social Work Initiative. (2013). Experience exciting careers in social work and aging. Retrieved from http://www.gswi.org/CSW0908.pdf

Kane, R. A. (2006). Standardized measures commonly used in geriatric assessment. In B. Berkman (Ed.), *Handbook of social work in health and aging* (pp. 737–748). New York, NY: Oxford University Press.

G

Kass-Bartelmes, B. L., & Hughes, R. (2003, March). Advance care planning: Preferences for care at the end of life. *Research in Action, 12*, 1–18.

Lee, M. J. (2017, February 27). GOP returns to daunting task of dismantling Obamacare, selling its plan to Trump. *CNN National Politics Reporter.* Retrieved from http://www.cnn.com/2017/02/27/politics/gop-dismantling-obamacare

Lubben, J., Blozik, E., Gillmann, G., Iliffe, S., Kruse, W. R., Beck, J. C., & Stuck, A. E. (2006). Performance of an abbreviated version of the Lubben Social Network Scale among three European community-dwelling older adult populations. *The Gerontologist, 46*(4), 503–513.

Lubben, J., Gironda, M., Sabbath, E., Kong, J. & Johnson, C. (2015). *Social isolation presents a grand challenge for social work. Grand Challenges for Social Work Initiative Working Paper No. 7.* Columbia, SC: American Academy of Social Work and Social Welfare.

Mahoney, K. J. (2011). Person-centered planning and participant decision making. *Health & Social Work, 36*(3), 233.

Matz-Costa, C., Besen, E., James, J., & Pitt-Catsouphes, M. (2014). Differential impact of multiple levels of productive activity engagement on psychological well-being in middle and later life. *The Gerontologist, 54*(2), 277–289. doi:10.1093/geront/gns148

Matz-Costa, C., Carr, D., McNamara, T., & James, J. (2016). Physical, cognitive, social, and emotional mediators of activity involvement and health in later life. *Research on Aging, 28*(7), 791–815. doi:10.1177/0164027515606182

McInnis-Dittrich, K. (2009). *Social work with elders: A biopsychosocial approach to assessment and intervention* (3rd ed.). Boston, MA: Allyn & Bacon.

Morrow-Howell, N., Gonzales, E., Matz-Costa, C., & Greenfield, E. A. (2015). *Increasing productive engagement in later life. Grand Challenges for Social Work Initiative Working Paper No. 8.* Columbia, SC: American Academy of Social Work and Social Welfare.

Reisch, M. (2012). The challenges of health care reform for hospital social work in the United States. *Social Work in Health Care, 51*(10), 873–893. doi:10.1080/00981389.2012.721492

Social Work Policy Institute. (2011). *Investing in the social work workforce.* Washington, DC: National Association of Social Workers.

Uehara, E., Flynn, M., Fong, R., Brekke, J., Barth, R. P., Coulton, C., … Walters, K. (2013). Grand challenges for social work. *Journal of the Society for Social Work and Research, 4*(3), 165–170. doi:10.5243/jsswr.2013.11

World Health Organization. (2002). *Active aging: A policy framework.* Geneva, Switzerland: Author.

Web Resources
Age Source Worldwide: http://www.aarpinternational.org/resource-library/agesource-agestats
Alzheimer's Disease Education and Referral Center: http://www.nia.nih.gov/alzheimers
Association for Gerontology Education in Social Work: http://www.agesocialwork.org
CSWE Gero-Ed Center, National Center for Gerontological Social Work Education: http://www.cswe.org/CentersInitiatives/GeroEdCenter.aspx
Geriatric Social Work Initiative: http://www.gswi.org
Hartford Partnership Program for Aging Education (HPPAE): http://www.hartfordpartnership.org
Merck Manual of Geriatrics: http://www.merck.com/mrkshared/mmg/sec1/ch7/ch7a.jsp

GERONTOLOGICAL SOCIETY OF AMERICA

The Gerontological Society of America (GSA) is dedicated to promoting the scientific study of aging. It encourages exchanges among researchers and practitioners and fosters the use of gerontological research in forming public policy. It is a leader in the advancement of knowledge, the generation of new ideas, and the translation of research findings into practice.

GSA was founded in 1945 and is the oldest and largest national multidisciplinary scientific organization devoted to the advancement of gerontological research. Its membership includes some 5,500 researchers, educators, practitioners, and other professionals in the field of aging. The society's principal missions are to promote research and education in aging and to encourage the dissemination of research results to other scientists, decision makers, and practitioners. It achieves this by disseminating information; providing networking opportunities; linking research with policy, practice, and education; advocating for increased public and private funding for research on aging; and promoting career development and advancement of its members and development of the next generation of leaders. To further fulfill its mission, GSA assembles more than 4,000 professionals from around the world to an annual scientific meeting. This event features more than 500 sessions each year.

PUBLICATIONS

In 70 years, GSA has moved from publishing one journal to publishing five. In 1946, the *Journal of Gerontology* was the first and, for many years, the only U.S. gerontological research journal. In 1995, it became four journals, each with a separate editor and published under two covers: *Journals of Gerontology: Biological Sciences and Medical Sciences* and *Journals of Gerontology: Psychological Sciences and Social Sciences*. In June 1954, the society first published the "Newsletter of the Gerontological Society" followed by *The Gerontologist* in 1965, which has evolved into a journal of applied research and analysis in gerontology, including social policy, program development, and service delivery. Other regular features of the journal include essay-style book reviews, audiovisual reviews, practice concepts, and the Forum, which features review articles or well-documented arguments on a topical issue. The society's *The Public Policy and Aging Report* was added in 1995. The *Report*, a quarterly policy newsletter published by the National Academy on an Aging Society (GSA's independent policy institute), examines policy issues associated with the aging society. The publication is targeted to those outside the academic and traditional aging communities. *Innovation in Aging* is an open access journal of GSA that publishes research studies that describe innovative theories, research methods, interventions, evaluations, and policies relevant to aging and the life course. Journal content reflects the wide-ranging research interests of GSA members. *Gerontology News* is the organizations' monthly newsletter that covers GSA's events (including the annual scientific meeting), news on members, funding opportunities, resources for aging researchers, policy issues, and legislative actions.

Elizabeth A. Capezuti

Web Resource
Gerontological Society of America: http://www.geron
  .org

GEROPSYCHIATRIC ADVANCED PRACTICE NURSING

Despite the long recognition that older men have the highest suicide rates in the United States and that the number of persons with dementia and other cognitive disorders is increasing dramatically worldwide, mental health and substance use disorders in older adults remains a hidden crisis in the United States, and they represent a vulnerable and underserved population. Not only is the number of older adults with mental health issues increasing, so is their diversity. In the face of this increasing need for services, the number of mental health specialists who focus chiefly on the mental health and substance use disorders in older adults is very limited and declining (Bartels & Naslund, 2013; Institute of Medicine, 2012). In response, The John A. Hartford Foundation Geropsychiatric Nursing Collaborative (GPNC) at the American Academy of Nursing carried out a 4-year project (2008–2012) to strengthen geropsychiatric nursing (GPN) education and the mental health workforce in the United States (Beck, Buckwalter, Dudzik, & Evans, 2011). They defined GPN as nurses capable of providing holistic support, care, and culturally sensitive treatment for older adults with mental health concerns or psychiatric/substance use disorders, as well as their families, across a wide range of health and mental health care settings. Adequately prepared geropsychiatric nurses are able to address psychiatric disorders, cognitive changes, and the medical disorders most common in later life. Geropsychiatric nurses and geropsychiatric advanced practice registered nurses (APRNs) are able to help off-set the shortage of geriatric mental health specialists in medicine, psychology, and social work (Bartels & Naslund, 2013; Institute of Medicine, 2012).

The GPNC made specific recommendations and developed educational resources to encourage schools of nursing, hospitals, nursing homes, and community agencies to enhance geropsychiatric competencies for two subtypes of APRNs: gerontological clinical nurse specialist (GCNS) and geropsychiatric nurse practitioner (GPNP). The chief difference between these two types of APRNs as described by the GPNC in regards to their geropsychiatric-focused competencies is that GCNSs are described as expert in providing direct care, consultation, systems leadership, and research with older adults and their families, whereas GPNPs are able to diagnosis health status, plan care, and implement treatment, as well as ensure the quality of health care services (see the Portal of Geriatrics Online Education [POGOe] for the key documents and resources generated by the GPNC). Both types of APRNs are essential members of the interdisciplinary health care team. Both are able to provide comprehensive assessment, management and evaluation of care, as well as teach health professionals regarding the mental health issues facing older adults. Although not as expert in using clinical evaluation tools as psychologists or working with families and agencies as social workers, they do have overlapping expertise in these areas as well. The level of autonomy of practice and prescriptive authority of APRNs varies across states and employers; in general GPNPs are more likely to have prescriptive ability, including for controlled substances, than GCNSs. In light of the APRN Consensus Work Group and the National Council of State Boards of Nursing APRN Advisory Committee's (2008) efforts to include gerontological education and competencies in all CNS and NP certifications, except those limited to children, adolescents, or school health, the recommendations and resources of the GPNC remain very relevant and valuable.

At this time, there is no certification or licensure specific for GPN or advanced practice nursing, and there is no evidence suggesting that more schools of nursing should include more geropsychiatric content in their advanced practice programs than they did 10 years ago, before the work of the GPNC and the implementation of the APRN Consensus Model (Stephens, Harris, & Buron, 2015). In their survey of 363 graduate nursing programs in the United States, 138 of the 202 schools that responded to their survey reported that they included GPN content in one or more of

their courses in their APRN programs, but only 17 reported a geropsychiatric program, track or minor (Stephens et al., 2015, p. 389). Likewise, there are also very few primary or acute care NP programs that adequately integrate psychiatric content or facilitate dual specialization, such as adult/gerontological primary care and psychiatric/substance use disorder. This lack suggests that program planners, funders, and students continue to be influenced by the double invisibility of the need that exists in the community and the double stigma of being elderly and suffering from mental illness or substance use disorders. It is unclear whether the implementation of parity legislation designed to improve insurance coverage for mental health services will be effective and help recruit additional clinicians to get the training they need to serve this population well.

See also Mental Health Services.

Steven L. Baumann

Advanced Practice Registered Nursing Consensus Work Group & National Council of State Boards of Nursing APRN Advisory Committee. (2008). Consensus model for APRN regulation: Licensure, accreditation, certification & education. Retrieved from https://www.ncsbn.org/Consensus_Model_for_APRN_Regulation_July_2008.pdf

Bartels, S. J., & Naslund, J. A. (2013). The underside of the silver tsunami: Older adults and mental health care. *New England Journal of Medicine, 363*, 493–496. doi:10.1056/NEJMp1211456

Beck, C., Buckwalter, K., Dudzik, P. M., & Evans, L. (2011). Filling the void in geriatric mental health: The geropsychiatric nursing collaborative as a model for change. *Nursing Outlook, 59*, 236–242.

Institute of Medicine. (2012). *The mental health and substance abuse workforce for older adults: In whose hands?* Washington, DC: National Academies Press.

Stephens, C. E., Harris, M., & Buron, B. (2015). The current state of U.S. geropsychiatric graduate nursing education: Results of the national geropsychiatric graduate nursing education survey. *Journal of the American Psychiatric Nurses Association, 21*, 385–394.

Web Resources
American Psychiatric Nurses Association's Geropsychiatric Nursing Resources: http://www.apna.org/i4a/pages/index.cfm?pageid=4291

POGOe Geropsychiatric Nursing Competency Enhancements: https://www.pogoe.org/productid/20660

GRANDPARENTS AS FAMILY CAREGIVERS

More than 2.5 million children in the United States were being raised by grandparents and other relative caregivers between 2013 and 2015 (Kids Count Data Center, 2016). Grandparents who are the primary caregivers of children face the joys of a close relationship with their grandchildren, as well as the struggles to keep their families together. The reasons for caregiving include death, incarceration, teen pregnancy, mental illness, abuse and neglect, HIV/AIDS, and active duty in the military. One of the most common reasons for caregiving is substance abuse, and the rise in heroin and other opioid use has resulted in more relatives stepping up to raise children whose parents have died or are incarcerated, using drugs, in treatment, or otherwise unable to care for them (Generations United [GU], 2016). The challenges of raising children, especially those with mental or physical disabilities, can be overwhelming. The inability to access child care is a barrier to much-needed doctor's visits, socialization, and employment. These issues are compounded when grandparents live in rural areas, isolated from social service providers, and lack information or transportation to access available services.

PHYSICAL AND MENTAL HEALTH

Caring for related children can be very rewarding. However, chronic health problems have been reported in studies of Hispanic, White, and African American grandparents raising grandchildren (Goodman & Silverstein, 2002; Whitley, Kelley, & Sipe, 2001). Caregiving grandparents often neglect their own physical health by skipping or postponing medical appointments. In addition to the stress on their physical health, caregivers and children have mental health needs (Langosch, 2012). A high level of depression among Native American grandparents who are raising their grandchildren has been reported (Letiecq, Bailey, & Kurtz, 2008). Grandparents care for children who have behavioral, physical, and emotional issues; who suffer from separation anxiety, loss, grief, and feelings of abandonment; whose parents have AIDS or are substance abusers; and who have witnessed violence or experienced abuse or neglect and act out as a result of this trauma (Kelley, Whitley, & Campos, 2011). Access to available health insurance may also affect the ability of the family to attend to these complex issues (Kelley et al., 2011). While trying to address their own anger, depression, resentment, and embarrassment, grandparents may also be faced with trying to restore parent–child relationships in a positive way that nurtures the entire family (Letiecq, Bailey, & Porterfield, 2008).

LEGAL ISSUES

Although caregivers are often able to make day-to-day decisions without a legal relationship, they may face challenges around enrolling children in school, accessing school records, or consenting to their medical care (Letiecq, Bailey, & Porterfield, 2008). These challenges can be especially difficult for caregivers who are responsible for children with mental or physical impairments that require medical assessment and treatment, hospitalization, or special education. Grandparents, with or without a legal relationship to the children in their care, need information and education about available benefits and about their legal decision-making authority. They may also require assistance to obtain that legal authority when necessary.

ECONOMIC CHALLENGES

Grandparent caregivers may be retired or live on limited incomes. Although children may be eligible for child-only Temporary Assistance to Needy Families (TANF) grants, Supplemental Nutrition Assistance Program (SNAP; formerly Food Stamps) benefits, Medicaid, State Children's Health Insurance Program (SCHIP), or Social Security benefits, grandparents may find it difficult to navigate a system of public benefits that was not intended to assist nonparents. This often results in difficulties in accessing much-needed financial assistance. Other possible sources of support, such subsidized guardianships or adoption subsidies, are usually limited to children who have been in the foster care system.

HOUSING NEEDS

Finding quality, affordable housing is a significant challenge for grandparents who are primary caregivers with limited incomes that may need larger living quarters to accommodate the children in their care. Grandparents who live in housing for the elderly are especially vulnerable because children are not allowed in these senior housing complexes and may face eviction for lease violations.

RESPITE

Respite, a break from the challenges of caregiving, is also greatly needed. Respite provides an opportunity for socialization, doctor's appointments or other self-care activities, or rest. The provision of recreational and educational activities for children can provide grandparents with the time off they need to "recharge their batteries," and intergenerational activities can provide grandparents and grandchildren with a break from their day-to-day activities and an opportunity to enjoy some fun together. When clearly defined, easily accessible, creative, and flexible, respite programs can help caregivers face their caregiving responsibilities.

COLLABORATIVE PARTNERSHIPS

With the growing awareness of grandparents as parents, a number of resources and services have been developed to address their distinct needs. Collaborations at the local, state, and national levels with public, private, and nonprofit groups have also helped the creation or expansion of programmatic opportunities for caregivers. The Brookdale Foundation Group's Relatives as Parents Program (RAPP) has a network of community based nonprofit organizations and state public agencies that provide direct services and stimulate the creation and expansion of services to grandparents and other relatives raising children. The network provides supportive services, including support groups, the most widespread method for addressing the support and educational needs of grandparent caregivers. Rural Development Cooperative Extension Programs are publicly funded and delivered through an educational network: U.S. Department of Agriculture, land-grant universities in every state and territory. Local extension educators at the community level provide programmatic initiatives, including support groups, to improve the quality of life of relative caregiver families across the nation. They have also created eXtension, a website that features articles, information, and resources on a wide range of topics, including family caregiving.

The National Center on Grandfamilies of GU is a valuable resource for educating policy makers and the public about the economic and social needs of grandparent caregivers and their families. Their reports, fact sheets, conferences, and newsletters help identify key issues faced by this special population of caregivers. GrandRallies, held in Washington, DC, and sponsored by national organizations such as GU, AARP, the Children's Defense Fund, the Child Welfare League of America, and the National Committee of Grandparents for Children's Rights, educate members of Congress and their staff about needed supportive services for grandparents and other relative caregivers.

The U.S. Census Bureau and others, such as the Annie E. Casey Foundation Kids Count Data Center, have contributed to the growing awareness of the unmet needs of relative caregivers by providing data on the number of caregivers at the state, local, and county levels. These data allow advocates, researchers, and service providers to document the need for services in the communities they serve. State Fact Sheets, a collaboration of national organizations such as GU, AARP, Children's Defense Fund, the Brookdale Foundation Group, Casey Family Programs, and the Child Welfare League of America, provide state-specific information on the issues, needs, and programs available to assist grandparents and other relative caregivers. The Grandfamilies State Law and Policy Resource Center, a collaboration of the American Bar Association's Center on Children and the Law, GU and Casey Family Programs, has a searchable database of laws, legislation, relevant resources, and publications to help relative caregivers and their advocates.

LEGISLATION

The Administration on Aging's National Family Caregiver Support Program (NFCSP) was established as part of the 2000 Amendments to the Older Americans Act. The NFCSP specifically designates funding, a maximum of 10%, for supportive services to grandparents and other relatives 55 years of age and older who are raising children. Services include information and referral, individual counseling, support groups, caregiver training, respite care, and supplemental services.

In response to the lack of affordable housing, several organizations have partnered to create housing opportunities for grandparents raising grandchildren. Some examples are GrandFamilies House, the first housing complex for grandparents and their grandchildren, in Dorchester, Massachusetts, as well as GrandParent Family Apartments in the Bronx, New York, sponsored by Presbyterian Senior Services, West Side Federation for Senior and Supportive Housing, and Calvary Baptist Church Senior Housing, with units set aside for grandparent caregivers and their families, in Queens, NY. A critical component for any intergenerational housing is the provision of in-house supportive services, including case management, for both seniors and children.

Federal law has also recognized the housing needs of grandparents who are primary caregivers of their grandchildren. The Living Equitably: Grandparents Aiding Children and Youth (LEGACY) Act of 2003 enabled the U.S. Department of Housing and Urban Development (HUD) to implement pilot programs to create affordable-housing opportunities for grandparents and other relatives aged 62 years and older who are raising children, to educate and train housing officials on policies that affect these families, and to work with the U.S. Census Bureau to conduct a national study of the housing needs of relative caregiver families.

Some states make it easier for caregivers to provide support and care for the children they are raising. Consent laws give caregivers without a legal relationship the authority to enroll children in school and/or obtain medical care, and Kinship Navigator programs, available in some states, help caregivers identify and apply for eligible benefits and services. Many programs funded at the federal, state, and local levels have created or expanded services to address the needs and issues identified here, but much remains to be done to ensure that this special population of relative caregivers and the children they are raising receive the support needed to keep their families together.

See also Family Care for Elders With Dementia; Family Care for Frail Elders; Intergenerational Programs; Respite Care; Support Groups.

Melinda Perez-Porter and Rolanda Pyle

Generations United. (2016). State of grandfamilies 2016: Raising children of the opioid epidemic: Solutions and supports for grandfamilies. Retrieved from http://www.gu.org/Portals/0/documents/Reports/16-Report-State_of_Grandfamiles.pdf

Goodman, C., & Silverstein, M. (2002). Grandmothers raising grandchildren: Family structure and well-being in culturally diverse families. *The Gerontologist, 42*(5), 676–689.

Kelley, S. J., Whitley, D. M., & Campos, P. E. (2011). Behavior problems in children raised by grandmothers: The role of caregiver distress, family resources, and the home environment. *Children and Youth Services Review, 33*, 2138–2145.

Kids Count Data Center. (2016). Children in kinship care. *Annie E. Casey Foundation.* Retrieved from http://datacenter.kidscount.org/data/bar/7172-children-in-kinship-care?loc=1&loct=1#1/any/false/1564/any/14207

Langosch, D. (2012). Grandparents parenting again: Challenges, strengths, and implications for practice. *Psychoanalytic Inquiry, 32*(2), 163–170.

Letiecq, B. L., Bailey, S. J., & Kurtz, M. A. (2008). Depression among rural Native American and European American grandparents rearing their grandchildren. *Journal of Family Issues, 29*, 334–356.

Letiecq, B. L., Bailey, S. J., & Porterfield, F. (2008). "We have no rights, we get no help": The legal and policy dilemmas facing grandparent care-givers. *Journal of Family Issues* (Special collection: Transforming the discussion on diversity: The influence of policies and law on families), *29*(8), 995–1012.

Whitley, D. M., Kelley, S. J., & Sipe, T. A. (2001). Grandmothers raising grandchildren: Are they at increased risk of health problems? *Health & Social Work, 26*(2), 105–114.

Web Resources

eXtension: http://www.eXtension.org

Generations United's National Center on Grand-families: http://www.gu.org/OURWORK/Grandfamilies.aspx

Grandfamilies State Law and Policy Resource Center: http://www.grandfamilies.org

State Grandfact Sheets: http://www.grandfamilies.org/State-Fact-Sheets

GREEN HOUSE PROJECT

The Green House Project offers a radically new national model for long-term care that returns control, dignity, and a sense of well-being to elders, their families, and direct care staff (Bowers & Nolet, 2011; Jenkens, Sult, Lessell, Hammer, & Ortigara, 2011; Kane, Lum, Cutler, Degenholtz, & Yu, 2007; Thomas, 1994, 1996). Elders live in small, self-contained homes where individuality and choice are honored, quality of care is a priority, and people have more satisfying and meaningful lives, work, and relationships. The model was created by Dr. Bill Thomas (2004) and originally described in the book *What Are Old People for? How Elders Will Save the World*. *Provider* called the Green House model the pinnacle of culture change (LaPorte, 2010), whereas *The New York Times* hailed it as the "most comprehensive effort to reinvent the nursing home" (Gustke, 2011, para. 9).

Through an intensive process, The Green House Project team partners with organizations to support their unique culture change journey. The initial feasibility phase ensures that organizations are set up for success with a shared vision, viable financial structure, and strong leadership (Jenkens et al., 2011). Comprehensive technical assistance, led by an expert project guide, empowers teams with knowledge, resources, and relevant experience at every step of the way. Support in areas such as finance, regulations, and design facilitate successful implementation and sustainability of the model. Through innovative education programs and coaching, staff develop the skills needed to achieve the Green House values and outcomes (Kane et al., 2007). Model fidelity is assessed annually through the Model Enrichment Resource and Integrity Tool (MERIT). Partners enjoy continued support and education from a national organization, including an extensive peer network of Green House organizations.

See also Culture Change; Nursing Homes; Pioneer Network.

Marla DeVries

Bowers, B., & Nolet, K. (2011). Empowered direct care workers: Lessons Learned from THE GREEN HOUSE® model. *Seniors Housing and Care Journal, 19*(1), 109–120.

Gustke, C. (2011, October 31). A nursing home shrinks until it feels like a home. *The New York Times*. Retrieved from http://www.nytimes.com/2011/11/01/health/shrinking-the-nursing-home-until-it-feels-like-a-home.html

Jenkens, R., Sult, T., Lessell, N., Hammer, D., & Ortigara, A. (2011). Financial implications of THE GREEN HOUSE® model. *Seniors Housing and Care Journal, 19*(1), 3–22.

Kane, R. A., Lum, T. Y., Cutler, L. J., Degenholtz, H. B., & Yu, T.-C. (2007). Resident outcomes in small-house nursing homes: A longitudinal evaluation of the initial Green House program. *Journal of the American Geriatrics Society, 55*, 832–839.

LaPorte, M. (2010, May). Culture change goes mainstream. *Provider, 36*(5), 22–33.

Thomas, W. H. (1994). *The Eden Alternative: Nature, hope and nursing homes*. Columbia: University of Missouri Press.

Thomas, W. H. (1996). *Life worth living: How someone you love can still enjoy life in a nursing home: The Eden Alternative in action*. Acton, MA: VanderWyk & Burnham.

Thomas, W. H. (2004). *What are old people for? How elders will save the world.* Acton, MA: VanderWyk & Burnham.

Web Resource
The Green House Project: http://www.thegreen houseproject.org

GUARDIANSHIP AND CONSERVATORSHIP

One of the most difficult situations for family members or health care providers to face is older adults who have become unable to make day-to-day decisions, potentially making them vulnerable to abuse, neglect, or financial exploitation by family members or strangers. This is especially true when they have not expressed their medical wishes in writing using a health care directive or advance directive for health care or if they have not created a power of attorney to allow others to handle financial matters. Aside from the anguish the impairment of the older adult may cause involved parties, the issue can quickly become one of providing sufficient but unintrusive assistance once the adult's ability to make financial and/or medical decisions is compromised. Guardianship is one of society's most drastic interventions because it represents the partial or total removal of older adults' civil rights and the appointment of others (surrogates) to make decisions on their behalf. Nevertheless, for people who need such services, guardianships can provide essential decision-making support.

Guardianship, also called *conservatorship* in some states, is usually divided into two types: personal and financial (or property). The terminology differs from state to state, although results of the Third National Guardianship Summit (TNGS) include recommendations that the term *guardianship* be used for the personal and *conservatorship* for the financial (National Guardianship Association [NGN], 2011). For purposes of this chapter, the term *guardianship* is used to refer to a surrogate decision-maker for both the person (the ward) and the property.

All jurisdictions are empowered to appoint a guardian for adults who are determined to lack the ability to make their own decisions, but the standards for that determination differ. For example, in a recent survey about circumstances under which judges and attorneys would recommend the appointment of a guardian, the study participants clearly indicated the desire for documentation showing more than just compromised decision-making capacity (Gavisk & Greene, 2007). In many states, a court investigator or an examining committee makes a formal assessment based on the adult's functional and cognitive capacity. If a person is judged to lack the capacity to make personal or financial decisions and has not already designated a surrogate through an advance directive, a guardian will be appointed for the person and/or the property, as the circumstances warrant.

There is increasing recognition that older adults may be able to make some decisions but lack the capacity to make others. For example, older adults may not be able to make medical treatment decisions but may be capable of determining where they would like to live. Guardianship can be tailored to the individual's abilities, with most states allowing for the appointment of a limited guardianship, removing the right to make only certain decisions. However, the limited guardianship option is used with varying frequency because some courts believe the older adult's condition will continue to deteriorate, eventually requiring full (i.e., plenary) guardianship (Wilber & Reynolds, 1995). Additional rights for wards, including those who have an intellectual (or developmental) disability, have been enumerated in state Bill of Rights statutes and at the Fourth World Congress on Guardianship (see "Guidelines on Article 14 of the Convention on the Rights of Persons with Disabilities," September 2015).

INITIATING GUARDIANSHIP PROCEEDINGS

An older adult with impaired capacity often comes to the attention of a family member or a neighbor, who notifies the police or adult protective services. The precipitating factor can be elder maltreatment, undue influence, or inability to perform activities of daily living (ADL) or pay bills, for example. In these cases, the need for medical or financial decision making often prompts the petition for guardianship.

When a guardian is believed necessary, a petition is filed with the probate court or its equivalent (e.g., Surrogate's Court in New York). The petition provides information to the court on the person's physical and mental condition. The petition to establish a guardianship may include the designation of the person to be appointed as guardian, but in some states (e.g., Florida), a separate application for an individual to be appointed as guardian is required.

Once a petition is filed, the probate court holds a hearing to rule on whether to appoint a guardian and who it will be. Many states have a process in which formal assessment of the proposed ward is ordered, before the hearing. The adult in question, family members, and any attorneys involved receive notice of the hearing and have the right to be present, to approve of or contest the guardianship, and/or to assert their desire to serve as the guardian for the older adult.

APPOINTING A GUARDIAN

Most often, the family member closest to the adult in question, either emotionally or geographically, is appointed as the guardian. In many cases, however, adult children do not live nearby or get along with one another. Appointing an adult child as guardian in such circumstances can become problematic, particularly in cases in which the child's qualifications are in doubt. In fact, many states require a background check to be completed before a guardian performs any duties related to the ward, some states offer a form of certification process for appointed guardians, and other states conduct a credit check on guardians (U.S. Government Accountability Office [GAO], 2010).

Many states provide for the appointment of a public or professional guardian if there is no one else to act in this role and/or the older adult is indigent (falls below a designated income level). Professional guardians can be a geriatric care manager, an individual or corporate professional guardian, or a social services agency. For older adults with sufficient funds, a bank trust department, attorney, or professional guardian can be hired to act as guardian. These services tend to be expensive and are clearly not accessible to everyone. Standards for expertise of family versus nonfamily guardians vary widely, leading the TNGS to recommend the adoption of similar standards for conduct, although retaining the higher standard of expertise required of professional guardians (NGN, 2011).

Appropriate guardianship varies with the circumstances of the person who needs protection. In some states, older adults can file pre-need guardian statements, informing the court which individual they would choose to serve as guardian should one ever be needed. Otherwise, two factors are paramount when appointing the guardian: the nature of the relationship between the guardian and ward and any potential conflicts of interest. In the former case, the issue of emotional closeness and trust must be weighed against family dynamics and the guardian's ability to manage finances and proximity to the ward. (Stiegel [2012], and Wilber & Reynolds [1996] discuss familial relationships and potential maltreatment.) In the latter, the person or entity appointed as guardian should not also be providing medical or social services, nor should the guardian have any personal or agency interest that could be perceived as self-serving or adverse to the interests of the ward (National Guardianship Association, 2013; Teaster, Schmidt, Wood, Lawrence, & Mendiondo, 2010).

RESPONSIBILITIES OF A GUARDIAN

Guardians of the person must make decisions regarding all kinds of health care, as well as place of residence and other aspects of the person's social life. Their duties typically include, but are not limited to, the following:

- Complying with all necessary filing requirements (the probate court will inform individuals of the specifics in each state)
- Complying with the rules of the jurisdiction for procedures such as changing the residence of the ward, charging a guardian's fee, or any other action that requires court approval (this varies by state and county)

- Determining where the ward will live and under what circumstances (e.g., at home or in an assisted-living facility, nursing home, or other placement; alone or with others; receiving or not receiving home- or community-based services)
- Consenting to or refusing on behalf of the ward any medical, surgical, or behavioral treatments recommended by the ward's medical providers
- Terminating life support, which can require court approval in some states

Most courts require an annual filing describing any actions the guardian has taken to protect, maintain, or improve the ward's quality of life. In addition, the TNGS recommends these reports include person-centered care plans based on the principles of substituted-judgment to ensure that the ward receives the care he or she would want (NGN, 2011).

Even when a guardian of the person has been appointed, there is no substitute for the vigilance of a caring family member or professional. Although a particular guardian may infrequently interact with the ward, the guardian can still be an advocate for the person. For instance, a geriatric care manager, who identifies a ward as overmedicated but lacks the authority to change clinicians or suggest a specialist referral, could involve the guardian in developing a plan of care. By combining the professional's knowledge of the ward and the advocacy role of the guardian, the best outcome for the ward can be ensured.

Guardians of the property have similar filing requirements to guardians of the person. They are charged with receiving all assets and filing an inventory of the ward's property as soon as possible following the appointment. Many states require the filing of an inventory of the ward's assets and a periodic accounting of all income received, bills paid, and property bought and sold on behalf of the ward. In addition to these duties, the guardian of the property is charged with preserving the assets of the estate; paying the ward's living expenses; investing the assets according to the prudent person rule; employing attorneys, investment advisers, and other professionals as needed; buying and selling property, including real estate; potentially

applying to serve as representative payee for federal benefits; and paying burial and funeral expenses (some states consider this the duty of the executor, not the guardian). Many of these actions require prior approval of the court, and many states allow the ward to petition the court when a decision by the guardian is undesirable.

CONCLUSIONS

The role of the guardian is critical and highlights the importance of having a caring professional, family member, or friend who is alert to the situation and the unique needs of the ward. Although the guardian is responsible to the court and to the ward for any decisions made and often has much of the decision-making authority for the ward, it takes a petition to the probate court and a subsequent hearing to replace guardians who make poor decisions or abuse their decision-making responsibility. As a result of the TNGS and research from the U.S. Government Accountability Office (2011), efforts to improve the guardianship process and oversight of appointed guardians have advanced under the multidisciplinary Working Interdisciplinary Networks of Guardianship Stakeholders (WINGS) (Wood, 2014). Members of WINGS include "judges and court staff, the aging and disability networks, the public and private bar, mental health agencies, advocacy groups, medical and mental health professionals, service providers, family members, and individuals affected by guardianship," among others (NGN, 2017). The WINGS initiatives are further complemented by various other reforms to substitute decision-making laws and laws protecting vulnerable adults taking place across the country (Nack, Dessin, & Swift, 2012).

Fortunately, the majority of guardians are diligent, caring, and careful individuals who treat their wards well and endeavor to make responsible decisions that benefit them. Under the right circumstances, having a guardian for an impaired older adult can be an enormous relief to the family, to providers, and most important, to the ward.

See also Advance Directives; Competency and Capacity; Elder Mistreatment: Overview; Elder

Neglect; Financial Abuse; Mental Capacity Assessment; Money Management.

Kevin E. Hansen

Gavisk, M., & Greene, E. (2007). Guardianship determinations by judges, attorneys, and guardians. *Behavioral Sciences and the Law, 25,* 339–353.

Nack, J. R., Dessin, C. L., & Swift, T. (2012). Creating and sustaining interdisciplinary guardianship committees. *Utah Law Review, 3,* 1667–1690.

National Guardianship Association. (2013). *Standards of Practice.* Bellefonte, PA: Author. Retrieved from http://www.guardianship.org/documents/Standards_of_Practice.pdf

National Guardianship Network. (2011). *Third National Guardianship summit releases standards and recommendations.* Vienna, VA: Author. Retrieved from http://www.americanbar.org/content/dam/aba/uncategorized/2011/2011_aging_gship_sumt_stmnt_1111.authcheckdam.pdf

National Guardianship Network. (2017). *Court-community reform through WINGS.* Retrieved from http://www.nationalguardianshipnetwork.org/NGN/WINGS/Court-Community_Reform_Through_WINGS/NGN/WINGS/Court-Community_Reform.aspx?hkey=7d32011f-2ac5-461a-9b4a-5636722c4914

Stiegel, L. A. (2012). An overview of elder financial exploitation. *Generations, 36*(2), 73–80.

Teaster, P. B., Schmidt, W. C., Wood, E. F., Lawrence, S. A., Mendiondo, M. S. (2010). *Public guardianship: In the best interests of incapacitated people?* Santa Barbara, CA: Praeger/ABC-CLIO.

U.S. Government Accountability Office. (2010, September). *Guardianships: Cases of financial exploitation, neglect, and abuse of seniors.* Washington, DC: Author. Retrieved from http://www.gao.gov/assets/320/310741.pdf

U.S. Government Accountability Office. (2011, July). *Oversight of federal fiduciaries and court-appointed guardians needs improvement.* Washington, DC: Author. Retrieved from http://www.gao.gov/assets/330/321761.pdf

Wilber, K. H., & Reynolds, S. L. (1995). Rethinking alternatives to guardianship. *The Gerontologist, 35,* 248–257.

Wilber, K. H., & Reynolds, S. L. (1996). Introducing a framework for defining financial abuse of the elderly. *Journal of Elder Abuse & Neglect, 8*(2), 61–80.

Wood, E. F. (2014). *WINGS: Court-community partnerships to improve adult guardianship.* Williamsburg, VA: National Center for State Courts. Retrieved from http://www.ncsc.org/~/media/Microsites/Files/Future%20Trends%202014/Wings-Court%20Community%20Partnerships_Erica%20Wood.ashx

World Congress on Adult Guardianship. (2015). *Fourth World Congress on Adult Guardianship: Committee on the Rights of Persons with Disabilities.* Bochum, Germany: Author. Retrieved from http://www.wcag2016.de/fileadmin/Mediendatenbank_WCAG/Tagungsmaterialien/Guidelines_Article14.pdf

Web Resources

American Bar Association: Commission on Law and Aging

Capacity Definition and Initiation of Guardianship Proceedings: http://www.americanbar.org/content/dam/aba/administrative/law_aging/chartcapacityandinitiation.authcheckdam.pdf

Guardianship Law and Practice: http://www.americanbar.org/groups/law_aging/resources/guardianship_law_practice.html

National Academy of Elder Law Attorneys: http://cqrcengage.com/naela/guardianship

National Guardianship Association: http://www.guardianship.org

National Guardianship Network: http://www.nationalguardianshipnetwork.org

State Adult Guardianship Legislation: Directions of Reform (2016): http://www.americanbar.org/content/dam/aba/administrative/law_aging/2016_final_guardianship_legislative_update.authcheckdam.pdf

H

HEADACHE

Headache is not usually associated with significant underlying pathology. Occasionally, however, underlying disease is undetected because headache is such a common complaint, with a prevalence as high as 51% in some populations (Prencipe et al., 2001). Despite its benign nature, headache often has a significant impact on quality of life (QOL) and productivity.

Although headache in older and younger adults is similar in most respects, there are some notable differences in symptomatology and epidemiology. Some causes are unique to the elderly, such as temporal arteritis. Signs and symptoms of the underlying cause may also be different, such as the absence of fever and neck stiffness in meningitis. Thus it is important to take the complaint of headache seriously and begin evaluation with the idea that the headache could be secondary to an underlying disease. The most important tools for evaluating headache in geriatric patients are the history and the physical and neurological examinations. Subsequent diagnostic testing should be guided by the information gained during the clinical evaluation. Careful clinical assessment may obviate the necessity of imaging, which is over utilized.

SECONDARY HEADACHE

During the initial evaluation, the physician must differentiate underlying pathology causing a symptomatic headache (i.e., secondary headache) from the more benign primary headache, in which the headache itself is the primary problem. There is an increase in the prevalence of secondary headache with an increase in age (Lipton, Pfeffer, Newman, & Solomon 1993).

Therefore underlying causes should be considered before diagnosing the more benign primary headache (e.g., tension-type headache).

Giant cell arteritis is a granulomatous vasculitis involving large arteries, including the carotid, vertebral, and temporal arteries. It classically presents with scalp tenderness; temporal headache with tender, enlarged temporal arteries; and jaw claudication. It may occur in association with polymyalgia rheumatica, with a history of several months of malaise, weight loss, generalized weakness, myalgias, and low-grade fever. Supported by an elevated erythrocyte sedimentation rate and C-reactive protein, diagnosis is based on clinical suspicion and confirmed by temporal artery biopsy. Expeditious treatment with corticosteroids is imperative to prevent compromise of vision (Gonzalez-Gay et al., 2005).

Other central nervous system pathologies that cause headache include intracranial hemorrhage, mass lesions, and meningitis. It is important to keep in mind that in the elderly, subdural hematoma can be present in the absence of focal neurological signs or a history of identifiable trauma. Signs and symptoms suggestive of secondary headache that require further investigation include new headache; significant change in preexisting headache, such as severity, frequency, characteristics, or location; any focal neurological signs or symptoms; nausea and vomiting without a history of migraine; fever; meningismus; prior history of malignancy; sudden, severe, explosive headache; personality change or drowsiness; progressively worsening headache; and seizures.

Causes outside the nervous system that should be kept in mind during the initial evaluation include referred pain from dental disease, sinusitis, glaucoma, and other disorders of the head and neck. Medication-induced headaches always need to be considered and can be caused

H

by the introduction of a new drug or the withdrawal of certain substances (Lipton et al., 1993).

PRIMARY HEADACHE

Primary headache is categorized into definable entities that suggest the prognosis and can facilitate appropriate treatment.

Cervicogenic headache is pain originating primarily from disease in the neck. Pain due to disease in the upper cervical regions can be referred to all parts of the head, not only the occipital region, but also the frontal, temporal, parietal, and even orbital regions. Neck pain may not be a prominent complaint in some patients; direct questioning is necessary to elicit these symptoms and a history of neck trauma. Neck crepitus and cervical paraspinal tenderness are usually present. Results of cervical spine imaging must be interpreted carefully, taking into consideration the clinical picture. Patients with significant cervical-related head pain can have normal radiographic studies, whereas asymptomatic patients can have significant cervical spondylosis.

In patients with headache associated with cervical spine dysfunction, treatment involves explaining the cause of the pain, prescribing physiotherapy, and educating the patient about ergonomics, such as using a firm pillow or a cervical collar. The patient should be taught how to avoid holding the neck in one position for long periods, especially in positions in which there is an excessive neck flexion, extension, or torsion. Pain can be initiated or exacerbated by long-distance driving or prolonged time spent typing or using a computer. Analgesic therapy includes nonsteroidal anti-inflammatory drugs (NSAIDs) and muscle relaxants, which can be given in topical form when appropriate. Treatment of coexisting depression or sleep disorders can also relieve pain.

Tension-type headache is a common diagnosis. Criteria that were established by the Headache Classification Committee of the International Headache Society (1988) have recently been updated (Olesen, 2013). Symptoms include mild to moderate, bilateral, nonpulsating, pressing or tightening pain that does not inhibit activity. There is no associated nausea or vomiting

and no aggravation of symptoms with routine physical activity. Secondary headache must be excluded to make this diagnosis. Treatment should be multidimensional, including pharmacological and psychological interventions. Medications to be taken as needed may include acetaminophen, NSAIDs, or other pain medications. However, overuse of analgesics can lead to rebound headaches and conversion of episodic headaches to a chronic form. Prophylactic therapy may be considered because headache frequency increases. Some examples include tricyclic antidepressants, valproic acid, topiramate, and propranolol. Patients can be referred to a comprehensive pain-management center with expertise in several areas, including neurology, anesthesia, rehabilitation medicine, psychology, and occupational and physical therapy. These centers may also offer alternative treatments not otherwise available to patients.

Migraine incidence peaks at about age 40 years and subsequently declines with age. Therefore new-onset migraine is rare in the geriatric population. The suggestion of this diagnosis should prompt an evaluation to rule out secondary causes. Patients with a history of migraine who continue to have headaches through their geriatric years should be treated appropriately. Tricyclic antidepressants, valproic acid, topiramate, and propranolol are used for migraine prophylaxis. Great care should be taken to be aware of side effects and drug interactions. Most medications should be started at lower doses and increased slowly (Landy & Lobo, 2005).

Trigeminal neuralgia causes severe pain and has an increased incidence in the elderly. It is characterized by paroxysms of high-intensity, stabbing pain lasting several seconds, with intervening periods of relief. Usually triggered by minimal stimulation of the face, episodes of pain usually last 1 to 2 hours and may occur over weeks to months, followed by a long period without painful episodes. The pain may be described as "electric," is unilateral, and is usually in the distribution of the second or third division of the trigeminal nerve (i.e., over the cheekbone and jaw). Carbamazepine has been the first line of treatment in the past. Oxcarbazepine is as effective and has a better side effect profile. Other medications that can also be effective include gabapentin, phenytoin, baclofen, pregabalin, and duloxetine. If multiple drug regimens fail, referral for surgery may be considered.

TREATMENT PRINCIPLES

Headaches can be treated with medication, but drugs should be only a small part of the overall management. A multidisciplinary approach to treatment of primary headache is not only warranted, but also preferred in the elderly because of an increase in the potential for drug interactions and side effects. Alternative treatments such as biofeedback and cognitive-behavioral therapies can be effective (Middaugh & Pawlick, 2002). Situational, social, and psychological triggers should be addressed. Once a secondary headache is ruled out, the patient needs reassurance that there is no serious underlying pathology causing the headache. This alone may provide symptomatic improvement by relieving anxiety, which can exacerbate pain. A "headache diary" can help improve symptoms by giving the patient a sense of control and might identify triggers. All patients should be carefully assessed for common comorbid conditions—depression, anxiety, and sleep disorders—that can exacerbate headache symptoms. Appropriate treatment can significantly improve symptoms and potentially obviate the need for analgesics. The National Headache Foundation (2009) released a brochure summarizing alternative therapies for headache treatment.

Ingested substances that can trigger headache include prescription medications, alcohol, nitrites in hot dogs and processed meats, and monosodium glutamate (e.g., in Chinese food). Carbon monoxide can induce headaches, as can environmental changes (e.g., bright lights; odors; changes in humidity, air pressure, or temperature), hormonal changes, and emotional stress. The patient should be educated about these potential triggers and avoid them if possible. Other triggers may be delayed or missed meals, fatigue, exercise, and sexual activity. Changes in sleep patterns, such as insomnia or excessive sleeping, may contribute to symptoms of pain.

Although headache is a benign condition, it is associated with significant morbidity that is underestimated by the medical community. Sufferers of chronic headache disorders can have a lower level of function than patients with other chronic medical illnesses (Solomon, Skobieranda, & Gragg, 1993). With appropriate treatment, QOL can improve significantly, not only for the patient, but also for the family or caregivers.

Cary Buckner

Gonzalez-Gay, M. A., Barros, S., Lopez-Diaz, M. J., Garcia-Porrua, C., Sanchez-Andrade, A., & Llorca, J. (2005). Giant cell arteritis: Disease patterns of clinical presentation in a series of 240 patients. *Medicine, 84*(5), 269–276.

Headache Classification Committee of the International Headache Society. (1988). Classification and diagnostic criteria for headache disorders, cranial neuralgias and facial pain. *Cephalgia, 8*(Suppl. 7), 1–96.

Landy, S. H., & Lobo, B. L. (2005). Migraine treatment throughout the lifecycle. *Expert Review Neurotherapeutics, 5*(3), 343–353.

Lipton, R. B., Pfeffer, D., Newman, L. C., & Solomon, S. (1993). Headaches in the elderly. *Journal of Pain and Symptom Management, 8,* 87–97.

Middaugh, S. J., & Pawlick, K. (2002). Biofeedback and behavioral treatment of persistent pain in the older adult: A review and a study. *Applied Psychophysiology and Biofeedback, 27*(3), 185–202.

National Headache Foundation. (2009). Alternative headache therapies. Retrieved from http://www.headaches.org/2009/11/09/alternative-headache-therapies

Olesen, J. (2013). Headache Classification Committee of the International Headache Society. The International Classification of Headache Disorders (3rd edition; beta version). *Cephalgia, 33*(9), 629–808.

Prencipe, M., Casini, A., Ferretti, C., Santini, M., Pezzella, F., Scaldaferri, N., & Culasso, F. (2001). Prevalence of headache in an elderly population: Attack frequency, disability, and use of medication. *Journal of Neurology, Neurosurgery, and Psychiatry, 70*(3), 377–381.

Solomon, G. D., Skobieranda, F. G., & Gragg, L. A. (1993). Quality of life and well-being of headache patients: Measurement by the medical outcomes study instrument. *Headache, 33*(7), 351–358.

H

HEALTH PROMOTION SCREENING

Health promotion screening covers a broad range of health care services (tasks and tests) designed to prevent or limit disease and disability and maximize independence and quality of life (QOL) in older adults. Screening is only one aspect of health maintenance and promotion; others include vaccinations, prophylactic medications (e.g., aspirin), and a health-promoting lifestyle (e.g., balanced diet, regular physical and mental activity). Evidence of the effectiveness of screening older people is often lacking because older adults are often excluded from clinical trials. Nonetheless, different organizations have guidelines for screening older adults for modifiable risk factors for disease and for the diseases themselves in the early stages. At the same time, screening may not always be recommended in certain circumstances in which the risks may outweigh the benefits. Certain screening can cause harm psychologically and physically and lead to unnecessary biopsies and procedures with higher complication risks. This is especially true when life expectancy is less than 10 years. Therefore a more judicious approach should be taken when reviewing screening methods and recommendations.

DEPRESSION SCREENING

Clinical depression is common in older adults, and the suicide rate is twice as high as in the younger population. Depression is associated with increased morbidity and mortality from other physical illnesses, such as cardiovascular disease. Once depression in an older adult is identified, treatment can reduce the associated morbidity. In clinical trials, treatment of depression led to better levels of physical functioning.

In older adults, risk factors for depression include disability from medical illness, grief, sleep disturbance, loneliness, and poor social support. Common screening instruments include the Patient Health Questionnaire and the Geriatric Depression Scale. The U.S. Preventive Services Task Force (USPSTF; 2017) recommends screening all adults and no longer advises selective screening.

ALCOHOLISM SCREENING

Although moderate levels of alcohol consumption have been associated with improved cardiovascular outcomes, heavy drinking by older adults is associated with increased disability and even mortality. Alcohol counseling can reduce heavy drinking and may prevent the associated harm. In clinical trials, counseling (15 minutes) and follow-up led to a 13% to 34% reduction in the amount of drinking that was maintained in a follow-up 4 years later. The USPSTF (2013) recommends screening for alcoholism because there is moderate net benefit to such screening in adults aged 18 years and older. Single-question screening has adequate sensitivity and specificity for alcohol misuse in adults older than 65 years and takes less than 1 minute to administer: "How many times in the past year have you had 4 or more drinks in a day?" (Moyer, 2013).

SCREENING FOR FALLS

Of the 250,000 hip fractures every year in the United States, almost all occur when an elderly person falls during regular activities. Approximately half of older patients with hip fracture do not regain their prior level of physical functioning and lose independence. An intervention, such as the use of vitamin D supplementation (800 IU daily), has proven effective in reducing hip fractures in older adults at risk for falls. A meta-analysis demonstrated that multifactorial interventions (including home safety evaluation and physical therapy) reduce falls by 12 per 100 adults per month. The American Geriatrics Society (AGS) recommends screening older adults annually for fall risk. In addition, the USPSTF (2012) recommends exercise or physical therapy and vitamin D supplementation for fall prevention in community-dwelling adults aged 65 years or older who are at increased risk for falls.

OTHER SCREENING QUESTIONS

The USPSTF (2017) recommends asking about claudication (i.e., pain in calf muscles with walking), a symptom of peripheral atherosclerotic occlusive disease that is also a marker for increased risk for heart attacks and strokes and would trigger more aggressive use of aspirin and cholesterol-lowering drugs (i.e., statins). The USPSTF recommends screening for new difficulties with mobility and activities of daily living (ADL) and unintentional weight loss of 5% or 20 lb or more in 6 months.

SCREENING FOR SENSORY DEFICITS AND EARLY SENSORY CHANGES

Hearing loss affects 40% of adults aged 65 years or older and 80% of those aged 85 years and older. It leads to social isolation, depression, and reduced QOL and has been associated with falls, cognitive decline, physical decline, and increased mortality. Easy and effective screening tests are available; the whispered voice test has a sensitivity of 94%. Hearing aids can improve hearing and normalize QOL and mortality risk. However, for asymptomatic individuals, the USPSTF (2012) concludes that there is insufficient evidence for hearing screening.

Approximately 16% of 75- to 84-year-olds and 27% of those 85 years and older are unable to read newsprint (even with glasses). It has been shown that up to one third of geriatric clinic patients had undiagnosed yet correctable loss of vision. In addition, older adults with cataracts may have 2.5 times increased risk for motor vehicle accidents. Vision loss is also a risk factor for hip fractures and is associated with faster physical decline and greater mortality.

Screening for (and correcting) vision loss may prevent these effects (Kass et al., 2002).

Age-related macular degeneration (ARMD) is the leading cause of blindness in elderly White Americans. About a quarter of those aged 75 years or older have early ARMD. Early laser photocoagulation in such individuals improves visual outcomes (Wormald, Evans, Smeeth, & Henshaw, 2005). The cost of laser therapy per quality-adjusted life-year (QALY) gained is only $5,600. Although visual acuity testing may be adequate for identifying refractive error, it is not sufficient for identifying early ARMD or early cataracts. With regard to primary open-angle glaucoma, the USPSTF (2013) concludes that there is insufficient evidence for screening.

BLOOD PRESSURE SCREENING

Hypertension (high blood pressure) increases with age, and one in two adults aged 70 years or older has high blood pressure. Treatment of hypertension strives to prevent heart attack, strokes, and heart failure. Several studies report that healthy older adults with hypertension can be treated with modest doses of blood pressure medications that substantially decrease the risk of strokes, stroke-related mortality, coronary artery disease mortality, and mortality overall. The cost of treatment in women aged 70 years and older is $1,300 for every year of life gained. The efficacy of treatment is even greater in those aged 80 years and older. Unfortunately, many patients are not treated because of failure to identify hypertension and institute treatment. The USPSTF (2017) recommends screening every 2 years and at every clinic visit. Obtaining blood pressure measurements outside of the clinical setting (i.e., at home) for diagnostic confirmation of hypertension is recommended by the USPSTF (2017) before starting medications.

OTHER SCREENING EXAMINATIONS

The USPSTF recommends annual monitoring of height and weight to screen for silent vertebral fractures and unintentional weight loss, full skin examination in those with previous history of skin cancer or extensive skin damage from sun exposure, an oral examination in smokers and

H

alcoholics, and a thyroid examination in those with history of exposure to radiation. Unless there are symptoms, screening for cognitive impairment in older adults is not recommended by the USPSTF (2013).

BLOOD GLUCOSE SCREENING

Diabetes mellitus is present in one of every 10 adults 65 years of age or older, and one of four adults aged 85 years or older. Diabetes is a major risk factor for heart attacks and strokes and is responsible for substantial morbidity and increased mortality in older adults. The fasting blood glucose level is the main test for the screening and diagnosis of diabetes, with a value of 126 mg/dL or greater meeting the criterion for diabetes. Levels between 100 and 125 mg/dL indicate a prediabetic stage, with an increased risk for developing overt diabetes. Clinical trial data suggest (albeit in younger adults) that early interventions in those at increased risk for diabetes can prevent its onset (Siu, 2015)

Early and aggressive treatment to control blood glucose levels reduces the long-term complications of diabetes—retinopathy, nephropathy, neuropathy, cardiovascular disease, and peripheral vascular disease. The USPSTF (2015) recommends screening all obese adults because obesity, especially abdominal obesity—waist girth greater than 40 in. for men and 36 in. for women—is a risk factor for diabetes; those from high-risk ethnic groups (i.e., African Americans, Native Americans, Hispanic Americans, Alaskan Natives, Asian Americans, Pacific Islanders); and those with other risk factors for cardiovascular disease (i.e., hypertension and/or hyperlipidemia).

SERUM CHOLESTEROL SCREENING

Several observational studies have found that high levels of serum cholesterol are associated with increased risk for cardiovascular events (e.g., heart attacks, strokes, peripheral arterial occlusions). Analysis of data from elderly subgroups in clinical trials shows that treatment with statins (i.e., the most effective class of cholesterol-lowering drugs) significantly reduces this risk.

Hypercholesterolemia screening is indicated in people with evidence of coronary artery disease (e.g., previous heart attack, coronary bypass or angioplasty, known angina pectoris), other atherosclerotic vascular disease (e.g., stroke, transient brain ischemia, or leg claudication [pain in calf muscles with walking]), or diabetes mellitus. According to the National Cholesterol Education Program Adult Treatment Panel III (ATP III), which were last updated in 2013, all three groups of adults were recommended to keep their low-density lipoprotein (LDL) cholesterol levels below 100 mg/dL, and statins should be instituted if LDL levels rise above that (Grundy et al., 2004; National Cholesterol Education Program (NCEP) ATP III, 2001). There is no age cutoff for cholesterol screening and treatment with statins for these individuals. In some very-high-risk individuals (e.g., those with a recent cardiovascular event, diabetics or smokers with known cardiovascular disease), the target LDL cholesterol level is even lower: 70 mg/dL (NCEP ATP III 2001). In 2013, the American College of Cardiology (ACC) and the American Heart Association (AHA) issued guidelines for the treatment of high blood cholesterol (Stone, Robinson, & Lichenstein, 2014) that updated the previous report of the National Cholesterol Education Program (NCEP). The ACC/AHA (Stone et al., 2014) provide a very different perspective for cholesterol management, in that LDL is not the central goal but rather focus on statin treatment instructions (Grundy, 2013).

In older adults who do not fall into one of the three high-risk groups, evidence is not as strong for the screening and treatment of elevated cholesterol levels. Based primarily on evidence from clinical trials in younger adults, the NCEP recommends cholesterol screening and treatment (if indicated) to bring LDL levels below 100 mg/dL in all older adults who smoke, have metabolic syndrome, or have serum C-reactive protein (CRP) levels higher than 3 mg/dL. The target LDL level is 130 mg/dL in older adults with either hypertension or low levels of high-density lipoprotein (HDL) cholesterol (i.e., below 40 mg/dL).

According to Walsh and Pignone (2004), there is insufficient evidence for benefit from screening and treating older men who have no cardiovascular risk factors, and there is no benefit from treatment with statins in older women (Walsh & Pignone, 2004). The USPSTF (2008), however, recommends screening for lipid disorders in women aged 45 years and older who are at increased risk for coronary heart disease and in all men aged 35 years and older. The ACP does not recommend screening for primary prevention in men and women 75 years of age and older who have no risk factors for cardiovascular disease.

The 10-year risk of heart disease or stoke can be determined using the Arteriosclerotic Cardiovascular Disease (ASCVD) Risk Estimator Calculator, which is available on the American College of Cardiology (ACC) and American Heart Association (AHA) website (tools.acc.org/ASCVD-Risk-Estimator). This calculator, which was released in 2013, can help guide decision making about whether to start statin therapy. New guidelines in 2013 from the ACC/AHA abandon the traditional LDL and non-HDL targets, and physicians are no longer asked to treat patients who have cardiovascular disease with an LDL of less than 100 mg/dL or an optional goal of less than 70 mg/dL. Instead, the new guidelines identify four categories of patients for primary and secondary prevention and recommend that patients with a 10-year risk of atherosclerotic cardiovascular disease of greater than 7.5% be treated with a high-intensity statin to achieve at least a 50% reduction in LDL cholesterol. For patients who have contraindications to high-intensity statins or have statin-associated adverse events, a moderate-intensity statin can be tried instead (Nayor & Vasan, 2016).

URINE SCREENING TESTS

Neither the ACP nor the USPSTF recommends routine urinalysis screening in asymptomatic older adults. However, it can be cost-effective to screen older adults for microalbuminuria and treat those with a urine albumin-to-creatinine ratio greater than 30 with a kidney-protective agent (e.g., angiotensin-converting enzyme [ACE] inhibitor, angiotensin receptor blocker). Everyone with diabetes mellitus should be screened annually and treated. In addition, it appears cost-effective to annually screen and treat all older adults irrespective of their diabetes status; the cost of such a screening and treatment practice in adults aged 60 years and older with hypertension is $19,000 per QALY saved and $54,000 per QALY saved in adults who are aged 60 years or older and who do not have either hypertension or diabetes mellitus (Boulware, Jarr, Tarver-Carr, Brancati, & Powe, 2003).

AORTIC ANEURYSM SCREENING

There are 15,000 deaths related to abdominal aortic aneurysms (AAAs) every year in the United States. Approximately 1% of adults aged 60 years and older have an AAA 5 cm or larger. In the United Kingdom, a clinical trial of ultrasound imaging screened for AAAs in asymptomatic individuals aged 65 years and older, preventing AAA-related deaths in men but not in women (Wilmink, Forshaw, Quick, Hubbard, & Day, 2002). The USPSTF (2014) recommends a one-time screening of male smokers 65 to 75 years of age; for female smokers in the same group, there is an insufficient evidence for screening.

BONE DENSITY SCREENING

The lifetime risk of an osteoporotic fracture in American women is 50%. Bone-mineral density in the femoral neck is an excellent predictor of hip fracture risk, and treatment of high-risk women with bisphosphonates reduces their risk for hip fractures. The USPSTF recommends screening every woman older than 65 years of age (USPSTF, 2017). The ACP recommends that physicians periodically evaluate older men for osteoporosis risk factors (i.e., age greater than 70, low body mass index [BMI] less than 20–25 kg/m², weight loss, androgen deprivation therapy, corticosteroid use, prior history of fragility fracture) and obtain dual-energy x-ray absorptiometry (DXA) scan for those who are at an increased risk for osteoporosis and who are candidates for drug treatment (Qaseem et al., 2008).

Vitamin D deficiency also affects bone health and has been associated with poor health outcomes. There are associations between low

25-hydroxy vitamin D levels and risk for falls, fractures, cardiovascular disease, colorectal cancer, diabetes, depression, and cognitive decline. Generally, levels lower than 50 nmol/L are associated with decreased bone health. Overall, conclusions indicate that treating vitamin D deficiency can reduce mortality risk in elderly individuals and their risk for falls but not for fractures (USPSTF, 2015).

SCREENING MAMMOGRAMS

In the United States, 45% of new breast cancer cases and 56% of breast cancer deaths occur in women aged 65 years and older. Clinical trial data show that in 50- to 74-year-old women, screening mammograms reduce breast cancer deaths by 25% and overall mortality by 2%; there was no difference between annual and biennial (i.e., every 2 years) screening strategies with respect to benefits (USPSTF, 2017). The USPSTF recommends a biennial screening mammogram in women aged 50 to 74 years. However, the American Cancer Society recommends biennial screening mammograms in older women until remaining life expectancy is 5 years or less.

However, breast cancer screening is not without harm. One in 10 mammograms give a false-positive result, and after 10 screening mammograms, there is a 50% chance of a false-positive finding and an 18% chance of an unnecessary biopsy with the accompanying anxiety about cancer. Recently, there has been controversy about whether the benefits from regular screening mammograms really exceed the harm. According to a recent study in the *New England Journal of Medicine*, women were more likely to have breast cancer that was over-diagnosed than to have earlier detection of a tumor that was destined to become large; the decline in breast cancer mortality after screening mammography is due to improved systemic treatment (Welch, Prorok, O'Malley, & Kramer, 2016).

LUNG SCREENING

Lung cancer is the leading cause of cancer death in the United States, with 85% of lung cancers due to smoking. The USPSTF (2017) recommends lung cancer screening in asymptomatic, older adults aged 55 to 80 years who have a 30-pack-year smoking history and currently smoke or have quit smoking within the past 15 years. Annual screening with low-dose CT (LDCT) has shown moderate net benefit. The Canadian Task Force on Preventative Health Care (CTFPHC, 2016) recommends screening with LDCT, however, for only three consecutive times. Screening should be discontinued in those who have not smoked for 15 years (USPSFT, 2013)

Chronic obstructive pulmonary disease (COPD) is a leading cause of death in the United States. However, screening for COPD in asymptomatic individuals does not improve QOL, morbidity, or mortality and is not recommended by the USPSTF (2016).

COLON SCREENING

The lifetime risk of colon cancer is 5%, and 94% of new cases are in adults aged 65 years and older. Colorectal cancer is the second leading cause of cancer deaths and is responsible for 60,000 deaths every year in the United States. The USPSTF (2017) recommends colorectal cancer screening in all older adults by using one of five strategies: (a) annual occult blood testing on six stool specimens from three different days, followed by colonoscopy on those testing positive; (b) flexible sigmoid examination of the distal colon every 5 years with fecal occult blood testing every 3 years; (c) colonoscopy every 10 years; (d) multitargeted stool DNA testing; or (e) CT colonography. A single fecal blood test during a routine clinic visit is inadequate; its sensitivity is less than 5% (Collins, Lieberman, Durbin, & Weiss, 2005). The USPSTF (2017) recommends against routine screening after 85 years of age in high-risk individuals. For those aged 76 to 85 years, colorectal cancer screening should be individualized; those who have never been screened may benefit if they are healthy enough to undergo treatment if cancer is found.

It is also important to consider when to discontinue screening. In general, one should consider stopping screening when life expectancy is less than 10 years or if the consequence of screening results in interventions and treatments that are of higher risk than benefit.

OTHER SCREENING LABORATORY TESTS

Screening for prostate cancer remains a controversial topic; the USPSTF (2012) recommends against prostate-specific antigen–based screening for prostate cancer. A clinician who decides to screen should ensure that the patient is advised of the benefits and harms of screening. Screening for hepatitis C virus infection is recommended in all high-risk individuals, with one-time screening to be offered to all those born between 1945 and 1965 (USPSTF, 2013).

SCREENING TESTS OF THE FUTURE

Several new laboratory and imaging tests may have potential as screening tests but have not yet been perfected or adequately evaluated for screening effectiveness and cost. Among them are coronary calcium measurements by high-resolution imaging (as a screen for coronary artery disease), helical CT for screening of smokers for lung cancer, MR mammography, and PET imaging of the brain to screen for Alzheimer's disease.

Despite the availability of national screening guidelines, health care providers must individualize the use of screening tasks and tests based on the older patient's existing medical conditions, beliefs and value system, and personal preferences.

See also Gait Assessment Instruments.

Hong-Phuc T. Tran, Susan D. Leonard, and Arun S. Karlamangla

Boulware, L. E., Jaar, B. G., Tarver-Carr, M. E., Brancati, F. L., & Powe, N. R. (2003). Screening for proteinuria in U.S. adults: A cost-effectiveness analysis. *Journal of the American Medical Association, 290*(23), 3101–3114.

Canadian Task Force on Preventive Health Care. (2016). Recommendations on screening for lung cancer. *Canadian Medical Association Journal, 188*(6), 425–432.

Collins, J. F., Lieberman, D. A., Durbin, T. E., & Weiss, D. G. (2005). Veterans Affairs Cooperative Study #380 Group. Accuracy of screening for fecal occult blood on a single stool sample obtained by digital rectal examination: A comparison with recommended sampling practice. *Annals of Internal Medicine, 142*(2), 81–85.

Grundy, S. M. (2013). Then and now: ATP III vs. IV. Retrieved from http://www.acc.org/latest-in-cardiology/articles/2014/07/18/16/03/then-and-now-atp-iii-vs-iv

Grundy, S. M., Cleeman, J. I., Bairey Merz, C. N., Brewer, H. B., Jr., Clark, L. T., Hunninghake, D. B., ... Stone, N. J., for the Coordinating Committee of the National Cholesterol Education Program. (2004). Implications of recent clinical trials for the National Cholesterol Education Program Adult Treatment Panel III Guidelines. *Circulation, 110,* 227–239.

Kass, M. A., Heuer, D. K., Higginbotham, E. J., Johnson, C. A., Keltner, J. L., Miller, J. P., ... Gordon, M. O. (2002). The Ocular Hypertension Treatment Study: A randomized trial determines that topical ocular hypotensive medication delays or prevents the onset of primary open-angle glaucoma. *Archives of Ophthalmology, 120*(6), 701–713.

Moyer, V. (2013). Screening and behavioral counseling interventions in primary care to reduce alcohol misuse: U.S. Preventive Services Task Force Recommendation Statement. *Annals of Internal Medicine, 159,* 210–218.

National Cholesterol Education Program Adult Treatment Panel III. (2001). Executive summary of the third report of the National Cholesterol Education Program (NCEP) Expert Panel on Detection, Evaluation, and Treatment of High Blood Cholesterol in Adults (Adult Treatment Panel III). *Journal of the American Medical Association, 285,* 2486–2497.

Nayor, M., & Vasan, R. S. (2016). Recent update to the US cholesterol treatment guidelines. *Circulation, 133,* 1795–1806.

Preventive Health Care. (2016). Recommendations on screening for lung cancer. *Canadian Medical Association Journal, 188*(6), 425–432.

Qaseem, A., Snow, V., Shekelle, P., Hopkins, R., Jr., Forciea, M. A., & Owens, D. K. (2008). Screening for osteoporosis in men: A clinical practice guideline from the American College of Physicians. *Annals of Internal Medicine, 148*(9), 680–684.

Siu, A. (2015). Screening for abnormal blood glucose and type 2 diabetes mellitus: U.S. Preventive Services Task Force Recommendation Statement. *Annals of Internal Medicine, 163,* 861–868.

Stone, N. J., Robinson, J. G., & Lichtenstein, A. H. (2014). 2013 ACC/AHA guideline on the treatment of blood cholesterol to reduce atherosclerotic cardiovascular risk in adults: A report of the American College of Cardiology/American Heart Association Task Force on Practice Guidelines.

Journal of the American College of Cardiology, 63(25), 3024–3025.

U.S. Preventive Services Task Force. (2014). The guide to clinical preventive services 2014. *Agency for Health care Research and Quality*. Retrieved from https://www.uspreventive servicestaskforce.org/Page/Name/tools-and -resources-for-better-preventive-care

U.S. Preventive Services Task Force. (2017). Published recommendations. Retrieved from https://www .uspreventiveservicestaskforce.org/BrowseRec/ Index

Walsh, J. M., & Pignone, M. (2004). Drug treatment of hyperlipidemia in women. *Journal of the American Medical Association, 291*(18), 2243–2252.

Welch, H. G., Prorok, P. C., O'Malley, A. J., & Kramer, B. S. (2016). Breast-cancer tumor size, overdi-agnosis, and mammography screening effec-tiveness. *New England Journal of Medicine, 375*, 1438–1447.

Wilmink, A. B., Forshaw, M., Quick, C. R., Hubbard, C. S., & Day, N. E. (2002). Accuracy of serial screening for abdominal aortic aneurysms by ultrasound. *Journal of Medical Screening, 9*(3), 125–127.

Wormald, R., Evans, J., Smeeth, L., & Henshaw, K. (2005). Photodynamic therapy for neovascu-lar age related macular degeneration. *Cochrane Database of Systematic Reviews, 2005*(4), CD002030. doi:10.1002/14651858.CD002030.pub2

Web Resources

Agency for Healthcare Research and Quality: http:// www.ahcpr.gov/clinic/uspstfix.htm

American Geriatrics Society: http://www.american geriatrics.org

American Heart Association: http://www.american heart.org

American Medical Association: http://www .ama-assn.org/ama

Arteriosclerotic Cardiovascular Disease (ASCVD) Risk Estimator Calculator: http://tools.acc .org/ASCVD-Risk-Estimator

Canadian Task Force on Preventive Health Care: http://canadiantaskforce.ca

Centers for Disease Control and Prevention: http:// www.cdc.gov

National Heart, Lung, and Blood Institute: http:// www.nhlbi.nih.gov

National Institute of Diabetes and Digestive and Kidney Diseases: http://www.niddk.nih.gov

U.S. Preventive Service Task Force: http://www .uspreventiveservicestaskforce.org/Page/Name/ recommendations

HEARING AIDS

Hearing aids, also referred to as *amplification*, are devices that allow individuals with hearing loss to receive auditory information at adjusted levels in the presence of a deficit in hearing sen-sitivity. Although human hearing spans the fre-quencies from 20 to 20,000 Hz, it is the range of speech from 500 to 6,000 Hz for which hear-ing aids are manufactured, thus assisting opti-mal communication efforts (Brant et al., 1996). Hearing aids can boost a signal's loudness from as softly as 20 decibels (dB) to as much as 120 dB or more.

Per statistics from the Centers for Disease Control and Prevention published in 2014, approximately 15% of adults older than 18 years indicate difficulty hearing (Carroll et al., 2017). Furthermore, between two and three out of every 1,000 infants born in the United States have some form of hearing loss caused by syn-dromes, hereditary sources, or disease processes (Blackwell, Lucas, & Clarke, 2014). The numbers of individuals experiencing significant hearing loss in the United States alone can conserva-tively be estimated at 38 million, or 10% of the population.

The most likely common causes of hearing loss in the adult demographic that are not a direct result of diseases process or syndromes are aging, noise, and chemical exposure to the auditory systems. The elderly and the so-called Baby Boomer generation are popu-lations in which research demonstrates that deficits in audition can cause declines in emo-tional health and cognitive function (Lin et al., 2013).

SELECTION PROCESS

Protocols to improve functional communication for the patient demonstrating a significant hear-ing loss are consistently used by audiologists and hearing instrument specialists. The steps they utilize are testing to document the degree of hearing loss, appropriate referrals to medi-cal professionals to determine the cause of and medical treatment for hearing loss, prescription of correct amplification and its options, and verification and validation of the prescribed instrument's benefits (Jorgensen, 2016; Valente et al., 1998).

1. Evaluation—Hearing loss is first documented via an audiogram, which is a record of behavioral and objective measures. The audiologist examines the auditory system and records for each ear, the degree of hearing loss and affected frequencies, and ways that the patient can discriminate the spoken word. These behavioral measures are confirmed via objective tests of middle and inner ear function.
2. Medical clearance—Appropriate care of the patient with hearing loss dictates that medical clearance be performed prior to the prescription of amplification.
3. Prescription—Consideration in selecting the appropriate style of hearing aid is made at the time of service with respect to the patient's physical, social, and vocational needs (see Components and Styles/Types in the following text). Notably, two of the key elements of successful dispensing and use of amplification is (a) the patient's realistic expectations about the instrument (what it can and cannot do in performance) and (b) the level of motivation the patient has to use the instrument. This often requires counseling from hearing health care and other health care professionals, as well as support from family and social systems.
4. Verification—The dispensing audiologist measures the usefulness of the prescribed amplifier via objective assessment, such as the real ear measurement, and/or behaviorally via performance in the sound field. This process helps ensure that the patient is optimally assisted with considerations to the physical condition of the ear and style of hearing aid.
5. Validation—After a short period of initial use, perhaps 1 or 2 weeks, the patient returns to the audiologist for adjustments and further measures to ensure best performance of the hearing aid. One or two further adjustment visits to the audiologist are not uncommon.

COMPONENTS AND STYLES/TYPES

The components of a hearing aid are straightforward in theory but complicated in execution. All hearing aids are powered by batteries, which vary in size depending on style; the smaller the hearing aid, the smaller the battery. Regarding the function of the instrument, digital circuitry has vastly improved the benefit that came with analog circuits 40 years ago. Whether analog or digital, the theoretical amplification process is the same: Sound (the acoustical signal) enters the instrument through a microphone, which converts it into an electronic signal. An amplifier enhances the electrical signal, sending it to the receiver, which delivers the modified sound either directly into the ear canal or through an earmold that rests in the ear canal. Usually, the hearing aid also has a volume control for adjusting the loudness of the signal entering the ear.

The complexities of an appropriate hearing aid fitting arise from several sites on the instrument itself and within its circuitry. For instance, the microphone location can affect what the patient hears. When microphone placement is designed close to the opening of the ear canal rather than elsewhere on the hearing aid casing, the acoustic signal begins to assume similar properties to the natural configuration of the ear. Furthermore, binaural amplification offers the advantage of avoiding auditory deprivation (Gelfand, Silman, & Ross, 1987). Analog or digital technology on which the amplifier is constructed allows for numerous modifications of the electronic signal and its enhancement.

Hearing aid types and styles that are currently available on the market are greatly varied, making the selection of the appropriate instrument an important process. This is based on physical dexterity, cosmetic concerns, and availability of advanced circuitry, which can allow for programmability and connection to Bluetooth technology. Notably, these considerations also make for more expensive instruments.

Batteries

The energy source that supplies the power to a hearing aid, the battery has advanced; it offers more power in a smaller size, thus enabling a revolution in hearing aid design. In this age of heightened eco-friendly mindfulness, rechargeable hearing aids have now allowed for environmental and financial conservation.

Earmolds

Every ear is different in terms of its shape and size. Customized earmold fittings have the advantage of physically comfortable seating in the outer ear (concha) and entry into the ear canal. Properly fit earmolds reduce feedback and improve clarity of sound. Hearing aid manufacturers have also introduced excellent noncustomized earmolds especially advanced behind-the-ear (BTE) aids.

Body Hearing Aids

The first electrical type of hearing aid, the body or pocket aid, was invented in the late 19th century. It was an instrument designed for placement on the body in a harness or pocket. Today, it is less often prescribed due to technological advances in miniaturizing components. As the amplifier's components are placed at a distance from ear level, the directionality of sound is lost to the user.

BTE Hearing Aids

BTE hearing aids were introduced in the 1950s due to the benefits of mass-produced transistors. Throughout the years, the BTE aid has advanced in terms of reduction of size because of smaller batteries and, most important, the introduction of digital technology. Today's BTE aids allow for programming by the audiologist via advanced, but proprietary, software from each manufacturer. The BTE aid can closely assume the natural process of the human ear hearing sound via receiver-in-canal (RIC) technology. Paired with digital technology in the amplifier, the RIC type of BTE aids offers superior benefit to the user. With BTE aids becoming smaller, the manufacturers have also started to offer more cosmetically appealing instruments with a variety of colors and sleek encasement of the components.

In-the-Ear, In-the-Canal, and Completely In-Canal Hearing Aids

In the late 20th century, in-the-ear (ITE), in-the-canal (ITC), and completely-in-canal (CIC) hearing aids were introduced as yet another benefit to the consumer as a result of miniaturization of components. The complete units fit entirely in the ear, offering the user a sense of confidence with regards to cosmetic appeal as well as improved microphone placement at the opening of the ear canal. This style of hearing aid accounts for about 80% of hearing aids in North America according to the Better Hearing Institute (2016).

With these styles, the user must compare the benefits of cosmetic appeal with sound quality; patients are best served by consulting with the audiologist to acquire the best compromise between the two.

FEEDBACK

A whistling sound may be generated when an uninterrupted signal produced by the receiver feeds back into the microphone. Feedback generally occurs from improper hearing aid fitting or poor placement in the ear, along with increased volume. Ensuring that the instrument is correctly seated in the ear and lowering the volume can usually remedy feedback.

TINNITUS AND AMPLIFICATION

Tinnitus, when not part of a disease process or physically induced, is the perception of a phantom sound by the brain which is likely caused by damaged inner ear cells. According to the Mayo Clinic (2016), one in five people suffer from tinnitus, with a large number of them able to tolerate the problem. Although many people learn to ignore tinnitus, others at the opposite end of the spectrum are troubled to the point of requiring psychiatric support. Because the majority of tinnitus sufferers also have some degree of hearing loss, amplification has demonstrated an advantage in terms of offering some relief from the problem.

Hearing aids offer a passive mechanism of benefit by, in some cases, masking the tinnitus. This is found when the acoustic signal delivered to the ear via the amplifier is louder than the perceived phantom sound. The tinnitus becomes less noticeable when the amplified sound is introduced into the auditory system.

Some manufacturers have specially designed hearing aids that can be further customized for the tinnitus sufferer. Research suggests that these hearing aids, along with counseling techniques known as *sound therapy*, are successful for this segment of the hearing loss population (Del Bo & Ambrosetti, 2007).

HEARING AID COST AND INSURANCE COVERAGE

The cost of amplification has increased somewhat with the emergence of advanced hearing aid technologies over the past several decades. A binaural hearing aid fitting (two hearing aids) may range from approximately $3,000 to $7,000. Notably, many insurance plans do not routinely cover the cost of amplification, nor does Medicare. The expense of hearing aids, items that typically have a 5-year life span, requires financial planning for a population that is increasing in size.

CONCLUSION

Although amplification has a number of technical drawbacks, it is far more advanced now than it was even 20 years ago. Manufacturers and professionals in the industry understand the current limitations of amplification and are working to generate even more advances in coping with issues regarding the user understanding speech in noisy environments—the most common complaint of hearing aid users. There are noteworthy accomplishments in digital technology and even cosmetics, which make hearing aids both socially acceptable, as well as highly functional.

Hearing aids offer a significant value to the population that requires improved social, vocational, or academic communication. The complexities of hearing aid fittings are best resourced to professionals who are experienced in communication; these specialists understand the needs of various populations experiencing hearing loss, as well as the causes of hearing loss.

Donald A. Vogel

Better Hearing Institute. (2016). Understanding hearing aids. Retrieved from http://www.better hearing.org/hearingpedia/hearing-aids

Blackwell, D. L., Lucas, J. W., & Clarke, T.C. (2014). Summary health statistics for U.S. adults: National Health Interview Survey, 2012. National Center for Health Statistics. *Vital Health Statistics, 10*(260), 1–61.

Brant, L. J., Gordon-Salantt, S., Pearson, J. D., Klein, L. L., Morrell, C. H., Metter, E. J, & Fozard, J. L. (1996). Risk factors related to age-associated hearing loss in the speech frequencies. *Journal of the American Academy of Audiology, 7*(3), 152–160.

Carroll, Y. I., Eichwald, J., Scinicariello, F., Hoffman, H. J., Deitchman, S., Radke, M. S., … Breysse, P. (2017). Vital signs: Noise-induced hearing loss among adults—United States 2011–2012. *Morbidity and Mortality Weekly Report, 66*(5), 139–144. Retrieved from https://www.cdc.gov/mmwr/volumes/66/wr/mm6605e3.htm

Del Bo, L., & Ambrosetti, U. (2007). Hearing aids for the treatment of tinnitus. *Progress in Brain Research, 166*, 341–345.

Gelfand, S., Silman, S., & Ross, L. (1987). Long-term effects of monaural, binaural and no amplification in subjects with bilateral hearing loss. *Journal of Scandinavian Audiology, 16*(4), 201–207.

Jorgensen, L. E. (2016) Verification and validation of hearing aids: Opportunity not an obstacle. *Journal of Otology, 11*(2), 57–62.

Lin, F. R., Yaffe, K., Xia, J., Xue, Q., Harris, T. B., Purchase-Helzner, E., … Simonsick, E. M. (2013). Hearing loss and cognitive decline in older adults. *JAMA Internal Medicine, 173*(4), 293–299. Retrieved from http://archinte.jamanetwork.com/article.aspx?articleid=1558452&resultclick=1

Mayo Clinic. (2016). Tinnitus. Retrieved from http://www.mayoclinic.org/diseases-conditions/tinni tus/symptoms-causes/dxc-20180362

Valente, M., Bentler, R., Kaplan, H. S., Seewald, R., Trine, T., van Vliet, D., & Higdon, L. W. (1998, March). Guidelines for hearing aid fitting for adults. *American Journal of Audiology, 7*(1), 5.

HEARING IMPAIRMENT

Hearing impairment is one of the most common chronic health conditions affecting older adults. Among noninstitutionalized elderly, hearing loss is the third most common condition after hypertension and arthritis. Approximately one third of the U.S. population older than 65 years has some degree of hearing loss. In nursing homes, 70% of residents have significant hearing loss (Warshaw & Moqeet, 1998). Gates, Cooper, Kannel, and Miller (1990) noted that only 10% of those in the Framingham cohort (1983–1985) who were likely to benefit from amplification had acquired hearing aids. Despite its prevalence, hearing impairment and its impact on quality of life often go unnoticed. Hearing impairment has been associated with social isolation, depression, and decreased cognitive functioning in the elderly. The relationship between such impairment and Alzheimer's dementia has been increasingly researched (Lin, Ferucci, et al., 2011a; Lin, Metter, et al., 2011b; Peracino, 2014).

Auditory function is dependent on the total functioning of the auditory pathways, from the external auditory canal to the auditory centers of the brain. The peripheral hearing apparatus—external ear, middle ear, inner ear, and the eighth cranial nerve—composes the conductive and sensorineural components of hearing. The external ear, containing the auricular concha and external auditory canal, directs sound medially to the tympanic membrane. When sound waves reach the tympanic membrane, the vibration sets into motion the three middle-ear ossicles: malleus, incus, and stapes. The middle ear acts as an impedance-matching mechanism and transmits acoustic energy from the air to the fluid of the inner ear, where the cochlea converts the sound from mechanical to electrical energy. This electrical energy, or nerve impulse, is transmitted via the eighth cranial nerve to the brainstem and central nervous system.

There are several age-related physiological changes taking place within the hearing apparatus. The external auditory canal is affected by atrophy of the cerumen glands, resulting in drier cerumen and an increasing risk of impaction in the elderly. Tympanosclerosis, or atrophic and sclerotic changes of the tympanic membrane itself, caused by previous middle-ear infections, are common. The effects of these changes are generally negligible with respect to hearing. Otosclerosis, the fixation of the stapes footplate to the oval window, causes conductive hearing loss in up to 10% of the elderly population, but its hearing-loss effects are usually present from earlier in life. Aging changes that may occur in the inner ear include atrophy of the basal end of the cochlea (the area responsible for high-frequency sounds), loss of hair cells, and loss of neurons in the auditory centers of the cortex and brainstem

TYPES

There are four types of hearing loss: conductive, sensorineural, mixed, and central auditory processing disorder (CAPD). *Conductive hearing loss* is impairment in the mechanical mechanisms of the outer and middle ear by which sound reaches the cochlea. It is characterized by disorders that impede the normal transmission of sound waves though the external canal, tympanic membrane, or middle ear. Thus there is a reduction in air-conducted, but not in bone-conducted, sounds. Conditions that frequently result in conductive hearing loss include impacted cerumen, tympanic membrane perforation, otitis media, and discontinuity or fixation of the middle-ear ossicles (e.g., otosclerosis, Paget's disease)

Sensorineural hearing loss occurs when the cochlea or the auditory nerve is not functioning properly and therefore is characterized by equal reduction in air and bone conduction. This type of hearing loss can be either congenital or acquired. The cochlea is the most common site of damage secondary to hair cell damage or ganglion cell loss.

The most common cause of sensorineural hearing loss in the aged is presbycusis, which affects one third of those older than 75 years of age. Presbycusis is an insidious hearing loss that initially is most pronounced at higher frequencies. Some few patients exhibit a flat configuration, with loss of hearing sensitivity essentially equal at all frequencies across the audiometric range (250–8,000 Hz). High-frequency hearing loss affects the ability to recognize or discriminate speech sounds especially in environments with background noise. Persons with presbycusis usually know when they are being spoken to, but they may not always understand what is said; they can hear the low-frequency and more acoustically powerful vowels but find distinctions among higher-frequency consonant sounds such as *f*, *s*, *th*, *h*, and *sh* difficult. The cause of presbycusis remains unclear. Studies have attempted to link the effects of metabolism, arteriosclerosis, smoking, noise exposure,

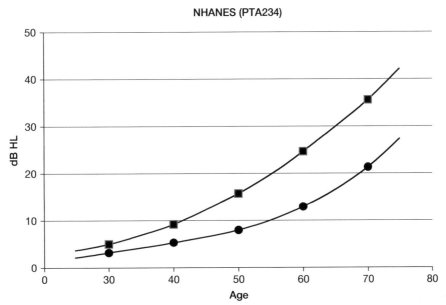

FIGURE H.1 Age-related change in the median threshold values of high-frequency sensitivity (2,000, 3,000, and 4,000 Hz) from the National Health and Nutrition Examination Survey (NHANES) 1999–2006.

Note: Squares indicate hearing loss in men; circles indicate hearing loss in women.

dB HL, decibels of hearing loss.

Source: Agrawal, Platz, and Niparko (2008).

genetics, diet, and stress. Presbycusis remains a diagnosis of exclusion; other causes of bilateral, progressive sensorineural hearing loss must be ruled out before the diagnosis can be made. This age-related change is demonstrated by the median threshold values of high-frequency sensitivity (2,000, 3,000, and 4,000 Hz) per the National Health and Nutrition Examination Survey (NHANES) 1999 to 2006 (Figure H.1).

Mixed hearing loss is a combination of conductive and sensorineural hearing loss. Air and bone conduction are both reduced, but loss of air conduction is greater.

A *CAPD* is a deterioration of auditory perceptual abilities that may be associated with the aging process, which is separate from the loss of hearing sensitivity associated with changes in the peripheral auditory mechanism, particularly the cochlea. An example of CAPD is a disproportionate reduction of the ability to understand speech in the presence of background noise or the inability to understand distorted or rapid speech. A CAPD is often mistaken for cognitive decline.

DIAGNOSIS

The first step in identifying hearing loss is obtaining information about its onset, character, and progression. Was the onset sudden, gradual, or insidious, unilateral or bilateral? Does it fluctuate, is it static, or is it progressive? A complaint of adult-onset unilateral hearing loss at any age raises suspicion of eighth cranial nerve compromise, whereas symmetrical, bilateral hearing loss of gradual onset in persons older than the age of 60 years is most often associated with presbycusis. Méniére's disease is associated with tinnitus, episodic vertigo, and fluctuating, rather than progressive, hearing loss.

It is necessary to inquire about predisposing factors such as head trauma, exposure to noise (industrial, environmental, or recreational), involvement of a neoplastic process, or family history of hearing loss. Medications must be carefully reviewed because commonly used drugs, such as the aminoglycoside antibiotics, loop diuretics, salicylates, antineoplastic agents

H

(e.g., cisplatin, oral or parenteral erythromycin), and many others, have ototoxic properties. Complaints similar to those encountered in presbycusis may accompany hearing loss secondary to excessive noise exposure, and such exposure, along with aging, may play a significant role in an individual's total hearing loss. On physical examination, any disfigurement of the ear architecture, including the auricle and external auditory canal, should be noted. The tympanic membrane should be closely observed for foreign body, impacted cerumen, perforation, tympanosclerosis, effusion, or infection. A complete head and neck, cranial nerve, and if indicated, neurological examination should be performed.

Screening techniques include simple tuning fork tests, such as the Rinne and Weber tests, although they provide qualitative rather than quantitative data. The Rinne test is performed by placing the stem of a vibrating tuning fork on the mastoid process (i.e., bone conduction) and then suspending the fork adjacent to the ear canal (i.e., air conduction). The patient is asked to determine in which position the sound is louder. Normally, air conduction is greater than bone conduction, so the sound would be louder with the tuning fork placed in front of the ear. The Weber test is performed by placing a vibrating tuning fork on the midline of the forehead and asking the patient which ear perceives the sound. In conductive hearing loss, the sound is louder in the affected ear; in sensorineural hearing loss, the sound is louder in the unaffected ear.

Audiometric screening in the office is recommended. Basic pure tone audiometers for manual screening or automatic audiometers that allow a patient to self-test (and provide more useful threshold data) should be part of a geriatric assessment. A relatively quiet location in the examination facility should be used for a reasonable assessment of auditory sensitivity. If hearing impairment is suspected after an office-based screening, referral to an audiologist for formal assessment is recommended.

Loss of hearing sensitivity is measured in units of sound known as decibels (dB). The greater the intensity of sound (in dBs) required for a person to hear, the poorer the hearing. Pure tone thresholds higher than 25 dB in the speech frequencies (500 through 3,000 Hz) are generally satisfactory for routine listening needs, whereas significant sensitivity loss in this range or more commonly at 3,000 Hz and above may suggest the need for intervention with prosthetic amplification.

Pure tone audiograms reflect the type of hearing loss (i.e., sensorineural, conductive, or mixed), magnitude of the loss, and unilateral or bilateral nature of the loss (i.e., including symmetry), as well as the frequencies at which the loss occurs. Speech sound discrimination or recognition, tested for each ear, identifies the degree to which a person understands spoken words (i.e., word intelligibility) in quiet and possibly in noise.

A tympanogram, which is generally part of the routine audiological test battery, provides a measure of tympanic membrane mobility and assesses middle-ear pressure. This analysis, often in conjunction with acoustic reflex assessment, can assist in the diagnosis of tympanic membrane perforation, effusion, ossicular fixation, ossicular discontinuity, and other causes of conductive hearing loss. Measurement of the brainstem auditory evoked response and/or otoacoustic emissions may be useful in older patients who may be unable to respond appropriately to classical testing techniques. These electrophysiological tests require only that the patient be cooperative and quiet during the procedure.

CT without contrast and MRI with gadolinium contrast are the radiological tests of choice for assessing the integrity of the auditory pathways. CT is particularly useful for identifying bony lesions of the temporal bone and mastoid process. MRI is the "gold standard" in the diagnosis of retrocochlear lesions such as acoustic schwannomas and is often used when results of the brainstem auditory evoked response are abnormal. When a patient complains of sudden or unilateral hearing loss, a draining ear, or signs of conductive hearing loss; is vertiginous; or has a significant reduction in hearing loss and/or speech discrimination, a prompt referral to neuro-otologist is strongly recommended.

MANAGEMENT

A simple procedure such as cerumen extraction may be all that is needed to restore adequate hearing. Antibiotic therapy can be used in infectious processes such as otitis media.

Corticosteroids have been used to treat immune-related or viral hearing loss. Surgical intervention is generally successful in many cases of conductive hearing losses and in the removal of acoustic schwannomas.

A hearing aid should be considered only after a complete otological and audiological evaluation has confirmed medically untreatable hearing loss. Hearing aids remain the most common treatment option for patients with hearing loss. The success of hearing aid intervention depends primarily on residual auditory and physical capabilities, which may include manual dexterity and mobility, and level of social activity; success is most highly dependent on individual motivation and adaptability.

Federal law once restricted the sale of hearing aids to individuals who had obtained a medical evaluation from a licensed physician, but that is no longer the case. Federal law did permit a fully informed adult to sign a waiver declining medical evaluation for religious or personal beliefs, which precluded consultation with a physician. They indicated, "The exercise of such a waiver is not in your best health interest and its use is strongly discouraged" (21 C.F.R. § 801.420, 2017).

They had recommended that in cases in which a waiver is invoked and the dispenser becomes aware of one of the following conditions, the individual should seek medical (preferably otologic) consultation. Although no longer required by the Food and Drug Administration (FDA), utilization of these guidelines as indicators of the appropriateness for referral to an otolaryngologist appears justified.

- Visible congenital or traumatic deformity of the ear
- History of active drainage from the ear within the previous 90 days
- History of sudden or rapidly progressive hearing loss within the previous 90 days
- Acute or chronic dizziness
- Unilateral hearing loss of sudden or recent onset within the previous 90 days
- Audiometric air–bone gap equal to or greater than 15 dB at 500, 1,000, and 2,000 Hz

- Visible evidence of significant cerumen accumulation or a foreign body in the ear canal
- Pain or discomfort in the ear

Although the major factor in the failure to acquire amplification has been its rather exorbitant cost, the perceived stigma of utilizing prosthetic amplification apparently plays a significant role, as evidenced by failure to acquire rates being similar in countries where hearing aids are made free to cost. Relatively recent changes in distribution paradigms have made these instruments available at more reasonable prices. In many locations, hearing aids are dispensed in "big box" stores by state licensed hearing instrument dispensers or audiologists. Although still not available under Medicare, many insurance policies include provision for partial or total hearing aid coverage. The President's Council of Advisors on Science and Technology (PCAST) has provided the president with recommendations regarding the future role of the FDA regarding hearing aids and personal sound-amplification products (PSAPs; see President's Council of Advisors on Science and Technology, 2015). Among their recommendations is a new class of amplification, PSAPs, that would be appropriate for individuals with mild or moderate hearing losses and that would be made available on an over-the-counter basis. Although a generic or semi-generic choice of such devices may prove to be of significant benefit to many who require prosthetic amplification, some undoubtedly will need the traditional personal interaction and expertise of audiologists or other hearing aid dispensers.

Although hearing aids play an integral part in hearing rehabilitation, other interventions, including speech-reading training, listening training, and lip-reading instruction, play a role in helping many elderly overcome their auditory difficulties. Many hearing-impaired individuals benefit from assistive listening devices in certain surroundings. For example, inexpensive amplifiers are available for use with the television or telephone. Infrared devices are particularly effective adjuncts when attending the theater, motion pictures, and lectures or when viewing television. Other

H

services include closed-captioned entertainment, vibrating alarm clocks, fire alarms that flash or vibrate the bed, accessory headsets for television or radio, and telephone- and doorbell-signaling devices.

See also Hearing Aids.

Marc B. Kramer

Agrawal, Y., Platz, E. A., & Niparko, J. K. (2008). Prevalence of hearing loss and differences by demographic characteristics among US adults: Data from the National Health and Nutrition Examination Survey, 1999–2004. *Archives of Internal Medicine, 168*(14), 1522–1530.

Gates, G. A., Cooper, J. C., Jr., Kannel, W. B., & Miller, N. J. (1990). Hearing in the elderly: The Framingham cohort, 1983–1985. Part I. Basic audiometric test results. *Ear and Hearing, 11*(4), 247–256.

Lin, F. R., Ferucci, L., Metter, E. J., An, Y., Zonderman, A. B., & Resnick, S. M. (2011a). Hearing loss and cognition in the Baltimore Longitudinal Study of Aging. *Neuropsychology, 25*(6), 763–770.

Lin, F. R., Metter, E. J., O'Brien, R. J., Resnick, S. M., Zonderman, A. B., & Ferrucci, L. (2011b). Hearing loss and incident dementia. *Archives Neurology, 68*(2), 214–220.

Peracino, A. (2014). Hearing loss and dementia in the aging population. *Audiology and Neurotology, 19*(Suppl. 1), 6–9.

President's Council of Advisors on Science and Technology. (2015). Retrieved from http://hearingloss.org/sites/default/files/docs/PCAST_Hearing_Tech_LetterReport_FINAL.pdf

21 C.F.R. § 801.420(c)(3) (2017).

Warshaw, G., & Moqeet, S. (1988). Hearing impairment. In T. T. Yoshikawa, E. L. Cobbs, & K. Brummel Smith (Eds.), *Practical ambulatory geriatrics* (2nd ed., Vol. 16, pp. 118–125). St. Louis, MO: Mosby Year-Book.

Web Resources

American Academy of Audiology: http://www.audiology.org

American Academy of Otolaryngology—Head and Neck Surgery: http://www.entnet.org/patient

American Speech-Language-Hearing Association: http://www.asha.org

American Tinnitus Association: http://www.tinnitus.org

Self-Help for Hard-of-Hearing People: http://www.shhh.org

HISPANIC AND LATINO ELDERS

Latinos make up the largest and fastest growing ethnic group in the United States, at 17.6% of the population, and are among the most rapidly aging Americans. In 2014, approximately 8% of the estimated 46 million people aged 65 years or older living in the United States identified as Hispanic or Latino. By 2050, the older Latino population is projected to increase by over 200%—with an estimated 15.4 million individuals representing almost 20% of the older population—as compared to a 59% increase for White non-Hispanics older adults (U.S. Census Bureau [Census], 2016).

Hispanic or Latino older adults in the United States are a heterogeneous population, representing a wide range of nationalities and ethnicities and encompassing many social, cultural, historical, economic, and political differences. The terms *Hispanic* and *Latino* are often used interchangeably in the literature; however, there are regional and cultural perspectives on and preferences for the terms (Alcoff, 2005). The U.S. Census moved in 2000 from "Hispanic" to "Spanish, Hispanic, or Latino," which includes Cubans, Mexican Americans, Puerto Ricans, South or Central Americans, and other Spanish cultures or origins, regardless of race. Understanding the diversity of Latino older adults is central to understanding and meeting the health and social care needs of aging Americans of Mexican, Puerto Rican, Cuban, Central and South American, and Spanish descent.

HEALTH AND HEALTH DISPARITIES

The National Healthcare Disparities Report (NHDR) illustrates significant health inequities among Latinos of all ages (Agency for Healthcare Research and Quality [AHRQ], 2012). Although, there is broad heterogeneity with respect to health indicators, Latinos are three times more likely than non-Hispanic Whites to lack a primary health care provider (Schiller, Lucas, Ward, & Peregoy, 2012) and are at greater risk than non-Hispanic peers for diabetes, cardiovascular disease, cancer, and HIV disease (Vega, Rodriguez, & Gruskin, 2009). In 2012, Latino older adults reported poorer scores on 76 health care measures than their non-Hispanic peers, including access to providers, difficulty and delays in obtaining care due to financial and insurance constraints, and quality of communication with providers (AHRQ, 2012). Cardiovascular disease, stroke, and cancer account for approximately 45% and 54% of deaths in Latino males and females, and hypertension, especially untreated hypertension, is alarmingly high (American Heart Association [AHA], 2013). Despite the existence of effective treatments, only 39% of Mexican Americans, for example, are estimated to have appropriate blood pressure control. Long-standing uncontrolled hypertension significantly increases chances of and represents the primary risk factor for stroke. According to the U.S. Census Bureau, the incidence of stroke in Latinos has increased 34% since 1980 and tends to occur at a younger age when compared to non-Hispanic Whites (AHA, 2013).

Cancer is also highly prevalent in Latino elders, with pancreatic, liver, gallbladder, uterine, cervical, and stomach cancers diagnosed at almost twice the rate as among non-Hispanic White older adults (American Cancer Society [ACS], 2013). Screening tests to detect breast, colon, cervical, and prostate cancer early are less used by Latinos than by non-White Hispanics and African Americans. Of note, mammography, Pap smears, colonoscopy, and digital rectal exams are partially or fully reimbursed by Medicare, but older Latinos rarely take advantage of these tests. Research suggests Latino women are traditionally the least likely population to take advantage of cancer screening and early detection opportunities (ACS, 2013).

Healthy People 2020 (U.S. Department of Health and Human Service [DHHS], 2010) highlighted the importance of reducing health disparities and increasing health equity among all Americans and of addressing social determinants of health, "conditions in the social, physical, and economic environment in which people are born, live, work, and age." This emphasis on addressing the structural and environmental correlates of health such as poverty, safe housing, and access to health care echoes current health initiatives such as the World Health Organization (WHO, 2008) and the National Prevention and Health Promotion Strategy (U.S. Centers for Disease Control and Prevention [CDC], 2014).

SOCIAL DETERMINANTS OF HEALTH

Income insecurity, a key determinant of access to quality health care, treatment, and medication, is a pervasive and challenging public health concern for Latino older adults. According to the U.S. Census, the poverty rate among older Latinos was 17.5% in 2015, approximately twice the poverty rate of all older adults (8.8%; Proctor, Semega, & Kollar, 2015). Latino elders are at high risk for poverty due to long-term income inequities, and are disproportionately vulnerable to economic fluctuations and policy changes in federal programs including Medicare and Social Security. The percentage of Latinos with health insurance coverage in 2015 (84%) was lowest of all ethnic/racial groups, compared with non-Hispanic Whites (93%), Blacks (89%), and Asians (92%; Barnett & Vornovitsky, 2016).

Educational levels vary widely among Latino groups, but completion of secondary and higher education is among the lowest among ethnic/racial groups. In 2014, an estimated 15% of adult Latinos had a bachelor's degree or higher, as compared to 41% of White non-Hispanics, 22% of Blacks, and 63% of Asians.

Lower levels of educational attainment, in turn, predisposes people to having higher rates of unemployment and lower wage jobs. Latino and African American households have significantly less in retirement savings than White households, and older Latinos are more likely to be highly dependent on Social Security than other racial/ethnic groups; about half of older Latinos receive more than 90% of their income from Social Security (Morrissey & Sabadish, 2013).

LANGUAGE AND CULTURAL BARRIERS

Although English language proficiency among Latinos is rising, more than one third report that they are not proficient in English, and those aged

H

65 years and older are the most likely to communicate only in Spanish (Krogstad, Stepler, & Lopez, 2015). Older Latinos with limited English proficiency or limited literacy face complex obstacles when accessing and using the health care system. Primary care providers must be cautious and judicious in the use of oral translation because the translators, who are often family members of the older patient, may have varying levels of fluency in Spanish. These relatives may edit, filter, or otherwise misconstrue important information necessary for a complete patient evaluation. Also, imposition of the interpreter's beliefs or self-perception into the interaction also influences the information exchange. Finally, cultural perceptions, such as the stigmatization of mental illness, may result in poor communication. Effective communication requires that clinicians providing care to Latino older adults be conversant in Spanish or have trained medical translators or bilingual staff.

The frequency with which individuals use the services of unlicensed healers, herbalists, and spiritual healers varies among the Latino subgroups, but is higher than among non-Hispanic adults. Alternative health practices include the use of Curanderos in the Mexican American communities, Santeria among Cuban Americans, and Espiritismo among Puerto Ricans (Ortiz, Shields, Clauson, & Clay, 2007). Health providers should ask older patients about their use of alternative healers (i.e., *verbas medicinales*) and traditional or herbal medicines. Additionally, providers should ascertain where medications are purchased because many Mexican Americans who live in the Southwest cross into Mexico, where medications can be bought without a prescription.

Living arrangements, gender, marital status, and literacy levels may contribute to poorer health outcomes among Latino elders. More than half of male Hispanics are married whereas only 38% of the women are married; approximately two thirds live with a spouse or relative. Extended-family support systems and a strong value of *familismo* among Latinos may lessen caregiver burden and maintain older adults in the community. Despite a traditional emphasis and reliance on family support, however, research on caregivers of older Latinos with

dementia documenting low levels of social support and high levels of distress among Latino family caregivers suggests the need for further study (Gelman, 2014).

HEALTH PROMOTION, DISEASE PREVENTION, AND HEALTH EDUCATION

Older adults and ethnic/racial "minority" populations have been identified as priority populations by the AHRQ because their unique health needs require special attention to ensure accessible, affordable, and quality health care (AHRQ, 2012). The majority of chronic diseases prevalent among Latino older adults require self-management of diet, exercise, medication adherence, and substantial modifications in lifestyle behaviors to promote health (i.e., smoking and alcohol cessation, stress reduction, and increased physical activity). Special outreach activities and bilingual educational campaigns are needed in Latino communities to teach the importance of medical screening and health management to Hispanics who are monolingual or prefer to speak in Spanish. Additionally, establishing effective protocols for referring individuals to screening centers would benefit Hispanics who commonly receive health care from large public hospitals and rarely experience continuity care. The National Hispanic Council on Aging (NHCOA) proposes increasing health outreach and services at community-based centers, the use of culturally sensitive and appropriate care, peer health educators, and increased inclusion of Latinos in long-term research programs to assess the effectiveness of current disease prevention and health promotion programs in order to increase the awareness and use of services (NCHOA, 2017).

Optimal health care for older Latinos requires that health care providers embrace and understand the cultural diversity of the populations they serve. Culturally appropriate health education, risk reduction, and health promotion interventions are particularly important considering the high incidence of cancer, diabetes, hypertension and cardiovascular disease among older Latinos. Given significant health disparities and barriers to health care access and utilization, health care providers are encouraged to focus on increasing multilingual access, developing and providing cultural sensitive services, and attending to social determinants in order to improve minority health and well-being. Priorities identified by the NHCOA include economic security, health promotion, disease prevention, education and community outreach, and adequate and affordable housing (NHCOA, 2017). Understanding culturally specific characteristics of Latino elders can enhance the quality of health care services, facilitate meaningful and culturally appropriate interventions, and promote healthy aging and longevity.

Daniel S. Gardner

Agency for Healthcare Research and Quality (AHRQ). (2012). *National healthcare disparities report*. Rockville, MD: U.S. Department of Health and Human Services. Publication Number 13–0003. Retrieved from https://archive.ahrq.gov/research/findings/nhqrdr/nhdr12/2012nhdr.pdf

Alcoff, L. M. (2005). Latino vs. Hispanic: The politics of ethnic names. *Philosophy & Social Criticism, 31*(4), 395–407.

American Cancer Society (ACS). (2013). Cancer facts & figures. Retrieved from https://www.cancer.org/content/dam/cancer-org/research/cancer-facts-and-statistics/annual-cancer-facts-and-figures/2013/cancer-facts-and-figures-2013.pdf

American Heart Association (AHA). (2013). Statistical fact sheet 2013 update Hispanics/Latinos & cardiovascular diseases. Retrieved from https://www.heart.org/idc/groups/heart-public/@wcm/@sop/@smd/documents/downloadable/ucm_319572.pdf

Barnett, J., & Vornovitsky, M. (2016). *Current population reports, P60-257(RV), Health insurance coverage in the United States: 2015*. Washington, DC: U.S. Government Printing Office. Retrieved from https://www.census.gov/content/dam/Census/library/publications/2016/demo/p60-257.pdf

Gelman, C. R. (2014). Familismo and its impact on the family caregiving of Latinos with Alzheimer's disease: A complex narrative. *Research on Aging, 36*(1), 40–71. doi:10.1177/0164027512469213.

Krogstad, J. M., Stepler, R., & Lopez, M. H. (2015). *English proficiency on the rise among Latinos; U.S. born driving language changes*. Washington, DC: Pew Research Center.

Morrissey, M., & Sabadish, N. (2013). *Retirement inequality chartbook*. Washington, DC: Economic Policy Institute. Retrieved from http://www.epi.org/publication/retirement-inequalitychartbook

National Hispanic Council on Aging (NHCOA). (2017). Priorities. Retrieved from http://www.nhcoa.org/priorities

Ortiz, B. I., Shields, K. M., Clauson, K. A., & Clay, P. G. (2007). Complementary and alternative medicine use among Hispanics in the United States. *The Annals of Pharmacotherapy, 41*(6), 994–1004. doi:10.1345/aph.1H600

Proctor, B., Semega, J., & Kollar, M. (2015). *Income and poverty in the United States: 2015. U.S. Census Bureau, Current Population Reports, P60-256(RV)*. Washington, DC: U.S. Government Printing Office 2016. Retrieved from https://www.census.gov/content/dam/Census/library/publications/2016/demo/p60-256.pdf

Schiller, J. S., Lucas, J. W., Ward, B. W., & Peregoy, J. A. (2012). Summary health statistics for US Adults: National health interview survey, 2010. Data from The National Health Survey. *Vital and Health Statistics, 10*, (252), 1–207. Retrieved from https://www.cdc.gov/nchs/data/series/sr_10/sr10_252.pdf

U.S. Census Bureau (Census). (2016). Annual estimates of the resident population by sex, age, race, and Hispanic origin for the United States and States: April 1, 2010 to July 1, 2015 U.S. Census Bureau, Population Division. Retrieved from https://factfinder.census.gov/faces/tableservices/jsf/pages/productview.xhtml?src=bkmk

U.S. Centers for Disease Control and Prevention (CDC). (2014). The national prevention strategy: America's plan for better health and wellness. Retrieved from https://www.cdc.gov/features/preventionstrategy

U.S. Department of Health and Human Service (DHHS). (2010). *Healthy People 2020: An opportunity to address the* societal determinants of health in the United States. Secretary's Advisory Committee on Health Promotion and Disease Prevention Objectives for 2020. Retrieved from http://www.healthypeople.gov/2010/hp2020/advisory/SocietalDeterminantsHealth.htm

Vega, W. A., Rodriguez, M. A., & Gruskin, E. (2009). Health disparities in the Latino population. *Epidemiologic Reviews, 31*, 99–112. doi:10.1093/epirev/mxp008

World Health Organization (WHO). (2008). Commission on Social Determinants of Health. Closing the gap in a generation: Health equity through action on the social determinants of health. Retrieved from http://www.who.int/social_determinants/en

Web Resources

Diverse Elders Coalition: http://www.diverseelders.org/who-we-are/diverse-elders/hispanic-elders

National Association for Hispanic Elderly/Asociación Nacional Pro Personas Mayores: https://nei.nih.gov/content/national-association-hispanic-elderly-asociacion-nacional-pro-personas-mayores

National Hispanic Council on Aging: http://www.nhcoa.org

HIV, AIDS, AND AGING

At the beginning of the AIDS epidemic in the United States, those infected with HIV were typically young, gay, White men. In the subsequent 30 years, the demographics of the epidemic have shifted as increasing numbers of women, minorities, and older adults have become infected. With the introduction of successful combination antiretroviral therapy in the 1990s, the life span for those living with HIV/AIDS has dramatically increased. In addition, as the general population continues to age, the percentage of older adults newly infected and living with HIV will also continue to rise. According to the Centers for Disease Control and Prevention (CDC, 2015), there were more than 44,000 new HIV diagnoses and almost 21,000 new AIDS diagnoses in the United States in 2014. Those aged 50 years and older accounted for 17% of new HIV diagnoses and 28% of new AIDS diagnoses; they also accounted for 42% of the 934,000 living with HIV, 50% of the 516,000 living with AIDS, and 62% of all deaths of persons with HIV/AIDS. Adults aged 65 years and older accounted for 6% of those living with HIV, 7% of those living with AIDS, and 14% of all deaths of persons with HIV.

Older adults share the same risk factors as younger adults for acquiring HIV, with risky sexual behavior remaining the most common, although active or former intravenous drug use is also an increasingly prevalent method of transmission among older adults. Unfortunately, older adults often perceive themselves, or are perceived by health care providers, to be at low risk of infection and are therefore less likely to be tested for HIV than younger adults. Awareness of the risk of HIV transmission is important for older adults and their care providers, who are remiss about discussing sexual issues and often underestimate the sexual activity of their older patients.

Many older adults are not aware that they or their partners are at risk from prior exposure or from a current relationship, despite the fact that 60% of men and 45% of women aged 60 to 69 years and 30% of men and 14% of women aged 70 years and above continue to be sexually active (Fisher, 2010). Some older adults may also not be willing to discuss their previous drug use or their sexuality and sexual behavior due to stigma or denial. Older men may be diagnosed more frequently because of the increased request for and use of medications to alleviate erectile dysfunction. Older women, however, may be particularly uncomfortable discussing their sex lives. In addition, they have less concern of pregnancy and/or may view condom use as too awkward or difficult to manage, contributing to less condom use. In a 2009 AARP survey on sexual activity and relationships among adults aged 50 years and older, only 8% reported using protection "all the time," with just an additional 4% using protection "usually, but not all the time." At the same time, a large majority of older individuals with an acknowledged risk for HIV have never been tested for the virus. Although current CDC guidelines recommend routine testing of patients aged 13 to 64 years, some organizations, such as the American College of Physicians, are recommending routine screening up to age 75 (Qaseem, Snow, Shekelle, Hopkins, & Owens, 2009).

Educational programs about HIV risk factors are only beginning to target the elderly as a risk group. As older patients fail to self-identify or are completely unaware of possible risks, HIV has become a silent epidemic in this population. Also, older adults diagnosed with HIV may face embarrassment and shame and may deal with their disease in isolation. They may be reluctant to discuss their illness with their sexual partners or their families. They may also avoid disclosing their diagnosis to other providers such as their dermatologist, podiatrist, or gynecologist—all of whom should know so that universal precautions can be reinforced and treatment-related effects and potential drug–drug interactions can be adequately evaluated.

HIV can present in myriad ways in elderly patients, particularly those with other comorbidities. Combining this issue with the lack of identified risk and adequate screening, HIV may not even be a consideration for providers when signs and symptoms do present. In later stages, HIV can present with weight loss, anemia or thrombocytopenia, dementia or other neurological problems, pneumonia, hair loss, or simple fatigue. Any of these complaints can be ascribed to other illnesses or can be associated with phenomena of aging. Providers, however, must consider and treat all possible etiologies, including HIV/AIDS and related opportunistic infections. Often when an HIV diagnosis is finally made in an older adult, the disease is frequently at a later stage than it would be in a younger adult at diagnosis. Among adults aged 50 years and older who were newly diagnosed with HIV from 2005 to 2010, almost 14% died within 12 months of diagnosis, compared with less than 4% for those younger than 50 years (CDC, 2015). For those aged 65 years and older, 26% died within 12 months of infection diagnosis.

Advancing age can exacerbate or accelerate the course of HIV infection, and in turn, HIV and use of HIV medications may accelerate the course of aging. Aging is associated with a decline in humoral and cellular immune function, and HIV can accelerate this decline. Elderly patients may have diabetes or renal insufficiency, which can also adversely affect immune function. In addition, some patients may be coinfected with hepatitis B or C. It is well recognized that HIV contributes to an earlier progression of fibrosis in the liver of patients who are coinfected. Osteopenia and mitochondrial toxicity are both consequences of aging and occur in HIV as well. Untreated HIV can also contribute to or exacerbate cardiovascular diseases,

neurocognitive defects and dementia, and both AIDS-related and non–AIDS-related cancers. HIV medications can also have significant effects on the aging body. HIV-positive patients who take nucleoside reverse transcriptase inhibitors for extended periods are vulnerable to the effects of mitochondrial toxicity, which include impaired organ function and chronic fatigue. Use of protease inhibitors can lead to many metabolic complications, including dyslipidemia, insulin resistance, kidney stones, gallstones, and hepatotoxicity. Integrase inhibitors can exacerbate renal impairment.

The latest guidelines for antiretroviral treatment for adults and adolescents with HIV favor initiating combination antiretroviral therapy in all adults aged 50 years and older regardless of the presenting CD4 cell count (U.S. Department of Health and Human Services [USDHHS], 2016). There are concerns that older adults do not experience immune recovery (namely, an increase in CD4 cell count) that younger adults experience; thus prompt initiation of therapy is preferred. Also, older adults are at much higher risk of opportunistic infections and serious non–AIDS-related events, necessitating early initiation of antiretroviral therapy. Unfortunately, doses and medication combinations have not been rigorously evaluated in elderly patients, including evaluations of long-term safety. However, data still suggest using treatment and evaluation recommendations that have been provided for all adults and adolescents.

Because of the complicated nature of treating older adults with HIV, particularly regarding concomitant treatments of other chronic conditions, providers should focus on potential adverse events pertaining to cardiovascular, metabolic, renal, hepatic, and bone disorders. Drug–drug interactions remain an ongoing aspect of HIV therapy in all patients, making therapeutic management more complex. Older adults may not only be taking medications for other conditions, but may also be adding medications for treatment-related side effects, such as gastrointestinal complaints or pain syndromes. Some of these medications may be supplements or other over-the-counter medicines, further complicating pharmacological management in the older adults with HIV. Chronic liver disease

H

and renal insufficiency are also factors that must be considered in calculating medication dosage for an effective and safe regimen.

Preventive care for older adults with HIV includes the same recommendations as for uninfected elderly patients, with a few additions. All older adults are advised to have yearly influenza vaccines and timely vaccinations against pneumococcal pneumonia. Hepatitis vaccines are recommended. In HIV patients, additional recommendations include a tetanus booster, an annual tuberculosis skin test (purified protein derivative [PPD] without anergy panel), and a regular ophthalmologic examination. Women should have yearly Papanikolaou (Pap) tests. In addition, everyone should have regular dental checkups. Recommendations for patients of any age and any health status include good nutrition, regular exercise, enough sleep, smoking cessation, limited alcohol intake, and elimination of recreational drug use.

Care and treatment of older adults with HIV/AIDS require a multidisciplinary approach combining medical, nursing, nutritional, social service, and mental health support. Patients may benefit from referral to an HIV specialist at the time of diagnosis because specialists can provide the expertise related to HIV medications and care that primary care providers may be lacking. Also, HIV care providers often have multidisciplinary resources that allow them to network for specific patient needs. Some HIV care providers, however, may lack the clinical skills and expertise for treatment of geriatric patients. Therefore they should continue to work closely with the patient's primary care provider; if the patient relies solely on the HIV provider for primary care, the HIV provider may need to seek additional education in the treatment of geriatric patients to adequately manage their patients' complex, chronic conditions.

Case management should facilitate access to appropriate benefits that cover medications, nutritional support, social services, mental health services, and where appropriate, physical therapy and spiritual supports. It is essential that all providers, including pharmacists, communicate with one another, especially when patients have complicated medical problems involving more than one subspecialty and

multiple therapeutic regimens. HIV is a treatable, although not yet curable, disease. The physical and psychosocial burden of HIV on the elderly population requires special attention and awareness to best care for patients.

See also Coping With Chronic Illness; and Physical and Mental Health Needs of Older LGBTQ Adults.

Larry Z. Slater

Centers for Disease Control and Prevention. (2015). *HIV surveillance report, 2014*. 26. Retrieved from http://www.cdc.gov/hiv/library/reports/surveillance/

Fisher, L. (2010). Sex, romance, and relationships: AARP survey of midlife and older adults. Retrieved from http://www.aarp.org/research/topics/life/info-2014/srr_09.html

Qaseem, A., Snow, V., Shekelle, P., Hopkins, R., Owens, D. K., & Clinical Efficacy Assessment Subcommittee of the American College of Physicians. (2009). Screening for HIV in health care settings: A guidance statement from the American College of Physicians and HIV Medicine Association. *Annals of Internal Medicine, 150*(2), 126–131. doi:10.7326/0003-4819-150-2-200901200-00300

U.S. Department of Health and Human Services, Panel on Antiretroviral Guidelines for Adults and Adolescents. (2016). Guidelines for the use of antiretroviral agents in HIV-1-infected adults and adolescents. Retrieved from https://aidsinfo.nih.gov/guidelines/html/1/adult-and-adolescent-treatment-guidelines/0

Web Resources
AIDS Community Research Initiative of America (ACRIA), Center of HIV and Aging: http://www.acria.org/aging

Centers for Disease Control and Prevention: HIV/AIDS: https://www.cdc.gov/hiv

Health Resources and Services Administration HIV/AIDS Bureau: https://www.hab.hrsa.gov

Medscape: HIV/AIDS: http://www.medscape.com/hiv

National Association on HIV Over Fifty (NAHOF): http://hivoverfifty.org/about/hof/national.html

The Body: The Complete HIV/AIDS Resource, Resource Center for Aging with HIV: http://www.thebody.com/index/whatis/older.html

HOME HEALTH CARE

Before the advent of Medicare home health benefits in 1965, approximately 1,400 visiting nurse associations and local health departments provided family-focused health promotion and sickness care services. In 2010, it was estimated that more than 30,000 agencies offered services to nearly 12 million clients (National Association for Home Care & Hospice [NAHC], 2010). According to 2014 estimates, 12,253 of those were Medicare-certified home health agencies, and 5,800 were hospice programs (Harris-Kojetin et al., 2016). The remaining agencies offered private duty, homemaker, companion, and personal care services. Many newer providers are hospital-based or proprietary, for-profit agencies. The dramatic escalation is in response to the reduced length of hospital stays, wider acceptance of home health and hospice care, and an aging population.

Agencies have diversified their programs, services, and staff to meet the needs of clients, families, and referral sources, and have added high-tech procedures, 24-hour care, hospice programs, pharmacy services, durable medical equipment, and telehealth programs.

Persons 65 years of age and older constitute approximately 70% of all home health clients, and those older than 85 years of age constitute an additional 17%. Circulatory system disease accounts for about 26% of referrals; neoplasms and endocrine diseases, especially diabetes, are common primary medical diagnoses. Approximately 92,000 RNs, 45,000 licensed practical nurses, 65,000 home care aides, 13,000 physical therapists, 8,000 occupational therapists, and 5,000 social workers are employed by Medicare-certified home health agencies (Harris-Kojetin et al., 2016; NAHC, 2010).

The average number of home health visits (all disciplines) per client increased from 33 in 1990 to 74 in 1996; the number decreased to 35 visits by 2008 and 18.31 by 2013 (NAHC, 2010; Visiting Nurses Association of America [VNAA], 2013). Regulations and reimbursement often determine whether clients are admitted to services, how frequent and how long the visits are, which disciplines provide services, and when patients are discharged.

PRACTICE

Core principles of home health practice are constant, but other aspects of practice are changing dramatically. Effective home health nurses and other clinicians have always needed extensive technical, interpersonal, and critical-thinking skills. They need to embrace a spirit of client-centered care and interprofessional collaboration to provide the highest quality care. When clinicians work in a hospital or nursing home, colleagues, technology, supplies, and references are nearby. When clinicians make a visit to a home, clinic, or other site, they are usually alone. Home health clinicians need to be creative and well informed about community resources; they need to have contingency plans for their daily schedules and for their clients' and their own safety. They need to work as partners with diverse clients (e.g., diversity in age, medical and nursing diagnoses, race, language, religion, culture, income, and values) to help them attain their maximal levels of self-care and independence. As part of that partnership, clinicians help clients follow regulations, including those that involve reimbursement.

Many clinicians provide generalized home health services involving chronic illnesses. Increasingly, others have specialized skills involving cardiovascular disease, diabetes, infusion therapy, wound care, hospice, parent–child, and HIV/AIDS and other infectious conditions. Some larger agencies employ staff members who have advanced nursing practice credentials, such as geriatric nurse practitioners or clinical specialists.

Most agencies use diverse technology in response to increasing communication, distance, clinician safety, client complexity, and outcome-management challenges. Agencies are implementing standardized terminologies, electronic clinical information systems, and telehealth to improve the quality of practice, documentation, and information management. As

H

part of the federal information technology (IT) and electronic health record (EHR) initiative, SNOMED CT, LOINC, and HL7 were selected as reference terminologies for promoting the standardization and exchange of clinical data (American Nurses Association [ANA], 2015; Martin, 2005; Martin, Monsen, & Bowles, 2011). Telemonitoring offers an additional way for clinicians to track vital signs and blood pressure, weight, oxygen saturation, and other data that suggest early changes in client status. Telehealth encourages clients to become more involved in and informed about their own care and decrease rates of rehospitalization and emergency room use (Institute of Medicine [IOM], 2012; Woods & Snow, 2013).

DESCRIPTION AND MEASUREMENT OF PRACTICE

Recent developments, including the use of technology, have helped home health agencies collect more accurate clinical data and convert those metrics documenting quality. In addition, Medicare publicizes agency-quality indicator data and is proposing pay-for-performance and value-based initiatives that would offer financial incentives for exceeding established levels of quality. Medicare's home health reimbursement regulations continue to change and increase regularly.

Problem-Solving Process

Home health clinicians are interested in evidence-based practice. The six steps of the problem-solving process offer a useful strategy for describing and measuring their practice, especially when these steps are combined with standardized vocabularies and automated clinical information systems. The steps are assessment, problem identification/diagnosis, plans, interventions, evaluation, and outcome management. One research-based method, the Omaha System, illustrates the application of this process in home health practice (Omaha System, 2016).

Assessment and Problem Identification/Diagnosis

When home health clients are referred for service, assessment and diagnostic information should accompany the referral. However, as part of the admission process, a focused and comprehensive assessment needs to be completed to address environmental, psychosocial, physiological, and health-related issues. Since 1999, the Centers for Medicare & Medicaid Services mandated that the staff of Medicare-certified home-care agencies complete an Outcome and Assessment Information Set (OASIS) as one part of the comprehensive assessment. OASIS consists of more than 100 items when staff members admit new clients; children and pregnant women are excluded. OASIS data must also be submitted at interim periods and discharge.

The assessment should involve interprofessional collaboration, with members of various disciplines communicating and contributing relevant data. Often, a case manager is responsible for obtaining additional information from the referral source and communicating pertinent information to the client's home health care physician and insurance or health-plan case manager.

After reviewing referral data and physicians' orders, nurses identify the home health client's problems (e.g., income, circulation, nutrition, medication regimen; Martin et al., 2011; Omaha System, 2016). Nurses then prioritize the problems in partnership with clients and families—a crucial step in determining the problems on which they will actively work.

Plans and Interventions

Just as clients' assessments and diagnoses need to be focused, so do care plans and interventions. Interventions used frequently by the home health interprofessional team include health teaching, guidance, and counseling; treatments and procedures; case management; and surveillance (Martin et al., 2011; Omaha System, 2016). Nurses may instruct clients about new medications and the use of a glucometer, give injections, collaborate with physical and occupational therapists about clients' poststroke needs, refer clients to Meals on Wheels or registered dieticians, or monitor environmental modifications to decrease the risk of falling.

The average duration of home health care services has been decreasing because of regulations and reimbursement, even though the complexity of clients' needs is increasing. Thus care plans and interventions should be selected for the client's priority problems. Ideally, the client, family, and health care team members share the goal of self-care or achieving the greatest degree of independence possible. Clinicians need to anticipate whether other types of services will be required after discharge from home health care services.

Evaluation and Outcome Management

Simple, valid, and reliable instruments are needed to evaluate which home health practices are best. Increasingly, third-party payers and accreditors require home health agencies to provide quantitative data that describe the clients they serve, the types of services they provide, the effects of those services on clients, and the costs of services. OASIS data can be used as one approach for evaluating home-care effectiveness, as can hospitalization rates. Client records are a major source of clinical data for an outcome-management program if agencies have automated clinical information systems. Clinicians need to ask and document the following: What works best? Has the client improved? By how much? From what perspective? A second approach is to use the Omaha System's Problem Rating Scale of Outcomes, a 5-point Likert-type scale designed for use with specific client problems. It includes three separate numeric subscales for knowledge, behavior, and status (Martin et al., 2011; Omaha System, 2016). Ratings offer cues to help clinicians select the most appropriate interventions for the client and provide a baseline for tracking knowledge, behavior, and status data throughout the duration of service. Data collection is repeated at established intervals and at discharge. The clinical data produced by the ratings can be analyzed in conjunction with

staffing, length of service, cost, and other statistical data.

Related Research

Data analysis, surveys, and research offer important strategies for identifying best practices and disseminating the benefits of home health services. Although agencies regularly collected extensive clinical data, those data usually remain in data cemeteries. Only recently have agencies introduced the needed rigor, methods, and technology to use their data and to consider the value of "big data" (Martin et al., 2011; Westra & Choromanski, 2014).

More than 1,100 agencies participated in a 2013–2014 national study (Fazzi Associates, 2013). The survey was designed to identify IT use and satisfaction trends, specifically the use of electronic billing and financial systems, IT in hospice programs, EHRs and point-of-care technology, telehealth, and quality and productivity measurement.

An extended series of funded studies have focused on the Transitional Care Model and interventions provided by advanced practice nurses. Earlier research addressed the needs of clients who had cardiac conditions; more recent studies involved clients who were cognitively impaired, had mental illness, or were dying, as well as their caregivers. All clients were at high risk of rehospitalization (Naylor et al., 2007, 2013).

A study published in 2012 (Monsen, Swanberg, Oancea, & Westra 2012) focused on the risk of rehospitalization using data available in EHRs. The sample included the EHRs of 14 home health agencies and represented 1,643 episodes of care. The authors identified some predictors to help agency providers reduce their clients' rehospitalization.

Sockolow, Bowles, Adelsberger, Chittams, and Liao (2014) designed a pre-postobservational study to compare workflow, financial billing, and patient outcomes before and after EHR implementation. Postimplementation findings were positive and suggest that EHRs can be beneficial.

See also Medicaid; Medicare; Mild Neuro-cognitive Disorder.

Karen S. Martin

American Nurses Association. (2015). Inclusion of recognized terminologies within EHRs and other health information technology solutions. Retrieved from http://www.nursingworld.org/MainMenuCategories/Policy-Advocacy/Positions-and-Resolutions/ANAPositionStatements/Position-Statements-Alphabetically/Inclusion-of-Recognized-Terminologies-within-EHRs.html

Fazzi Associates. (2013). 2013 national state of the home care industry study. Retrieved from https://www.fazzi.com/2013-national-state-of-the-home-care-industry-study

Harris-Kojetin, L., Sengupta, M., Park-Lee, E., Valverde, R., Caffrey, C., Rome, V., & Lendon, J. (2016). Long-term care providers and services used in the United States: Data from The National Study of Long-Term Care Providers, 2013-2014. *National Center for Health Statistics, Vital Health Statistics, 3*(38), x–xii.

Institute of Medicine. (2012). *The role of telehealth in an evolving health care environment: Workshop summary.* Washington, DC: National Academies Press. Retrieved from http://books.nap.edu/openbook.php?record_id=13466

Martin, K. S. (2005). *The Omaha System: A key to practice, documentation, and information management* (Reprinted 2nd ed.). Omaha, NE: Health Connections Press.

Martin, K. S., Monsen, K. A., & Bowles, K. H. (2011). The Omaha System and meaningful use: Applications for practice, education, and research. *Computers, Informatics, Nursing, 29*(1), 52–58.

Monsen, K. A., Swanberg, H. L., Oancea, S. C., & Westra, B. L. (2012). Exploring the value of clinical data standards to predict hospitalization of home care patients. *Applied Clinical Informatics [Online], 3*(3), 419–436.

National Association for Home Care & Hospice. (2010). *Basic statistics about home care.* Retrieved from http://nahc.org/facts/10HC_Stats.pdf

Naylor, M. D., Bowles, K. H., McCauley, K. M., Maccoy, M. C., Maislin, G., Pauly, M. V., & Krakauer, R. (2013). High-value transitional care: Translation of research into practice. *Journal of Evaluation in Clinical Practice, 19*(5), 727–733.

Naylor, M. D., Hirschman, K. B., Bowles, K. H., Bixby, M. B., Konick-McMahan, J., & Stephens, C. (2007). Care coordination for cognitively impaired older adults and their caregivers. *Home Health Care Services Quarterly, 26* (4), 57–78.

Omaha System. (2016). Retrieved from http://www.omahasystem.org

Sockolow, P. S., Bowles, K. H., Adelsberger, M. C., Chittams, J. L., & Liao, C. (2014). Impact of homecare electronic health record on timeliness of clinical documentation, reimbursement, and patient outcomes. *Applied Clinical Informatics, 5*(2), 445–462.

Visiting Nurses Association of America. (2013). New comparative home health data available on reimbursements, visits and therapy. Retrieved from http://www.vnaa.org/article_content.asp?article=185

Westra, B. L., & Choromanski, L. (2014). Amazing news for sharable/comparable nursing data to support big data science. *Computers, Informatics, Nursing, 32*(6), 255–256.

Woods, L. W., & Snow, S. W. (2013). The impact of telehealth monitoring. *Home Healthcare Nurse, 31*(1), 39–45.

Web Resources

American Nurses Association: Recognized terminologies that support nursing practice: http://www.nursingworld.org/terminologies

Centers for Medicare & Medicaid Services: http://www.cms.gov

National Association for Home Care & Hospice: http://www.nahc.org

Office of the National Coordinator Health Information Technology: http://healthit.gov

Visiting Nurses Association of America: http://www.vnaa.org

HOMELESS ELDERS

A key issue in studying and understanding the magnitude of elder homelessness in the United States is the challenge of defining the population. In light of the prevalence of chronic illness, disability, and early mortality associated with homelessness, individuals experiencing homelessness may look and behave 10 to 20 years older than their chronological age (Brown, Kiely, Bharel, & Mitchell, 2013; Salem et al., 2013). Thus most researchers, policy makers, and advocacy groups define homeless individuals over the age of 50 as homeless elders.

Data from the U.S. Department of Housing and Urban Development (HUD) reveal that homelessness among older adults is on the rise. In 2014, adults aged 51 years and above accounted for 31.1% of all individuals in homeless shelters, an 8.6% increase from 2007 (HUD, 2015). Adults aged 51 to 61 years make up the largest portion of the homeless older adult population, accounting for 25.4% of the sheltered population (HUD, 2015). Although individuals aged 62 years and older accounted for only 5.7% of the total number of individuals in shelters in 2014, this is an increase from 4.1% in 2007. As the Baby Boomer generation continues to age, it is anticipated that the number of homeless individuals over the age of 50 years will continue to rise, doubling by 2050 (National Health Care for the Homeless Council [NHCHC], 2013). At the same time, the number of persons aged 65 years and older who are homeless is expected to rise only modestly, in part because of social welfare programs (including housing subsidies, Medicare, and Social Security benefits) that provide a financial safety net for people aged 65 years and above (National Leadership Initiative to End Elder Homelessness [NLIEEH], 2011). In addition, high early mortality rates among adults experiencing homelessness result in few individuals reaching age 65 years (Culhane, Metraux, & Bainbridge, 2010). Thus it is imperative that nurses, social workers, physicians, and others caring for adults experiencing homelessness be prepared to meet the complex health and social needs of the population.

The causes of homelessness among older adults are complex and varied, although the primary contributors are the lack of affordable housing and poverty (National Coalition for the Homeless [NCH], 2009). Housing assistance programs across the country are overwhelmed with applications, resulting in long wait lists and even closing of program wait lists due to excessive demand (HUD, n.d.). For example, the Houston Housing Authority (n.d.) notes that the standard wait time for public housing is between 18 and 24 months for persons under the age of 62 years and 6 to 9 months for seniors

aged above 62 years. The wait list for housing assistance of the Chicago Housing Authority (2016) closed in 2014 after 280,000 applications were received, resulting in a lottery system to distribute housing subsidies. These affordable housing shortfalls are often compounded for older adults because of relationship changes (e.g., death of a spouse, partner, or relative), physical and/or mental illness, job insecurity, and increased health expenditures. Individuals between the ages of 51 and 61 years are particularly vulnerable to these threats because they are not yet eligible for Social Security, Medicare, senior housing subsidies, or other social support systems available to those aged above 62 years (NCH, 2009). Although some individuals resort to sleeping on the street, many more find shelter in temporary accommodations, such as the home of a friend or family member, welfare hotels, congregate shelters, and transitional housing. Older adults facing homelessness also remain homeless longer than their younger peers; more than 30% of individuals staying in emergency shelters for longer than 180 days are aged above 50 years, reflecting the complex nature of and absence of resources available to older adults with unstable housing (NCH, 2009). Efforts to utilize permanent supportive housing have shown promise in reducing elder homelessness over the last several years, although the needs continue to outnumber available resources (NLIEEH, 2011).

Older adults experiencing homelessness are most often men, White, and unpartnered (Gordon, Rosenheck, Zweig, & Harpaz-Rotem, 2012). Given this male predominance, most studies of homeless elders' health and social needs have focused on small convenience samples of homeless older men. However, more studies are emerging that include female participants (Brown et al, 2013; Salem et al., 2013), expanding the understanding of the unique needs of older women who are experiencing homelessness. It is unclear whether these emerging findings are translating into practice for this population.

Numerous studies have established that older homeless persons suffer substantially more physical illness than younger homeless adults and domiciled elders. For example, studies have found a high incidence of frailty and geriatric syndromes among adults aged 50 years and above experiencing homelessness (Brown et al., 2013; Salem et al., 2013). Brown et al. (2013) found not only that homeless older adults experience disproportionate rates of falls, cognitive impairment, depression, sensory impairment, and urinary incontinence compared with their housed peers, but also that these geriatric syndromes were associated with difficulty in performing activities of daily living (ADL), diabetes, and arthritis. Many health problems experienced by older homeless persons are also exacerbated by chronic alcoholism and drug addiction (Brown et al., 2013; Gordon et al., 2012). Although they are slightly less likely to abuse substances than younger homeless adults, older homeless adults are also less likely than their younger peers to engage in and successfully complete substance abuse recovery programs (Gordon et al., 2012). Although alcoholism and prescription drug dependence are more typical among older adults, the prevalence of heroin, crack cocaine, and other substance abuse has also been reported (Substance Abuse and Mental Health Services Administration, 2002). The shift in geriatric substance abuse creates new challenges for health care professionals.

There is also compelling evidence that homeless elders have higher overall rates of mental illness than the general older population, as well as limited access to mental health care services (Gordon et al., 2012). An estimated 10% to 15% of homeless elders have a serious or chronic mental illness, including alcohol and drug abuse and dependency, anxiety disorders, depression, and schizophrenia. Despite this prevalence, few studies address the mental health needs in this population, provide information about assessing the possibility of alcohol-related dementia among older homeless persons, or consider the long-term effects of drug misuse on the individual's physical, psychosocial, and/or spiritual health.

Housing programs alone cannot solve the problems of homeless elders. Although stable housing is crucial to the well-being of older homeless persons, recent intervention strategies have included community-based interdisciplinary programs whose focus is on housing and case management. The number of permanent supportive housing units in the United States is increasing, although not yet keeping pace with demand. Permanent supportive housing is a critical first step in stabilizing the lives of older adults experiencing homelessness so that the complex needs underlying their housing instability can be addressed. Thus there is growing recognition that older homeless men and women have unique and complex needs that span the gamut from health factors to safety issues.

Laura E. Gultekin and Barbara L. Brush

Brown, R. T., Kiely, D. K., Bharel, M., & Mitchell, S. L. (2013). Factors associated with geriatric syndromes in older homeless adults. *Journal of Health Care for the Poor and Underserved, 24*(2), 456–468.

Chicago Housing Authority. (2016). 2014 housing waitlist information. Retrieved http://www.the cha.org/residents/update-waitlist-information

Culhane, D. P., Metraux, S., & Bainbridge, J. (2010). The age structure of contemporary homelessness: Risk period or cohort effect? Penn School of Social Policy and Practice Working Paper, 1–28. Retrieved from http://repository.upenn.edu/cgi/view content.cgi?article=1148&context=spp_papers

Gordon, R. J., Rosenheck, R. A., Zweig, R. A., & Harpaz-Rotem, I. (2012). Health and social adjustment of homeless older adults with a mental illness. *Psychiatric Services, 63*(6), 561–568.

Houston Housing Authority. (n.d.). Apply for public housing. Retrieved from http://www .housingforhouston.com/public-housing/apply -for-public-housing.aspx

National Coalition for the Homeless. (2009). Homelessness among elderly persons. Retrieved from http://www.nationalhomeless.org/fact sheets/elderly.html

National Health Care for the Homeless Council. (2013). Aging and housing instability: Homelessness among older and elderly adults. *In Focus, 2*(1), 1–5. Retrieved from http://www.nhchc.org/ wp-content/uploads/2011/09/infocus_september 2013.pdf

National Leadership Initiative to End Elder Homelessness. (2011). Ending homelessness among older adults and elders through permanent supportive housing. Retrieved from http:// www.csh.org/wp-content/uploads/2012/01/ Report_EndingHomelessnessAmongOlder AdultsandSeniorsThroughSupportiveHousing_ 112.pdf

Salem, B. E., Nyamathi, A. M., Brecht, M. L., Phillips, L. R., Mentes, J. C., Sarkisian, C., & Leake, B. (2013). Correlates of frailty among homeless adults. *Western Journal of Nursing Research, 35*(9), 1128–1152. doi:10.1177/0193945513487608

Substance Abuse and Mental Health Services Administration. (2002). *Substance use by older adults: Estimates of future impact on the treatment system.* Rockville, MD: Author.

U.S. Department of Housing and Urban Development. (n.d.). Housing First Vouchers fact sheet. Retrieved from http://portal.hud.gov/hud portal/HUD?src=/program_offices/public_indian_housing/programs/hcv/about/fact_sheet

U.S. Department of Housing and Urban Development. (2015). The 2014 Annual Homeless Assessment Report to Congress, Part 2. Retrieved from https://www.hudexchange.info/onecpd/assets/File/2014-AHAR-Part-2.pdf

Web Resources

Corporation for Supportive Housing (CSH)—The Source for Housing Solutions: http://www.csh.org/csh-solutions/serving-vulnerable-populations/older-adults

Hearth—Ending Elder Homelessness: http: //hearth-home.org

National Health Care for the Homeless Council: http://www.nhchc.org

HOSPICE

Hospice care is specialized end-of-life care that focuses on maximizing quality of life rather than curing illness or prolonging life. It is delivered to those in the final stages of a life-limiting illness. The goals of hospice care are to provide excellent pain and symptom management, improve comfort, and deliver emotional, psychosocial, and spiritual support to allow for a death with dignity. This focus helps patients and families experience improved-quality end-of-life closure. The term *hospice* may refer to this philosophy of care, the Medicare benefit that pays for this model of care, the agency providing these services, or the facility where this type of care is delivered.

Hospice services developed in response to the improvement of life-prolonging and curative interventions, which moved end-of-life care from the home to the acute care setting. British physician Dame Cicely Saunders began the work in the United Kingdom in the late 1940s. The nurse Florence Wald, dean of Yale School of Nursing, invited Dame Cicely Saunders to the United States in the mid-1960s to teach this philosophy of care to an interdisciplinary group of students from medicine, nursing, social work, and chaplaincy. The work was further developed by the psychiatrist Elisabeth Kübler-Ross. The Medicare hospice benefit was established in 1983.

Hospice care may be provided across a variety of settings and is based on the understanding that dying is a normal part of the life cycle. It provides interdisciplinary and comprehensive medical and supportive services in the home, residential facilities, hospitals and nursing facilities, and other settings (e.g., homeless shelters, prisons). Hospice care supports the patient through the dying process and the surviving family through the dying and bereavement process.

ELIGIBILITY

For a patient to be eligible for the Medicare-reimbursed hospice benefit, two physicians must certify that to the best of their knowledge, the patient has a life expectancy of 6 months or less, if the illness takes its natural course. This requirement is often responsible for a delay in hospice referral; physicians may be reluctant to estimate life expectancy, especially with regard to nononcological diseases. People who use the hospice benefit for the last 7 to 8 weeks of life (a) maximize cost savings to the Medicare program and (b) receive the full benefits of hospice care, such as bereavement counseling, palliative care, and respite for caregivers (National Hospice and Palliative Care Organization [NHPCO], 2015a).

HOSPICE SERVICES

At the time of admission, the hospice agency obtains the necessary medical information from the referring physician. The hospice medical

H

director must concur with the diagnosis of a terminal illness. Most hospices welcome the opportunity to include primary care physicians on the hospice interdisciplinary teams, which establishes the plan of care. The hospice team and the patient's physician work together to maximize quality of life. They jointly develop the plan of care based on the patient's diagnosis, symptoms, and other needs. The hospice program and the patient's physician must together approve any proposed tests, treatments, and services. In general, only treatments that are necessary for palliation and/or management of the terminal illness are approved.

Hospice care is directed primarily at symptom control, not disease control. Pain management is one of the measures taken to maintain the patient's quality of life. Hospice care also takes into consideration concurrent stressful symptoms, such as loss of appetite, nausea, vomiting, hiccups, itching, labored breathing, coughing, insomnia, depression, anxiety, incontinence, constipation, and difficulty swallowing. Eliminating pain and physical symptoms are only two aspects of the hospice concern for maintaining quality of life.

One of the most important cornerstones of a hospice program is a dedicated team of care providers. The team usually consists of a physician, nurses, social workers, clergy, home health aides, and volunteers; other participants might include a dietician, physical therapist, occupational therapist, speech and swallowing therapist, and bereavement counselor. The patient and family are also important members of the team and are encouraged to participate in decision making and formulation of a plan of care oriented to the patient's comfort. A nursing evaluation is done within the first 24 hours and covers not only physical status, but also psychosocial and spiritual needs. Although nurses work under a physician's supervision, the specially designed system of protocols and as-needed orders allows them greater independence in symptom management.

Hospice care can be provided in a variety of settings, most frequently in the patient's home but also in acute care settings (i.e., hospitals), long-term care institutions (i.e., assisted-living facilities, nursing homes), and hospice residential facilities. In addition to making frequent visits, team members are available by telephone 24 hours a day. Care can be provided at different levels of intensity, ranging from brief daily visits to continuous home care, depending on the patient's needs (NHPCO, 2015b).

Bereavement support is a vital component of hospice care; end-of-life care does not end with the death of the patient. Grief and bereavement interventions begin at admission with attention to anticipatory needs and multiple losses of both patient and family. Bereavement support is provided to help the family work to normalize grief, access needed services, and refer high-risk families to specialists.

REIMBURSEMENT

Medicare Part A, Medicaid, and most private insurance policies cover hospice care. For the first 90 days of hospice coverage, the hospice must obtain a certification that the patient is terminally ill from both the medical director of the hospice or the physician member of the hospice interdisciplinary group and the individual's attending physician (if he or she has an attending physician) no later than two calendar days after hospice care is initiated. An attending physician is a doctor of medicine or osteopathy or a nurse practitioner (NP) who is identified by patients, at the time that they elect to receive hospice care, as having the most significant role in the determination and delivery of medical care. The statute allows only a medical doctor or a doctor of osteopathy to certify or recertify that the patient is terminally ill.

Since January 2011, a hospice physician or hospice NP must have a face-to-face encounter with hospice patients prior to, but not more than 30 days prior to, the third benefit period recertification, as well as prior to, but not more than 30 days prior to, each recertification thereafter, to determine continued eligibility for hospice benefit (Centers for Medicare & Medicaid Services, 2015).

Medicare pays for covered services, at a slightly lower rate if required quality data are not submitted, using a per-diem capitated arrangement in one of the following four categories:

- *Routine home care* ($190.55/day for the first 60 days, then $149.82/day): care at home or nursing home
- *Inpatient respite care* ($170.97/day): care in an inpatient setting (nursing home or hospital) for short periods (up to 5 days) to give caregivers a rest
- *General inpatient care* ($734.94/day): acute inpatient care for conditions related to the terminal illness (e.g., pain and symptom control, caregiver breakdown, impending death)
- *Continuous home care* ($964.63/day): acute care at home with around-the-clock care for a crisis that might otherwise lead to inpatient care (U.S. Department of Health and Human Services, 2016).

Medicare beneficiaries are required to sign a statement electing hospice care, thus waiving traditional Medicare benefits covering curative treatment for the terminal disease. Patients can be hospitalized or undergo surgery to palliate their symptoms, but this care is expected to be coordinated through the hospice nurse. A do-not-resuscitate (DNR) order is optional; however, many patients elect not to be resuscitated.

The Medicare hospice benefit covers medications, durable medical equipment, treatments related to the terminal diagnosis, nursing visits, home health aide visits, social worker visits, and bereavement care. It does not cover aggressive curative treatment of the terminal illness, services that are not part of the palliative plan of care or are not preapproved by the interdisciplinary hospice team, or services that duplicate hospice care and are provided by a facility that does not have a contract with the hospice. The patient can revoke the hospice service at any time and for any reason. After a patient signs a written consent indicating a wish to revoke hospice care, regular Medicare benefits are reinstated (Centers for Medicare & Medicaid Services, 2015).

Hospice providers remain under scrutiny in light of the industry's history of Medicare fraud and abuse. The Office of the Inspector General provides oversight of hospice marketing practices and relationships with other providers, such as skilled nursing facilities or hospitals. Hospice and palliative care services

offer aggressive noncurative treatments and interventions. Patients and families across diverse life-threatening illnesses receive support and care based on their unique goals and needs.

See also Access to Hospice Care; Death and Dying; Palliative Care; Primary Palliative Care.

Lara Wahlberg

Centers for Medicare & Medicaid Services. (2015). *Medicare benefit policy manual.* Retrieved from https://www.cms.gov/Regulations-and-Guidance/Guidance/Manuals/downloads/bp102c09.pdf

National Hospice and Palliative Care Organization. (2015a). *The Medicare hospice benefit.* Alexandria, VA: Author. Retrieved from http://www.nhpco.org/sites/default/files/public/communications/Outreach/The_Medicare_Hospice_Benefit.pdf

National Hospice and Palliative Care Organization. (2015b). *NHPCO facts and figures: Hospice care in America.* Alexandria, VA: Author. Retrieved from http://www.nhpco.org/sites/default/files/public/Statistics_Research/2015_Facts_Figures.pdf

U.S. Department of Health and Human Services. (2016). *Medicare learning network: Updates to the hospice payment rates, hospice cap, hospice wage index, and hospice pricer for fiscal year 2017.* Washington, DC: U.S. Department of Health and Human Services, Centers for Medicare & Medicaid Services. Retrieved from https://www.cms.gov/Outreach-and-Education/Medicare-Learning-Network-MLN/MLNMattersArticles/Downloads/MM9729.pdf

Web Resources
American Academy of Hospice and Palliative Medicine: http://www.aahpm.org
Hospice: http://hospicenet.org
Hospice and Palliative Nurses Association: http://www.hpna.org
Hospice Association of America: http://www.nahc.org/haa
Hospice Foundation of America: http://www.hospicefoundation.org
Medicare: How hospice works: https://www.medicare.gov/what-medicare-covers/part-a/how-hospice-works.html

Medicare Hospice Benefits: Centers for Medicare & Medicaid Services: https://www.medicare.gov/Pubs/pdf/02154-Medicare-Hospice-Benefits.PDF

National Hospice and Palliative Care Organization: http://www.nhpco.org

HOSPITAL-BASED SERVICES

In nonfederal hospitals, patients 65 years of age and older account for 38% of all discharges and 45% of inpatient days of care. Rates of hospitalization are more than twice as high for patients aged 85 years and older compared with patients aged 65 to 74 years. Older patients have longer hospitalizations, higher mortality rates, and higher rates of nursing home placement. Furthermore, hospitalization is associated with the risk of functional decline or physical disability during the course of treatment for an acute medical illness (Malone, Capezuti, & Palmer, 2015). Functional decline during hospitalization occurs more often in patients who are older than age 75 years, cognitively impaired, and dependent at baseline (before the acute illness) in two or more instrumental activities of daily living (IADL).

Clinical studies demonstrate that at least some of the poor functional outcomes of hospitalization can be attenuated through improved processes and systems of care. Several promising models of hospital care are potentially applicable to most hospitals in the United States. Most of the successful models have been nurse driven, often employing an advanced practice nurse. Interdisciplinary models are common and frequently include geriatricians, nurse specialists, physical and occupational therapists, speech therapists, social workers, and dieticians. The usual objectives are to improve functional outcomes, reduce hospital length of stay, prevent nursing home admissions, and prevent unplanned rehospitalization (Malone et al., 2015).

ACUTE CARE FOR ELDERS UNITS

An acute care for elders (ACE) unit may be either a discrete nursing unit (all beds) or a "virtual unit" with a mixed population of elderly and nonelderly patients. The goal of an ACE unit is to prevent functional decline that results from processes of care (e.g., polypharmacy, imposed bed rest, inadequate medical standards of care, uncoordinated care) and patient characteristics (e.g., depression, cognitive impairment, physical disability) that often go undetected or untreated. Although the model fidelity of ACE units may vary considerably, they have in common four main components: a prepared environment, patient-centered care, interdisciplinary team rounds and discharge planning, and medical care review. The physical environment of the ACE unit is designed to enhance the patient's independent functioning in activities of daily living (ADL) and mobility. For example, ACE units avoid clutter in hallway corridors and low-risk (for injury) flooring but have grab bars in bathrooms, handrails in hallways, and common activity areas to permit dining outside of rooms or socializing with family. Patient-centered care includes a multidimensional assessment at the time of admission and an interdisciplinary team care plan to maintain or restore the patient's independent functioning in basic ADL and to coordinate transitions of care. Acute geriatric units deploying ACE components identified improved health outcomes, including reduced incidence of falls, delirium, functional decline, and discharges to nursing facilities, as well as reduction in 30-day hospital readmissions, reduced costs, and increased discharges to home (Malone, Capezuti, & Palmer, 2014).

GERIATRIC CARE PROGRAM

A gerontological clinical nurse specialist working with geriatric resource nurses—RNs with additional training in geriatrics—focuses nursing care on patients at high risk for functional decline. Interventions include identification and monitoring of frail older patients by a multidisciplinary geriatric care team and a nursing-centered educational program. The training of resource nurses has been fostered by the program Nurses Improving Care for Healthsystem Elders (NICHE), which serves as a technical resource center and a catalyst for collaboration among facilities to provide quality geriatric care (Capezuti et al., 2012).

HOSPITAL ELDER LIFE PROGRAM

The goal of the Hospital Elder Life Program (HELP) is to prevent incident delirium. Patients at risk of incident delirium are identified shortly after hospital admission using the Confusion Assessment Method (HELP; Inouye, Bogardus, Jr., Baker, Leo-Summers, & Cooney, Jr., 2000). An array of protocols targeted at specific risk factors (e.g., sensory deprivation, cognitive impairment) serve to optimize cognitive function (e.g., reorientation, therapeutic activities), prevent sleep deprivation (e.g., relaxation, noise reduction), avoid immobility (e.g., ambulation, exercises), improve vision (e.g., visual aids, illumination), improve hearing (e.g., hearing devices), and treat dehydration (e.g., volume repletion). The HELP program employs volunteers and activities coordinators. HELP reduces the incidence of delirium in medically ill patients at risk for delirium. The intervention is cost-effective when it targets patients at moderate risk for delirium. Components of the intervention are inexpensive and are easily incorporated into standard medical and nursing care in most hospitals and have generated cost savings (Rubin, Neal, Fenlon, Hassam, & Inouye, 2011).

TRANSITIONAL CARE INTERVENTIONS

Improving transitions of care across all settings of health care has the potential to improve patient safety and health outcomes. Several care transitions models targeted at elderly adults have been implemented in an effort to reduce hospital and emergency room readmissions and to decrease health care costs. In one model of care, the Transitional Care Model (TCM; Naylor, Aiken, Kurtzman, Olds, & Hirschman, 2011), an advanced practice nurse (or a trained RN) implements comprehensive discharge planning for patients with common diagnoses, conducts short-term home care, maintains close collaboration with the patient's attending physician, provides patient/caregiver education in the hospital and at home, and remains available by telephone following the patient's discharge to

home. The intervention reduces readmissions at 24 weeks and reduces reimbursements (costs) of health services. Comprehensive discharge planning plus postdischarge support also reduces readmission rates for older patients with congestive heart failure (CHF).

A Care Transitions Intervention the Transitional Care Program (TCP; Coleman, Parry, Chalmers, & Min, 2006) prepares patients and their caregivers to participate in care delivered across health care settings. A transition coach (e.g., geriatric nurse practitioner) meets patients in the hospital or after discharge and enables them to create a personal health record and to understand their medications, prepares them for talking to their primary care physician or specialists, and teaches them about indications that their condition is worsening and ways to respond. The TCP reduces hospital readmission rates for patients at risk for readmission and reduces total costs of care.

A related quality-improvement intervention, Project BOOST (Better Outcomes for Older Adults through Safe Transitions), was developed by the Society of Hospital Medicine to improve planning for care transitions with the goal of reducing 30-day readmissions.

POST-ACUTE SERVICES

Closely aligned to the acute-care hospital, post-acute services include subacute units, skilled nursing facilities (SNFs), geriatric evaluation and management (GEM) units, and in-patient rehabilitation hospitals (American Hospital Association [AHA], 2015). Subacute units are SNFs that provide short-term, goal-oriented, and intensive rehabilitative or skilled nursing services. Medicare patients are often transferred to subacute units of SNFs for continuing care after their clinical status has been stable for at least 72 hours in the hospital. Patients with Medicare-managed care benefits can be admitted directly to the SNF or subacute unit from the community. Rehabilitation hospitals are appropriate sites for patients with a categorical illness (e.g., hip fracture, acute stroke) who can tolerate physical therapy and are likely to return to a community residence. In Veterans Affairs hospitals, elderly patients who remain

H

functionally impaired following admission to an acute-care hospital might be eligible for transfer to a GEM unit for further assessment and rehabilitation.

CURRENT TRENDS

As financial incentives align to reduce the costs of care and improve quality, the acute care hospital is evolving into an integrated health system in which the most cost-effective services are applied to targeted patients in various subsystems of care. The subsystems of geriatric care in a growing number of medical centers include acute care units (e.g., ACE, HELP, stroke), and inpatient palliative care and hospice programs. The Medicare Innovations Collaborative (Leff et al., 2012) demonstrated the feasibility of bundling models of care (NICHE, ACE, HELP, palliative care, care transitions) to address the needs of older patients in health care systems. Furthermore, these programs may be viewed by health care systems as cost-effective models of patient safety and quality care; the Centers for Medicare & Medicaid Innovation Center, mandated in the Patient Protection and Affordable Care Act, promotes care coordination and transitions to improve quality of care and decrease Medicare costs.

Recently the President and Senior Program Officer of The John A. Hartford Foundation (Fulmer & Berman, 2016) asked, "How do we move from a model at a time to a set of strategies that transform systems, drive improved health and cost outcomes, efficiently utilize available resources, deploy them strategically to those at greatest risk, and create the least amount of stress on the care delivery system?" The John A. Hartford Foundation, along with the Institute for Healthcare Improvement and the American Hospital Association, has launched a new Age-Friendly Health Systems Initiative. This $3.19 million, 42-month grant focuses on initiating and evaluating a health systems–wide prototype model of care for older adults. The overall goal is that 20% of hospitals and health systems in the United States will be "age friendly" by 2020.

See also Clinical Pathways; Discharge Planning; Geriatric Evaluation and Management Units; Geriatric Resource Nurse; Hospital Elder Life Program; Nurses Improving Care for Healthsystem Elders (NICHE).

Marissa Galicia-Castillo

American Hospital Association. (2015). The role of post-acute care in new care delivery models. *Trendwatch.* Retrieved from http://www.aha.org/research/reports/tw/15dec-tw-postacute.pdf

Capezuti, E., Boltz, M., Cline, D., Dickson, V., Rosenberg, M., Wagner, L., ... Nigolian, C. (2012). NICHE—A model for optimizing the geriatric nursing practice environment. *Journal of Clinical Nursing, 21,* 3117–3125.

Coleman, E. A., Parry, C., Chalmers, S., & Min, S. J. (2006). The care transitions intervention: Results of a randomized controlled trial. *Archives of Internal Medicine, 166*(17), 1822–1828.

Fulmer, T., & Berman, A. (2016, November 3) Age-friendly health systems: How do we get there? [Health Affairs Blog]. Retrieved from http://healthaffairs.org/blog/2016/11/03/age-friendly-health-systems-how-do-we-get-there

Inouye, S. K., Bogardus Jr., S. T., Baker, D. I., Leo-Summers, L., & Cooney Jr, L. M. (2000). The Hospital Elder Life Program: A model of care to prevent cognitive and functional decline in older hospitalized patients. *Journal of the American Geriatrics Society, 48*(12), 1697–1706.

Leff, B., Spragens, L. H., Morano, B., Powell, J., Bickert, T., Bond, C., ... Siu, A. L. (2012). Rapid reengineering of acute medical care for Medicare beneficiaries: The Medicare innovations collaborative. *Health Affairs, 6,* 1204–1215.

Malone, M. L., Capezuti, E., & Palmer, R. (Eds.). (2014). *Acute care for elders—A model for interdisciplinary care.* Cham, Switzerland: Springer International.

Malone, M. L., Capezuti, E., & Palmer, R. M. (2015). *Geriatrics models of care—Bringing "Best Practice" to an Aging America.* Cham, Switzerland: Springer International.

Naylor, M. D., Aiken, L. H., Kurtzman, E. T., Olds, D. M., & Hirschman, K. B. (2011). The importance of transitional care in achieving health reform. *Health Affairs, 30*(4), 746–754.

Rubin, F. H., Neal, K., Fenlon, K., Hassam, S., & Inouye, S. K. (2011). Sustainability and scalability of the Hospital Elder Life Program at a community hospital. *Journal of the American Geriatrics Society, 59,* 359–365.

Web Resources

Care Transitions Program (Coleman): http://www
.caretransitions.org

Hospital Elder Life Program (Inouye): http://www
.hospitalelderlifeprogram.org/public/public
-main.php

Nurses Improving Care for Healthsystem Elders
(NICHE): http://nicheprogram.com

Society of Hospital Medicine BOOST: http://www
.hospitalmedicine.org/BOOST

Transitional Care Model (Naylor): http://www
.transitionalcare.info

Hospital Elder Life Program

The *Hospital Elder Life Program* (HELP; www
.hospitalelderlifeprogram.org) is a unique multidisciplinary approach to caring for older hospitalized patients at risk for delirium or functional
decline, with proven effectiveness and cost-
effectiveness. HELP was originally tested in the
Yale Delirium Prevention Trial involving 852
patients aged 70 years and older. Half received
the HELP intervention, and the remainder
received usual hospital care. The intervention resulted in a 40% reduction in the risk of
delirium (Inouye et al., 1999). In more than 35
studies to date, HELP has repeatedly demonstrated effectiveness in diverse settings and
populations. Multicomponent interventions for
delirium prevention have been recommended
in guidelines developed by the American
Geriatrics Society and National Institute for
Health and Care Excellence (NICE), and HELP
is the most widely studied program. In 2013,
protocols were updated to enhance the scope of
HELP and to allow fulfillment of the NICE clinical guidelines on delirium. The NICE guidelines
included 10 recommendations for delirium prevention. HELP provided the basis for seven of
the recommendations; three additional protocols were developed for HELP to address hypoxia, infection, and pain (Yue et al., 2014).

A key feature of the program is that it does
not rely on a dedicated hospital unit. The program provides a real-world approach that can
be integrated into usual care on any hospital
unit and has been successfully implemented
in medical, surgical, geriatric, telemetry, intensive care, emergency department, and nursing
home settings. HELP is designed to deliver
geriatric expertise throughout the institution,
thereby broadening its impact to a larger percentage of patients. Goals of the program are
to (a) maintain physical and cognitive functioning throughout hospitalization, (b) maximize
independence at discharge, (c) assist with transition from hospital to home, and (d) prevent
unplanned readmission.

PROGRAM DESCRIPTION

Enrollment and Intervention

On admission, patients aged 70 years and older
are screened for the presence of at least one of
five delirium risk factors, including cognitive
impairment, functional or mobility impairment,
dehydration, vision impairment, and decreased
hearing. Interventions that target these and
six other risk factors—sleep deprivation, poor
nutrition, polypharmacy, pain, hypoxia, and
infection—are implemented by the HELP team
and tracked for adherence.

HELP Team Roles and Responsibilities

Elder Life nurse specialist (ELNS). The ELNS is a
master's-prepared nurse with experience and
knowledge in geriatrics. The ELNS performs
patient assessments and interventions using
standardized protocols targeting geriatric care
issues and delirium risk factors. The ELNS is
also an educational resource for nursing staff
and other hospital staff via daily rounds and
regular in-services. The ELNS acts as a liaison
between the HELP program and hospital staff,
communicating recommendations and ensuring
follow-up.

Elder Life specialist (ELS). The ELS is a unique
role created for HELP, requiring a bachelor's or
master's degree in human services or health
care, experience working with older patients,
and excellent communication skills. The ELS
screens and enrolls patients, orients patients and
families to the program, and develops care plans
for volunteer interventions. Although the care
plans are individualized to each patient's risk

factors, the interventions consist of standardized protocols. The ELS supervises volunteers and the day-to-day operations of the program.

Geriatrician. The HELP geriatrician participates in interdisciplinary rounds and provides medical expertise and back-up for HELP staff. The geriatrician also provides ongoing educational programs and consultations. The geriatrician may serve as program champion and clinical director, but these roles may also be performed by the ELNS, ELS, or another HELP team member.

Volunteers. Volunteers are a unique aspect of HELP. Trained volunteers have been found to provide added value to the HELP program, reducing patient loneliness and enhancing participant satisfaction (Steunenberg, van der Mast, Strijbos, Inouye, & Schuurmans, 2016). Volunteers are recruited and screened for characteristics such as maturity, respect for older patients, and enthusiasm. A time commitment of 6 months is required. Volunteer training is extensive and encompasses a minimum of 16 hours of classroom learning, 16 hours of one-on-one training on the nursing units, and completion of competency-based checklists. These interventions include daily visits with orienting techniques, therapeutic activities, early mobilization, and vision and hearing enhancement. All interventions are tracked by the ELS for adherence.

Interdisciplinary expertise. Critical to the effectiveness of HELP is a skilled interdisciplinary team. The HELP program conducts twice-weekly interdisciplinary care rounds on all HELP patients to coordinate the program and interventions. In addition to the HELP staff, participants include primary nurses and physicians, as well as rehabilitation therapy (physical, occupational, speech therapy), clinical pharmacy, nutrition, chaplaincy, social work, and discharge-planning services.

OUTCOMES AND BENEFITS

Acute Care

Over the past 16 years, multiple studies have found that HELP prevents delirium, falls, and cognitive and functional decline and decreases institutionalization, use of sitters, and length of stay. Overall, absolute risk reduction for incident delirium ranged from 5% to 32% (Inouye et al., 1999; Hshieh, Saczynski, et al., 2017; Hshieh, Yue, et al., 2015; Zaubler et al., 2013). A few studies found significant reduction in rate of institutionalization after discharge and a decreased incidence of falls by 2% to 13% (Hshieh, Yue, et al., 2015). HELP has also been modified for the emergency room setting, using volunteers to prevent avoidable complications, including falls, delirium, restraint use, and functional decline, while improving patient satisfaction with care (Sanon, Baumlin, Kaplan, & Gruzden, 2014).

Long-Term Care

The patients in the initial Yale Delirium Prevention Trial were followed for 1 year after discharge. The intervention was associated with a 15.7% decrease in long-term care costs, with an average savings of $9,446 per patient. Furthermore, HELP has been adapted by a number of sites for long-term care settings and has been found to be feasible (Huson, Stolee, Pearce, Bradfield, & Heckman, 2016).

Potential Health Care Savings

HELP is highly cost-effective. In large implementation of HELP at a community hospital, the cost savings for hospital care alone were estimated at $7.3 million per year, or more than $1,000 per patient served. The costs of implementing the program were more than offset by the cost savings from the program, and patients in HELP reported greater satisfaction with their quality of care (Rubin, Neal, Fenlon, Hassan, & Inouye, 2011). Contributing to the program's cost-effectiveness were decreased length of stay, falls, and sitter use among HELP patients.

The 1-year health care costs for a delirious patient were calculated at $120,349 compared with $59,833 for nondelirious patients, or $60,516 per case prevented (Leslie, Marcantonio, Zhang, Leo-Summers, & Inouye, 2008). In 2008, there were 13.2 million hospital discharges of older patients in the United States and at least 3.96 million cases of delirium. Based on a 40% reduction in delirium incidence provided by

Table H.1
HELP PROGRAM INTERVENTIONS

Interventions	Description
Core interventions	
—Orientation/therapeutic activities	Orientation board with names of care team members and daily schedule. Cognitive stimulation activities.
—Sleep enhancement	At bedtime, warm milk or herbal tea, relaxation tapes or music, and back massage. Unit-wide noise reduction and schedule adjustments to allow uninterrupted sleep.
Early mobilization	Ambulation or active range-of-motion exercises; minimize use of immobilizing equipment.
Vision protocol	Daily reinforcement of visual aids and adaptive equipment.
Hearing protocol	Portable amplifying devices and special communication techniques; ear wax clearing as needed.
Fluid repletion	Encourage fluids; promote mobility and regular toileting.
—Feeding assistance	Feeding assistance and encouragement during meals.
Other program interventions	
Other geriatric nursing assessments and interventions	
—Delirium protocol	Create calm, orienting environment; communicate with patients clearly and pleasantly; encourage family involvement; refer to physicians if needed.
—Dementia protocol	Collaborate with medical staff and family; avoid psychoactive medications.
—Psychoactive medications	Screen medication list daily for medications associated with delirium; collaborate with interdisciplinary team about potential/actual adverse medication outcomes; make recommendations.
—Discharge planning	Assess home environment and social supports for possible discharge needs.
—Optimizing length of stay	Identify risk factors indicating a need for intensive discharge planning; anticipate discharge needs.
—Additional areas	Nursing assessment and interventions for emotional health, nutrition, functional status, incontinence and elimination issues, skin, and social issues.
Interdisciplinary interventions	
—Interdisciplinary rounds	Twice-weekly rounds to discuss each Elder Life patient, set goals, and review all Elder Life issues with interdisciplinary input; track/recommend interventions.
—Interdisciplinary consultation	Provide as-needed consultation and input about Elder Life patients on referral by staff.
—Geriatrician consultation	Targeted consultation on Elder Life issues, as referred by program staff. Formal geriatric consultation on a limited basis.
Discharge and postdischarge procedures	
—Community linkages and… Telephone follow-up	Referrals and communication with community agencies to optimize transition to home. Telephone follow-up phone call within 7 days after discharge for all patients.
Educational interventions	
—Education program	Formal didactic sessions, one-on-one interactions, and resource materials to educate nursing and physician staff about Elder Life issues.

HELP, Hospital Elder Life Program.

HELP, approximately 2.38 million cases of delirium could be prevented annually, resulting in Medicare cost savings of approximately $14 billion per year (Leslie et al., 2008).

DISSEMINATION

HELP continues to be actively disseminated worldwide, and there are currently more than 200 active sites in the United States, Canada, Australia, United Kingdom, Singapore, Netherlands, Japan, and Taiwan. Implementation of the HELP program is rewarding, but presents some challenges. Although some hospitals have implemented the program in its entirety, others have implemented certain components or made adaptations. With adaptations, it is important to demonstrate continued effectiveness, as has

H

been done in other countries; it is also important to demonstrate feasibility and scalability in other specialty settings (e.g., surgery, emergency medicine).

Staff from nine hospitals who implemented HELP were asked to describe the challenges faced while starting and sustaining the program (SteelFisher, Martin, Dowal, & Inouye, 2013). Challenges included gaining internal support for the program despite differing requirements and goals of administration and clinical staff, ensuring effective clinician leadership, integrating with existing geriatric programs, balancing program fidelity with hospital-specific circumstances, documenting and publicizing positive outcomes, and maintaining the momentum of implementation in the face of difficult time frames and limited resources. Long-term follow up of 19 successful programs showed that maintaining a strong HELP program requires sustained and meaningful communication with hospital administration, effective documentation of day-to-day operational success, metrics that align with institutional priorities, and continued support from clinical staff (SteelFisher et al., 2013).

HELP incorporates practical, hands-on patient interventions with geriatric-focused oversight, resulting in improved quality of care for hospitalized older patients and improved patient and family satisfaction with care. HELP also plays an important role in improving nursing satisfaction, retention, and skills in caring for older persons. Close communication between patients, families, and caregivers allows changes in a patient's status to be addressed expeditiously. The use of volunteers is cost-effective, and patients and staff relate well to the human element that they provide. HELP raises visibility for geriatrics, often bringing widespread recognition to affiliated hospitals as geriatric centers of excellence or magnet status. The HELP website provides detailed dissemination materials, information for health care professionals, patients and families and a searchable reference database that has been widely used for implementation, adaptation, and educational efforts.

HELP's patient-centric approach generates benefits beyond the basic goal of delirium prevention by enhancing overall geriatric care and contributing to system-wide change. By emphasizing a humanistic approach to medical care, the HELP model provides the means to improve the quality and effectiveness of hospital care for older persons and prepares our health care system to cope with our aging society (Table H.1).

ACKNOWLEDGMENTS

This work is dedicated to the memory of Joshua Bryan Inouye Helfand. The authors wish to thank the HELP Advisory Board, the HELP Dissemination Team, the Centers of Excellence, and the community of HELP clinicians for their unflagging dedication to improving care for seniors worldwide.

Tammy T. Hshieh, Sarah L. Dowal,
Jaclyn R. Freshman, and Sharon K. Inouye

Hshieh, T. T., Saczynski, J., Gou, R. Y., Marcantonio, E., Jones, R. N., Schmitt, E., … Inouye, S. K. (2017). Trajectory of functional recovery after postoperative delirium in elective surgery. *Annals of Surgery, 265*(4), 647–653. doi:10.1097/sla.0000000000001952

Hshieh, T. T., Yue, J., Oh, E., Puelle, M., Dowal, S., Travison, T., & Inouye, S. K. (2015). Effectiveness of multicomponent nonpharmacological delirium interventions: a meta-analysis. *JAMA Internal Medicine, 175*(4), 512–520. doi:10.1001/jamainternmed.2014.7779

Huson, K., Stolee, P., Pearce, N., Bradfield, C., & Heckman, G. A. (2016). Examining the Hospital Elder Life Program in a rehabilitation setting: A pilot feasibility study. *BMC Geriatrics, 16*, 140. doi:10.1186/s12877-016-0313-3

Inouye, S. K., Bogardus, S. T., Jr., Charpentier, P. A., Leo-Summers, L., Acampora, D., Holford, T. R., & Cooney, L. M., Jr. (1999). A multicomponent intervention to prevent delirium in hospitalized older patients. *New England Journal of Medicine, 340*(9), 669–676. doi:10.1056/nejm199903043400901

Leslie, D. L., Marcantonio, E. R., Zhang, Y., Leo-Summers, L., & Inouye, S. K. (2008). One-year health care costs associated with delirium in the elderly population. *Archives of Internal Medicine, 168*(1), 27–32. doi:10.1001/archinternmed.2007.4

Rubin, F. H., Neal, K., Fenlon, K., Hassan, S., & Inouye, S. K. (2011). Sustainability and scalability of the hospital elder life program at a community hospital. *Journal of the American Geriatrics Society, 59*(2), 359–365. doi:10.1111/j.1532-5415.2010.03243.x

H

Sanon, M., Baumlin, K. M., Kaplan, S. S., & Grudzen, C. R. (2014). Care and Respect for Elders in Emergencies program: A preliminary report of a volunteer approach to enhance care in the emergency department. *Journal of the American Geriatrics Society, 62*(2), 365–370. doi:10.1111/jgs.12646

SteelFisher, G. K., Martin, L. A., Dowal, S. L., & Inouye, S. K. (2013). Learning from the closure of clinical programs: a case series from the Hospital Elder Life Program. *Journal of the American Geriatrics Society, 61*(6), 999–1004. doi:10.1111/jgs.12274

Steunenberg, B., van der Mast, R. C., Strijbos, M. J., Inouye, S. K., & Schuurmans, M. J. (2016). How trained volunteers can improve the quality of hospital care for older patients. A qualitative evaluation within the Hospital Elder Life Program (HELP). *Geriatric Nursing, 37*(6), 458–463. doi:10.1016/j.gerinurse.2016.06.014

Yue, J., Tabloski, P., Dowal, S. L., Puelle, M. R., Nandan, R., & Inouye, S. K. (2014). NICE to HELP: Operationalizing National Institute for Health and Clinical Excellence guidelines to improve clinical practice. *Journal of the American Geriatrics Society, 62*(4), 754–761. doi:10.1111/jgs.12768

Zaubler, T. S., Murphy, K., Rizzuto, L., Santos, R., Skotzko, C., Giordano, J., … Inouye, S. K. (2013). Quality improvement and cost savings with multicomponent delirium interventions: Replication of the Hospital Elder Life Program in a community hospital. *Psychosomatics, 54*(3), 219–226. doi:10.1016/j.psym.2013.01.010

Web Resources

HELP Program: http://www.hospitalelderlifeprogram.org

National Health Service, National Institute for Health and Care Excellence (NICE) guidelines for delirium: http://www.nice.org.uk/cg103

National Quality Measures Clearinghouse (NQMC): Delirium Quality Measure: http://www.quality measures.ahrq.gov/content.aspx?id=27635

I

IATROGENESIS

Iatrogenic illness is any illness that results from a diagnostic procedure or therapeutic intervention and is not a natural consequence of the patient's disease. In general, iatrogenic illness is one that results from medication, diagnostic or therapeutic procedures, nosocomial infections, or environmental hazards. A broader definition includes a complication related to the diagnosis and treatment of disease, regardless of whether the condition occurs as a known risk of a procedure or through errors of omission or commission. Most studies of iatrogenesis have been conducted in acute care hospitals. Older patients are predisposed to iatrogenic illness because of reduced homeostatic reserves, high levels of comorbid illnesses, and polypharmacy, which increases the probability of adverse drug events.

A related concept, medical error, overlaps with iatrogenic illness. Medical errors are mistakes committed by health professionals that result in harm to the patients. Recent analyses suggest that medical errors account for an estimated 210,000 to 400,000 deaths per year in the U.S. hospitals (Markay & Daniel, 2016), making errors the third most common cause of death. The high rates of iatrogenesis, medical error, and negligence reported in hospitalized patients led the Institute of Medicine (IOM) to release a report, *To Err Is Human: Building a Safer Health System*. This monograph advocated for dramatic, system-wide changes to reduce these rates (Kohn, Corrigan, & Donaldson, 1999). A subsequent publication from the IOM, the Quality Chasm report (2001), describes broader quality issues and defines six aims: Care should be (a) safe, (b) effective, (c) patient centered, (d) timely, (e) efficient, and (f) equitable. In response, The Joint Commission established National Patient Safety Goals that include correctly identifying patients, preventing surgical errors, improving staff communication, preventing infections (hospital acquired, central line, catheter related), identifying patient-safety risks, and using medicines safely (The Joint Commission, 2017). Per the Centers for Medicare & Medicaid Services (CMS), hospitals do not receive a higher payment for cases in which one of the selected conditions is acquired during hospitalization. These hospital-acquired conditions (HACs) that are particularly relevant to elderly inpatients are falls with trauma, catheter-associated urinary tract infections, and pressure injuries stages 3 and 4.

ADVERSE DRUG EVENTS

Adverse drug events in hospitalized patients are associated with significantly prolonged lengths of stay, higher costs, and increased risk of death. Polypharmacy, prescribing potentially inappropriate medications (American Geriatrics Society, 2015), and prescribing errors are common preventable causes of iatrogenic illness, with psychotropic and anticholinergic effects among the highest-risk medications.

Adverse drug events are commonly because of medical errors. The American Hospital Association (n.d.) lists the following as some common types of medication errors:

- Incomplete patient information (e.g., not knowing about patients' allergies, other medicines they are taking, previous diagnoses, and laboratory results)
- Unavailable drug information (e.g., lack of up-to-date warnings)
- Miscommunication of drug orders, which can involve poor handwriting, confusion among drugs with similar names, misuse of zeroes and decimal points, confusion of metric and other dosing units, and inappropriate abbreviations

- Lack of appropriate labeling as a drug is prepared and repackaged into smaller units
- Environmental factors, such as lighting, heat, noise, and interruptions, which can distract health professionals from their medical tasks

The prevention of adverse drug events in older hospitalized patients can include a variety of strategies, including guidelines for appropriate drug prescribing and the use of electronic medical records with educational supports.

DIAGNOSTIC AND THERAPEUTIC PROCEDURES

Common medical complications of diagnostic studies include anemia from extensive venipunctures, urinary tract infections from bladder catheterizations, and contrast-induced nephropathy. Patients at high risk of contrast nephropathy include those with diabetes mellitus and preexisting renal insufficiency. The patient's hydration should be maintained before and after a diagnostic study is performed with intravenous radiocontrast dyes. Contrast should be avoided if patients have baseline renal insufficiency. If possible, nonsteroidal anti-inflammatory drugs and diuretics should be withheld before and after exposure to contrast medium.

Functional decline, delirium, pressure injuries, and trauma (e.g., falls) may occur because of inadequate processes of care or poor environmental conditions. Pneumothorax and hematomas from arterial lines placed during surgical or invasive procedures have been reported in hospitalized patients. Complications of immobility, including physical disability, deep vein thrombosis/thromboembolism, and pressure injuries, are potentially preventable through greater attention to patient mobility and exercise, avoidance of physical restraints, and interdisciplinary care (Agency for Healthcare Research and Quality [AHRQ], 2016). Patients should be assessed for the risk of pressure injuries, with attention to nutritional repletion, mobility, and skin lubrication.

Standardized protocols can improve surgical outcomes. Attention to blood pressure regulation, oxygen supplementation, and the avoidance of anticholinergic agents in the perioperative period appear to reduce the incidence of postoperative delirium. Anticoagulation with low-molecular-weight, unfractionated heparin or a vitamin K antagonist reduces the incidence of venous thrombosis in elderly patients undergoing elective or emergent hip or knee surgery (Maynard, 2015). The use of intermittent pneumatic compression is also an option, especially in patients with high bleeding risk.

NOSOCOMIAL INFECTIONS

Nosocomial, or hospital-acquired, infections are common causes of iatrogenic illness in both hospitalized and institutionalized elderly patients; they increase the length of stay and the costs of hospitalization and increase overall morbidity and mortality. Common nosocomial infections often resistant to usual antibiotics include methicillin-resistant *Staphylococcus aureus* (MRSA), vancomycin-resistant enterococci (VRE), extended spectrum beta-lactamase *Escherichia coli*, and *Clostridium difficile* colitis. These infections are potentially preventable through best practices that avoid the overuse of antibiotics and use universal handwashing and antibacterial skin sanitizers.

Bacterial resistance to usual antibiotic therapy results from interaction among microorganisms, patients, antibiotics, and infection-control practices. The factors that contribute to antibiotic resistance are frequent prescribing of antibiotics, intrainstitutional transmission of resistant bacteria by cross-colonization of patients because of poor handwashing practices of health care workers, and transfer of colonized patients between institutions. Colonization and infection with VRE have been associated with exposure to antibiotics and environmental contamination. Infection and antibiotic control procedures, including restriction of vancomycin use, better selection of empirical antibiotics, education of hospital personnel, early detection and reporting of vancomycin resistance, isolation of colonized patients, and appropriate cleansing of the environment, may prevent the spread of VRE in health care settings.

Resistant urinary tract infections are common in elderly patients following prolonged

I

indwelling urinary catheterization. The incidence of infection increases by approximately 5% per day, although the rate of bacteremia is lower. Chronic catheter use should be limited to patients with incurable urinary retention who cannot be kept clean and dry with standard nursing measures. Patients who are critically ill, whose precise measurement of urine output is important, are candidates for temporary catheter placement for the shortest duration possible. Prophylactic antimicrobial therapies and routine catheter replacement are not recommended.

Nosocomial pneumonia results from colonization of the upper respiratory and gastrointestinal tracts and occurs most often in critically ill patients who are ventilator dependent. The factors promoting nosocomial pneumonia include gastric aspiration, spread of pathogens on the hands of medical and nursing personnel, fecal–oral spread of pathogens, and cross-contamination from other patients. Prevention includes proper cleaning of respiratory equipment at timely intervals, consistent handwashing between patient contacts, cleaning of mechanical equipment between patient contacts, and maintenance of the patient in a semi-upright position to minimize the risk of gastric aspiration.

Intravascular infections, most often related to central intravenous or intraarterial lines, are associated with the duration and site of catheter use. To reduce the risk of infection, the patient's skin should be disinfected with chlorhexidine gluconate before catheterization, triple-lumen catheters impregnated with antimicrobial should be used when a multilumen catheter is necessary, and the line should be removed when there is clinical evidence of infection from the catheter (Mermel et al., 2009). Outcomes are improved with a checklist of standardized behaviors that decrease the incidence of infections during central line insertion.

Improving the use of antibiotics is an important patient-safety issue to prevent iatrogenic illness and control emergence of multi-drug-resistant organisms in health care settings. A growing interest is hospital-based programs dedicated to improving antibiotic use (antibiotic stewardship programs) that recognize the frequent overuse of antibiotics (Barlam et al., 2016)

ENVIRONMENTAL HAZARDS

The physical environment of the hospital can contribute to the risk of iatrogenic illness. Most older hospitals were not designed to foster the independent functioning of older patients. Shiny and slippery-appearing floors can discourage walking, and various tethers such as physical restraints and intravenous lines can limit mobility. Likewise, the noise and frequent interruptions of meals and sleep can increase the risks of delirium, falls, and functional decline. Aspects of the physical environment should be modified to reduce the potential for an iatrogenic event while enhancing the patient's independent functioning in activities of daily living and mobility. The desirable features of the environment include clutter-free corridors equipped with handrails, low-gloss floors in hallways and rooms, diffuse lighting, quiet rooms at night, appropriate signage, and grab bars in bathrooms. The physical barriers to patient mobility, including restraints, should be minimized.

See also Environmental Modifications: Home; Polypharmacy; Polypharmacy: Drug–Drug Interactions; Pressure Injury Risk Assessment; Restraints; Signage.

Robert M. Palmer

Agency for Healthcare Research and Quality. (2016). Patient safety and medical errors. Retrieved from http://www.ahrq.gov/legacy/qual/patient safetyix.htm

American Geriatrics Society. (2015). Updated Beers criteria for potentially inappropriate medication use in older adults. *Journal of the American Geriatrics Society, 63,* 2227–2246.

American Hospital Association. (n.d.). Improving medication safety. Retrieved from http://www.aha.org/advocacy-issues/tools-resources/advisory/96-06/991207-quality-adv.shtml

Barlam, T. F., Cosgrove, S. E., Abbo, L. M., MacDougall, C., Schuetz, A. N., Septimus, E. J., ... Trivedi, K. K. (2016). Implementing an antibiotic stewardship program: guidelines by the Infectious Diseases Society of America and the Society for Healthcare Epidemiology of America. *Clinical Infectious Diseases, 62*(10), e51–e77.

Institute of Medicine. (2001). *Crossing the quality chasm: A new health system for the 21st century.* Washington, DC: National Academies Press. doi:10.17226/10027

The Joint Commission. (2017). National patient safety goals. Retrieved from https://www.joint commission.org/assets/1/6/NPSG_Chapter_HAP_Jan2017.pdf

Kohn, L., Corrigan, J., & Donaldson, M. (Eds.). (1999). *To err is human: Building a safer health system.* Committee on Quality of Health Care in America, Institute of Medicine. Washington, DC: National Academy Press.

Markay, M. A., & Daniel, M. (2016). Medical error: The third leading cause of death in the US. *British Medical Journal, 353,* i2139.

Maynard, G. (2015). *Preventing hospital-associated venous thromboembolism: A guide for effective quality improvement* (2nd ed.). Rockville, MD: Agency for Healthcare Research and Quality. Retrieved from http://www.ahrq.gov/professionals/quality -patient-safety/patient-safety-resources/ resources/vtguide/index.html

Mermel, L. A., Allon, M., Bouza, E., Craven, D. E., Flynn, P., O'Grady, N. P., …. Warren, D. K. (2009). Clinical practice guidelines for the diagnosis and management of intravascular catheter-related infection: 2009 update by the Infectious Diseases Society of America. *Clinical Infectious Disease, 49,* 1–45.

Web Resources

Centers for Disease Control and Prevention (CDC). (2016). *Healthcare-associated infections*: https://www .cdc.gov/hai/bsi/bsi.html

Centers for Medicare & Medicaid Services (CMS). *Hospital-acquired conditions*: http://www.cms.gov/ Medicare/Medicare-Fee-for-ServicePayment/ HospitalAcqCond/Downloads/HACFactsheet .pdf

IMMIGRANT ELDERS

The World Health Organization (WHO) identifies that older people of ethnic and migrant background face significant challenges in accessing health services as they live longer (WHO, 2015). Cultural diversity must therefore be considered as a key aspect for clinicians working with older adults. In current estimates, this will become an ever-increasing issue over time. By 2020, the number of people aged 60 years and older will outnumber children younger than 5 years (WHO, 2015). In addition:

- In 2050, 80% of older people will be living in low-and middle-income countries.
- In the developed world, the "very old" (age older than 80 years) is the fastest growing population group.
- Women outlive men in virtually all societies; in very old age, the ratio of women: men is 2:1.

With the unprecedented increase in refugee and displaced populations around the world since 2015, the number of older adults who migrate is likely to increase. The future projections of aging populations in the United States, Canada, Australia, and across Europe reveal increasing heterogeneity of immigrant elders, and it is anticipated that the numbers will increase even more extensively than that of nonimmigrant elders. In Australia, for example, the population is ageing at a fast rate and it is estimated that by 2056, 23% to 25% of the population will be older than the age of 65 years (Australian Bureau of Statistics, 2008). These statistics are similar to those of other Western nations.

Thus people working in health and human services face two intertwined challenges: how to assist immigrant elders with their health needs and how to develop the cultural competence skills to meaningfully engage, assess, and treat patients, accepting both the challenges and opportunities posed by diversity.

Cultural competence with immigrant elders involves the clinical use of a set of behaviors, attributes, and policy infrastructure that come together in a system or organization or among professionals to enable that system or organization or those professions to work effectively in cross-cultural situations. In addition, it is also important to mobilize strengths inherent in health systems to improve health and well-being by valuing cultural perspectives. The importance of cultural competency in clinical elder care is particularly relevant to the management of chronic physical conditions such as diabetes, heart disease, musculoskeletal conditions, and cancer. In each condition, the ability of the provider to create and deliver a specific intervention depends on cultural competence.

Cultural competence also goes a long way in promoting positive health and well-being and reduce suffering. A culturally competent approach to immigrant elder care takes into account the nature and scope of family supports through family and community infrastructure, meaningful social interaction, improved nutrition, and moderate physical activity. These factors provide substantial insight into the role of risk and protective factors in the developmental pathways for health problems and illness.

Practical work with immigrant elders requires service providers to understand the concept of culture, its impact on human behavior, and the interpretation and evaluation of behavior. At the core of engaging immigrant elders in a culturally competent manner is understanding issues such as stigma, isolation, communication and language difficulties, and sensitivity to specific problems, as well as the way that they are experienced and understood.

In addition, the importance of churches, synagogues, temples, mosques and prayer rooms is also important and, more broadly, the means for immigrant elders to engage in their religious practices in the host society. Religion and spirituality are important to consider in the planning and provision of care and support to immigrant elders. For example, for older migrants who identify as Muslim, a strong preference for care staff of the same sex may be present (Guintoli & Cattan, 2012).

The combined elements of social and interpersonal factors lead practitioners to consider the deeper-meaning structures held by immigrant elders. This means clinicians must be open to the way of examination in which symptoms of health and illness are understood and presented, the way help is sought, and the way that care is evaluated by those who receive it. The clinical work of any health professional—no matter how willing or keen to help—is compromised if it does not consider how patients understand health difficulties and what practitioners themselves see as differently perceived causes of illness, optimal care, and culturally appropriate support and treatment. This is particularly so

in the mental health arena. Chiriboga, Yee, and Jang (2005) suggest mental health problems and mental illness for immigrant elders arrive in circumstances often associated with depression, and their problems can be accentuated by their experience in the new culture.

ISOLATION

Despite living in the host country for many years, immigrant elders who live in cultural enclaves are more likely to have problems understanding the language of the host country. Immigrant older adults also appear to be at risk of social isolation because traditional intergenerational relationships are rapidly disappearing. Taken in combination, social isolation and perceived burdensomeness are known risk factors for suicide among immigrant elders (Deuter & Procter, 2015). Urban sprawl results in social dislocation of young and old, without adequate social-support measures and extended family in place. In the case of a refugee or displaced person, the immigrant elder is likely to arrive with only a few members of the extended family for support. As time goes on, the elder may also find that younger generations are reluctant to provide the kind of support the elder expects (Chiriboga et al., 2005). Immigrant elders have described the unavailability of members from their own community of origin with whom to socialize as a profound loss (Guintoli & Cattan, 2012).

TRAUMATIC STRESS

Immigrants who leave their homelands involuntarily as a result of wars, social and political unrest, personal loss, and the loss of loved ones may create a context for trauma. Health professionals providing treatment to older people from culturally and linguistically diverse backgrounds should have and display respect for their cultural heritage, provide services in their preferred language if they are limited in English proficiency, and understand how the cultural background of the patient might affect symptom manifestation, significance, and treatment.

Clinical assessment, health, and helping strategies for immigrant elderly must incorporate personal reflection, therapeutic sensitivity, compassion, patience, and understanding. Effective communication with immigrant elders, an important basis for building trust, means that health professionals should ascertain the person's preferred language and determine whether an interpreter is necessary. Lack of English proficiency should not be assumed to be the result of poor language attainment; it could be associated with dysphasia because of a current or previous stroke or other neuromuscular disease or the loss of an acquired language because of a cognitive decline such as dementia. Care should be individualized according to a patient's customs and beliefs, as well as practices regarding health, illness, and death, and patients should be asked what *they believe* is the cause of their problem. The clinician should specifically encourage older patients to talk about any issues, needs, or problems they may be experiencing in the hospital or community setting. Health care professionals should allow each patient to decide the level of family involvement and the additional networks that may be available for informal support, such as religious groups or friends.

Assessment of these issues should be interlinked with, and used to improve, clinical care situations. Cultural sensitivity should frame how the older person is interviewed. Simply asking a question can be an opportunity for the development of a trusting and effective therapeutic relationship. To achieve these aims and ideals, health care professionals must also identify what their own prejudices and biases are and what is suggested by them. The following questions can guide this reflective process:

- What are my own feelings toward migrants and refugees? Am I comfortable working with those who are distressed and noncommunicative? Do I fear or dislike them? Do they unsettle me? Am I ambivalent toward them and, if so, why?
- How are my ideas, thoughts, and feelings about working with immigrant elders manifested during clinical practice?
- How do media and popular opinions regarding particular immigrant and religious groups shape my views?
- To what extent do I encourage and allow immigrant elderly patients and their families, where appropriate, to make decisions about their care?

Perhaps the most challenging aspect of health care practice with immigrant elderly is that they tend to access the health care system at the very point of their distress. Nevertheless, from migration to resettlement, health care professionals can assist immigrant elders to make sense of an increasingly globalized and at times hostile world, better understand and respond to individual need, develop culturally competent problem-solving abilities, and appreciate the factors that can promote health and comfort. With an informed knowledge base of background issues in the wider world—including the sociopolitical—clinicians, immigrant elders, their families, and significant networks can work together to target strategies and support programs that seek to maximize ongoing coping and health choices.

See also Asian American and Pacific Islander Elders; Cultural Competence and Aging.

Nicholas G. Procter and Amy E. Z. Baker

Australian Bureau of Statistics. (2008). *Population projections, Australia (2006–2011)* (Report No. 3222.0). Canberra, Australia: Australian Government.

Chiriboga, D. A., Yee, B. W. K., & Jang, Y. (2005). Minority and cultural issues in late-life depression. *Clinical Psychology: Science and Practice, 12*(3), 358–363.

Deuter, K., & Procter, N. G. (2015). Attempted suicide in older people: A review of the evidence. *Suicidologi, 20*(3), 4–13.

Guintoli, G., & Cattan, M. (2012). The experiences and expectations of care and support among older migrants in the UK. *European Journal of Social Work, 15*(1), 131–147.

World Health Organization. (2015). Fact sheet 404 ageing and health. Retrieved from http://www.who.int/mediacentre/factsheets/fs404/en

Web Resources

Centre for Cultural Diversity and Ageing: http://www.culturaldiversity.com.au

U.S. Department of Health and Human Services. *Curriculum in ethnogeriatrics*: http://www.stanford.edu/group/ethnoger/index.html

World Health Organization. *Ageing and health:* http://www.who.int/topics/ageing/en

I

IMMUNIZATION

Prevention of infectious disease is an essential component of primary health care for older adults. Immunity to diseases can decline after time within older adults, making it vital to take the precaution of receiving vaccinations when necessary. It is important for the health professional to inform the patient about how vaccines are used to prevent important and common illnesses. Table I.1 summarizes recommendations regarding indications and timing for immunizations. Although it is challenging to definitively establish the benefits of vaccines in older adults in terms of morbidity and mortality outcomes, these vaccines help with prevention of future illnesses. The influenza vaccine, for example, is 60% effective in reducing hospitalizations in older adults (Talbot et al., 2011). Influenza vaccination remains a cost-saving intervention in older adults and provides clinical protection against illness and hospitalization. Tetanus vaccination effectively decreases all cases, and the cases that do occur are in undervaccinated older adults. Likewise, vaccination for shingles among older adults shows a 60% reduction in burden of illness, a 50% decrease in cases of shingles, and a 66% reduction in cases of postherpetic neuralgia

(Oxman et al., 2005). Unfortunately, older adults do not routinely get immunized at a rate consistent with children. Barriers to immunization include beliefs about the effectiveness, access, and cost, among others. Ongoing initiatives are working toward addressing barriers and increasing use and efficacy of vaccines among older individuals.

PATIENT INVOLVEMENT AND CONSENT

The purpose of immunization should be explained, and the patient should be allowed to define their preferences. For older adults living in the community, signed consent should be obtained before immunization. Nursing home residents with decision-making capacity should participate in the choice whether to be immunized. For those unable to make their own decisions, consent should be obtained from the health care power of attorney.

RISK FACTORS

Compliance with recommended immunization guidelines has improved; however, the goal set in Healthy People 2010 of 95% adherence to immunization has not been met. To facilitate compliance, the federal government in 2002

Table I.1
RECOMMENDED IMMUNIZATIONS FOR OLDER ADULTS IN 2016

Vaccine	Recommendations	Notes
Tetanus, diphtheria, pertussis (Tdap/Td)	One-time substitute Tdap for Td and then Td every 10 years. For age 65 years and older	1 dose Td/Tdap if there is the risk of exposure to an infant
Influenza	1 dose annually	High-dose vaccine recommended
Pneumococcal	1 dose of PCV13 and PPSV23 1 year apart	1 dose of PPSV23 after 5 years
Zoster	1 dose	May be repeated after 20 years
Varicella	2 doses needed has never had varicella	
Measles, mumps, and rubella	1 dose if never had the diseases; adults born before 1957 assumed to be immune	
Hepatitis A and B	Vaccinate only if at high risk (behavioral risk factors; occupational risk factors; relevant travel)—see text	

Note: Substitute Tdap for Td.
PVC13, pneumococcal conjugate vaccine (Prevnar 13 [Pfizer]); PPSV23, pneumococcal polysaccharide vaccine (Pneumovax [Merck]).

approved standing orders for annual influenza vaccinations and pneumococcal pneumonia vaccination for older adults in institutional settings and home health agencies for all Medicare and Medicaid beneficiaries. As noted, there is much misconception about the efficacy and benefits of vaccination for older adults. Education about the benefits versus risks of vaccines is essential to patients, providers, and caregivers. It should be explained that vaccines are safe. One may, however, have mild systemic reactions such as generalized weakness, fever, transient local pain, or reddened skin. As with any vaccine, there is the rare possibility of a serious anaphylactic reaction. Influenza and pneumonia vaccinations should not be administered to individuals who are allergic to any component of the vaccine or to anyone with an acute infection.

REIMBURSEMENT

Medicare Part B covers influenza, pneumococcal, and hepatitis B vaccines. Providers purchase the vaccines and, after their administration, Medicare reimburses the cost at 95% of the average wholesale price. Medicare, however, does not provide tetanus-diphtheria (Td) vaccination as a covered preventive service. Older adults have to pay for this vaccine and its administration out of pocket. Zoster (shingles) and tetanus-diphtheria and acellular pertussis (Tdap) vaccines were issued after the Medicare prescription drug benefit program (Medicare Part D) was enacted and are therefore both covered by this program. Medicare beneficiaries who do not participate in Part D must pay for these vaccines themselves. As of the time of this writing, Medicare beneficiaries covered by Medicare part B receive a cost-free recommended vaccines, including (Stewart, Richardson, Cox, Hayes, & Rosenbaum, 2010) influenza, pneumococcal and hepatitis B vaccines. For vaccines covered by Medicare Part D, some cost will remain.

INFLUENZA VACCINE

Approximately 36,000 deaths and more than 186,000 hospitalizations occur each year because of influenza (Rolfes et al., 2016). This vaccine is available in standard or high doses and must be received annually. Ideally, the vaccine is given just before flu season starts. The immune response is delayed for 3 to 4 weeks, and antibody titers decline rapidly. A high-dose influenza vaccine is now available for people older than the age of 65 years, having four times the amount of antigen compared with a standard shot. This vaccine benefits older adults because their immune systems weaken and are at higher risk of contracting the flu. The high-dose vaccine is 24.2% more effective compared with the standard shot in older adults (DiazGranados et al., 2014). High-dose vaccines cost approximately $32, and standard vaccines cost approximately $12. Influenza vaccines are reformulated annually and are trivalent (i.e., contain inactivated viruses from three strains: two type A strains and one type B strain). Efficacy of the vaccine is challenging to establish because it would be unethical to withhold vaccine from an older individual.

PNEUMOCOCCAL VACCINE

Pneumococcal disease is a common cause of hospitalization and death in persons aged 65 years and older. There are two vaccines available for adults older than 64 years: pneumococcal conjugate vaccine (PCV13) and pneumococcal polysaccharide vaccine (PPSV23). PCV13 is recommended for adults who have not received this vaccine before, with a follow up of the PPSV23 a year later. However, if adults have received the PPSV23 vaccine before, then they should get the PCV13 a year later. The PPSV23 vaccine contains materials from the 23 types of pneumococcal bacteria that cause 88% of pneumococcal infections and is effective in preventing pneumococcal bacteremia in older adults. Antibody responses are similar in healthy young and older adults, but opsonophagocytic activity (which is what clears pneumococci) declines after approximately 6 years. All high-risk older adults (above the age of 65 years) who have received both vaccines previously should receive another PPSV23 pneumococcal vaccination 5 years or more after their first immunization. Side effects are generally limited to pain, erythema, and swelling at the injection site, lasting no longer than 48 hours; fever and myalgia are rare (Htar et al., 2017).

TETANUS AND DIPHTHERIA

Because pertussis is underdiagnosed and underreported substantially in all age groups, the actual burden of disease in adults aged 65 years and older is unknown (Centers for Disease Control and Prevention, 2015). It is anticipated that pertussis incidence in older adults is much higher than reported. Thus the addition of the tetanus-diphtheria and acellular pertussis is recommended as a one-time substitute for the standard booster every 10 years of Td. Generally, there is no greater risk of side effects from vaccination among older adults than in younger individuals. Neurological reactions and severe hypersensitivity after a previous dose are contraindications for repeat vaccinations.

HEPATITIS A AND B

Vaccination is recommended for high-risk patients as described in Table I.1. Preexposure immunization for hepatitis A is recommended for individuals at risk of exposure: those who live in or travel to countries where the rate of hepatitis A virus is high, homosexual persons, intravenous drug users, and individuals with liver disease. At this time, data are insufficient with regard to periodic booster immunization.

VARICELLA

The varicella vaccine live is approved by the Food and Drug Administration (FDA) to prevent varicella. Many adults with no history of chickenpox have immunity to varicella; fewer than 10% of adults in the United States are susceptible to the disease. These people should receive two doses of the vaccine 4 weeks apart to increase immunity. Individuals who were born before 1980 are assumed to be immune (Hendriksz, Malouf, & Foy, 2011). Varicella is a primary infection of the zoster virus; when reactivated it may lead to herpes zoster. If it is contracted, the disease is more severe than in children. One option, therefore, is to obtain titers

and vaccinate if there is an inadequate antibody titer of varicella in an older individual who may not be certain about prior exposure.

HERPES ZOSTER

In the summer of 2006, the FDA approved a new vaccine, zoster vaccine live, for the prevention of herpes zoster (shingles) in individuals aged 60 years and older. Currently, this is the only medical option that may prevent shingles. Shingles affects approximately 600,000 to 1 million Americans diagnosed each year (Oxman et al., 2005). Some 90% of adults aged 60 years and older have not been vaccinated against herpes zoster (Weaver, 2011). It is also suggested that they receive a booster shot every 20 to 30 years. Side effects of the vaccine are similar to those associated with other vaccines and include local reactions (including small vesicles), headache, itching, and mild discomfort.

Saffia Bajwa and Michael L. Malone

Centers for Disease Control and Prevention. (2015). Tdap (tetanus, diphtheria, pertussis) VIS. Retrieved from https://www.cdc.gov/vaccines/hcp/vis/vis-statements/tdap.html

DiazGranados, C. A., Dunning, A. J., Kimmel, M., Kirby, D., Treanor, J., Collins, A., ... Talbot, H. K. (2014). Efficacy of high-dose versus standard-dose influenza vaccine in older adults. *New England Journal of Medicine, 371*(7), 635–645. doi:10.1056/NEJMoa1315727

Hendriksz, T., Malouf, P., & Foy, J. E.; Advisory Committee on Immunization Practices of the Centers for Disease Control and Prevention. (2011). Vaccines for measles, mumps, rubella, varicella, and herpes zoster: Immunization guidelines for adults. *Journal of the American Osteopathic Association, 111*(10, Suppl. 6), S10–S12.

Htar, M. T. T., Stuurman, A. L., Ferreira, G., Alicino, C., Bollaerts, K., Paganino, C., ... Ansaldi, F. (2017). Effectiveness of pneumococcal vaccines in preventing pneumonia in adults, a systematic review and meta-analyses of observational studies. *PLOS ONE, 12*(5), e0177985. doi:10.1371/journal.pone.0177985

Oxman, M. N., Levin, M. J., Johnson, G. R., Schmader, K. E., Straus, S. E., Gelb, L. D., ... Weinberg, A. (2005). A vaccine to prevent herpes zoster and postherpetic neuralgia in older adults. *New England Journal of Medicine, 352*(22), 2271–2284.

Rolfes, M. A., Foppa, I. M., Garg, S., Flannery, B., Brammer, L., Singleton, J. A., … Bresee, J. (2016). Estimated influenza illnesses, medical visits, hospitalizations, and deaths averted by vaccination in the United States. Retrieved from https://www.cdc.gov/flu/about/disease/2015-16.htm

Stewart, A. M., Richardson, O. L., Cox, M. A., Hayes, K. J., & Rosenbaum, S. J. (2010). The Affordable Care Act: US vaccine policy and practice. Retrieved from http://hsrc.himmelfarb.gwu.edu/cgi/viewcontent.cgi?article=1168&context=sphhs_policy_facpubs

Talbot, H. K., Griffin, M. R., Chen, Q., Zhu, Y., Williams, J. V., & Edwards, K. M. (2011). Effectiveness of seasonal vaccine in preventing confirmed influenza-associated hospitalizations in community dwelling older adults. *Journal of Infectious Diseases, 203*(4), 500–508.

Weaver, B. A.; Advisory Committee on Immunization Practices of the Centers for Disease Control and Prevention. (2011). Update on the Advisory Committee on Immunization Practices' recommendations for use of herpes zoster vaccine. *Journal of the American Osteopathic Association, 111*(10, Suppl. 6), S31–S33.

INFORMATION TECHNOLOGY

Interactive technology, specifically the Internet, has radically altered the way individuals communicate, interact, access information, and make health care decisions. Nowhere is this change more dramatic than in the older population. Fifty-eight percent of senior citizens in 2015 used the Internet, compared with 14% in 2000 (Perrin & Duggan, 2015). Almost half (47%) of older adults report having a high-speed broadband connection at home and 77% a cell phone (Pew Research Center, 2014). Research delineates two groups of older adult technology users. The first group (younger, more highly educated, more affluent) has relatively substantial technology resources and a more positive attitude toward the use of technology; the second group (older, fewer financial resources, with more physical disabilities) tend to be less connected to the digital world. Some older adults have physical conditions, chronic illnesses, and disabilities that present challenges to using technology; a recent study demonstrated that approximately 39% of older adults fell into this category. Many older adults report needing assistance in learning how to use technology devices and digital services and cite this as a barrier to using more technology (Pew Research Center, 2014).

A recent systematic review (Kampmeijer, Pavlova, Tambor, Golinowska, & Groot, 2016) demonstrated that older adults use e-health and m-health tools in a variety of health-promotion and formal health programs to monitor and improve their health. As the older cohort approaches retirement, the numbers of seniors using telecommunication and the Internet to access health care information is expected to grow. They use technology to manage their health care, research treatment options, investigate health care policies, and connect with health care providers.

INTERACTIVE HEALTH COMMUNICATION AND OLDER ADULTS

As a result of the rapid technological advances and ease of use of the Internet, the World Wide Web has become a most important resource in education, communication, and information dissemination. As the population ages and the number of individuals with chronic illnesses increases, individuals are going to be called on to manage their health more independently. Online health-management tools have the potential to meet this need. Online health-management tools provide a low-cost, accessible means to take control of health. These technologies also allow consumers to tailor their communication with health care providers based on their needs. In turn, health care providers have the aggregate electronic data to pick up care at the point and time of contact. Seniors, the most vulnerable population for many illnesses, functional disabilities, and social isolation, stand to benefit the most from effective interactive communication and access to Internet resources.

The proliferation of websites geared specifically to the needs of older adults attests to the important role this technology can play in the lives of the people aged 65 years and older. This technology has the potential to ensure autonomy and care independence far longer than the current care modalities. Older adults have lagged behind younger adults in their adoption, but now a clear majority (58%) of senior citizens uses the Internet. Despite the significant increase in internet use among older adults, there remains an opportunity to reach out to this population to promote computer literacy and competency. Studies support that seniors would benefit from free computer classes, financial assistance, helplines for technical difficulties, and volunteer visits for technical problems.

There is a "digital divide" between the income groups and access to telecommunication services. The disparity of income affects all ages, but it is most pronounced among seniors (Choi & Dinitto, 2013). In addition, as in younger populations, level of education and literacy, household income, and urban living have all been demonstrated to be indicators of Internet use. The "wired seniors" are at an advantage, but it is the seniors in the lower income group who could most benefit from access and familiarity with telecommunication. Providing outreach to the most disadvantaged seniors is a challenge to policy makers, health care providers, and community organizations.

REMOTE MONITORING FOR HEALTH CARE

The use of electronic information and communication technologies to provide and support health care when distance separates participants has gained prominence because of the accessibility and flexibility of technology. Success in remote monitoring of specific populations has significant implications for improved health care outcomes. Potential benefits include early management of impending medical emergencies, home monitoring of patients posthospital stay, and mobility monitoring for elderly patients with dementia and functional disabilities (Gellis et al., 2012). Telemonitoring has the potential to provide cost-effective care, as well as improved outcomes, particularly in patients with chronic obstructive pulmonary disease (COPD), congestive heart failure (CHF), and hypertension. In addition to improved patient outcomes, other benefits include decreased rehospitalizations, reduced hospital stays, improved vitality, and patient-perceived quality of life (Gellis et al., 2012).

The Internet allows for personal communication between caregivers and patients, which may be particularly important in regions with less access to personal and information communication. Studies of remote monitoring reported decreased incidence of depression and isolation among the homebound elderly, as well as an improved lifestyle and functional outcomes. Web-based remote monitoring applications have customized features such as e-mail, health reminders, diaries, and health information. All of these have the potential to increase on the frequency and quality of communication. Seniors are able to communicate their wishes and needs accurately and in a timely fashion. Even older seniors (i.e., 75 years and older) demonstrate a remarkable facility to adapt and use computer-based communications and interactions when provided the opportunity.

FUTURE OF THE INTERNET AND ELDERS

The group aged 50 years and older is the fastest-growing segment of the population to use the Internet. This cohort is three times more likely to have Internet access than those older than 65 years. This "silver tsunami" of soon-to-be seniors revolutionize how the Internet is used for e-health, recreation, business, socialization, and communication. There are thousands of websites devoted to seniors; SeniorNet, for example, has introduced more than 1 million older adults to computers and the Internet and supports 240 SeniorNet Learning Centers across the country (www.seniornet.org). Studies indicate that older adults use computers for peer support, health care information, and professional advice. As a result, individuals using the Internet feel empowered, are more informed, and are better equipped to participate in decision making about their health care. Older adults also extol the social benefits of the Internet, which include discussion groups, contact with children and grandchildren, recreation ideas, and learning activities. Heinz et al. (2013) found that many older adults were eager to learn how to use technology in their everyday life, despite the fact that some reported usability issues. The researchers suggested that technology companies actively seek the input of older adults to improve their product use.

With the proliferation of websites for older adults, caution must be taken to ensure that the sites are valid and provide the most accurate and current information. This is especially true of health care sites. The interpretation and use of Internet information in the senior population may need the support and guidance of health care providers. There are also health care sites that advise seniors and older seniors how to navigate websites; these include www.healthfinder .gov, www.aarp.org, and www.nihseniorhealth .gov.

PROVIDER AND CONSUMER ISSUES

The Internet can be a powerful tool for health care providers in communicating with patients and improving consumer health care outcomes. Web-based technology can integrate knowledge sources, clinician expertise, and patient-based preferences. How health care professionals incorporate the medium into their practice and use it as a major source of communication and interaction raises many issues, such as response turnaround time, type of transaction (e.g., prescription, appointment, advice), authentication and confidentiality of communications, and the incorporation of e-mail as part of the medical record.

The proliferation of Internet-based health care networks also challenges providers because the expansion of electronic health tools and e-health enables the public to monitor their health status, report health data, access disease prevention information, and purchase health care products. The professional educational system has to change to produce and support professional practice in a dynamic, digital society. The fastest growing segments of the population (i.e., those older than 50 years) are enthusiastic about using electronic communication in creative and beneficial ways to improve the quality of their life. Professionals also need to demonstrate competence in incorporating technology into their care protocols and patient interactions.

See also Technology.

Sharon Stahl Wexler and
Marie-Claire Rosenberg Roberts

Choi, N. G., & Dinitto, D. M. (2013). Internet use among older adults: Association with health needs, psychological capital, and social capital. *Journal of Medical Internet Research, 15*(5), e97. doi:10.2196/jmir.2333

Gellis, Z. D., Kenaley, B., McGinty, J., Bardelli, E., Davitt, J., & Ten Have, T. (2012). Outcomes of a telehealth intervention for homebound older adults with heart or chronic respiratory failure: A randomized controlled trial. *The Gerontologist, 52*, 541–552.

Heinz, M., Martin, P., Margrett, J. A., Yearns, M., Franke, W., Yang, H., … Chang, C. K. (2013). Perception of technology among older adults. *Journal of Gerontological Nursing, 39*(1), 42–45.

Kampmeijer, R., Pavlova, M., Tambor, M., Golinowska, S., & Groot, W. (2016). The use of e-health and m-health tools in health promotion and primary prevention among older adults: A systematic literature review. *BMC Health Services Research, 16*(5), 467–479. doi:10.1186/s12913-016-1522-3

Perrin, A., & Duggan, M. (2015). *Americans' Internet access: 2000–2015.* Washington, DC: Pew Research Center. Retrieved from http://www.pewinternet .org/2015/06/26/americans-internet-access -2000-2015

Pew Research Center. (2014). Older adults and technology use. Retrieved from http://www/pewinternet .org/2014/04/03/older-adults-and-technology -use

Web Resources
AARP: http://www.aarp.org
Health Finder, Office of Disease Prevention and Health Promotion, U.S. Department of Health and Human Services: http://www.healthfinder.gov
NIH Senior Health – National Institute on Aging: http://www.nihseniorhealth.gov

Older Adults Technology Services (OATS): http://oats.org

Pew Research Center's Internet and American Life Project: http://pewinternet.org

Senior Net Learning Centers: http://www.seniornet.org

Senior Planet: http://seniorplanet.org

Staying Connected: Technology Options for Older Adults. *Eldercare.gov, a project of the Administration on Aging*: http://www.eldercare.gov/eldercare.net/public/Resources/Brochures/docs/N4A_Tech_Brochure_P06_high.pdf

INJURY AND TRAUMA

Traumatic injury, occurring in all age groups with varying degrees of frequency and severity, is a significant public health problem in the United States costing $671 billion annually (National Trauma Institute, 2016). As the population ages, increasingly more patients of advanced age are seeking care because of injury. It is estimated that 40% of all trauma center admissions will be older than 65 years by 2050 (Campbell, DeGolia, Fallon, & Rader, 2009). The most common causes of injury in older adults is associated with falls or motor vehicle/traffic events.

The current cohort of older adults are healthier and more active and therefore increasingly more exposed to injury. For all severity levels of injury, older adults suffer negative outcomes, including functional decline, which is disproportionately more serious than in younger patients with similar injuries; they also die more often than their younger counterparts. The worse outcomes are attributable to the severity of the injury compounded by the physiologic changes associated with aging and the toll of preexisting medical conditions common to most older adults. Age alone, however, is not an accurate predictor of discharge outcomes. Functional status and multiple comorbidities are also important indicators of outcomes in older adults. An active, healthy 75-year-old man can be at much less risk for poor outcomes from injury than a sedentary 65-year-old man with multiple comorbidities. However, recent data demonstrate that the adverse outcomes in older adults may often be minimized by focused interdisciplinary care.

MECHANISMS OF INJURY

The most common mechanisms of injury in older adults are falls and motor vehicle collisions as passengers or pedestrians (American College of Surgeons, 2015). Falls are multifactorial, often associated with normal changes of aging such as muscle weakness, loss of balance or coordination, orthostatic hypotension, and decreased acuity of sight or hearing. Falls may also be associated with preexisting conditions such as cardiovascular disease, stroke, diabetes, poor nutrition, or anemia associated with chronic diseases. Alcohol use or prescription medications can also alter cognition, awareness, or gait. The other leading causes of injury include assault (including abuse) and thermal injuries.

Comorbid illness is more often the initiating event for injury in older adults than for younger adults. More than 70% of those aged 65 years and older have one or more chronic diseases; the most common include hypertension, arthritis, heart disease, cancer, diabetes, stroke, asthma, and chronic bronchitis or emphysema (Administration on Aging, 2015). These conditions can also contribute to judgment decisions that result in injury. Some examples include miscalculations of distance and speed of oncoming traffic, inadequate ability to negotiate curbs at street crossings, and injuries resulting from ambulating or ascending and descending too rapidly.

ASSESSMENT

Diagnostic workups for injured older adults should include not only history and physical assessment, but as many details related to the injury as are available (e.g., motor vehicle speed, fall height, and position; consciousness status of the injured at the site). Data demonstrate that the perceived severity of injury should not be the sole screening criterion for determining the intensity of treatment needed for injured older adults. The usual criteria for determining severity of injury, such as blood pressure and heart rate, are not as predictive of injury severity in older adults as in those who are younger. For older adults, the cardiovascular system may be unable to respond to physical insult because of physiologic changes or because of cardiovascular medications, such as beta-blockers. Delayed or inadequate resuscitation because of a misleading clinical picture of stability is known to result in poorer outcomes.

Trauma assessment scoring indices, such as the Injury Severity Score (ISS) and the Glasgow Coma Scale (GCS), are routinely documented by trauma centers and have been shown to predict functional outcomes and discharge disposition. These parameters, however, are limited because they are based on injury severity or presentation without factoring in a patient's preinjury physiologic reserve. More recently, frailty determination is being recognized as an important predictor of functional discharge outcomes in injured older adults (Joseph et al., 2014).

There is a growing evidence that frailty, a measurable syndrome, contributes significantly to worse outcomes in injured older patients. Frailty, as defined by an assessment of physiologic reserve and/or degree of physiologic impairment, has been associated with adverse health outcomes. Validated frailty scales integrate mobility and endurance assessment, evaluate elements of patient performance (observed and self-reported), and incorporate predicted effects of comorbidities and medication use. The calculated frailty outcome categories range from very fit to very frail, including terminally ill (McDonald et al., 2016).

MANAGEMENT

In the United States, the American College of Surgeons, Committee on Trauma (2014), establishes guidelines for management of the injured and now has recommended the transport of all injured people aged 55 years and older to trauma centers. Multiple studies have demonstrated that outcomes for all injured patients are better when they are managed in trauma centers, where current management recommendations are more likely to be implemented. The goals of prehospital care (whether by emergency medical services or other first responders) are to prevent further injury, initiate resuscitation, and provide safe and timely transport of injured patients. On arrival to the hospital, a primary assessment to determine critical injuries that require immediate intervention and stabilization is performed. Then a secondary survey is performed for more detailed assessment.

The ABCs of trauma management include maintaining airway, supporting breathing, and ensuring adequate circulation (generally by stopping bleeding and assessing/restoring circulatory volume). Maintaining an airway may be complicated by a weakened gag reflex or by dentures in older adults. Blood pressure and heart rate may not be reliable predictors of volume status in this group because these indicators may be affected by chronic medication use or be more reflective of comorbidities (such as congestive heart failure or renal disease) than circulatory volume status.

Fluid resuscitation needs to be more judicious in older adults, depending on their preinjury status and response to therapy. Traditionally, initial fluid resuscitation involved the administration of 1 to 2 L of crystalloids, followed by blood (packed red blood cells), if a patient had signs of ongoing hemorrhagic shock. In recent years, the standard approach for volume resuscitation in a bleeding patient required giving blood products first and avoiding the initial administration of crystalloids. Several studies have demonstrated improved survival in severely injured patients after initial resuscitation with blood products that include a high ratio of platelets and fresh frozen plasma (FFP) to packed red blood cells. This specific combination helps control the acute coagulopathy associated with massive blood loss (Inaba et al., 2010; Shaz et al., 2010).

Continued management varies depending on the type and extent of injury and preexisting medical condition of the patient. All efforts should be focused, however, on preventing further deterioration and maximizing functional outcomes. As with any age group, this is best managed by coordinated, interdisciplinary team efforts.

IMPROVING DISCHARGE OUTCOMES

Improving outcomes and preserving the preinjury functional status of older adults are goals of both the trauma and geriatric health care communities in the United States. Fewer preventable complications are now expected by, and acceptable to, the Centers for Medicare & Medicaid Services (CMS) and other regulatory and reimbursing agencies. Many hospital-acquired conditions in older patients (such as delirium, pressure injuries, pneumonia, urinary tract infections, nutrition-related issues, and functional decline) are now recognized as preventable complications. An expanding body of evidence suggests that early and preventive interventions can improve outcomes (Bolz, Capezuti, Fulmer, & Zwicker, 2012). Identifying at-risk older adults requires early and targeted assessment and demands interdisciplinary intervention with oversight by those knowledgeable about older adult management.

Geriatricians can positively impact hospital care and improve transition of care issues such as extended lengths of stay and readmissions. Additional assessment and intervention techniques related to injury prevention include ongoing sensory evaluation (vision, hearing, and balance), evaluation of medications that affect coordination and balance, safety assessment of the home environment, strength and balance conditioning and ongoing safety-awareness education.

There are individual, societal, and economic costs to serious injury. Because the older adults are more prone to injury and can have poorer outcomes when it occurs, ongoing injury-prevention measures must continue beyond the hospital experience. The goals of the treatment of injury and trauma in older adults are prevention of functional decline and effective transition of care back to the community, as well as an ongoing safety-awareness education for this growing group of vulnerable Americans.

Christine Cutugno and Melvin E. Stone

Administration on Aging. (2015). Aging statistics. *U.S. Department of Health and Human Services.* Retrieved from https://www.acl.gov/sites/default/files/news%202017-03/A_Statistical_Profile_of_Older_Americans.pdf

American College of Surgeons. (2015). *National trauma data bank: Annual report.* Retrieved from https://www.facs.org/~/media/files/quality% 20programs/trauma/ntdb/ntdb%20annual%20 report%202015.ashx

American College of Surgeons, Committee on Trauma. (2014). *Resources for optimal care of the injured patient.* Chicago, IL: Author.

Bolz, M., Capezuti, E., Fulmer, T., & Zwicker, D. (Eds.). (2012). *Evidence-based geriatric nursing protocols for best practice* (4th ed.). New York, NY: Springer Publishing.

Campbell, J., DeGolia, P., Fallon, W., & Rader, E. (2009). In harm's way: Moving the older trauma patient toward a better outcome. *Geriatrics, 64,* 8–13.

Inaba, K., Lustenberger, T., Rhee, P., Blackbourne, L., Shulman, I., Nelson, J., ... Demetriades, D. (2010). The impact of platelet transfusion in massively transfused trauma patients. *Journal of the American College of Surgery, 211,* 573–579.

Joseph, B., Pandit, V., Rhee, P., Aziz, H., Sadoun, M., Wynne, J., ... Randall, F. (2014). Predicting hospital discharge disposition in geriatric trauma patients: Is frailty the answer? *Journal of Trauma and Acute Care Surgery, 76*(1), 196–200.

McDonald, V., Thompson, K., Lewis, P., Sise, C., Sise, M., & Shackford, S. (2016). Frailty in trauma: A Systematic review of the surgical literature for clinical assessment tools. *Journal of Trauma and Acute Care Surgery, 80,* 824–834.

Shaz, B., Dente, C., Nicholas, J., MacLeod, J., Young, A., Easley, K., ... Hillyer, C. D. (2010). Increased number of coagulation products in relationship to red blood cell products transfused improves mortality in trauma patients. *Transfusion, 50*(2), 493–500.

Web Resources
Administration for Community Living: https://www.acl.gov
National Resource Center on Safe Aging: http://www.safeaging.org
National Trauma Institute: https://www.nattrauma.org

INSTITUTIONAL MISTREATMENT: ABUSE AND NEGLECT

Institutional mistreatment generally refers to abuse and neglect that occurs in acute care facilities, nursing homes, or residential facilities (i.e., foster homes, group homes, personal care homes, assisted-living facilities, domiciliary care homes, adult congregate living facilities, adult care homes, shelter care homes). It is perpetrated by those who have a legal or contractual obligation to provide elder victims with care and protection (Hawes & Kimbell, 2010; McDonald et al., 2012). Institutional mistreatment includes harm caused by individual staff members, as well as ownership/managerial failures in which the administration of the facility contributed to or caused abuse or neglect. The legal definitions of *abuse* and *neglect* vary widely from state to state, since various regulatory, law-enforcement, and social-service entities possess the authority to address the abuse and neglect of older adults (Castle, Ferguson-Rome, & Teresi, 2015); the following are, however, generally accepted definitions (Post et al., 2010).

- *Physical abuse*: Contact with an older adult's body such as hitting, punching, slapping, pinching, and kicking.
- *Sexual abuse:* Any form of nonconsensual sexual contact, sexual coercion, sexual harassment, or sexual assault, ranging from rape to unwanted touching or indecent exposure.
- *Verbal abuse:* Use of oral, written, or gestured language that includes disparaging or derogatory terms to a resident or in the resident's hearing, regardless of the resident's age, ability to comprehend, or disability, such as threats of harm or statements intended to frighten an older adult.
- *Involuntary seclusion:* Separation of residents from others or from their rooms opposed to their will or the will of their legal representative.
- *Mental/psychological abuse*: Action or verbal communication directed toward a resident that is threatening or menacing and results in fear or emotional or mental distress.
- *Financial abuse:* Theft of the resident's personal belongings or money; changes in the resident's will or other financial documents without the resident's permission.
- *Neglect:* Per section 2011(16) of the Social Security Act (as added by section 6703[a][1][C] of the Patient Protection and Affordable Care Act), (a) the failure of a caregiver or fiduciary to provide goods or services that are necessary to maintain the health or safety of an elder or (b) self-neglect, in which an individual neglects to attend appropriately to their own needs or physical well-being (Elder Justice Act, 2009). In general, neglect is considered the failure of a caregiver to fulfill his or her legal obligations or duties to an older person, including providing food, clothing, medicine, shelter, supervision, medications and medical care, and services that are essential for the health and well-being of the older adult. Recent federal regulations for nursing homes specify broader accountability, describing neglect as the "failure of the facility, its employees or service providers to provide goods and services to a resident that are necessary to avoid physical harm, pain, mental anguish or emotional distress" (*Federal Register*, 2016, p. 68825).

RISK FACTORS

Older adults who reside in nursing homes and residential settings are particularly vulnerable to mistreatment because most suffer from several chronic diseases that lead to limitations in physical and cognitive functioning and are, to some extent, dependent on others. In addition, many residents are either unable to report abuse or neglect or are fearful of retaliation. Social isolation, mental health challenges, behavioral problems, and poverty are additional risk factors for mistreatment (Post et al., 2010). Organizational risk factors for abuse and neglect include low staffing numbers, inadequate supervision of staff, and high staff turnover (Castle & Beech, 2011; Castle et al., 2015; Schiamberg et al., 2011).

INCIDENCE

The number of older adults who have been abused or neglected in institutions is not known. However, there is significant evidence that institutional mistreatment is a pervasive problem. Some 7% of all complaints regarding institutional facilities reported to long-term care ombudsmen (advocates for residents' rights and access to resources) are complaints of abuse, neglect, or exploitation (National Center on Elder Abuse, 2012). A large multisite study showed that more than 50% of nursing home staff admitted to mistreating (e.g., physical violence, mental abuse, neglect) older patients in the previous year (Natan & Lowenstein, 2010). In addition, a U.S. House of Representatives (2001) report stated that 10% of nursing homes in the United States were cited for abuse violations that caused harm to residents or placed them in immediate jeopardy of death or serious injury. The cases involving abuse included physical and sexual abuse, as well as verbal abuse involving threats and humiliation. Similarly, elder mistreatment in assisted-living facilities is considered to be seriously under-identified, even by state inspectors (Phillips, Guo, & Kim, 2013).

Government and ombudsman reports suggest the most common problems in nursing homes include lack of appropriate attention to dramatic, unplanned weight loss; failure to properly treat pressure injuries; inadequate care to maximize physical functioning in activities of daily living (ADL); lack of adequate supervision to prevent accidents; and failure to manage chronic or severe pain. Unsanitary conditions and unsafe medication practices are the most commonly cited problems in residential-care facilities (Hawes, 2002).

SIGNS

The signs of physical abuse include bruising, fractures, burns, lacerations, subdural hematomas, and pain. Accidental bruises occur in a predictable location pattern in older adults and rarely occur on the neck, ears, genitalia, buttocks, or soles of the feet. Other signs of potential mistreatment include unexplained or inconsistent explanations for injuries; heavy sedation; rapid weight change; pressure injuries; unexplained functional decline; repeated illnesses; failure to contact the family about trips to the emergency room, illnesses, or accidents; and unexplained or unanticipated death. In addition, unexplained loss or transfer of belongings or funds or a transfer inconsistent with the older

adult's previous wishes may suggest financial exploitation. The signs of mistreatment can also be emotional, including social withdrawal, isolation, agitation, unusual behaviors, and threats or ignoring by family and friends.

PROTECTION FROM MISTREATMENT: REGULATORY REQUIREMENTS

Federal regulations require nursing homes to develop and implement written policies and procedures that prohibit the mistreatment, neglect, and abuse of residents and the misappropriation of resident property. These requirements mandate staff and resident education on abuse and neglect and procedures to follow in the event of suspected mistreatment, including investigative procedures, reports to regulators, and protection and treatment of the resident. Furthermore, the law requires that the facility must not employ individuals who have been found guilty of abusing, neglecting, or mistreating residents or who have had a finding in the state nurse aide registry concerning the abuse, neglect, or mistreatment of residents or the misappropriation of their property (42 CFR Section 488.301, 2010). Most states require assisted-living and personal-care homes to adhere to similar regulations. The administration of the facility serving older adults is responsible not only to ensure that these regulations are followed, but also to employ adequate numbers of sufficiently trained and supervised staff to prevent mistreatment of residents.

In addition, federal law requires states to establish a nurse's aide registry and investigate all complaints of abuse, neglect, and misappropriation of resident property by any nurse's aide in any nursing home that participates in the Medicare or Medicaid program. If a state finds that a nurse's aide has neglected or abused a nursing facility resident or misappropriated property of a resident, the law requires the state to include such information in the state's nurse's aide registry and to bar the aide from nursing-home employment. In addition, under federal regulations, states are obligated to determine whether facility practices or policies caused or contributed to the substantiated abuse, neglect, or misappropriation (42 CFR Section 488.301, 1998).

An investigation by the Office of the Inspector General in 2009 was conducted in a stratified random sample of 260 nursing facilities to determine whether and to what extent they employed individuals with criminal convictions. The findings show that 92% of nursing facilities employed at least one individual with at least one criminal conviction, and nearly half the facilities employed five or more individuals with at least one conviction (Levinson, 2011).

INVESTIGATIONS OF MISTREATMENT

Reporting suspected cases of elder mistreatment is required in most states under mandatory elder-abuse reporting laws. The Patient Protection and Affordable Care Act [Section 6703 (b)(3)] mandates the reporting of any reasonable suspicion of a crime against a resident in a nursing home to law enforcement in 24 hours and in 2 hours in the event of serious bodily injury. Although there are multiple agencies with some responsibility for investigating cases of abuse or neglect, often there is little or no coordinated effort to address these allegations. For residents in nursing homes and residential-care facilities, responsible agencies differ across states but typically include long-term-care ombudsmen, adult protective services, state agencies responsible for licensing nursing homes, state agencies responsible for operation of the nurse aide registry, Medicaid Fraud Control Units in state attorney general offices, and professional licensing boards (e.g., board of nursing or boards of nursing home administrators; Hawes, 2002). There is no federal patient abuse and neglect statute; therefore government attorneys have effectively used a financial fraud statute, the federal False Claims Act, to address failure of care cases across the country.

Several factors complicate the task of adequately assessing for abuse and neglect. First, the signs that may indicate mistreatment tend to be attributed to the normal processes of aging or to the chronic diseases and disabilities experienced by many frail older adults. Care needs to be taken by clinicians to secure a thorough medical history, including baseline conditions, and to conduct a careful, comprehensive physical examination. Moreover, the monitoring of additional signs such as fear, confusion, and depression over a reasonable period may be warranted. Another barrier for identifying mistreatment is that evidence of potential abuse or neglect is lost or mishandled by facility staff who perform the initial investigation into abuse and neglect allegations. The responsibility for investigating elder mistreatment falls initially to providers, who may not have adequately trained their staff on how to perform an investigation into abuse or neglect. A lack of knowledge regarding evidence preservation makes the task of taking appropriate action against potential abusers difficult for law enforcement or facility administrators (Caceres & Fulmer, 2016).

Facility managers are responsible for protecting the residents from future mistreatment during and after an investigation and to ensure proper and timely treatment of the resident's medical and psychological needs. How older adults are protected after abuse and neglect has been alleged is critical to ensuring the safety and rights of not only the alleged victim, but also all older adults residing in the institutional setting (Charpentier & Soulières, 2013).

The Elder Justice Roadmap (Connolly, Brandl, & Brekman, 2014), developed with support from the U.S. Department of Justice (USDOJ) and the U.S. Department of Health and Human Services (USDHHS), provides guidance for advancing strategic policy, practice, education, and research initiatives that address elder abuse and neglect.

See also Aging Agencies: Federal Level; Aging Agencies: State Level; Elder Mistreatment: Overview; Elder Neglect; Nursing Homes.

Marie Boltz and David R. Hoffman

42 CFR Section 488.301 [42 CFR Ch. IV (10-1-98 Edition), §483.13 (c) (1) (ii) (A) (B)]. (2010). *Elder Justice Act. Public Act 111–148. Patient Protection and Affordable Care Act*. Retrieved from https://www.gpo.gov/fdsys/pkg/PLAW-111publ148/pdf/PLAW-111publ148.pdf

Caceres, B., & Fulmer, T. (2016). Mistreatment detection. In M. Boltz, E. Capezuti, D. Zwicker, & T. Fulmer (Eds.), *Evidence-based geriatric nursing protocols for best practice* (5th ed., p. 725). New York, NY: Springer Publishing.

Castle, N., & Beech, S. (2011). Elder abuse in assisted living. *Journal of Applied Gerontology, 32*(2) 248–267.

Castle, N., Ferguson-Rome, J. C., & Teresi J. A. (2015). Elder abuse in residential long-term care: An update to the 2003 National Research Council report. *Journal of Applied Gerontology, 34*(4), 407–443.

Charpentier, M., & Soulières M. (2013). Elder abuse and neglect in institutional settings: The resident's perspective. *Journal of Elder Abuse & Neglect, 25*(4), 339–354.

Connolly, M.-T., Brandl, B., & Brekman, R. (2014). *Elder Justice Roadmap report.* Washington, DC: U.S. Department of Justice.

Federal Register. (2016, October 4). *Medicare and Medicaid programs; reform of requirements for long-term care facilities.* Centers for Medicare & Medicaid Services.

Hawes, C. (2002). Elder abuse in residential long-term care settings: What is known and what information is needed? In R. Bonnie & R. Wallace (Eds.), *Elder mistreatment: Abuse, neglect, and exploitation in an aging America* (pp. 446–500). Washington, DC: National Academies Press.

Hawes, C., & Kimbell, A. (2010). *Detecting, addressing and preventing elder abuse in residential care facilities* [Report to the National Institute of Justice, U.S. Department of Justice]. Retrieved from https://www.ncjrs.gov/pdffiles1/nij/grants/229299.pdf

Levinson, D. R. (2011). Nursing facilities' employment of individuals with criminal convictions. Retrieved from https://oig.hhs.gov/oei/reports/oei-07-09-00110.pdf

McDonald, L., Beaulieu, M., Harbison, J., Hirst, S., Lowenstein, A., Podnieks, E., & Wahl, J. (2012). Institutional abuse of older adults: What we know, what we need to know. *Journal of Elder Abuse & Neglect, 24*(2), 138–160.

Natan, B. M., & Lowenstein, A. (2010). Study of factors that affect abuse of older people in nursing homes. *Nursing Management, 17*(8), 20–24.

National Center on Elder Abuse. (2012). *Fact sheet: Abuse of residents of long-term care facilities.* Retrieved from http://www.centeronelderabuse.org/docs/Abuse_of_Residents_of_Long_Term_Care_Facilities.pdf

Patient Protection and Affordable Care Act. 42 U.S.C. § 18001. (2010). Retrieved from http://www.gpo.gov/fdsys/pkg/BILLS-111hr3590enr/pdf/BILLS-111hr3590enr.pdf

Phillips, L. R., Guo, G., & Kim, H. (2013). Elder mistreatment in U.S. residential care facilities: The scope of the problem. *Journal of Elder Abuse & Neglect, 25*(1), 19–39.

Post, L., Page, C., Conner, T., Prokhorov, A., Fang, Y., & Biroscak, B. (2010). Elder abuse in long-term care: Types, patterns, and risk factors. *Research on Aging, 32*(3), 323–348.

Schiamberg, L. B., Barboza, G. G., Oehmke, J., Zhang, Z., Griffore, R. J., Weatherill, R. P., . . . Post, L. A. (2011). Elder abuse in nursing homes: An ecological perspective. *Journal of Elder Abuse & Neglect, 23*(2), 190–211.

U.S. House of Representatives. (2001). *Committee on Government Reform, Special Investigations Division, Minority Staff. Abuse of residents is a major problem in U.S. nursing homes.* Retrieved from http://www.canhr.org/reports/2001/abusemajorproblem.pdf

Web Resources

Elder Abuse and Neglect: In search of solutions, American Psychological Association: http://www.apa.org/pi/aging/resources/guides/elder-abuse.aspx

Elder Justice Roadmap: https://www.justice.gov/file/852856/download

Elder Mistreatment: Abuse, Neglect, and Exploitation in an Aging America, The Committee on National Statistics, National Academies Press: https://www.nap.edu/catalog/10406/elder-mistreatment-abuse-neglect-and-exploitation-in-an-aging-america

National Center on Elder Abuse, Administration on Aging: http://www.ncea.aoa.gov

National Consumer Voice for Long-Term Care: http://www.theconsumervoice.org

Nursing Home Abuse and Neglect Resource Center for Older Adults and Their Families: http://www.NursingHomeAlert.com

State Elder Abuse Hotline: Where to Report Abuse: https://www.seniorhomes.com/p/elder-abuse-hotlines

INSTITUTIONALIZATION

Institutionalization refers to the placement of an individual in a long-term care facility. The setting in which long-term care is provided is determined by the individual patient's medical, psychological, and social needs. The patient's financial status also affects placement. Long-term care may be provided in a nursing home, assisted-living facility, life-care community, or at home. This chapter focuses on institutionalization in nursing homes.

A nursing home can provide patients with skilled nursing care, rehabilitation, and other medical and social services. In the United States, as of 2014, there were 15,600 nursing homes containing 1.7 million beds with an 86% occupancy rate (Centers for Disease Control and Prevention [CDC], 2017). Twenty five percent of people who stay in nursing homes for 3 months or fewer are largely there for rehabilitation or end-of-life care. About half of residents are there for at least a year, and as many as 21% are there for approximately 5 years (HealthinAging, 2017). It is estimated that by 2030, the number of individuals residing in nursing homes could double or triple (Administration on Aging [AOA], 2016). Placement in a nursing home occurs more frequently when individuals have limited social and financial resources. Additional factors that increase the likelihood of a nursing home admission include older age, low social activity, and functional and/or mental health problems. Nursing home residents are likely to have at least one impairment that affects their ability to perform activities of daily living (ADL), more than half have either bowel or bladder incontinence, and 50% to 70% may be affected by dementia. Approximately one third of the residents experience vision or hearing problems. More than 70% of nursing home residents are female and about half are 85 years or older (HealthinAging, 2017).

Both patients and families can experience considerable emotional stress when an older loved one moves into an institution (Ellis, 2010). The transition from the community to an institution is associated with high mortality rates for new residents, even when other factors are controlled, suggesting that the transition process itself is difficult to cope with and life altering (Ferrah, Ibrahim, Kipsaina, & Bugeja, 2017). The decision by the family to institutionalize a relative is difficult as well (Church, Schumacher, & Thompson, 2016). Many family members continue to provide some care to the resident even after nursing home placement and must contend with the nursing home administration and staff, new decision-making responsibilities, and end-of-life care decisions (Schulz et al., 2014).

Although medical care is a major concern in the nursing home, a nursing home is more than just a medical facility; it is a place where individuals live their daily lives. Goffman (1961), in his early and seminal work, *Asylums*, described how "total institutions" limit "inmate" autonomy and independence, and control the day-to-day existence of residents. Indeed, in one study, researchers found that the lack of autonomy and interpersonal complications were the key concerns of nursing home residents (Bradshaw, Playford, & Riazi, 2012). In the medicalized environment of a nursing home, the "personhood" of the resident may be secondary. The experience of institutionalization for the older patients is often accompanied by a sense of loss. Privacy, personal possessions, access to resources, autonomy, and control are lost to a degree that varies with the organization and structure of the nursing home. Society's negative attitude about nursing home placement may accentuate the new resident's feelings of loss and failure. Moreover, in settings where private rooms are possible, meals are usually communal.

Today, although nursing homes have some of the characteristics that Goffman enumerates, many long-term care facilities strive to optimize residents' sense of control and maintain their individual sense of self. To improve the quality of nursing homes, some long-term care facilities are embracing person-centered long-term care models (Crandall, White, Schuldheis, & Talerico, 2007). This approach recognizes the importance of autonomy and individual choice for residents. Residents participate in decision making about their services, and a home, rather than an institutional, environment, is fostered. A 2006 group of stakeholders of a person-centered care culture change for nursing homes proposed that an "ideal institution" would include resident direction; a homelike atmosphere; close relationships among patients, family, and staff; staff empowerment; collaborative decision making; and quality-improvement processes. Limited research suggests the success of this effort to move toward a more person-centered care model is mixed, with adoption lagging behind awareness (Koren, 2010). However, many nursing homes encourage residents to decorate their rooms with their own furniture, pictures, and mementos. By encouraging familiarity and comfort, the nursing home can foster an enhanced sense of belonging. To empower residents, some nursing homes have a resident council, where residents meet regularly for discussion of concerns related to living in the facility.

It is critical that the residents' primary aide, nurse, and physician know their life histories and the values that have guided them so that these health care providers can ascertain what is meaningful to them, including spiritual needs. An interdisciplinary approach is necessary for delivering quality care in the long-term care setting. To respond sensitively to psychosocial and medical needs, all disciplines must communicate regularly about individual residents. It is also imperative that advance directives be discussed and clarified on admission by the resident (or health care proxy if the resident is cognitively impaired) to ensure that medical staff act in accordance with such wishes and stated goals of care.

Residents with dementia have special needs in the nursing home, depending on the severity of their cognitive loss. In 2012, the Centers for Medicare & Medicaid Services (CMS) announced a new program to improve care for nursing home patients, with a special focus on the appropriate use of antipsychotic medications and rethinking the standard approach to dementia care, including an emphasis on person-centered care (CMS, 2017). When the program began, 23.9% of nursing home residents received antipsychotic medication; by mid-2016, the national prevalence had decreased to 16.1% (CMS, 2016).

With the majority of nursing home residents dying within a year of placement and many in the first 6 months (National Hospice and Palliative Care Organization [NHCPO], 2017), it is important to establish the presence of palliative care and hospice services in the nursing home. Nursing home patients are undertreated for pain (Teno, Weitzen, Wetle, & Mor, 2001). The research demonstrates that analgesic management of daily pain is better for nursing home residents enrolled in hospice than for those not enrolled in hospice (Miller, Mor, Wu, Gozalo, & Lapane, 2002). Palliative care programs in nursing homes can proactively evaluate patients for pain and other symptoms. If a patient has cognitive loss and is not able to provide a history, the nursing aide and other professionals can observe behavioral changes, grimacing, and other possible signs that may indicate pain and should prompt evaluation. Proactive care to anticipate a range of symptoms may do much to spare residents unnecessary suffering.

There are many guides developed by the federal government, voluntary agencies, and consumer groups to assist in identifying quality nursing homes. The CMS website on long-term care includes a booklet, *Your Guide to Choosing a Nursing Home or Other Long-Term Care*, with helpful guidelines to help in choosing a facility (www.medicare.gov/Pubs/pdf/02174 .pdf). Given the demographic inevitability of an increasing number of older people requiring long-term care, there is an unparalleled opportunity to create nursing homes that respond more and more to their vulnerable residents. The challenge ahead is formidable.

Michele G. Greene, Ronald D. Adelman,
and Mara A. G. Hollander

Administration on Aging. (2016). *Aging into the 21st century.* Washington, DC: U.S. Department of Health & Human Services, Administration on Community Living. Retrieved from http://www .aoa.acl.gov/Aging_Statistics/future_growth/ aging21/health.aspx#Nursing

Bradshaw, S. B., Playford, E. D., & Riazi, A. (2012). Living well in care homes: A systematic review of qualitative studies. *Age and Ageing, 41*(4), 429–440.

Centers for Medicare & Medicaid Services. (2016, December). *National partnership to improve dementia care in nursing homes: Antipsychotic medication use data report.* Washington, DC: U.S. Department of Health & Human Services. Retrieved from https://www .nhqualitycampaign.org/files/AP_ package_20170112.pdf

Centers for Medicare & Medicaid Services. (2017). *National Nursing Home Quality Improvement (NNHQI) Campaign.* Washington, DC: U.S. Department of Health & Human Services. Retrieved from https://www .nhqualitycam- paign.org/dementiaCare.aspx

Church, L. L., Schumacher, K. L., & Thompson, S. A. (2016). Mixed-methods exploration of family caregiver strain in the nursing home. *Journal of Hospice & Palliative Nursing, 18*(1), 46–52.

Crandall, L. G., White, D. L., Schuldheis, S., & Talerico, K. A. (2007). Initiating person-centered care practices in long-term care facilities. *Journal of Gerontological Nursing, 33*(11), 47–56.

Ellis, J. M. (2010). Psychological transition into a residential care facility: Older people's experiences. *Journal of Advanced Nursing, 66*(5), 1159–1168.

Ferrah, N., Ibrahim, J. E., Kipsaina, C., & Bugeja, L. (2017). Death following recent admission into nursing home from community living: A systematic review into the transition process. *Journal of Aging and Health*, 1–21. Advance online publication. doi:10.1177/0898264316686575

Goffman, E. (1961). *Asylums: Essays on the social situation of mental patients and other inmates.* New York, NY: Doubleday.

HealthinAging. (2017). *Aging & health A to Z: Nursing homes.* New York, NY: Health In Aging Foundation. Retrieved from http://www.healthinaging.org/aging-and-health-a-to-z/topic:nursing-homes

Koren, M. (2010). Person-centered care for nursing home residents: The culture-change movement. *Health Affairs, 29*(2), 312–317.

Miller, S. C., Mor, V., Wu, N., Gozalo, P., & Lapane, K. (2002). Does receipt of hospice care in nursing homes improve the management of pain at the end of life? *Journal of the American Geriatrics Society, 50*(3), 507–515.

National Hospice and Palliative Care Organization. (2017). Retrieved from http://www.nhpco.org/sites/default/files/public/palliativecare/PALLIATIVECARE_PC_NursingHome.pdf

Schulz, R., Rosen, J., Klinger, J., Musa, D. Castle, N., & Kane, A. L. (2014). Effects of a psychosocial intervention on caregivers of recently placed nursing home residents: A randomized controlled trial. *Clinical Gerontologist, 27*, 347–367.

Teno, J. M., Weitzen, S., Wetle, T., & Mor, V. (2001). Persistent pain in nursing home residents. *Journal of the American Medical Association, 285*(16), 2081. doi:10.1001/jama.285.16.2081-a

Web Resources

Administration for Community Living: https://aoa.acl.gov

HealthinAging: http://www.healthinaging.org/aging-and-health-a-to-z/topic:nursing-homes

Medicare: www.Medicare.gov/nursinghomecompare/search.html

National Center for Health Statistics: Nursing home care: http://www.cdc.gov/nchs/fastats/nursing-home-care.htm

National Nursing Home Quality Improvement Campaign: https://www.nhqualitycampaign.org

National Partnership to Improve Dementia Care in Nursing Homes: Antipsychotic medication use data report: https://www.nhqualitycampaign.org/files/AP_package_20170112.pdf

INTERDISCIPLINARY TEAMS

Older people often have multiple illnesses and conditions, sometimes with cognitive loss, which may result in an increased loss of function and isolation. Frequently, each medical condition requires a specific treatment or medication regimen that is difficult to adhere to—remembering to take it at the right time and in the appropriate way. In addition, prescriptions and over-the-counter (OTC) medications may interact, causing negative side effects. Thus older patients with a number of chronic or acute conditions benefit when they receive coordinated care from several disciplines working together. However, these professionals must be able to work together effectively, create an integrated plan, and coordinate the patient's care on an ongoing basis. When multiple health care practitioners administer uncoordinated care, services can be at odds with one another, and the patients often suffer. The "layering" of recommendations, orders, and medications, one on another, is *multidisciplinary* care. This is in sharp contrast to *interdisciplinary* care—that is, coordinated care developed by skilled clinicians who jointly agree on a care plan and work together to implement that plan.

Not all older patients require the care of an interdisciplinary team, and even patients who benefit from teams do not require a team review at every visit. The needs of the patient should drive the number and types of providers delivering care. Generally, patients with complex physical, emotional, social, and economic issues need, at a minimum, medical, nursing, social work, and pharmacy services to develop or alter a care plan. Other practitioners, such as psychology, chaplaincy, and nutrition, are often part of the team as well. Studies of the clinical and cost effectiveness of teams generally demonstrate that the patients are helped by an initial comprehensive geriatric assessment conducted by multiple disciplines (Deschodt et al., 2016).

Transitions between levels of care are particularly important points where patients can benefit from interdisciplinary care. Frequently cited benefits of teams include a patient-centered focus that engages the patient as a partner in care and improved communication among providers, resulting in better patient outcomes. Among the successful collaborative-practice models were nurses and physicians working together to monitor at home patients who had chronic and unstable medical conditions such as congestive heart failure, hypertension, and diabetes.

Teams, as opposed to independent practitioners, are distinguished by agreement to work together and coordinate care. The focus on the patient requires that team members reach consensus on the goals of care, the priorities of treatment, and the ongoing measurement of the plan's outcomes. Sometimes a full and heated discussion of the patient's needs is required to recognize the trade-offs inherent in the plan of care. Effective health care teamwork requires agreement, and agreement requires keen interpersonal skills so that all members freely contribute to and feel accountable for the plan. The other characteristics of effective teams include a clear division of labor, training for members, and an administrative system that supports coordinated care and creates synergy among the providers.

STAGES OF TEAM DEVELOPMENT

Becoming a team requires work. Teams generally move through five stages of development that can vary in duration from days to weeks; these stages are fluid and the teams frequently move from stage to stage. These phases, conceptualized by Drinka and Clark (2000), are as follows:

Stage 1—Forming. During this period, members are tentative and want to learn about one another and the reasons they became members of the team. Effective tasks in this stage include icebreakers to help members get to know one another and discussions about the purpose and goals of the health care team.

Stage 2—Norming. Team ground rules are agreed on, and members now have a sense of cohesion and membership. Members know what to expect at meetings and share responsibility for the team process.

Stage 3—Confronting. This is considered the "difficult" stage by many, but in fact it can be a productive stage in that it brings issues and conflicts to the fore. This is the phase when members develop and implement criteria for decision making, leadership, and protocols for the team processes, often through exchanges that are confrontational and challenging. However, conflict, particularly in an environment that is somewhat safe, can lead to a fine-tuning of the team goals and process because the underpinning assumptions are hammered out.

Stage 4—Performing. The roles, process, and structure are so well honed in this phase that the team is "humming along"—it is truly a team, more than the sum of its members. Although the group does need to monitor its progress to avoid "group think," the close working relationship and excellent communication among members allow the team to provide well-coordinated care for patients.

Stage 5—Leaving. This is an intermittent stage that reflects unavoidable turnover on the team. Leaving can involve one or many members (e.g., when a team downsizes because of organizational cutbacks). How the team reacts to the departure of one or more members varies but inevitably result in team readjustment.

Meeting Ground Rules

The team must establish its own rules or norms. Examples include attendance policy, promptness, types of permitted interruptions (e.g., patient emergencies only), confidentiality, protocol for patient presentations, breaks, premeeting preparation, completion of work between meetings, and rules on side conversations and digressions from the topic. Agreement about such standards usually prevents misunderstandings and improves team members' behavior.

Teaching Team Skills

The Geriatric Interdisciplinary Team Training (GITT) program, a large initiative sponsored by The John A. Hartford Foundation, focuses on the experience of 13 universities and health care organizations that developed innovative programs to educate and train health personnel and students to work in geriatrics interdisciplinary teams (Schultz, Keyser, & Pincus, 2011). It provides a practical approach to team development in different settings that includes setting up a team-training program, implementing a specific curriculum, and examining the challenges of teamwork in different organizational environments. The GITT program reinforces the importance of having students participate on well-functioning teams. Interdisciplinary teams allow students to witness professionals working together to solve patient problems, share expertise, create a plan of care, and resolve conflicts. Students see the rigor involved in productive meetings and can observe the interpersonal dynamics of teams.

The teaching of team skills should focus on the attitudes, knowledge, and skills that team members must learn:

Attitudes. How much respect is there for the roles of all health professionals in the care of older adults and their families or caregivers? Are members willing to collaborate with all health care professionals? Is there an appreciation for the interdisciplinary team approach, especially for patients with functional and psychosocial disabilities? Studies have shown that work is needed in this area because trainees in some disciplines, such as medicine, are less inclined to embrace teamwork.

Knowledge. Team members need to learn about the skills, education, and training of their teammates. In GITT programs, trainees shadow members from other disciplines or interview team members about education and license requirements. Team members also benefit from learning about formal and informal community support services and how to access services such as home health care, hospice, mental health services, care management, telephone reassurance, visitors, companions, homemakers, chore services, meal programs, transportation services, senior centers, adult day care, respite care, and local area agencies on aging.

Skills. Effective teams improve patient care and meet the patient's needs. By identifying the myriad problems and issues involved in elder care, the team is better able to prioritize concerns and galvanize treatments and services. Focusing on the patient and family is a key skill. Other communication skills that are important include active listening, succinct presentations, summary of discussions, testing for agreements, focused questions, probes to clarify issues, and willingness to sacrifice autonomy to group consensus.

Effective and patient-centered teamwork is not happenstance. It involves patience, commitment, and flexibility. Practitioners and educators should make every effort to pass on teamwork knowledge, attitudes, and skills through active engagement of new team members and trainees.

Elizabeth A. Capezuti

Deschodt, M., Claes, V., Van Grootven, B., Van den Heede, K., Flamaing, J., Bolands, B., & Milisen, K. (2016). Structure and processes of interdisciplinary geriatric consultation teams in acute care hospitals: A scoping review. *International Journal of Nursing Studies, 55,* 98–114.

Drinka, T. J. K., & Clark, P. G. (2000). *Health care teamwork.* Westport, CT: Auburn House.

Schultz, D., Keyser, D., & Pincus, H. A. (2011). Developing interdisciplinary centers in aging: Learning from the RAND/Hartford Building Interdisciplinary Geriatric Health Care Research Centers Initiative. *Academic Medicine, 86,* 1318–1324.

Web Resource
American Geriatrics Society: http://www.american geriatrics.org/pha/partnership_for_health_in_aging/interdisciplinary_team_training_statement

INTERGENERATIONAL PROGRAMS

Intergenerational programming was pioneered in 1965 with the development of the Foster Grandparent Program (FGP), a federally funded project that paired low-income adults older than the age of 60 years with children who had special needs or experienced circumstances that limited academic, social, or economic development. The program sought to reduce poverty and isolation of participating older adults while providing needed support and services to children in institutional group settings (Corporation for National & Community Service [CNCS], 2017; Generations United, 2007). The model established mutually beneficial partnerships; older adult participants experienced a sense of purpose and social connections and were able to contribute to the community while earning an hourly stipend, and the children received tutoring, mentorship, and needed attention. The FGP eventually expanded its services to include children and youth in public schools and other settings. In 2009, they lowered the eligibility age for adult volunteers from 60 to 55 years and increased the eligibility for a stipend to 200% more than the poverty level (CNCS, 2017). The FGP remains an active program even today, administered through the Senior Corps of the CNCS.

Since the FGP was launched, intergenerational programming has expanded to bring together participants across the life span to engage in activities that meet a variety of social needs (Generations United, 2007). These programs provide opportunities for the participants to give and receive knowledge and skills, build social capacity, and improve physical and emotional health. They reduce age segregation and have the potential to address ageist assumptions through age-diverse spaces and interaction and acknowledgment of the value that older adults contribute as important and productive members of the community. Intergenerational programs have taken shape as friendly visiting projects, in which younger or older volunteers visit homebound older adults in the community; lifelong learning programs that bring together participants of multiple ages to enhance knowledge and skills on a range of topics; community service projects designed to support improvement of the built environment; and colocated programs such as day-care facilities for children in long-term care facilities for adults.

KEY COMPONENTS

Intergenerational programming is found on a belief that individuals of all ages have valuable resources to share with one another. To develop programs that operationalize this fundamental philosophy and are sustainable, a thoughtful planning process should be undertaken. The best practices for planning and implementing intergenerational programming include (Bishop & Moxley, 2012; New York City Department for the Aging [NYC DFTA], 2010):

- Involving all stakeholders (e.g., future program participants, intra-agency departments, community resources, organizations) in the planning process
- Conducting a needs assessment
- Defining a need and rationale for the program
- Establishing measurable and well-defined goals
- Developing planned activities and materials
- Developing an evaluation plan
- Creating a realistic budget
- Developing an outreach and recruitment plan and corresponding promotional materials
- Training the project coordinators/managers and direct-service staff
- Providing training for program participants that includes sensitivity training with culturally competent curricula
- Making time for reflection during the planning period, implementation phase, and evaluation process

Generations United serves as a member organization that works to improve the lives of all people and strengthen communities through intergenerational collaboration, public policy, and programs. It serves as a key resource for service providers, program managers, advocates, and policymakers who are interested in building and growing intergenerational initiatives.

CHALLENGES

To ensure the success of intergenerational programs, it is important that organizations commit to collaboration, planning, and training. In doing so, the challenges in developing and managing intergenerational programs, as well as barriers to full implementation and sustainability, will more likely be addressed and overcome. The common challenges to be aware of include limited or loss of funding for programs; lack of knowledge and skills related to intergenerational program planning; difficulty engaging stakeholders in the planning process; insufficient time allocated to developing the program; staff turnover, which can result in the loss of a program's "champions"; inadequate administrative support; generational differences and misconceptions, both among the participants and in the program staff; scheduling that meets the needs of all participants; recruitment and retention of volunteers and participants; ability to measure outcomes of programs; and appropriate physical space for programming (NYC DFTA, 2010; Jarrott, 2007).

PROGRAM EXAMPLES

Intergenerational programs can address a variety of issues and be held in a range of settings. The FGP is just one of the many programs that bring children and youth together with older adults for mutually beneficial interactions. The Habitat Intergenerational Program (HIP), launched in 1997 by Mass Audubon Habitat Wildlife Sanctuary, organizes a community of people of all ages and backgrounds and engages them in environmental education and community service projects. Together, participants are committed to nurturing intergenerational connections and learning about and protecting the environment. Providence Mount St. Vincent, a longtime provider of assisted living and skilled nursing units for older adults in Seattle, determined that its housing community needed the presence of children to bring more joy to their residents. In the 1990s, "The Mount" opened its Intergenerational Learning Center (ILC), a licensed child care provider for community members and employees of Providence Mount St. Vincent. Five days a week, the children in the colocated ILC interact with older adults living at The Mount through planned activities and everyday encounters. The Intergenerational Work Study Program (IWSP) in New York, New York is a collaboration between the City's DFTA and the Department of Education. The program, established in 1987 as an effort to prevent high school dropout, has broadened its mission to now focus on college enrollment of youth participants and postgraduation readiness for careers in health and social services. During their time in the program, youth participants provide needed services to the older adults in senior centers, nursing facilities, and home care settings. It is expected that more intergenerational programs like these will emerge in response to shifting demographics and community need and in light of the reported benefits experienced by youth, older adults, and communities engaged with intergenerational programming (Bishop & Moxley, 2012; Generations United, 2007).

LOOKING AHEAD

Innovation in the implementation of intergenerational programming is needed because communities are increasingly age diverse and funding constraints remain a challenge. A closer look at programing across racially/ethnically diverse communities and in urban and nonurban settings would allow for culturally competent best practices. The studies that explore outcomes—changes in individuals, organizations, communities, and the environment—should be conducted. The movement for evidence-based practice models demands additional research. An increased body of knowledge and evidence that intergenerational programming generates physical, emotional, and economic benefits to the community and cost-savings in other programs would strengthen the potential for future funding mechanisms that support this program.

Daniel S. Gardner and Rebekah Glushefski

Bishop, J. D., & Moxley, D. P. (2012). Promising practices useful in the design of an intergenerational program: Ten assertions guiding program development. *Social Work in Mental Health, 10,* 183–204.
Corporation for National and Community Service. (2017). *FGP operations handbook.* Retrieved from https://www.nationalservice.gov/documents/2016/fgp-operations-handbook

Generations United. (2007). Fact sheet: The benefits of intergenerational programs. Retrieved from http://www.gu.org/LinkClick.aspx?fileticket=71wHEwUd0KA%3D&;tabid=157&mid=606

Jarrott, S. E. (2007). *Tried and true: A guide to successful intergenerational activities at shared site programs.* Retrieved from http://www.intergenerational.clahs.vt.edu/pdf/jarrotttriedtrue.pdf

New York City Department for the Aging. (2010). *Good practices in intergenerational programming: Models advancing policy, practice and research.* Retrieve from http://www.nyc.gov/html/dfta/downloads/pdf/publications/good_practices.pdf

Web Resources

Corporation for National and Community Service: https://www.nationalservice.gov

Generations United: http://www.gu.org

Habitat Intergenerational Program (HIP): http://www.massaudubon.org/get-outdoors/wildlife-sanctuaries/habitat/get-involved/intergenerational-program

Intergenerational Work Study Program (IWSP): http://www.nyc.gov/html/dfta/html/community/intergenerational.shtml

Providence Mount St. Vincent (The Mount): http://washington.providence.org/senior-care/mount-st-vincent

INTERNATIONAL PSYCHOGERIATRIC ASSOCIATION

The International Psychogeriatric Association (IPA), founded in 1982, is recognized as the world's leading multidisciplinary, nonprofit organization providing health care professionals and scientists with information about behavioral and biological geriatric mental health. With more than 1,100 IPA members from approximately 68 countries, IPA includes most of the world's preeminent professionals and scientists interested in psychogeriatrics. The IPA is also committed to fostering education, facilitating the advancement of research, and promoting international consensus and understanding in psychogeriatric issues through its innovative educational programs, regional initiatives, scientific congresses, regional meetings, peer-reviewed quarterly journal (i.e., *International Psychogeriatrics*, published by Springer Publishing, New York), special-focus supplements, quarterly newsletter (i.e., IPA *Bulletin*), and website. IPA's goals are to:

- Promote awareness of issues related to mental health of the elderly, including diagnosis, assessment, treatment, and rehabilitation
- Provide an international forum for the exchange of information by professionals in all relevant disciplines on matters pertaining to the mental health of the elderly
- Encourage the development of educational resources in basic and applied research in the field of psychogeriatics
- Support the development of services for maximizing the potential of elderly persons in the community and in institutions
- Support the role of families and professional caregivers
- Encourage affiliation to IPA by related organizations

IPA's scientific meetings are educational vehicles that bring together opinion leaders from around the world to hear and present research papers, often before publication. Through plenary sessions, symposia, debates, and poster presentations, IPA meetings cover a vast array of topics, including anxiety, depression, dementia (i.e., Alzheimer's, Lewy body, and other types), behavioral and psychological symptoms of dementia, delirium, cognitive and noncognitive impairment, suicide, schizophrenia, transcultural issues, models of service delivery, and caregiver issues.

Elizabeth A. Capezuti

Web Resource

International Psychogeriatric Association: http://www.ipa-online.org

INTERVIEWING

Highly developed interviewing skills are needed for effective and empathic communication between health care professionals and older patients. Research has shown that the quality of communication between health professionals and patients significantly influences patient satisfaction, adherence to medication regimens, recommendations for changes in lifestyle and diagnostic tests, recall of information, anxiety, safety, and health status (Stewart, Meredith, Brown, & Galajda, 2000). Communication also influences the health professionals' ability to diagnose and treat, their satisfaction with the encounter, and the risk of malpractice suits.

The barriers to quality communication may derive from the health professional, the older patient, or the medical care system. Health professionals may not have sufficient training in communication or geriatric care. For example, they may not have been taught how to raise difficult subjects, such as advance directives, sexual dysfunction, and cognitive impairment, in a sensitive and effective manner (Adelman, Greene, Friedmann, & Cook, 2008), depression, bereavement, and elder abuse. In addition, practitioners' ageist beliefs may interfere with accurate diagnosis and treatment (e.g., misdiagnosis of cognitive impairment when depression is the underlying problem). In many care settings, health professionals are under enormous time constraints and financial incentives that conspire to undermine communication between health professionals and patients. Unfortunately, diminished dialogue makes it unlikely for health professionals to reach the "personhood" of the patient. Patients themselves may have ageist biases, attributing symptoms to the natural processes of aging. These misperceptions may result in older patients who do not discuss potentially serious problems with clinicians. The symptoms that may be embarrassing to older people, including urinary incontinence, sexuality, or memory loss, may also inhibit patient disclosure. In addition, some older patients are fearful about the meaning of new symptoms and may not reveal their presence. The lower health literacy of some older patients (Chesser, Woods, Smothers, & Rogers, 2016) may translate into inadequate reporting of symptoms, poor elaboration of complaints, poor questioning of the

clinician, and patient inability to adhere to the health professionals' recommendations.

One way to transcend an ageist perspective is to conduct a life history (or, if time does not permit, a modified life review) to learn about the patient's past and present circumstances, values, and goals. A life history can explore an individual's identity, dispel ageist stereotypes, and enable the health care professional to provide effective and sensitive care. The acquisition of this information does not have to occur at one visit. It may take multiple interactions to develop a complete knowledge of the patient's lifeworld. When a comprehensive understanding of the geriatric patient is unrealized, the patient and provider lose an opportunity to collaborate in the healing process (Adelman, Greene, & Ory, 2000).

Interviewing older patients requires many of the same skills required for interviewing younger adults. Practitioners must be attentive listeners and adept at identifying the patient's agenda for the visit. Interviews should be patient centered and address the patient's major concerns. Open-ended questions to facilitate the patient-centered interview may be helpful but may also be inadequate. They may set the stage for an effective, empathic encounter, but practitioners must also carefully attend to patients' responses and listen to what is said, as well as what is unsaid. To improve communication, it may be helpful for clinicians to elicit the older patient's agenda for the visit and incorporate these topics, when feasible, into the overall agenda for the visit. Questioning is just one component of good interviewing skills. Providing sufficient information to the patient in language that is free of technical jargon and responding to the older patient's level of health literacy are also important keys.

In recent years, clinicians have been using motivational interviewing to promote health behavior change in adults. This patient-centered approach focuses on the patient's own motivation to change and plans for actual behavior change. There is some early evidence that motivational interviewing techniques may be effective in influencing health behavior, such as diet and physical activity, of elderly patients (Purath, Keck, & Fitzgerald, 2014).

It is important to realize that interactions between physicians and older patients may be significantly different from interactions with younger patients. The "old-old" (individuals aged 85 years and older) grew up in an age of deep respect for the authority of the physician and may not desire to participate as fully in the medical encounter as "young-old" or "middle-old" patients. The health care professional must determine the patient's wishes for participation in decision making (Arora & McHorney, 2000). Research indicates that overall physician responsiveness (i.e., the quality of questioning, informing, and support) is better with younger patients than with older patients. Physicians are less likely to be egalitarian, patient-centered, respectful, and engaged to demonstrate therapeutic optimism with older patients than with younger patients. The research has also shown that older patients are less assertive than younger patients (Greene, Adelman, & Rizzo, 1996).

When interviewing older patients, attention must be paid to numerous factors that influence communication: the presence of multiple chronic conditions, sensory deficits, cognitive limitations, and the presence of an accompanying individual during the medical encounter. These issues may make interviews long and complex. Thus health care professionals must be skilled at focusing the interview and getting to the immediate issues at hand while achieving and maintaining the relationship's interpersonal aspects. There does not have to be a choice between providing effective care and maintaining a warm interpersonal relationship. Coordinating a medically efficient and interpersonally warm patient-centered visit constitutes the art of medicine. Although more medical schools and residency programs address training in communication skills, these efforts, in general, remain suboptimal and are not usually focused on older patient–health professional interaction.

Sensory deficits (i.e., problems with hearing and vision) are likely to influence communication in medical encounters. Approximately one third of individuals aged 65 to 74 years have hearing loss, and approximately half of individuals aged more than 75 years have problems with hearing (National Institute on Deafness and Other Communication Disorders, 2016). To facilitate communication, health care professionals can try several approaches, including identifying the patient's specific needs in this area, reducing background noise in the office, speaking at a slightly louder level (without shouting), establishing good visual contact, rephrasing rather than repeating misunderstood phrases, pausing at the end of a topic to allow for questions, and amplifying with a microphone and headset (Cobbs, Duthie, & Murphy, 1999).

Vision loss may also affect practitioner–patient interactions. It is estimated that 6.5 million people in the United States aged more than 65 years have severe visual impairments (American Foundation for the Blind, 2016). Individuals older than 65 years are more likely than younger individuals to experience a decrease in visual acuity, contrast sensitivity, and visual fields. Sitting close to the older patient and providing environmental supports, such as improved illumination in the office, can facilitate communication with patients with vision problems. In the appropriate context, it may helpful to let the patient know who is in the room and when they enter or depart. Describing the room may also assist the patient in accommodating to the environment.

Although the incidence of dementia increases with age, it should *not* be assumed that all older people have a cognitive impairment. Inappropriately stereotyping patients with any cognitive dysfunction as being incompetent and incapable of participating in their care must be avoided (Adelman et al., 2000); each patient must be individually assessed. Given the different communication and language impairments over the course of dementia, health care providers must become adept at identifying the needs of the patient at the particular stage of the illness (Orange & Ryan, 2000).

Older patients are often accompanied to the medical visit by a third party (e.g., spouse, adult child, or hired professional caregiver), who may significantly affect communication between the health care professional and the patient (Greene & Adelman, 2013; Ishikawa, Roter, Yamazaki, & Takayama, 2005; Schilling et al., 2002; Wolff, Boyd, Gitlin, Bruce, & Roter, 2012). One study found that in three-person encounters, older patients were often referred to as "he" or "she" (making the patient an outsider to the interaction). Indeed, exclusion of the older patient in triadic interaction is a not-so-subtle manifestation of ageism in the medical encounter. Moreover, when comparing two- and three-person interactions, it was found that although the content of the physicians' discussion was no different, older patients were less responsive and assertive and there was less shared laughter and joint decision making, in triadic visits (Greene, Majerovitz, Adelman, & Rizzo, 1994). Research in a primary care setting has shown that older patients are often accompanied by two or three other individuals who participate in the medical interview. Thus the health care professional must also become adept at facilitating small group discussions. However, the health care professional should spend some time alone with older patients to give them the opportunity to express concerns and problems that may be highly personal. Research continues in the investigation of older patient–physician–companion triadic encounters (Wolff et al., 2016).

One task of communication in the physician–older patient relationship is to determine the patient's wishes concerning advance directives. As there may be disagreement between the patient and the health care proxy, it is important that the practitioner help the patient–health care proxy achieve concordance on this difficult subject (Fins et al., 2005).

The provision of quality medical care to older patients requires sensitive communication skills on the part of health care professionals and a health care system that supports a patient-centered approach. Recognition of the interdependence of medical care and interpersonal care is essential for the practice of effective and compassionate health care.

Michele G. Greene, Ronald D. Adelman,
and Mara A. G. Hollander

Adelman, R., Greene, M., Friedmann, E., & Cook, M. (2008). Discussion of depression in follow-up medical visits with older patients. *Journal of the American Geriatrics Society, 56*(1), 16–22.

Adelman, R., Greene, M., & Ory, M. (2000). Communication between older patients and their physicians. *Clinics in Geriatric Medicine, 16*(1), 1–24.

American Foundation for the Blind. (2016). Aging and vision loss fact sheet. Retrieved from http://www.afb.org/section.aspx?SectionID=68&TopicID=320&DocumentID=3374&rewrite=0

Arora, N., & McHorney, C. (2000). Patient preferences for medical decision making: Who really wants to participate? *Medical Care, 38*(3), 335–341.

Chesser, A. K., Woods, N. K., Smothers, K., & Rogers, N. (2016). Health literacy and older adults. *Gerontology and Geriatric Medicine, 1,* 1–13.

Cobbs, E., Duthie, E., & Murphy, J. (1999). *Geriatrics review syllabus: A core curriculum in geriatric medicine.* Dubuque, IA: Kendall Hunt.

Fins, J., Maltby, B., Friedmann, E., Greene, M., Norris, K., Adelman, R., & Byock, I. (2005). Contracts, covenants and advance care planning: An empirical study of the moral obligations of patient and proxy. *Journal of Pain and Symptom Management, 29*(1), 55–68.

Greene, M., & Adelman, R. (2013). Beyond the dyad: Communication in triadic (and more) medical encounters. In L. Martin & R. DiMatteo (Eds.), *Oxford handbook of health communication, behavior change, and treatment adherence.* New York, NY: Oxford University Press.

Greene, M., Adelman, R., & Rizzo, C. (1996). Problems in communication between physicians and their older patients. *Journal of Geriatric Psychiatry, 29,* 13–32.

Greene, M., Majerovitz, D., Adelman, R., & Rizzo, C. (1994). The effects of the presence of a third person on the physician-older patient medical interview. *Journal of the American Geriatrics Society, 42,* 413–419.

Ishikawa, H., Roter, D. L., Yamazaki, Y., & Takayama, T. (2005). Physician-elderly patient-companion communication and roles of companions in Japanese geriatric encounters. *Social Science & Medicine, 60*(10), 2307–2320.

Mishler, E. (1984). *The discourse of medicine.* Norwood, NJ: Ablex.

National Institute on Deafness and Other Communication Disorders. (2016). *Hearing loss and older adults.* NIH Publication No. 01-4913. Retrieved from https://www.nidcd.nih.gov/sites/default/files/Documents/health/hearing/HearingLossOlderAdults-12-07-16.pdf

Orange, J., & Ryan, E. (2000). Alzheimer's disease and other dementias: Implications for physician communication. *Clinics in Geriatric Medicine, 16*(1), 153–173.

Purath, J., Keck, A., & Fitzgerald, C. (2014). Motivational interviewing for older adults in primary care: A systematic review. *Geriatric Nursing, 35*(3), 219–224.

I

Schilling, L., Scatena, L., Steiner, J., Albertson, G., Lin, C., Cyran, L., … Anderson, R. (2002). The third person in the room: Frequency, role, and influence of companions during primary care medical encounters. *Journal of Family Practice, 51*(8), 685–690.

Stewart, M., Meredith, L., Brown, J. B., & Galajda, J. (2000). The influence of older patient-physician communication on health and health-related outcomes. *Clinics in Geriatric Medicine, 16*(1), 25–37.

Wolff, J. L., Boyd, C. M., Gitlin, L. N., Bruce, M. L., & Roter, D. L. (2012). Going it together: Persistence of older adults' accompaniment to physician visits by a family companion. *Journal of the American Geriatrics Society, 60*(1), 106–112

Wolff, J. L., Guan, Y., Boyd, C. M., Vick, J., Amjad, H., Roth, D. L., … Roter, D. L. (2016). Examining the context and helpfulness of family companion contributions to older adults' primary care visits. *Patient Education Counseling 100*(3), 487–494. doi:10.1016/j.pec.2016.10.022

Web Resources

Alzheimer's Association, Communication and Alzheimer's: http://www.alz.org/care/dementia-communication-tips.asp

Family Practice Management: http://www.aafp.org/fpm/2006/0900/p73.html

Institute for Healthcare Communication, Impact of Communication on Health Care: healthcarecomm.org/aboutus/impact-of-communication-in-healthcare

NIA, Talking With Your Doctor: A guide for older people: https://www.nia.nih.gov/health/talking-your-doctor-presentation-toolkit

NIA. Talking With Your Older Patient: https://www.nia.nih.gov/sites/default/files/talking_with_your_older_patient.pdf

U.S. Department of Health and Human Services (USDHHS). Administration for Community Living: https://aoa.acl.gov/AoA_Programs/Tools_Resources/Older_Adults.aspx

JOINT REPLACEMENT

Joint disease is one of the major causes of morbidity in older adults. Joints can be damaged by osteoarthritis, rheumatoid arthritis, and traumatic injuries such as falls and motor vehicle accidents. These conditions may result in joint dysfunction and in some cases, extreme pain with activity and at rest. Often, pain motivates the patient to avoid using the joint, resulting in weakness and atrophy of the muscles that surround and stabilize it. This leads to further pain and deterioration. Likewise, joint disease may limit physical activity and precipitate a sedentary lifestyle. Joint replacement may be an option for maintaining mobility and function and reducing the pain of disease or fracture.

The prevalence of total hip replacement (THR) and total knee replacement (TKR) among adults aged 50 years and older is as high as 2.3% and 4.6%, respectively. The prevalence of THR rises to nearly 6% by the age of 80 years. The prevalence of TKR rises to nearly 10% by 80 years of age. The states with the highest number of THR and TKR patients are California, Florida, and Texas; the two states with the lowest numbers are Alaska and Hawaii. Approximately 168,000 THR procedures and 385,000 TKR procedures were performed in patients aged 65 years and older in America in 2010 (Williams, Wolford, & Bercovitz, 2015). The rate of primary joint-replacement surgery from 1991 to 2010 among Medicare beneficiaries has increased, and the rate of revision has likewise increased.

Joints in the lower extremities that are commonly replaced include the hip and knee, which function by different mechanisms. The hip is a simple ball-and-socket joint, and the knee is a complex hinge-like joint. Both diarthrodial joints allow free motion about a cartilage-lined interface separated by a thin layer of synovial fluid enclosed by an impermeable joint capsule. Problems occur when cartilage breaks down because of disease or joint integrity is lost because of a fracture, although cartilage is avascular and does not contain nerves that convey pain but underlying subchondral bone does. Pain in advanced joint disease occurs with an excessive load on, and sometimes exposure of, subchondral bone. During joint-replacement surgery, the damaged joint is removed and replaced by an artificial device designed to replicate normal joint function (Reininga et al., 2012).

Indications for joint-replacement surgery include severe pain that restricts activities of daily living (ADL) and cannot be resolved by a combination of conservative approaches such as oral medications, steroid injections, assistive devices, and weight reduction. The extent of bone damage can be evaluated through x-rays to determine the appropriate level of treatment. Because joint-replacement surgery has little impact on the physical demands required for the joint to function, patients aged 55 years and older may be considered good candidates. When acute trauma damages a joint, emergency joint replacement may be necessary (unless contraindicated by poor medical condition, significant peripheral vascular disease, neuropathy affecting the joint, or an active infection).

The hip joint consists of the femoral head (the ball) and a cup-shaped bone in the pelvis, called the *acetabulum* (from the Latin for "vinegar cup"). Depending on the extent of bone damage, hip reconstruction may involve replacement of either the femoral head (i.e., hemiarthroplasty) or the head and acetabulum (i.e., total hip arthroplasty). Hemiarthroplasty is restricted to fracture treatment. In hip-replacement surgery, the native femoral head is replaced by a prosthetic metal stem that inserts into the shaft of the femur. The acetabular component is a metal hemisphere attached to polyethylene, ceramic, or highly polished metal liner. The optimal interface (i.e., polyethylene cup on a steel head, metal-on-metal, or ceramic-on-ceramic) is under debate and may depend on the patient's activity level and age (Grover, 2005; McMinn, Daniel, & Ziaee, 2005; Sandhu & Middleton, 2005).

The knee joint acts as a hinge between the femur and the tibia. The movement of the knee joint can be very complex, combining flexion, rotation, and medial or lateral motion. As the knee flexes, the femur rolls back on the tibia, increasing the potential flexion of the knee. It is necessary to duplicate this complex motion in the artificial joint to ensure effective muscle contraction and maximum angular motion of the joint.

The artificial joint consists of a femoral component, a tibial component, and an optional patellar replacement. Total knee arthroplasty may involve replacement of the entire knee or only the medial or lateral compartment. In TKR, the worn articulating surfaces of the patella, tibia, and femur are cut at distinct angles, exposing the underlying bone. These surfaces are oriented to provide proper alignment of the implants. The metal implants are then fitted over the surfaces and fixed to the bone by either a bone cement or a porous coating on the devices.

The joint-replacement rehabilitation process begins even before the elective surgery. Many programs offer an engaging patient education program, called *joint camp*, to prepare the patient and family for the procedure. Recovery efforts commence immediately following the surgery. A successful outcome requires both replacements of the joint and strengthening of the surrounding muscles. Therefore strengthening exercises are an important component of rehabilitation. Initially, the rehabilitation program includes exercises specific to the joint that was replaced, with weight bearing as tolerated using crutches or a walker. A continuous passive motion machine is commonly used early in the recovery of a patient who has had a TKR. The immediate goals of rehabilitation are using an assistive device and functioning independently in performing one's self-care. Gait training gradually continues with a walker, crutches,

or a cane until the patient can walk without these assistive devices. *Optimal Perioperative Management of the Geriatrics Patient*, published by the American College of Surgeons/National Surgical Quality Improvement Program and the American Geriatrics Society, is available online.

The benefits of total joint-replacement surgery are pain relief and restoration of joint function. Joint replacement allows patients to carry out many daily activities that were previously restricted by pain. Although these artificial devices improve the functioning of the joint, they do not provide the same range of motion as a normal, healthy joint. The patient's goals may include being able to walk, sit, climb stairs, put on socks or shoes, and enter a car, but patients should not perform activities involving repetitive impact. Factors that may affect the outcome of rehabilitation include age, weight, the level of activity, frailty, and postoperative delirium.

There are relatively few complications from total joint-replacement surgery, considering the magnitude of the operation. The rate of infection after THR is 0.2% to 1.1%, and the rate of infection complicating TKR is 1% to 2%. A septic or aseptic loosening may occur in one or more of the components, causing pain. This happens with cemented implants because of degradation of the bone cement. Excessive wear of the device can generate particulate debris and accelerate implant failure. Other complications may include nerve damage from the surgery, dislocation of the joint, bone fracture, and infection of the joint. Depending on the level of failure and complication, revision surgery may be required.

As with any major surgery, there are potential systemic complications, including infection and thromboembolic diseases. Heart failure and chronic obstructive pulmonary disease increase the risk of a postoperative adverse event. Postoperative delirium poses a challenging complication. Proactive geriatrics consultation reduces delirium among older patients who required surgical repair of hip fracture (Marcantonio, Flacker, Wright, & Resnick, 2003). An interdisciplinary approach to treatment and rehab holds the key to a good outcome. A study of perioperative mortality after total knee and total hip arthroplasty reviewed all these procedures in the United States between 1998 and

2003 (Memtsoudis et al., 2012). The incidence of deep infection has declined since the early years of joint-replacement surgery. Currently, the infection rates are low, around 1% for primary knee replacements and 0.3% to 0.6% for hip replacements. The average mortality rate for total knee arthroplasty is 0.13%, and the average mortality rate for total hip arthroplasty is 0.18%. Factors associated with increased risk of in-hospital death include age, male gender, ethnic minority background, emergency admission, the number of comorbidities, and a number of complications.

Total joint replacements of the hip and knee are among the most common orthopedic procedures performed in older adults. The patient can expect the implant to last 10 to 15 years or more and provide pain-free functioning that would not otherwise be possible. Advances in the field of orthopedics are increasing the functional level of artificial joints and extending their longevity. Minimally invasive joint replacement is a technique that is being evaluated. It is designed to generate a smaller scar, less soft tissue disruption, less postoperative pain, and faster recovery than conventional approaches. Surgical exposure is compromised, and the technique is challenging. It remains controversial whether radiographic and clinical outcomes of minimally invasive hip and knee replacement are superior to conventional approaches (Ranawat & Ranawat, 2005; Stulberg, 2005).

A retrospective study described a cohort of 1,792 adult patients who had received TKR and THR surgery at the University of Iowa Hospital (Fang, Noiseux, Linson, & Cram, 2015). Their findings were remarkable for the low in-hospital complication rates. These complications did, however, increase with advancing age, as did the rate of need for intensive care during the hospital stay. Furthermore, older patients had longer hospital stays and were more likely to require posthospital care in a subacute care setting. There was no difference with the increased age in the 30-day readmission rate, mortality rate, or total costs.

TKR and THR surgery can improve the quality of life of older adults who have pain and functional limitations related to joint diseases. These procedures can be done safely in older adults. Although the rate of common hospital complications is remarkably low, older individuals may stay in the hospital longer than middle-aged adults and may need intensive care during the perioperative period. Older patients commonly recover in local subacute nursing facilities. The Centers for Medicare & Medicaid Services have bundled payments to stimulate better coordination of care between the hospital and the post-acute care setting.

See also Osteoarthritis; Osteoporosis; Rheumatoid Arthritis.

Laila M. Hasan, Saima T. Akbar,
and Michael L. Malone

Fang, M., Noiseux, N., Linson, E., & Cram, P. (2015). The effect of advancing age in total joint replacement outcomes. *Geriatric Orthopaedic Surgery & Rehabilitation, 3,* 173–179.

Grover, M. L. (2005). Controversial topics in orthopedics: Metal-on-polyethylene. *Annals of the Royal College of Surgeons of England, 87*(6), 416–418.

Marcantonio, E. R., Flacker, J. M., Wright, R. J., & Resnick, N. M. (2003). Reducing delirium after hip fracture: A randomized trial. *Journal of the American Geriatrics Society, 49*(5), 516–522.

McMinn, D. J., Daniel, J., & Ziaee, H. (2005). Controversial topics in orthopedics: Metal-on-metal. *Annals of the Royal College of Surgeons of England, 87*(6), 411–415.

Memtsoudis, S. G., Pumberger, M., Ma, Y., Chiu, L. Y., Fritsch, G., Gerner, P., ... Della Valle, A. G. (2012). The epidemiology and risk factors for perioperative mortality after total hip and knee arthroplasty. *Journal of Orthopedic Research, 30*(11), 1811–1821.

Ranawat, C. S., & Ranawat, A. S. (2005). A common sense approach to minimally invasive total hip replacement. *Orthopedics, 28*(9), 937–938.

Reininga, I., Stevens, M., Wagenmakers, R., Bulstra, S. K., & van den Akker-Scheek, I. (2012). Minimally invasive total hip and knee arthroplasty: Implications for the elderly patient. *Clinical Geriatric Medicine, 28,* 447–458.

Sandhu, H. S., & Middleton, R. G. (2005). Controversial topics in orthopedics: Ceramic-on-ceramic. *Annals of the Royal College of Surgeons of England, 87*(6), 415–416.

Stulberg, S. D. (2005). Minimally invasive navigated knee surgery: An American perspective. *Orthopedics, 28*(10, Suppl.), S1241–S1246.

J

Williams, S. N., Wolford, M. L., & Bercovitz, A. (2015). Hospitalization for total knee replacement among inpatients aged 45 and over: United States, 2000–2010. NCHS Data Brief No. 210. Retrieved from https://www.cdc.gov/nchs/data/databriefs/db210.pdf

Web Resources
American Academy of Orthopaedic Surgeons: http://orthoinfo.aaos.org

Optimal Perioperative Management of the Geriatrics Patient: http://www.facs.org/quality-programs/acs-nsqip/geriatric-periop-guideline
U.S. Department of Health and Human Services, Conditions & Treatments: Joint-Replacement Surgery: http://www.hss.edu/Conditions/Joint-Replacement-Surgery

L

LEADINGAGE

LeadingAge, formerly the American Association of Homes and Services for the Aging, is the national nonprofit organization representing more than 6,000 nonprofit nursing homes; continuing care retirement communities; and assisted-living, housing, and community service organizations serving older adults. Through advocacy, grassroots action, and coalition work, LeadingAge influences public policy pertaining to health, housing, community, and related services to ensure that aging populations receive the services they need and to protect and enhance the viability of nonprofit providers. LeadingAge also offers members information and assistance in interpreting relevant bills, laws, and regulations. LeadingAge offers timely newsletters, publications, and other communications to keep members up to date on congressional and regulatory actions and other trends and issues in the field of aging services.

LeadingAge provides education and training in a variety of formats designed to meet the diverse informational needs of professionals in the aging services field. Its annual meeting/exposition is highly acclaimed for its extensive curriculum. The continuing education program offers more than 200 concurrent sessions, special symposia, and intensive workshops. The exposition enables participants to view hundreds of the latest products and services. LeadingAge's annual spring conference and exposition, held in Washington, DC, combines reports on the latest developments in public policy with intensive educational programs. The public policy and educational components are enhanced by visits to members of Congress. Stand-alone seminars focus on topics of major concern to members and permit comprehensive examination of issues vital to the effective management of nonprofit organizations. The Retirement Housing Professionals Certification Program provides professional recognition and management training in the administrative, property management, and human services aspects of retirement housing.

The LeadingAge Development Corporation provides consultation to members on development planning and assists members in obtaining project financing. Its publications and educational programs keep members informed on various capital formation techniques and resources. Launched in 2012, the LeadingAge Center for Housing Plus Services serves as a national catalyst for the development, adoption, and support of innovative housing solutions that enable low- and modest-income seniors to age safely and successfully in their homes and communities.

See also Assisted Living; Continuing Care Retirement Communities; Nursing Homes.

Elizabeth A. Capezuti

Web Resource
LeadingAge: http://www.leadingage.org

LEISURE PROGRAMS

As people enter late adulthood, they generally experience dramatically increased free time due to retirement from their primary career. As leisure occurs mostly during this free time, how they engage in and experience leisure could be a crucial determinant for their health and well-being in later life. Baby boomers, who are becoming the overwhelming majority in late adulthood, are particularly paying close attention to their health and well-being. Moreover, they are likely to be active and engage in meaningful activities, and leisure has been a leading issue for them in later life. In fact, they are interested in active travel and hosteling, adventure tourism, dining out, sports leagues, exercise classes, adult education, and connections with others on the Internet, to name a few. In addition, they are passionately engaging in volunteering. They desire to feel that they can be of service and make significant contributions to the greater good in unlimited ways, from serving meals to the homeless to knitting newborn caps for a women's shelter, raising scholarship monies for a local college, delivering cards and books to hospitalized patients, and tutoring in afterschool programs.

Also, previous research showed empirical evidence that leisure plays important roles, especially those who are functionally independent and living in their homes as well as those in senior day care, retirement homes, or assisted living (Janke, Davey, & Kleiber, 2006). Specifically, while leisure engagement strengthens physical functioning (e.g., flexibility, balance) and biological health (e.g., glucose metabolism, physical stamina), it enhances happiness and life satisfaction but decreases cognitive decline, depression, and stress. In addition, as leisure is social in nature, leisure activities encourage meaningful social interaction that provides companionship for older adults. At the same time, seniors often need opportunities for structured solitude in which to foster a creative, self-expressive nature through activities such as painting. Furthermore, emphasis on a contemplative life that stresses spiritual health is a valuable benefit of well-designed leisure activities for older adults. Activities such as prayer, meditation, yoga, and journaling are valuable opportunities for personal growth and renewed sense of meaning. Rather than being passive, escapist, or diversionary such as while watching television or napping, an intentional pursuit of a contemplative lifestyle is critically vital for dealing with stressful and disruptive life changes natural to the aging process.

Despite the benefits and importance of leisure engagement in late adulthood and more discretionary time for leisure pursuits, older adults are less likely to engage in a larger number of leisure activities and higher frequency after retirement (Nimrod, Janke, & Kleiber, 2009). In addition, many retirement-planning programs are focused on financial issues and overlook the leisure aspect. Although very few leisure-centered programs exist for older adults, the leisure component is handled only as a section in the retirement-planning programs at the most. Therefore, more diverse and well-designed leisure-related programs should be developed and offered.

When leisure programs are designed, they should be holistic, using a whole-person approach that is both person-centered and lifestyle-focused rather than activity-focused. Participants need activities that are intrinsically rewarding, give them a sense of control, provide an opportunity for intergenerational interaction, and maximize successful participation across multiple physical and cognitive abilities. This means that the leisure-program planning must revolve around the needs, interests, and abilities of the participant rather than those of the staff or facility. In this regard, structured programming is less important than the ability of the program to induce a sense of "flow," in which participants find activities rewarding and meaningful in ways that create energy, focus, and satisfaction. In short, people of any age who find themselves in "flow" are engaged in activities that give meaning and purpose to life.

Furthermore, what matters is how actively older adults are involved in leisure activities and how they perceive their experiences, rather than the activities in which they are engaged. This is because older adults could have entirely different tastes of leisure depending on their physical, social, emotional, intellectual, ethnic/cultural, and spiritual background. Hence, leisure programs should go beyond simply providing information or teaching skills on a specific activity. It is also necessary to focus on nurturing positive attitudes toward overall leisure and development of older adults' leisure repertoires and leisure skills because attitudes and self-efficacy are closely related to leisure involvement and satisfaction. In this way, participants can engage in leisure activities more actively and be more satisfied with their experiences.

Besides, as with any other age, older adults value the concept of belonging and the virtue of being instrumental in their families and communities. Indeed, the social aspects have been pointed out as one of the most paramount motivators behind older adults engaging in leisure activities (Beggs, Kleparski, Elkins, & Hurd, 2014; Toepoel, 2013). Also, there is a growing need for programs that help older adults discover or rediscover the idea of living a full and resilient life grounded in the belief that the end of life is to be lived just as intentionally and transformatively as any other life stage. As a result, it is crucial that intergenerational programming is always a part of the leisure activities mix, with components that frequently allow participants to feel integrated into the social fabric of a community. This is particularly important as sectors of age segregation continue to grow, as evidenced by the proliferation of retirement homes and communities across the country.

In conclusion, leisure experiences continue to provide the single most important ingredient for adjustment to and enjoyment of the later years of life. Practitioners must consider the role that leisure has played and continued to play in the lives of older adults if they hope to contribute to their quality of life. As a matter of fact, residential retirement communities with more physical activity opportunities, more physical activity–related staff, better facilities, and multiple channels for communicating available activities have the most physically active residents (Barnett, van Sluijs, & Ogilvie, 2012). This shows the importance of establishing leisure programs that are accessible, affordable, frequently offered, flexible, modifiable, well communicated, well staffed, and relevant to older adults, so that leisure engagement can be encouraged and benefits can be obtained from it.

See also Adult Day Services; Creativity; Retirement; Technology; Therapeutic Recreation Specialists and Recreation(al) Therapists.

Chungsup Lee and Jinmoo Heo

Barnett, I., van Sluijs, E. M., & Ogilvie, D. (2012). Physical activity and transitioning to retirement: A systematic review. *American Journal of Preventive Medicine, 43*(3), 329–336.

Beggs, B., Kleparski, T., Elkins, D., & Hurd, A. (2014). Leisure motivation of older adults in relation to other adult life stages. *Activities, Adaptation & Aging, 38*(3), 175–187. doi:10.1080/01924788.2014.935910

Janke, M., Davey, A., & Kleiber, D. (2006). Modeling change in older adults' leisure activities. *Leisure Sciences, 28*, 285–303.

Nimrod, G., Janke, M. C., & Kleiber, D. A. (2009). Expanding, reducing, concentrating and diffusing: Activity patterns of recent retirees in the United States. *Leisure Sciences, 31*(1), 37–52. doi:10.1080/01490400802558087

Toepoel, V. (2013). Ageing, leisure, and social connectedness: How could leisure help reduce social isolation of older people? *Social Indicators Research, 113*(1), 355–372. doi:10.1007/s11205-012-0097-6

LIFE EVENTS

Occasionally, a concept or theory is so irresistible that it takes the scientific community by storm. Introduction of the concept of life events to the social and biomedical sciences had precisely that effect. Life events remain a major topic in aging research. Life events are identifiable, discrete changes in life patterns that create stress and can lead to illness onset or the exacerbation of preexisting illness.

Why was the concept of life events so compelling? Numerous other variables are equally powerful predictors of physical and mental illness. Primarily, life events offered a potential social risk factor compatible with epidemiological theories of illness onset. Although the consensus is that social environments play powerful roles in health and illness, isolating relevant parameters of social environments and documenting their effects has been a difficult challenge. Life events are especially attractive because they represent a social risk factor rivaling physical risk factors in terms of being objective (i.e., occurrence of the event can be verified), potentially quantifiable, and occurring prior to illness onset (thus clarifying causal order). A broad body of research examines the effects of life events on health in later life. The life events perspective is compatible with the crisis orientation that characterizes much research on aging, focusing on losses that are common in later life. Many of those losses (e.g., widowhood or widowerhood, economic problems) are, in fact, life events. Research shows that older adults experience fewer life events than younger adults. Interest in the impact of life events on health in late life continues because of evidence that (a) life events experienced by older adults are more likely than those experienced by younger adults to involve major losses, especially bereavement, and (b) resources for coping with stress typically decrease in later life. Thus older adults may be more vulnerable than younger adults to the adaptive challenges posed by life events.

EVOLUTION OF THE LIFE EVENTS PERSPECTIVE

Initially, research emphasized only one element of life events: the degree to which they disrupt established behavior patterns. Early research stated that subjective perceptions of stress are unimportant and that degree of change calibrates the stressfulness of life events. Later research demonstrated convincingly, however, that change itself is not the *active ingredient* in the link between life events and illness. Rather, life events have negative health consequences only if they are perceived as negative and stressful. Thus measures of life events now are routinely restricted to events that are perceived as negative or stressful by the individuals who experience them.

Life events were initially considered synonymous with social stress. It is now clear, however, that they are but one category of stressful experiences. Also important are chronic stressors, which are ongoing stressful experiences that persist over a long time (e.g., chronic poverty, provision of long-term care for an impaired relative). Thus social stress is a broad concept, with life events representing only one important area of inquiry.

MAJOR ISSUES IN LIFE EVENTS RESEARCH

Research on life events covers a broad range of issues. Two major research areas of special relevance to late life are mediators and moderators and life course perspectives.

Mediators and Moderators

A major focus of life events research has been identifying the conditions under which life events do and do not place health at risk. Life events have variable outcomes; although they are statistically significant predictors of illness, most individuals who experience life events do not become ill. More than three decades of research has focused on the causal pathways between stress and illness. It is now clearly documented that whether or not stressful life events harm health is a function of both the strength of the life event (e.g., death of a loved one poses a greater threat than retirement) and the resources available to the individual for responding to the stress. Two major types of social resources are especially powerful in offsetting the effects of stress: economic resources and social support. The value of economic resources is straightforward: Many stressful situations can be remedied or diminished by adequate financial resources (e.g., the economic consequences of widowhood or widowerhood are minimized). Social support, which refers to the tangible and intangible forms of assistance provided by family and friends, is a broader resource. Most research now focuses on three types of social support: (a) instrumental support, which refers to the provision of tangible assistance (e.g., transportation or personal care); (b) informational support, which refers to the provision of information about resources external to the support system (e.g., information about relevant community services); and (c) emotional support, which refers to the comfort, self-validation, and companionship offered by intimate others.

Although both economic resources and social support have been shown to mediate the effects of stress on health outcomes, other research suggests that social support is statistically interactive rather than mediating. The idea that social support interacts with stress is known as the stress-buffering hypothesis (Avison & Cairney, 2003). Its proponents suggest that social support protects health only under conditions of stress, rather than having a more general protective effect that exists independent of stress. Research provides empirical confirmation for both the stress-buffering hypothesis and the hypothesis that social support mediates the effects of stress. Either way, social support plays a vital role in reducing the negative effects of life events on health. Psychosocial resources such as self-esteem and a sense of mastery also mediate some of the effects of life events on health (Pearlin & Bierman, 2013).

Life events (and stressors more generally) also partially mediate the effects of status characteristics—including race, sex, and socioeconomic status—on health outcomes. This is a complex research literature; nonetheless, the general pattern of findings suggests that life events mediate some, but not all, of the effects of demographic characteristics and socioeconomic status on health. Thus racial, socioeconomic, and sex health disparities are due in part to the higher levels of stress exposure experienced by the socially disadvantaged.

Biological processes also mediate the relationships between life events and health outcomes. Biological pathways linking stress and health include the endocrine system, inflammation, and immune function (Dhabhar, 2014).

Life Events in Life Course Perspective

Studies that examine life events in life course perspective have greatly enriched understanding of the long-term consequences of stressful life events. Traumas and other important life events experienced in childhood and early adulthood are associated with poor health decades later. The relationships between childhood traumas (e.g., physical abuse, parental divorce) and late life health are especially strong. Most studies document the strong effects of early life events on mental health outcomes. Recent studies demonstrate that early traumas also have negative effects on physical illness, cognitive status, and disability/frailty (Peek, Howrey, Ternent, Ray, & Ottenbacher, 2012). In general, the economic resources and social support acquired throughout adulthood mediate some, but not all, of the negative effects of early traumas and events.

After more than 40 years, the antecedents and consequences of life events continue to engage the energies of social, behavioral, and biomedical scientists. The core of this research has been the links between stress and illness. More recently, the life course perspective has highlighted that life events often have demonstrable health consequences even decades after they occur.

Linda K. George

Avison, W. R., & Cairney, J. (2003). Social structure, stress, and personal control. In S. H. Zarit, L. I. Pearlin, & K. W. Schaie (Eds.), *Personal control in social and life course contexts* (pp. 127–164). New York, NY: Springer Publishing.

Dhabhar, F. S. (2014). Effects of stress on immune function: The good, the bad, and the beautiful. *Immunologic Research, 58*(2–3), 193–210.

Pearlin, L. I., & Bierman, A. (2013). Current issues and future directions in research into the stress process. In C. S. Aneshensel, J. C. Phelan, & A. Bierman (Eds.), *Handbook of the sociology of mental health* (pp. 325–340). Dordrecht, Netherlands: Springer Publishing.

Peek, M. K., Howrey, B. T., Ternent, R. S., Ray, L. A., & Ottenbacher, K. J. (2012). Social support, stressors, and frailty among older Mexican American adults. *Journal of Gerontology: Social Sciences, 67,* 755–764.

Web Resources

AARP: http://healthtools.aarp.org/learning-center/featured/depression-anxiety?lcStart=1

National Institute of Mental Health: http://www.nimh.nih.gov/health/topics/older-adults-and-mental-health/index.shtml

LIFE REVIEW

In 1963, Robert Butler postulated that reminiscence in the older adult was part of a normal life review process brought about by the realization of approaching dissolution and death. It is characterized by the progressive return to consciousness of past experiences and particularly the resurgence of unresolved conflicts for reexamination and reintegration. If the reintegration is successful, such reminiscence can give new significance and meaning to life and prepare the person for death by mitigating fear and anxiety. There has been some confusion surrounding the two mental processes because life review and reminiscence are often used interchangeably and inconsistently in the literature. Researchers have attempted to define the concepts and improve study methodologies to understand the phenomena. Although life review is defined as systematic and more evaluative in nature, reminiscence is part of and can facilitate life review.

The evaluative process of the life review is believed to occur universally in all persons in the final years of their lives, although they may not be totally aware of it and may in part defend themselves against realizing its presence. It is spontaneous, unselective, and seen in other age groups as well (e.g., adolescence, middle age), especially when individuals are confronted by death or a major crisis. However, the intensity and emphasis on putting one's life in order are most striking in older adults. In late life, people have a particularly vivid imagination and memory for the past and can recall with sudden and remarkable clarity early life events. They often experience a renewed ability to free-associate and to bring up material from the unconscious. Individuals realize that their own personal myth of invulnerability and immortality can no longer be maintained. All this results in a reassessment of life, which, depending on the individual, may bring depression, acceptance, or satisfaction.

The life review can occur in a mild form through, for example, mild nostalgia, mild regret, and a tendency to reminisce or tell stories. Often, the life story will be told to anyone who will listen. At other times, it is conducted in monologue in private and is not meant to be overheard. It is in many ways similar to the psychotherapeutic situation in which a person is reviewing his or her life to understand present circumstances.

As part of the life review, one may experience a sense of regret that is increasingly painful. In severe forms, it can lead to anxiety, guilt, despair, and depression. In extreme cases, if a person is unable to resolve problems or accept them, terror, panic, and suicide can result. The most tragic life review is one in which a person decides that life was a failure.

Some of the positive results of a life review can be the righting of old wrongs, making up with enemies, coming to accept mortality, and gaining a sense of serenity, pride in accomplishment, and a feeling of having done one's best. Life review gives people an opportunity that allows them to decide what to do with the time left to them and work out emotional and material legacies. People begin to accept death with a sense of readiness. Possibly the qualities of serenity, philosophical development, and wisdom observable in some older people reflect a state of resolution of their life conflicts. This is usually accompanied by a lively capacity to live in the present, including the direct enjoyment of elemental pleasures such as nature, children, forms, colors, warmth, love, and humor. Some become more capable of mutuality, with a comfortable acceptance of the life cycle, the universe, and the generations. Creative works such as memoirs, art, music, and blogging or other Internet activities may result. People may put together videos, family albums, and scrapbooks and study their genealogies.

RESEARCH AND BEST PRACTICES

Since Butler proposed life review more than 50 years ago, the field of reminiscence and life review has made significant progress in research, practice, and theory. Reminiscence research advanced with the empirically validated taxonomy of reminiscence functions. Webster (1993) developed the Reminiscence Functions Scale to assess how often the individual reminisces and for what purpose. The reminiscence functions identified through Webster's work are boredom reduction, problem solving, teaching, intimacy maintenance, conversation, identity, death preparation, and bitterness revival. Researchers have utilized the scale to develop an empirical model demonstrating links between reminiscence functions and well-being (Cappeliez & O'Rourke, 2006; O'Rourke, Cappeliez, & Claxton, 2011). Practitioners find the Reminiscence Functions Scale useful in promoting the mental health and well-being of their patients. Understanding the function reminiscence serves the individual assists the practitioner in encouraging the older adult to interpret experiences in a positive way and improve mental health. Another growing area of research pertinent to practice is the examination of cultural differences in reminiscence. Comparisons of reminiscence functions across cultural groups indicate the following: (a) the way that culture influences how memories are interpreted, (b) differences in the underlying reasons why the older adult reminisces, and (c) the willingness of the older adult to reminisce. For instance, the strong oral traditions of Black older adults are an example of a cultural tradition that facilitates their willingness to share memories and traditions with younger generations.

Reminiscence scholars continue to examine the effects of life review and reminiscence on quality of life outcomes such as depression, anxiety, life satisfaction, and self-esteem. One significant contribution to the field of life review and reminiscence is the development of an overarching conceptual model created by Webster, Bohlmeijer, and Westerhof (2010). The heuristic model identifies process, content, and outcome variables of life review and reminiscence to guide research and practice. Westerhof and Bohlmeijer (2014) utilized the model in a review of reminiscence research and applications over the past 50 years to identify personal characteristics and contextual factors related to social, positive, and negative reminiscence functions that influence psychological resources such as social support, coping, and self-esteem. In turn, the psychological resources impact the mental health and well-being of the older adult. In addition, results from the review show increasing evidence that reminiscence interventions foster positive mental health outcomes in older adults with therapeutic and preventive effects. Other researchers have postulated that younger adults, such as nursing students reminiscing with an older adult, learn about and appreciate the life of the individual and thus decrease feelings of ageism. Interventions that promote reminiscence between older adults and nursing students facilitate interactions that increase trust and communication so that students effectively gather information regarding older adults' health beliefs, coping skills, and cultural perspectives.

Research and practice over the years has led to the realization that facilitating reminiscence as part of the life review has benefits for practitioners as well as older adults. For example, incorporating group reminiscence sessions in nursing homes and senior centers, implementing reminiscence with dementia patients and their caregivers, educating nursing students to facilitate reminiscence with their patients, and encouraging families to be part of this process are just some of the best practices that can be used when an individual is receiving care. Intergenerational reminiscence programs implemented in high schools, churches, and other community organizations are ways of increasing an understanding between generations. As the field of life review and reminiscence matures, it is becoming increasingly clear that facilitating these reflective processes improves the quality of life for older adults, and keeps their legacies alive.

See also Creativity; Patient–Provider Relationships.

Juliette Shellman

Butler, R. N. (1963). The life review: An interpretation of reminiscence in the aged. *Psychiatry, 26*, 65–76.

Cappeliez, P., & O'Rourke, N. (2006). Empirical validation of a model of reminiscence and health and later life. *Journal of Gerontological Sciences, Social Sciences, 61*(4), 237–244.

O'Rourke, N., Cappeliez, P., & Claxton, A. (2011). Functions of reminiscence and the psychological well-being of young-old and older adults over time. *Aging and Mental Health, 15*, 271–281.

Webster, J. D. (1993). Construction and validation of the Reminiscence Function Scale. *Journal of Gerontology: Psychology Sciences, 48*, P256–P262.

Webster, J. D., Bohlmeijer, E., & Westerhof, G. (2010). Mapping the future of reminiscence: A conceptual guide for research and practice. *Research on Aging, 32*(4), 527–564.

Westerhof, G., & Bohlmeijer, E. (2014). Celebrating fifty years of research and application in reminiscence and life review: State of the art and new directions. *Journal of Aging Studies, 29*, 107–114.

L

Web Resources
International Institute for Reminiscence and Life
     Review: http://reminiscenceandlifereview.org
The International Journal of Reminiscence and Life Review:
     http://www.ijrlr.org/ojs/index.php/IJRLR/
     index

LONG-TERM CARE POLICY

Long-term care is the term used to describe
extended care provided to individuals who
need additional assistance managing the activities of daily living. These services can be costly
and therefore call on considerable public and
private resources to meet the growing needs of
those with functional disabilities. Public policy addressing long-term care tends to focus
on financing and managing costs, balancing
institutional and home- and community-based
services (HCBS), and improving the quality of
care. In recent years, health care cost and system
reform have been leading topics in public policy debate. The federal government has taken
interest in containing the cost and improving
the quality of long-term services and support
(LTSS). The Patient Protection and Affordable
Care Act (PPACA) of 2010 made substantial
changes to LTSS programs, which incentivized
states to improve their HCBS. In 2013, the U.S.
Senate Commission on Long-Term Care was
established to evaluate the system and present a
detailed vision for a coordinated system of high-
quality long-term care for the elderly and people with disabilities.

MANAGING RISING DEMAND

The need for long-term-care services affects persons of all ages, but the prevalence of disability
increases sharply with age. People older than 65
years are currently the largest group receiving
LTSS. People aged 85 years and older, the population most likely to need long-term care services, will increase from 6.2 million in 2014 to
14.6 million in 2040 (U.S. Department of Health
and Human Services, Administration on Aging,

2015). About half of all people aged 85 years and
older have a disability in the community or are
in a nursing home. Over the next few decades,
the health care system will have to accommodate a growing number of people likely to need
long-term care and manage the cost of providing
care for people with multiple chronic illnesses
and functional disabilities. Total (i.e., public and
private) long-term care expenditure in 2012 was
$219.9 billion, and if present trends continue, this
figure will reach $346 billion by 2040 (National
Health Policy Forum, 2014). Most cannot afford
the high cost of long-term care services, so individuals and families can easily exhaust their
savings and other resources to pay for even a
brief period of uncovered care. Because private
insurers and Medicare typically do not pay for
the nonmedical aspects of long-term care, the
majority (65%) of all LTSS expenditures are paid
for by Medicaid (U.S. Senate Commission on
Long-Term Care, 2013). These estimates do not
take into account the vast amount of unpaid
labor provided by family caregivers, which constitutes the bulk of total care.

Long-term care insurance is an underutilized market-based mechanism that can help
offset the cost of long-term care for both private
individuals and public insurance plans. Policy
makers have proposed strengthening the incentive for private individuals to invest in long-
term care insurance by enhancing the associated
tax benefits and by increasing the variety of
plans available on the market. They propose an
awareness-raising educational campaign on the
importance of planning for long-term care needs
and purchasing financial protection (U.S. Senate
Commission on Long-Term Care, 2013).

BALANCE BETWEEN
INSTITUTIONAL CARE AND HCBS

Historically, nursing-facility care has been the
predominant long-term care service covered
by public funds. However, widespread policy
initiatives at the federal and state levels intend
to shift the balance of care toward that delivered in the home and community. The 1999 U.S.
Supreme Court ruling in *Olmstead v. LC* accelerated the move toward increasing home- and
community-based care by requiring states to

make accommodations for people with disabilities, which would allow them to live in the least restrictive, most integrated setting. Because states have tended to vary widely in their investment in HCBS, the PPACA of 2010 established two new federal matching programs and enhanced existing programs that offered states additional incentives for improving their HCBS infrastructure. States wishing to take advantage of the PPACA-enhanced programs are encouraged to expand access to HCBS by reexamining their existing criteria for eligibility to allow more people to take advantage of available services. Participating states are also expected to improve their procedures for tracking and reporting data on the quality of services to the federal government (U.S. Government Accountability Office, 2012).

Residential care alternatives have been developed in response to the need for less restrictive congregate living options. Assisted living, Green House homes, adult foster care, board and care homes and continuing care retirement communities are all examples of residential arrangements that can provide more intensive support for people with functional care needs who may not be able to remain in their homes. Policy makers and older people hope that these facilities will be able to provide services in a more home-like environment that provides greater personal autonomy and more personal choice than nursing homes. Although most residential care facility residents pay privately, Medicaid and Supplemental Security Income are increasingly important sources of payment.

QUALITY IN LONG-TERM CARE

Nursing homes have been dogged by concerns about poor quality care for decades (D. B. Smith & Feng, 2010). One of the key policy rationales for expanding HCBS is that the quality of life for beneficiaries is better than in nursing homes. Although increasing numbers of people are receiving services in the home, there is insufficient evidence to believe that their care is superior in quality or safety to residential care. People who use home care typically report high levels of satisfaction; however, it is difficult to measure the quality of care in the home and community

setting because providers tend to work independently and without intensive supervision (D. B. Smith & Feng, 2010). The Centers for Medicare & Medicaid Services, as well as the National Quality Forum, have embarked on intensive efforts to develop and validate measures of quality in HCBS. Quality measures should focus on health outcomes, processes, utilization, consumer and family experience (U.S. Senate Commission on Long-Term Care, 2013).

To improve quality in both HCBS and residential care, policy makers have emphasized the importance of person-centered care, a principle of care delivery that allows the individuals who receive services to have maximal control over who provides their services, as well as when and how they are delivered. In this model of care, consumers are actively engaged in developing their own service plan in a way that highlights their preferences and values. Some programs allow consumers to spend their budgeted Medicaid/Medicare dollars in ways that best meet their needs, allowing them to select and pay their care providers independently. In this arrangement, sometimes the preferred care provider is an existing family caregiver who can now be reimbursed for their labor (U.S. Senate Commission on Long-Term Care, 2013).

A key to empowering consumers is ensuring that they have adequate, detailed information about long-term care options and support in making decisions about their care. Fragmentation of services and lack of coordination across settings have been a major problem for people seeking services. For this reason, Aging and Disability Resource Centers (ADRCs) were established in 2009 to serve as a single point of entry to LTSS programs in each state. The No Wrong Door System is a federal initiative that supports states in coordinating their LTSS systems to optimize consumer choice and access to high-quality care.

WORKFORCE

Long-term care workers, such as certified nurse assistants, home health aides, and personal care attendants, are the backbone of the formal long-term care delivery system, providing the majority of paid assistance to people with functional care needs. Direct care workers provide needed assistance with activities of daily living, such as eating, bathing, and dressing, as well as instrumental activities of daily living such as medication management and meal preparation. The central role of these workers in providing "hands on" services makes them the key factor in determining the quality of paid long-term care.

Long-term care providers report that workforce shortages and turnover rates may be reaching crisis proportions. These shortages are likely to worsen over time in the face of increased demand for services. High turnover and understaffing compromise the quality and safety of the care provided. The low status, low pay, and lack of benefits associated with these direct-care jobs have negative implications for job satisfaction. Paraprofessional long-term care workers receive low wages and often live close to poverty (K. Smith, 2012). Many home care aides work part time, further reducing their earnings and access to benefits such as health insurance and pension plans. Policies that promote career advancement, training, and worker protections for long-term care workers are needed. Direct-care workers can be integrated into care team decision making and given other opportunities to develop skills and relationships throughout their careers. Furthermore, because family caregivers provide the majority of long-term care, their needs should be assessed and accommodated through long-term care policy development.

CONCLUSION

Long-term care is an important policy issue that affects billions of dollars in public expenditures and millions of people. Long-term care is a rising topic on the national political agenda, as evidenced by the array of new political initiatives developed to evaluate and prepare the LTSS infrastructure for the imminent expansion in demand for services.

See also Assisted Living; Medicare; Medicaid; Nursing Homes; Veterans and Veteran Health.

Meredith Doherty

National Health Policy Forum. (2014). The basics: National spending for long-term services and supports. Retrieved from http://www.nhpf.org/library/the-basics/Basics_LTSS_03-27-14.pdf

Olmstead v. LC, 527 US 581 (1999).

Smith, D. B., & Feng, Z. (2010). The accumulated challenges of long-term care. *Health Affairs, 29(1),* 29–34.

Smith, K. (2012). Lack of protections for home care workers: Overtime pay and minimum wage. *The Carsey Institute at the Scholars' Repository.* Retrieved from http://scholars.unh.edu/carsey/158

U.S. Department of Health and Human Services Administration on Aging. (2015). A profile of older Americans. Retrieved from http://www.aoa.acl.gov/aging_statistics/profile/2015/docs/2015-Profile.pdf

U.S. Government Accountability Office. (2012). *States' plan to pursue new and revised options for home- and community-based services* (GAO-12-649). Washington, DC: Author. Retrieved from https://www.gao.gov/products/GAO-12-649

U.S. Senate Commission on Long-Term Care. (2013). *Report to the Congress.* Washington, DC: US Government Printing Office.

Web Resources

AARP Public Policy Institute: http://www.aarp.org/research/ppi/ltc

Aging and Disability Resource Centers: No Wrong Door: https://www.adrc-tae.acl.gov/tiki-index.php?page=HomePage

Clearinghouse for the Community Living Exchange Collaborative: http://www.hcbs.org

Kaiser Family Foundation: http://kff.org/infographic/visualizing-health-policy-a-short-look-at-long-term-care-for-seniors

The Commonwealth Fund: http://www.commonwealthfund.org/Topics/Long-Term-Care-Quality.aspx

MEALS ON WHEELS

Senior nutrition programs (SNPs) play a vital role in enhancing health, independence, and quality of life in older adults. An estimated 17% of seniors face hunger (Meals on Wheels America, 2016). There is a great deal of evidence that SNPs improve the nutritional health of the individuals who participate in the programs. Improving or maintaining nutritional health of older adults is critically important to promoting their health and well-being; poor nutritional status and physical inactivity are considered the second leading cause of death—behind smoking—in the United States.

There are more than 5,000 SNPs in the United States, providing more than 2.4 million senior meals each year. *Meals on Wheels* meal programs (i.e., Meals on Wheels) and (b) congregate meal programs. These two types of nutrition program have similar objectives, but there are differences— some obvious, some subtle—between the programs, and between the populations they serve. Home-delivered meal programs deliver meals directly to the homes of elders whose mobility is limited. Congregate meal programs are offered in community settings such as senior centers and adult day centers, where older adults can assemble and partake in meals together. Both SNPs are provided to, individuals aged 60 years or older (and their spouses, in home-delivered meal programs) and adults with disabilities who live in facilities where there are congregate meal programs. Because demand far outstrips available services, both programs are targeted, by law, to prioritize serving those in greatest economic and social need.

The Older Americans Act of 1965 (OAA), most recently reauthorized in 2016, is the principal law governing the operation and practices of SNPs and is the primary source of federal funding. The National Resource Center on Nutrition and Aging (NRC) is a cooperative initiative of the Administration on Aging and the Meals On Wheels America, and is designed to assist the national aging network in implementing the nutrition portions of the OAA. The primary objective of home-delivered and congregate meal programs is to furnish hot, nutritious meals to needy seniors at least 5 days per week. Each meal must meet the minimum standard of furnishing at least one third of the recommended dietary allowances (RDAs) of key nutrients. Most meals actually exceed this RDA minimum, approximating 40% to 50% of the daily requirement, and typically the meals are "nutrient dense" (i.e., their ratios of nutrients to calories are high). As a result, the daily intake of key nutrients is greater for program participants than it is for similar individuals who do not participate in the program.

SNPs provide program participants with more than a meal. Over half of all programs provide nutrition screening and education, and more than a third also include nutrition assessment and counseling. Although it is accomplished in different ways and to a different degree in congregate programs and in the home-delivered meals, socialization—or at least the reduction of social isolation—is a critical benefit that all SNP participants enjoy (Timonen & O'Dwyer, 2010). Older adults participating in senior meal programs have more social contact than similarly situated nonparticipants. This is true, even though older adults who participate in SNPs are more than twice as likely as elders in the general population to reside alone.

Other than setting, programs differ in the demographic characteristics of program participants. Program participants in all SNPs are older, more likely to be female, a member of a racial/ ethnic minority group, and poorer than the overall population of like-aged peers. Moreover, home-delivered meal recipients are, on average, older, poorer, and frailer than their counterparts in congregate programs. An estimated 63% of older adults receiving home-delivered meals have six or more chronic conditions, compared with 45% of those receiving congregate meals (Kowlessar, Robinson, & Schur, 2015). In addition, the majority of homebound participants have some type of functional disability.

Demographic forecasts of aging into the next century suggest that demand for the nutritional services will continue to increase. Historically, policies supporting SNPs have been sensitive and responsive to the changing and growing needs of an ever-burgeoning cohort of aging Americans. However, the degree to which SNPs continue to contribute to the health and well-being of America's older adults is dependent on public support in the form of federal, state, and local funding; financial support from individuals, the corporate sector, and private foundations; and the investment of the time and personal resources of volunteers and staff who prepare, serve, and deliver meals. SNPs are one of the most prudent, economical investments the public sector can make to promote health in later life. The cost of providing a senior citizen with Meals on Wheels for a year is roughly equivalent to the cost of a hospital day for a Medicare patient.

SNPs are well-established, effective, and valuable national programs that provide a broad range of nutrition services and interventions for vulnerable adults. By preventing, reducing, and postponing of the onset of chronic diseases and functional disabilities in older adults, SNPs, including Meals on Wheels, can enhance quality of life, delay individual institutionalization, and reduce overall national health care costs.

See also Aging Agencies: City and County Level; Nutritionists; Senior Centers; Senior Hunger.

Caitlin McAfee

Kowlessar, N., Robinson, K., & Schur, C. (2015). *Older Americans benefit from Older Americans Act nutrition programs. Administration for Community Living.* OnlineResearch Brief No. 8. Retrieved from https://www.acl.gov/sites/default/files/programs/2016-11/AoA-Research-Brief-8-2015.pdf

Meals on Wheels America. (2016). Meals on Wheels fact sheet. Retrieved from http://www.mealsonwheelsamerica.org/docs/default-source/fact-sheets/2012/mow-factsheet-national2016.pdf?sfvrsn=2

Older Americans Act of 1965. 42 U.S.C., As amended through Pub.L. No. 114-144, §§ 101-765. (2016). Retrieved from http://www.aoa.gov/AOA_programs/OAA/Reauthorization/2016/docs/Older-Americans-Act-of-1965-Compilation.pdf

Timonen, V., & O'Dwyer, C. (2010). "It is nice to see someone coming in": Exploring the social objectives of Meals-on-Wheels. *Canadian Journal on Aging/La Revue canadienne du vieillissement, 29,* 399–410.

Web Resources
Administration on Aging: http://www.aoa.org
Meals on Wheels America: http:// www.mowaa.org
National Resource Center on Nutrition and Aging: http://www.nutritionandaging.org

MEASUREMENT

Passage of the Patient Protection and Accountable Care Act in 2010—in tandem with other key developments such as the widespread diffusion of electronic health records and utilization of practice (EBP)—requires greater accountability and demonstration of clinical, fiscal, and organizational outcomes. Providers across the entire health care spectrum have embraced EBP and adhere to a wide range of reporting requirements established by insurers, government agencies, agency-specific mandates, and professional standards. These trends have had a significant impact on the current health care delivery system, requiring use of clearly defined and standardized measures and tools for sound, data-driven decision-making, as well as effective action and strategic plans. Whether for clinical decisions, quality performance and improvement activities, or research purposes, there is little doubt that all health care providers will be involved in measurement activities in their daily practices.

Measurement is defined as the use of standard definitions and empirical measures to identify, monitor, and interpret observable behaviors and phenomena. It is widely understood that the availability of empirical (i.e., observable) and objective data enhances scientific credibility, and the ability to perform statistical procedures is dependent on measurement. Statistics, from basic "descriptive statistics" to elaborate algorithms or models, would not be possible without the ability to quantify. Measurement also refers to the process of observing and recording observations that are collected and aggregated as part of research studies.

Measurement is the process of assigning numerical values to concepts, phenomena, or events. Numerical values offer objectivity and standardization that allow individuals to examine and interpret events, concepts, and phenomenon using common understanding and expectations. Many types of standard measures may be used in daily life and clinical practice; for example, clocks measure time, scales measure weight, thermometers measure temperature, and rulers measure distance. The use of common measures increases the reliability and validity of information in that each event or phenomenon with an assigned number is similar to others with the same assigned number. Measurements of quality—such as benchmarks, scorecards, and dashboards—depend on agreed-on definitions and rely on numerical data to compare and contrast indicators across settings, time intervals, or patient populations.

LEVELS OF MEASUREMENT

One approach to understanding measurement is to focus on the four levels of measurement: nominal/categorical, ordinal, interval, and ratio. Each of the levels reflects a different type of data used for measuring a behavior, concept, or phenomenon. In addition, each level of measurement and its corresponding data have implications for the appropriate statistics available for analysis. Understanding the relationship between levels of measurement and types of statistics is particularly important for effective statistical analyses in research studies and big data analytics.

One of the most commonly used measurement tool is the checklist approach, which often serves as a reminder for clinicians to perform steps in protocols and standards of care. The checklist is an example of *nominal/categorical* measurement; for instance, numbers may be assigned to clinical activities performed for a patient: for example, 1 = *yes, documented* and 0 = *no, not documented*. These numerical values make it possible to aggregate the data and determine how often activities are performed or documented. The resulting data then can be further analyzed to examine similarities and differences between responses or groups of responses. These assessments are conducted by scoring data and performing statistical analyses, most typically frequencies and percentages.

The values assigned in *nominal/categorical* measurement are arbitrary. There is no intrinsic value to the 1, 2, or 3. *Nominal* data are purely for categorization or classification purposes. Some demographic data is nominal/categorical; for example, with reference to "state of residence," there is no inherent value to assigning numbers to each state in alphabetical order (i.e., Alabama = 1, Alaska = 2, Arkansas = 3, … Wyoming = 50). Wyoming is no "better" or "worse" for having been assigned a value of 50.

With ordinal, interval, and ratio measurements, however, each numeric value has significance. *Ordinal measures* show the relative ranking of people, objects, or events. The classic example of ordinal data is the class ranking of students. One student is ranked higher than another, but the actual difference between the students may differ more widely than the ranking. Another example is "highest earned degree"; when someone moves up the educational ladder from baccalaureate to master's to doctoral degree, each educational achievement is "higher" than the previous. However, the amount of time or the level of difficulty between the educational degrees is not equal.

Ordinal measures can be aggregated to produce cumulative tallies, which characterize many scores associated with assessment tools.

Scales are among the most familiar forms of interval measurement in nursing practice and provide an easy method for measuring the magnitude of a phenomenon, attitude/perception, or event. The Braden Scale is one example. There are six items in the scale and each item has corresponding, hierarchical values that are aggregated to determine a patient's risk for developing a pressure injury. In the Braden Scale, the lower the cumulative score, the higher the risk.

Likert scales are often used to measure attitudes, behaviors, or practices. Familiar in staff satisfaction and staff surveys, Likert scales offer a range of intervals to distinguish one level to another—for example, 1 = *very satisfied*; 2 = *satisfied*; 3 = *not satisfied*; 4 = *very unsatisfied*—but there is no level that reflects absolute zero (or nothing). The items in Likert scales are often aggregated to create a cumulative score.

Ratio scales, on the other hand, measure phenomena that may register zero and include intervals that are equal to each other. Patient pain assessment scales that ask patients to rate their pain from 0 to 10 illustrate *ratio* measurement. The numbers used in the pain scale have intrinsic value: a score of 1 means less pain than 2 and 0 means no pain. A pain score of 8 is understood as twice as painful as a score of 4. Scales that measure height or weight are ratio in that each pound or inch is equal to another and there is theoretical possibility on zero weight; that is, it is nonexistent. When exploring the pros and cons of using an instrument for possible use, clinicians should be aware of whether the measure uses categorical, ordinal, interval, or ratio data because the selection of appropriate statistical analyses depends on the type of measurement data.

INTERPRETATION OF NUMERICAL VALUES

The primary benefit of measuring people, phenomena, and events using numerical values is the ability to quantify the results using statistical methods. Very fundamentally, there would be no statistics if there were no measures. The use of frequencies, which provides total numbers and percentages of varying response grouping, is the most basic statistic for aggregation and analysis.

Statistical procedures used to interpret numerical data are predicated on measures of central tendency, and they describe the "middle" or the "average" among the group of responses. The *mean* is the arithmetic average of all the numerical responses. The *median* is the middle score, or the number at which 50% of the responses are above it and 50% are below it. The *mode* is the most frequent score or response. It is possible to have more than one mode.

Each measure of central tendency is suitable for different types of data. The mean is commonly used for establishing averages for *ordinal, interval,* and *ratio* data, such as test scores, performance on an assessment tool, or analysis of height and weight data among patients. However, the median is more appropriate for data that have a wide range, such as salaries or length of stay or for developing quartiles. Modes are most suitable for *nominal* data; determining which value garners the most responses. Basic statistics, such as modes and frequencies that summarize data by describing observations numerically, are known as *descriptive statistics*. Most complex statistical procedures, such as analysis of variance (ANOVA), *t*-test, and multiple regressions, build on the mean. It is useful to examine the standard deviations in addition to the mean to understand the variation of responses/results. "Inferential statistics" use patterns of data to draw inferences about populations, including testing hypotheses, describing associations, and extrapolating future trends, and predictive models. Use of scales and measures can be critical elements in research. Whether a protocol proposes to examine differences between an intervention and control group or whether the protocol calls for comparison between preintervention and postintervention, it is critical that appropriate measures are selected to measure variations across groups and across time.

ASSESSMENT TOOL IN GERIATRICS

Standardized assessment tools permit practitioners to assess, evaluate, and measure where a particular patient fits on any number of clinical, administrative, and educational variables. Once a patient has been assessed, the practitioner can proceed with appropriate interventions. There are many good measures in geriatrics. However, a particular measure is selected, it is necessary to evaluate its appropriateness for one's specific needs. It is also important to consider the potential of the tool or instrument for research or analytic purposes.

First, the practitioner must decide what exactly he or she wants to measure and determine who or what is being measured. For example, is it the needs of a patient with a particular diagnosis, the evaluation of a program, or staff satisfaction? If a type of person is being assessed, is it a patient with a specific diagnosis, in an age group, in a particular setting? In addition, the clinician must decide how much detail is wanted or needed from a measurement tool. It is important to balance the pros and cons of using more detailed instruments, which are more time-consuming, or using shorter measures that may provide less detail but are more efficient. It is not advisable to use a tool that was developed for a purpose or population different than the one you are interested in. For example, fall-assessment tools designed for home should not be used for hospitals or long-term care facilities. Similarly, surveys of RN satisfaction would not be effective for measuring satisfaction among MDs or other professionals.

When selecting an appropriate measure, clinicians should get as much background information as possible about the development and application of the instruments. This information is often available in the published literature. When reviewing written material, it is important to examine the size of the group on which the instrument was tested and the type of population on which the instrument was used. Ideally, a measure that has been used extensively with the same population the clinician plans to assess should be selected. In short, if the clinician plans to assess nursing home residents, it would be best to use a measure developed for this population rather than selecting one for home care or acute care.

Evaluating the validity and reliability of a measurement tool is important, although potentially difficult. There are several general guidelines to follow when considering which tools to use in clinical practice. Tools that have been used repeatedly are usually reliable. In many instances, the creator of a scale or index provides a "score" or statistical coefficient to summarize the level of confidence of the measure. Many different statistical techniques are used for these purposes. As a general rule, the higher the score, the more confidence one should have in the measure; for example, 0.83 reflects strong confidence, 0.53 reflects moderate confidence, and under 0.50 is usually considered unacceptable.

In addition, the user should consider the method for scoring and interpreting the results when selecting a tool. Difficult scoring methods and complicated statistical interpretations can be too time-consuming for a busy clinician. In some cases, copy-written instruments may require a fee for scoring and interpreting the results.

Finally, the data obtained through different measurements are rich sources for statistical analyses to better monitor trends, understand root causes of problems, and ascertain effectiveness of interventions among larger groups of individuals. The ability to aggregate standardized data from many patients is key to answering a wide range of research questions, as well as devising quality-improvement initiatives.

Measurement is fundamental to nursing practice, research, and management. Assigning numerical values to events, practices, perceptions, and behaviors allows nurses to quantify their impact on patient care, their workplaces, and the American health care system. With heightened attention to the use of data in all aspects of nursing practices, an appreciation and understanding of measurement is critical to success of individual RNs and the nursing profession.

Peri Rosenfeld

MEASURING PHYSICAL FUNCTION

Choosing an appropriate outcome measure to assess physical functioning can be a daunting

M

task for physicians, nurse practitioners, physical and occupational therapists. The need to utilize objective, reliable, and valid measures of physical function cannot be overstated. Assessment of a person's physical performance should be included in any evaluation to establish a baseline. It is important for health care providers to select the most appropriate physical measures of functional performance for the geriatric population in the setting in which they practice. The selection of appropriate measures of gait and balance is important for determining the effectiveness of reducing morbidity in the geriatric population. Measures of physical performance are utilized to determine fall risk, mobility limitations, cardiovascular tolerance, and impairments in activities of daily living (ADL). Interpreting the results of physical function measurements lead to interventions, which might include referral to other health care professionals such as social services for community-based resources, an occupational therapist for ADL impairments, or a geriatrician to manage medical needs.

A compilation of physical performance measures (instruments) can be found on the website www.rehabmeasures.org. The website includes information such as the title of the assessment, acronym, link to the tool, length of time it takes to perform the test, diagnoses in which there are evidence-based summaries, and psychometric properties of the instruments,

The physical performance measures described here were chosen because they have been shown to be valid and reliable instruments and can be performed quickly and in any clinical settings in which the older adult may be seen. They require no special equipment, are easy to administer, and can be performed by nonskilled personnel (i.e., a research assistant). They are the Timed Up and Go (TUG) Test" (Podsiadlo & Richardson, 1991), Tinetti Gait and Balance Test (Tinetti, 1986), 2-Minute Walk Test (Stewart, Burns, Dunn, & Roberts, 1990), Functional Reach Test (Duncan, Weiner, Chandler, & Studenski, 1990), and Five Times Sit to Stand Test.

TIMED UP AND GO TEST

The Timed Up and Go (TUG) Test measures mobility, balance, and motor performance

in the older adult with balance impairments (Podsialdo, 1991). It has shown to be a valid and reliable instrument in people with Parkinson's disease and elderly people with and without cognitive impairments. Other groups that have been studied utilizing the TUG are lower extremity amputees; patients with total joint arthroplasty, cerebral vascular accident, hip fracture, and rheumatoid and osteoarthritis; frail elderly; deconditioned, community-dwelling elderly; and those with vestibular impairments. The TUG test is performed by timing individuals as they stand from an 18-inch chair, walk 3 m, turn 180 degrees, return to the chair, and sit down. The score on this test is the time it takes in seconds to complete the task. The test takes 2 to 3 minutes to complete. Interrater reliability, criterion, and construct validity are high, correlating well with laboratory and clinical measures of gait and balance. A score of less than 10 sec is normal. Cut off scores in seconds indicating risk of falls by population are as follows: community-dwelling adults, greater than 13.5; older patients who have sustained a stroke, greater than 14; seniors with Parkinson's disease, greater than 11.5; and older adults with vestibular disorders, greater than 11.1. Relating the score of the TUG test to a functional mobility skill, it has been demonstrated that a score of less than 20 seconds indicates independence for basic transfers, and greater than 30 seconds indicates dependence on transfers and a need for help to enter/exit the shower or tub.

TINETTI GAIT AND BALANCE TEST

The Tinetti Gait and Balance Test, also referred to as the Performance Oriented Mobility Assessment (POMA), identifies mobility impairments. It utilizes an ordinal scale, made up of two sections. The balance section rates the ability to maintain postural stability during various activities (e.g., sit-to-stand transfers, standing balance, 360-degree turns). The gait section consists of mobility tasks, such as initiation of gait, step length, step height, and path deviation. Both sections are scored on a scale of 0 to 28. The maximum score is 28/28. It takes approximately 10 minutes to complete and is widely used in a variety of clinical settings, with diversified patient populations. It has been shown to be a reliable instrument with good sensitivity. A score of less than 19/28 indicates a fall risk (see Gait Assessment Instruments).

2-MINUTE WALK TEST

The 2-Minute Walk Test (2MWT) is a performance-based measure where the distance walked in 2 minutes is recorded in feet or meters (Stewart et al., 1990). The patient may stop and rest as many times as necessary. The patient may use an assistive device, which should be kept consistent from test to test. The patient should be able to ambulate without physical assistance. The total distance walked is recorded. The greater the distance, the better the performance. The 2MWT was adapted from the 6MWT, which assessed exercise tolerance in individuals with respiratory disease. Performance on the 2MWT can be used to determine an individual's capacity for community ambulation to complete essential activities such as crossing the street in the time of a walk signal or walking the distance required to complete grocery shopping.

The populations tested were: chronic obstructive pulmonary disease, multiple sclerosis, and neurological impairment; those who have had cardiac surgery; and older adults/geriatric patients. Normative data for the 2MWT distance (with accompanying standard deviation in parentheses reported by Connelly, Thomas, Cliffe, Perry, and Smith (2009) were 77.5 (25.6) m for the long-term care group, 150.4 (23.1) m for retirement-home dwelling older adults, and 149 (48) m for patients who had a stroke (chronic) 149 (48) m. For patients who underwent coronary artery bypass graft surgery, mean distance covered was 151 (31) m.

FUNCTIONAL REACH TEST

The Functional Reach (FR) Test (Duncan et al., 1990) is a clinical test of dynamic postural control that addresses limits of postural stability. It quantifies the maximal distance one can reach forward beyond arm's length (in the horizontal plane) while maintaining a fixed base of support in the standing position. The following groups have been tested utilizing the FR test: community-dwelling elderly, frail elderly, and those with

cerebrovascular accident (CVA), hemiparesis, traumatic brain injury, low back pain, and Parkinson's disease. A reach performed at less than 6 inches is a high risk for falls. A reach performed greater than 12 inches without external support is normal.

FIVE TIMES SIT TO STAND TEST

The Five Times Sit to Stand Test (5TSST) was described by Csuka and McCarty (1985) to assess lower extremity strength and balance. The groups that have been studied utilizing the 5TSST were healthy older adults and patients with renal disease, stroke, osteoarthritis and rheumatoid arthritis, Parkinson's disease, and total knee arthroplasty. The 5TSST test is performed by timing the individual perform sitting to standing five times. The patient sits with arms folded across chest with the back against a standard arm chair (43–35 cm). The patient is instructed to stand up and sit down five times as quickly as possible after the tester says "go." Patients are instructed not to use their hands, to keep their arms folded across their chest, and to fully stand up between repetitions. Normative data for 60- to 69-years-olds was 11.4 seconds; for 70- to 79-year-olds, 12.6 seconds; and for 80 to 89-year-olds, 14.8 seconds. Increased fall risk was identified in older adults when the score was greater than 12 seconds, in patients with vestibular disorders when it was greater than 15 seconds, and in patients with Parkinson's disease when it was greater than 16 seconds.

See also Gait Assessment Instruments; Occupational Therapy Assessment and Evaluation; Physical Therapy Services.

Sandy B. Ganz

Connelly, D. M., Thomas, B. K., Cliffe, S. J., Perry, W. M., & Smith, R. E. (2009). Clinical utility of the 2-minute walk test for older adults living in long-term care. *Physiotherapy Canada, 61*(2), 78-87.

Csuka, M., & McCarty, D. J. (1985) Simple method for measurement of lower extremity muscle strength. *American Journal of Medicine, 78*, 77–81.

Duncan, P. W., Weiner, D. K., Chandler, J., & Studenski, S. (1990). Functional reach: A new clinical measure of balance. *Journals of Gerontology, Series A, 45*(6), M192–M197.

M

Podsiadlo, D., & Richardson, S. (1991). The timed "Up & Go": A test of basic functional mobility for frail elderly persons. *Journal of the American Geriatrics Society, 39*(2), 142–148.

Stewart, D. A., Burns, J. M. A., Dunn, S. G., & Roberts, M. A. (1990). The two-minute walking test: a sensitive index of mobility in the rehabilitation of elderly patients. *Clinical Rehabilitation, 4*(4), 273–276.

Tinetti, M. E. (1986). Performance-oriented assessment of mobility problems in elderly patients. *Journal of the American Geriatrics Society, 34*(2), 119–126.

Web Resources (Instructions For Administering Tests)

5 times Sit to Stand Test: http://www.rehabmeasures .org/Lists/RehabMeasures/DispForm.aspx? ID=1015

Functional Reach Test: http://www.rehabmeasures .org/Lists/RehabMeasures/DispForm.aspx? ID=950

National Institutes of Health Toolbox: http://www .nihtoolbox.org/WhatAndWhy/Assessments/ E-learning%20files/player.html

Timed Up and Go Test: http://www.rehab measures .org/Lists/RehabMeasures/DispForm.aspx? ID=903, with link to administration of test

Tinetti Gait and Balance Test: http://www.bhps.org .uk/falls/documents/TinettiBalanceAssessment.pdf

2-Minute Walk Test: http://www.archives-pmr.org/ article/S0003-9993(04)00280-1/pdf

MEDICAID

Medicaid was enacted in 1965 as Title XIX of the Social Security Act to assist states in paying for the health care of the very poor. By setting minimum standards, Medicaid was designed not only to give states flexibility in their programs, but also to ensure that specific groups of people would be assisted and that particular core services would be provided across the country.

Medicaid was originally tied to eligibility for other public assistance programs such as Aid to Families with Dependent Children (AFDC) and Supplemental Security Insurance (SSI) cash assistance programs. However, beginning in 1984, a series of expansions in Medicaid coverage reflected a significant shift in the philosophical underpinnings of the program. In 1984, changes were made to provide coverage to pregnant women before their receipt of AFDC to ensure the coverage of prenatal care. In 1989, Medicaid eligibility was expanded to cover pregnant women and children, and the link to other public-assistance programs was dropped entirely. In 1990, federal law expanded Medicaid coverage to children younger than 6 years, pregnant women whose income falls below 133% of poverty (at a minimum), and children aged 7 to 19 years whose family income is less than 100% of poverty.

The Children's Health Insurance Program (CHIP) was created under the Balanced Budget Act in 1997. The CHIP, also known as Title XXI of the Social Security Act, enables states to initiate and expand health care to uninsured, low-income children. States may either create a new health insurance coverage program that defines the amount, duration, and scope of benefits, expand eligibility for children under the state's current Medicaid program, or both.

Prior to enactment of the Patient Protection and Affordable Care Act of 2010 (PPACA), eligibility for Medicaid was based on both falling into a "categorically needy" eligibility group and meeting a financial needs test. Historically, individuals have had to be low-income and either aged, blind, disabled, pregnant, a dependent child, or a parent of a dependent child to qualify for Medicaid. Pursuant to the PPACA, states could pursue Medicaid expansion eligibility beginning in 2014 based on income alone. Thirty-two states and the District of Columbia have opted to expand Medicaid under the PPACA to working-age adults who do not currently meet categorical requirements but whose income falls at or below 138% of the federal poverty level (Centers for Medicare & Medicaid Services, 2016a, 2016b).

States have a tremendous amount of latitude in determining how the program will be structured, what is covered, how much and by what method providers will be paid, how the state will calculate income and assets for program eligibility, and whether optional categories of services will be covered. Consequently, the 50 states, the District of Columbia, and the five American territories have different Medicaid programs. Someone who is eligible in one state may not be eligible in another state.

States receive federal matching funds for every dollar spent on Medicaid services. The precise federal match, or participation rate, is inversely related to the state's fiscal capacity (based primarily on per capita income), ranging from 74.6% in Mississippi in 2017 to no less than 50% for the richest states (The Henry J. Kaiser Family Foundation, 2016).

In 2016, approximately 71.1 million people were enrolled in Medicaid and an additional 6 million children and pregnant women were covered by the CHIP (CMS, 2016a). Children accounted for the largest proportion (43%) of Medicaid beneficiaries, followed by adults in families (22%), nonelderly blind and disabled (14%), adults in expansion states (13%), and the elderly (8%). Medicaid spending (both federal and state) totaled $496 billion in 2014; the federal government financed approximately 62% and the remainder was financed by states and local governments (Martin, Hartman, Benson, Catlin, & National Health Expenditure Accounts, 2016).

Although children and adults in families comprise the largest proportion of enrollees, they tend to have fewer health needs relative to low-income elderly and nonelderly disabled beneficiaries, and therefore they incur a relatively smaller proportion of Medicaid expenditures. During 2012, Medicaid and CHIP expenditures were incurred by children (26%), adults in families (13%), the nonelderly disabled (41%), and elderly Medicaid enrollees (17%; Centers for Disease Control and Prevention [CDC], National Center for Health Statistics, 2015).

At a state's discretion, people with income that is above the threshold for Medicaid eligibility but who face relatively high medical expenses (such as due to nursing home residence) may receive eligibility for Medicaid by "spending down" to a state-set eligibility standard under the optional "medically needy" program. A total of 34 states operate medically needy programs. Beneficiaries who are eligible through the medically needy pathway account for approximately 5% of Medicaid enrollment, but 11% of spending (The Henry J. Kaiser Family Foundation, 2012b).

Mandatory health services provided under Medicaid include inpatient and outpatient hospital care, physician services, laboratory and x-ray services, primary and preventive care, nursing facility and home health care, and other medically necessary services. In addition, states have the option of providing additional covered services, such as prescription drugs, dental services and dentures, rehabilitation services, intermediate care facilities for individuals with mental retardation, and personal care services to individuals in noninstitutional settings.

For individuals enrolled in both Medicare and Medicaid (the dually eligible population), Medicaid covers cost sharing related to the Medicare Part B premium, deductibles, and copayments, as well as some health-related services that are not covered by Medicare. In 2011, Medicaid provided supplemental health coverage for about 9.4 million Medicare beneficiaries. Although individuals who were eligible for both Medicare and Medicaid accounted for only 15% of all Medicaid enrollees, they incurred 38% of overall Medicaid expenditures (The Henry J. Kaiser Family Foundation, 2013a). Approximately two-thirds of overall Medicaid spending for the dually eligible population was related to long-term care services.

Long-term services and support comprise 28% of Medicaid spending (Reaves & Musumeci, 2015). In 2013, Medicaid was estimated to pay for 51% of long-term services and supports expenses nationally, making it the single largest source of long-term care financing.

Individuals who require long-term care services are quite diverse, and Medicaid's beneficiary population receiving long-term care services reflects this diversity, including older adults with age-related physical and cognitive impairments, children and adults with mental retardation and developmental disabilities, individuals with severe mental illness, individuals with traumatic brain and spinal cord injuries, and individuals with debilitating illnesses. Recent estimates suggest that approximately 1.3 million Medicaid beneficiaries receive long-term care within institutional settings and an additional 3.2 million receive home and community-ba care services (The Henry J. Kaiser Family Foundation, 2015).

The high costs of long-term care, along with growing interest in integrating individuals with disability in the community, have led states to experiment with new models of providing

M

long-term care in the home and in the community, as alternatives to nursing homes. Waiver programs that afford states the flexibility to expand home and community-based services in a more limited way have been expanded in recent years. Medicaid beneficiaries who are older are more likely to receive institutional long-term care; those with disabilities are more likely to receive long-term care services through home and community-based programs. A provision in the PPACA permits states to establish Community First Choice programs with a six-percentage-point enhanced federal match to cover personal care and other home and community-based services for Medicaid beneficiaries who would otherwise require institutional care (Burwell, 2015).

The Congressional Budget Office (CBO) estimates that spending on long-term care will continue to rise as the U.S. population ages, putting significant strain on Medicaid, Medicare, and private payers and eventually comprising up to 3.3% of the U.S. gross domestic product (CBO, 2013).

Although the majority of Medicaid services were traditionally delivered on a fee-for-service basis, managed care has been increasingly adopted by Medicaid. States have long been able to voluntarily enroll Medicaid beneficiaries into managed care, and the 1997 Balanced Budget Act afforded states greater ability to expand managed care within Medicaid, including the ability to mandate enrollment in managed care for most categories of beneficiaries (excluding dual eligibles, some children with special needs, and Native Americans). Managed care greatly expanded throughout Medicaid in the 1990s and 2000s, and by 2011, three quarters of Medicaid beneficiaries were covered fully or partially by managed care organizations (The Henry J. Kaiser Family Foundation, 2013a). Most states require managed care enrollment for Medicaid beneficiaries who are children with disabilities, children with special health care needs, and older adults and adults with disabilities who are not also eligible for Medicare. Approximately half of all states enroll dually eligible beneficiaries in managed care (The Henry J. Kaiser Family Foundation, 2012a).

In response to rising Medicaid costs, state budgetary constraints, and federal efforts to reduce spending, states have been actively experimenting with a variety of mechanisms to hold down program costs. Cost-containment efforts vary by state, but restricting provider payments and controlling expenses related to prescription drugs and disease management are being widely implemented. On a more limited basis, increases in cost sharing and cuts in benefits and eligibility are also being used to control expenses.

A total of 31 states and the District of Columbia have expanded Medicaid coverage under the PPACA. The Supreme Court ruling on the constitutionality of the PPACA in June 2012 curtailed universal expansion of Medicaid, effectively converting Medicaid expansion to a state option. For states electing to pursue Medicaid expansion, the federal government will finance the first 3 years of Medicaid expansion at 100% and at 90% or more thereafter based on a state's matching rate (The Henry J. Kaiser Family Foundation, 2013b).

Although surveys and studies of this expansion are ongoing, studies to date find large increases in Medicaid enrollment, and large reductions in the uninsured in Medicaid expansion states (The Henry J. Kaiser Family Foundation, 2016). The sharp declines in uninsured rates among the low-income population in expansion states are widely attributed to gains in Medicaid coverage. Studies confirm that Medicaid expansion has improved access to care and utilization of services among low-income populations. Additional research also suggests that Medicaid expansion has helped to reduce income- and race-based coverage disparities. Medicaid expansion improves the affordability of care and financial security among the low-income population. Some research shows that improved access to care and utilization is leading to increased diagnoses of certain chronic conditions. A recent study suggests that Medicaid expansion may promise meaningful health benefits in the future (Antonisse, 2016; Sommers, Baicker, & Epstein, 2012), but additional research is needed to provide longer-term insight into expansion's effects on health outcomes.

See also Pensions and Financing Retirement; Long-Term Care Policy; Medicare Managed Care; Program of All-Inclusive Care for the Elderly (PACE).

Karen Davis

Antonisse, L., Garield, R., Rudowitz, R., & Artiga, S. (2016). *The effects of Medicaid expansion under the ACA: Findings from a literature review.* Menlo Park, CA: Kaiser Family Foundation.

Burwell, S. M. (2015). Report to Congress: Community First Choice: Final report to Congress as required by the Patient Protection and Affordable Care Act of 2010 (P.L. 111–148). Retrieved from https://www.medicaid.gov/medicaid/hcbs/downloads/cfc-final-report-to-congress.pdf

Centers for Disease Control and Prevention, National Center for Health Statistics. (2015). Health US 2015. Retrieved from http://www.cdc.gov/nchs/data/hus/2015/109.pdf

Centers for Medicare & Medicaid Services. (2016a). CMS fast facts. Retrieved from http://www.cms.gov/fastfacts

Centers for Medicare & Medicaid Services. (2016b). Medicaid coverage expansion as of July 2016. Retrieved from https://www.medicaid.gov/medicaid-chip-program-information/program-information/downloads/medicaid-expansion-state-map.pdf

Congressional Budget Office. (2013). Rising demand for long-term services and support for elderly people, 2013. Retrieved from http://www.cbo.gov/sites/default/files/cbofiles/attachments/44363-LTC.pdf

The Henry J. Kaiser Family Foundation. (2012a). Medicaid managed care: Key data, trends, and issues. Retrieved from http://kaiserfamilyfoundation.files.wordpress.com/2013/01/8046-02.pdf

Martin, A. B., Hartman, M., Benson, J., Catlin, A., & National Health Expenditure Accounts Team (2016). National health spending in 2014: Faster growth driven by coverage expansion and prescription drug spending. *Health Affairs, 35*(1). Retrieved from http://content.healthaffairs.org/content/early/2015/11/25/hlthaff.2015.1194.full.html

Reaves, E. L., & Musumeci, M. B. (2015). Kaiser Family Foundation, Medicaid and long-term services and supports. Retrieved from http://kff.org/medicaid/report/medicaid-and-long-term-services-and-supports-a-primer

Sommers, B. D., Baicker, K., & Epstein, A. M. (2012). Mortality and access to care among adults after state Medicaid expansions. *New England Journal of Medicine, 367*(11), 1025–1034.

The Henry J. Kaiser Family Foundation. (2012b). The Medicaid medically needy program: Spending and enrollment update. Retrieved from http://kaiserfamilyfoundation.files.wordpress.com/2013/01/4096.pdf

The Henry J. Kaiser Family Foundation. (2013a). Medicaid: A primer—Key information on the nation's health coverage program for low-income people. Retrieved from http://kff.org/medicaid/issue-brief/medicaid-a-primer

The Henry J. Kaiser Family Foundation. (2013b). Visualizing health policy: Medicaid expansion under the Affordable Care Act, 2013. Retrieved from http://kff.org/infographic/visualizing-health-policy-medicaid-expansion-under-the-affordable-care-act

The Henry J. Kaiser Family Foundation. (2016). Federal Medical Assistance Percentage (FMAP) for Medicaid and multiplier. Retrieved from http://kff.org/medicaid/state-indicator/federal-matching-rate-and-multiplier

Web Resources
Centers for Disease Control and Prevention, National Center for Health Statistics: http://www.cdc.gov/nchs/data/hus/2015/109.pdf

Centers for Medicare & Medicaid Services: http://www.cms.hhs.gov/home/medicaid.asp

Congressional Budget Office: http://www.cbo.gov/topics/health-care/medicaid-and-chip

The Henry J. Kaiser Family Foundation: http://www.kaiserfamilyfoundation.org/medicaid/index.cfm

MEDICARE

Medicare was enacted in 1965 as Title XVIII of the Social Security Act. This federal program of health insurance was originally developed to provide health coverage for persons aged 65 years or older who are eligible for Social Security benefits. In addition, in 1972 the program was extended to people under age 65 years who were entitled to federal disability benefits for at least 2 years and to certain individuals with end-stage renal disease. Medicare was enacted in response to a growing awareness of the need to help older persons obtain and pay for necessary medical care. In the early 1960s, only about half of older Americans had any health insurance (compared with 75% of those aged under 65 years). Those seeking to purchase private coverage were often denied on the basis of age or pre-existing conditions or found private insurance unaffordable (Blumenthal, Davis, & Guterman, 2015).

Medicare is a federal entitlement program that pays for medical care delivered by private health care providers. Eligibility is linked to Social Security through workforce participation (either employment or through marriage). Unlike Medicaid, Medicare is not subject to tests of financial need. Today, the Medicare program covers approximately 56.5 million Americans. Most beneficiaries are elderly. Approximately 16% of beneficiaries are younger than 65 years of age (Centers for Medicare & Medicaid Services [CMS], 2016).

Medicare expenditures in 2015 totaled $634 billion (Congressional Budget Office, 2016). Of this spending, about 27% of the Medicare Advantage program (Medicare managed care), 23% went toward inpatient hospital care, 11% for physician services, 7% for outpatient prescription drugs, and the remainder toward skilled nursing facilities, home health, hospital outpatient and other services. Total Medicare spending is projected to nearly double by 2026 due to the influx of retirees from the Baby Boomer generation and rising costs of health care (Congressional Budget Office, 2016). Prescription drug prices have driven much of this growth in recent years, increasing at a higher rate than other services (Martin, Hartman, Benson, & Catlin, 2016).

Medicare consists of four programs: hospital insurance (known as Part A), supplementary medical insurance (known as Part B), Medicare Advantage (known as Part C), and prescription drug insurance (known as Part D). Medicare Part A covers hospital services and post-acute care and is primarily financed by current workers and their employers through a payroll tax. Beneficiaries who age into the program are automatically enrolled at the time that they begin to receive Social Security benefits. The payroll tax rates for Part A are 1.45% of payroll each for workers and their employers. Individuals and couples earning $200,000 and $250,000 per year, respectively, are subject to an additional 0.9% on earned income above the threshold. The remainder of Part A funding comes from a tax on Social Security benefits, interest, and other sources.

Although most beneficiaries elect to participate in both Medicare Parts A and B, participation in Part B is voluntary. Part B covers physicians' services and other ambulatory care services and is financed through a different mechanism than Medicare Part A. A fourth is financed through premiums paid by the beneficiaries (typically deducted from their monthly Social Security payments), and the remaining 75% is financed through general tax revenues, interest, and other sources. In 2016, the standard monthly Part B premium was $104.90. However, beneficiaries whose individual incomes exceeded $85,000 paid incrementally higher Part B premiums, up to a maximum of $389.80 per month for those whose individual income exceeded $214,000.

Medicare Part C, the Medicare Advantage program, has its origins in Medicare + Choice, which resulted from legislation in 1997 that allowed the CMS to pay managed care plans a fixed monthly amount per enrollee to cover the same basic benefits package offered under the traditional program. Enrollees in Medicare Advantage plans pay the monthly Medicare Part B premium and, depending on the health plan, may also be responsible for additional monthly premiums. Approximately 17.6 million or 31% of Medicare beneficiaries were enrolled in managed care plans in 2013, an increase from 16% in 2006 (The Henry J. Kaiser Family Foundation, 2016a). The majority of Medicare beneficiaries are enrolled in the fee-for-service (FFS) program.

Part D is a voluntary prescription drug insurance program that is delivered through a variety of private vendors. The program was created under the 2003 Medicare Prescription Drug, Improvement, and Modernization Act (MMA) and began in 2006. It is funded through general tax revenues (74%), beneficiary premiums (15%), and payments made by states for beneficiaries dually eligible for Medicare and Medicaid (The Henry J. Kaiser Family Foundation, 2016b).

Although Medicare provides significant coverage for health care services, beneficiariesare still left with a significant out-of-pocket contribution. The largest sources of out-of-pocket expenses have historically been for services not covered by Medicare—most notably, extended long-term care (e.g., nursing home care beyond 100 days, assisted-living facility care, personal care and supportive services in private homes) and dental, vision, and hearing services. Co-payments and deductibles, particularly for multiple hospital admissions, can also result in extensive out-of-pocket medical expenses.

Most Medicare-covered services are subject to cost-sharing and time constraints. For example, after beneficiaries have paid their deductible ($1,288 in 2016), Medicare Part A reimburses inpatient hospital care during the first 60 days of each benefit period (period associated with one acute illness). For days 61 and beyond, beneficiaries are responsible for co-payments of $322 per day until day 90, and for stays beyond 90 days in a benefit period, an insured person may elect to draw on a 60-day lifetime reserve that requires a co-payment of $644 per day. Following a hospitalization of at least 3 days, Part A will reimburse services delivered during the subsequent 100 days of skilled nursing care or skilled rehabilitation services; however, only the first 20 days in the skilled nursing facility are free from cost sharing and the remaining 80 days involve a $161/day co-pay.

Part B of Medicare pays 80% of physicians' fees set by the Medicare Fee Schedule for most covered services in excess of an annual $166 deductible. Covered services include medically necessary physician services, laboratory and other diagnostic tests, x-ray and other radiation therapy, outpatient services at a hospital or comprehensive outpatient rehabilitation facility, rural health clinic services, home dialysis supplies and equipment, prostheses (other than dental), physical and speech therapy, and ambulance services.

To augment the health care coverage provided by Medicare, most beneficiaries carry supplemental health insurance in addition to Medicare. Some beneficiaries purchase private supplemental policies, called Medigap plans, to cover coinsurance, co-payments, and deductibles for Medicare services. Historically, retiree benefits have also provided supplemental health care coverage, although there is evidence—and concern—that these benefits are eroding. Beneficiaries with incomes below the poverty level meeting asset tests are "dually eligible" for both Medicare and Medicaid, and state Medicaid programs pay the Medicare Part B premiums and all other deductibles and co-payments for Medicare-covered services. Medicaid also covers the Part B premium for beneficiaries with incomes up to 135% of poverty. Nonetheless, only 65% of Medicare beneficiaries with incomes below poverty and 38% of those with incomes between 100% and 149% of poverty are covered by Medicaid (Schoen, Davis, & Willink, 2016).

Efforts to control Medicare costs have taken many forms over the years, including prospective payments to hospitals, home health agencies, and skilled nursing facilities, as well as relative value payments to physicians. The 2003 MMA enacted the most widespread changes to Medicare since its inception. In addition to creating Medicare Part D, the MMA called for income-relating for preventive services and further extended coverage for preventive services, including tobacco cessation and yearly wellness visits. It also expanded prescription drug benefits to offer discounts on medications and to reduce the out-of-pocket burden to individuals who reach the "donut hole" for medications. In addition, the PPACA contained numerous provisions to reduce Medicare spending growth, including reduced payments to hospitals and post-acute care providers and Medicare Advantage plans and greater sharing of beneficiary Part B premiums (The Henry J. Kaiser Family Foundation, 2013). Accountable care organizations (ACOs), groups of coordinated health care providers, were developed to be accountable for the quality, cost, and overall care of Medicare beneficiaries in FFS Medicare. These ACOs can participate in the shared savings achieved through the provision of appropriate and more coordinated care. The PPACA introduced a 15-member Independent Payment Advisory Board to recommend changes to

Medicare if projected per-beneficiary spending growth exceeds specified targets, although this provision has not been implemented. The PPACA also mandated a Center for Medicare & Medicaid Innovation to test cost-saving models of care delivery and a Federal Coordinated Health Care Office to align and coordinate benefits between Medicare and Medicaid (The Henry J. Kaiser Family Foundation, 2013).

Although these changes are positive steps toward bringing Medicare's benefit package in line with contemporary standards and the health needs of its beneficiary population, several issues remain. In particular, the fiscal challenges facing the Medicare program have grown more formidable in recent years, in large part due to demographic trends and rising costs of technology. Medicare now accounts for more than 15% of overall federal expenditures and is anticipated to compose 16.8% by 2023. It is projected that the Part A trust fund will be depleted by 2028 unless changes are made to the program's benefit structure or financing (The Henry J. Kaiser Family Foundation, 2016c). At the same time, lower-income Medicare beneficiaries not covered by Medicaid and those with multiple chronic conditions and physical or cognitive impairment causing out-of-pocket costs for covered and noncovered services represent a high proportion of income, reflecting limitations in the Medicare benefit package.

See also Long-Term Care Policy; Medicaid.

Amber Willink

Blumenthal, D., Davis, K., & Guterman, S. (2015). Medicare at 50: Origins and evolution. *New England Journal of Medicine, 372*(5), 479–486.

Centers for Medicare & Medicaid Services. (2016). CMS fast facts. Retrieved from http://www.cms .gov/fastfacts

Congressional Budget Office. (2016). Congressional Budget Office's March 2016 Medicare baseline. Retrieved from https://www.cbo.gov/sites/ default/files/51302-2016-03-Medicare.pdf

The Henry J. Kaiser Family Foundation. (2013). Summary of the Affordable Care Act. Retrieved from http://kaiserfamilyfoundation.files.word press.com/2011/04/8061-021.pdf

The Henry J. Kaiser Family Foundation. (2016a). Medicare advantage 2016 spotlight: Enrollment market update. Retrieved from http://kff.org/ medicare/issue-brief/medicare-advantage-2016 -spotlight-enrollment-market-update

The Henry J. Kaiser Family Foundation. (2016b). The Medicare prescriptive drug benefit. Retrieved from http://kff.org/medicare/fact-sheet/the -medicare-prescription-drug-benefit-fact-sheet

The Henry J. Kaiser Family Foundation. (2016c). Medicare spending and financing fact sheet. Retrieved from http://kff.org/medicare/issue -brief/the-facts-on-medicare-spending-and -financing

Martin, A. B., Hartman, M., Benson, J., & Catlin, A. (2016). National health spending in 2014: Faster growth driven by coverage expansion and prescription drug spending. *Health Affairs, 35*(1), 150–160.

Schoen, C., Davis, K., & Willink, A. (2016). Medicare beneficiaries often face high out-of-pocket costs-profile of cost burdens and unmet need by income and health status. Retrieved from http://www.commonwealthfund.org/publi cations/issue-briefs/2017/may/medicare-out-of -pocket-cost-burdens

Web Resources
Centers for Medicare & Medicaid Services Homepage: http://www.cms.hhs.gov/home/medicare.asp
HealthCare.gov: Affordable Care Act consumer page: https://www.healthcare.gov
The Henry J. Kaiser Family Foundation: http://www .kaiserfamilyfoundation.org/medicare/index.cfm

MEDICARE MANAGED CARE

Medicare managed care is a means of delivering the Medicare program through private health insurance companies. The primary method for achieving this is through Medicare Advantage plans. Individuals in the Medicare program can elect to have their coverage managed by a Medicare Advantage plan or to remain in the traditional Medicare program. Approximately 31% of all Medicare beneficiaries, or 17.6 million individuals, are enrolled Medicare Advantage plans (The Henry J. Kaiser Family Foundation, 2016). This reflects a continued trend in an increasing number of people receiving their Medicare benefit through managed care.

Medicare Advantage is administered by the Centers for Medicare & Medicaid Services (CMS) as part of the Medicare program. Also known as Medicare Part C, Medicare Advantage is an alternative to the Original Medicare fee-for-service program. Medicare Advantage plans are managed by private health insurance companies that contract with the CMS to provide an individual's Medicare Parts A and B benefits. CMS pays the health plans on a capitated basis, meaning that they pay the plan per enrollee to manage their care.

Medicare Managed Care began in 1973 with the Health Maintenance Organization Act, which amended the Medicare program to allow beneficiaries to enroll in a health maintenance organization (CMS, 2015a). The Balanced Budget Act of 1997 further established new managed care options for Medicare beneficiaries. The name Medicare Advantage was established through the Medicare Prescription Drug, Improvement, and Modernization Act (MMA) of 2003.

There are different types of Medicare Advantage plans, including health maintenance organizations, preferred provider organizations, and special needs plans (SNPs), among others. The benefits of Medicare Advantage plans must be at least the same as Original Medicare, but they can also provide services not traditionally covered by Original Medicare, such as glasses, dental services, hearing aids, and health and wellness programs.

A Medicare SNP is a specific type of Medicare Advantage plan that is not open to all Medicare beneficiaries. Medicare SNPs are limited to individuals with certain diseases or conditions. These plans then tailor the treatment and care that individuals receive based on these conditions. This includes a network of providers, a benefit package, and drug formularies. There are also different types of SNPs. These include chronic condition SNPs for people with conditions such as dementia or diabetes. There are institutional SNPs for people who live in institutions such as nursing homes or who need nursing care at home. There are also dually eligible SNPs for people who are dually eligible for Medicare and Medicaid. All of an individual's care is coordinated through the SNP.

There are also demonstration programs underway through CMS. One such example is the fully integrated duals advantage (FIDA) program in New York. It is focused on managing the care of those who are dually eligible for the Medicare and Medicaid programs. Through the Patient Protection and Affordable Care Act, CMS established the Medicare-Medicaid Coordination Office to explore opportunities to better manage the care for the 10.7 million individuals who are enrolled in both programs (CMS, 2015b). Reviewing opportunities in managed care is one dimension of their work.

Each year in the fall, individuals in the Medicare program have the opportunity to change the way that they receive their Medicare benefit. Individuals can also change the specific Medicare Advantage or prescription drug plan that they are enrolled in. In 2016, the annual open enrollment period was from October 15 through December 7. New coverage begins on January 1. Individuals can receive assistance in determining what option best meets their health and financial needs by speaking with a State Health Insurance Assistance Program (SHIP) counselor.

Thomas Bane

Centers for Medicare & Medicaid Services. (n.d.). Costs in the coverage gap. Retrieved from https://www.medicare.gov/part-d/costs/coverage-gap/part-d-coverage-gap.html

Centers for Medicare & Medicaid Services. (2015a). Milestones 1937–2015. Retrieved from https://www.cms.gov/About-CMS/Agency-Information/History/Downloads/Medicare-and-Medicaid-Milestones-1937-2015.pdf

Centers for Medicare & Medicaid Services. (2015b). Medicare-Medicaid Coordination Office fiscal year 2015 report to Congress. Retrieved from https://www.cms.gov/Medicare-Medicaid-Coordination/Medicare-and-Medicaid-Coordination/Medicare-Medicaid-Coordination-Office/Downloads/MMCO_2015_RTC.pdf

The Henry J. Kaiser Family Foundation. (2015). The Medicare Part D prescription drug benefit. Retrieved from http://files.kff.org/attachment/fact-sheet-the-medicare-part-d-prescription-drug-benefit

The Henry J. Kaiser Family Foundation. (2016). Medicare Advantage. Retrieved from http://files.kff.org/attachment/Fact-Sheet-Medicare-Advantage

M

MEDICARE PART D BENEFIT

Medicare coverage is composed of four parts: A, B, C, and D. The Medicare Part D benefit provides coverage for prescriptions medications. Medicare Part D was an expansion of the original benefits beyond hospital and provider coverage. Similar to the Medicare Advantage program, the Medicare Part D benefit is managed by private health insurance companies, which are called prescription drug plans. An individual who has Original Medicare (Parts A and B) can enroll in a stand along prescription drug plan. The Part D drug benefit can also be managed through a Medicare Advantage plan. The Part D program is a voluntary program for those enrolled in the Medicare program.

The MMA of 2003 established the Medicare Part D benefit (CMS, 2015a). People could first enroll into the Medicare Part D program in 2006. Prior to this, many people on Medicare experienced challenges in affording their prescription medications. This led to unhealthy behaviors such as sharing pills, splitting dosages, or even skipping medications that were critical to health.

Individuals enrolled in a Medicare prescription drug plan pay a monthly premium, as well as co-payments or coinsurances, and may also have a deductible associated with their plan. Different prescription drug plans may have corresponding levels, or tiers, on which co-payments and coinsurances are based. Individuals who have higher yearly incomes may also pay more for their Medicare Part D benefit, which

is called the Part D income-related monthly adjustment amount (Part D-IRMAA).

Most Medicare prescription drug plans also have a coverage gap, which is sometimes referred to as the *donut hole*. The coverage gap refers to the period of time when an individual's prescription drug plan temporarily limits what they pay for medications. Not everyone enrolled in a prescription drug plan will reach this coverage gap. It is based on the cost of their prescription medications. In 2016, the coverage gap was entered when individuals and their plan spent $3,310 on prescription drugs (CMS, n.d.). While in the coverage gap, an individual does not pay more than 45% of the cost for brand name medications and 58% for generic medications in 2016. Once $4,850 in out-of-pocket costs is spent, individuals enter catastrophic coverage and are no longer in the coverage gap. This means that a Medicare beneficiary spends only a small co-pay or coinsurance for prescriptions for the rest of the year. As part of the Patient Protection and Affordable Care Act, the coverage gap is decreasing each year. By 2020, no more than 25% for covered brand-name and generic medications will be paid until individuals reach catastrophic coverage.

Individuals in the Medicare Part D program can also receive premium and cost-sharing assistance based on their income and assets through the Low-Income Subsidy program. This is also sometimes referred to as the Extra Help program. It is for people who have an income of less than 150% of the federal poverty level, which in 2015 was $17,655 (The Henry J. Kaiser Family Foundation, 2015). A total of 12 million individuals are enrolled in the Low-Income Subsidy program.

Individuals who do not enroll into Medicare Part D when they are first eligible may face a late enrollment penalty when they enroll later. Individuals who receive Extra Help or are enrolled in creditable coverage do not face the penalty. Individuals may receive creditable coverage through an employer or a union's prescription drug coverage that meets the standard of a Medicare prescription drug plan. Individuals may have to pay the penalty if they go 63 consecutive days without this type of creditable coverage. The penalty is calculated by multiplying the number of full, uncovered months by 1% of a national base premium.

Each year in the fall, individuals in the Medicare program have the opportunity to change the way that they receive their Medicare Part D benefit. Individuals can change the specific Prescription Drug Plan that they are enrolled in. In 2016, the Annual Open Enrollment period was from October 15 through December 7. New coverage begins on January 1st each year. Individuals can receive assistance in determining what option best meets their health and financial needs by speaking with a State Health Insurance Assistance Program (SHIP) counselor.

Thomas Bane

Centers for Medicare & Medicaid Services. (2015). Milestones 1937-2015. Retrieved from https://www.cms.gov/About-CMS/Agency-Information/History/Downloads/Medicare-and-Medicaid-Milestones-1937-2015.pdf

Centers for Medicare & Medicaid Services. (n.d.). Costs in the coverage gap. Retrieved from https://www.medicare.gov/part-d/costs/coverage-gap/part-d-coverage-gap.html

The Henry J. Kaiser Family Foundation. (2015). The Medicare Part D prescription drug benefit. Retrieved from http://files.kff.org/attachment/fact-sheet-the-medicare-part-d-prescription-drug-benefit

Web Resources

Centers for Medicare & Medicaid Services: https://www.medicare.gov/part-d

The Henry J. Kaiser Family Foundation: http://www.kff.org

Social Security Administration: http://www.ssa.gov/medicare/prescriptionhelp

MEDICATION ADHERENCE

Increasing age is associated with a higher prevalence of chronic diseases requiring long-term medication intake. Patients older than 65 years are the largest consumers of medications, receiving nearly half of all prescribed medicines. *Polypharmacy*, traditionally defined as taking more than five medications simultaneously, is highly prevalent in this age group.

Supporting patients to take their medications correctly is a high priority as "drugs do not work in patients who do not take them" (C. Everett Koop, in Osterberg & Blaschke, 2005). This implies supporting patients in obtaining medications at the pharmacy and starting treatment (*initiation*), supporting correct dosing (taking and timing) while on the treatment regimen (*implementation*), as well as support with continuing to take the medication until it is no longer prescribed (*persistence*). Medication adherence (previously called *compliance*; Figure M.1) entails all three phases of the medication-taking process as described earlier (Vrijens et al., 2012). It is important to clearly discern which phase of medication adherence is the focus in clinical practice or research because each phase has distinct definition, measurement, and analysis considerations.

MEASUREMENT

Assessing medication adherence should also focus on the three aspects of *initiation, implementation*, and *persistence*. Initiation is a dichotomous variable (yes/no). Implementation is time series and represents patient's dosing history over time (e.g., taking errors, timing errors, dosing errors), whereas persistence is a time-to-event variable. Measurement methods need to fit the adherence phase assessed. Direct and indirect methods exist to assess adherence; some are more suited to assess a specific adherence phase than others.

Direct methods include assays of medication, medication by-products, or tracers (e.g., digoxin) in bodily substances, as well as observation of medication administration. Repeated direct methods can have value for assessing the implementation phase. The reliability of assays for adherence assessment depends on the half-life of the substance under scrutiny and the unobtrusiveness of the assessment method (e.g., Hawthorn effect). Observation allows evaluation of complex medication behaviors such as insulin injection, inhalers, or eye drops (Osterberg & Blaschke, 2005). Observation also permits assessment of elders' ability to independently

M

ABC Taxonomy: **Medication Adherence**

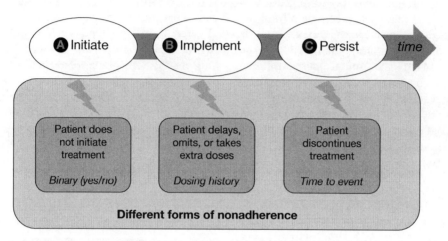

The process by which patients take their medication as prescribed

FIGURE M.1 Components of medication adherence.

Source: Adapted from Vrijens et al. (2012).

manage medications despite visual or physical impairments. Such observation can be accomplished during a clinical encounter or using electronic communication methods and is an option for assessing implementation, especially in case of repeated assessments such as in directly observed therapy.

Indirect measurement methods are self-report, collateral report by a family member or caregiver, pill count, prescription refills, and electronic monitoring. *Self-reports* have value when asked in a nonthreatening, nonaccusatory, and approach, yet correlate only moderately with more reliable assessment methods such as electronic event monitoring. For instance, clinicians can ask: "We know that taking medications correctly every day, at the same time, can be difficult for many patients. Do you remember missing a dose of any of your medications in the past 4 weeks?" Assessing adherence using *prescription refill records* is most feasible in centrally managed pharmacy systems and is particularly helpful in assessing initiation and persistence. Electronic monitoring uses a pill bottle that is fitted with a cap containing a microelectronic circuit that registers the date and time of each bottle opening. Recorded data

can be downloaded to a computer, and medication dynamics can be visualized in listings and graphics, thus creating time-series data representing medication-taking dynamics adequate for assessing the implementation phase of medication adherence. Electronic monitoring has superior sensitivity compared with other direct and indirect methods (Osterberg & Blaschke, 2005).

None of the assessment methods can be regarded as a gold standard for any given adherence phase to be routinely used in practice, and therefore a combination of different assessment approaches is most valuable (Osterberg & Blaschke, 2005).

PREVALENCE

Prevalence of nonadherence is high and universal. This includes issues with initiation, such as not filling prescriptions, which was recently found to average 16.4% but has been reported to be as high as 57% of patients (da Costa et al., 2015; McHorney, 2015). Evidence also highlights that persistence issues are prominent with 55% of patients having stopped their regimen by 1 year after initiation. *Implementation* issues regard about 10% of nonadherence over time (Vrijens, Vincze, Kristanto, Urquhart, & Burnier, 2008).

CONSEQUENCES

Medication nonadherence has been recognized as an important risk factor jeopardizing the efficacy and effectiveness of long-term drug regimens. Medication nonadherence is associated with poor clinical outcomes (e.g., higher mortality) and higher costs. Given the magnitude of the problem of nonadherence and given its negative consequences, the WHO deemed nonadherence a major public health problem (WHO, 2003).

RISK FACTORS/CORRELATES

Risk factors or correlates for nonadherence can be categorized as socioeconomic, patient-related, treatment-related, condition-related, and health care team– and health care system–related factors (WHO, 2003) and should be assessed separately for each phase of medication adherence. The relevance of health care system factors, although understudied, emerges increasingly as important in explaining nonadherence. Indeed, the quality of communication between health care providers and patients, health care providers' expertise in adherence management, the way that adherence strategies are incorporated in the care processes in health care organizations (e.g., hospitals, pharmacies, outpatient clinics), and the degree of financial coverage for prescription medications all influence medication adherence (WHO, 2003).

Older age per se is not associated with a higher risk for medication nonadherence, but a number of processes associated with aging may negatively influence patients' ability to manage medications independently and correctly. These include functional, sensory, and cognitive impairment; social isolation; depression; and marginal functional health literacy. Moreover, physiological effects of aging in combination with polypharmacy make older patients more susceptible to medication-related adverse events (De Geest et al., 2004). A complex medication regimen of long duration with troublesome side effects (e.g., beta-blockers can induce fatigue, impotence, and sleeplessness)

also hinders good adherence. Although simple forgetfulness is a common reason for nonadherence in all age groups, dementia becomes more prevalent with advanced age and may further impede independent medication management (WHO, 2003).

Mistaken illness representations or health beliefs (e.g., concerns about medications) can threaten adherence (Ruppar, Dobbels, & De Geest, 2012). Barriers to medication adherence in elderly patients can include changes in the prescription, complexity of the regimen, or changes in routine. The risk for nonadherence is also higher in patients who are depressed. Modifiable factors can be targeted for intervention.

ADHERENCE INTERVENTIONS

Preventing and remediating nonadherence to medication regimens is a high priority in health care delivery. For maximum effectiveness, adherence interventions should target not only the patient but also the health care provider, the care processes, the health care organization, and the health care system (National Institute for Health and Care Excellence [NICE], 2013; WHO, 2003). Interventions may differ for the three different phases of medication adherence, and nonadherence may be intentional or unintentional.

The available evidence derived from studies testing the efficacy of adherence interventions remains meager compared to the magnitude of the issue. Successful interventions have combined several strategies over a sustained time at different levels of the health care system (Conn et al., 2009; NICE, 2013; WHO, 2003). Very limited work has been done to specifically apply intervention strategies for each separate phase of medication adherence.

An electronic medical record can be used to track the patient's adherence to medications. Likewise, this record can help each of the patient's providers (e.g., family physician, home health nurse, specialist physicians, hospital, nursing home) to view a single medication list, thus avoiding prescribing errors. Good communication skills and competencies of health professionals can support patients in medication adherence, but interventions should not focus solely on health care provider knowledge or

M

behavior. Implementation of adherence strategies can be included in the multiple processes of the patient's care. Full insurance coverage of medications is likewise an effective intervention to improve adherence (NICE, 2013; WHO, 2003).

At the patient level, one can monitor adherence, with regular assessment of the older patient's ability to independently manage a medication regimen. Functional and sensory abilities, cognition, literacy, knowledge, motivation, illness representations, sources of social support, and financial status should be carefully evaluated during a standard clinical assessment (De Geest et al., 2004).

Adherence interventions at the patient level combine educational/cognitive, behavioral/counseling, and social support/affective strategies. *Patient education*, traditionally an interventional approach in which the most time and effort are invested, increases knowledge yet has limited value to change behavior (Conn et al., 2009). Information transfer to patients is best targeted and personalized to the patient's situation. Most important, education, whether provided by individual or group session or via video or Internet modules, should be combined with other interventional approaches to be effective for behavioral change.

Behavioral strategies/counseling strategies include tailoring the regimen to patients' lifestyles, teaching patients self-monitoring strategies (e.g., medication booklet), suggesting the use of medication aids (e.g., pill box) or reminders (e.g., alarm on cell phone), and cueing (e.g., leaving containers in a particular location). Monitoring by an electronic monitoring system and providing feedback has shown to be very efficacious in improving adherence. Most effective interventions to improve older adults' medication adherence include self-monitoring of medication effects, dosing cues or stimuli, adherence-enhancing packaging (e.g., pillboxes, color-coded labeling), and/or succinct written instructions (Conn et al., 2009).

Social support from caregivers may involve preparing the patient's medication, reminding the patient to take the medicine, refilling prescriptions, and helping the patient decide to contact a health care worker if a problem arises.

Simplification of the regimen is always a goal. Clinicians should also assess the patient's ability to pay for needed medications and utilize the lowest-cost medication options when possible. A variety of local, state, and federal programs may be available to assist with medication costs. Finally, investing in good patient–provider relationships and developing a system of care in which adherence is regularly assessed and the behavioral aspects of medication management are incorporated further contribute to improved adherence (NICE, 2013; WHO, 2003).

See also Assistive Devices; Medicaid; Medicare; Polypharmacy; Social Supports: Formal and Informal.

Todd Ruppar, Sabina M. De Geest, and Sandra Schönfeld

Conn, V. S., Hafdahl, A. R., Cooper, P. S., Ruppar, T. M., Mehr, D. R., & Russell, C. L. (2009). Interventions to improve medication adherence among older adults: Meta-analysis of adherence outcomes among randomized controlled trials. *The Gerontologist, 49*(4), 447–462.

da Costa, F. A., Pedro, A. R., Teixeira, I., Bragança, F., da Silva, J. A., & Cabrita, J. (2015). Primary nonadherence in Portugal: Findings and implications. *International Journal of Clinical Pharmacy, 37*(4), 626–635.

De Geest, S., Steeman, E., Leventhal, M. E., Mahrer-Imhof, R., Hengartner-Kopp, B., Conca, A., … Brunner-La Rocca, H. (2004). Complexity in caring for an ageing heart failure population: Concomitant chronic conditions and age related impairments. *European Journal of Cardiovascular Nursing, 3*(4), 263–270.

McHorney, C. (2015). Patient-centered reasons for primary non-adherence as derived from the peer-reviewed literature. *Value in Health, 18*(7), A737.

National Institute for Health and Care Excellence. (2013). Medication adherence: Involving patients in decisions about prescribed medicines and supporting adherence. NICE clinical guidelines. Retrieved from http://publications.nice.org.uk/medicines-adherence-cg76/#close

Osterberg, L., & Blaschke, T. (2005). Adherence to medication. *New England Journal of Medicine, 353*(5), 487–497.

Ruppar, T. M., Dobbels, F., & De Geest, S. (2012). Medication beliefs and antihypertensive

M

adherence among older adults: A pilot study. *Geriatric Nursing*, 33(2), 89–95.

Vrijens, B., De Geest, S., Hughes, D. A., Przemyslaw, K., Demonceau, J., Ruppar, T., … Urquhart, J. (2012). A new taxonomy for describing and defining adherence to medications. *British Journal of Clinical Pharmacology*, 73(5), 691–705.

Vrijens, B., Vincze, G., Kristanto, P., Urquhart, J., & Burnier, M. (2008). Adherence to prescribed antihypertensive drug treatments: Longitudinal study of electronically compiled dosing histories. *British Medical Journal*, 336(7653), 1114–1117.

World Health Organization. (2003). Adherence to long-term therapies: Evidence for action. Retrieved from http://www.who.int/chp/knowledge/publications/adherence_report/en

Web Resources

American College of Preventive Medicine: http://www.acpm.org/?MedAdhereTTProviders

American Society on Aging and the American Society of Consultant Pharmacists Foundation: http://www.adultmeducation.com

Apps to support medication adherence: http://www.prnewswire.com/news-releases/new-medication-management-and-adherence-app-mymeds-introduced-for-iphone-android-web-unites-consumers-pharmacists-caregivers-physicians-214893981.html

Medication reminders: http://www.epill.com

National Consumers League—medication adherence campaign: http://www.scriptyourfuture.org/hcp

MENTAL CAPACITY ASSESSMENT

Mental capacity refers to the ability to make a reasoned decision, such as for general self-care, medical treatment, or the drafting and execution of a legal document. A person is assumed to have adequate capacity until there is enough compelling evidence to the contrary that warrants further investigation (Berghmans, 2008). Questions about mental capacity and its assessment are increasing as the aging population grows.

The most important consideration in the assessment of an elder's mental capacity is the person's observable behavior, or "clinical findings." It is a mistake to rely primarily, or solely, on test results to make a determination of mental capacity. All cognitive tests require comparison to the elder's observable behavior to ensure proper interpretation. With this understanding, mental capacity instruments may be divided into four categories: (a) behavior-based assessments, (b) screening tests, (c) semistructured interviews, and (d) neuropsychological test batteries. The last category refers to combinations of statistically standardized tests for assessing specific cognitive functions. Specialized training is necessary to properly administer, score, and interpret the results. This chapter reviews some of the assessment tools that may be used by a variety of medical and nonmedical personnel and do not require specialized training. These are not meant to represent all possible tests, merely a few of the more commonly utilized ones.

BEHAVIOR-BASED ASSESSMENTS

Most behavior-based assessments may be used by nonmedical professionals to identify potentially problematic behaviors in elderly clients and serve as gateway assessments for determining whether more detailed evaluation is necessary by a medical professional. There are many variations, but two common assessments are the PARADISE-2 protocol and the Lichtenberg Financial Decision Screening Scale.

PARADISE-2 PROTOCOL

The PARADISE-2 protocol was originally created for attorneys and other nonmedical professionals and uses six categories to evaluate mental capacity through behavioral observations: cognition, emotion, language, consistency with prior acts and beliefs, mitigating factors such as medical considerations, and personal and interpersonal disruptions. The administrator reviews specific behaviors and functions to identify whether any of these categories or subcategories are potentially impaired in the elder (Blum, 2000).

Lichtenberg Financial Decision Screening Scale

The Lichtenberg Financial Decision Screening Scale (LFDSS) is a brief 10-item screening tool for

M

determining the elder's understanding, appreciation, reasoning, choice, and susceptibility to undue influence by using a specific real-life financial decision to determine whether the elder is impaired. Its primary use is to assess financial decision-making capacity. The scale was created for adult protective services workers and other nonmedical professionals as an alternative to the Lichtenberg Financial Decision Making Rating Scale (LFDRS), a 77-item tool for mental health professionals that require a level of training and an administration and scoring time commitment impractical for use by nonmedical professionals (Lichtenberg et al., 2016).

SCREENING TESTS

These short, standardized tests may be administered quickly and provide rapid, rough assessments across multiple cognitive domains, including executive functioning, to assess whether further evaluation may be needed. Although cognitive deficits are known to be strongly correlated with decision-making capacity, these tests do not directly assess decision-making capacity or executive functioning (Palmer & Harmell, 2016). In one study, nearly 25% of partners with dementia maintained decisional capacity, the ability to make a decision, even in the absence of executional capacity, the ability to execute the decision (Boyle, 2013). In addition, tests of executive function are limited due to lack of an operational or conceptual definition and poor ecological validity (Barkley, 2012).

Mini-Mental State Examination

The Mini-Mental State Examination (MMSE) is a 30-point questionnaire that includes questions about orientation, registration and recall, language, attention, and calculation. According to the creator, the MMSE does not discriminate well between people who have intact versus impaired executive functions (Holzer, Gansier, Moczynski, & Folstein, 1997). The test is arguably the most widely used cognitive screening method and has multiple culturally and linguistically adapted versions. A standardized MMSE is available and includes preadministration guidelines to increase reliability (Molloy, Alemayehu, & Roberts, 1991.) MMSE scores are not directly correlated with decision-making capacity and must be added to the clinical history. Elders deemed impaired by the MMSE have demonstrated intact decision-making capacity, and conversely, those evaluated to be cognitively intact have exhibited impaired capacity (Holzer et al., 1997; Whitlatch, 2013). In addition, there is an inherent bias for cortical neurodegenerative disease, so it may not be as sensitive for other causes of cognitive impairment (Royall, Cordes, & Polk, 1998). Results have also been shown to be affected by educational, racial, and language disparity (Crowe, Clay, Sawyer, Crowther, & Allman, 2008; Ramirez, Teresi, Holmes, Gurland, & Lantigua, 2006).

Executive Interview

The Executive Interview (EXIT25) is a 25-item brief, bedside standardized clinical interview for assessing executive function (Royall, Mahurin, & Gray, 1992). The test has exhibited sensitivity to differences in etiology and severity of neurocognitive disorders, including early cognitive impairment, HIV dementia, and bipolar disorder (Berghuis, Uldall, & Lalonde, 1999; Gildengers et al., 2004; Royall et al., 1992). Compared with other assessment tools, EXIT25 may exhibit increased sensitivity and specificity for impaired decision-making capacity (Holtzer et al., 1997). Given arguments that the test has a lengthy administrative time and poor face and content validity of some items, multiple studies maintained or improved internal consistency and validity while reducing to 14, 9, or 8 items (Jahn, Dressel, Gavett, & O'Bryant, 2015; Larson & Heinemann, 2010; Mujic, Lebovich, Von Heisin, Clifford, & Prince, 2014).

Clock Drawing Executive Task

The Clock Drawing Executive Task (CLOX1/CLOX2) is a rapid, widely used clock-drawing test for evaluating working memory, executive function, receptive language, and visuospatial and visuoperceptive skills. In CLOX1, a novel clock is drawn to evaluate executive functioning, and in CLOX2, a clock is copied to determine visuospatial abilities (Shon et al., 2013).

Each drawing is evaluated by its elements, size, form, position, and distractions. The test is well validated in multiple culturally and linguistically diverse populations (Royall et al., 2003; Yap, Ng, Yeo, & Henderson, 2007) The test may be more sensitive to executive dysfunction than the MMSE in subclinical and reversible forms of cognitive impairment (Royall et al., 1998). However, in practical terms, the degree of impairment required may be quite significant and correspond with a normal elementary-age level of functioning (Cohen, Ricci, Kibby, & Edmonds, 2000). Results may also be limited by racial and reading abilities (Crowe et al., 2008).

SEMISTRUCTURED INTERVIEWS

More formalized than screening tools, semistructured interviews consist of standardized vignettes or clinical interview based on four elements of decisional capacity commonly found in U.S. state statutes: the ability to (a) understand alternatives, (b) appreciate the consequences of a choice, (c) provide reasoning for the choice, and (d) express a choice (Grisso & Appelbaum, 1998). It has been shown with greater standardization; there is higher validity, inter-rater reliability, and test–retest reliability (Anastasi & Urbina, 1997).

Capacity to Consent to Treat Instrument

The Capacity to Consent to Treat Instrument (CCTI) is a widely utilized semistructured interview consisting of two hypothetical vignettes for determining decisional capacity for treatment-related decisions. The test is well validated and utilized on diverse populations. Its creators published age-adjusted and age-independent normative data to improve results. One the other hand, some elders may demonstrate rational decision-making abilities with the clear, simple standardized vignettes yet exhibit impairment with complex, multistep decisions. In addition, standardized vignettes ignore situationally dependent factors, such as an alternative that is inherently incompatible with the elder's values (Palmer & Harmell, 2016).

MacArthur Competence Assessment Tools

The MacArthur Competence Assessment Tools (MacCAT) is one of the original, and most widely utilized, semistructured interviews dedicated to the assessment of decision-making ability and often described as the gold standard for capacity assessment. There are now various theme-specific versions to allow for greater contextual assessment, such as consenting to a specific treatment or research protocol, a Spanish version, and a manual to guide its use (Palmer & Harmell, 2016). The test has shown high validity and reliability on diverse populations, and one study found that in conjuncture with a clinical interview, the MacCAT can produce highly reliable capacity judgments (Cairns et al., 2005). One drawback of the MacCAT is that it does not produce a global rating of competency, but rather provides information about each of the four criteria mentioned (Breden & Vollmann, 2004).

CONCLUSION

Assessment of decision-making capacity is an important component of proper elder care. In fact, ensuring the elder is capable of informed decision making is one of the ethical foundations of care. The aging of society, increasingly sophisticated and sometimes dangerous medical treatment alternatives, increasingly complex research proposals involving human subjects, and increasing rates of elder financial exploitation make it clear that mental capacity assessment is a critical skill for all care providers. Even the most skilled professionals can struggle to provide a reliable mental capacity determination without a structured assessment. Yet, even with the most standardized assessment method, results are often limited by the elder's emotional state, values, preferences, and culture. Most important, capacity instruments can only guide capacity assessment and must be balanced with behavioral observations, the nature of the decision, and intra-individual factors (Palmer & Harmell, 2016). Finally, decision-making capacity can change over time based on cognitive fluctuations or decision complexity (Trachsel, Hermann, & Biller-Andorno, 2015). Elders previously deemed to have intact or impaired decision-making capacity still require decisional capacity assessment if enough compelling evidence of impairment is present.

R. Bennett Blum and Jill Spice

Anastasi, A., & Urbina, S. (1997). *Psychological testing* (7th ed.). Upper Saddle River, NJ: Prentice Hall.

Barkley R. A. (2012). *Executive functions—What they are, how they work, and why they evolved.* New York, NY: Guilford.

Berghmans, R. L. (2008). Informed consent and decision-making capacity in neuromodulation: Ethical considerations. *Neuromodulation: Journal of the International Neuromodulation Society, 11*(3), 156–162.

Berghuis, J. P., Uldall, K. K., & Lalonde, R. (1999). Validity of two scales in identifying HIV-associated dementia. *Journal of Acquired Immune Deficiency Syndromes, 12*(2), 134–140.

Blum, B. (2000). Forensic issues. In B. J. Sadock & V. A. Sadock (Eds.), *Kaplan and Sadock's comprehensive textbook of psychiatry* (8th ed.). Philadelphia, PA: Lippincott Williams & Wilkins.

Boyle, G. (2013). "She's usually quicker than the calculator:" Financial management and decision-making in couples living with dementia. *Health & Social Care in the Community, 21*(5), 554–562.

Breden, T. M., & Vollmann, J. (2004). The cognitive based approach of capacity assessment in psychiatry: A philosophical critique of the MacCAT-T. *Health Care Analysis, 12*(4), 273–283.

Cairns, R., Maddock, C., Buchanan, A., David, A. S., Hayward, P., Richardson, G., ... Hotopf, M. (2005). Reliability of mental capacity assessments in psychiatry in-persons. *British Journal of Psychiatry, 187*(4), 372–378.

Cohen, M. J., Ricci, C. A., Kibby, M. Y., & Edmonds, J. E. (2000). Developmental progression of clock face drawing in children. *Child Neuropsychology, 6*, 64–76.

Crowe, M., Clay, O. J., Sawyer, P., Crowther, M. R., & Allman, R. M. (2008). Education and reading ability in relation to differences in cognitive screening between African American and Caucasian older adults. *International Journal of Geriatric Psychiatry, 23*(2), 222–223.

Gildengers, A. G., Butters, M. A., Seligman, K., McShea, M., Miller, M. D., Mulsant, B. H., ... Reynolds, C. F. (2004). Cognitive functioning in late-life bipolar disorder. *American Journal of Psychiatry, 161*(4), 736–738.

Grisso, T., & Appelbaum, P. S. (1998). *Assessing competence to consent to treatment: A guide for physicians and other health professionals.* New York, NY: Oxford University Press.

Holzer, J. C., Gansier, D. A., Moczynski, N. P., & Folstein, M. F. (1997). Cognitive functions in the informed consent evaluation process: A pilot study. *Journal of the American Academy of Psychiatry and the Law, 25*(4), 531–540.

Jahn, D. R., Dressel, J. A., Gavett, B. E., & O'Bryant, S. E. (2015). An item response theory analysis of the Executive Interview and development of the EXIT8: A Project FRONTIER Study. *Journal of Clinical and Experimental Neuropsychology, 37*(3), 229–242.

Larson, E. B., & Heinemann, A. W. (2010). Rasch analysis of the Executive Interview (The EXIT-25) and introduction of an abridged version (The Quick EXIT). *Archives of Physical Medicine and Rehabilitation, 91*(3), 389–394.

Lichtenberg, P. A., Ficker, L., Rahman-Filipiak, A., Tatro, R., Farrell, C., Speir, J. J., ... Jackman, J. D. (2016). The Lichtenberg Financial Decision Screening Scale (LFDSS): A new tool for assessing financial decision making and preventing financial exploitation. *Journal of Elder Abuse & Neglect, 28*(3), 134–151.

Molloy, D. W., Alemayehu, E., & Roberts, R. (1991). Reliability of a Standardized Mini-Mental State Examination compared with the traditional Mini-Mental State Examination. *American Journal of Psychiatry, 148*(1), 102–105.

Mujic, F., Lebovich, E., Von Heisin, M., Clifford, D., & Prince, M. J. (2014). The Executive Interview (EXIT25) as a tool for assessing executive functioning in older medical and surgical inpatients referred to a psychiatry service: feasibility of creating a brief version. *International Psychogeriatrics, 26*(6), 935–941.

Palmer, B. W., & Harmell, A. L. (2016). Assessment of healthcare decision-making capacity. *Archives of Clinical Neuropsychology, 31*(6), 530–540.

Ramirez, M., Teresi, J. A., Holmes, D., Gurland, B., & Lantigua, R. (2006). Differential item functioning (DIF) and the Mini-Mental State Examination (MMSE): Overview, sample, and issues of translation. *Medical Care, 44*(11, Suppl. 3), S95–S106.

Royall, D. R., Cordes, J. A., & Polk, M. J. (1998). CLOX: An executive clock drawing task. *Journal of Neurology, Neurosurgery, and Psychiatry, 64*(5), 588–594.

Royall, D. R., Espino, D. V., Polk, M. J., Verdeja, R., Vale, S., Gonzales, H., ... Markides, K. P. (2003). Validation of a Spanish translation of the CLOX for use in Hispanic samples: the Hispanic EPESE study. *International Journal of Geriatric Psychiatry, 18*(2), 135–141.

Royall, D. R., Mahurin, R. K., & Gray, K. F. (1992). Bedside assessment of executive cognitive impairment: the executive interview. *Journal of the American Geriatrics Society, 40*(12), 1221–1226.

Shon, J. M., Lee, D. Y., Seo, E. H., Sohn, B. K., Kim, J. W., Park, S. Y., … Woo, J. I. (2013). Functional neuroanatomical correlates of the executive clock drawing task (CLOX) performance in Alzheimer's disease: A FDG-PET study. *Neuroscience, 246*(29), 271–280.

Trachsel, M., Hermann, H., & Biller-Andorno, N. (2015). Cognitive fluctuations as a challenge for the assessment of decision-making capacity in patients with dementia. *American Journal of Alzheimer's Disease and Other Dementias, 30*(4), 360–363.

Whitlatch, C. J. (2013). Person-centered care in the early stages of dementia: Honoring individuals and their choices. *Generations, 37*(3), 30–36.

Yap, P. L., Ng, T. P., Yeo, D., & Henderson, L. (2007). Diagnostic performance of clock drawing test by CLOX in an Asian Chinese population. *Dementia and Geriatric Cognitive Disorders, 24*(3), 193–200.

Web Resources
American Bar Association Commission on Law and Aging: Resources for lawyers, judges, and mental health professionals regarding capacity assessment: http://www.americanbar.org/groups/law_aging/resources/capacity_assessment.html

Mini-Mental State Examination: http://www.ncbi.nlm.nih.gov/pubmed/1202204 (Note that the MMSE is protected under U.S. copyright and should be purchased for use.)

National Center on Elder Abuse: https://ncea.acl.gov

National Centre for the Protection of Older People: http://ncpop.ie/educationandtraining_onlinemodules

National Committee for the Protection of Elder Abuse: http://www.preventelderabuse.org

PARADISE-2 protocol: http://www.bennettblummd.com/id15.html

MENTAL HEALTH SERVICES

The prevalence of most mental illnesses, including substance abuse, is lower among older adults than among younger adults. However, research also indicates that rates for cognitive disorders, particularly dementias caused by Alzheimer's disease, are higher for older adults than for younger adults (Hudson, 2012) and that older adults complete suicide more often than younger adults (WHO, 2014). Despite older adults' experiences with mental illness and suicidality, persons over 65 years of age are less likely to utilize mental health services than younger adults, particularly in rural areas (Karel, Gatz, & Smyer, 2012; Stewart, Jameson, & Curtin, 2015).

When older adults do seek care, they use a variety of mental health services. Traditional services include those provided through community-based agencies and through total and partial hospitalization (Schneider, Kropf, & Kisor, 2000). Many of these programs treat mental illness through medication and counseling techniques such as psychoanalysis, group therapy, and cognitive and behavioral therapies. Elders with more severe, persistent mental illness may use case management, in which a caseworker coordinates services within a network of providers.

Community-watch systems have been developed, whereby workers who have regular contact with older adults are trained to look for potential problems. For instance, mail carriers are asked to watch for uncollected mail or other signs that a resident may have a problem. If a problem is suspected, the carrier contacts a participating state or community agency, which checks on the resident. This system supports elders who are living alone and may have difficulties that affect their daily functioning. Many communities use telephone contact programs through which a worker maintains contact with elders known to be at risk for mental health or other problems. Many senior centers offer daycare programs for those with cognitive impairments. These programs offer services such as recreation, personal care, and nutrition management. Finally, many health clinics and senior and drop-in centers screen for mental illness. To prevent problems, these sites often provide educational workshops to inform elders of risk factors associated with mental illness. If mental health problems are identified, older adults must be referred to a mental health professional.

Several residential programs serve elders with mental illness. In addition to services provided at inpatient psychiatric and state hospital settings, older adults living in skilled nursing facilities can receive mental health treatment as part of their care plan. Many Alzheimer's disease units or campuses have been developed for patient care as the disease progresses. Thus patients can be admitted during the early stages of the disease and be moved to specialized units on the campus to provide support as the disease becomes more debilitating.

PROFESSIONALS AND PROGRAMS

Physicians, psychiatrists, psychologists, social workers, and psychiatric nurse practitioners are some of the professionals who offer geriatric mental health care. Professionals in these disciplines may choose to obtain specialized training in gerontology. Services provided include referral, advocacy, psychotherapy, medication, and service coordination and management. Also, many master's-level programs in gerontology exist. Graduates of these courses provide mostly management services and are generally involved in developing and administering mental health service programs for older adults rather than providing direct mental health services.

Medicare and Medicaid are the two programs that provide coverage for the majority of elders needing mental health services. Medicare, the main health insurance program for people aged 65 years and above, covers a limited amount of mental health services. Part A (hospital insurance) pays 80% of the costs for inpatient psychiatric care, up to a lifetime limit of 190 days. Part B (medical insurance) pays 50% of outpatient mental health services. However, older adults must pay a monthly premium for Part B coverage, as well as extra costs for prescription medications. Medicare Part D program provides coverage for prescription medications, including those prescribed for behavioral health needs. Seniors can record their medications in the online programs during enrollment periods to choose plans that match their needs. Several supplemental insurance programs (e.g., Medigap) provide varying coverage for mental health services not covered by the basic Medicare program. These supplemental programs also require elders to pay monthly premiums (Centers for Medicare & Medicaid Services [CMS], 2012).

Medicaid, the health insurance program for low-income individuals, pays for nursing home care if older adults cannot afford these services. Medicaid also pays for a variety of mental health services, including medication costs, but the type of services covered, the amount paid, and eligibility for services vary from state to state (CMS, 2012). Medicare and Medicaid programs have moved toward a managed care model of providing services in many communities. In these instances, the older adult must obtain a referral from a primary care physician to receive mental health services. A patient not participating in a managed care program needs to seek a provider who accepts Medicare or Medicaid payments.

Many older adults rely on private insurance for their health care. Most health insurance companies offer limited mental health services, and some cover the costs of medications. Older adults also can elect to obtain mental health services through a fee-for-service agreement. Finally, many community mental health centers offer services based on a sliding fee scale for elders who have low incomes, fixed budgets, or both.

Older adults can complete advance directives for mental health care. These directives enable them to specify the type and scope of treatment they would desire if they were unable to articulate their wishes.

GAPS IN AVAILABILITY AND COVERAGE

A major concern about elders with mental illness is their low rate of service use. Many do not seek services from mental health professionals because of the stigma attached to receiving such services (Webb, Jacobs-Lawson, & Waddell, 2009). Consequently, many elders visit their primary care physicians complaining of symptoms that may be caused by mental illness. Unfortunately, many health care providers are not trained to recognize symptoms of mental illness in older adults or to differentiate between behavioral health and other health problems. Health care providers holding stereotypical views of aging may assume that symptoms of mental illness are part of normal aging (Pepin, Segal, & Coolidge, 2009). For this reason, elders with mental illness may be misdiagnosed or not referred to mental health specialists. Furthermore, there is a lack of communication and collaboration between professionals in health care settings and community mental health centers, so many seniors are not receiving comprehensive care (Cummings & Kropf, 2009). When referred for mental health problems, they find few agencies specializing in treating older adults. Many agencies focus on programs for children and young adults with chronic mental illness. Moreover, many agencies lack outreach services, and many older adults who are ill, frail, disabled, or home-bound or who lack transportation cannot access services. Programs that offer outreach services, such as home health care and delivered meals, do not offer mental health services. Finally, many of the mental health services that are available are cost prohibitive to elders on fixed incomes.

Although Medicare and Medicaid cover some mental health services, these programs are designed to focus on health and long-term care. If older adults use Part B for mental health services, the cost can be prohibitive because they must pay 50%. Furthermore, if older adults suffer from severe or persistent mental illness, a limit of 190 days for hospitalization is usually not sufficient for adequate treatment. Purchasing supplemental insurance is not an option for many low-income seniors.

Elders can choose to participate in managed care plans, which often provide some mental health benefits. However, managed care programs are designed for physically functional individuals who have acute health problems. Also, the emphasis in managed care is on cost containment. Thus managed care systems tend to restrict access to specialized psychiatric care or to limit the type and scope of treatment that individuals can receive. Furthermore, many mental health providers outside the managed care system cannot survive financially, which limits elders' choice of providers.

Some legislation has addressed mental health service coverage among health insurance companies, but gaps in coverage still exist. The Mental Health Parity Act requires that all group health plans, and insurance coverage offered in connection with group plans, place dollar limits on mental health benefits equal to those placed on medical and surgical benefits. However, this act does not require health plans to provide mental health services. It also does not mandate guidelines on cost sharing, types of mental health services available, or amount of mental health services one can receive. The Patient Protection and Affordable Care Act addresses some cost issues in Medicare to help make medications and other services more affordable, which may benefit some older adults with mental health needs.

See also Cognitive Changes in Aging; Medicaid; Medicare; Psychotropic Medication Use in Long-Term Care.

Anissa T. Rogers and Ashley B. Kinnaman

Centers for Medicare & Medicaid Services. (2012). What Medicare covers. Retrieved from https://www.medicare.gov

Cummings, S. M., & Kropf, N. P. (2009). Formal and informal support for older adults with severe mental illness. *Aging & Mental Health, 13*(4), 619–627.

Hudson, C. G. (2012). Declines in mental illness over the adult years: An enduring finding or methodological artifact? *Aging and Mental Health, 16*(6), 735–752.

Karel, M. J., Gatz, M., & Smyer, M. (2012). Aging and mental health in the decade ahead: What psychologists need to know. *American Psychologist, 67*, 184–198.

Pepin, R., Segal, D. L., & Coolidge, F. L. (2009). Intrinsic and extrinsic barriers to mental health care among community-dwelling younger and older adults. *Aging & Mental Health, 13*(5), 769–777.

Schneider, R. L., Kropf, N. P., & Kisor, A. J. (2000). *Gerontological social work: Knowledge, service settings, and special populations* (2nd ed.). Belmont, CA: Brooks/Cole.

Stewart, H., Jameson, J. P., & Curtin, L. (2015). The relationship between stigma and self-reported willingness to use mental health services among rural and urban older adults. *Psychological Services, 12*(2), 141–148.

Webb, A. K., Jacobs-Lawson, J. M., & Waddell, E. L. (2009). *Older adults' perceptions of mentally ill older adults. Aging & Mental Health, 13*(6), 838–845.

World Health Organization. (2014). *Preventing suicide: A global imperative*. Geneva, Switzerland: Author.

Web Resources
Administration on Aging: http://www.aoa.dhhs.gov
Alzheimer's Association: http://www.alz.org
Centers for Medicare & Medicaid Services: http://www.medicare.gov
Health Care Financing Administration: http://www.hcfa.gov
National Institute on Aging: http://www.nih.gov

Mild Neurocognitive Disorder

Mild neurocognitive disorder (NCD) is a phase of cognitive dysfunction defined by clinical, intellectual, and functional criteria. Although there is a lack of consensus on how best to characterize mild NCD subjects, studies have revealed several clinical subtypes, including those with impaired memory, those with impairments in multiple cognitive domains with or without memory, and those with impairment in a single nonmemory domain. Efforts to identify the minority of persons whose mild NCD will lead to dementia are intense but far from definitive. Presumptive treatment with medication approved for Alzheimer's disease (AD) does not delay the conversion of mild NCD to dementia and risks adverse reactions (Birks & Flicker, 2006).

Echoing the criteria as discussed by Stokin, Krell-Roesch, Petersen, and Geda (2015); the *Diagnostic and Statistical Manual of Mental Disorders* (5th ed.; *DSM-5*; American Psychiatric Association, 2013); and Ganguli and colleagues' (2011) criteria for *Mild NCD*, the National Institute on Aging–Alzheimer's Association (NIAAA) workgroup proposed revised criteria to diagnose mild NCD due to AD (Sperling et al., 2011): (a) The patient, close associate, or clinician recognizes a change in the patient's cognition. (b) In one or two cognitive domains typically including but not limited to memory, the patient demonstrates decreased performance compared with that of someone with similar age and educational background. Other affected cognitive domains include executive function, attention, language, and visuospatial skills. (c) The patient performs basic activities of daily living despite inefficiently performing complex functional tasks such as paying bills, shopping, and preparing a meal. (d) The patient is not noticeably impaired in social and occupational functioning. In addition, vascular, traumatic, and medical causes must be ruled out. To increase the likelihood that the mild NCD is due to AD, other types of dementia must be ruled out and history consistent with AD genetic factors reported (Albert et al., 2011).

However, the criteria are defined, mild NCD is consistently associated with an increased risk of subsequent dementia. Nonetheless, in a meta-analysis of 41 studies, the overall annual conversion rate from mild NCD to dementia was only 5% to 10% of persons observed. By implication even after 10 years of observation, most individuals labeled with mild NCD do not become demented (Mitchell & Shiri-Feshki, 2009). In contrast, Koepsell and Monsell (2012) cite studies that reveal varied estimates of remission to normal or near-normal cognition ranging from 4% to 15% in clinic-based studies and 29% to 55% in population-based studies. Persons who experienced remission were more likely to exhibit nonamnestic, single-domain mild NCD, less severe cognitive impairment, and absence of the *APOE* e4 allele and to have had a comorbid illness or medication that was associated with intellectual impairment. Interest in establishing criteria for mild NCD is sustained by consensus that the disease process is well underway by the time cognitive symptoms manifest and that disease-modifying interventions, once available, would be most effective when used prior to symptom onset.

BIOMARKERS OF DEMENTIA

There exists a growing body of research on neuropathological features that precede the onset of cognitive impairments and may predict its course. The NIAAA (Sperling et al., 2011) gave considerable importance to the diagnostic role of biomarkers and identified five (Table M.1) that

Table M.1
CEREBROSPINAL FLUID AND BRAIN IMAGING
BIOMARKERS IN ALZHEIMER'S DISEASE

Brain Aβ-plaque deposition
CSF Aβ42
PET Aβ Imaging
Neurodegeneration
CSF tau
Fluorodeoxyglucose-PET
Structural MRI

Aβ, beta-amyloid; CSF, cerebrospinal fluid.
Source: Adapted from Jack et al. (2010).

have been sufficiently examined to be used in observational studies and in therapeutic trials.

It is recognized that low cerebrospinal fluid (CSF) beta-amyloid (Aβ42) is secondary to Aβ accumulation in plaques, leading to its reduced diffusion into the CSF. During the asymptomatic phase of AD, individuals may have biological signs of Aβ accumulation as reflected in low Aβ42 in CSF and/or increased uptake of amyloid PET tracers, such as carbon 11-labeled Pittsburgh compound B (PiB) that labels fibrillar Aβ deposits (Jagus, 2009). Several multicenter studies have shown that decreased Aβ42 displayed good diagnostic performance. In one such study (Shaw et al., 2009), Aβ42 levels were significantly decreased when comparing normal controls (NC) with patients with mild NCD, and patients with mild NCD with those with AD. The same trend was evident in premortem obtained from patients with autopsy-confirmed AD and NCs who were matched for age. In another study (Mattsson et al., 2009), patients with mild NCD that progressed to AD had significantly decreased levels of Aβ42 compared with NCs, patients with stable mild NCD, and patients with mild NCD and other dementias.

When comparing Aβ deposition as reflected in PiB uptake among NCs, patients with mild NCD, and patients with AD, on average the amount of tracer uptake is highest in patients with AD, with decreased amounts seen in mild patients with NCD, and even lower amounts seen in normal older people. Although conclusive results are lacking to establish an association between PiB uptake and cognition, evidence thus far suggests that the relationship is stronger in earlier disease stages and relatively weak

in AD (Koepsell & Monsell, 2012), implying that Aβ deposits may be an early event that plateaus at an early stage.

The second category of biomarkers includes those downstream from neuronal injury. It is thought that increased CSF levels of phospho-tau (P-tau) and total tau (T-tau) occur after their intracellular accumulation disrupts neuronal activity and leads to their release from damaged neurons into the extracellular space. Thus one would see increases in tau in ischemic and traumatic brain injury, and in Creutzfeldt-Jakob disease (Jack et al., 2010). Several studies show high correlations between increased CSF T-tau and P-tau in mild NCD that has progressed to AD. Increased CSF T-tau, P-tau, and decreased Aβ42 were found in mild NCD that progressed to AD after 3 to 6 years, with close to 90% sensitivity. A large multicenter study concluded that the combined measurement of Aβ42, T-tau, and P-tau provided good accuracy in predicting mild NCD progression to AD (Henry et al., 2013).

Brain glucose metabolism as measured by fluorodeoxyglucose-PET (FDG-PET) uptake reflects synaptic activity. FDG-PET studies of patients with AD demonstrate reduced glucose metabolism in the parietotemporal and posterior cingulate cortices, which are involved in memory and other cognitive processes. In mild NCD progressing to AD, greater decreases in FDG uptake correlated with greater cognitive impairment. In contrast, Landau and Mintun (2012) found that among NCs, amyloid deposition was associated with ongoing cognitive decline.

Finally, gray matter loss or hippocampal atrophy seen on structural MRI likely is the last biomarker to become abnormal, reflecting decreased synaptic density, neuronal loss, and cell shrinkage. There is strong evidence that changes in brain structure can be detected with MRI in NCs progressing to mild NCD and AD. Tondelli and Wilcock (2012) found that brain volume differences were present in NCs who did not have memory complaints or cognitive impairments and later progressed to mild NCD and AD. In addition, Jack et al. (2010) found, at 3-year follow-up, significant increases in annualized hippocampal atrophy rates in NCs progressing to mild NCD or AD compared with

NCs who remained stable. Structural MRI measures of atrophy retain highly significant correlations with observed clinical impairment in both the mild NCD and dementia phases of AD. In summary, the sequence of biomarker emergence begins with Aβ deposits followed by tau, hypometabolism, and finally anatomic shrinkage.

Limitations

Unfortunately, the available array of biomarkers has several limitations for both research and clinical purposes. One limitation is the lack of standardization. A second is that the data on potential markers are derived from correlation studies, which may or may not indicate a causal relationship between a marker and the disease. Biomarker comparison studies, studies using a combination of biomarkers, predictive studies in unselected populations, postmortem studies, and studies on the evolution of the marker during disease progression may ultimately determine the utility of biomarkers for the diagnosis of mild NCD.

Clearly, biomarkers are present in mild NCD that progresses to AD, yet the time of onset and points of transition within the disease process remain elusive. The goal of combining clinical and neuropsychological features with biomarkers and neuroimaging is the identification of individuals for whom disease modifying treatments will halt the progression of mild NCD to dementia.

NEUROIMAGING

Many imaging methods have been developed in an attempt to understand disease progression, as well as the pathogenesis of neurocognitive disorders. MRI volumetry has been used extensively in both the diagnosis of mild NCD and Alzheimer's dementia. Prominent volume reduction of the entorhinal cortex and hippocampus have been well established in AD, as shown by MRI volumetry studies. Volume reduction in these regions in patients with mild NCD appears to be intermediate, falling between those of healthy subjects and those with AD. Volume of the superior temporal

sulcus and anterior cingulate cortex have also been demonstrated to differ between patients with mild NCD and age-matched healthy controls (Yin, Li, Zhao, & Feng, 2013). Of particular interest is the idea that MRI volumetry can aid in predicting the conversion of mild NCD to AD. A study by DeToledo-Morrell et al. (2004) examined 27 subjects diagnosed with mild NCD. These patients received a high-resolution MRI scan at baseline and were followed with yearly clinical evaluations. Hippocampal and entorhinal cortex volumes at baseline were compared to determine which of these regions could best differentiate between subjects who converted to AD from those who did not. It was found that the right hemisphere entorhinal volume best predicted conversion to AD (DeToledo-Morrell et al., 2004). MRI volumetry remains valuable in identifying disease process at a preclinical stage of cognitive impairment and may be useful in identifying those at higher risk of developing Alzheimer's dementia.

Voxel-based morphometry (VBM) has also been useful in assessing regional gray matter atrophy. A study by Whitwell et al. (2008) followed 28 patients diagnosed with mild NCD. Patients progressing to AD within 18 months of follow-up showed greater baseline gray matter loss in the medial and inferior temporal lobes, the temporoparietal neocortex, posterior cingulate, precuneus, anterior cingulate, and frontal lobes, as demonstrated by VBM. VBM has been particularly useful in identifying multiple areas of the brain that may play a role in the pathogenesis of mild NCD and AD (Whitwell et al., 2008).

Functional imaging, particularly proton magnetic resonance spectroscopy (MRS), has become increasingly important in clinical settings because it detects metabolic changes due to neurodegenerative disease. Recent MRS studies have investigated patients with both mild NCD and AD. Both subsets of patients showed metabolic disturbances in the left temporal lobe, posterior cingulate cortex, and medial occipital lobe. Significantly lower ratios of myoinositol/creatine-phosphocreatine were seen in patients with mild NCD than in patients with AD, suggesting that increased myoinositol may indicate early pathological changes. Another feature of mild NCD found on MRS is reduced *N*-acetyl aspartate/creatine-phospho-creatine ratio in the left medial temporal lobe and right hippocampus. This finding becomes more widespread in patients who progress to AD. This change is thought to be transitional between normal older adults and those with AD (Yin et al., 2013).

GAIT ABNORMALITIES

Gait dysfunction has been reported to predict progression to dementia in cognitively normal older adults, as well as in those with mild NCD. This area of research may very well provide insight into another aspect of brain function in mild NCD. A 2008 study by Verghese et al. examined 527 subjects aged 70 years and older, 116 of whom met criteria for mild NCD, over a 15-month period. Several standardized gait parameters were measured in these patients and in healthy controls. Quantitative testing (blinded to cognitive assessments and mild NCD diagnosis) revealed more gait dysfunction in subjects with amnestic and nonamnestic mild NCD subtypes than in healthy controls, even after accounting for potential confounders. In addition, gait abnormalities differed between amnestic and nonamnestic subtypes of mild NCD; those with amnestic mild NCD had worse swing time and stride length variability compared with healthy controls, whereas subjects with nonamnestic mild NCD were found to have worse cadence, swing time, and double support time than controls (Verghese et al, 2008). Of particular importance is the effect of gait disturbance on major noncognitive outcomes in this population: falls, loss of functional independence, and disability. Gait abnormalities were indeed found to predict a greater risk of disability in this population. Defining gait function in mild NCD could have utility in clinical settings, by helping to identify patients at risk of developing a greater burden of disability (Verghese et al., 2008).

Michelle Kaplan, Janella Hong, and
Gary J. Kennedy

Albert, M. S., DeKosky, S. T., Dickson, D., Dubois, B., Feldman, H. H., Fox, N. C., ... Phelps, C. H. (2011). The diagnosis of mild cognitive impairment due to Alzheimer's disease: Recommendations from the National Institute on Aging—Alzheimer's Association workgroups on diagnostic guidelines for Alzheimer's disease. *Alzheimer's & Dementia, 7,* 270–279.

American Psychiatric Association. (2013). *Diagnostic and statistical manual of mental disorders* (5th ed.). Arlington, VA: American Psychiatric Publishing.

Birks, J., & Flicker, L. (2006). Donepezil for mild cognitive impairment. *Cochrane Database of Systematic Reviews, 19*(3), CD006104.

DeToledo-Morrell, L., Stoub, T. R., Bulgakova, M., Wilson, R. S., Bennett, D. A., Leurgans, S., ... Turner, D. A. (2004). MRI-derived entorhinal volume is a good predictor of conversion from MCI to AD. *Neurobiology of Aging, 25,* 1197–1203.

Ganguli, M., Blacker, D., Blazer, D. G., Grant, I., Jeste, D. V., Paulsen, J. S., ... The Neurocognitive Disorders Work Group of the American Psychiatric Association's (APA) DSM5 Task Force. (2011). Classification of neurocognitive disorders in DSM-5: A work in Progress. *The American Journal of Geriatric Psychiatry: Official Journal of the American Association for Geriatric Psychiatry, 19*(3), 205–210.

Henry, M. S., Passmore, A. P., Todd, S., McGuinness, B., Craig, D., & Johnston, J. A. (2013). The development of effective biomarkers for Alzheimer's disease: A review. *International Journal of Geriatric Psychiatry, 4,* 331–340.

Jack, C. R., Knopman, D. S., Jagust, W. J., Shaw, L. M., Aisen, P. S., Weiner, M. W., Petersen, R. C., & Trojanowski, J. Q. (2010). Hypothetical model of dynamic biomarkers of the Alzheimer's pathological cascade. *Lancet Neurology, 9,* 119–128.

Jagus, W. (2009). Mapping brain amyloid. *Current Opinion in Neurology, 22,* 356–361.

Koepsell, T. D., & Monsell, S. E. (2012). Reversion from mild cognitive impairment to normal or near-normal cognition: Risk factors and prognosis. *Neurology, 79*(15), 1591–1598.

Landau, S. M., & Mintun, M. A. (2012). Amyloid deposition, hypometabolism, and longitudinal cognitive decline. *Annals of Neurology, 72,* 578–586.

Mattsson, N., Zetterberg, H., Hansson, O., Andreasen, N., Parnetti, L., Jonsson, M., ... Blennow K. (2009). CSF biomarkers and incipient signature in Alzheimer's disease in patients with mild cognitive impairment. *Journal of the American Medical Association, 302*(4), 385–393.

Mitchell, A. J., & Shiri-Feshki, M. (2009). Rate of progression of MCI to dementia—Meta-analysis of 41 robust inception cohort studies. *Acta Psychiatrica Scandinavica, 119,* 252–265.

M

Shaw, L. M., Vanderstichele, H., Knapik-Czajka, M., Clark, C. M., Aisen, P. S., & Petersen, R. C. (2009). Cerebrospinal fluid biomarker signature in Alzheimer's disease neuroimaging initiative subjects. *Annals of Neurology, 65*(4), 403–413.

Sperling, R. A., Aisen, P. S., Beckett, L. A, Bennnett, D. A., Craft, S., Fagan, A. M., … Phelps, C. H. (2011). Toward defining the preclinical stages of Alzheimer's disease: Recommendations from the National Institute on Aging—Alzheimer's association workgroups on diagnostic guidelines for Alzheimer's disease. *Alzheimer's & Dementia, 7,* 280–292.

Stokin, G. B., Krell-Roesch, J., Petersen, R. C. & Geda, Y. E. (2015). Mild neurocognitive disorder: Anold wine in a new bottle. *Harvard Review of Psychiatry, 23* (5), 368–376. doi:10.1097/HRP.0000000000000084

Tondelli, M., & Wilcock, G. K. (2012). Structural MRI changes detectable up to ten years before clinical Alzheimer's disease. *Neurobiology of Aging, 33,* e25–e36.

Verghese, J., Robbins, M., Holtzer, R., Zimmerman, M., Wang, C., Xue, X., & Lipton, R. B. (2008). Gait dysfunction in mild cognitive impairment syndromes. *Journal of the American Geriatrics Society, 56*(7), 1244–1251.

Whitwell, J. L., Shiung, M. M., Przybelski, S. A., Weigand, S. D., Knopman, D. S., Boeve, B. F, … Jack, C. R. (2008). MRI patterns of atrophy associated with progression to AD in amnestic mild cognitive impairment. *Neurology, 70*(7), 512–520.

Yin, C., Li, S., Zhao, W., & Feng, J. (2013). Brain imaging of mild cognitive impairment and Alzheimer's disease. *Neural Regeneration Research, 8*(5), 435–444.

MONEY MANAGEMENT

The elderly population in the United States continues to grow, with 20% of the population expected to be older than 65 years by 2030. Likewise, life expectancy of the elderly is projected to improve. Elders older than 85 years are at greater risk for cognitive impairment and are more likely to require assistance. If elders are to continue to live independently in the community, they must be able to manage their financial affairs and avoid financial exploitation, which is quickly becoming recognized as a significant social phenomenon among vulnerable elderly (Peterson et al., 2014). The ability to carry out the daily money management (DMM) tasks of managing a budget and paying bills are essential tasks of independence. The ability to maintain the tasks of DMM or to find the right person to assist with them, can determine whether a person continues to live independently at home or is left with the only option of institutional care.

DMM assistance to manage financial affairs can range from education and advocacy to guardianship. Factors contributing to a senior's inability to handle day-to-day finances can include visual impairment, physical frailty, and emotional illness. An unsafe neighborhood, lack of transportation, or mobility issues can prevent a person from going to the bank. Memory problems, ranging from forgetfulness to dementia, can lead to self-neglect. Immigrants or elderly with limited literacy in English, as well as lack of familiarity with standard banking, credit, or tax practices, may also need DMM assistance (National Center on Elder Abuse, 2003).

Too often, families do not become aware of the need for money management assistance until they are faced with a crisis. For example, failure to pay bills may trigger an eviction proceeding or a utility company threatening to shut off service. Collection letters, irregularities in payments to credit card companies, unusually large donations, or frequent withdrawals of money are additional signs of self-neglect or a manifestation of financial exploitation (Lachs & Pillemer, 2015).

Seniors who require financial assistance often rely on family or friends, but for many, families are often inaccessible or the senior has outlived all individuals who would have been entrusted with personal affairs. Resources such as automatic check deposit and online bill payment may not be enough to help families in caring for their elder relative's money management needs. DMM services are an important and cost-effective resource for keeping elders in the community (Sacks et al., 2012). Most do not know where to start looking for assistance, and finding programs or private help varies greatly, depending on where they live and what they can afford. Services are not standardized or well publicized, and the absence of regulation allows almost anyone to offer DMM assistance and does little to protect elders from those who would exploit them.

DMM services vary widely, and when families are seeking assistance, they are looking for someone to help with any or all of the tasks of DMM, including:

- Sifting through letters and bills
- Helping with medical insurance claims and advocating for proper payment
- Assisting with paying bills, which includes writing checks for the senior to sign and arranging for automatic bill payment or online bill payment
- Helping with banking: transferring money between accounts, arranging for direct deposits, and balancing checkbooks
- Setting up a method for the senior to access cash for daily expenses
- Determining budgets and tracking expenditures
- Filling out forms and entitlement applications and advocating for the senior
- In some instances, serving as representative payee, power of attorney, or guardian with authority to handle financial transactions, administer benefits, and make decisions as needed

Good DMM, no matter who provides it, begins with a thorough assessment. It includes the identification and evaluation of existing supports, an analysis of available financial resources and entitlements, financial responsibilities and expenditures, and evidence of possible financial exploitation (National Center on Elder Abuse, 2003), as well as a full assessment of the person's health and functional abilities. The daily money manager must distinguish between the inability to handle money tasks and the inability to make decisions about money. If there are questions about the senior's cognitive capacity, a psychiatric assessment is necessary to determine whether the elder is an appropriate candidate for DMM. Only in instances in which a senior is able to understand and work with the DMM professional or program should DMM be considered. If a person lacks capacity for decision making, a referral to adult protective services

or other legal intervention, such as the appointment of a guardian, may be necessary (Lachs & Pillemer, 2015).

Many senior citizens needing DMM need additional social services, and money-management problems are often early signs that they need other support. Thus DMM assistance should not preclude the need for other professionals. A DMM provider should be a part of the interprofessional long-term care team.

The number of nonprofit agencies, for-profit agencies, and public agencies providing DMM continues to grow, although a small number of agencies nationwide provide these services. Some agencies provide DMM exclusively, whereas others offer it as a continuum of health and social services, and the scope of DMM services offered varies widely among service providers. There is no governmental oversight of DMM providers. The National Resource Center for Services (NRCPDS) assists states, agencies, and organizations in offering services to people with disabilities, including older adults. These programs have been introduced into Medicaid programs in 15 states through the Cash & Counseling grant.

Despite the recognized value of DMM, many community agencies have chosen not to provide it because of its labor-intensive costs, insufficient funding to subsidize DMM programs, and fear of liability or because seniors are reluctant or cannot afford to pay for these services. To assist in the development of DMM programs, the Brookdale Center for Healthy Aging's Sadin Institute for Law and Public Policy in New York City developed the Daily Money Management Assistance Program to encourage and assist care-management agencies to offer DMM services safely and effectively. Research supports the efficacy of this program (Sacks et al., 2012) and demonstrates that the combined DMM and comprehensive case-management services is a cost-effective alternative that enables elders to age in place.

To fill the need for DMM assistance, a new type of practitioner, the daily money manager, has become available in many parts of the United States. Professional qualifications of the daily money manager may vary as well.

The American Association of Daily Money Managers (AADMM) has a website to assist in locating a manager. The AADMM, with over 700 members, has published a code of ethics and standards of practice. The site also guides the consumer with questions to ask when interviewing a perspective manager. The charge for DMM services is dependent on location and the complexity of the situation.

Although all successful relationships are built on trust, it is essential that all parties entering into a formal DMM relationship do so with written contracts that delineate the roles and responsibilities of the daily money manager. Only accurate records about all transactions and strict adherence to written policies and procedures can hope to protect the parties against misunderstandings and potential lawsuits. DMM programs or practitioners should be bonded or insured, although experts report that lawsuits are rare (National Center on Elder Abuse, 2003).

A money manager should use the least restrictive interventions available to help the senior manage financial affairs. A senior with a trusted family member or friend should consider establishing a durable power of attorney to prevent the need for a guardian if they lose capacity. The powers can be broad or limited by the elder. A power of attorney could also be abused because there is no real legal oversight. For those who have lost the capacity to handle their finances, additional tools such as representative payee or guardianship should be considered. Although guardianship is the most restrictive measure (because it takes away the older person's rights), it also provides the most protection with the court's oversight of the elder's affairs.

As seniors age and find it more difficult to manage their financial affairs, they risk financial exploitation and institutionalization. DMM is becoming an essential component of any successful long-term care system and has the goal of helping seniors live safely in the community.

See also Adult Protective Services; Crime Victimization; Elder Mistreatment: Overview; Elder Neglect; Financial Abuse.

Janet M. Bairardi

Lachs, M., & Pillemer, K. (2015). Elder abuse. *New England Journal of Medicine, 373,* 1947–1956. doi:10.1056/NEJMra1404688

National Center on Elder Abuse. (2003, June). *Daily money management programs: A protection against elder abuse.* Washington, DC: Author. Retrieved from http://www.ncea.aoa.gov/Resources/Publication/docs/DailyMoneyManagement.pdf

Peterson, J., Burnes, D., Caccamise, P., Mason, A., Henderson, C., Wells, M., & Lachs, M. (2014). Financial exploitation of older adults: a population-based prevalence study. *Journal of General Internal Medicine, 29*(12), 1615–1623. doi:10.1007/s11606-014-2946-2

Sacks, D., Das, D., Romanick, R., Caron, M., Morane, C., & Fahs, M. C. (2012). The value of daily money management: An analysis of outcomes and costs. *Journal of Evidence-Based Social Work, 9,* 498–511. doi:10.1080/15433714.2011.581530

Web Resources

American Association of Daily Money Managers: http:// www.aadmm.com

Brookdale Center for Health Aging: https://brookdale.org/policy/daily-money-management-assistance-program

Elder Justice Roadmap: https://www.justice.gov/elderjustice/research/roadmap.html

Federal Deposit Insurance Corporation: Money Smart—A Financial Education Program: http://www.fdic.gov/consumers/consumer/money smart/OlderAdult.html

National Center on Elder Abuse: https://ncea.acl.gov

National Committee for the Prevention of Elder Abuse: http://www.preventelderabuse.org/elderabuse/fin_abuse.html

National Council on Aging: Money Management: https://www.ncoa.org/economic-security/money-management

National Resource Center for Participant-Directed Services (NRCPDS): http://www.bc.edu/schools/gssw/nrcpds

N

NATIONAL ASIAN PACIFIC CENTER ON AGING

Web Resource
National Asian Pacific Center on Aging: http://www
.napca.org

In 1979, the specific needs of the aging Asian American and Pacific Islander (AAPI) population were recognized at the federal level. The National Asian Pacific Center on Aging (NAPCA) has directly served tens of thousands of AAPI seniors who represent the fastest-growing segment of the aging population in the country. The AAPI aging community is faced with many unique challenges, including cultural and language barriers and access to services and employment opportunities. NAPCA has brought critical issues impacting the AAPI aging community to the forefront of national debates.

NAPCA is committed to the dignity, well-being, and quality of life of Asian Pacific Americans (APAs) in their senior years. The goals of NAPCA are as follows:

- To advocate on behalf of the AAPI aging community at the local, state, and national levels
- To educate AAPI seniors and the general public on the needs of the APA aging community
- To empower AAPI seniors and the aging network to meet the increasing challenges facing the AAPI aging community.

The organization operates employment programs for older workers and conducts policy and research projects among 10 geographic multiethnic and multilingual AAPI elder communities. They develop useful, accessible, and accurate information on health care access. Materials on Medicare, Medicaid, and dual-eligible state buy-in programs and affordable health care for low-income elders and other information are available on its website.

Elizabeth A. Capezuti

NATIONAL CONSUMER VOICE FOR QUALITY LONG-TERM CARE

The National Consumer Voice for Quality Long-Term Care ("Consumer Voice") is the leading national organization representing consumers in issues related to long-term care, facilitating them to be empowered to advocate for themselves. They are a primary source of information and tools for consumers, families, caregivers, advocates, and ombudsmen to help ensure quality care for the individual. The activities of the Consumer Voice include:

- Advocate for public policies that support quality care and quality of life responsive to consumers' needs in all long-term care settings
- Empower and educate consumers and families with the knowledge and tools that they need to advocate for themselves
- Train and support individuals and groups that empower and advocate for consumers of long-term care
- Promote the critical role of direct-care workers and best practices in quality-care delivery.

The Consumer Voice was originally formed as the National Citizens' Coalition for Nursing Home Reform (NCCNHR) to address public concerns about poor quality care in nursing homes. It was the culmination of advocacy works by those working for Ralph Nader and later for the Gray Panthers. Elma Holder, NCCNHR founder, was working with the Gray Panthers when she organized a group meeting of advocates from across the country to attend a nursing home

N

industry conference in Washington, DC, in 1975. Representatives of 12 citizen action groups met and spoke collectively to the industry about the need for serious reform in nursing home conditions. The consumer attendees were inspired to develop a platform of common concerns and formed a new organization to represent the consumer's voice at the national level. Most of the original members had witnessed and endured personal experiences with substandard nursing home conditions.

The Consumer Voice's current 20-member board, which includes residents of nursing homes, represents the grassroots membership of concerned advocates of quality long-term care nationwide. Consumer-controlled member groups elect the board and meet quarterly to establish policies and help direct financing and programming issues.

The Consumer Voice has 200 member groups, with a growing individual membership of more than 2,000. Members and subscribers to the Consumer Voice compose a diverse and caring coalition of local citizen action groups, state and local long-term care ombudsmen, legal services programs, religious organizations, professional groups, nursing home employees' unions, concerned providers, national organizations, and growing numbers of family and resident councils in nearly all 50 states.

The Consumer Voice provides information and leadership on federal and state regulatory and legislative policy development and models and strategies to improve care and life for residents of nursing homes and other long-term care facilities. Ongoing work addresses issues such as the following:

- Inadequate staffing in nursing homes, particularly all levels of nursing staff
- Poor working conditions, salaries, and benefits for long-term care workers
- Maintenance of residents' rights and empowerment of residents
- Support for family members and development of family councils
- Development and support for the long-term care ombudsman program
- Minimization of the use of physical and chemical restraints

- High cost of poor care, such as pressure injuries, dehydration, incontinence, and contracture of residents' muscles
- Accountability to taxpayers for nursing home expenditures and failure to fulfill government contracts.

Elizabeth A. Capezuti

Web Resource
National Consumer Voice for Long-Term Care: http://www.theconsumervoice.org

NATIONAL COUNCIL ON AGING

The National Council on Aging (NCOA) is the nation's first association of organizations and professionals dedicated to promoting the dignity, self-determination, well-being, and contributions of older persons. NCOA's 2,000 partners include senior centers, area agencies on aging, adult day service centers, faith-based service organizations, senior housing facilities, employment services, consumer groups, and leaders from academia, business, and labor.

Founded in 1950, NCOA helps community organizations enhance the lives of older adults, turns creative ideas into programs and services that help older people in hundreds of communities, and is a national voice and powerful advocate for public policies, societal attitudes, and business practices that promote vital aging. NCOA was instrumental in the development of Foster Grandparents, Meals on Wheels, Family Friends, and dozens of other innovative programs for older adults.

NCOA provides leadership, technical assistance, tools, and training to community-service organizations. It conducts research and demonstration projects on the impact of promising innovations and supports the adaptation of proven interventions. NCOA also cosponsors community service jobs for low-income seniors.

Elizabeth A. Capezuti

Web Resource
The National Council on Aging: http://www.ncoa.org

NATIONAL GERONTOLOGICAL NURSING ASSOCIATION

The National Gerontological Nursing Association (NGNA) was founded in 1984 and is dedicated to the clinical care of older adults across diverse care settings. Members include clinicians, educators, and researchers with vastly different educational preparation, clinical roles, and interest in practice issues. Many NGNA members are active participants in their local/state chapters of NGNA.

The purpose of NGNA is to improve nursing care given to older adults. Among some of the values described are:

- *Inclusiveness:* Evidenced in appreciation of the importance of diverse perspectives and experience
- *Respect:* Evidenced in constructive attitude and behavior among all who are dedicated to quality nursing care for older adults
- *Innovation:* Evidenced in creative thinking and flexibility in the continuous pursuit of effective responses to ever-changing conditions
- *Responsiveness:* Evidenced in the commitment to knowledgeable practices that make a positive difference.

Elizabeth A. Capezuti

Web Resource
National Gerontological Nursing Association: http://www.ngna.org

NATIONAL INDIAN COUNCIL ON AGING

The National Indian Council on Aging, Inc. (NICOA) was founded in 1976 by members of the National Tribal Chairmen's Association that called for a national organization to advocate for improved, comprehensive health and social services to American Indian and Alaska Native elders. NICOA provides leadership and advocacy for Indian aging issues and has been actively involved in public policy and research efforts on federal, state, and local levels. NICOA also acts as a National Sponsor of the federal Senior Community Service Employment Program (SCSEP) in 14 states through a grant from the U.S. Department of Labor. SCSEP is part of a network of national organizations and state governments that offer the only federally assisted job-training program focused on the needs of low-income older adults. The NICOA SCSEP mission is to provide opportunity for low-income elders through paid training, meaningful community service, and skills development.

A 13-member board of directors composed of American Indian and Alaska Native Elders, representing each of the 12 Bureau of Indian Affairs regions, and the National Association of Title VI Grantees govern NICOA. The voting membership consists of American Indian and Alaska Native Elders aged 55 years and older.

NICOA's overall objectives are as follows:

- Enhance communications and cooperation with organizations that represent and advocate for Native American elders
- Provide information and technical assistance for Native American communities to improve health care for elders
- Network to maximize resources and increase the efficiency and effectiveness of the service-delivery systems for elders
- Provide information, reports, and expert testimony requested by Tribal Nations and the U.S. Congress
- Provide a clearinghouse for information on issues affecting American Indian and Alaska Native Elders

Elizabeth A. Capezuti

Web Resource
National Indian Council on Aging: http://www.nicoa.org

N

NATIONAL INSTITUTE ON AGING

The National Institute on Aging (NIA), one of the 27 institutes and centers of the National Institutes of Health, leads a broad scientific effort to understand the nature of aging and to extend the healthy, active years of life. In 1974, Congress granted authority to form NIA to provide leadership in aging research, training, health-information dissemination, and other programs relevant to aging and older people. Subsequent amendments to this legislation designated the NIA as the primary federal agency on Alzheimer's disease research.

NIA's mission is to improve the health and well-being of older Americans through research and, specifically, to:

- Support and conduct high-quality research on aging processes, age-related diseases, and special problems and needs of the aged
- Foster the development of research and clinician scientist in aging
- Provide research resources
- Disseminate information about aging and advances in research to the public, health care professionals, and scientific community, among a variety of audiences.

NIA sponsors research on aging through extramural and intramural programs. The extramural program funds research and training at universities, hospitals, medical centers, and other public and private organizations nationwide. The intramural program conducts basic and clinical research in Baltimore, MD, and on the NIH campus in Bethesda, MD.

Elizabeth A. Capezuti

Web Resource
The National Institute on Aging: http://www.nia.nih
.gov/AboutNIA

NATIONAL LONG-TERM CARE OMBUDSMAN PROGRAM

Long-term care ombudsmen are advocates for older adults who reside in nursing homes, board and care homes, assisted-living facilities, and other adult care facilities. Their responsibilities, described in Title VII of the Older Americans Act (OAA), include representing residents' interests before government agencies and seeking administrative, legal, and other means to ensure the health, safety, welfare, and rights of residents. They are also responsible for providing consumer and public education on issues and concerns related to long-term care and facilitating public discussion on related laws, policies, and actions. In addition, they promote citizen organization and participation through various programs; offer technical support for the development of resident and family councils; protect the well-being and rights of residents; identify, investigate, and resolve complaints made by or on behalf of residents; and provide information to residents about long-term care services.

The growing elderly population residing in long-term care facilities, especially the oldest of this demographic, has had a significant impact on the ombudsman program. The ombudsman program serves the vital public purpose of contributing to the well-being of long-term care residents and their families. Many long-term care residents are frail or disabled, have Alzheimer's disease or other dementias, or have other limitations of communication, which may limit the ability to ascertain their informed consent and care preferences. Although many residents receive quality care in long-term care facilities, some suffer neglect or are victims of mental, physical, and other kinds of abuse. Each state is required by the OAA to have trained staff and volunteer ombudsmen visit long-term care facilities to monitor conditions and provide a voice for those unable to speak for themselves.

The Long-Term Care Ombudsman Program (LTCOP) is funded under Title VII (i.e., Vulnerable Elder Rights Protection Activities), with additional funding provided by state and local governments and community agencies. The legislation also funds training and technical assistance to state and local ombudsmen. Within each state, the LTCOP operates within the state unit on aging. Each state designates a long-term care ombudsman to develop a statewide program for the identification, investigation, and submission of complaints on behalf of residents. For example, in California, state ombudsmen must, "represent the interests of the residents before governmental agencies and seek administrative, legal, and other remedies to protect the health, safety, welfare, and rights of the residents" (Office of the State Long-Term Care Ombudsman, 2012). When ombudsmen express resident needs and interests, residents are empowered with choice and dignity. The OAA also has a provision that protects ombudsmen from threats of willfulinterference from any state or federal government agencies.

The word *ombudsman*, which derives from the Swedish language, refers to a public official who is appointed to investigate citizens' complaints concerning local or national government agencies. More generally, ombudsmen act as liaisons, supporters, and friends who can provide information and guidance. The LTCOP first began in 1972 as a five-state pilot program in response to widespread reports of poor quality in nursing homes. Today, the program is active in all 50 states administered by the Administration on Aging (AoA). The mission of the program, as mandated by the OAA, is to seek the resolution of problems and advocate for the rights of residents of long-term care facilities with the goal of enhancing their quality of life and care.

Program data for the year 2013 indicate that 1,233 full-time equivalent staff and 8,290 volunteers were trained and certified to investigate and resolve complaints, highlighting the extensive services provided to residents in long-term care facilities. In their role as ombudsmen, these staff members worked to resolve 592 complaints initiated by residents, their families, and other concerned individuals. Of these, 73% were resolved or partially resolved to the satisfaction of the resident or complainant. Furthermore, 335,088 consultations with individuals were performed across 70% of all nursing homes and

29% of all board and care, assisted-living and other homes at least quarterly, and 5,417 training sessions were conducted in facilities on topics such as residents' rights.

The most frequently lodged complaints were about the quality, quantity, variation and choice of food; poor staff attitudes; violations of residents' rights; lost items; premature discharge or eviction notices; the administration and organizations of medications; and the disrepair and or hazardous aspects of buildings and equipments. If a problem is not resolved, the ombudsman can suggest alternatives, such as filing a complaint with the state's regulatory agency. Ombudsmen are not regulators or surveyors, but rather meet with facility staff members and residents to educate them about residents' rights. They can attend resident and family councils within a facility and encourage residents and families to do so as well. A resident or family member's name cannot be used in the follow-up of a complaint unless permitted by the resident or person acting on the resident's behalf. Ombudsman records are confidential and cannot be read by facility staff.

Ombudsmen encourage residents and families to use the care-planning process to ensure that residents receive individualized care. Care-planning sessions are held quarterly or when changes in the resident's condition warrant them and include facility staff (including nursing assistants), family, and the resident. An ombudsman can suggest how to make these sessions more productive and how to use the sessions to address various problems. At the resident's request, the ombudsman may attend a care-planning session to advocate for and assist them. In addition, ombudsmen work to address systemic issues to improve quality of care.

The effectiveness of the ombudsman program varies from state to state. Across states, there is significant variety in the interpretation and implementation of certain provisions of the act related to the ombudsman program, which has resulted in residents of long-term care facilities receiving inconsistent services from ombudsman programs in some states. The efforts of the long-term care ombudsmen, summarized in the National Ombudsman Reporting System (see the AoA website), include a number of facilities visited, types of complaints handled, and the kinds of complaints filed with ombudsmen. This data which has been collected since 2013, offers a clear picture of the extent of ombudsman activities both nationally and within each state.

Margaret Salisu

Office of the State Long-Term Care Ombudsman, SB-345. (2012). Retrieved from https://leginfo.legislature.ca.gov/faces/billTextClient.xhtml?bill_id=201120120SB345

Web Resources
Administration on Aging: LTC Ombudsman National and State Data: http://www.aoa.gov/aoa_programs/elder_rights/Ombudsman/National_State_Data/index.aspx
Consumer Coalition on Assisted Living: http://www.ccal.org
Eldercare Locator: http://www.eldercare.gov/eldercare.NET/Public/index.aspx
National Consumer Voice for Quality Long-Term Care: http://www.theconsumervoice.org
National Long-Term-Care Ombudsman Resource Center: http://www.ltcombudsman.org
Nursing Home Compare, Health Care Financing Administration: http://www.medicare.gov/NHCompare

NATURALLY OCCURRING RETIREMENT COMMUNITIES (NORCs)

The term naturally occurring retirement community (NORC) was first introduced in the early 1980s by Michael E. Hunt to describe age-integrated housing developments, buildings, and neighborhoods that were not planned or designed for older people but evolved to house large heterogeneous concentrations of people 60 years of age or older who are aging in place (Hunt & Hunt, 1985). As such housing configurations of older adults have proliferated, advocates have developed and promoted the NORC Supportive Service Program (NORC-SSP) model and integrated service delivery systems to transform communities and enhance the provision of programs and services that support aging-in-place.

The Older American Act Amendments of 2006 (42 U.S.C. § 3032k, Title IV, §422) defined the NORC as a community with a concentrated population of older individuals, which may include a residential building, a housing complex, an area (including a rural area) of single family residences, or a neighborhood composed of age-integrated housing (where 40% of the heads of households are older individuals). It can also be where a critical mass of older individuals exists, based on local factors that, taken in total, allow an organization to achieve efficiencies in the provision of health and social services to older individuals living in the community. It is not an institutional care or assisted-living setting.

Unlike purpose-built senior-housing or retirement communities, NORCs cannot be built or developed. NORCs evolve over time as people age in place or can emerge as a result of in-migration, when people at or near retirement relocate. NORCs can develop in communities that have experienced significant out-migrations of younger people, leaving behind older residents who cannot leave their homes and/or desire to remain in their homes. As the number of people older than the age of 65 years increases, NORCs will be more prevalent throughout the United States as increasing numbers of people age in place. This has the potential to change the composition of many American communities, many of which are or will become NORCs as the proportion of older residents living in them grows.

NORC SUPPORTIVE SERVICE PROGRAM MODEL

The NORC-SSP is a partnership between housing entities or neighborhoods, residents, health and social service providers, governments, and philanthropies to (a) organize a range of coordinated health, social services and (b) integrate community-building activities on-site, with the goal of promoting "healthy" and "successful" aging and providing calibrated supports as individual needs evolve. The model builds on the critical role that communities play in how well people age and the important resources that must be arranged to support people of all functional abilities. NORCs are staffed by multi-disciplinary teams of social workers and nurses, with the older residents carrying multiple volunteer and advisory roles. Residents are eligible for participation on the basis of age (i.e., 60 years and older) and residence (i.e., live in the NORC-designated area).

NORC-SSP services are designed to meet the needs of the residents of the NORC. The Jewish Federations of North America identify the core component services of a NORC to include:

- Case management, assistance, and social work services
- Health care management, assistance, and prevention programs
- Education, socialization, and recreational activities
- Volunteer opportunities for program participants.

Social work services provide information and referral, benefits and entitlements advocacy, biopsychosocial assessment and casework support, individual and family counseling, service coordination, monitoring for changing status of clinically complex or fragile individuals, assistance negotiating the systems and services available under the public programs, and education and support for clients, family members, and paid and unpaid caregivers.

Health care-related services utilize both population-based community health principles and individual care-management protocols. Services include individual care management to help individuals live with and manage chronic conditions and address acute situations, nonreimbursable but necessary monitoring; care coordination; support to maintain frail individuals at home; physical assessments, regular blood pressure monitoring, and individual instruction; advocacy in negotiating the myriad health care systems; coordination with primary care physicians and on-site social workers; and health promotion, prevention, and wellness programs.

Diverse educational and recreational opportunities are designed to engage a broad mix of the older residents and include lectures on many topics, an array of classes, discussion and support groups, and health talks with health care professionals. Many of these activities are identified and led by residents.

Community engagement through volunteer opportunities makes it possible for older people to take on new community roles as program ambassadors, leaders, and program extenders, in addition to that of consumers of service. Their knowledge and understanding of their communities are essential to informing the planning process during a program's formative stages, setting priorities as programs evolve, and identifying the resources, talents, and skills within each community that can be harnessed.

Ancillary services are often developed in response to the unique needs or local conditions of the NORC. Programs have the flexibility to develop additional supports and services that draw on the social capital found within the NORC as well as leverage the resources found in the larger surrounding community.

CURRENT EFFORTS

The prototype of the NORC-SSP housing-based model was developed in 1986 in a moderate-income high-rise housing development in New York City. Based on successful replication in two other housing developments, New York State enacted the legislation and funding to establish the first public policy to encourage the development of NORC-SSPs in housing developments that met state-specific older-population density requirements in 1995. New York City followed suit with similar policies in 1999. In 2005, New York State modified legislation to add the neighborhood-based model to its public policy approach to address the need for NORC-SSPs in suburban or rural low-rise and single-family homeowner neighborhoods.

In 2006, the United Hospital Fund and New York City's Department for the Aging began the "Health Indicators in NORC Programs Initiative." This initiative identifies significant health issues in particular communities and designs programs of intervention to proactively target the issues. The aim of the health indicator program is to improve the management of chronic disease among NORC members. Baseline data have been collected on more than 6,000 older adults living in NORCs, and the health-based interventions are underway.

The NORC-SSPs have triggered other community aging initiative work. In 2015, the White House Conference on Aging discussed age-friendly community initiatives (AFCIs). The goal is for future work to capitalize on creating living environments that will support the booming aging population. Some concepts of NORC-SSP will be included. A major tenet of AFCIs is to build on the community relationships to grow services and resources. Greenfield (2014) conducted a qualitative research study in 10 NORC-SSP programs in New Jersey, which reinforced the importance of social capital in enhancing community-based services.

Today, more than 80 programs across the country have received public support. The majority of the NORC-SSPs are in New York. NORC-SSP legislation has been enacted and ongoing funding has been established by both New York state's and New York City's governments to support both housing and neighborhood-based NORC-SSPs. An equal amount of private support rounds out the budgets of these programs. Other states are considering similar approaches.

Interest in this model has also taken hold at the federal level. Recognizing that aging-in-place is occurring across the country and innovations are needed to manage the aging population boom, congressional grants have been awarded to nonprofit agencies in 42 different localities (located in 25 states) for NORC program development. Administered through the Administration on Aging (AoA) in the U.S. Department of Health and Human Services, these efforts are underway in many housing developments and neighborhoods.

See also Retirement.

Donna E. McCabe

Greenfield, E. A. (2014). Community aging initiatives and social capital developing theories of change in the context of NORC Supportive Service Programs. *Journal of Applied Gerontology, 33*(2), 227–250.

Hunt, M. E., & Hunt, G. (1985). Naturally occurring retirement communities. *Journal of Housing for the Elderly, 3*(3/4), 3–21.

Web Resources

2015 White House Conference on Aging: https://whitehouseconferenceonaging.gov

Administration on Aging Initiatives for Aging in Place: https://aoa.acl.gov/AoA_Programs/HCLTC/CIAIP/index.aspx

NORC Blueprint: A Guide to Community Action: http://www.norcblueprint.org/faq

Older Americans Act Amendments of 2006: http://www.gpo.gov/fdsys/pkg/PLAW-109publ365/html/PLAW-109publ365.htm

United Hospital Fund Aging in Place: http://www.uhfnyc.org/initiatives/aging-in-place

United Hospital Fund: Health Indicators: https://www.uhfnyc.org/initiatives/aging-in-place/health-indicators

NEUROPSYCHOLOGICAL ASSESSMENT

DEFINITIONS AND HISTORY

Neuropsychology involves the study of brain–behavior relationships. Clinical neuropsychology focuses on the behavioral consequences of disordered brain function. Although the brain bases of behavior have been a topic of great interest to poets, philosophers, and scientists for centuries, the modern discipline of clinical neuropsychology is relatively new, having emerged from the disciplines of neurology and psychology in the mid-20th century. Pioneering work by A. R. Luria, a Russian neurologist, focused on qualitative analysis and detailed observation of individual behavior, and this method was further developed by American psychologists such as Ralph Reitan, with an emphasis on psychometrics. Both approaches inform current neuropsychological assessment, with rigorous statistical and operational approaches being blended with careful observation of the individual; the generated information is interpreted within the context of that individual's medical history, mood, education, occupation, and general life experiences.

A clinical neuropsychological evaluation, then, involves a detailed interview and the administration of tasks assessing various aspects of cognitive function in the attempt to make statements about the integrity of those functions. The strength of such detailed assessment derives not only from the unique perspective of the psychologist trained in behavioral observation, but also from the fact that the tests are reliable and valid measures of the abilities in question and that normative data are available to aid interpretation: Most neuropsychological tests have been given to a large number of healthy men and women of different ages, educational levels, and even cultural backgrounds. As such, a given individual's performance can be compared with that of similar individuals and is judged according to statistically defined criteria for distinguishing what is likely to be normal from that which is abnormal. Normal age-related changes in some abilities, such as memory, are thus taken into account when interpreting test performance. Readers can refer to detailed resources for more information about areas assessed and tests used (Lezak, Howieson, Bigler, & Tranel, 2012; Strauss, Sherman, & Spreen, 2006), as well as issues relating to neuropsychological assessment and intervention in older adult populations (Ravdin & Katzen, 2013).

PURPOSES AND OUTCOMES

A clinical neuropsychological assessment may serve a variety of purposes. Although modern neuroimaging techniques can readily detect medical conditions such as strokes and tumors, neuropsychological assessment can aid in diagnosis of other conditions such as progressive neurological disorders, in which early and subtle brain changes, not yet detectable on routine imaging, may be evident in the pattern of neuropsychological strengths and weaknesses. For example, the preclinical phase of dementia is associated with certain subtle changes in cognition that can only be detected by careful assessment of a broad range of cognitive skills, interpreted with an understanding of what constitutes a change for that individual. An assessment may also address which among a group

of possible explanations for cognitive change is most likely. As there is not always a direct correspondence between neuroimaging findings of brain atrophy, structural lesions, or metabolic change and the level or type of cognitive impairment, neuropsychological assessment can serve the basic purpose of detecting the presence of cognitive impairment with identified disorders. Such detection can be crucial in determining functional status and subsequent treatment.

Another purpose of neuropsychological assessment is to aid in treatment planning after injury or illness. This may involve generating an informed discharge plan after hospitalization or developing an appropriate rehabilitation program or behavioral management plan. Information about and training in appropriate intervention or lifestyle strategies may be offered to clients and caregivers. Whenever interventions are offered, assessment results can serve to evaluate treatment efficacy and guide adjustments to the treatment plan as the client's needs or capabilities change.

Related to treatment efficacy is another purpose for neuropsychological assessment, the measurement of change over time. For older individuals having sustained a stroke, who are undergoing surgery for tumor removal or shunt insertion or in whom an early neurodegenerative process is suspected, an initial assessment may serve as a baseline against future comparison. Follow-up assessments can be used by the rehabilitation team for on-going guidance of effective treatment or by the referring physician to enhance diagnostic confidence.

Assessments can also be requested for financial or forensic purposes, such as when the information will be used for assistance with decisions about competence in decision making, suitability for disability or other compensation, or medicolegal purposes in civil or criminal suits. Finally, neuropsychological tests are useful research in brain–behavior relationships that will ultimately inform not only knowledge but also future clinical practice.

The typical outcome of an assessment is a report that integrates information from interviews, medical documents, and the evaluation. A conclusion or overall interpretation of the findings is provided, often with recommendations for further steps in the diagnostic process

N

or in treatment of symptoms. Statements about vocational impact, implications for daily living, or driving safety may be made, to the extent that a neuropsychological assessment can provide valid information about these activities.

PROCESS

A typical evaluation includes a clinical interview, test administration, and feedback. Multiple cognitive domains, including attention, processing speed, verbal and visual memory, language, perception and spatial abilities, and executive skills (i.e., planning/organization, attention management, generation of novel ideas, abstract thinking, and flexibility of problem solving), are assessed. In many cases, aspects of sensory and motor skills are also evaluated. The exact nature of the assessment is informed by the possible diagnosis, the reason for the evaluation, and the limitations of the individual. The tests are scored along relevant dimensions, including speed and accuracy, and the result is compared with norms appropriate for that individual. In addition to the neuropsychological domains evaluated, measures of mood and/or academic skill are often obtained. In an interprofessional setting, the neuropsychologist may work with other health professionals such as occupational therapists to obtain an understanding of how the pattern of strengths and weaknesses observed in the test situation translate to daily function.

MAKING REFERRALS

How does a health care professional know whether a neuropsychological assessment will be useful in a given case? Neuropsychological assessments may serve a variety of purposes, but not everyone needs, or is appropriate for, such intensive assessment. When considering elder individuals, one must keep in mind factors that limit the use of this type of evaluation. These include sensory limitations such as compromised vision or hearing; decreased facility in the language in which the client is tested; severe cognitive impairment such as delirium or clear dementia; severe mood disorder or psychosis, which should be treated before referral; and decreased stamina that precludes tolerance of a lengthy assessment.

In addition to people for whom an assessment could benefit from a treatment planning/efficacy perspective, individuals who complain of cognitive problems but do well on typical cognitive screens may also benefit from more detailed examination of various skills to aid diagnosis and guide treatment.

WHAT THE CLIENT CAN EXPECT

A person referred for a neuropsychological evaluation should normally expect the appointment to last several hours. Given the length of the evaluation, clients are given breaks when needed, and in some cases appointments can be conducted over multiple days.

An evaluation typically consists of a clinical interview, testing, and feedback. During the interview, the neuropsychologist explains the reasons for the referral, the nature of the testing, and the person who will receive the results of the evaluation. The client will be asked about their background, health history, and cognitive concerns. The bulk of the appointment consists of testing. The neuropsychologist or an associate administers paper-and-pencil or computerized question-and-answer tests that may involve defining words, reproducing drawings, remembering lists of words, solving problems, and/or completing questionnaires. Questions usually range from simple to complex, and clients are asked simply to put forth their best effort on all tasks. At some point after the assessment is completed, the neuropsychologist may provide feedback about the client's cognitive strengths and weaknesses, implications for diagnosis, and recommendations for interventions, as appropriate. The client and any accompanying family members are typically given the opportunity to ask questions to ensure that they have a full and accurate understanding of the information provided. Clients and families often find education around the factors contributing toward cognitive problems reassuring and empowering.

NEUROPSYCHOLOGICAL INTERVENTIONS

Neuropsychological evaluations may be followed by interventions to address cognitive, emotional, and/or behavioral changes that can accompany brain-related injuries and illness. For older clients, interventions may include:

- Psychoeducational groups to enable clients to learn about cognitive changes and compensation strategies and/or to enhance coping with cognitive disorders
- Lifestyle interventions that focus on cognitive engagement, physical exercise, nutrition, and stress management to maximize brain health and minimize risk of further cognitive decline
- Cognitive rehabilitation for focal cognitive impairments such as visual neglect, memory impairment, or problems with executive skills and planning
- Management of challenging behaviors associated with severe cognitive impairments such as dementia or delirium

Kathryn A. Stokes and Angela K. Troyer

Lezak, M. D., Howieson, D. B., Bigler, E. D., & Tranel, D. (2012). *Neuropsychological assessment* (5th ed.). New York, NY: Oxford University Press.
Ravdin, L. D., & Katzen, H. L. (2013). *Handbook on the neuropsychology of aging and dementia: Clinical handbooks in neuropsychology.* New York, NY: Springer Publishing.
Strauss, E., Sherman, E. M., & Spreen, O. (2006). *A compendium of neuropsychological tests: Administration, norms, and commentary* (3rd ed.). New York, NY: Oxford University Press.

Web Resources
International Neuropsychological Society: http://www.the-ins.org
Neuropsychology Central: http://www.neuropsychologycentral.com

NEUROPSYCHOLOGY

Neuropsychology is the study of the brain and behavior. Neuropsychologists are interested in how changes in the brain, whether because of injury, disease, or maturation, affect thinking abilities. In practice, clinical neuropsychologists administer formal measures of cognition to assess the integrity of brain function and provide insight into aspects of cognitive functioning. Of particular interest to elder care providers, information from a neuropsychological evaluation can be especially useful in identifying the early stages of dementia, differentiating dementia from depression, and identifying patterns of performance that can be useful in the differential diagnosis of age-related cognitive disorders.

Neuropsychology has its roots in both psychometrics and behavioral neurology. Techniques include both formal standardized tests, as well as informal measures of assessing behavior, the results of which are interpreted in the context of the patient's history, estimated premorbid abilities, and symptom presentation. Before modern neuroimaging, neuropsychology answered the question of whether or not brain damage was present. Now in the era of advanced imaging, the primary purpose of the neuropsychological evaluation provides both quantitative and qualitative information about the individual's cognitive abilities. Some common reasons for neuropsychological evaluation include:

- Quantify changes in mental status
- Differentiate cognitive decline because of dementia versus depression
- Determine the nature and severity of cognitive and behavioral manifestation of head injury
- Establish a cognitive baseline before pharmacotherapy or surgical intervention (e.g., temporal lobectomy for epilepsy, deep brain stimulation for Parkinson's disease)
- Inform treatment planning and determine recovery of function
- Answer questions regarding cognitive capacity for issues regarding safety, supervision, or legal decision making (e.g., capacity to write a will)
- Determine an individual's mental ability to adequately perform a job (i.e., fitness for duty evaluation).

CLINICAL NEUROPSYCHOLOGICAL EVALUATIONS

A comprehensive neuropsychological evaluation includes standardized tests of thinking abilities including measures of basic and complex

4

attention, language, visuospatial skills, new learning and memory, and neurobehavioral and emotional symptoms. Test scores and performance are compared to normative data that adjust for various demographic factors such as age, gender, and level of education. Tests used for neuropsychological assessments should have acceptable levels of test reliability and validity. Noncognitive indices, such as measures of performance validity and symptom validity, can add to the value of the conclusions based on cognitive tests.

Formal testing follows standard protocols as identified in the administration manuals. The neuropsychologist attempts to obtain the examinee's best performance by promoting an environment and tone that encourages engagement in the testing procedures. The data must be interpreted in the context in which they are obtained, with attention to factors such as premorbid abilities, alertness/stamina, language and cultural factors, and sensory impairments that may otherwise impact performance.

WORK SETTINGS

Neuropsychologists often work in university hospitals or academic medical centers and can be found in departments of psychology, neuropsychology, neurology, rehabilitation, and psychiatry. Many are private practitioners, and many neuropsychologists are also involved in forensic work, applying the principles of cognitive assessment to assist in issues involving legal decisions.

TRAINING IN NEUROPSYCHOLOGY

Neuropsychology is a specialty of psychology. Aspirational guidelines for a well-integrated education and training model in neuropsychology are widely recognized and include a program of study highlighting a scientist practitioner model with training throughout graduate school, an internship, and the residency levels.

There are a number of clinical psychology programs with specialized training in clinical neuropsychology at the doctoral level, and specialized training has become far more common in recent years. In the fall of 1997, the University of Houston was the site for a meeting convened for the purpose of establishing a model for training

and education in the field of clinical neuropsychology, and the outcome of this event lead to guidelines referred to as the Houston Conference Policy Statement (Hannay et al., 1998).

Training in neuropsychology includes attainment of a doctoral degree in psychology from an accredited university training program, an internship in a clinically relevant area of professional psychology, and the equivalent of 2 years of experience and specialized training, at least one of which is at the postdoctoral level, in the study and practice of clinical neuropsychology and related neurosciences. These 2 years include supervision by a clinical neuropsychologist. More recently, formal practicum guidelines have also been developed (Nelson et al., 2016). Ultimately, licensure in psychology is required for independent clinical practice.

The guidelines delineating the specialized training in neuropsychology were originally designed as aspirational training standards, yet data suggest that the Houston Conference has had a significant impact on the course of training for clinical neuropsychologists across the country (Sweet, Benson, Nelson, & Moberg, 2015). The American Board of Clinical Neuropsychology (ABCN) has endorsed the Houston Conference guidelines for specialty training in clinical neuropsychology for individuals who completed their neuropsychological training on or after January 1, 2005. A listing of self-declared doctoral programs in clinical neuropsychology, as well internships and residencies, can be found at the website for the American Psychological Association's Division on Neuropsychology, the Society for Clinical Neuropsychology.

BEST-PRACTICE PARAMETERS

In 1989, the definition of a clinical neuropsychologist was published in *The Clinical Neuropsychologist*, followed by the statement, "Attainment of the ABCN/ABPP Diploma in Clinical Neuropsychology is the clearest evidence of competence as a Clinical Neuropsychologist." The American Board of Professional Psychology (ABPP) is the primary organization for specialty board certification across all areas in psychology, and ABCN is the member board that establishes criteria for education, training, and competency for board certification in clinical neuropsychology. Board certification by ABPP/ABCN is viewed by many as the final step in professional credentialing for neuropsychologists.

There is also a subspecialty board certification in pediatric neuropsychology for those who are already ABPP/ABCN board certified but want to add this voluntary credential signifying their focus on pediatric populations.

Lisa Ravdin Rosenberg

Hannay, J., Bieliauskas, L., Crosson, B., Hammeke, T., Hamsher, K., & Koffler, S. (1998). Proceedings of the Houston conference on specialty education and training in clinical neuropsychology. *Archives of Clinical Neuropsychology, 13*, 157–250.

Nelson, A. P., Roper, B. L., Slomine, B. S., Morrison, C., Greher, M. R., Janusz, J., … Wodushek, T. R. (2015). Official position of the American Academy of Clinical Neuropsychology (AACN): Guidelines for practicum training in clinical neuropsychology. *Clinical Neuropsychologist, 29*(7), 879–904.

Sweet, J. J., Benson, L. M., Nelson, N. W., & Moberg, P. J. (2015). The American Academy of Clinical Neuropsychology, National Academy of Neuropsychology, and Society for Clinical Neuropsychology (APA Division 40) 2015 TCN Professional Practice and 'Salary Survey': Professional practices, beliefs, and incomes of U.S. neuropsychologists. *Clinical Neuropsychologist, 29*(8), 1069–1162.

Web Resources
American Academy of Clinical Neuropsychology: https://theaacn.org
American Board of Clinical Neuropsychology: https://theabcn.org
International Neuropsychological Society: http://www.the-ins.org
National Academy of Neuropsychology: https://nanonline.org
Society for Clinical Neuropsychology: http://www.scn40.org

Normal Pressure Hydrocephalus

Normal pressure hydrocephalus (NPH) is largely a progressive disorder characterized by (a) a clinical triad of urinary dysfunction, gait disturbance, and cognitive impairment; (b) radiological findings of increased size of the cerebral ventricles; and (c) laboratory findings of normal cerebrospinal fluid (CSF) pressure on lumbar puncture in the absence of papilledema (Siraj, 2011).

HISTORY

NPH was first identified by the Colombian neurosurgeon Salomon Hakim in his 1964 thesis, "Some Observations on Cerebrospinal Fluid (CSF) Pressure: Hydrocephalic Syndrome in Adults with 'Normal' CSF Pressure" (Hakim, 1964). The following year, Adams described the same syndrome in older adults with increased cerebral ventricles without increased intracranial pressure, along with gait difficulty, cognitive disturbance, and urinary incontinence. With the advent of procedures to remove CSF via intracranial shunts, NPH became the first cause of dementia that could be fully reversed (Rosseau, 2011).

ETIOLOGY

NPH usually occurs as idiopathic (iNPH) or secondary (sNPH). sNPH may occur because of subarachnoid or intraventricular hemorrhage caused by trauma or aneurysms. Infections such as meningitis and inflammatory conditions may also lead to sNPH. The pathophysiology of iNPH is not fully understood, but impairment in absorption and drainage of CSF leading to gradual accumulation and dilation of the cerebral ventricles, rather than excess production, is the suspected mechanism (Siraj, 2011). Other rare causes include Paget's disease of the skull, mucopolysaccharidosis of the meninges, and achondroplasia.

EPIDEMIOLOGY

The incidence of NPH varies from 2 to 20 per million per year. Hospital discharge rates suggest that about 11,500 patients in the United States are diagnosed with NPH annually. It is estimated to be the cause of about 5% of cases

N

of dementia (Siraj, 2011). iNPH occurs more commonly in the sixth or seventh decade of life, whereas sNPH may occur in all age groups. NPH occurs with equal frequency in male and female patients (Siraj, 2011).

CLINICAL FEATURES

The triad of gait abnormality, urinary incontinence, and cognitive impairment are the salient signs of the illness. Gait abnormality is the most frequent symptom in the early stages of NPH and is described as magnetic gait with the appearance of the patient's feet being stuck to the ground. Alternately the gait is described as gait apraxia or frontal ataxia. The patient finds it difficult to initiate movement and walks with short steps and outwardly rotated feet. Gait abnormality is the clinical feature most responsive to treatment by ventricular shunting (Siraj, 2011). Cognitive impairment is characterized by prominent loss of subcortical and frontal functions, with inertia, forgetfulness, and poor executive function appearing early in the course (Bradley, 2000). The slowness and lack of interest may be mistakenly regarded as signs of mood disorder, but these patients lack depressive thoughts (Shprecher, Schwalb, & Kurlan, 2008). Urinary incontinence is usually seen in the advanced stage of the disease and appears to occur as a result of disruption of periventricular pathways to the sacral bladder center, leading to urgency. Incontinence may also result from gait disorder impeding access to the toilet or lack of concern for micturition because of impaired cognition (Siraj, 2011).

DIAGNOSIS

The importance of diagnosing NPH lies in the opportunity to identify that minority of dementia patients whose illness, if discovered early, can at least partially be reversed. Differentiating the cognitive impairment of NPH from other types of dementia is complicated by the fact that three quarters of patients with NPH severe enough to require treatment also suffer from another neurodegenerative disorder (Kiefer & Unterberg, 2012). Ventriculomegaly on CT or MRI may be misinterpreted as primary

age-related brain atrophy, which normally occurs after age 60 years. Atrophy associated with age or neurodegenerative dementia produces a proportionate enlargement of both ventricular and sulcal size and is often called *hydrocephalus ex vacuo*. The criteria for diagnosis, as well as for selecting patients for shunt placement, remain imperfect. To date, no clinical picture or diagnostic test has definitively differentiated iNPH from other dementias that occur in old age. The "gold standard" for diagnosis remains clinical improvement with CSF withdrawal (Hebb & Cusimano, 2001).

Diagnostic Tests

Imaging—The hallmark finding on MRI or CT is ventriculomegaly in the absence of, or out of proportion to, sulcal enlargement. Ventriculomegaly is said to be present if the modified Evans' ratio is greater than 0.31. This is calculated by measuring the maximal diameter of the frontal horns of the lateral ventricles (at the slice where the frontal horns are largest) to the maximum width of the cranial cavity measured at the inner tables of the skull at the same level. Both MRI and CT can assess sulcal and ventricular size, but MRI is superior to CT in the evaluation of patients with probable NPH. MRI allows visualization of other markers of NPH and provides additional information that can rule out other possible causes in the differential diagnosis.

MRI may also show a characteristic high signal abnormality around the ventricles, which is thought to represent transependymal fluid diffusion. However, it remains a challenge to distinguish this finding from the age-related white matter changes or from subcortical vascular dementia. The association between white matter lesions and the response to shunting has been variable.

CSF tap test—The tap test is also known as the *Miller Fisher test* and is named after the neurologist who first described it. It involves drainage of 40 to 50 mL of CSF from the lumbar cistern or the ventricles and simulates shunt placement. The cutoff level of CSF flow for shunt surgery is controversial and varies between 8 and 18 mmHg/mL/min, with many centers using 12 mmHg/mL/min. Abnormal CSF dynamics (i.e., high resistance to outflow or improvement after CSF drainage) indicate good effects of shunt surgery (Tisell et al., 2011). Carotid blood flow measured using Doppler sonography before and after the tap test has shown that increased flow after CSF drainage correlates with clinical improvement. Extended external lumbar drainage and controlled-resistance continuous lumbar drainage techniques may prevent patients from being exposed to an unnecessary operation (Hebb & Cusimano, 2001).

TREATMENT

The basis of therapy for NPH is CSF diversion via a shunt to add additional capacitance to the system, increasing perfusion but not decreasing the pressure, which is already normal (Bradley, 2000). Procedures, including ventriculoperitoneal, ventriculopleural, and ventriculoatrial shunting, lead to significant improvement in approximately 60% of patients (Shprecher et al., 2008). Lumboperitoneal (LP) shunts with horizontal–vertical valves (HVVs) are an alternative for CSF diversion that avoids direct cerebral injury and may reduce the risk of overdrainage (Bloch & McDermott, 2012). Lumboperitoneal shunts are increasingly used in Japan (Kazui, 2016). The CSF excess is managed using a passive pressure or flow-regulated mechanical shunt. It is desirable to have a shunt valve that responds dynamically to the changing needs of the patient, opening and closing according to a dynamic physiological pattern, rather than simply to the hydrostatic pressure across the valve. The constant-resistance or differential-pressure valve systems are classified according to their opening pressure: low, medium, or high. Low-pressure valves are more consistently associated with decreased ventricular size postoperatively, but there is no difference in clinical outcome several months after surgery. They are associated with more marked improvement in dementia but with more complications as well (Hebb & Cusimano, 2001). In more recent studies, however, shunt surgery is most sensitive for improving global cognition, learning and memory, and psychomotor speed in patients with NPH (Peterson et al., 2016). However, the association between white matter lesions and the response to shunting has been variable. Nevertheless, vascular white matter changes should not exclude patients from shunt surgery (Tullberg, Jensen, Ekholm, & Wikkelsø, 2001).

COMPLICATIONS

The perioperative and long-term morbidity and mortality of CSF shunting procedures are significant. A meta-analysis of 44 articles found that the pooled mean rate of shunt complications, including death, infection, seizures, shunt malfunction (overdrainage or underdrainage), subdural hemorrhage, and effusion was 38%, with 22% of patients requiring additional surgery (Shprecher et al., 2008).

PROGNOSIS

Ventriculoperitoneal shunting is less successful in iNPH (30%–50%) than in sNPH (50%–70%). Patients whose gait disturbance, dementia, and/or urinary incontinence have lasted 2 years or less tend to be more responsive (Rosseau, 2011). Although the cognitive impairment of iNPH may initially improve with placement of the shunt, cognitive decline because of concurrent degenerative brain disease is not uncommon (Koivisto et al., 2013).

CONCLUSION

The diagnosis and management of NPH remains a challenge. There are not enough current evidence-based guidelines for treatment. Controversy exists as to whether shunting consistently improves cognition and whether some form of quantified intracranial pressure monitoring can predict postoperative benefits. Patients with enlarged cerebral ventricles secondary to cerebral atrophy (hydrocephalus ex vacuo) and with no impediment to CSF do not benefit from shunt procedures. Those whose NPH is secondary to an acute event such as trauma, hemorrhage, or infection are more likely to benefit from shunting. However, the frequency of postoperative complications is not trivial. The natural course of either type of NPH has not been fully studied. To maximize the benefits of shunt treatment, surgery should be performed as soon

N

as the diagnosis is made (Andrén, Wikkelsø, Tisell, & Hellström, 2014). Nevertheless, NPH remains largely underdiagnosed and remains a potential cause of reversible dementia if recognized and discovered early.

Uchechukwu Nnamdi, Anneline Kingsley,
and Gary J. Kennedy

Andrén, K., Wikkelsø, C., Tisell, M., & Hellström, P. (2014). Natural course of idiopathic normal pressure hydrocephalus. *Journal of Neurology, Neurosurgery and Psychiatry, 85*(7), 806–810.

Bloch, O., & McDermott, M. W. (2012). Lumboperitoneal shunts for the treatment of normal pressure hydrocephalus. *Journal of Clinical Neuroscience, 19*(8), 1107–1111.

Bradley, W. G. (2000). Normal pressure hydrocephalus: New concepts on etiology and diagnosis. *American Journal of Neuroradiology, 21,* 1586–1590.

Hakim, S. (1964). Some observations on C.S.F. pressure: Hydrocephalic syndrome in adults with "normal" C.S.F. pressure. Retrieved from http://www.hydroassoc.org/docs/KB%20Articles/Hakim_Thesis_1964.pdf

Hebb, A. O., & Cusimano, M. D. (2001). Idiopathic normal pressure hydrocephalus: A systematic review of diagnosis and outcome. *Neurosurgery, 49,* 1166–1184.

Kazui, H. (2016). Current state of diagnosis and treatment of idiopathic normal pressure hydrocephalus. *Brain and Nerve, 68*(4), 429–440.

Kiefer, M., & Unterberg, A. (2012). The differential diagnosis and treatment of normal-pressure hydrocephalus. *Deutsches Ärzteblatt International, 109*(1–2), 15–26.

Koivisto, A. M., Alafuzoff, I., Savolainen, S., Sutela, A., Rummukainen, J., Kurki, M., … Kuopio NPH Registry. (2013). Poor cognitive outcome in shunt-responsive idiopathic normal pressure hydrocephalus. *Neurosurgery, 72*(1), 1–8.

Peterson, K. A., Savulich, G., Jackson, D., Killikelly, C., Pickard, J. D., & Sahakian, B. J. (2016). The effect of shunt surgery on neuropsychological performance in normal pressure hydrocephalus: A systematic review and meta-analysis. *Journal of Neurology, 263*(8), 1669–1677.

Rosseau, G. (2011). Normal pressure hydrocephalus. *Disease-a-Month, 57*(10), 615–624.

Shprecher, D., Schwalb, J., & Kurlan, R. (2008). Normal pressure hydrocephalus: Diagnosis and treatment. *Current Neurology and Neuroscience Reports, 8*(5), 371–376.

Siraj, S. (2011). An overview of normal pressure hydrocephalus and its importance: How much do we really know? *Journal of the American Medical Directors Association, 12*(1), 19–21.

Tisell, M., Tullberg, M., Hellström, P., Edsbagge, M., Högfeldt, M., & Wikkelsö, C. (2011). Shunt surgery in patients with hydrocephalus and white matter changes. *Journal of Neurosurgery, 114,* 1432–1438.

Tullberg, M., Jensen, C., Ekholm, S., & Wikkelsø, C. (2001). Normal pressure hydrocephalus: Vascular white matter changes on MR images must not exclude patient from shunt surgery. *American Journal of Neuroradiology, 22*(9), 1665–1673.

NURSES IMPROVING CARE OF HEALTHSYSTEM ELDERS (NICHE)

Nurses Improving Care of Healthsystem Elders (NICHE) is a program at New York University's Rory Meyers College of Nursing (NYU Meyers). NICHE functions as both a not-for-profit professional membership organization and a professional collaborative. NICHE designation entails an organizational commitment, including participation of senior personnel in the NICHE Leadership Training Program and ongoing documentation of active geriatric programming through an annual self-evaluation (Boltz et al., 2013). Currently NICHE is composed of approximately 500 NICHE active member sites, representing individual hospitals and almost 100 health systems in North America.

The national office coordinates a centralized, web-based portal for members to access educational, clinical, and operational tools (Capezuti et al., 2012). The extensive learning management system provides courses for advanced practice nurses and RNs, patient care associates, the interdisciplinary team, and families. The NICHE benchmarking service provides member sites access to several survey instruments that are used to evaluate organizational attributes such as perceived work environment, knowledge competencies, and unit-level patient outcomes. Members access these via a web-based data entry that provides automated benchmarking reports of several valid and reliable instruments, including the NICHE Geriatric Institutional Assessment Profile (Capezuti, Boltz, et al., 2013). Also, a web-based discussion forum and annual conference provide a catalyst for networking among facilities committed to quality geriatric care.

NICHE is associated with positive nurse, patient, and organizational outcomes. A key component of the success of NICHE is the positive influence of NICHE on the geriatric nursing practice environment (specifically, the focus of NICHE on nurse involvement in hospital decision making regarding care of older adults). NICHE principles and resources are consistent with professional nursing practice models (Boltz, Capezuti, & Shabbat, 2010; Capezuti et al., 2012), and NICHE hospitals are also more likely to have Magnet® designation.

NICHE is supported by numerous foundations that have facilitated a business model in which health systems or other health care entities pay membership fees to access the NICHE network of resources and participate with other NICHE members. This has led to financial sustainability for the program to ensure its growth (Capezuti, Bricoli, & Boltz, 2013).

See also Advanced Practice Nursing; Geriatric Resource Nurse; Hospital-Based Services.

Elizabeth A. Capezuti

Boltz, M., Capezuti, E., & Shabbat, N. (2010). Building a framework for a geriatric acute care model. *Leadership in Health Services*, 23, 334–360.

Boltz, M., Capezuti, E., Shuluk, J., Brouwer, J., Carolan, D., Conway, S., … Galvin, J. E. (2013). Implementation of geriatric acute care best practices: Initial results of the NICHE SITE self-evaluation. *Nursing & Health Sciences*, 15(4), 518–524.

Capezuti, E., Boltz, E., Cline, D., Dickson, V., Rosenberg, M., Wagner, L., … Nigolian, C. (2012). NICHE—A model for optimizing the geriatric nursing practice environment. *Journal of Clinical Nursing*, 21, 3117–3125.

Capezuti, E., Boltz, M., Shuluk, J., Denysyk, L., Brouwers, J., Roberts, M. C., … Secic, M. (2013). Utilization of a benchmarking database to inform NICHE implementation. *Research in Gerontological Nursing*, 6(3), 198–208.

Capezuti, E., Bricoli, B., & Boltz, M. (2013). NICHE: Creating a sustainable business model to improve care of hospitalized older adults. *Journal of the American Geriatrics Society*, 61(8), 1387–1393.

Web Resource
NICHE Program: http://nicheprogram.org

NURSING HOME MANAGED CARE

BACKGROUND

In the early 1900s, managed care emerged in various settings across the country as prepaid medical care in which, for a set monthly premium, subscribers' health care needs were met by participating providers. These early managed-care programs were typically started by physicians who collected a monthly premium in exchange for care, but as the concept developed, so did the organizations' corporate structures (Tufts Managed Care Institute, 2006). The monthly premium arrangement proved cost effective for the subscribers and alleviated the stress of financial burden resulting from illness. The financial risk of providing care shifted from the individual to managed care organizations (MCOs) operating the program. Throughout the 20th century, managed care became known by employers as a less expensive yet comprehensive and quality form of insurance to offer their employees. Although managed care grew in this private environment, the publicly funded Medicare and Medicaid programs insured the indigent, frail, and elderly population in a traditional fee-for-service environment where the government held the financial risk. In 2015, these two public programs accounted for 37% of national health expenditures, up from 36% in 2011. With increasing financial pressure on the Medicare and Medicaid programs beginning in the 1970s, the state and federal governments also looked to the privately operated managed care system as a way to control the escalating health care costs. As a result, the MCOs from the private insurance market were introduced and tested in the public sector.

NURSING HOME REVENUE

Nursing homes provide patients and residents with services that include medical and nursing care, room and board, and social activities. Some of these services are skilled, such as physical rehabilitation and skilled nursing, and others are long-term residential or custodial care. The reimbursement structure for these services is primarily two-pronged, as follows:

- Reimbursement for skilled services is covered by Medicare Part A, Medicare MCOs (under a Part A benefit), and commercial insurances when eligibility criteria for a specific skilled need are met. This is generally covered for a short time until improvement has plateaued or the benefit is exhausted. Medicare reimburses nursing homes for these services at federally established Medicare reimbursement rates determined by the complexity of skilled need or resource utilization groups (RUGs). Medicare MCOs and commercial insurances reimburse at negotiated rates established through a contractual agreement between the insurer and provider. In many cases, these rates mirror the federally established Medicare RUG rates. When a patient qualifies for a nursing facility stay under Medicare, Medicare and Medicare MCOs cover the cost of room and board, skilled services, and medically necessary supplies. They cover 100% of the costs for the first 20 days. Beginning on day 21 of the facility stay, there is a significant copayment ($161 a day in 2016). Coverage is exhausted after 100 days, at which point the individual is responsible for payment (Medicare.gov).
- Custodial services, such as room and board, are covered through Medicaid, Medicaid MCOs, and private payments. Medicaid and Medicaid MCOs typically reimburse at a state-defined daily rate. For private pay, the nursing homes typically charge what the market will bear. Medicare and Medicare MCOs do not cover custodial care if it is the only type of care that is needed. Custodial care, however, is covered along with a skilled benefit and is included in that reimbursement rate.

Medicare and Medicaid programs remain the dominant funding sources for nursing home care. The National Investment Center for Senior Housing and Care's *Skilled Nursing Data Report on Key Occupancy and Revenue Trends* (2016) reports that although Medicare occupancy has declined from 2011 through 2015, Medicare managed care has increased. Furthermore, although Medicare rates have stayed relatively flat, Medicaid rates have increased 5.5% and Medicare Advantage (MA) rates have decreased 10.1% over that same period. According to the report, Medicare covers 13.7% of nursing home patient days, with an average revenue of $497/day, MA covers 6.1% with an average revenue of $434/day, Medicaid covers 65.3% of nursing home patient days with an average revenue of $196/day, and 9.8% is paid for privately with an average revenue of $245/day.

According to National Health Expenditure Accounts data, total national spending on long-term services and supports was $310 billion in 2013, with Medicaid covering 51% of that total (The Henry J. Kaiser Family Foundation, 2015a, 2015b) and The Henry J. Kaiser Family Foundation reports that 5% of the total Medicare expenditures of $536 billion is spent on skilled nursing facility services (The Henry J. Kaiser Family Foundation, 2015c). These long-term services and supports benefits included spending on nursing home services, home health care, intermediate care facility services, and home and community-based services (HCBS).

NURSING HOME MANAGED CARE

Nursing home costs under both Medicare and Medicaid programs have increased significantly in recent decades. In 2015, Medicaid spent just more than $45 billion (combined state and federal funds) on nursing homes. Spending increases averaged 1.7% annually between 2002 and 2010, for a total of 16% more than the measurement period (Medicare Payment Advisory Commission [MedPAC], 2012). With this increasing fiscal pressure, state and federal governments turned to managed care programs to control the cost escalation related to nursing home care. Under managed care, the federal and state governments pay a monthly capitation to private MCOs, who in turn accept the financial risk for the health care services used by the consumers covered under the plans. The MCOs are then responsible for managing those services, within defined benefits. Under these arrangements, MCOs offer the federal and state governments a level of cost predictability.

MEDICARE MANAGED CARE

Medicare managed care has been in existence since the 1970s and was expanded as a voluntary Medicare option, called Medicare + Choice, with the Balanced Budget Act in 1997. The Medicare Modernization Act (2003) further expanded the Medicare managed care options, now called MA plans, and created special needs plans (SNPs) for certain groups, including the institutionalized nursing home population. These plans are voluntary alternatives to traditional Medicare fee-for-service plans and provide all of the traditional services covered by Medicare Parts A, B, and D. Many MA plans also offer additional supplemental benefits such as preventive dental coverage. The Centers for Medicare & Medicaid (CMS) oversees the MA plans. Of the 57 million individuals who receive their health benefits through the Medicare program, 31% are covered by private MA plans, which is increased from 24% in 2010 (The Henry J. Kaiser Family Foundation, 2016). SNPs, specifically, are "intended to encourage more choices for certain populations by allowing organizations that specialize in the treatment of beneficiaries with particular needs to have MA contracts" (*Federal Register*, 2005, pp. 4587–4741). The concept is that the market will drive participating organizations to develop expertise and efficiencies in caring for groups with special health care needs, such as institutionalized elderly. SNPs can, for example, provide coverage for more preventative and primary care services, thus reducing the expected rate of costlier hospitalizations. CMS had approved 83 institutional SNPs by January 2017, covering 62,775 beneficiaries (National Health Policy Group, 2017). The SNPs, like other MA plans, receive a monthly, fully capitated, risk-adjusted premium that covers all contractually covered health care services. The risk-adjustment reimbursement formula results

in higher payments for those with costlier conditions. There is an additional allowance for the institutionalized status. Nursing homes must enter into a contractual relationship with the SNPs and other MA plans to be network providers and serve plan members.

LONG-TERM MEDICAID MANAGED CARE

Medicaid managed care programs, like traditional Medicaid, are designed and maintained by states with approval from the CMS. These managed care programs are implemented in a variety of ways, most commonly section 1115 demonstrations or 1915(b) waivers with a combination of state and federal funding. These waivers provide flexibility to states by offering an avenue for testing new approaches for structuring the long-term care services available through Medicaid that differ from traditional federal rules.

Long-term services and supports (LTSS) are long-term HCBS and long-term nursing home services that are included in a LTSS Managed Medicaid program designed to serve the long-term care population. The CMS reports that states are increasingly turning toward managed long-term care (MLTC) and managed long-term service and supports (MLTSS) options to support alternatives to long-term nursing home care, "as a strategy for expanding HCBS, promoting community inclusion, ensuring quality, and increasing efficiency" (CMS, 2013, p. 1). The number of states engaged in MLTSS programs has increased from 9 in 2006 to 22 in 2015 (National Association of States United for Aging and Disabilities, 2015), with an additional 11 states expressing interest and submitting waiver applications.

Under these MLTC and MLTSS programs, MCOs receive an actuarially determined monthly payment to cover long-term care services, including custodial nursing home care and HCBS. Accordingly, managed LTSS spending increased 55% in 2014, up to $22.5 billion, 15% of the total spent (CMS, 2016) Currently 64% of LTSS dollars are spent on nursing facility care (CMS, 2013). Although the majority of those who receive these services are still funded

N

through traditional fee-for-service programs, as states shift to MLTC and MLTSS options, CMS believes that it "could increase the breadth, availability, and quality of LTSS available to those who require them" (CMS, 2013, p. 17).

Programs are either mandatory or voluntary. Mandatory programs direct that all eligible Medicaid beneficiaries join a managed care plan, whereas voluntary programs give it only as an option as an alternative to fee-for-service. In the states where the programs are mandatory, the MCOs achieve significant negotiating leverage with providers because they control such a significant portion of the potential Medicaid revenue. In mandatory and voluntary states, the providers have incentives to contract with MCOs based on market share. Government cost predictability appears to be the main driver for program expansion.

CONSUMER IMPACT

Managed care plans characteristically provide a richer selection of covered benefits for nursing home residents compared with traditional public plans. Managed care plans also offer reduced premiums and other out-of pocket costs. In exchange, the enrollee must go through the MCO provider network and preauthorization requirements to receive the benefits. Opponents of the privatization of public nursing home funding programs believe that the closed networks of managed care programs will result in restriction of provider choice and access to care. It is important that consumers understand any in-network or out-of-network restrictions before joining a plan. Evidence suggests that both Medicare and Medicaid managed care plans can improve quality outcomes for nursing home residents (National Health Policy Forum Issue Brief, 2005). The federal government and state licensing authorities monitor quality, cost-effectiveness, and enrollee satisfaction of MCOs through their contractual agreements. These organizations ensure that enrollees covered by Medicaid and Medicare MCOs are able to receive professional care that meets the set standards. In addition, MCOs may participate in a voluntary national accreditation program that requires them to meet certain standards, including National Committee

for Quality Assurance (NCQA) accreditation. In 2013, CMS issued guidance to states that outline best practices for designing and implementing these programs with respect to quality measurement. Per the guidance, states implementing managed LTSS programs must include a quality strategy for assessing and improving care and quality of life for all beneficiaries, including those that are in nursing homes, to align with existing Medicaid quality initiatives (CMS, 2013).

See also Medicaid; Medicare; Nursing Homes.

Elizabeth M. Miller

Centers for Medicare & Medicaid Services. (2013). *Guidance to states using 1115 demonstration or 1915(b) waivers for managed long-term services and supports programs.* Baltimore, MD: Author.

Centers for Medicare & Medicaid Services. (2016). Medicaid expenditures for long-term services and supports (LTSS) in FY 2014. Retrieved from https://www.medicaid.gov/medicaid/ltss/downloads/ltss-expenditures-2014.pdf

Federal Register. (2005, January 28). Medicare program; Establishment of the Medicare Advantage Program; Final rule. 70(18), 4587–4741.

The Henry J. Kaiser Family Foundation. (2015a). Distribution of fee-for-service Medicaid spending on long term care. Retrieved from http://kff.org/medicaid/state-indicator/spending-on-long-term-care/?currentTimeframe=0

The Henry J. Kaiser Family Foundation. (2015b). Medicaid and long-term services and supports: A primer. Retrieved from http://kff.org/medicaid/report/medicaid-and-long-term-services-and-supports-a-primer

The Henry J. Kaiser Family Foundation. (2015c). Medicare spending and financing fact sheet. Retrieved from http://kff.org/medicare/fact-sheet/medicare-spending-and-financing-fact-sheet

The Henry J. Kaiser Family Foundation. (2016). Medicare advantage. Retrieved from http://kff.org/medicare/fact-sheet/medicare-advantage

Medicare Payment Advisory Commission: Report to Congress: Medicare Payment Policy. (2012). Chapter 7, Skilled nursing facility services. Retrieved from http://www.medpac.gov/chapters/Mar12_Ch07.pdf. Entire Report available at http://www.medpac.gov/documents/Mar12_EntireReport.pdf

National Association of States United for Aging and Disabilities. (2015). state of the states in aging and disability: 2015 Survey of state agencies. Retrieved from http://www.nasuad.org/sites/nasuad/files/NASUAD%202015%20States%20Rpt.pdf

National Health Policy Forum. (2005). National health policy forum IssueBrief. Retrieved from http://www.nhpf.org/pdfs ib/IB808 SNP11–11-05.pdf

National Health Policy Group. (2017). Special needs plan comprehensive report. Retrieved from http://www.nhpg.org/media/24535/snp_2017_01.pdf

National Investment Center for Senior Housing and Care. (2016). Skilled nursing data report key occupancy and revenue trends. Retrieved from http://info.nic.org/hubfs/Skilled_Nursing_Data_Report_December_2015_Final.pdf

Tufts Managed Care Institute. (2006). A brief history of managed care. Retrieved from http://www.thci.org/downloads/BriefHist.pdf

Web Resources

AARP: http://www.aarp.org

American Health Care Association: http://www.ahca.org

Centers for Medicare & Medicaid Services: http://www.cms.hhs.gov/SpecialNeedsPlans http://www.cms.hhs.gov/MedicaidDataSourcesGenInfo/01Overview.asp

National Health Expenditure Fact Sheet: https://www.cms.gov/research-statistics-data-and-systems/statistics-trends-and-reports/national healthexpenddata/nhe-fact-sheet.html

The Henry J. Kaiser Family Foundation: http://www.kff.org

National Health Policy Forum: http://www.nhpf.org

Tufts Managed Care Institute: http://www.thci.org

U.S. House of Representatives: http://www.cbo.gov

NURSING HOME REFORM ACT

As part of the Omnibus Budget Reconciliation Act (OBRA) of 1987, Pub. L. No. 100–203, Congress enacted the Nursing Home Quality Reform Act [codified at 42 U.S.C. §§1395i-3(a)-(h) and 1396r(a)-(h)]. This Act contains many of the recommendations made in a 1986 Institute of Medicine report (Institute of Medicine, 1986) that Congress had directed the U.S. Department of Health and Human Services (USDHHS) to commission. OBRA 87 amended the Social Security Act, Titles XVIII (Medicare) and XIX (Medicaid), to require substantial upgrades in nursing home quality and enforcement. Passage of this act demonstrated the impatience of Congress and the courts with what they, and the public, perceived as ineffectual regulation of nursing homes by USDHHS's Health Care Financing Administration (now the Centers for Medicare & Medicaid Services [CMS]).

Under the Nursing Home Reform Act, each nursing facility is required to "care for its residents in such a manner and in such an environment as will promote maintenance or enhancement of the quality of life of each resident" and to "provide services and activities to attain or maintain, for each resident, the highest practicable physical, mental, and psychological well-being." For each admitted resident, a facility must collect information according to a defined minimum data set (MDS), using a Resident Assessment Instrument (RAI), about an individual's physical, mental, and emotional condition. Using this information, facilities must develop and implement an individualized plan of care for each resident.

To implement this legislation, the USDHHS published a series of regulations that has been codified at 42 Code of Federal Regulations Part 483. Nursing homes must comply with very specific mandates set forth in these requirements for participation. These federal requirements, for which nursing homes are surveyed, concern (a) resident rights; (b) admission, transfer, and discharge rights; (c) resident behavior and facility practices; (d) quality of life; (e) resident assessment; (f) quality of care; (g) nursing services; (h) dietary services; (i) physician services; (j) rehabilitation services; (k) dental services; (l) pharmacy services; (m) infection control; (n) physical environment; (o) administration; (p) laboratory; and (q) other. There are more than 185 individual survey items within those 17 categories.

On July 16, 2015, CMS published in the *Federal Register* a proposed rule that would substantially reform Medicare/Medicaid

N

requirements for long-term care facilities. In the preamble to the proposed regulations, CMS stated that "we are reviewing regulations in an effort to improve the quality of life, care and services in LTC facilities, optimize resident safety, reflect current professional standards, and [to] improve the logical flow of the regulations" (CMS, 2015, p. 42169).

Among the specific proposed changes were provisions for making sure that nursing home staff is properly trained on caring for residents with dementia and in preventing elder abuse; ensuring that nursing homes take into consideration the health of residents when making decisions on the kinds and levels of staffing a facility needs to properly take care of its residents; ensuring that staff have the right skill sets and competencies to provide person-centered care to residents, considering a resident's goals of care and preferences; and strengthening rights of nursing home residents, including limits on when and how binding arbitration agreements may be used in the nursing home context. Subsequent to publication of the proposed rule, there was an extended public comment period.

The federal government contracts with the states to assess, through its survey agencies (usually the state health department), whether nursing homes meet these standards through annual surveys and complaint investigations. The annual standard survey, which must be conducted on average every 12 months and no less than once every 15 months at each facility, entails teams of state surveyors arriving without prior notice and spending several days in a facility. Their purpose is to determine whether care and services meet the assessed needs of residents and whether a facility is in compliance with other regulatory requirements. Through its *State Operations Manual* (SOM; containing interpretive guidelines and survey protocols), CMS establishes specific protocols, or investigative procedures, for state surveyors to use in conducting the surveys. In contrast, complaint investigations, also conducted by state surveyors but following the individual state's procedures (within certain federal guidelines and time frames), usually target a single alleged problem in response to a complaint filed against a facility

by a resident, a resident's family or friends, or nursing home employees. Quality-of-care problems identified during either standard surveys or complaint investigations are classified into 1 of 12 categories according to their scope (i.e., the number of residents potentially or actually affected) and their severity (i.e., extent of possible harm).

Addressing documented deficiencies is a shared federal–state responsibility. CMS is responsible for enforcement actions involving nursing homes with Medicare certification. The scope and severity of a deficiency determines what the applicable enforcement action is and whether it is optional or mandatory. Enforcement sanctions can involve, among other options: compelling corrective action plans; levying civil monetary fines; denying a facility new Medicare and Medicaid payments; mandating directed staff training on particular aspects of care; imposing a receivership arrangement to manage a facility; forcing the transfer of residents out of an offending facility; and ultimately, decertifying a facility from (kicking it out of) participation in the Medicare and Medicaid programs altogether. Sanctions may be applied retroactively for the period since the last standard survey. CMS ordinarily accepts a state's recommendation for sanctions or other corrective actions but has the authority to modify those recommendations.

In addition to the Nursing Home Reform Act, there are other federal laws that regulate nursing homes in the United States, including the False Claims Act, 31 United States Code §§ 3729–3732; the Mail and Wire Fraud Acts, 18 United States Code §§ 1341 and 1343; the Americans with Disabilities Act (ADA), 42 U.S.C. §§12101–12213; and the Rehabilitation Act, 29 U.S.C. §794. Moreover, the Patient Protection and Affordable Care Act (PPACA), signed into law in 2010, incorporated the Nursing Home Transparency and Improvement Act of 2009. This set of statutory provisions establishes requirements for nursing facilities regarding public disclosure of, among other things, facility ownership, administration, and staffing levels (The Henry J. Kaiser Family Foundation, 2013). The act also expanded the information available on the CMS Nursing Home Compare website (Koehler, 2016) and included enhanced mechanisms for enforcing applicable standards of practice. The PPACA incorporated provisions pertaining to mistreatment of nursing home residents contained in the Elder Justice Act and the Patient Safety and Abuse Prevention Act.

In addition to these federal laws, the quality of care delivered to nursing home residents is governed by state professional and institutional licensure statutes and regulations; standards of private accrediting bodies such as The Joint Commission (TJC); state elder abuse and neglect laws; private civil litigation for malpractice; and state legislative counterparts to the False Claims Act, ADA, and Rehabilitation Act.

See also Americans With Disabilities Act; Nursing Homes.

Marshall B. Kapp

Centers for Medicare & Medicaid Services. (2015). Medicare and Medicaid programs; reform of requirements for long-term care facilities; proposed rule. *Federal Register, 80*(136), 42169.

The Henry J. Kaiser Family Foundation. (2013). *Issue paper: Implementation of Affordable Care Act provisions to improve nursing home transparency, care quality, and abuse prevention* (Pub. #8406). Washington, DC: Author.

Institute of Medicine. (1986). *Improving the quality of care in nursing homes.* Washington, DC: National Academies Press.

Koehler, K. (2016). Comparative shopping in nursing homes. *Journal of Health & Biomedical Law, 11,* 439–474.

Web Resources
American Health Care Association: http://www .ahcancal.org
American Health Lawyers Association: http://www .healthlawyers.org
American Medical Directors Association: The Society for Post-Acute and Long-Term Care Medicine: http://www.paltc.org
Centers for Medicare & Medicaid Services: https:// www.cms.gov/Medicare/Provider-Enrollment -and-Certification/CertificationandComplianc/ NHs.html
LeadingAge: http://www.leadingage.org
National Academy of Elder Law Attorneys: http:// www.naela.org
National Consumer Voice for Quality Long-Term Care: http://www.theconsumervoice.org
Nursing Home Compare: http://www.medicare .gov/nursinghomecompare
Pioneer Network: http://www.pioneernetwork.net

NURSING HOMES

The nursing home (NH) industry remains an important part of the health care continuum, providing housing and health care services to more than 1.4 million older adults (Centers for Disease Control and Prevention [CDC], 2014). As the population continues to age at an unprecedented rate, the typical NH resident demonstrates higher acuity, more comorbid conditions, and higher care needs than ever before (Mor, Caswell, Littlehale, Niemi, & Fogel, 2009). NHs care for an old, frail population and are devoting more resources to the care and treatment of persons needing short-term rehabilitation, persons needing continuous medical monitoring, persons with profound dementia/cognitively impaired and functional disabilities, and the terminally ill. Resident acuity, or intensity of need, has increased since the 1990s, with many NHs providing services and care previously provided only in acute care facilities.

FACILITY CHARACTERISTICS

As of 2014, there were approximately 16,000 NHs in the United States with almost 1.6 million Medicare and/or Medicaid certified beds (CDC, 2014). Overall, the number of NHs has declined over the past 10 years, but the number has stabilized within the past 5 years (Centers for Medicare & Medicaid [CMS], 2015). In 2014, the number of dually certified NHs for both Medicare and Medicaid continued to increase to almost 95%, whereas the number of Medicare-only and Medicaid-only have decreased. On average, 67% of NHs are for-profit; 25%, nonprofit; and 8%, government and other (CMS, 2015). Approximately 55% of for-profit homes are group or chain affiliated, compared with 46% of nonprofit homes.

Despite a reduced bed supply relative to those aged 65 years and older (e.g., in 2005: 45.7

N

beds/1,000 older adults; in 2014: 36 beds/1,000 older adults), occupancy rates continue to gradually fall from 85% occupancy in 2005 to 82.4% occupancy in 2014 (CMS, 2015). The decline is attributed to reductions in reimbursements, as well as increasing home care options and less restrictive environments such as assisted-living residences (Castle & Engberg, 2009). Of the 1.4 million current NH residents, 77% are 65 years and older, and 8% are 95 years and older (CDC, 2014). These statistics can be explained by the fact that people are living longer and NH care has become more medically sophisticated over the last 15 years.

RISK FACTORS FOR ADMISSION AND SERVICES PROVIDED

Approximately 1.4 million people (approximately 12% of the population aged 65 years and older) are in a NH on any given day, with 36% admitted from a hospital (CDC, 2014). Risk factors for admission are primarily advanced age, medical diagnosis, living alone, loss of self-care ability, mental status, race, lack of informal supports, poverty, hospital admission, bed immobility, and female gender. Mentally ill, developmentally disabled, or mentally retarded individuals cannot be admitted to a NH unless the type or intensity of services needed, determined through a formalized screening process, can be provided.

NH goals of care are to maintain or improve physical and mental function, eliminate or reduce pain and discomfort, offer social involvement and recreational activities in a safe environment, reduce unnecessary hospitalizations and emergency room use, and ensure a dignified death. As of 2014, 19.8% of all NH residents received no assistance in activities of daily living (ADL), compared with 15% receiving assistance in five ADL domains (CMS, 2015). NHs must provide dental, podiatric, and medical-specialty consultation services; social services; and mental health and nutrition services. Some homes have fully equipped dental, podiatric, and x-ray suites; laboratory facilities; and pharmacies.

All NHs provide care at the end of life. Approximately 78% of NHs provide hospice care, although this can vary from a consultative relationship with a certified hospice agency to one in which the resident's care is planned, managed, and monitored by the hospice agency in the NH (CMS, 2015). Residents receiving hospice services have better pain management, fewer hospitalizations, and less use of feeding tubes than residents receiving standard end-of-life care.

Virtually all homes provide rehabilitative services (i.e., physical therapy, occupational therapy, speech, hearing), but the intensity of the service varies with the home's program operation and Medicare participation. Slightly more than 15% of NHs have formally designated special care units (SCUs), constituting approximately 7% of all NH beds. These units care for residents with dementias, hospice, rehabilitation, and ventilator-dependent residents.

RESIDENT CHARACTERISTICS

Most NH residents are White (78%) and female (65.5%); 15% are younger than 65 years (CMS, 2015). Black residents were twice as likely as White residents to be younger than 65 years. The most frequent admission diagnoses were related to diseases of the circulatory system, mental disorders, and diseases of the nervous system (CMS, 2014). As of 2015, more than one third of residents were incontinent of bowel or bladder.

Approximately 50.4% of NH residents have Alzheimer's disease or another type of dementia; 48.7% have a diagnosis of depression, and 32.4% have a diabetes mellitus. The percentage of residents receiving psychoactive medication at least once in the past 7 days decreased from 63% in 2004 to 21.7% in 2014 (CMS, 2015). One third of residents exhibit inappropriate or dangerous behavior. The use of physical restraints in the past 7 days has decreased to 1% in 2014 from 7.5% in 2004 and is attributed to increased regulatory oversight and staff education (CMS, 2015).

According to Wang, Shah, Allman, and Kilgore (2011), NH residents are prominent users of the emergency department, accounting for more than 2.2 million visits annually. Also, NH residents had higher acuity than non-NH residents, were more likely to be admitted to the hospital, exhibited higher mortality, and were more likely to have been discharged from the hospital within the prior 7 days. Influences on hospitalization decisions include physician practice pattern in the NH and local area, hospital vacancy rate, Medicare eligibility, staff and family pressure, and NH resources (e.g., diagnostic services, intravenous therapy, insufficient RNs, systemic infectious processes, cost of antibiotic therapy, pulmonary disease, payment source, advanced age). In 2011, one fourth of NH patients were transferred for inpatient admissions, accounting for $14.3 billion of Medicare spending. The most common reason for admission, was septicemia. On comparison, for-profit NHs had higher rates of hospital transfers than nonprofit (Harrington, Carillo, & Garfield, 2015).

Of all NH residents, 65% have some form of advance directive (including do not resuscitate [DNR] orders); 66% of all residents die in the NH. An anticipated increase in do-not-hospitalize (DNH) requests (currently, 4%–6% of NH residents) and refusal of life-sustaining interventions will likely result in fewer hospitalizations and more "planned deaths" in NHs.

The average length of stay (LOS) for long-term residents is 835 days. Justification of continued-stay review, intensive rehabilitation, and aggressive outplacement to cheaper, lesser levels of care, such as assisted-living or home care, are resulting in shorter NH LOS. Increasingly, more residents are being discharged back to the community, "recovered or stabilized."

STAFFING

Of the 1.7 million full-time equivalent (FTE) employees in NHs in 2014, almost two thirds were nursing staff (i.e., RN, licensed practical nurse [LPN], certified nurse assistant [CNA]). Nursing staff turnover is pervasive and costly and impacts negatively on quality of care. In some states, CNA turnover exceeds 100% annually. Turnover is associated with staffing levels lower than in comparable NHs, poor quality of care, larger facilities, and for-profit ownership (Castle & Engberg, 2009). The "interdisciplinary team" consisting of nursing and social services, activities, dietician services, rehabilitation

therapy, and physician services, are accountable for resident care and outcomes.

NHs with 60 or more residents require that an RN must be that on duty 8 consecutive hours per day, 7 days per week. An RN or LPN must be used for the remaining 16 hours. Total nursing care hours per resident day increased from 3.7 hours in 2004 to 3.8 hours in 2014 (American College Health Association [ACHA], 2016). On average, current staffing per resident day is RNs, 0.6 hour; LPNs, 0.7 hour; and CNAs, 2.3 hours. Several studies found a positive relationship between RN staffing and quality outcomes. The Patient Protection and Affordable Care Act (PPACA) implemented a requirement in 2015 to include dementia and resident abuse training as part of 12 hours per year of continuing education training for nurse aides (Harrington et al., 2015).

Every resident must have a physician who is legally responsible for the plan of care. Few NH physicians are certified geriatricians. A full-time NH physician can have 60 to 80 residents and also serve as the medical director. Every NH is required to have a medical director on-site a minimum of 20 hours per week, with responsibilities that include quality improvement, patient services, resident rights, and administration (U.S. Office of Inspector General [USOIG], 2012).

Some 12% of NHs have no physical therapists, 20% have no occupational therapist, and 26% have no speech/language therapist. The number of social workers, activity therapists, and nutritionists varies with facility size. NH administrators must be licensed and, in most states, have a bachelor's degree in long-term care administration or a related health field.

COSTS AND REIMBURSEMENT

Approximately 65 of NH residents are dually eligible (Medicare/Medicaid) beneficiaries; 29.7% have Medicare only, and less than 5% have Medicaid only. Medicaid is the primary payer for approximately 63% of NH residents. Historically, nursing facilities have preferred Medicare rates and private-pay rates. Higher Medicaid reimbursement rates have been associated with high staffing and higher care quality

N

(Harrington et al., 2015). Private pay accounted for 44% of NH revenue in 1985, 28% in 1996, and 23% in 2014. Whereas at time of admission a dual-beneficiary resident is likely to be Medicare covered, Medicaid is likely to cover the extended-stay non-Medicare portion of NH residence. The Medicare component of the NH program remains essentially restricted to 100 days of only posthospital skilled nursing and/or skilled rehabilitation. A year of long-term care in a nursing facility costs approximately $80,000. In 2013, national spending on skilled nursing facility care cost approximately $155.8 billion (Harrington et al., 2015).

Implementation of a prospective payment system (PPS) for Medicare reimbursement in 1998 (Balanced Budget Act [BBA] Pub. L. No. 105–33) placed NHs under increasing pressure to maximize revenue and reduce costs. This system shifted payment from a cost-based system with limits for routine operating costs to a per-diem payment system based on a resident's resource utilization group (RUG) defined by the types of services required and other resident characteristics (Huckfeldt, Sood, Romley, Malchiodi, & Escarce, 2013). At least 17 states are using some kind of case-mix reimbursement system that classifies residents into homogeneous RUGs and links reimbursement to residents' characteristics and resource use. Almost two thirds of Medicare-covered NH stays in 1999 were provided to residents in three of the five Rehabilitation RUG-III groups and in the Extensive Care RUG-III Group (Centers for Medicare & Medicaid Services, 2011).

QUALITY OF CARE MONITORING

In 1987, NHs were subject to sweeping reforms contained in the Omnibus Budget Reconciliation Act of 1987 (Pub. L. No. 100-203, 101 Stat. 1330) or the Nursing Home Reform Law. NHs have an unannounced survey every 9 to 15 months by a state's health department acting as agents for the CMS. There can be a "look-behind" survey by federal Medicare surveyors. The CMS Nursing Home Compare website provides NH-specific data that include 12 long-term and 3 short-stay quality measures and that compares NHs within states and with national benchmarks (CMS,

2016). Review and accreditation by The Joint Commission is optional for all NHs but mandatory for hospital-based NHs and those seeking managed-care contracts or affiliations. The Joint Commission's Nursing Care Center (NCC) is an accreditation program launched to replace the Long-Term Care Accreditation program. In 2014, new requirements regarding memory care have been implemented to improve care for residents with cognitive impairment (The Joint Commission, 2015). In 2015, CMS added new measurements to the star rating system to make a five-star rating more difficult to obtain (Harrington et al., 2015).

Quality-of-care and quality-of-life deficiencies are characterized by their scope (i.e., number of residents potentially or actually affected) and severity. The most frequently cited deficiencies in 2014 were related to infection control (42.6%), accident environment (39.7%), food sanitation (38.9%), quality of care (33.1%), and unnecessary drugs (25.6%). More than one in five facilities received a deficiency for actual harm or jeopardy (Harrington et al., 2015). The top 10 deficiencies concerned accidents, resident dignity, pressure injuries, and comprehensive care planning (CMS, 2014). Pain management has improved significantly. Reduction in problems with quality, since 1999, might be attributable to inconsistencies in how states conduct surveys and understatement of serious deficiencies (U.S. Government Accountability Office, 2010). In 2015, the PPACA proposed regulations to outline standards for quality-assurance and performance-improvement programs. These regulations built on the existing requirements to address quality deficiencies. The new requirements also focus on food services and residents' rights to address common deficiencies in these areas (Harrington et al., 2015).

FUTURE TRENDS

At least 46% of the older adults in the United States spend some time in a NH as they age. The potential for technology to improve quality of care and quality of life in NHs includes fall prevention (e.g., chair alarms, rehabilitation equipment to improve strength), wandering management (i.e., low- or high-tech), incontinence care (e.g., voiding reminders), and passive call systems. Barriers to implementation include lack of experience and skill in application of advanced technologies, absence of industry standards and applicable regulations regarding use of the technologies, and insufficient financing. To improve quality of care, the Improving Medicare Post-Acute Care Transformation (IMPACT) Act of 2014 (Pub. L. No. 113-118; 128 Stat. 1952) was passed to standardize the clinical assessment data reported by all post-acute care providers, and requires hospitals to provide consumers with information on the quality of post-acute providers before discharge.

The notion of *culture change*, articulated by the Pioneer Network in the late 1990s, has captured the attention of the NH industry, as well as industry regulators; the movement seeks to improve quality of care and quality of life in NHs and creates a model for and sets policies that support resident growth and creativity through person-centered care and staff empowerment. NHs are reinventing themselves so that resident dependency, in part a product of the institutional model, is less likely to occur in the future. Emerging best practices in NHs include mentoring programs, staff involvement in decision making, flexible work schedules, data-driven plan of care, family involvement, and a home-like environment that includes resident choices and input into facility operations (USOIG, 2009). In 2015, the USDHHS announced a goal to link 90% of Medicare payments to quality- or value-based payments. These goals have the potential to create stronger initiatives for NHs to partner with organizations to improve quality, reduce readmissions, and lower costs.

See also Advance Directives; Assisted Living; Dementia: Special Care Units; Nursing Home Managed Care; Nursing Home Reform Act.

Susan M. Renz and Emily C. Stout

Castle, N. G., & Engberg, J. (2009). Factors associated with increasing nursing home closures. *Health Services Research, 44*, 1088–1109.

Centers for Medicare & Medicaid Services. (2011). Medicare and Medicaid statistical supplement. Retrieved from https://www.cms.gov/Research -Statistics-Data-and-Systems/Statistics-Trends -and-Reports/Archives/MMSS/index.html

Centers for Medicare & Medicaid Services. (2015). Nursing home data compendium, 2015. Retrieved from https://www.cms.gov/Medicare/Provider -Enrollment-and-Certification/Certification andComplianc/Downloads/nursinghome datacompendium_508-2015.pdf

Centers for Medicare & Medicaid Services. (2016). Nursing home compare. Retrieved from https:// www.medicare.gov/nursinghomecompare/ search.html?

Harrington, C., Carillo, H., & Garfield, R. (2015). *Nursing facilities, staffing, residents, and facility deficiencies, 2009 through 2014.* Menlo Park, CA: The Henry J. Kaiser Family Foundation.

Huckfeldt, P. J., Sood, N., Romley, J. A., Malchiodi, A., & Escarce, J. J. (2013). Medicare payment reform and provider entry and exit in the post-acute care market. *Health Services Research, 48*(5), 1557–1580.

The Joint Commission. (2015). Facts about the nursing care center (NCC) accreditation program. Retrieved from https://www.jointcommission .org/facts_about_ncc_accreditation

Mor, V., Caswell, C., Littlehale, S., Niemi, J., & Fogel, B. (2009). Changes in the quality of nursing homes in the U.S.: A review and data update. Retrieved from http://www.ahcancal .org/research_data/quality/Documents/ ChangesinNursingHomeQuality.pdf

U.S. Government Accountability Office. (2010). Some improvement seen in understatement of serious deficiencies, but implications for the longer-term trend are unclear. [GAO-10-434R]. Retrieved from http://www.gao.gov/products/GAO-10-434R; http://www.gao.gov/new.items/d07794t.pdf

U.S. Office of Inspector General. (2009). *Emerging practices in nursing homes.* Washington, DC: U.S. Department of Health and Human Services.

U.S. Office of Inspector General. (2012). *National medical director survey.* Washington, DC: U.S. Department of Health and Human Services.

Wang, H. E., Shah, M. N., Allman, R. M., & Kilgore, M. (2011). Emergency department visits by nursing home residents in the United States. *Journal of the American Geriatrics Society, 59*, 1864–1872.

Web Resources

American Association of Homes and Services for Aging: http://www.aahsa.org

American Health Care Association: http://www .ahca.org

National Center for Health Statistics: http://www
.cdc.gov/nchs

Nursing Home Compare: http://www.medicare
.gov/NHCompare

Pioneer Network (Culture Change): http://www
.pioneernetwork.org

Burwell, S., Secretary, U.S. Department of Health
and Human Services, January 26, 2015 [Press
statement]: http://www.hhs.gov/about/news/
2015/01/26/better-smarter-healthier-inhistoric
-announcement-hhs-setsclear-goals-and-timeline
-for-shifting-medicare-reimbursements-from
-volume-to-value.html

NUTRITIONISTS

A registered dietician nutritionist (RDN) or registered dietician (RD) is the nutrition professional
most commonly employed in health care facilities and community nutrition programs. The
two designations are interchangeable and reflect
the same level of education and training. The
RDN is a designated member of the health care
team responsible for nutrition care as defined
by the Health Care Financing Administration
standards for Medicare and Medicaid and recognized by The Joint Commission. In 2016, there
were more than 96,000 RDNs in the United
States (www.cdrnet.org/about). The Academy
of Nutrition and Dietetics (AND; formerly the
American Dietetic Association) is the primary
professional organization for dietetic professionals, with more than 100,000 members in 2015 to
2016 (www.eatright.org/resources/about-us).

ACADEMIC AND CLINICAL
PREPARATION OF THE RD

The Commission on Dietetic Registration (CDR)
of the AND confers the RDN credential on an
individual who meets specific academic and
supervised practice requirements and passes a
national registration examination.

An RDN must have a minimum of a bachelor's degree with a curriculum accredited
by the Accreditation Council for Education
in Nutrition and Dietetics (ACEND) of AND.

Academic requirements include physiology,
anatomy, biochemistry, the psychosocial sciences, management, and nutrition and food
science. Courses must include information
about assessment of nutritional status of the
elderly; age-related effects on metabolism,
nutrition needs, and food choices; adaptive
feeding techniques and alternative feeding
modalities; medical nutrition therapy for
a range of diseases and conditions; nutrition counseling; and the effects of socioeconomic, cultural, and psychological factors on
food and nutrition behavior. Courses are also
required in economics, organizational management, large-volume feeding, and foodservice management. Approximately 50%
of AND members have master's or doctoral
degrees (Rogers, 2016).

In addition to academic education, a minimum of 1,200 hours of supervised clinical
practice in an ACEND-accredited program is
required. Experiences are planned for developing basic skills in nutritional assessment and
management of food and nutritional needs for
people across the life span. Supervised practice programs may include experiences in
acute and ambulatory care settings, skilled
nursing facilities, home-care programs, congregate feeding and home-delivered meal programs for the elderly, and other community
programs. Following completion of the supervised practice experience, the person is eligible
to take the national registration examination
and obtain the RDN certification. In addition
to national registration, 36 states have licensure statutes for dieticians and nutritionists
(www.cdrnet.org).

OTHER NUTRITION PROVIDERS

A certified nutrition specialist (CNS) has a graduate degree in nutrition or a related field or is a medical doctor or doctor of osteopathic medicine and
has completed 1,000 hours of supervised practice
and passed a certification examination administered by the Certification Board for Nutrition
Specialists (www.nutritionspecialists.org). The
same organization administers the certified nutrition specialist–scholar (CNS-S) credential for
individuals who have a doctoral degree in a field

of clinical health care; meet minimum requirements for nutrition coursework, experience, and scholarship; and pass a certification examination. The Certification Board for Nutrition Specialists requirements for these credentials can be met through the professional education obtained for a variety of health professions.

A nutrition and dietetic technician, registered (NDTR) must complete an ACEND-accredited associate of science degree in dietetics or a bachelor's degree in dietetics and pass a national registration examination. The NDTR works under the supervision of the RDN and may provide the following services: screening for nutrition risk, intervention for patients with less complex nutrition problems, and preventive nutrition services.

A certified dietary manager, certified food protection professional (CDM, CFPP) is trained to manage food services including menu planning, food purchasing and preparation, and to ensure food safety. The educational preparation typically is provided through a community college program [Association of Nutrition and Foodservice Professionals (www.anfponline.org)] to prepare for a national examination. Individuals with the CDM, CFPP credential often work in a skilled-nursing or long-term care facility, or a small acute care facility under the supervision of an RDN.

SPECIALTY PRACTICE

RDN may obtain a specialty credential in geriatric nutrition through the CDR. The Board Certified Specialist in Gerontological Nutrition (CSG) credential requires 2 years of experience as an RDN, a minimum of 2,000 hours in geriatric nutrition practice, and a passing grade on a national examination. RDNs and NDTRs must complete continuing education to maintain their credential. Requirements for continuing education include a periodic self-assessment of learning needs and a plan to update needed knowledge and skills. An RDN working with the geriatric population could establish a CPE goal related to geriatric nutrition and seek CPE opportunities that address this topic.

ROLE OF NUTRITIONIST IN HEALTH CARE

Data from 2015 indicate that 57% of RDNs work in clinical health care, comprised of 32% in acute-care hospitals, 17% in ambulatory settings, and 8% in long-term care. In addition, 10% worked in community and public health programs (including congregate feeding and home-delivery meals for the elderly) and 8% as consultants or in private practice (Rogers, 2016). The U.S. Bureau of Labor Statistics (2017) projects that employment for dieticians will grow 16% by 2024 because of an increasing emphasis on health promotion and disease prevention. By 2022, the supply of dieticians may be inadequate to meet demand. The growing aging population, health care reform, increased prevalence of certain chronic conditions, and evolution of personalized nutrition drive increased demand, whereas attrition in the dietetics profession causes a gap in professionals to meet future demands (Hooker, Williams, Papneja, Sen, & Hogan, 2012).

RDNs, as members of integrated multidisciplinary teams, play a key role in supporting successful aging through research, education, and practice. They are uniquely qualified to apply evidence-based nutrition interventions that are essential for health in later life and for mitigation of chronic health conditions. Older adults experience higher risk of chronic conditions and functional impairments that interfere with maintenance of good nutritional status. Almost 80% of older adults have one chronic condition, and half have two or more (Bernstein & Munoz, 2012). Lack of attention to dietary intake and poor nutritional status can have a negative impact on common age-related diseases and contribute to declining health. Daily eating habits change as people age. Food intake typically declines, even in healthy older adults (Nieuwenhuizen, Weenan, Rigby, & Hetherington, 2010). The MyPlate for Older Adults delivers easy, actionable ways for older adults to adjust their diet and lifestyle to correspond with the federal government's 2015 to 2020 Dietary Guidelines for Americans (www.choosemyplate.gov/older-adults).

Physiological and functional changes that occur with aging can further affect nutrient needs (Wernette, White, & Zizza, 2011). Numerous national clinical practice guidelines are available for the management of chronic diseases such as those for cardiovascular disease, diabetes, renal failure, hypertension, obesity and osteoporosis. These include a medical nutrition therapy (MNT) component and recommend RDNs for their recognized expertise in delivering these services. Consistent evidence has confirmed positive outcomes and the cost-effectiveness of RDN-provided nutrition intervention as therapy for chronic diseases (Cody & Tuma, 2013; Bernstein & Munoz, 2012).

In addition to helping prevent or manage chronic conditions, adequate and proper nutrition ensures that older adults maintain a healthy, replete nutritional status critical for optimal aging (Moats & Hoglund, 2012; Pray, Boon, Miller, & Pillsbury, 2010). Although the Institute of Medicine (IOM) has cited obesity as the most common nutritional disorder in older adults, malnutrition, continues to be a pervasive problem. Malnutrition affects an estimated 30% to 50% of hospitalized adults and affects both overweight and underweight individuals (Corkins et al., 2013). With the high prevalence of malnutrition in the older population and its link to poor functional status and dependency (Bernstein & Munoz, 2012), greater health services utilization, and higher likelihood of mortality (Buys et al., 2014), assessment of nutritional status has become a standard of care for older adults in all health care settings. The RDN's role is to assess nutritional risk and in collaboration with other health care professionals, plan interventions that are consistent with the overall plan of care, and evaluate the outcome of care. Interventions may include individual or group counseling to promote improved nutritional intake, prevent disease, or reduce the effects and progression of disease; addressing food insecurity; recommending and providing modified diets; supplementing energy and nutrient intake; and recommending and monitoring nutrition support (via enteral and parenteral routes). In some settings, particularly home care, the RDN may educate other health professionals, such as nurses and other caregivers who provide direct care to patients.

The AND published several evidence-based position papers to address the importance of nutrition and the role of RDNs in the care of older adults over a continuum of living situations, including principles of healthy aging and age-related changes in nutrition needs (Bernstein & Munoz, 2012) in community-residing older adults (Kamp, Wellman, & Russell, 2010) and older adults in health care communities (Dorner, Friedrich, & Posthauer, 2010), as well as health promotion (Slawson, Fitzgerald, & Morgan, 2013).

There is little direct reimbursement by third-party payers for nutrition services at present. In the acute care setting and in skilled nursing facilities, care and services provided by RDNs are part of the daily costs, which also include other basic services such as nursing and food service. In home care, RDNs' services are required for patients at high nutrition risk, but there is no additional reimbursement for this service. In the ambulatory setting, insurance coverage for nutrition counseling varies widely among insurance plans and may not be covered at all. One exception is that beginning in 2002, Medicare Part B coverage was modified to include reimbursement for medical nutrition therapy for diabetes and renal disease (nondialysis) when the services are provided by an RDN. Medicare reimbursement is also available for diabetes self-management and requires that an RDN be part of the teaching team. Some private insurance plan benefits include nutrition counseling for medical nutrition management of some chronic conditions.

See also Oral Health Assessment.

Patricia Booth and Marian C. Devereaux

Bernstein, M., & Munoz, N. (2012). Position of the Academy of Nutrition and Dietetics: Food and nutrition for older adults: Promoting health and wellness. *Journal of the Academy of Nutrition and Dietetics, 112*(8), 1255–1277.

Buys, D. R., Roth, D. L., Ritchie, C. S., Sawyer, P., Allman, R. M., Funkhouser, E. M., ... Locher, J. L. (2014). Nutritional risk and body mass index predict hospitalization, nursing home admissions, and mortality in community-dwelling older adults: Results from the UAB Study of Aging with 8.5 years of follow-up. *Journal of Gerontology: Biological Science and Medical Science, 69*(9), 1146–1153.

N

Cody, M. M., & Tuma, P. A. (2013). The Academy of Nutrition and Dietetics' public policy priorities overview. *Journal of the Academy of Nutrition and Dietetics, 113*(3), 392–394.

Corkins, M. R., Guenter, P., DiMaria-Ghalili, R. A., Jensen, G. L., Malone, A., Miller, S., … American Society for Parenteral and Enteral Nutrition. (2013). Malnutrition diagnosis in hospitalized patients: United States, 2010. *Journal of Parenteral Enteral Nutrition, 38*(2), 186–195.

Dorner, B., Friedrich, E. K., & Posthauer, M. E. (2010). Position of the American Dietetic Association: Individualized nutrition approaches for older adults in health care communities. *Journal of the American Dietetic Association, 110*, 1549–1553.

Hooker, R. S., Williams, J. H., Papneja, J., Sen, N., & Hogan, P. (2012). Dietetics supply and demand: 2010–2020. *Journal of the Academy of Nutrition and Dietetics, 112*(Suppl. 1), S75–S91.

Kamp, B. J., Wellman, N. S., & Russell, C. (2010). Position of the American Dietetic Association, American Society for Nutrition, and Society for Nutrition Education: Food and nutrition programs for community-residing older adults. *Journal of the American Dietetic Association, 110*, 463–472.

Moats, S., & Hoglund, J. (2012). *Nutrition and healthy aging in the community: Workshop summary.* Washington, DC: National Academies Press. Retrieved from http://www.ncbi.nlm.nih.gov/books/NBK91530/pdf/TOC.pdf

Nieuwenhuizen, W. F., Weenan, H., Rigby, P., & Hetherington, M. M. (2010). Older adults and patients in need of nutritional support: Review of current treatment options and factors influencing nutritional intake. *Clinical Nutrition, 29*(2), 160–169.

Pray, L., Boon, C., Miller, E. A., & Pillsbury, L. (2010). *Providing healthy and safe foods as we age: Workshop summary.* Washington, DC: National Academies Press. Retrieved from http://www.ncbi.nlm.nih.gov/books/NBK5187/pdf/TOC.pdf

Rogers, D. (2016). Compensation and benefits survey 2015. *Journal of the Academy of Nutrition and Dietetics, 116*, 370–388.

Slawson, D., Fitzgerald, N., & Morgan, K. (2013). Position of the Academy of Nutrition and Dietetics: The role of nutrition in health promotion and chronic disease prevention. *Journal of the Academy of Nutrition and Dietetics, 113*(7), 972–979.

U.S. Bureau of Labor Statistics, U.S. Department of Labor. (2017). *Occupational outlook handbook, 2016–17 edition.* Retrieved from http://www.bls.gov/ooh/healthcare/dietitians-and-nutritionists.htm

Wernette, C. M., White, B. D., & Zizza, C. A. (2011). Signally proteins that influence energy intake may affect unintentional weight loss in elderly persons. *Journal of the American Dietetic Association, 111*(6), 864–873.

Web Resources

Academy of Nutrition and Dietetics: http://www.eatright.org

American Society for Parenteral and Enteral Nutrition: http://www.nutritioncare.org

Association of Nutrition and Foodservice Professionals (ANFP): http://www.anfponline.org

Centers for Disease Control and Prevention: http://www.cdc.gov/chronicdisease/overview/index.htm

Certifying Board for Dietary Managers: http://www.cbdmonline.org

Commission on Dietetic Registration: https://www.cdrnet.org

Hunger in America 2014: http://www.feedingamerica.org/research/hunger-in-america

MyPlate for Older Adults: http://hnrca.tufts.edu/myplate/what-is-myplate-for-older-adults

Society for Nutrition Education and Behavior: http://www.sneb.org

U.S. Department of Health and Human Services: HealthyPeople 2020: http://www.healthypeople.gov/2020/default.aspx

O

OBESITY

Obesity, overweight, and their consequences are major public health concerns in the United States and around the world (World Health Organization [WHO], 2016). Prevalence rates of overweight and obesity have escalated in the past years and have reached epidemic proportions in the United States, where more than 28% of adults are obese nationally and 35% are overweight (National Center for Chronic Disease Prevention and Health Promotion, 2015). The fundamental causes of the obesity epidemic are sedentary lifestyles and consumption of foods high in sugar, fat, and salt. Although there was no change in the prevalence of obesity from 2007 to 2010, there continues to be an alarming trend toward obesity in older adults. In fact, rates of obesity increase with age from 32.6% in persons aged 20 to 39 years to 39.7% in persons aged 60 years and older (Fakhouri, Ogden, Carroll, Kit, & Flegal, 2012). Both overweight and obesity are most prevalent among non-Hispanic Blacks and persons with lower income and less education.

Historically, criteria defining undesirable or unhealthy weight—overweight and obesity—were derived from studies on health risks and excess mortality conducted by the Metropolitan Life Insurance Company. The studies set a body mass index (BMI), calculated as weight in kilograms divided by height in meters squared (kg/m²), as undesirable if greater than 27.2 for men and 26.9 for women. Current standards adopted by WHO (2016) and the Centers for Disease Control and Prevention (National Institutes of Health, 1998), define healthy weight as a BMI of 18.5 to 24.9, overweight as a BMI of 25.0 kg/m² or greater, and obesity as a BMI of 30.0 kg/m² or greater, with extreme or class III obesity constituting a BMI of at least 40.0 kg/m². Recognizing that relative weight does not reflect fat distribution, particularly in the abdominal region, waist circumference also has been utilized as an indicator of excess adiposity, with cut points of 102 cm (40 inches) for men and 88 cm (35 inches) for women used to define high-risk status (Expert Panel on the Identification, Evaluation and Treatment of Overweight in Adults, 1998).

With growing prevalence, there has been increased recognition of obesity-related health risks, which include hypertension, dyslipidemia, type 2 diabetes, coronary heart disease, stroke, gallbladder disease, osteoarthritis, sleep apnea and respiratory problems, and endometrial, breast, prostate, and colon cancers (Inelmen, Sergi, Coin, Miotto, Peruzza, & Enzi, 2003; National Institute of Diabetes and Digestive and Kidney Diseases [NIDDK], 2012; Patterson, Frank, Kristal, & White, 2004; U.S. Department of Health and Human Services [USDHHS], 2001). In fact, the American Medical Association reclassified obesity as a disease in of itself (American Medical Association, 2013). Higher body weight is also associated with substantial limitations in physical functioning and increased disability in older persons (Ferraro, Ya-Ping, Gretebeck, Black, & Badylak, 2002; Inelmen et al., 2003) and greater all-cause mortality across the age spectrum (Expert Panel, 1998; Manson, Skerrett, Greenland, & VanItallie, 2004). Evidence linking obesity to cognitive impairment and dementia independent of associated vascular disease risk factors (e.g., hypertension, type 2 diabetes) has begun to emerge as well, although studies have not been well replicated (Elias, Elias, Sullivan, Wolf, & D'Agostino, 2003; Gustafson, Rothenberg, Blennow, Steen, & Skoog, 2003).

The relationship between overweight and obesity and health outcomes, including mortality in older adults and particularly the oldest old, is complex. Two age-associated factors account for much of the difficulty in understanding the impact of excess weight and adiposity in older age. First, since weight loss frequently occurs in response to disease processes, weight in older age may not accurately reflect lifelong obesity status. That is, persons with low to normal weight in older age comprise those who have maintained a healthful weight throughout their lives and those who have lost weight because of severe debilitating illness. Second, older adults typically experience loss of appendicular lean mass, or sarcopenia, and increased deposition of fat in the abdominal region. This alteration in body composition, which has known weight-related health consequences, may not be apparent from measures of relative weight (NIDDK, 2012; USDHHS, 2001). In other words, normal-weight older persons may have unhealthy levels of adiposity and an undesirable weight distribution. For this reason, some suggest further consideration of appropriate measures of obesity in older adults (Kennedy, Chokkalingham, & Srinivasan, 2004). In general, older persons who remain weight stable—that is, who do not experience illness-related weight loss—exhibit the best health profile. Nevertheless, within weight-stable older adults, overweight and obesity confer similar risks of cardiovascular disease and associated conditions, as observed in the general population.

Although the need to develop effective preventive and treatment programs for overweight and obesity for both children and adults has been promoted worldwide (Expert Panel, 1998; WHO, 2016) and the efficacy of weight loss has been established for key cardiovascular disease risk factors, including hypertension, hyperlipidemia, and type 2 diabetes (Manson et al., 2004; NIDDK, 2012; USDHHS, 2001), the issues of whether and how to treat obesity in older adults remain controversial. Many studies have found increased mortality associated with weight loss in older adults, so the merits and safety of weight reduction have been questioned. In consideration of the potential hazards of weight loss in the elderly, the Expert Panel (1998) issued the following statement regarding weight loss in older adults:

> A clinical decision to forego obesity treatment in older adults should be guided by an evaluation of the potential benefits of weight reduction for day-to-day functioning and reduction of the risk of future cardiovascular events, as well as the patient's motivation for weight reduction. Care must be taken to ensure that any weight reduction program minimizes the likelihood of adverse effects on bone health or other aspects of nutritional status. (p. xxi)

Alternately, a review of obesity in older adults focused on energy use and recommended increased physical activity, particularly resistance training, as an effective approach to combat excess adiposity and preserve muscle mass and strength (Kennedy et al., 2004).

Overweight and obesity constitute a major and growing threat to the health and functioning of older persons worldwide because many manifestations of excess energy intake and inadequate energy expenditure begin to emerge in early to late old age. Improved identification of older persons at risk and the development of safe and effective treatments that combine dietary modification and activity promotion appear to be key antidotes to the obesity epidemic.

April Bigelow

American Medical Association House of Delegates. (2013). *Resolution: 420 (A-13). Recognition of obesity as a disease.* Retrieved from http://media.npr.org/documents/2013/jun/ama-resolution-obesity.pdf

Elias, M. F., Elias, P. K., Sullivan, L. M., Wolf, P. A., & D'Agostino, R. B. (2003). Lower cognitive function in the presence of obesity and hypertension: The Framingham Heart Study. *International Journal of Obesity, 27,* 260–268.

Expert Panel on the Identification, Evaluation and Treatment of Overweight in Adults. (1998). *Clinical guidelines on the identification, evaluation, and treatment of overweight and obesity in adults.* Bethesda, MD: National Heart, Lung, and Blood Institute.

Fakhouri, F., Ogden, C. L, Carroll, M. D., Kit, B. K., & Flegal, K. M. (2012). *Prevalence of overweight and obesity among adults: United States, 2007–2010.* (National Center of Health Statistics Data Brief, No 106). Atlanta, GA: Centers for Disease Control and Prevention.

Ferraro, K. F., Ya-Ping, S., Gretebeck, R. J., Black, D. R., & Badylak, S. F. (2002). Body mass index and disability in adulthood: A 20-year panel study. *American Journal of Public Health, 92,* 834–840.

O

Gustafson, D., Rothenberg, E., Blennow, K., Steen, B., & Skoog, I. (2003). An 18-year follow-up of overweight and risk of Alzheimer disease. *Archives of Internal Medicine, 163*, 1524–1528.

Inelmen, E. M., Sergi, G., Coin, A., Miotto, F., Peruzza, S., & Enzi, G. (2003). Can obesity be a risk factor in elderly people? *Obesity Reviews, 4*, 147–155.

Kennedy, R. L., Chokkalingham, K., & Srinivasan, R. (2004). Obesity in the elderly: Who should be treating and why, and how? *Current Opinion in Clinical Nutrition and Metabolic Care, 7*, 3–9.

Manson, J. E., Skerrett, P. J., Greenland, P., & VanItallie, T. B. (2004). The escalating pandemics of obesity and sedentary lifestyle. *Archives of Internal Medicine, 164*, 249–258.

National Center for Chronic Disease Prevention and Health Promotion. (2015). *Nutrition, physical activity and obesity data, trends and maps web site.* Atlanta, GA: Centers for Disease Control and Prevention.

National Institute of Diabetes and Digestive and Kidney Diseases. (2012). *Health risks of being overweight.* Bethesda, MD: National Institutes of Health.

National Institutes of Health. (1998). Clinical guidelines on the identification, evaluation, and treatment of overweight and obesity in adults—The evidence report. *Obesity Research, 6*(Suppl. 2), 51S–209S.

Patterson, R. E., Frank, L. L., Kristal, A. R., & White, E. A. (2004). Comprehensive examination of health conditions associated with obesity in older adults. *American Journal of Preventative Medicine, 27*, 385–390.

U.S. Department of Health and Human Services. (2001). *The Surgeon General's call to action to prevent and decrease overweight and obesity.* Rockville, MD: U.S. Department of Health and Human Services, Public Health Service, Office of the Surgeon General.

World Health Organization. (2016). *Obesity and overweight* (Fact Sheet No. 311). Geneva, Switzerland: Author.

OCCUPATIONAL THERAPISTS

Occupational therapists provide skilled services using day-to-day activities that are valued, important, and meaningful (i.e., occupation) to facilitate desired levels of function. Occupations are how people "occupy" their time (Boyt Schell, Scaffa, Gillen, & Cohn, 2014) in everyday living that includes looking after oneself, enjoying life and being socially and economically productive. A core philosophical assumption is that people of all ages and abilities require occupation to grow and thrive (American Occupational Therapy Association [AOTA], 2014). Hence, active participation in occupation supports health and well-being. For example, older adults who participate in occupation-based programs, compared with simply social programs or no activity, have less pain, higher life satisfaction, diminished depressive symptoms, and better general health and physical function (Clark et al., 2012).

DOMAIN OF PRACTICE

The focus of occupational therapy intervention is "supporting health, well-being, and participation in life through engagement in occupation" (AOTA, 2014, p. S2). The context that supports participation in occupation includes not only the physical and social environments, but also the cultural, personal, temporal, and virtual contexts. Occupational therapists address occupations for activities of daily living (ADL) such as bathing, dressing, and eating; instrumental activities of daily living (IADL) such as meal preparation, medication management, community mobility; and other occupations including rest and sleep, education, work, play, leisure, and social participation (AOTA, 2014). To assist an older individual's return to a preferred *occupational performance*, occupational therapists may address motor skills, process skills, or social interaction skills (*performance skills*) while embedding these skills in the return or development of functional habits, routines, rituals, and roles (*performance patterns*). "Occupational performance is the accomplishment of the selected occupation resulting from the dynamic transaction among the client, the context and environment, and the activity or occupation" (AOTA, 2014, p. S14). For full participation, the client may need to work on motor skills such as posture, coordination, or strength; process skills such as problem solving, organization, adaptation, or attention; and social interaction skills such as orientation or verbal expression.

EVALUATION AND INTERVENTION APPROACHES

Best practice begins with an evaluation process that develops an *occupational profile* of the client's history, skills, factors (values, beliefs, spirituality, and body traits), problems, and concerns, all of which drive the choice of assessments to analyze performance. The intervention plan is then developed collaboratively with the client and incorporates a variety of approaches designed to meet the client's needs. Beyond functional restoration and adaptation, approaches may include self-management, educational services, environmental modifications, and health-promotion activities (AOTA, 2014).

Self-management may be promoted through the restoration of skills following a cerebral vascular accident (CVA). As a result of a CVA, client may have physical limitations in upper-extremity strength and sensation (Hayner, Gibson, & Giles, 2010), cognitive impairments that affect problem solving, and situational depression because of the impact on their abilities. The occupational therapist addresses range of motion, strength, and coordination in preparation for the functional performance needed to engage in everyday tasks. As part of therapy, the occupational therapist identifies cognitive deficits as well as compensatory strategies needed for safety in the home and community. For example, an occupational therapist may use a cooking task as a modality for addressing the client's strength and problem-solving ability, with the goal of returning to independence in meal preparation. Engagement in occupation is both the means and the ends of therapy.

An important concern for many older adults is to remain living in their own homes. Occupational therapists engage homeowners in assessments that evaluate how they live in their homes. Therapists educate clients and families and provide recommendations for home modifications based on current and predicted functional performance (Chase, Mann, Wasek, & Arbesman, 2012). Examples of home modifications include changing faucets to levers, doorknobs to lever handles, adding grab bars and shower chairs, adding ramps, moving the washer/dryer to the main level of the home,

changing lighting in the home, and adding non-skid stair treads. Programs run by occupational therapists address prevention by mediating risk factors that could lead to impairment (Leland, Elliott, O'Malley, & Murphy, 2012). For example, falls can lead to significant loss of function, independence, or life. Occupational therapists address balance, flexibility, vision, fear of falling, and personal efficacy through individualized or group education and treatment such as the Matter of Balance programs (Smith, Jiang, & Ory, 2012).

Healthy habits and routines are at the core of successful aging. Occupational therapists help older adults develop or reestablish routines (Hayner et al., 2010), enabling efficiency and healthy patterns to promote health and self-management (e.g., integrating medication management into daily routines to minimize medication errors). Healthy routines may also include mental and physical exercise and social participation.

A foundation of occupational therapy is *activity analysis*. In analyzing tasks and activities, occupational therapists address the person–environment–occupation fit. Occupational therapists break down the tasks to determine the required motor, process, and interaction skills required for successful completion of the task. In addition, the occupational therapist addresses the values, interests, skills, and abilities of the person engaged in the task. How do the activity demands meet the abilities of the person? How do the environment and context support the task performance? Is the selected occupation valued or interesting? These questions lead the occupational therapist to modify either the task or the environment or address remediation of client skills. Goals are collaborative in nature and are driven by the client's values, interests, and desire to return to or acquire skill in occupations.

CONDITIONS AND DISABILITIES

Occupational therapists work with clients throughout the life span as individuals, groups, or populations. Comorbidities often accompany a new illness or disability and affect an older adult's function. Occupational therapists work with clients with neurological, cardiac, and orthopedic impairments or other medical conditions, such as cancer, joint replacements, arthritis, dementias, and depression. Occupational therapists may work with older adults and their families in institutional settings such as hospitals, skilled nursing facilities, hospice programs, and community-based programs such as daycare programs, home care, and wellness centers. Special areas of practice include fall prevention, home modification, low vision, driver assessment and rehabilitation, retirement transition, successful aging, and occupational justice (i.e., removing barriers for engagement in occupations). Because occupational therapists are trained in the physical, biological, and psychological sciences, they are well suited for meeting the holistic needs of an aging population.

EDUCATION AND TRAINING

Entry-level practice requires either a master's degree or a clinical doctorate in occupational therapy. Bachelor-level–prepared practitioners graduating before 2007 continue to serve as master-clinicians (Leland et al., 2012). To practice in the United States, occupational therapists must graduate from a school accredited by the Accreditation Council for Occupational Therapy Education (ACOTE) and receive initial certification from the National Board for Certification in Occupational Therapy (NBCOT). Most states also require additional state licensure or certification to demonstrate continuing competence.

See also Physical Therapists; Rehabilitation; Speech and Language Problems.

Carol Getz Rice and Noralyn Davel Pickens

American Occupational Therapy Association. (2014). Occupational therapy practice framework: Domain and process. *American Journal of Occupational Therapy, 68*, S1–S48.

Boyt Schell, B., Scaffa, M., Gillen, G., & Cohn, E. (2014). Contemporary Occupational Therapy Practice. In B. A. B. Schell, G. Gillen, & M. E. Scaffa (Eds.), *Willard and Spackman's occupational therapy*

(12th ed., p. 50). Philadelphia, PA: Lippincott Williams & Wilkins.

Chase, C. A., Mann, K., Wasek, S., & Arbesman, M. (2012). Systematic review of the effect of home modification and fall prevention programs on falls and the performance of community-dwelling older adults. *American Journal of Occupational Therapy, 66*, 284–291.

Clark, F., Jackson, J., Carlson, M., Chou, C., Cherry, B. J., Jordan-Marsh, M., ... Azen, S. (2012). Effectiveness of a lifestyle intervention in promoting the well-being of independently living older people: Results of the Well Elderly 2 Randomized Controlled Trial. *Journal of Epidemiology and Community Health, 66*, 782–790.

Hayner, K., Gibson, G., & Giles, G. (2010). Comparison of constraint-induced movement therapy and bilateral treatment of equal intensity in people with chronic upper-extremity dysfunction after cerebrovascular accident. *American Journal of Occupational Therapy, 64*, 528–539.

Leland, N. E., Elliott, S. J., O'Malley, L., & Murphy, S. L. (2012). Occupational therapy in fall prevention: Current evidence and future directions. *American Journal of Occupational Therapy, 66*, 149–160.

Smith, M., Jiang, L., & Ory, M. (2012). Falls efficacy among older adults enrolled in an evidence-based program to reduce fall-related risk: Sustainability of individual benefits over time. *Family & Community Health, 35*, 256–263.

Web Resources
American Occupational Therapy Association (AOTA): https://www.aota.org
American Occupational Therapy Foundation (AOTF): http://www.aotf.org
Canadian Association of Occupational Therapists: http://www.caot.ca
National Board for Certification in Occupational Therapy: https://www.nbcot.org

OCCUPATIONAL THERAPY ASSESSMENT AND EVALUATION

Occupational therapists (OTs) evaluate clients' abilities to perform meaningful daily life activities. OTs have a distinct role in determining a client's functional diagnosis (i.e., the daily activities they have difficulty performing and the reasons why). In the profession of occupational therapy, activities that have meaning to the client are referred to as *occupations*. These are activities that a client needs or wants to do and can include activities of daily living (ADL; e.g., bathing, dressing, feeding); instrumental activities of daily living (IADL; e.g., caring for a spouse or grandchild, preparing meals, moving around the community); work (e.g., participating in paid or volunteer work); education (e.g., auditing a college course, seeking health information on the Internet); social participation (e.g., socializing with a friend); leisure; play; and rest/sleep. The goal of occupational therapy is the achievement of health, well-being, and participation in life for persons, groups, and populations through engagement in *occupation* (American Occupational Therapy Association [AOTA], 2014).

The first step in the occupational therapy evaluation process is to complete an occupational profile. Using an interview format, the OT ascertains the occupational history, past experiences, and patterns of daily living (e.g., routines and habits) both before and after an illness, disability, or injury. Types of questions include why the client might be seeking services as well as areas of occupation that are successful and those that are causing difficulty. A clear picture of the client's and environment, including the physical, social, virtual, temporal, personal and cultural components, is key to the occupational profile and necessary for formulating realistic and relevant goals in conjunction with the client and family (AOTA, 2014). For example, a client who lives alone in a walk-up apartment in an urban environment will have different goals and occupational therapy needs than a one who lives with a caregiving spouse, in a ranch home in the suburbs. The occupational profile thus includes questions pertaining to environments that help or hinder occupational performance.

OTs evaluate the client's skills and ability to perform meaningful activities as well as the underlying factors and environmental features that may impact performance. For example, OTs may evaluate the ability to complete meal preparation but will also assess the underlying factors that might impact the activity (e.g., cognition, affect, joint mobility, sensory function,

pain). They will also consider how the environment, such as the height of the shelves where frequently used kitchen items are stored, affects performance, as well as cultural expectations for meal preparation within the home.

OTs use a variety of assessment tools and measures, including interviews, checklists, rating scales, questionnaires, paper-and-pencil tasks, and measurement tools and devices (e.g., specialized equipment to measure grip strength, range of motion, useful field of view, light touch). Both strengths and deficits are assessed. Information from the occupational profile and the assessments that follow, as well as information from the health care team, including the family, are used in planning interventions to address goals.

Repeat assessments of actual performance are valuable for monitoring progress and identifying the effects of multidisciplinary interventions on function. For example, the Barthel Index (Eichhorn-Kissel, Dassen, & Lohrmann, 2011; Mahoney & Barthel, 1965) can be administered using direct observation and measures a client's level of independence in ADL. Areas assessed include self-care, bowel and bladder management, transfers, mobility, and stairs. This rating scale allows OTs and other members of the health care team to monitor progress.

OTs modify and adapt the activity or the environment to promote optimal functionality. They also work with clients to restore, maintain, promote, and prevent loss of function. Examples of prevention programs carried out by OTs include fall-prevention programs, driver-safety programs, and self-management programs that help prevent exacerbation of chronic conditions such as diabetes and respiratory disease.

OTs assist older adults to "age in place," or remain in their home and/or community safely and independently. When supportive housing, such as assisted-living or nursing home placement, is needed, OTs have a role in helping older adults enhance or maintain function and improve overall quality of life.

Assessment and treatment of older adults by OTs can occur in acute care, subacute/skilled nursing centers, nursing homes, home care, adult day health care centers, and other community-based settings such as Program of

O

All-Inclusive Care for the Elderly (PACE) program sites. The following case study illustrates an evaluation performed by an OT in a skilled nursing facility.

CASE STUDY

As per a chart review, Mr. Clay is an 87-year-old man who was admitted for short-term rehabilitation because of a recent fall and hip fracture. His past medical history includes osteoarthritis, hypercholesterolemia, and macular degeneration.

According to the results of an initial interview, which are used to formulate an occupational profile, before his recent fracture, Mr. Clay was living alone in a building with an elevator. He was independent in all his ADL and most IADL, including bathing, dressing, grooming, meal preparation, and community mobility (he walked to the corner store and used taxis if traveling more than a few blocks). Mr. Clay had assistance twice a month for housekeeping and had most of his groceries delivered. He used a cane for mobility. He mentions that he had experienced several falls before this one but that this was the first time he sustained a serious injury. The OT asks about the circumstances surrounding these falls. For leisure, Mr. Clay reports he enjoys reading and meeting with friends for lunch at local restaurants. His goals are to be able to return home and be independent in all his ADL. His priority is to be able to take himself to the bathroom independently. When asked about his mood, he reports that it is "not good" and that he has been feeling demoralized and very discouraged lately because of his declining health.

As per the bedside evaluation, he currently requires contact guard for bed mobility and minimal assistance for transfers and functional mobility tasks. Setup is needed for upper body dressing and grooming, and minimal assistance and the use of adapted devices are needed for lower body dressing. Using a pain scale, he reports his pain as 4/10 in his left hip. He is alert and oriented to person, place, and time and is able to follow multistep directions during the evaluation. Mr. Clay also demonstrates the ability to retain information provided by the OT,

including her name and his therapy schedule for the coming week. Although he has crepitus and minimal limits in active range of motion in bilateral shoulders, they do not interfere with his ability to carry out any of his daily activities.

Mr. Clay asks about going to the bathroom by himself. The OT discusses with the client that based on his current functional status, she recommends that he call for assistance to ensure his safety until his functional mobility improves. Results of the assessment, including his need for assistance to go to the bathroom, are discussed with both the nurses after the initial evaluation and the rest of the team during a team meeting.

Mr. Clay is able to read large-print material. He demonstrates the ability to read small print, including newsprint and a restaurant menu, with the use of a magnifier. When asked, he reports that, at times, he has difficulty recognizing faces of people he knows.

A standardized depression screening measure, the Geriatric Depression Scale (Yesavage et al., 1982–1983), is administered by the OT, if not completed by another team member. Results of the screening are discussed with Mr. Clay and the health care team, and a referral for further evaluation is requested if needed.

During a subsequent therapy visit, a performance-based assessment reveals that Mr. Clay is able to complete, with minimal assistance and the use of a mobility device, light meal preparation of his preferred lunch foods. His standing balance and standing tolerance affect his ability to perform this activity independently. The placement of items on the top shelf of the fridge as opposed to the lower shelf greatly improves his performance because it is less of a challenge for his standing balance. Given his regular use of taxis for community mobility, his ability to complete car transfers is also assessed.

Once Mr. Clay no longer requires physical assistance for transfers and mobility, the OT administers the Timed Up and Go Test, which is a standardized assessment of functional mobility (Podsiadlo & Richardson, 1991). This same tool is used in subsequent reevaluations to monitor his progress.

As Mr. Clay continues to progress with therapy, an evaluation of community mobility and shopping is planned. Mr. Clay's goal is to be able to walk a few blocks to buy milk and bread from the local store. The assessment will include Mr. Clay's ability to navigate curbs and cross the street safely within the time allotted for the traffic light as well as his ability to carry a small bag of groceries. A backpack is suggested to promote hands-free carrying of grocery items. This evaluation may be completed with the physical therapist.

Given his history of multiple falls and low vision, research evidence suggests that Mr. Clay would benefit from a home evaluation (Gillespie et al., 2012). If scheduling permits, this is completed by the OT before his discharge or he is referred to home care for further evaluation. Examples of home evaluations include the Centers for Disease Control and Prevention (CDC) Check for Safety and the In-Home Occupational Performance Evaluation (I-HOPE), a standardized, performance-based assessment that examines the effects of environmental barriers on occupational performance (Stark, Somerville & Morris, 2010).

SUMMARY

OTs assess the ability to perform the daily activities that a client needs and wants to do, using standardized and nonstandardized assessment tools. They examine the underlying reasons why difficulties may occur, including client and environmental factors that help or hinder occupational performance. They work with the client and health care team to establish functional goals.

Referral to occupational therapy is indicted when older adults are demonstrating early functional decline, are at risk for increased morbidity or dependency, or have sustained an injury or illness. OTs can determine how much assistance is needed for ADL and how much improvement is possible. Using remediation or compensation, OTs can help clients remain as independent as possible and help prevent functional decline. They can also implement evidenced-based programs to promote healthy and productive aging.

Tracy L. Chippendale

American Occupational Therapy Association. (2014). Occupational therapy practice framework: Domain and process (3rd ed.). *American Journal of Occupational Therapy, 68*(Suppl. 1), S1–S48. doi:10.5014/ajot.2014.682006

Eichhorn-Kissel, J., Dassen, T., & Lohrmann, C. (2011). Comparison of the responsiveness of the Care Dependency Scale for rehabilitation and the Barthel Index. *Clinical Rehabilitation, 25,* 760–767. doi:10.1177/0269215510397558

Gillespie, L. D., Robertson, M. D., Gillespie, W. J. Sherrington, C., Gates, S., Clemson, M., & Lamb, S. E. (2012). Interventions for preventing falls in older people living in the community. *The Cochrane Library, 11.* doi:10.1002/14651858.CD007146.pub3

Mahoney, F. L., & Barthel, D. W. (1965). Functional evaluation: The Barthel Index. *Maryland State Medical Journal, 14,* 61–65.

Podsiadlo, D., & Richardson, S. (1991). The Timed Up and Go: A test of basic functional mobility for frail elderly persons. *Journal of the American Geriatrics Society, 39,* 142–148.

Stark, S. L., Somerville, E. K., & Morris, J. C. (2010). In-Home Occupational Performance Evaluation (I-HOPE). *American Journal of Occupational Therapy, 64,* 580–589. doi:10.5014/ajot.2012.08065

Yesavage, J. A., Brink, T. L., Rose, T. L., Lum, O., Huang, V., Adey, M., & Leirer, V. O. (1982–1983). Development and validation of a geriatric depression screening scale: A preliminary report. *Journal of Psychiatric Research, 17,* 37–49.

Web Resources
American Occupational Therapy Association: http://www.aota.org
Centers for Disease Control and Prevention: Check for safety: A home fall prevention checklist for older adults: http://www.cdc.gov/homeandrecreationalsafety/pubs/english/booklet_eng_desktop-a.pdf

OLDER AMERICANS ACT

The federal Older Americans Act (OAA; Pub. L. No. 89–73, 79 Stat. 218) was enacted on July 14, 1965, the year during which three programs that are cornerstones of the nation's support and protection of its older citizens were established. Amendments to the Social Security Act on July 30, 1965 (Pub. L. No. 89–97, 79 Stat. 286;

O

Title XVIII and Title XIX, respectively) created two new national health entitlement programs, Medicare and Medicaid. Parts of the Medicare health insurance program are funded by a payroll tax, by premiums paid by beneficiaries who are citizens or permanent legal residents, and/ or by general fund revenues. Means-tested and restricted to eligible citizens and permanent legal residents, Medicaid is funded jointly by the federal and state governments. Unlike Medicare and Medicaid, the OAA programs are funded annually by discretionary congressional appropriations and matched by requisite state and local funds. OAA programs do not restrict access by level of income.

Medicare and Medicaid finance health care for older Americans. Medicare also provides assistance to disabled nonelderly persons who are Social Security disability insurance beneficiaries and to persons with certain medical conditions. The Centers for Medicare & Medicaid Services (CMS) in the U.S. Department of Health and Human Services (USDHHS) administer Medicare and, with the states, Medicaid. Medicaid finances health care for eligible low-income children, pregnant women, and disabled individuals. For low-income persons aged 65 years and older, it funds some home, community-based, and institutional long-term care.

The Administration on Aging (AoA), established in 1965, now resides within the Administration for Community Living (ACL), which was instituted on April 18, 2012, using the organization and delegation authority vested in the USDHHS Secretary. The AoA administers OAA programs, oversees the Aging Network (AN), and is the chief federal advocate for older Americans. Preventive and supportive home and community-based services (HCBS), including social, health, legal, nutrition, and other programs and services, are authorized for persons aged 60 years and older under the OAA, Title III. For the National Family Caregiver Support Program (Title IIIE), the age of eligibility of the recipient and the family caregivers varies.

The ACL also hosts the new Administration for Intellectual and Developmental Disabilities and aims to better coordinate services and supports and foster collaboration among entities that serve older Americans and persons with disabilities.

OAA VISION FOR OLDER AMERICANS

The OAA, Title I, details the nation's broad aspirations for its citizens aged 60 years and older. Dignity, self-determination, and independence are among the values championed, as are quality-of-later-life assurances such as protection from abuse and neglect and an adequate retirement income, housing, meaningful participation and activity, education, health and mental health, and the application of research evidence to promote optimal functioning and responsive programming. Recognizing its increasing significance, oral health was added as a disease-prevention and health-promotion priority for older Americans in the 2016 reauthorization.

AGING NETWORK

Title II of the OAA and subsequent amendments established the AoA and the national AN that is composed of state units on aging (56 SUAs), local area agencies on aging (629 AAAs), 244 Native American Indian tribal organizations representing 400 tribes, and two nonprofits serving Native Hawaiians. SUAs and AAAs coordinate community services and advocate for older persons. They and native organizations must develop and submit aging plans based on needs assessments informed by AN data sets, research by universities and others, and information from community residents, consumers of OAA services, and service providers. State and local assessments of their readiness to meet the challenges of an aging America are requisite. The 2016 amendments require AAA plans to specify public awareness, prevention, and investigation procedures and efforts related to elder abuse, neglect, and exploitation in coordination with their SUA and other AN partners.

More than 200 Aging and Disability Resource Centers (ADRCs), an AoA partnership with CMS, are access or single points of entry to long-term services and supports provided by more than 29,000 AN service providers nationwide. The 2016 amendments called for improvements to ADRC coordination with AAA and other community organizations around the provision of HCBS information to persons already in or at risk of institutional care.

MAJOR PROVISIONS OF THE OAA

Title II specifies the statutory roles and responsibilities of the Assistant Secretary for Aging, the AOA, and the AN and its structure. The responsibilities of the Assistant Secretary of the ACL were expanded in 2016 and include expectations pertaining to best-care coordination practices to benefit persons with multiple chronic illnesses, public education about older Americans' health and economic needs, service of Holocaust survivors, consumer guidance in selecting HCBS, best practices for the modernization of multipurpose senior centers, and person-centered transportation services.

A number of programs and centers are authorized in Title II: the Eldercare Locator; the Pension, Counseling, and Information Program; the National Center for Benefits Outreach and Enrollment; the National Center on Elder Abuse; the National Long-Term Care Ombudsman Resource Center; the ADRCs under the Nursing Home and Long-Term Care Initiative; and the Senior Medicare Patrol (permanently authorized in 2016 within Title IV). The 2006 Title II amendments spoke to elder justice, elder abuse, and mental health issues, adding at least one dedicated staff position each to focus within AOA on elder abuse prevention and services and mental health services. A secretary-level federal interagency coordinating council was added to address issues ranging from housing to technology for older persons. Title II 2006 amendments provided a National Center on Senior Benefits Outreach and Enrollment, along with provisions for better services to limited English-speaking populations by federal agencies, heightened evidence-based approaches to nutrition services, and the inclusion of private-pay options for older adults not typically served by the OAA programs.

Through a series of OAA reauthorizations, AoA's responsibilities for older persons and their families have expanded since 1965, with significant emphasis on assisting family caregivers and systematizing home and community-based supports. In 1975, amendments to the OAA mandated the inclusion and prioritization of HCBS such as transportation, home care, legal services, and home repair. Three years later, AAAs were authorized, and HCBS were consolidated under Title III, Grants for State and Community Programs on Aging. The OAA Grants to Indian Tribal Organizations was restructured under Title VI in the same year. Without means tests, the AN targets older Americans with the greatest economic or social need, particularly low-income minorities and older persons who reside in rural communities. Voluntary contributions by service recipients are now welcome.

The OAA authorization lapsed in 1996, but the proposal of a new National Family Caregiver Support Program (enacted as Title IIIE) garnered strong support for the OAA reauthorization in 2000. The act's authorization lapsed again in 2005 but was restored in 2006, adopting significant amendments focusing the AN on, for example, assessment of the aging preparedness of communities and evidence-based long-term care systems development.

Title III includes Supportive Services and Senior Centers (IIIB), and Congregate (Title IIIC-1) and Home-Delivered (Title IIIC-2) Nutrition Services, as well as Disease Prevention and Health Promotion Services (Title IIID, enacted in 1987). The 2006 amendments infused Title III with "principles of choice for independence," calling for consumer empowerment, healthy lifestyles, and community-based residential options for older adults needing supportive services. Persons with limited English-language proficiency and persons at risk of institutional care were also identified as potentially appropriate for OAA assistance.

The 2016 reauthorization provides appropriations for OAA health promotions programs that are evidence based. Health-promotion collaborations ongoing with the Centers for Disease Control and Prevention (CDC), CMS, and the Substance Abuse and Mental Health Services Administration (SAMHSA) should inform AN programs.

The National Family Caregiver Support Program (NFCSP, Title IIIE) utilizes evidence-based approaches and offers information and assistance, counseling and other support,

O

training and education for family caregivers, respite care, and specially tailored services. It was expanded and its funding was increased in 2016 to acknowledge the challenges associated with giving care to persons with Alzheimer's disease, adult children with disabilities, and minors younger than 18 years (by older relatives).

Title IV provided significant funding support for gerontology education, and demonstration programs in the 1970s and 1980s. Redesignated "Activities for Health, Independence, and Longevity" in 2006, it added naturally occurring retirement communities (NORCs), other long-term care services, and mental health services and screening as foci. The Computer Training, Multidisciplinary Centers and Multidisciplinary Systems, and Ombudsman and Advocacy Demonstration Projects were retired in 2016.

The Community Service Senior Opportunities Act (Title V, enacted in 1973), now the Senior Community Service Employment Program (2006), trains eligible unemployed adults aged 55 years and older and facilitates part-time community service employment. Performance outcomes and a more competitive funding award process were incorporated as requirements in 2006 to enable the U.S. Department of Labor Secretary to select contractors based on merit rather than service longevity.

Title VI, Grants for Native Americans, was authorized in 1978, and Native Hawaiian elders were added to the Title during the 1987 reauthorization.

In 2006, the Grants to Promote State Elder Justice Systems section was enacted under Title VII, Vulnerable Elder Rights Protection, and activities, resources, and accountability were specified in the Programs for Prevention of Elder Abuse, Neglect, and Exploitation. Significant elder abuse and ombudsman policy and program boosts were then authorized in 2016. Elder abuse terms were clarified, and public awareness, staff training, elder abuse data promotion, and the use of best practices were promoted. Long-term care ombudsman programs (LTCOPs) were directed to serve all long-term care (LTC) facility residents of all ages and to work for residents who lacked representatives and the ability to communicate. A

series of assurances were also specified: the barring of impediments to LTCOP access, authorization to serve residents in transition from institutions to home care, provision for disclosure of all program information, facilitation of the development of resident and family councils in institutions, authorization of the LTCOP to serve as a health oversight agency for the Health Insurance Portability and Accountability Act (HIPAA), protection against institutional and other conflicts of interest, and management of the LTCOP. The 2016 amendments acknowledged that LTCOs must possess a core set of knowledge and skills and noted that elder abuse, neglect, and exploitation best practices are available through trainings by the National Long-Term Care Ombudsman Resource Center.

The Alzheimer's Disease Support Services Program (421 U.S.C. 280_3 to 280 C-56) and the Lifespan Respite Care Program (Title XXIX, 42 U.S.C.30011–4) are administered by the AoA but are not OAA programs. Together with Title III services, they aid caregivers and others in need of support.

CHALLENGES AND OPPORTUNITIES

Nearly 70 years of lower birth rates, improvements in public health that have supported population aging, and the coming of age of the Baby Boomers should have resulted in the elimination of or declines in ageism. Congressional, state, and local funding for OAA's discretionary programs and services have not kept pace with the growing number of older Americans. Public policies continue to lean on families and their personal resources when a loved one needs care or support. The human and financial costs of care are commonly borne by the caregiver, whose health and earnings, benefits, and retirement security may be placed at risk as a consequence.

The Community Living Assistance Services and Supports (CLASS) program proposed by the AoA was enacted as part of the ACA, offering a brief moment of hope that supportive services could be financed as a universal national program. However, actuarial analyses concluded that CLASS was fiscally unsustainable because of the likely risk pool it would attract, and thus it was repealed on January 2, 2013, via the American Taxpayer Relief Act of 2012 budget agreement. A hastily organized national commission charged thereafter with formulating a financing and long-term care service delivery plan found itself at an impasse on the national financing model.

The flexing of institutional parameters to have the AoA lead in the development of CLASS demonstrated the capacity of the organization to serve as a site for innovative policy and program development. The OAA itself is a versatile policy tool for legislating responsive discretionary programs. At least one challenge and opportunity for the AN to resolve is how to enact policies and programs for older persons that do not rely so heavily on family caregivers, who commonly sacrifice their financial, social, and physical well-being while caring for another.

Jeanette C. Takamura

Web Resources
Administration for Community Living: http://www.acl.gov/About_ACL/Index.aspx
Historical Evolution of Programs for Older Americans: http://www.aoa.gov/AoARoot/AoA_Programs/OAA/resources/History.aspx
Outline of 2016 Amendments to the Older Americans Act: http://www.aoa.gov/AoA_programs/OAA/oaa.aspx#t4-OAA2016: changes

ORAL HEALTH ASSESSMENT

Despite increasing awareness of the need for dental care, many older people have poor oral health, inadequate oral hygiene, and carious teeth; are edentulous (i.e., toothless); and lack or have poorly fitting dentures. Oral health problems often affect an individual's well-being, self-esteem, and quality of life (Kayser-Jones, Bird, Paul, Long, & Schell, 1995). Maintaining oral health in old age is important because untreated dental problems can cause pain and discomfort that may interfere with eating and swallowing, resulting in inadequate nutritional intake. Poor

oral health can also lead to life-threatening conditions, including, for example, brain abscesses, vascular heart disease, renal disease, and respiratory infections such as hospital-acquired pneumonia (Kanzigg & Hunt, 2016; Ní Chróinín et al., 2016).

Oral carcinoma is a concern. In 2015, it was estimated that there were 45,780 cases of oral and pharyngeal cancer, resulting in an estimated 8,650 deaths (American Cancer Society, 2015). Most of these cases occurred in older people. Early detection and treatment are the most important factors in reducing oral-cancer morbidity and mortality (American Cancer Society, 2015).

Although edentulism has declined since the 1960s, about 19% of people aged 65 years and older and 26% of people aged 75 years and older are edentulous (Dye, Thorton-Evans, Li, & Iafolla, 2015). Lower socioeconomic status, geographical region, cultural factors, and education influence oral health. Among older Americans, 37% of those living at less than 100% of the poverty level were edentulous compared with 16% of people living at or more than 200% of the poverty level (Dye, Li, & Beltran-Aguilar, 2012).

Numerous studies document the high prevalence of oral disease among older people and the need for evaluation and treatment, particularly among those with dementia (Chen, Clark, & Naorungroj, 2013). Barriers to obtaining oral health care in nursing homes include a shortage of skilled geriatric dentists, lack of private dental insurance, and lack of Medicare coverage for routine dental care. The Patient Protection and Affordable Care Act required dental coverage for children on Medicaid but not for adults, resulting in varying coverage across the states, with 18 states covering only emergency services and 27 states covering preventive services (Medicaid and CHIP Payment and Access Commission [MACPAC], 2015).

Federal regulations state that nursing facilities must provide routine and emergency dental services (including an annual oral health examination), cleaning, repair, inspection for signs of dental disease, and radiographs or other procedures as needed, but only 80% of facilities reported providing dental care (Centers for Medicare & Medicaid Services, 2016; Dolan,

O

Atchison, & Huynh, 2005). Provision for dental care in long-term care communities varies from state to state. In most states, dentists are not employed on staff and dental services are provided by contract, usually during monthly visits. If emergency dental care is needed, it is provided only if the family, resident, or a nurse requests care. Nursing staff—RNs, licensed vocational nurses (LVNs), and certified nursing assistants (CNAs)—are responsible for providing oral hygiene and are therefore in a position to identify oral health problems. Most nursing staff, however, have limited or no preparation in assessing oral health, make it a low priority, and report resistance by residents as reasons oral care is not provided (Willumsen, Karlsen, Naess, & Bjørntvedt, 2012).

KAYSER-JONES BRIEF ORAL HEALTH STATUS EXAMINATION

The Kayser-Jones Brief Oral Health Status Examination (BOHSE) was designed to provide nursing home staff with a tool that could be used to assess oral health. It was developed based on recommendations from the American Dental Association, a review of available oral assessment guides, and consultation with dental-school faculty. Ten items reflect the status of oral health and function: lymph nodes; lips; tongue; tissue inside cheek, floor and roof of mouth; gums between teeth or under artificial teeth; saliva; condition of natural teeth; condition of artificial teeth; pairs of teeth in chewing position; and oral cleanliness. Each item has three descriptors and is rated on a 3-point scale (0, 1, 2)—0 indicating the healthy end and 2 the unhealthy end of the scale (see Figure O.1). The final score is the sum of the scores from the 10 categories and can range from 0 (*very healthy*) to 20 (*very unhealthy*; Kayser-Jones et al., 1995). It must be emphasized that the Kayser-Jones BOHSE is for screening purposes only; it is not a diagnostic tool and it does not replace the need for an annual examination by a professional dentist.

In performing the assessment when this instrument was being developed, several residents were referred for immediate dental care for conditions discovered during data collection, including an infected root tip, a moderately

severe case of lichen planus, a gum abscess, gingivitis, several cases of candidiasis, and poorly fitting or broken dentures. The residents with these conditions had not complained to staff; these problems were discovered only through participation in the research project (Kayser-Jones et al., 1995). In a study using the Kayser-Jones BOHSE with residents with Alzheimer's disease, the investigators found that the nursing staff was unaware that two of their residents wore dentures. The residents' dentures had never been removed although they had lived in the facility for several months (Lin et al., 1999).

Since the initial publication of this tool, the original or modified versions of the Kayser-Jones BOHSE have been used in numerous countries around the world, including Australia, Taiwan, China, Sweden, Germany, Turkey, Belgium, Indonesia, and Japan. It is also being used to assess oral health in hundreds of facilities in the United States and Canada, and it can be used in a variety of settings, including residential and acute care, and in the community (Johnson, 2012). Furthermore, it is useful with residents who are cognitively impaired and are unable to request dental services (Jablonski et al., 2011).

ADVANTAGES OF ORAL HEALTH EXAMINATIONS BY NURSING STAFF

Nurses are in an excellent position to conduct an oral health examination. They are well acquainted with residents and are familiar with their habits, behaviors, likes, and dislikes. A resident who refuses to be examined one day can be examined the following day. Nurses can examine residents on a regular basis, which is especially important for people with cognitive impairment and for non–English-speaking residents who may be unable to report pain or discomfort. Moreover, if there is a change in a resident's behavior, such as refusal to eat, the nurse can perform an examination to rule out oral disease. Involving the nursing staff leads to earlier recognition of problems and may prevent systemic infections or other situations such as weight loss. Furthermore, teaching nursing staff to perform an oral health assessment increases their awareness of the importance of dental health and oral hygiene.

Resident's Name _____   Date _____

Examiner's Name _____   TOTAL SCORE _____

CATEGORY	MEASUREMENT	0	1	2
LYMPH NODES	Observe and feel nodes	No enlargement	Enlarged, not tender	Enlarged and tender*
LIPS	Observe, feel tissue and ask resident, family or staff (e.g., primary caregiver)	Smooth, pink moist	Dry, chapped, or red at corners*	White or red patch, bleeding or ulcer for 2 weeks*
TONGUE	Observe, feel tissue and ask resident, family or staff (e.g., primary caregiver)	Normal roughness, pink and moist	Coated, smooth, patchy, severely fissured or some redness	Red, smooth, white or red patch; ulcer for 2 weeks*
TISSUE INSIDE CHEEK, FLOOR AND ROOF OF MOUTH	Observe, feel tissue and ask resident, family or staff (e.g., primary caregiver)	Pink and moist	Dry, shiny, rough, red, or swollen*	White or red patch, bleeding, hardness; ulcer for 2 weeks*
GUMS BETWEEN TEETH AND/OR UNDER ARTIFICIAL TEETH	Gently press gums with tip of tongue blade	Pink, small indentations; firm, smooth and pink under artificial teeth	Redness at border around 1-6 teeth; one red area or sore spot under artificial teeth*	Swollen or bleeding gums, redness at border around 7 or more teeth, loose teeth; generalized redness or sores under artificial teeth*
SALIVA (EFFECT ON TISSUE)	Touch tongue blade to center or tongue and floor of mouth	Tissues moist, saliva free flowing and watery	Tissues dry and sticky	Tissues parched and red, no saliva*
CONDITION OF NATURAL TEETH	Observe and count number of decayed or broken teeth	No decayed or broken teeth/roots	1-3 decayed or broken teeth/roots*	4 or more decayed or broken teeth/roots; fewer than 4 teeth in either jaw*
CONDITION OF ARTIFICIAL TEETH	Observe and ask patient, family or staff (e.g., primary caregiver)	Unbroken teeth, worn most of the time	1 broken/missing tooth, or worn for eating or cosmetics only	More than 1 broken or missing tooth, or either denture missing or never worn*
PAIRS OF TEETH IN CHEWING POSITION (NATURAL OR ARTIFICIAL)	Observe and count pairs of teeth in chewing position	12 or more pairs of teeth in chewing position	8-11 pairs of teeth in chewing position	0-7 pairs of teeth in chewing position*
ORAL CLEANLINESS	Observe appearance of teeth or dentures	Clean, no food particles/tartar in the mouth or on artificial teeth	Food particles/tartar in one of two places in the mouth or on artificial teeth	Food particles/tartar in most places in the mouth or on artificial teeth

Upper dentures labeled: Yes ☐ No ☐ None ☐   Lower dentures labeled: Yes ☐ No ☐ None ☐

Is your mouth comfortable? Yes ☐ No ☐ If No, explain: _____

_____

Additional comments: _____

_____

*Underlined = refer to dentist immediately

FIGURE O.1 Kayser-Jones Brief Oral Health Status Examination.

Source: © 1995, Regents of the University of California, San Francisco. All rights reserved. Used with permission. The author acknowledges the assistance of William F. Bird, DDS, Dr PH, in the development of this instrument.

Given the high level of unmet dental needs in nursing homes and the relationship among oral health status, physical health, and well-being, nurses, dentists, and physicians should collaborate in addressing this important problem.

See also Dentures; Geriatric Dentistry: Clinical Aspects; Oral Health Assessment; Xerostomia.

Tara Sharpp and Jeanie Kayser-Jones

American Cancer Society. (2015). *Cancer facts & figures 2015.* Atlanta, GA: Author.

Centers for Medicare & Medicaid Services. (2016). *State operations manual, Section 483.55, Appendix PP—Guidance to surveyors for long term care facilities.* Washington, DC: U.S. Department of Health and Human Services.

Chen, X., Clark, J. J., & Naorungroj, S. (2013). Oral health in older adults with dementia living in different environments: A propensity analysis. *Special Care Dentist, 33*(5), 239–247.

Dolan, T. A., Atchison, K., & Huynh, T. N. (2005). Access to dental care among older adults in the United States. *Journal of Dental Education, 69*(9), 961–974.

Dye, B., Li., X., & Beltran-Aguilar, E. D. (2012). *Selected oral health indicators in the United States, 2005–2008.* Hyattsville, MD: National Center for Health Statistics.

Dye, B., Thorton-Evans, G., Li, X., & Iafolla, T. J. (2015). *Dental caries and tooth loss in adults in the United States, 2011–2012.* Hyattsville, MD: National Center for Health Statistics.

Jablonski, R. A., Kolanowski, A., Therrien, B., Mahoney, E. K., Kassab, C., & Leslie, D. L. (2011). Reducing care-resistant behaviors during oral hygiene in persons with dementia. *BMC Oral Health, 11*, 30. doi:10.1186/1472-6831-11-30

Johnson, V. (2012). Evidence-based practice guideline: Oral hygiene care for functionally dependent and cognitively impaired older adults. *Journal of Gerontological Nursing, 38*(11), 11. doi:10.3928/00989134-20121003-02

Kanzigg, L. A., & Hunt, L. (2016). Oral health and hospital-acquired pneumonia in elderly patients: A review of the literature. *Journal of Dental Hygiene, 90*(Suppl. 1), 15–21.

Kayser-Jones, J., Bird, W. F., Paul, S. M., Long, L., & Schell, E. S. (1995). An instrument to assess the oral health status of nursing home residents. *The Gerontologist, 35*(6), 814–824.

Lin, C. Y., Jones, D. B., Godwin, K., Godwin, R. K., Knebl, J. A., & Niessen, L. (1999). Oral health

assessment by nursing staff of Alzheimer's patients in a long-term-care facility. *Special Care in Dentistry, 19*(2), 64–71.

Medicaid and CHIP Payment and Access Commission. (2015). *Medicaid coverage of dental benefits for adults, Report to Congress on Medicaid and CHIP.* Washington, DC: Author.

Ní Chróinín, D., Montalto, A., Jahromi, S., Ingham, N., Beveridge, A., & Foltyn, P. (2016). Oral health status is associated with common medical comorbidities in older hospital inpatients. *Journal of the American Geriatric Society, 64*(8), 1696–1700.

Willumsen, T., Karlsen, L., Naess, R., & Bjørntvedt, S. (2012). Are the barriers to good oral hygiene in nursing homes within the nurses or the patients? *Gerodontology, 29*(2), e748–e755.

Web Resources

American Dental Association: http://www.ada.org

International Association for Dental Research: http://www.iadr.com

National Institute of Dental and Craniofacial Research: http://www.nidcr.nih.gov

Oral Health America: http://www.oralhealthamerica.org

OSTEOARTHRITIS

Osteoarthritis (OA), with its prevalence reaching 40% of individuals older than 70 years, disproportionately affects older populations and is a major public health issue, given its contribution to long-term pain and disability. The most commonly affected sites include the hands, knees, hips, and spine, with radiographic changes typical of OA found in most people aged 65 years and older. Traditionally dismissed as an inevitable result of aging, it is now recognized as a complex interaction of cellular, biomechanical, and genetic factors. Although OA can affect any joint, those best studied in the literature include the hips, knees, and hands.

PATHOPHYSIOLOGY

OA can be viewed as the loss of homeostasis within the joint involving not only cartilage and bone, but also the synovium, ligaments, and muscles. This results in a net loss of articular cartilage with joint space narrowing, the remodeling of subchondral bone with both hypertrophy (sclerosis), and new bone formation (osteophytes) at the joint margins, as well as inflammation and hyperplasia of the synovial membrane and joint capsule.

The net loss of articular cartilage centers around the chondrocyte, the cell responsible for cartilage metabolism. It exists in a relatively acellular extracellular matrix consisting of proteoglycans, type II collagen and noncollagen matrix proteins. The proteoglycans present as large aggrecans that consist of hyaluronate, chondroitin sulfate, and keratin sulfate. Stimulated by a stressor such as biochemical–biomechanical strain or direct damage, the chondrocytes begin to proliferate, resulting in both increased matrix synthesis and production of proinflammatory cytokines (e.g., interleukin-1 and tumor necrosis factor-alpha [TNF-alpha]), accelerating the release of matrix-degrading enzymes (matrix metalloproteinases [e.g., stromelysin]). This imbalance between degradation and repair determines the progression from softening of cartilage to fibrillation, ulceration, and eventual cartilage loss.

Increasingly, the role of the synovium has also been recognized. Cartilage breakdown products may be considered foreign by synovial cells, stimulating both catabolic and proinflammatory mediators and leading to excess production of proteolytic enzymes that, in turn, promote further cartilage breakdown (Lories, Neerinckx, & Kloppenburg, 2015). In addition, it has been demonstrated that systemic metabolic abnormalities may play a role because adipokines secreted by adipose tissue such as leptin and adiponectin are found in synovial tissue and have been shown to increase the activity of matrix-degrading enzymes and key cytokines in the cartilage catabolic process.

RISK FACTORS

Most cases of OA are primary or idiopathic, especially in those of advancing age. Ethnicity has also been observed to be a factor; Southern Chinese and South African Blacks have a very low incidence of hip OA (Goodman,

2005). Secondary causes include prior trauma (including iatrogenic from surgical procedures), impact sports such as football, developmental dysplasia of the hip, inflammatory arthritis such as rheumatoid arthritis (RA), metabolic diseases such as hemochromatosis, and hypermobility and joint laxity. In terms of knee OA, increased incidence has been observed in obese women; in those with occupations that involve lifting, bending, kneeling, and squatting; and those who have local mechanical factors, such as malalignment and muscle weakness, leading to focal loading that accelerates progressive damage of the knee joint. Genetic factors also contribute, with ongoing research into candidate genes that have effects on skeletogenesis, ligament laxity and epigenetic regulation of matrix-degrading enzymes (Reynard & Loughlin, 2013). Recreational sports such as jogging do not increase the incidence of OA for those with normal joint-supporting structures such as tendons and menisci.

CLINICAL FEATURES

Patients with OA typically complain of gradual-onset joint pain that is worse with activity and relieved by rest. The pain is generally worse toward the end of the day and, as symptoms progress, may interfere with sleep. Stiffness after a period of immobility (gel phenomenon) is brief, as is morning stiffness, a complaint that helps distinguish OA from an inflammatory arthritis such as RA. Prolonged activity increases the symptoms of OA, whereas symptoms of an inflammatory arthritis are ameliorated by activity. Patients may note joint swelling and nodal disease (e.g., Bouchard's and Heberden's nodes of the proximal and distal interphalangeal joints, respectively), but the affected joint does not become inflamed, red, or hot. Range of motion may be affected with palpation of the joint during movement, eliciting crepitus. Careful evaluation is important to separate causes of pain because hip disease can cause referred pain to the knee and back disease can produce referred pain in distal limbs. Furthermore, a small subset of patients have "inflammatory OA" with inflammatory changes, erosions and medial or

O

lateral subluxation, commonly of the proximal and/or distal interphalangeal joints.

INVESTIGATIONS

Plain radiographs typically reveal joint-space narrowing alongside osteophyte formation, subchondral sclerosis, and subchondral bone cysts. However, patients may have radiographic evidence of disease, yet be asymptomatic. The correlation between standard radiographic changes and symptoms attributable to OA is greatest for the knee and least for the hands. Blood tests or advanced imaging are generally not required but can exclude other inflammatory entities when the history or examination is equivocal. Joint aspiration can distinguish OA from infection or inflammatory causes of arthritis via analysis of the joint fluid, which is typically clear/amber and has fewer than 2,000 white blood cells/mm^3.

MANAGEMENT

Managing OA requires early recognition and, like many conditions, includes lifestyle and nonpharmacologic management in addition to medical and surgical interventions. Treatment typically focuses on the relief of pain and improving function alongside potential disease-modifying OA drugs (DMOADs) that may attenuate the progression of cartilage loss. Given the prevalence of OA, it is not surprising that a number national and international societies have published guidelines for its treatment (American Academy of Orthopedic Surgeons [AAOS], 2013; Hochberg et al., 2012; McAlindon et al., 2014; National Institute for Health and Care Excellence [NICE], 2014).

Nonpharmacological Treatment

As always, management begins with patient and caregiver education about the disease and its prognosis and all published treatment guidelines emphasize the role of nonpharmacologic therapy, primarily exercise in various forms. A strengthening and conditioning program is strongly recommended. Effective physical therapy (PT) includes localized modalities such as heat, ultrasound, and ice, and a graduated exercise regimen to improve joint range of motion and motor strength. Tai Chi, a multicomponent traditional Chinese mind–body practice has been shown to be as beneficial for pain and function as standard PT in knee OA (Wang et al., 2016). A recent comparison of swimming versus cycling in a small cohort with predominantly knee OA for 3 months revealed significant reductions in joint pain, stiffness, and physical limitation compared to baseline, with no difference in the magnitude of improvement between the two modalities (Alkatan et al., 2016). Weight reduction is also important because it can decrease symptoms from OA of the weight-bearing joints and slow progressive joint damage.

Recent Cochrane Reviews have not been overly supportive of acupuncture (did not reach the investigators' threshold for clinical significance), therapeutic ultrasound (no clinically significant improvement), or electromagnetic therapy (no clinically significant improvement in physical function or quality of life; Li et al., 2013; Manheimer et al., 2010; Rutjes, Nüesch, Sterchi, & Jüni, 2010).

Patients with hip and knee OA should be advised about appropriate footwear with thick but soft soles and no raised heels. Both physical and occupational therapists can fit supportive devices that reduce pain and improve function, whereas adjunctive assistive devices such as enlarged grips on pens and cutlery can reduce mechanical loading and facilitate specific tasks. Those with knee OA may benefit from a knee brace, whereas those with thumb OA may benefit from splinting. A properly used cane can also provide effective "unloading" of an involved knee or hip. The cane length should be equal to the distance from the bottom of the shoe heel to the wrist crease when the arm is held at the side. For the cane to be effective, it must be used on the side opposite the involved leg.

Pharmacological Treatment

Analgesia

Traditionally, acetaminophen has been advocated as first-line pharmacologic therapy for OA. However, this has recently been questioned based on potential adverse effects such as liver toxicity as well as a recognition that its effect in chronic pain is small. A recent network meta-analysis found no role for single-agent acet-aminophen, given its nearly null effect on pain symptoms especially when compared with non-steroidal anti-inflammatory drugs (NSAIDs; da Costa et al., 2016).

NSAIDs and cyclo-oxygenase (COX-2) inhibitors provide both analgesic and anti-inflammatory activity and are effective at pro-viding pain relief from OA symptoms. However, significant potential side effects limit their wide-spread use. Gastrointestinal toxicity, including ulcer formation and risk of bleeding, is increased in patients who are older than 65 years. This is the most common reason for discontinuing NSAID use and can be decreased by the concomitant use of a proton pump inhibitor. Although COX-2 inhibitors confer less gastrointestinal risk, the substantial risk of cardiovascular events has limited their use. Additional contraindications to the long-term use of NSAIDs include hyper-tension, renal disease, and heart failure. Topical NSAIDs confer similar benefits while minimiz-ing toxicity and are recommended for patients who have only one or few symptomatic joints.

Other topical agents include capsaicin that can reduce the pain associated for hand and knee OA and is recommended for knee OA by the OA Research Society International (OARSI; McAlindon et al., 2014). However, it is not recommended by the American College of Rheumatology (ACR; Hochberg et al., 2012). Use of tramadol or centrally acting agents such as duloxetine may be helpful but may be limited by adverse effects, including nausea, somno-lence, and fatigue. However, opiate analgesics should be used only in cases in which pain remains severe after exhausting nonopioid anal-gesic therapies and the patient declines or is not a candidate for surgical therapy. If used, careful patient selection and monitoring are essential for avoiding adverse effects.

Intra-Articular Therapy

Judicious use of intra-articular corticosteroid injections (no more than three or four times a year) can be very effective in relieving pain, especially in patients with a single painful joint.

Commonly used preparations include triamcin-olone acetonide and methylprednisolone 40 mg, often mixed with 1 to 2 mL of 1% to 2% lido-caine for a large joint such as the knee. Efficacy is rarely sustained for longer than 1 to 4 weeks for knee OA and 8 weeks for hip OA, but the effect may be prolonged for individual patients. It is a safe and well-tolerated procedure, although patients should be warned about the potential for temporary exacerbation of pain in the first 24 to 48 hours.

Hyaluronic acid can be administered as a series of intra-articular injections, the ther-apeutic goal being the maintenance of intra-articular lubrication or "viscosupplementation." However, clinical evidence for its benefit in knee OA remains mixed and debated (Hunter, 2015). Given this uncertainty, hyaluronic acid is not recommended for knee OA by OARSI and only conditionally recommended by the ACR, if no relief is gained from acetaminophen or NSAIDs (Hochberg et al., 2012; McAlindon et al., 2014).

Disease-Modifying Therapy

As understanding of the molecular pathogenesis of OA has improved, a number of potential ther-apeutic targets have been identified. However, DMOADs have yet to be approved by any reg-ulatory agency. Doxycycline, which reduces matrix metalloproteinase (MMP) activity, decreased joint-space narrowing in knee OA in a clinical trial using standardized radiographs, although follow-up has not been encouraging (Brandt et al., 2005). Another medication stud-ied was risedronate, which did reduce cartilage degradation but did not have any significant effects on symptoms or structural progression of knee OA. Furthermore, clinical studies of inter-leukin-1 or TNF-α blockade have yet to show any impact on clinical outcomes.

Chondroitin sulfate and glucosamine sul-fate have been used to treat OA both individu-ally and in combination. However, systematic reviews and meta-analyses have failed to show consistent benefit in terms of symptom relief so they are not recommended for use in knee OA (AAOS, 2013; McAlindon et al., 2014). Trials of already available medications (meth-otrexate and hydroxychloroquine), as well as

O

newer agents (protease inhibitors), are ongoing (Paskins, Dziedzic, & Leeb, 2015).

Surgical Treatment

Arthroscopic lavage and/or debridement has been studied in knee OA. However, given its lack of efficacy compared to usual therapy in symptomatic patients, it is not recommended in treatment guidelines but can be considered in those with additional mechanical symptoms such as locking (AAOS, 2013; NICE, 2014).

Joint replacement is highly effective for end-stage hip and knee OA based on observational studies, large cohort studies, and a smaller number of randomized studies (Skou et al., 2015). It is indicated for patients who have continued pain and loss of function attributable to advanced radiographic OA, despite the non-surgical measures described previously. When surgery is appropriate, most patients report satisfactory results when pain, walking ability, and range of motion are assessed, with over 95% of joint replacements continuing to function well into the second decade after surgery. Complications include infection, leg-length discrepancy, dislocation, and persistent pain.

Jonathan T. L. Cheah and Susan M. Goodman

Alkatan, M., Baker, J. R., Machin D. R., Park, W., Akkari, A. S., Pasha, E. P., & Tanaka, H. (2016). Improved function and reduced pain after swimming and cycling training in patients with osteoarthritis. *Journal of Rheumatology, 43*(3), 666–672.

American Academy of Orthopaedic Surgeons. (2013). *Treatment of osteoarthritis of the knee.* Rosemount, IL: Author.

Brandt, K. D., Mazzuca, S. A., Katz, B. P., Lane, K. A., Buckwalter, K. A., Yocum, D. E., ... Heck, L. W. (2005). Effects of doxycycline on progression of osteoarthritis: Results of a randomized, placebo-controlled, double-blind trial. *Arthritis and Rheumatism, 52*(7), 2015–2025.

da Costa, B. R., Reichenbach, S., Keller N., Nartey, L., Wandel, S., Jüni, P., & Trelle, S. (2016). Effectiveness of non-steroidal anti-inflammatory drugs for the treatment of pain in knee and hip osteoarthritis: a network meta-analysis. *Lancet, 387*(10033), 2093–2105.

Goodman, S. M. (2005). Osteoarthritis. In S. Paget, & A. Yee (Eds.), *Expert guide to rheumatology.* Philadelphia, PA: American College of Physicians.

Hochberg, M. C., Altman, R. D., April, K. T., Benkhalti, M., Guyatt, G., McGowan, J., ... Tugwell, P. (2012). American College of Rheumatology 2012 recommendations for the use of nonpharmacologic and pharmacologic therapies in osteoarthritis of the hand, hip, and knee. *Arthritis Care & Research, 64*(4), 465–474.

Hunter, D. J. (2015). Viscosupplementation for osteoarthritis of the knee. *New England Journal of Medicine, 372*(26), 2570.

Li, S., Yu, B., Zhou, D., He, C., Zhuo, Q., & Hulme, J. M. (2013). Electromagnetic fields for treating osteoarthritis. *Cochrane Database of Systematic Reviews, 2013*(12), 1-47. doi:10.1002/14651858.CD003523.pub2

Lories, R., Neerinckx, B., Kloppenburg, M. (2015). Osteoarthritis: Pathogenesis and clinical features. In J. W. J. Bijlsma & E. Hachulla (Eds.), *EULAR textbook on rheumatic diseases* (2nd ed.). London, UK: BMJ.

Manheimer, E., Cheng, K., Linde, K., Lao, L., Yoo, J., Wieland, S., ... Bouter, L. M. (2010). Acupuncture for peripheral joint osteoarthritis. *Cochrane Database of Systematic Reviews, 2010*(1). doi:10.1002/14651858.CD001977.pub2

McAlindon, T. E., Bannuru, R. R., Sullivan, M. C., Arden, N. K., Berenbaum, F., Bierma-Zeinstra, S. M., ... Underwood, M. (2014). OARSI guidelines for the non-surgical management of knee osteoarthritis. *Osteoarthritis and Cartilage/OARS, Osteoarthritis Research Society, 22*(3), 363–388.

National Institute for Health and Care Excellence. (2014). *Osteoarthritis: care and management.* London, UK: Author.

Paskins, Z., Dziedzic, K., & Leeb, B. (2015). Osteoarthritis: Treatment. In J. W. J. Bijlsma, & E. Hachulla (Eds.), *EULAR textbook on rheumatic diseases* (2nd ed.). London, UK: BMJ.

Reynard, L. N., & Loughlin, J. (2013). Insights from human genetic studies into the pathways involved in osteoarthritis. *Nature Reviews Rheumatology, 9*(10), 573–583.

Rutjes, A. W., Nüesch, E., Sterchi, R., & Jüni P. (2010). Therapeutic ultrasound for osteoarthritis of the knee or hip. *Cochrane Database of Systematic Reviews, 2010*(1). doi: 10.1002/14651858.CD003132.pub2

Skou, S. T., Roos, E. M., Laursen, M. B., Rathleff, M. S., Arendt-Nielsen, L., Simonsen, O., & Rasmussen, S. (2015). A randomized, controlled trial of total knee replacement. *New England Journal of Medicine, 373*(17), 1597–1606.

Wang, C., Schmid, C. H., Iversen, M. D., Harvey, W. F., Fielding, R. A., Driban, J. B., ... McAlindon,

T. (2016). Comparative effectiveness of Tai Chi versus physical therapy for knee osteoarthritis: A randomized trial. *Annals of Internal Medicine,* 165(2), 77–86.

Web Resources
American Academy of Family Physicians: http://www.aafp.org/afp/2012/0101/p49.html
American College of Rheumatology: http://www.rheumatology.org/I-Am-A/Patient-Caregiver/Diseases-Conditions/Osteoarthritis
Arthritis Foundation: http://www.arthritis.org/about-arthritis/types/osteoarthritis
Hospital for Special Surgery: https://www.hss.edu/condition-list_osteoarthritis.asp

OSTEOPOROSIS

Osteoporosis is a systemic skeletal disorder characterized by microarchitectural disruption of bone and an increased susceptibility to fracture. Approximately 10 million men and women in the United States have osteoporosis, and an even greater number have osteopenia. Osteoporosis is four times more prevalent in women than in men. The most common types of osteoporotic fractures include vertebral, hip, and wrist. The yearly mortality rate associated with a hip fracture is 10% to 20%, and men have a higher mortality rate than women. Even if a patient does not die after hip fracture, the chance of significant disability (i.e., needing a cane or walker) indefinitely remains. Vertebral fractures can result in kyphosis, early satiety, abdominal complaints, and restrictive lung disease. All osteoporotic fractures can result in a fear of ambulation and a sense of loss of independence.

PATHOPHYSIOLOGY

Bone is composed of matrix, primarily type II collagen, and mineral, primarily hydroxyapatite. There are two types of bone, cancellous and cortical. Vertebral bodies are examples of cancellous bone. Because they have a large surface area, often bone loss or formation is first detected in these areas. Cortical bone, which is found in the hip, is denser.

There are three major cell types in bone. The osteoblast is responsible for bone formation, and the osteoclast is responsible for bone resorption; these processes are tightly coupled. The osteocyte is responsible for communication within the complex bony structure. Bone formation outpaces bone resorption until the age of 30 years, when bone resorption begins to outpace bone formation. Much research has focused on the receptor activator of nuclear factor-kappa B ligand (RANKL) and its receptor, RANK. This interaction promotes osteoclast differentiation. Osteoprotegerin (OPG) controls this system; when OPG binds to RANK, then osteoclast differentiation is abated. Understanding basic bone biology is helpful in understanding the current and proposed treatments of osteoporosis.

DIAGNOSIS

Dual energy x-ray absorptiometry (DEXA) is considered the gold standard for the measurement of bone mineral density. Lumbar spine and hip measurements are classically reported. Repeat densities should be done on the same machine type because different types (i.e., Lunar vs. Hologic) cannot be compared. Medicare permits a bone density test every 2 years and third-party payers every 1 to 2 years. The National Osteoporosis Foundation (NOF) recommends a baseline density at menopause and earlier if there are significant risk factors. Many recommend that men have a baseline bone-mineral density (BMD) test at the age of 70 years or earlier if there are risk factors.

Peak bone mass is reached at 30 years of age. The *T*-score represents a comparison of BMD to a healthy 30-year-old of similar gender and ethnicity. The Z-score is a comparison to an age-matched control. Risk of fracture is often expressed in terms of BMD. For every 1 standard deviation decrease in BMD, fracture risk is increased by 1.5- to 2.7-fold. In women, bone density decreases approximately 0.5% every year until menopause; then it decreases 2% to 5% for the 2 years before menopause, and for the 2 to 5 years after menopause, it decreases

O

0.5% to 1% per year. Men have a steady decline of 0.5% to 1% per year after the age of 30 years.

For men older than 50 years and postmenopausal women, a *T*-score greater than or equal to –2.5 defines osteoporosis. A *T*-score between –1.0 and –2.4 defines osteopenia, and a *T*-score less than –1.0 is considered normal. For premenopausal women and men younger than 50 years, a Z-score greater than or equal to –2.0 defines "low bone density."

RISK FACTORS

Major risk factors for osteoporosis are a personal history of fracture as an adult, history of a fragility fracture in a first-degree relative, female sex, weight less than 127 pounds, current tobacco use, and use of corticosteroid therapy for more than 3 months. Minor risk factors include any illness that is associated with an increased risk of falls, three or more alcoholic beverages per day in men and more than one per day in women, low calcium and vitamin D intake and low physical activity. Many medical conditions such as malabsorption states, rheumatoid arthritis, and multiple myeloma increase the risk of osteoporosis.

TREATMENT

The NOF recommends treating patients who have a diagnosis of osteoporosis. The Fracture Risk Assessment Tool (FRAX) is a WHO tool that predicts the risk of fracture over the next 10 years, if the patient is not treated. It is used to evaluate women and men with osteopenia. If the risk of fracture overall is greater than or equal to 20% or the risk of hip fracture is greater than or equal to 3%, treatment is recommended.

Calcium and Vitamin D

Secondary hyperparathyroidism may be associated with a lack of calcium and/or vitamin D intake or absorption and is felt to be deleterious to bone health. Many studies document low vitamin D levels in the population as a whole.

Treatment of osteoporosis should first focus on an appropriate amount of calcium and vitamin D. The NOF recommends a daily calcium intake of 1,000 mg for women less than or equal to 50 years and 1,200 mg for women greater than 50 years. For men aged 70 or younger, 1,000 mg is recommended, and 1,200 mg is recommended for those aged 70 years and older. A serum 25-hydroxy vitamin D level of 30 ng/mL or greater is desirable. Calcium citrate has less chance of precipitating calcium kidney stones than calcium carbonate. The official position statement of the American Society for Bone and Mineral Research (ASBMR) is that current evidence does not support the concept of calcium supplementation promoting atherosclerosis.

Exercise

Patients should get a regular amount of weight-bearing exercise. In addition to reducing the degree of osteoporosis, exercise promotes balance and agility, thereby reducing the risk of falls associated fractures. Clinicians should focus on maximizing correction of vision, reducing environmental fall risks, and encouraging the safe use of assistive devices. Patients with poor balance can be referred to physical therapy for balance training.

Pharmalogic Treatment

Pharmacologic treatment is either antiresorptive or anabolic. The common antiresorptive therapies include estrogen-replacement therapy, selective estrogen uptake modulators (SERMs), bisphosphonates, denosumab, and calcitonin. The available anabolic therapy is teriparatide, which is recombinant parathyroid hormone.

Hormone-Replacement Therapy/SERMs

Hormone-replacement therapy (HRT) was used for many years as a mainstay treatment for osteoporosis. In the Women's Health Initiative Study, there were eight fewer hip fractures in the women on HRT. Because of better appreciated side effects of an increased risk of breast cancer and an increased risk of myocardial infarction and stroke, HRT is no longer considered a preferred treatment of osteoporosis. Raloxifene, a SERM, has been shown to reduce the risk of vertebral fractures but not of hip fractures. Side effects include leg cramps, vasomotor symptoms, and increased risk of thrombosis.

Bisphosphonate Therapy

The bisphosphonates as a class are a potent inhibitor of bone resorption. The available oral agents include alendronate, risedronate, and ibandronate. All have the potential side effect of upper gastrointestinal irritation. Bisphosphonates reduce the risk of vertebral and hip fractures, an effect evident after 6 months of therapy. The available intravenous agents include ibandronate every 3 months and zolendronic acid every 12 months.

Bisphosphonates should not be used in patients with renal insufficiency or in women before conception. It is now recognized that prolonged therapy with bisphosphonates is associated with a small increase in atypical stress fractures of the femur, osteonecrosis of the jaw, and uveitis.

Therefore there has been concern about the prolonged use of bisphosphonates. The concern is that if bone resorption is turned off entirely, microdamage will result in an increased susceptibility to fracture and perhaps osteonecrosis of the jaw. Most recommend having a holiday off bisphosphonate therapy after 5 years of use. Others monitor the urine N-telopeptide (urine NTX), which measure bone resorption. If a low rate is obtained (i.e., less than or equal to 20 nmol bone collagen equivalent/mmol), bisphosphonate should be discontinued or teriparatide substituted.

Denosumab

Denosumab is a fully human monoclonal antibody against RANKL, a cytokine that is essential for the formation, function, and survival of osteoclasts. By binding RANKL, denosumab prevents osteoclast differentiation and bone resorption. It is a subcutaneous injection, given every 6 months and has been shown to prevent both hip and vertebral fractures. Studies demonstrate a slight increase in eczema in patients receiving this drug. There have also been case reports of osteonecrosis of the jaw and atypical femur fractures.

Calcitonin

Data supporting the efficacy of calcitonin are limited; therefore calcitonin is rarely used in the treatment of osteoporosis.

Teriparatide

This is a recombinant parathyroid hormone, which increase bone formation. It increases bone density and reduces the risk of vertebral and hip fractures. It is a subcutaneous (20 mcg) injection given daily for 2 years. It is generally very well tolerated. The primary concern has been an increased risk of osteosarcoma in rats. This has not been seen in humans, and the risk to humans is felt to be low. This agent seems to be more efficacious if not given with bisphosphonates. HRT or a SERM may be given simultaneously. Paget's disease and prior skeletal radiation are contraindications for the use of teriparatide; both have been associated with osteosarcoma.

Linda A. Russell

Miller, P. D., Hattersley, D., Riis, J., Williams, G., Lau, E., Russo, L. A., … for the ACTIVE Study Investigators. (2016). Effect of abaloparatide vs placebo on new vertebral fractures in postmenopausal women with osteoporosis. *Journal of the American Medical Association, 316*(7), 722–733.

Neer, R. M., Arnaud, C. D., Zanchetta, J. R., Prince, R., Gaich, G. A., Reginster, J.-Y., … Mitlak, B. H. (2001). Effect of parathyroid hormone (1–34) on fractures and bone mineral density in postmenopausal women with osteoporosis. *New England Journal of Medicine, 344*(19), 1434–1441.

Seeman, E., & Delmas, P. D. (2006). Bone quality—The material and structural basis of bone strength and fragility. *New England Journal of Medicine, 354*(21), 2250–2261.

Woo, S.-B., Hellstein, J. W., & Kalmar, J. R. (2006). Systematic review: Bisphosphonates and osteonecrosis of the jaws. *Annals of Internal Medicine, 144*(10), 753–761.

P

PAIN ASSESSMENT INSTRUMENTS

Assessing pain among older adults is an essential part of the pain-management process. Lack of systematic pain assessment places older adults at risk for undertreatment and persistent pain that can negatively impact their health, functioning, and quality of life (Herr, 2011). Effective pain management involves thorough assessment to understand the type of pain (e.g., nociceptive, neuropathic), duration (e.g., acute, persistent), and intensity of the pain to develop an appropriate treatment strategy. Because there are no objective biological markers of pain, the patient's self-report is the most reliable and accurate method of assessing pain (Hadjistavropoulos et al., 2007).

Pain is a multidimensional, subjective experience with sensory, cognitive, and emotional dimensions (Institute of Medicine [IOM], 2011). Few assessment tools, however, evaluate all of the different dimensions of pain. The most notable exception is the McGill Pain Questionnaire (Melzack, 1975), which measures pain affect and evaluation (based on 78 word descriptors), pain location (using a body map), and pain intensity (based on the Present Pain Intensity [PPI] subscale, a single-question rating subjective pain on a 6-point scale).

Intensity is the most commonly assessed aspect of pain and is typically measured using a numeric rating scale (NRS) or visual analog scale (VAS). The NRS is widely used in hospital and clinical settings, whereas the VAS is more commonly used in research. Patients are asked to verbally rate the intensity of their pain on a 0 to 10 (NRS) or 0 to 100 (VAS) scale. Both tools require the ability to discriminate subtle differences in pain intensity and may be difficult for some older adults to complete, particularly those with hearing loss or cognitive deficits.

The verbal descriptor scale (VDS) is an alternate measure of pain intensity recommended for use with older adults (Herr, 2002). The VDS measures pain intensity by asking participants to select a word that best describes their present pain (e.g., no pain to worst pain imaginable). This measure has been found to be a reliable and valid measure of pain intensity and is reported to be the easiest to complete and the most preferred by older adults (Herr, 2002).

Regardless of the self-report measure used, there is evidence that older adults often underreport the presence of pain (Gerontological Society of America [GSA], 2014; IOM, 2011). Some reasons for this phenomenon are the belief that pain is a normal part of aging, concern about being labeled a complainer, fear of the meaning of the pain in relation to disease progression or prognosis, fear of narcotic addiction and analgesics, and worry about health care costs (American Geriatrics Society [AGS], 2009). Other factors, such as hearing and speech difficulties, may prevent older adults from communicating pain to health care providers. Furthermore, cognitive impairment is an important factor in reducing older adults' reporting of pain (AGS, 2009).

Since the mid-1990s, there has been growing recognition of the challenges associated with assessing and managing pain in older adults with dementia. People with dementia lose the ability to self-report pain because of disease-related cognitive and verbal deficits, which worsen as the disease progresses. It may be assumed that because they cannot report pain, people with dementia no longer experience pain. In fact, recent evidence suggests that people with Alzheimer's dementia and vascular dementia, the two most common forms of dementia, are more susceptible to the development of central, neuropathic pain (Scherder

& Plooij, 2012). In addition to memory loss, dementia affects the pain pathways in the brain such that older adults with dementia may fail to interpret sensations as painful, are less able to recall pain, and are not able to verbalize it to care providers (Husebo, Achterberg, & Flo, 2016). Thus people with dementia are at increased risk for inadequately assessed and managed pain.

In patients with dementia who cannot provide self-report, other assessment approaches must be used to identify the presence of pain. A hierarchical pain-assessment approach is recommended that includes four steps: (a) attempt to obtain a self-report of pain; (b) search for an underlying cause of pain, such as surgery, procedure, or skin breakdown; (c) observe for pain behaviors; and (d) seek input from family and caregivers (Herr, Coyne, et al., 2006). Observational techniques for pain assessment focus on behavioral or nonverbal indicators of pain (Hadjistavropoulos et al., 2007; Herr, Coyne, et al., 2006; Horgas, Elliot, & Marsiske, 2009).

Many measurement tools have been developed to assess pain in persons with dementia over recent decades (Herr, Bjoro, & Decker, 2006; Taylor, Harris, Epps, & Herr, 2005). In general, the instruments are based on the recommendations of the AGS (2009) that pain can be expressed through facial expression (e.g., grimacing), body movements (e.g., guarding, bracing, rubbing, vocalizations [e.g., groaning, verbal expressions]). Persons with dementia may also express pain in atypical ways through behavioral changes. For instance, changes in interpersonal interactions (e.g., aggression, agitation, resisting care), activity patterns (e.g., wandering), and mental status (e.g., confusion, crying) may signal the presence of pain (Husebo et al., 2016).

Despite progress in this area, there is no consensus on which instrument should be used. Few of the tools have undergone complete reliability and validity testing, and most lack evidence to support sensitivity to change over time; thus the ability to detect treatment effects is undermined. One notable exception is the (Mobilization-Observation-Behaviour-Intensity-Dementia-2 [MOBID-2] Pain Scale; Husebo, Ostelo, & Strand, 2014). This tool has undergone the most extensive and rigorous

testing and has demonstrated reliable and sensitivity to treatment effects in several clinical trials (Husebo, Ballard, Sandvik, Nilsen, & Aarsland, 2011; Husebo et al., 2014; Husebo, Strand, Moe-Nilssen, & Ljunggren, 2010).

Other promising behavioral observation measures include the Pain Assessment in Advanced Dementia (PAINAD; Warden, Hurley, & Volicer, 2003) and the Pain Assessment Checklist for Seniors with Limited Ability to Communicate-II (PACSLAC-II). The PAINAD is a 5-item measure that has good reliability and validity, is widely used, has been translated into several languages, and is endorsed by professional medical organizations. The PACSLAC-II is a valid and reliable, 31-item tool designed to assess the presence or absence of pain (Chan, Hadjistavropoulos, Williams, & Lints-Martindales, 2013). The checklist is organized into conceptually based subscales reflecting social personality/mood indicators, facial expressions, activity/body movement, and physiological indicators/eating/sleeping changes/vocal behaviors. The total score is considered valid and reliable for clinical use. It is important to note that none of the currently available tools specifically address cultural aspects of pain expression and warrant further development in that regard (Booker & Herr, 2015).

One assessing pain in patients with advanced dementia cannot rely on behavior alone. Instead, behavioral expressions should be used to trigger a comprehensive pain assessment protocol. The American Society for Pain Management Nursing's Task Force on pain assessment in nonverbal patients (including patients with dementia) recommends a comprehensive, hierarchical approach, including the following: (a) ask for a self-report, (b) look for potential causes of pain, (c) observe patient's behavior, (d) obtain surrogate reports of pain or changes in patient's behaviors/activities, and (e) give pain medications and determine whether pain indicators are reduced or eliminated (Herr, Coyne, et al., 2006). The Multidimensional Objective Pain Assessment Tool (MOPAT) can be used to assess pain in unresponsive patients at the end of life (McGuire, Kaiser, Haisfield-Wolfe, & Iyamu, 2016; McGuire, Reifsnyder, Soeken, Kaiser, & Yeager, 2011).

P

In summary, pain is a complex experience that requires careful assessment to effectively manage it. A number of different pain measures can be used with older adults, including subjective measures of self-reported pain, as well as objective measures of behavioral expressions of pain. There is no one best measure of pain. Rather, it is recommended that the pain measure be the one that best fits patients' cognitive and physical abilities, the setting, and the situation. The most important recommendation for measuring pain in older adults is for clinicians to use a standardized pain assessment tool and to apply it consistently in assessing patient's pain and in evaluating the effectiveness of pain-management strategies.

Ann L. Horgas and Toni L. Glover

American Geriatrics Society. (2009). Pharmacological management of persistent pain in older persons. *Journal of the American Geriatrics Society, 57*(8), 1331–1346.

Booker, S. S., & Herr, K. (2015). The state-of "cultural validity" of self-report pain assessment tools in diverse older adults. *Pain Medicine, 16*(2), 232–239.

Chan, S., Hadjistavropoulos, T., Williams, J., & Lints-Martindales, A. (2013). Evidence-based development and initial validation of the Pain Assessment Checklist for Seniors with Limited Ability to Communicate-II (PACSLAC-II). *Clinical Journal of Pain, 30*, 816–824.

Gerontological Society of America. (2014). *From policy to practice: The health of an aging America: Focus on pain.* Washington, DC: Author.

Hadjistavropoulos, T., Herr, K., Turk, D., Fine, P., Dworkin, R. H., Helme, R., ... Williams, J. (2007). An interdisciplinary expert consensus statement on assessment of pain in older persons. *Clinical Journal of Pain, 23*(Suppl. 1), 1–43.

Herr, K. (2002). Chronic pain: Challenges and assessment strategies. *Journal of Gerontological Nursing, 28*(1), 20–27.

Herr, K. (2011). Pain assessment strategies in older adults. *Journal of Pain, 12*(3), S3–S13.

Herr, K., Bjoro, K., & Decker, S. (2006). Tools for assessment of pain in nonverbal older adults with dementia: A state-of-the-science review. *Journal of Pain and Symptom Management, 31*(2), 170–192.

Herr, K., Coyne, P. J., Key, T., Manworren, R., McCaffery, M., Merkel, S., ... Wild, L. (2006). Pain assessment in the nonverbal patient: Position statement with clinical practice recommendations. *Pain Management Nursing, 7*, 44–52.

Horgas, A. L., Elliott, A. F., & Marsiske, M. (2009). Pain assessment in persons with dementia: Relationship between self-report and behavioral observation. *Journal of the American Geriatrics Society, 57*(1), 126–132.

Husebo, B. S., Achterberg, W., & Flo, E. (2016). Identifying and managing pain in people with Alzheimer's disease and other types of dementia: A systematic review. *CNS Drugs, 30*, 481–497.

Husebo B. S., Ballard, C., Sandvik, R., Nilsen, O. D., & Aarsland, D. (2011). Efficacy of treating pain to reduce behavioural disturbances in residents of nursing homes with dementia: Cluster randomized clinical trial. *British Medical Journal, 343*, 1–10.

Husebo, B. S., Ostelo, R., & Strand, L. I. (2014). The MOBID-2 pain scale: Reliability and responsiveness to pain in patients with dementia. *European Journal of Pain, 18*, 1419–1430.

Husebo, B. S., Strand, L. I., Moe-Nilssen, R., & Ljunggren, A. E. (2010). Pain in older persons with severe dementia. Psychometric properties of the Mobilization-Observation-Behaviour-Intensity-Dementia (MOBID-2) Pain Scale in a clinical setting. *Scandinavian Journal of Caring Science, 2*, 380–391.

Institute of Medicine. (2011). *Relieving pain in America: A blueprint for transforming prevention, care, education, and research.* Washington, DC: National Academies Press.

McGuire, D. B., Kaiser, K. S., Haisfield-Wolfe, M. E., & Iyamu, F. (2016). Pain assessment in non-communicative adult palliative care patients. *Nursing Clinics of North America, 51*(3), 397–431. doi:10.1016/j.cnur.2016.05.009

McGuire, D. B., Reifsnyder, J., Soeken, K., Kaiser, K. S., & Yeager, K. A. (2011). Assessing pain in non-responsive hospice patients: Development and preliminary testing of the Multidimensional Objective Pain Assessment Tool (MOPAT). *Journal of Palliative Medicine, 14*(3), 287–292. doi:10.1089/jpm.2010.0302

Melzack, R. (1975). The McGill Pain Questionnaire: Major properties and scoring methods. *Pain, 1*(3), 277–299.

Scherder, E. J., & Plooij, B. (2012). Assessment and management of pain, with particular emphasis on central neuropathic pain, in moderate to severe dementia. *Drugs & Aging, 29*(9), 701–706.

Taylor, L. J., Harris, J., Epps, C. D., & Herr, K. (2005). Psychometric evaluation of selected pain intensity scales for use with cognitively impaired and cognitively intact older adults. *Rehabilitation Nursing, 30,* 55–61.

Warden, V., Hurley, A. C., & Volicer, L. (2003). Development and psychometric evaluation of the Pain Assessment in Advanced Dementia (PAINAD) scale. *Journal of the American Medical Directors Association, 4,* 9–15.

PAIN: ACUTE

The International Association for the Study of Pain (IASP) defines *pain* as "an unpleasant sensory and emotional experience associated with actual or potential tissue damage" (IASP, 2017). Acute pain is shorter in duration than chronic or persistent pain, usually lasting less than 3 months, and typically has an abrupt onset that corresponds to an event such a trauma or a known pathology. Acute pain is increasingly prevalent in older adults, and inadequate pain management is a significant problem, especially for hospitalized patients (Cullison, Carpenter, & Milne, 2016).

Both age-related physiological changes and comorbid diseases, such as pulmonary complications, decline in physical function, and thromboembolic events, increase the risk of harmful outcomes from unrelieved acute pain in older adults. Poorly controlled postoperative pain is associated with increased hospital stays, delayed healing, cognitive impairment, depression, functional decline, and increased need for services after discharge (Herr, 2011; Malcom, 2015). Severe pain compromises the ability to perform self-care activities and maintain the responsibilities of independent living. Untreated acute pain from acute tissue injury also leads to chronic pain states by evoking long-lasting disruptions in the neuromodulation of pain through the central nervous system.

Surgery, hip and long bone fractures; compression fractures; exacerbations of rheumatoid arthritis; herpes zoster; and peripheral neuropathy (often associated with diabetes) are some common causes of acute pain in older adults. Chronic health problems are often sources of daily discomfort. Osteoarthritis, the most common long-term painful condition in older adults, is characterized by episodes of both acute and chronic pain. Sudden and unpredictable atypical chest, jaw, or arm pain can occur with cardiac problems. Chronic diseases that compromise circulation, such as atherosclerosis and diabetes, result in peripheral vascular and acute ischemic pain. Not only do a large number of older adults suffer needless pain while in the hospital, but also many are discharged with pain still poorly controlled (Cullison et al., 2016; Platts-Mills et al., 2016).

Age-related biological and psychosocial factors greatly influence the perception and response to pain. For example, a woman with osteoporosis can fracture a rib with a vigorous sneeze or cough and have sudden point tenderness. Slowed neurological function with age can alter the nociceptive, or sensing, component of pain, leading to delayed pain, particularly in the case of trauma. It is not uncommon for older adults to experience a traumatic injury but fail to report pain until hours or even days after the event. Emotional states such as anxiety, fear, and worries about losing independence have a profound impact on how patients cope with pain.

Comorbid conditions, preexisting chronic pain states, complex pharmacological regimens, and cognitive impairment complicate the assessment of acute pain in older adults. Differentiating acute from chronic pain in older adults is challenging. Although sometimes present with acute pain, autonomic responses such as tachycardia, elevated or depressed blood pressure, diaphoresis, and pupillary changes are not always reliable indicators.

PAIN ASSESSMENT

Assessing pain in the older adult is a particular challenge for a variety of reasons, including atypical presentations. Acute confusion and chronic cognitive impairment also can damage the older adult's ability to localize, interpret, or communicate discomfort to caregivers.

Concerns about the opioid epidemic are complicating matters. In response to the undertreatment of pain, in the 1990s national organizations and accrediting bodies began recommending, and eventually requiring, health care organizations to document patients' pain as a vital sign. Pain scores are now included as a quality measure tied to reimbursement. These types of regulations have contributed to the overprescription of opioids as a quick fix to improve scores. The American Medical Association recently has proposed removing pain as the fifth vital sign precisely because it leads to providers treating a pain score, which is not an objective measure (Friedman, 2016). The American Academy of Pain Medicine suggests, instead, that uncontrolled pain scores not be tied to reimbursement because this incentivizes the overprescription of opioids. The American Society for Pain Management Nursing released a position statement recommending against the practice of treating patients' subjective pain scores. They recommend considering the entire clinical picture of the patient, including comorbidities, functional assessment, respiratory status and sedation level, to prescribe opioids safely and responsibly (Pasero, Quinlan-Colwell, Rae, Broglio, & Drew, 2016). This requires that providers have training and excellent clinical judgment. Removing pain as a vital sign could disproportionately negatively affect older adults who already have trouble reporting their pain.

Comprehensive tools such as the Brief Pain Inventory (BPI), which measures multiple dimensions of pain (i.e., intensity, relief, and pain interference with daily living), have been validated with older adults (Stubbs, Eggermont, Patchay, & Schofield, 2015). Descriptors such as *sore*, *hurt*, and *ache* should be used to overcome altered perceptions and beliefs about pain and elicit an accurate report. Structured questions about pain history, including duration, situations, or factors that increase or lessen pain and strategies used to manage pain (including nonprescription medications and complementary or alternative therapies), can be used to obtain information about a patient's pain. The effectiveness of each treatment strategy and the individual's daily routine for managing acute pain should be documented in the assessment. The onset of pain should be differentiated from preexisting chronic pain by the duration, pattern, and precipitating factors.

Older adults who are not able to communicate, because of cognitive impairment, delirium, or sensory deficits, are particularly vulnerable to having their pain left untreated. A variety of assessment tools offer ways to monitor and document changes in behaviors by observing for facial grimacing, splinting or guarding of painful areas, and reluctance to move or decline in activity (American Geriatrics Society [AGS], 2009; Herr, 2011). Agitation and delirium may also be caused by untreated pain.

MULTIMODAL APPROACH TO PAIN MANAGEMENT

Treatment of acute pain in older adults may require multimodal therapy, which combines analgesics with synergistic or additive effects and different actions on targets in the peripheral and central nervous system. Advantages of multimodal therapy include dose reductions of analgesics, decreased side effects, and improved pain relief. Analgesic regimens should be designed to prevent "analgesic gaps" that can occur at various times when (a) there are interruptions in analgesic therapy (e.g., transfers between services/hospital locations, transitions from one medication route to another such as switching from epidural to intravenous or intravenous to oral therapy, lapses or delays in medication administration); or (b) pain is exacerbated during and following a procedure and with activity.

The pharmacological treatment of pain in older adults is a challenge because of a decline in organ-system functions, resulting in altered responses to analgesic medications. Overall, older adults are more sensitive to the cognitive and sedating effects of opioid analgesics and are more likely to experience constipation and urinary retention. They are also more susceptible to hepatic toxicity from acetaminophen and gastrointestinal and renal toxicity from nonsteroidal anti-inflammatory drugs (NSAIDs). Standard analgesics used to treat acute mild to moderate pain include acetaminophen, NSAIDs, nonopioid and opioid combinations (i.e., acetaminophen plus tramadol, acetaminophen plus codeine, acetaminophen plus hydrocodone, acetaminophen plus oxy-codone). Hepatotoxicity can occur with doses of acetaminophen in excess of 3,000 mg/day. Because acetaminophen has different names, is available over the counter, and is often combined with other drugs, it is important that older adults understand the maximum dosing from all sources of acetaminophen. Gastric bleeding, renal impairment, and platelet dysfunction are associated with the use of some NSAIDs. Opioids (e.g., oxycodone, morphine) can be given for moderate to severe pain. Adverse effects of opioid analgesics include increased constipation, sedation, respiratory depression, and altered mental status that can lead to falls. The AGS recommends a "start low and go slow" approach. Evidence-based guidelines (National Guideline Clearinghouse, 2012) are available to assist clinicians with selecting appropriate analgesics, determining usual starting doses, and monitoring adverse effects (AGS, 2009).

In the acute care setting, when patients have severe pain, especially postsurgical or incident pain (that which comes on suddenly or is brought on by activity), intravenous patient-controlled analgesia (PCA) is safe and effective for older adults. PCA infusions allow for smaller doses to be given and for the patient to control the delivery. Older adults are more likely to experience higher analgesic peaks, longer duration of action, and increased side effects; therefore continuous background or basal infusion should not be used in opioid-naïve patients until opioid requirements and response to therapy are apparent. Morphine, hydromorphone, or fentanyl are generally used. Morphine has active metabolites that can reach toxic levels and generally should be avoided in those with renal dysfunction. Verbal and written information should be provided to emphasize the principles of PCA therapy, the need to self-medicate before the pain worsens, and the importance of reporting unrelieved pain. That only the patient is to press the PCA is of the utmost importance, as sedation precedes respiratory depression. If family members, friends or health aides are used to helping the older patient, they must be reminded to not override this important safety feature. Older patients may require more reinforcement of teaching to alleviate concerns of addiction and fear of administering too much.

Patient-controlled epidural analgesia (PCEA) is often used after surgery and is associated with improved pain relief at rest, coughing, earlier return of bowel function, and greater patient satisfaction compared with intravenous PCA (Zhu, Wang, Xu, & Qingpin, 2013). A combination of an opioid (e.g., morphine, fentanyl) and a local anesthetic (e.g., bupivacaine, ropivacaine) is administered by continuous infusion, although either may be administered alone. There is an increased risk of respiratory depression with concurrently administered epidural and systemic opioids. Altered cognitive status and urinary retention are also potential adverse effects of epidural analgesia. Patients receiving epidural therapy should be regularly monitored with hourly respiratory rates for the first 24 hours. Lower concentrations of a local anesthetic can be administered to limit the incidence and severity of orthostatic hypotension and lower motor weakness.

Interventional pain management is the use of injections (such as a femoral nerve block for hip fracture), catheters, spinal cord stimulation, and neuroablation techniques and can allow for more localized pain control and decreased need for systemic analgesics (Jones et al., 2016). Patients receiving a local anesthetic may need assistance getting out of bed or ambulating, especially for the first 24 hours. Frequent repositioning is necessary to prevent pressure injuries and to maintain circulation because patients may experience a decrease in sensation.

TRANSITIONS IN CARE

Older adults and their caregivers are often inadequately prepared to deal with post hospital needs; acute pain is frequently a problem after discharge and can prompt additional telephone calls and outpatient visits. Shorter hospitalizations have placed tremendous pressure on expediting discharge, causing insufficient time to evaluate analgesic regimens and teach patients about their medications and other pain-relieving methods. Nevertheless, realistic goals for pain control should be established, and patients should be instructed to report

P

increased levels of pain and any adverse effects of analgesics. Discharge instructions should stress expectations for pain relief, considering that pain may not steadily decline but could worsen with increased activity. Specific dosing guidelines for analgesics should be reviewed along with measures to manage side effects such as constipation from opioids. Patients should receive information regarding alternative methods of pain control, such as heat, massage, relaxation, proper alignment of body parts, and scheduling of alternating periods of rest and activity.

Home health nursing visits should be ordered to monitor pain levels and assess the response to analgesic therapy. If resources are available to help older adults with activities of daily living, a home health aide might reduce physical exertion that can exacerbate pain. Scheduling activities and structuring the environment to place minimal demands on an older adult with acute pain can conserve energy and promote recovery.

Lara Wahlberg

Cullison, K., Carpenter, C. R., & Milne, W. K. (2016). Hot off the press: Use of shared decision-making for management of acute musculoskeletal pain in older adults discharged from the emergency department. *Academic Emergency Medicine, 23*(8), 956–958. doi:10.1111/acem.12985

Friedman, J. (2016). *Remove pain as 5th vital sign, AMA urged—Making it part of quality measurement hurts reimbursement.* Retrieved from http://www.med pagetoday.com/meetingcoverage/ama/58486

Herr, K. (2011). Pain assessment strategies in older patients. *Journal of Pain, 12*(3), S3–S13.

International Association for the Study of Pain. (2017). IASP taxonomy. Retrieved from https://www.iasp-pain.org/Taxonomy

Jones, M. R., Ehrhardt, K. P., Ripoll, J. G., Sharma, B., Panos, I. W., Kaye, R., & Kaye, A. D. (2016). Pain in the elderly. *Current Pain and Headache Reports, 20*(23), 1–9. doi:10.1007/s11916-016-0551-2

Malcom, C. (2015). Acute pain management in the older person. *Journal of Perioperative Practice, 25*(7–8), 134–139.

National Guideline Clearinghouse. (2012). Pain management in older adults. Retrieved from https://www.guideline.gov/summaries/summary/43932

Pasero, C., Quinlan-Colwell, A., Rae, D., Broglio, K., & Drew, D. (2016). Prescribing and administering opioid doses based solely on pain intensity: A position statement by the American Society for Pain Management Nursing. *Pain Management Nursing, 17*(3), 170–180.

Platts-Mills, T. F., Flannigan, S. A., Bortsov, A. V., Smith, S., Domeier, R. M., Swor, R. A., … McLean, S. A. (2016). Persistent pain among older adults discharged home from the emergency department after motor vehicle crash: A prospective cohort study. *Annals of Emergency Medicine, 67*(2), 166–176. doi:10.1016/j.annemergmed.2015.05.003

Stubbs, B., Eggermont, L., Patchay, S., & Schofield, P. (2015). Older adults with chronic musculoskeletal pain are at increased risk of recurrent falls and the Brief Pain Inventory could help identify those most at risk. *Geriatrics and Gerontology International, 15*(7), 881–888. doi:10.1111/ggi.12357

Zhu, Z., Wang, C., Xu, C., & Qingping, C. (2013). Influence of patient-controlled epidural analgesia versus patient controlled intravenous analgesia on postoperative pain control and recovery after gastrectomy for gastric cancer: A prospective randomized trial. *Gastric Cancer, 16*(2), 193–200. doi:10.1007/s10120-012-0168-z

Web Resources
American Geriatrics Society: http://americangeriatrics.org
American Pain Society: http://www.ampainsoc.org
American Society for Pain Management Nurses: http://www.aspmn.org
Clinical Practice Guidelines: http://www.geriatricpain.org/Content/Resources/CPGuidelines/Pages/default.aspx

PAIN: CHRONIC/PERSISTENT

Chronic pain, also known as *persistent pain*, is pain that persists or recurs for longer than 3 to 6 months and may or may not be associated with a clearly understood disease process. It can fluctuate and change in character and intensity over time and is associated with functional and psychologic impairment (American Geriatrics Society [AGS], 2009; Reuben et al., 2015). Persistent pain is one of the most pervasive

P

yet undertreated problems in older adults. Physiological changes of aging, sensory deficits, cognitive impairment, and underreporting of pain complicate the recognition and treatment of painful conditions in this vulnerable population.

Unrelieved pain results in depression, decreased socialization, sleep disturbances, impaired ambulation, and increased health care utilization and costs. Care of the older adult with persistent pain requires an understanding of the differences in older adults' perceptions, beliefs, and coping styles (Molton & Terrill, 2014). The detection and management of pain must include routine pain assessment and reassessment, careful use of analgesic drugs, and a multidisciplinary, nonpharmacological approach that may include physical therapy, complementary and alternative modalities, psychological support, and engagement in a social support network (Makris, Abrams, Gurland, & Reid, 2014; Matos, Bernardes, & Goubert, 2016; Molton & Terrill, 2014).

DEFINITIONS

Persistent pain in older adults can be categorized as (a) nociceptive, (b) neuropathic, and (c) mixed or unspecified pain. *Nociceptive pain* is defined as a normal sensory process that is caused by stimulation of pain receptors in response to inflammation, tissue destruction, or ongoing injury. Nociceptive pain includes *somatic* pain, such as nonmalignant pain from musculoskeletal problems (e.g., osteoporosis, arthritis), peripheral vascular disease, myofascial pain syndromes, back pain, and fibromyalgia, as well as *visceral* pain, involving the organs or lining of the body cavities. Cancer-related pain such as bony or organ metastasis is also caused by activation of nociceptors.

Neuropathic pain is an abnormal response to pain stimuli resulting from damage to the central and peripheral nervous systems. Neuropathic pain syndromes include poststroke thalamic pain and pain from neurodegenerative disorders such as Parkinson's disease, multiple sclerosis, spinal-cord injury, and cancer. Examples of peripheral neuropathic pain are postherpetic neuralgia, phantom limb pain,

chemotherapy-induced neuropathy, and diabetic neuropathy (Bradford et al., 2015). Older adults may also experience mixed or unspecified pain of unknown origin, which can be difficult to assess and requires multiple trials of pain-relieving modalities (AGS, 2009).

PAIN ESTIMATES IN OLDER ADULTS

Persistent pain in older adults is a major public health problem, occurring in up to 35% to 48% of community-dwelling older adults and in 45% to 85% of nursing home residents (Herr, 2011). Undertreated pain has negative consequences such as depression, anxiety, falls, malnutrition, cognitive impairment, sleep disturbances, social isolation, functional decline, and poor quality of life (Herr, 2011), and unfortunately, persistent pain contributes to significant morbidity and mortality.

PERSISTENT PAIN ASSESSMENT

Current literature on the assessment of pain in older adults incorporates the evaluation of cognitive function to guide clinicians in selecting the most appropriate pain measures. Because pain is a subjective experience, a thorough pain history should include location, onset, duration, pattern, intensity, character and quality, and aggravating factors (e.g., movement, positioning, stressful events). Pain interference with sleep, eating, mood, social activities, relationships, and other aspects of quality of life should be assessed. A thorough health history is used to identify both medical and psychiatric comorbidities that may exacerbate pain. A risk assessment tool should be used to screen for substance abuse potential because addiction can significantly interfere with a clinician's ability to adequately treat pain (AGS, 2009; Bradford et al., 2015). A physical examination can provide additional information about pain locations, sensory disturbances associated with neuropathic pain, visual signs of swelling, limited range of motion, pain on palpation, and evoked pain or tenderness at trigger points (Bradford et al., 2015; Herr, 2011).

Because there are no objective biological markers of pain, self-report is the most effective method for information gathering regarding pain. Numerous patient-reported assessment scales are available; however, it is important to select appropriate pain measures that are interpretable and easy to use because the presence of pain can affect an older adult's ability to process and retain information. Unidimensional scales for pain intensity include visual analog scales (0- to 100-mm line scale), numeric rating scale (0, no pain, to 10, worst or unbearable pain), verbal descriptive scales (VDSs) with categories (no, mild, moderate, or severe pain), and Adult Faces Rating Scale (AFRS) with pictures of faces showing varying degrees of pain. The Brief Pain Inventory (BPI)—Short Form is a multidimensional tool that evaluates dimensions of pain intensity (present, average, worst, and least pain), location, pain relief, and pain interference with general activity (i.e., mood, walking ability, normal work, relationships with others, sleep, enjoyment of life).

Older adults with cognitive impairment may be unable to provide reliable estimates of pain, and alternative approaches such as behavioral observations should be used. Guidelines are available to assist with the clinical assessment of pain in older adults who are cognitively impaired secondary to disorders such as Alzheimer's disease, Lewy body dementia, and delirium (Herr, 2011).

When pain is assessed in cognitively impaired older adults, the same general principles for obtaining a health history and conducting a physical examination apply. Older adults with mild to moderate cognitive impairment may be able to accurately self-report pain intensity with the aid of AFRS and VDS scales and associated symptoms and cooperate with a physical examination. For those who are unable to verbalize or express pain and symptoms, it may be necessary to rely on a health history and physical examination alone. Past or current health problems can provide information about painful diseases or conditions. Obtaining information from a reliable source on falls or injuries can also yield important findings. Causes of acute pain, such as upper respiratory and urinary tract infections, should also be considered in the differential diagnosis (Herr, 2011). Common pain behaviors in older adults with

cognitive impairment include sad, frightened, and grimacing facial expressions; moaning, groaning, or verbally abusive language; guarded or rigid posture; rocking or pacing; diminished mobility; decreased socialization; socially inappropriate or aggressive behavior; diminished appetite; and increased or decreased sleep (AGS, 2009; Herr, 2011). A review of pain assessment instruments for nonverbal older adults with cognitive impairment has been published with criteria to determine the most appropriate methods for assessing pain (Herr, 2011; Herr, Coyne, McCaffery, Manworren, & Merkel, 2011).

MANAGEMENT OF PERSISTENT PAIN

Managing persistent pain in an older adult requires a combination of both pharmacologic and nonpharmacological approaches. The goal of therapy is to relieve pain and suffering, restore function, and improve quality of life, which can be gauged by the ability to maintain an optimal level of self-care and participation in social activities.

Pain management may be complicated by adverse drug reactions and sensitivity to analgesics. Safe, effective analgesic therapy requires in-depth knowledge of age-related changes in pharmacokinetics and pharmacodynamics. Critical changes that occur with aging must be considered when selecting analgesics and titrating doses. These include body composition (i.e., fat to water and muscle mass changing the distribution of drugs), gastrointestinal motility (i.e., decreases, leading to longer transit times), liver metabolism (i.e., decreased oxidation, leading to a prolonged drug half-life), renal clearance (i.e., decreases, leading to accumulation of active drug or metabolites), and central nervous system (i.e., increased susceptibility to sedation and altered mentation) (AGS, 2009; Bradford et al., 2015). The general rule is to "start low" with initial doses and "go slow" with titrating to therapeutic effect (AGS, 2009).

Nonopioid analgesics such as acetaminophen can be tried for mild to moderate pain, but caution should be used to avoid maximum daily doses of greater than 3 g. Nonsteroidal anti-inflammatory drugs (NSAIDs) can be administered on an as-needed basis to treat pain of musculoskeletal or inflammatory origin.

For neuropathic pain, certain antidepressants and anticonvulsants, such as duloxetine and gabapentin, are indicated. Tricyclic antidepressants may also be effective, but anticholinergic effects are much more common in older adults, so they should be used with caution (AGS, 2009; Bradford et al., 2015). There may be a role for interventional pain management strategies such as nerve blocks, injections, or other minimally invasive procedures (Abdulla et al., 2013).

The Centers for Disease Control and Prevention (CDC) recently recommended not using opioids for chronic, nonmalignant pain (Dowell, Haegerich, & Chou, 2016). However, earlier recommendations by the AGS included the use of opioids for persistent, nonmalignant pain if they achieved the desired effect of improving the patient's ability to function (AGS, 2009; Bradford et al., 2015). Universal precautions to deter and detect abuse or diversion should be used if treating older adults with opioids (Bradford et al., 2015). If opioids used for persistent nonmalignant pain do not improve functional status, the patient should be referred to a pain specialist.

For malignant, moderate to severe, persistent pain, short-acting opioid analgesics can be prescribed (e.g., hydrocodone/acetaminophen combinations, oxycodone, morphine, hydromorphone); however, they should be initiated at half the usual starting doses for adults. Patients must be monitored for sedation, changes in blood pressure and mentation, respiratory depression, fall risk, and opioid-induced constipation. A preventive bowel regimen with standing laxatives is recommended for older adults taking opioids.

Long-acting opioids may be appropriate but should only be started in patients who are not opioid naïve (i.e., have been tolerating short-acting opioid equivalents of oral morphine 30–60 mg/day on an around-the-clock schedule for a week or more). The transdermal fentanyl patch is a tempting treatment consideration in older patients to decrease pill burden or in patients with difficulty swallowing. However, transdermal fentanyl is a long-acting opioid and even at its lowest dose (12 mcg/hr) should not be used in opioid-naïve patients. Buprenorphine transdermal patch may be used in opioid-naïve patients in its lowest dosage form (5 mcg/hr) after other agents have been tried but is indicated only for severe, persistent pain requiring around-the-clock dosing. It should be prescribed only by experienced providers (Bradford et al., 2015; Reuben et al., 2015).

Nonpharmacological strategies should always be used with pharmacologic agents because of the physical, emotional, mental, social, and spiritual dimensions and effects of persistent pain. Patient education, physical therapy, exercise groups, and cognitive behavioral therapy have all been used successfully in pain-management programs. Distraction, humor, massage therapy, therapeutic touch, acupuncture, hypnosis, and imagery provide alternative means for pain relief. Physical deconditioning that can occur with persistent pain may result in limited activity and loss of muscle mass; therefore a structured physical therapy program helps the senior regain strength, balance, and flexibility. Cognitive behavioral interventions foster new coping mechanisms and adaptation to limitations imposed by pain (AGS, 2009).

Management of persistent pain may change as older adults reach the final months of life and treatment goals become more focused on comfort. It is important to balance good pain control with alertness and physical function according to what is important to the patient and to regularly readdress such goals. Such patients should be referred to palliative care providers who have expertise in helping patients balance these goals.

Lara Wahlberg

Abdulla, A., Bone, M., Adams, N., Elliott, A., Jones, D., Knaggs, R., … Schofield, P. (2013). Evidence-based clinical practice guidelines on management of pain in older people. *Age and Ageing*, 42(2), 151–153. doi:10.1093/ageing/afs199

American Geriatrics Society Panel on the Pharmacological Management of Persistent Pain in Older Persons. (2009). Pharmacological management of persistent pain in older persons. *Journal of the American Geriatrics Society*, 57, 1331–1346.

Bradford, E. M., Hartzell, M., Asih, S., Hulla, R., Gatchel, R., & Robeck, I. (2015). Pain management in the elderly: Treatment considerations. *Practical Pain Management*. Retrieved from http://www.practicalpainmanagement.com/treatments/pain-management-elderly-treatment-considerations?page=0,2

Dowell, D., Haegerich, T. M., & Chou, R. (2016). CDC guideline for prescribing opioids for chronic pain—United States, 2016. *MMWR Recommendations and Reports, 65*(1), 1–49. doi:10.15585/mmwr.rr6501e1

Herr, K. (2011). Pain assessment strategies in older patients. *Journal of Pain, 12*(3), S3–S13.

Herr, K., Coyne, P. J., McCaffery, M., Manworren, R., & Merkel, S. (2011). Pain assessment in the patient unable to self-report: Position statement with clinical practice recommendations. *Pain Management Nursing, 12*(4), 230–250.

Makris, U., Abrams, R., Gurland, B., & Reid, M. (2014). Management of persistent pain in the older patient: A clinical review. *Journal of the American Medical Association, 312*(8), 825–836.

Matos, M., Bernardes, S. F., & Goubert, L. J. (2016). The relationship between perceived promotion of autonomy/dependence and pain-related disability in older adults with chronic pain: The mediating role of self-reported physical functioning. *Journal of Behavioral Medicine, 39*(4), 704–715.

Molton, I. R., & Terrill, A. L. (2014). Overview of persistent pain in older adults. *American Psychologist, 69*(2), 197–207. doi:10.1037/a0035794

Reuben, D. B., Herr, K. A., Pacala, J. T., Pollock, B. G., Potter, J. F., & Selma, T. P. (2015). *Geriatrics at your fingertips: 2015* (17th ed.). New York, NY: American Geriatrics Society.

Web Resources

American Chronic Pain Association Resource Guide, 2016 Edition: https://theacpa.org/uploads/documents/ACPA_Resource_Guide_2016.pdf

American Geriatrics Society: http://www.americangeriatrics.org

American Pain Society: http://www.ampainsoc.org

National Institute for Neurological Disorders and Stroke: http://www.ninds.nih.gov/disorders/chronic_pain/chronic_pain.htm

National Institute on Aging: End of life: Providing comfort at the end of life: https://www.nia.nih.gov/health/what-end-life-care

National Institute on Aging: Pain: You can get help: https://www.nia.nih.gov/health/publication/pain

PALLIATIVE CARE

The focus of health care has changed over the past century. Advances in medical care, as well as in nutrition and public health, have led to longer life expectancy and a change in the way people die (Coyle, 2015). Medical advances also have led to the institutionalization of illness and death. Because people now live longer, they often experience multiple chronic or life-threatening diseases: heart disease, cancer, stroke, respiratory diseases, renal and liver failure, and progressive dementia. These life-threatening illnesses, which are often protracted and often involve predictable chronic deterioration, are frequently treated aggressively until their very late stages. Patients with chronic multiple comorbidities have complex needs for symptom management, psychosocial and spiritual support, and assistance in navigating the goals of care (Gorman, 2016).

Reports have documented that deficits exist in end-of-life care. The oft-cited landmark national SUPPORT study (SUPPORT Principal Investigators, 1995) first documented that people were dying with significant pain and other symptoms, in impersonal technological environments, and without their health care providers acknowledging their last wishes. Evidence continues to suggest that care for elders with advanced illness is often suboptimal, with poor symptom control and limited advance care planning (Institute of Medicine [IOM], 2016).

Professional concern and public demand have resulted in the evolution of palliative care, an approach to care that emphasizes quality of life throughout the disease trajectory. *Palliative care* is defined as patient- and family-centered care that optimizes quality of life by anticipating, preventing, and treating suffering. Palliative care throughout the continuum of illness involves addressing physical, intellectual, emotional, social, and spiritual needs and facilitating patient autonomy, access to care, and choice (Dahlin, 2013).

It is essential to differentiate between palliative care and hospice care. Hospice care was established to address the specific needs of patients at the very end of life. Hospice care is a part of palliative care, with similar aims of symptom management, family support, and emphasis on quality of life. However, hospice is directed toward care at the end of life. It is billed under a separate hospice benefit and is designated for patients with a life expectancy of 6 months or less (National Hospice and Palliative Care Organization [NHPCO], 2015). Palliative care evolved from the traditional hospice model by addressing quality-of-life concerns much earlier in the disease trajectory and by its integration into life-prolonging or curative treatment plans. Since elders now frequently live with prolonged, progressive chronic illness, skilled and compassionate care is needed at any stage of the illness continuum, regardless of prognosis, life-prolonging treatment, or proximity to death (Coyle, 2010). In a ground-breaking study, Temel et al. (2010) demonstrated that palliative care offered with active oncology treatment improved quality of life while also improving survival in patients with lung cancer. Ideally, patients should receive palliative care throughout the course of their illness to provide symptom management and family support and to optimize quality of life.

In 2001, five leading national organizations convened to develop the National Consensus Project Clinical Practice Guidelines for Quality Palliative Care to guide professional practice in this evolving specialty. Revised in 2013, the Consensus Guidelines continue to provide the standards of care, and define the characteristics of palliative care within eight domains (Dahlin & Lynch, 2013).

STRUCTURE AND PROCESSES

The guidelines call for care planned and delivered by an interdisciplinary team of health care professionals. Such a team typically includes a physician, nurse (including those in advanced practice), social worker, and spiritual care provider. Ideally, collaboration with other disciplines would include the involvement of psychologists, pharmacists, nutritionists, rehabilitation specialists, and practitioners trained in complementary therapies. The program must maintain a strong partnership with community resources, since palliative care is now offered in a variety of settings, such as in-patient units, ambulatory settings, community hospices, long-term care settings, and assisted-living facilities.

PHYSICAL ASPECTS OF CARE

Pain management has always been a cornerstone of palliative care, yet pain among older adults remains undertreated in many settings; barriers to adequate pain management may be multifactorial and include the following: misperceptions about the nature of pain in the elderly, patient underreporting of pain, comorbidities, cognitive losses that impede assessment, knowledge deficits on the part of care providers, and limited numbers of professional staff in long-term care facilities.

The first step in the successful management of pain is accurate assessment. Because pain is a subjective experience, asking—and believing—the patient is most crucial. Use of a visual analogue scale (0–10 pain scale) and the incorporation of pain assessment as the fifth vital sign can ensure the consistent measurement of pain frequency and intensity.

Pain assessment also includes identification of the location, duration, and quality of pain, as well as the exacerbating and alleviating factors, meaning of the pain, and its effect on activities of daily living (ADL). In the elder population, assessment can be complicated by coexisting cognitive impairment. Patients with mild impairment are often capable of reporting pain in the present moment. Pain in noncommunicative patients can be assessed through observation of body movement or with validated pain-assessment instruments such as the Checklist of Nonverbal Pain Indicators (Derby, 2013).

Basic principles of analgesic pharmacology can be applied successfully to treat an older adult in pain, although caution is warranted. Differences in drug distribution and metabolism may lead to a more profound analgesic effect or more side effects in the elderly (AGS, 2009). The "start low and go slow" philosophy is well suited to the pharmacologic treatment of pain in the elderly. Short-acting medications are more easily titrated, but once a stable dose is determined, longer acting drugs can be used successfully if carefully monitored.

The nonpharmacologic treatment of pain includes transcutaneous electrical nerve stimulation (TENS), acupuncture, and physical therapy. Cognitive-behavioral techniques such as progressive muscle relaxation and guided imagery are complementary therapies that can be taught to involved caregivers. Other complementary therapies are music and art therapy, aromatherapy, massage, therapeutic touch, and

P

the use of prayer and meditation (Derby, 2013). These complementary therapies are also being used to treat other distressful symptoms such as dyspnea, nausea, and anxiety.

Other Physical Symptoms

Symptoms experienced by severely ill older adults can be different from those in younger patients, with a higher incidence of delirium, sensory impairment, and incontinence. However, older patients also report difficulties with the most common symptoms: pain, constipation, anorexia, and dyspnea (Derby, Tickoo, & Salvidar, 2015).

Dyspnea, the subjective feeling of breathlessness, can be a frightening symptom. Constipation is a nearly universal problem in ill older adults and can lead to severe complications if left untreated. Confusion, a debilitating symptom that may develop from many different etiologies, often leads to hospitalization or institutionalization. The goal is the prevention and early treatment of symptoms, eliminating the underlying cause, if possible. Care providers must avail themselves of the growing number of resources available to guide them in implementing effective pharmacologic, nonpharmacologic, and complementary interventions.

PSYCHOLOGICAL ASPECTS OF CARE

The suffering associated with chronic life-limiting illness is multidimensional. Suffering affects the mind and spirit as well as the body. Issues such as self-esteem disturbance, anxiety, depression, and grief from multiple losses (real and anticipated) are all areas of concern. Spiritual concerns and existential distress may also contribute to patient suffering. With careful consideration of the patient's cultural and spiritual background and through contributions from psychology, social work, and pastoral care, these needs can be addressed.

SOCIAL ASPECTS OF CARE

The social needs of patients and families include financial hardship and caregiver burden. Often

the direct caregivers of these patients are elderly themselves, leading to significant personal and financial stress and consequent hospitalization or institutionalization. Interventions aimed at supporting direct caregivers can include using psychoeducational programs (e.g., support groups), increasing home care services, using volunteers and respite care, and maintaining open and direct lines of communication.

ETHICAL–LEGAL ASPECTS OF CARE

The preferences and goals of the patient and family must remain at the forefront of all care decisions. Advance care planning includes two common forms of medical advance directives: the identification of a health care proxy and the determination of treatment preferences (often known as a living will). It is imperative to remember that treatment preferences are often influenced by cultural considerations. Some older adults prefer family members to make decisions on their behalf, without completing written documents. Care planning is also complicated by cognitive decline and mental incapacity, leaving care providers to rely on surrogates (Derby et al., 2015). The practitioner providing palliative care must be aware of local regulations that govern advance directives. Important also is a familiarity with common ethical issues that may arise in the care of dying elderly, such as withdrawing or withholding artificial nutrition, hydration, or ventilation; implementing do-not-resuscitate (DNR) orders, and using palliative sedation at the end of life.

FUTURE OF PALLIATIVE CARE

The field of palliative care has been rapidly growing as a specialty within several disciplines. The Accreditation Council for Graduate Medical Education recognizes palliative care as a medical board specialty, granting official recognition for it. The Hospice and Palliative Credentialing Center now offers national board-certification examinations for a variety of nursing clinicians, including direct bedside care providers (nursing assistants), advanced practice nurses, and hospice palliative care administrators. Similar certification is available nationally for social workers and chaplains. The Joint Commission (TJC) now offers palliative care certification for hospitals.

Despite this expansion of services, the field is still evolving, and nowhere is this more evident than within geriatrics. The changing demographics and rapidly growing elderly population will tax the demands of specialists. Workforce capacity of palliative care specialists cannot meet all the needs of the growing population of patients with advanced progressive disease. Palliative care is increasingly being integrated into the primary care of elders (see Primary Palliative Care). The mandates of evolving health care reform will provide greater opportunity to introduce palliative care into all settings of elder care (Gorman, 2016). Increasing palliative care by all providers will ensure improved symptom management, appropriate care planning, and earlier utilization of specialist services, with the goal of enriched quality of life for elders with chronic illness.

See also Hospice; Primary Palliative Care.

Dorothy Wholihan

American Geriatrics Society Panel on the Pharmacological Management of Persistent Pain in Older Persons. (2009). Pharmacological management of persistent pain in older persons. *Journal of the American Geriatrics Society, 57,* 1331–1346.

Coyle, N. (2010). Introduction to palliative nursing care. *Oxford textbook of palliative nursing* (3rd ed., pp. 3–11). New York, NY: Oxford University Press.

Coyle, N. (2015). Introduction to palliative care nursing. In B. R. Ferrell, N. Coyle, & J. A. Paice (Eds.), *Oxford textbook of palliative nursing* (4th ed., pp. 3–10). New York, NY: Oxford University Press.

Dahlin, C. M. (2013). *Clinical practice guidelines for quality palliative care* (3rd ed.). Pittsburgh, PA: National Consensus Project for Quality Palliative Care. Retrieved from http://www.nationalconsensus project.org/NCP_Clinical_Practice_Guidelines_3rd_Edition.pdf

Dahlin, C. M., & Lynch, M. T. (2013). *Core curriculum for the advanced practice hospice and palliative registered nurse.* Pittsburgh, PA: Hospice and Palliative Nurses Association.

Derby, S., Tickoo, R., & Salvidar, R. (2015). Elderly patients. In B. R. Ferrell, N. Coyle, & J. A.

Paice (Eds.), *Oxford textbook of palliative nursing* (4th ed., pp. 592–605). New York, NY: Oxford University Press.

Gorman, R. (2016). Integrating palliative care into primary care. In J. Pace & D. Wholihan (Eds.), *Palliative and end-of-life care, An Issue of Nursing Clinics of North America, 51,* 367–380.

Institute of Medicine, Committee on Approaching Death. (2015). *Dying in America: Improving quality and honoring individual preferences near the end of life.* Washington, DC: National Academies Press.

National Hospice and Palliative Care Organization. (2015). NHPCO's facts and figures: Hospice care in America. Retrieved from http://www.nhpco.org/sites/default/files/public/Statistics_Research/2015_Facts_Figures.pdf

SUPPORT Principal Investigators. (1995). A controlled trial to improve care for seriously ill hospitalized patients. *Journal of the American Medical Association, 274,* 1591–1598.

Temel, J. S., Greer, J. A., Muzikansky, A., Gallagher, E. R., Admane, S., Jackson, V. A., … Lynch, T. J. (2010). Early palliative care for patients with metastatic bob-small cell lung cancer. *New England Journal of Medicine, 363,* 733–741.

Web Resources

American Academy of Hospice and Palliative Care Medicine: http://www.aahpm.org

American Geriatrics Society: http://www.american geriatrics.org

CAPC Center to Advance Palliative Care: http://www.capc.org

GeriPal: Geriatrics and Palliative Care Blog: http://www.geripal.org

Growthhouse: http://www.growthhouse.org

Hospice and Palliative Nurses Association: http://www.hpna.org

National Hospice and Palliative Care Organization: http://www.NHPCO.org

Palliative Care Fast Facts: http://www.PCNOW.org

PALLIATIVE HANDFEEDING IN DEMENTIA

Dementia is a neurodegenerative disease that progressively robs individuals of cognitive, verbal, and functional ability, creating a dependence on caregivers to provide assistance with

P

nutritional intake through handfeeding until death (DiBartolo, 2006; Palecek et al., 2010). Weight loss in dementia is a complex process but often is the first clinical sign that a person with dementia needs more support with meals. Mealtime difficulty is a concept for framing issues related to maintaining nutrition in dementia by considering multiple levels: the sociocultural and individual preferences of the person with dementia, the quality of interactions with caregivers, and the environment (Aselage & Amella, 2010).

RESEARCH AND BEST PRACTICES

As the assessment process begins, the C3P Model is a helpful problem-solving framework for identifying potentially reversible causes, by making changes in the person, people, or place (Amella & Batchelor-Aselage, 2014). The current clinical practice guidelines call for assessment and management by an interprofessional team consisting of the primary care provider, dietician, nurse, dentist, therapy (primarily occupational and speech), direct caregiver(s), and family members (Batchelor-Murphy & Crowgey, 2016). Optimal assessment includes an investigation into potentially reversible/modifiable physiological causes, as well as performance of a meal observation to determine the impact of any feeding behaviors such as turning the head away or not opening the mouth, and/or the impact of interactions with caregivers, and/or the environment (Batchelor-Aselage, Amella, Rose & Bales, 2014; Batchelor-Murphy & Crowgey, 2016; Lin, Watson, & Wu, 2010). Effective management is possible once the underlying issues are identified.

Change the person: Food intake problems may be because of *biological* issues of poor vision, swallowing disorders, poor dentition, pain, depression, urinary tract infection, lack of needed adaptive equipment, constipation, or other underlying issues (Aselage & Amella, 2012). Changes in vision may also make it more difficult for a person with dementia to understand and respond to *visual cues*. In addition, a myriad of problems related to *cognitive decline and functional ability* are highly likely to appear as the disease progresses: remembering to eat, recognizing food, changes in ability to transport

food to the mouth, performing the voluntary and involuntary stages of swallowing, and/or recognizing when to stop eating (Amella, 2004).

Change the people: Mealtimes are more than a time to ingest food, not simply a task to be completed. In every culture, the sharing of food has social and religious connotations. The relationship between a person with dementia and their caregiver has a profound impact during meals, when this fundamental social interaction occurs, regardless of where the meal takes place (Amella, 2002). The quality of this interaction has the potential to affect the amount of food consumed. Caregivers must be able to individualize needs of older adults, but this can be a monumental task, given issues of understaffing, inadequate training, and lack of cultural sensitivity in our nation's institutional settings.

Change the place: Environmental considerations for problem areas relate to the dining environment: too noisy, too much traffic, inadequate lighting, and/or inconsistent seating arrangements (Amella & Aselage, 2012). Mealtimes and mealtime environments are often institutionalized, bereft of social and cultural context and cues. Institutionalized persons with dementia are less likely to find environments that allow mealtimes to be enjoyed, as a lifelong pastime that promotes exchange.

Palliative handfeeding in dementia: Maintaining nutrition through the use of tube feeding has not demonstrated benefit in dementia but does have the potential to do harm (Finucane, Christmas, & Travis, 1999). In response to this resounding message in medicine, the numbers of feeding tube placements have steadily declined (Mitchell, Mor, Gozalo, Servadio, & Teno, 2016). The recommended option for care at end-of-life in dementia is palliative handfeeding (Mitchell et al., 2016). Providing handfeeding assistance to a person with dementia requires a unique set of skills to manage swallowing problems, feeding behaviors, and provision of enough support to compensate for functional deficits while promoting as much independence with meals as possible (Batchelor-Murphy et al., 2017). From physicians to direct care providers, education to recognize the risk for swallowing problems and management of these problems is provided in basic training programs; however, the complex skills needed to manage feeding behaviors and provide handfeeding support are still needed for optimizing meal intake in this population (Batchelor-Murphy, Amella, Zapka, Mueller, & Beck, 2015; Batchelor-Murphy & Crowgey, 2016).

Feeding Behaviors

As the ability to use and understand spoken language declines, persons with dementia may also lose the ability to interpret the *verbal cues* given by caregivers, leaving *nonverbal cues* as the primary form of communication for the dyad. Without language, persons with dementia use feeding behaviors to communicate preferences and may turn their head away, clamp their mouth shut, spit food out, or push away assistance. When feeding behaviors are interpreted by caregivers as "resistance," rather than need-driven, dementia-compromised behaviors, feeding assistance may cease, putting the person with dementia at greater risk of premature death. Emerging evidence supports that persons with dementia consume more food when feeding behaviors are responded to differently after trained staff spend time attempting determining what those behaviors mean (Batchelor-Murphy et al., 2015).

Handfeeding Techniques

Evidence is emerging to support the use of three handfeeding techniques: Direct Hand, Over Hand, and Under Hand (Batchelor-Murphy, 2015; Batchelor-Murphy et al., 2015, 2017; Batchelor-Murphy & Crowgey, 2016). Expanding the repertoire of basic nursing care related to providing feeding assistance, each technique has its own time/place for optimal use. The decision for how/when to use each technique should be based on (a) the person's functional ability related to holding a utensil and upper arm range of motion, (b) the person's energy level, and (c) individual preferences (Batchelor-Murphy et al., 2017). The least amount of support should be used to promote independence and to be fully supportive for a resident with late- or end-stage dementia.

Over Hand: If a person can hold the utensil and has adequate upper extremity range of motion, the Over Hand technique may be the best option for providing a little help guiding the utensil toward the mouth. From the perspective of the resident, the Over Hand technique may feel as if the feeding assistant is forcing the food toward the face; therefore care should be taken to use a gentle, guiding manner.

Under Hand: If the person is losing the ability to hold the utensil, using the Under Hand technique allows the care provider to compensate for this functional loss. The Under Hand technique taps into lifelong sensorimotor cues associated with eating, engages the resident in the meal experience, and allows the resident to control the pace of feeding assistance.

Direct Hand: If a resident is bedridden and in the very late stages of dementia, use of the Direct Hand technique may be the best option for avoiding fatiguing the person. Use of Direct Hand puts all of the effort and energy required for moving the food from the plate to the mouth on the care provider, rather than the person with dementia.

In the first efficacy study to experimentally compare the use of the handfeeding techniques, their use proved time neutral; 43 to 45 minutes is typically required to assist these residents with meals (Batchelor-Murphy et al., 2017; Simmons & Schnelle, 2004). This research also found that Under Hand and Direct Hand resulted in persons with dementia consuming more food, with less feeding behaviors, relative to Over Hand (Batchelor-Murphy et al., 2017).

Melissa Batchelor-Murphy

Amella, E. J. (2002). Resistance at mealtimes for persons with dementia. *Journal of Nutrition and Health Aging,* *6*(2), 117–122.

Amella, E. J. (2004). Feeding and hydration issues for older adults with dementia. *Nursing Clinics of North America, 39*(3), 607–623.

Amella, E. J., & Batchelor-Aselage, M. B. (2014). Facilitating ADLs by caregivers of persons with dementia: The C3P Model. *Occupational Therapy Health Care, 28*(1), 51–61. doi:10.3109/07380577.2013.867388

Aselage, M. B., & Amella, E. J. (2010). An evolutionary analysis of mealtime difficulties in older adults with dementia. *Journal of Clinical Nursing, 19*(1/2), 33–41. doi:10.1111/j.1365-2702.2009.02969.x

Aselage, M. B., & Amella, E. J. (2012). Response to Watson R (2011) Commentary on Aselage MB

(2010). Measuring mealtime difficulties: Eating, feeding, and meal behaviours in older adults with dementia. *Journal of Clinical Nursing, 19,* 621–631. *Journal of Clinical Nursing, 20,* 297–298. *Journal of Clinical Nursing, 21*(9–10), 1494–1495.

Batchelor-Aselage, M., Amella, E., Rose, S. & Bales, C. (2014). Dementia-related mealtime difficulties: Assessment and management in the long-term-care setting. In C. Bales, J. Locher, & E. Salzman (Eds.), *Handbook of clinical nutrition and aging* (3rd ed., pp. 287–301). New York, NY: Springer.

Batchelor-Murphy, M. (Producer). (2015, September 22). Handfeeding techniques for assisting persons with dementia. Retrieved from https://youtube/NYzH_B7XfjY

Batchelor-Murphy, M., Amella, E. J., Zapka, J., Mueller, M., & Beck, C. (2015). Feasibility of a web-based dementia feeding skills training program for nursing home staff. *Geriatric Nursing, 36*(3), 212–218.

Batchelor-Murphy, M., & Crowgey, S. (2016). Mealtime difficulties in dementia. In M. Boltz (Ed.), *Evidence-based geriatric nursing protocols for best practice* (pp. 417–429). New York, NY: Springer Publishing.

Batchelor-Murphy, M., McConnell, E., Amella, E., Anderson, R., Bales, C., Silva, S., ... Colon-Emeric, C. (2017). Experimental comparison of efficacy for three handfeeding techniques in dementia. *Journal of the American Geriatrics Society, 65*(4) e89–e94. doi:10.1111/jgs.14728

DiBartolo, M. C. (2006). Careful hand feeding: A reasonable alternative to PEG tube placement in individuals with dementia. *Journal of Gerontological Nursing, 32*(5), 25–35.

Finucane, T. E., Christmas, C., & Travis, K. (1999). Tube feeding in patients with advanced dementia: A review of the evidence. *Journal of the American Medical Association, 282*(14), 1365–1370.

Lin, L., Watson, R., & Wu, S. (2010). What is associated with low food intake in older people with dementia? *Journal of Clinical Nursing, 19*(1–2), 53–59. doi:10.1111/j.1365-2702.2009.02962.x

Mitchell, S. L., Mor, V., Gozalo, P. L., Servadio, J. L., & Teno, J. M. (2016). Tube feeding in U.S. nursing home residents with advanced dementia, 2000–2014. *Journal of the American Medical Association, 316*(7), 769–770. doi:10.1001/jama.2016.9374

Palecek, E. J., Teno, J. M., Casarett, D. J., Hanson, L. C., Rhodes, R. L., & Mitchell, S. L. (2010). Comfort feeding only: A proposal to bring clarity to decision-making regarding difficulty with eating for persons with advanced dementia. *Journal of the American Geriatrics Society, 58*(3), 580–584. doi:10.1111/j.1532-5415.2010.02740.x

Simmons, S. F., & Schnelle, J. F. (2004). Individualized feeding assistance care for nursing home residents: Staffing requirements to implement two interventions. *Journals of Gerontology: Series A, Biological Sciences & Medical Sciences, 59A*(9), 966–973.

Web Resources
Batchelor-Murphy, M. (2015). Feasibility of a web-based dementia feeding skills training program for nursing home staff. Retrieved from https://www.youtube.com/watch?v=1wKupHcuKIc
You Tube Channel: DementiaCareNP

PARKINSONISM

Parkinsonism is defined by a clinical constellation of motor signs including muscle rigidity, bradykinesia or slowed movement, and tremor. It arises from a diverse array of causes (Table P.1) but most commonly is due to idiopathic Parkinson's disease, an age-related, progressive, and incurable neurodegenerative disorder.

DIAGNOSIS

Parkinsonism is diagnosed mainly on clinical grounds: A detailed history and physical examination aid in formulating the most likely cause. Certain clinical features aid in the diagnosis. For example, a combination of symmetric parkinsonism, slow eye movements, and square wave jerks with early falls suggests the possibility of progressive supranuclear palsy (PSP). Asymmetrical apraxia and dystonia may suggest corticobasal syndrome. Prominent autonomic dysfunction raises the possibility of multiple system atrophy. Significant early cognitive decline is seen in dementia with Lewy bodies. Although these are the classic presentations, the various neurodegenerative parkinsonisms can often be misdiagnosed because of an overlap of symptoms. Each may have various subtypes, such as PSP cerebellar variant and PSP parkinsonism (Koga et al., 2015).

Although diagnosis remains primarily clinical, neuroimaging is invaluable in particular cases. For example, MRI aids evaluation in cases of parkinsonism resulting from masses, normal pressure hydrocephalus, or vascular parkinsonism. Detection of the dopamine transporter, with the ioflupane (^{123}I) ligand and single-photon emission CT (SPECT) is now available for use in clinical practice. To date, studies have demonstrated that they can aid in evaluating parkinsonian syndromes, distinguishing, for example, essential tremor or drug-related parkinsonism from Parkinson's disease (Cummings et al., 2011). However, SPECT cannot distinguish among the various neurodegenerative parkinsonisms (Bajaj, Hauser, & Grachev, 2013). PET scans measuring brain fluorodeoxyglucose (FDG) uptake have also been used to examine atypical cases of parkinsonism, but their use in this regard remains primarily in the research arena.

Genetic testing can be useful in certain conditions (e.g., Huntington's disease, which is associated with parkinsonism in a minority of cases). In Parkinson's disease itself, however, the role of genetic testing in diagnosis is limited. Fewer than 5% of cases of Parkinson's disease are attributable to single-gene mutations, although a monogenic cause is more likely in those with a strong family history and early age of onset. There are, as yet, no specific genetic tests for many of the conditions listed in Table P.1, such as multiple system atrophy or PSP.

PARKINSON'S DISEASE

Epidemiology

Population-based study estimates of the prevalence of Parkinson's disease vary, but in the United States, one-half to 1 million persons are believed to be affected, with a predicted doubling in that number by 2040 (Pringsheim, Jette, Frolkis, & Steeves, 2014). In general, the disease is unusual in persons younger than 50 years of age but affects approximately 1% of those older than 60 years and up to 4% of those older than 80 years. Most studies have found a slight male predominance (i.e., 1.2–1.7:1). The reason for this gender difference is unknown; however, some evidence suggests that estrogen may be protective and delay disease onset. Differences in symptoms and in treatment response between genders have also been described, but few studies have examined this to date.

Epidemiological studies have suggested rural residence, occupational exposures, lead exposure and pesticide exposure as possible environmental risk factors for Parkinson's disease. Coffee consumption, cigarette smoking, and high uric acid levels in men have been associated with a decreased risk of Parkinson's disease, whereas dairy consumption, high levels of inflammatory markers, and low cholesterol levels are associated with an increased risk (Tanner, 2010). Unfortunately, there are inconsistencies in these associations, and age remains the biggest factor in disease development (Kieburtz & Wunderle, 2013). However, genetic vulnerability combined with environmental exposures likely plays a greater role than any one risk factor alone.

Genetics

At the time of writing, there are 18 *PARK* loci identified, and multiple genes are known to modify the risk of Parkinson's disease (Kumar et al., 2011). The monogenic causes of Parkinson's disease include *LRRK2* (the most common genetic cause of autosomal dominant inherited Parkinson's disease), parkin (the most common genetic cause of autosomal recessive inherited Parkinson's disease) (alpha-synuclein, *PINK1*, and DJ-1. Glucocerebrosidase (traditionally studied in Gaucher's disease, a storage disorder) is an important genetic risk factor that is associated with the development of Parkinson's disease (Brockman & Gasser, 2015). *LRRK2*, *PRKN*, and *PINK1* mutations have also been identified in sporadic cases of Parkinson's disease. Testing for *SNCA* (alpha-synuclein), *LRRK2*, parkin, *PINK1*, and DJ-1 is now available in the clinic and may be considered in certain cases. Access to family counseling by a professional genetic counselor is then strongly advised.

Pathogenesis

Most neurodegenerative parkinsonian conditions result from loss of the effect of dopamine on the basal ganglia. In Parkinson's disease, this occurs from attrition of dopamine-producing neurons in the substantia nigra,

P

Table P.1
CONDITIONS ASSOCIATED WITH PARKINSONISM

Parkinson's disease

Parkinson's-plus disorders
   Progressive supranuclear palsy
   Corticobasal degeneration
   Multiple system atrophy

Dementing illnesses
   Alzheimer's disease
   Dementia with Lewy bodies
   Frontotemporal dementia

Heredodegenerative diseases
   Huntington's chorea
   Wilson's disease
   Spinocerebellar ataxias
   Lubag

Fragile-X tremor ataxia syndrome (FXTAS)

ATP1*A*3 mutation spectrum disorders—rapid-onset dystonia-parkinsonism

Drugs
   Neuroleptic medications (haloperidol and others, including atypical antipsychotics such as olanzapine)
   Antiemetic agents (prochlorperazine, metoclopramide)
   Dopamine-depleting agents (tetrabenazine, reserpine)
   Valproic acid
   Calcium channel-blocking agents

Infections and masses
   Postencephalitic parkinsonism
   Lesions (infectious or neoplastic) of the basal ganglia or midbrain
   HIV
   Prion disorders (e.g., Creutzfeldt-Jakob disease; rare)

Toxins
   MPTP
   Lead
   Manganese
   Organic solvents
   Cyanide
   Carbon monoxide
   Carbon disulphide

Other
   Vascular parkinsonism
   Normal pressure hydrocephalus

MPTP, 1-methyl-4-phenyl-1,2,3,6-tetrahydropyridine.

with intracytoplasmic inclusions, termed *Lewy bodies*, present in many of the surviving neurons. These Lewy bodies contain, among other constituents, aggregates of alpha-synuclein. Loss of dopaminergic neurons in the substantia nigra accounts for the majority of motor symptoms. However, Lewy bodies and related Lewy neurites are much more widespread in both the central nervous system (e.g., in the cerebral cortex) and the peripheral autonomic nervous system (e.g., involving the gastrointestinal tract, bladder, and other organs) (Jellinger, 2012). This widespread pathology likely accounts for some of the motor and many of the nonmotor symptoms that make Parkinson's disease so complex.

Mechanisms leading to neuronal damage and loss are believed to arise from the interplay of environmental and genetic causes. Accidental ingestion of a drug contaminant 1-methyl-4-phe-nyl-1,2,3,6 tetrahydropyridine (MPTP) by several individuals in the 1980s demonstrated that parkinsonism can arise from chemical exposure, and compounds such as rotenone and paraquat lead to parkinsonism in animal models of disease. Study of Parkinson's disease-associated genes has further fleshed out the understanding of pathogenesis and suggest that a complex network of cellular processes is disrupted in Parkinson's disease, including altered protein handling, lysosomal function, inflammation, altered calcium conductance leading to excessive reactive oxygen species, and altered energy metabolism with impaired mitochondrial function. Most recently, it has been proposed that misfolded alpha-synuclein will "self-propagate" from cell to cell, reminiscent of a prion-like protein (Abeliovich & Rhinn, 2016).

Clinical Manifestations

Although asymmetric resting tremor, muscle rigidity, bradykinesia (i.e., delayed or slowed execution of movement), and decline in postural reflexes are the cardinal features of Parkinson's disease, a wide array of both motor and nonmotor symptoms are recognized (Table P.2).

Resting tremor is a common initial symptom but is absent in approximately 30% of cases. Bradykinesia may manifest as hypophonia, hypomimia ("masked facies"), difficulty with fine coordination, micrographia, and slowed gait. Swallowing is affected in many, and dysphagia places the patient at risk of and contributes to bothersome drooling. Muscular rigidity is described as "lead pipe" in quality, meaning that it is independent of velocity of movement on passive motion. "Cogwheeling rigidity" describes a superimposed tremor leading to a ratchet-like movement. Patients may experience rigidity as stiffness and pain, and it is sometimes confused with musculoskeletal syndromes such as rotator-cuff tear. Impairment of postural reflexes, typically seen later in Parkinson's disease, leads to falls and is therefore a significant source of morbidity and mortality. Falls

Table P.2
CLINICAL FEATURES OF PARKINSON'S DISEASE

Motor Manifestations

Bradykinesia
  Delayed or slowed execution of movement
  Difficulty with fine motor coordination
  Micrographia
  Hypomimia or "masked facies"
  Hypophonia
Resting tremor
Rigidity, often with "cogwheeling"
Imbalance and falls
Freezing of gait
Festinating gait
Dysphagia
Dystonia

Nonmotor Manifestations

Cognitive:
  Mild cognitive impairment
  Dementia
Psychiatric:
  Depression
  Anxiety
  Impulse-control disorders
  Hallucinations, paranoid ideation—can be induced by
    medications or be intrinsic to disease pathology
Autonomic:
  Orthostatic hypotension
  Hyperhidrosis
  Urinary urgency, frequency, incontinence
  Sialorrhea
  Delayed gastric emptying
  Constipation
  Sexual dysfunction
Sleep disturbances:
  REM-behavior disorders
  Sleep apnea
  Restless legs syndrome
  Sleep fragmentation
  Excessive daytime drowsiness
Pain syndromes
Weight loss
Hyposmia

may result from a tendency to propel forward (i.e., propulsion) or backward (i.e., retropulsion), from festination (i.e., progressively faster and smaller steps) and from freezing, a sudden block of motor function. In addition to features already described, focal limb dystonia may be seen, particularly in younger patients with Parkinson's disease, resulting in a diagnostic challenge when it is the presenting sign.

Nonmotor symptoms are common in Parkinson's disease (Table P.2), occurring in more than 90% of patients at various stages of the disease (Chaudhuri, Odin, Antonini, & Martinez-Martin, 2011). In late disease, they may constitute the majority of burden on patient and caregiver. Nonmotor features include cognitive, behavioral, sleep, and autonomic manifestations. Mild cognitive impairment (MCI) may occur in 20% to 50% of individuals with Parkinson's disease, and point prevalence of dementia has been estimated at 40%, with up to 80% affected in longitudinal studies. However, although MCI may occur even in mild disease, the early presence of dementia would suggest an alternate diagnosis. Depression and anxiety are also common, with a prevalence of up to 40% each, and the clinical picture may also be complicated by apathy and fatigue. Hallucinations or paranoid ideation may be seen later in the disease, and although hallucinations are commonly associated with various medications, there is suggestion that the intrinsic disease-related pathology plays a role in their development (Pagonabarraga et al., 2016). Other behavioral disturbances related to medications include impulse-control disorders, which may manifest as compulsive gambling, hypersexuality, and compulsive eating, for example. Although most strongly related to treatment with dopamine agonists (Table P.3), they may also occur in the context of other Parkinson's disease medications. Autonomic dysfunction, including orthostatic hypotension, excessive sweating, sialorrhea, urinary frequency and incontinence, sexual dysfunction, and constipation, may occur. Disturbances of sleep are common and include REM-behavior disorder (RBD), sleep apnea, restless legs syndrome, and excessive daytime drowsiness.

A subset of nonmotor symptoms, including olfactory dysfunction, constipation, and RBD, may occur before the onset of motor symptoms, supporting the existence of premotor Parkinson's disease.

PHARMACOTHERAPY

There are many drugs for symptomatic treatment of Parkinson's disease, as listed in Table P.3. The choice of medication depends on the individual case, but published treatment recommendations aid in formulating an appropriate treatment strategy (Fox et al., 2011; Pahwa et al.,

2006). Unfortunately, other forms of neurodegenerative parkinsonism usually respond little, if at all, to these interventions.

Levodopa remains the cornerstone of therapy, significantly improves the reduced life expectancy associated with untreated Parkinson's disease, and is available in oral form as immediate- and extended-release tablets and as extended-release capsules. In general, levodopa is preferred in the elderly over other drugs because of its higher tolerability. There is also excellent tolerability data for rasagiline in the elderly. However, when making a treatment choice, it is important to consider a patient's "functional," rather than chronological, age; for example, if a young patient is considerably impaired, starting levodopa is warranted.

Unfortunately, after months to years, the majority of patients develop levodopa-related motor complications, including "wearing off" and dyskinesia. *Wearing off* describes the reemergence of symptoms at progressively shorter levodopa dosing intervals. Such individuals often experience fluctuations between the "on" state (symptoms controlled) and "off" state (symptoms not controlled). Switching from immediate-release carbidopa/levodopa tablets to extended-release capsules reduces the amount of time in the "off" state. However, although adjusting levodopa formulation, dose, and timing may help, adjunct medications provide additional and sometimes preferable options. For example, the addition of catechol-O-methyl transferase (COMT) inhibitors, monoamine oxidase-B (MAO-B) inhibitors, and dopamine agonists have been shown to reduce "off" time by 1 to 1.5 hours/day (Table P.3). Carbidopa/levodopa is also available as an enteral suspension, for infusion directly into the jejunum via a percutaneous endoscopic gastrostomy jejunostomy (PEG-J) tube, and decreases time in the "off" state by almost 2 hours over placebo. Dyskinesias are involuntary and sometimes disabling choreiform movements, most commonly seen as the levodopa effect peaks, although sometimes seen at levodopa dose onset or during wearing off. Sometimes these movements may be painful dystonic in quality. Management require balancing dyskinesia with "off" periods and can be challenging.

Decreasing the dose of levodopa may improve dykinesia, but may lead to more "off" periods that subsequently requires more frequent dosing. Adding amantadine, or decreasing the other medications, may also improve dyskinesia. However, in this phase of Parkinson's disease, the side effects of medications, particularly amantadine and dopamine agonists, may limit their use in the elderly, further reducing the options available.

Attention to nonmotor symptoms can significantly enhance a patient's quality of life, and a number of potential therapies have now been successfully tested in clinical trials (Seppi et al.,

2011). Serotonin reuptake inhibitors and tricyclic antidepressants have shown to be helpful for depression in Parkinson's disease. Symptoms of dementia may show a modest response to acetylcholinesterase inhibitors, and rivastigmine has demonstrated benefit in treating Parkinson's disease dementia. Unfortunately, fewer data support the use of other drugs, including donepezil and galantamine, for this purpose, although they can be used judiciously. Memantine also has insufficient data to support its utility in treating dementia in Parkinson's disease, although some data suggest benefit. Psychotic symptoms can be treated with

Table P.3
PARKINSON'S DISEASE MEDICATIONS

Medication Name	Class	Comments and Side Effects
Early Parkinson's Disease: Initial Treatment		
Carbidopa/levodopa	Dopamine "replacement"	Nausea and vomiting, hypotension, sleepiness, hallucinations Levodopa-associated "wearing off" and dyskinesia (long term)
Rotigotine, pramipexole, ropinirole	Dopamine agonist	Nausea, hallucinations, somnolence, and "sleep attacks," leg edema, postural hypotension, impulse-control disorders (e.g., pathologic gambling) Site reaction for rotigotine patch
Rasagiline, selegiline	MAO-B inhibitor	Generally mild Flu-like syndrome and arthralgias, nausea, dizziness
Amantadine	Multiple actions, including N-methyl-D-aspartate (NMDA) antagonist, anticholinergic, dopaminergic	Hallucinations, cognitive dysfunction and confusion, nausea, livedo reticularis
Moderate–Severe Parkinson's Disease: Adjunct Treatment to Levodopa		
Rotigotine, pramipexole, ropinirole, apomorphine	Dopamine agonist	Reduction of "off" time but possible increase in dyskinesias Nausea, hallucinations, somnolence and "sleep attacks," leg edema, postural hypotension, impulse-control disorders (e.g., pathologic gambling) Site reaction for rotigotine patch Nausea/vomiting, postural hypotension for apomorphine injection
Rasagiline, selegiline	MAO-B inhibitor	Reduction of "off" time, possible adjustment in levodopa dose if dyskinesias increase
Entacapone, tolcapone	COMT inhibitor	Reduction in "off" time but possible increase in dyskinesia Diarrhea and discolored urine (entacapone) Required monitoring of liver function (tolcapone) for rare association with liver failure
Amantadine	Multiple actions, including NMDA antagonist, anticholinergic, dopaminergic	Reduction in dyskinesia Hallucinations, cognitive dysfunction and confusion, nausea, livedo reticularis

COMT, catechol-O-methyl transferase; MAO-B, monoamine oxidase-B.

clozapine and quetiapine, but other antipsychotic medications (especially so-called typical antipsychotic medications such as halperidol) should be avoided because they worsen parkinsonian symptoms. Recently, pimavanserin, a serotonin 5-HT$_{2A}$ receptor inverse agonist, was by the U.S. Food and Drug Administration (FDA) for the treatment of Parkinson's disease psychosis (Markham, 2016). Orthostasis may require increased hydration, increased dietary salt intake, or medications that increase plasma volume (fludrocortisone, desmopressin), induce vasoconstriction (midodrine), or block vasodilation (indomethacin, octreotide). Droxidopa, which is peripherally and centrally converted to norepinephrine, was approved by the FDA in 2014 for the treatment of symptomatic neurogenic orthostatic hypotension (NOH) and has been shown to be effective in treating NOH without increasing supine hypertension (Strassheim, Newton, Tan, & Frith, 2016). Sialorrhea may respond to botulinum toxin injections. Urinary symptoms often respond to anticholinergic agents, and in some cases, a referral to a urologist for consideration of botulinum toxin injections is appropriate. Constipation should be aggressively treated with dietary changes, attention to adequate hydration, and medications. Treatment for sexual dysfunction in Parkinson's disease has been poorly studied, particularly in women, although it is a common problem for both genders. Some men benefit from phosphodiesterase inhibitors, testosterone, and other treatments, and some improvement may occur with dopaminergic therapy.

NONPHARMACOLOGIC TREATMENT

Attention to overall health and well-being is paramount in Parkinson's disease and parkinsonism in general. A variety of exercise and movement-based therapies are now being actively used and studied, including dance, weight training, aerobic exercise, yoga, and particularly tai chi, which has been demonstrated to improve balance. There is a strong case for considering physical therapy, occupational therapy, and speech therapy, including the Lee Silverman Voice Treatment, in patients with parkinsonism. Physical and occupational therapy

has been shown to improve motor symptoms and disability, building physical capability and teaching strategies to overcome impairments (such as sensory tricks to overcome freezing of gait). Physical activity has also shown to be inversely related to neuropsychiatric symptoms, especially fatigue. Tai chi is documented to improve balance.

Surgical treatment for Parkinson's disease has been increasingly utilized in the last few years. Most commonly, this involves the insertion of electrodes for continuous high-frequency deep brain stimulation (DBS). This approach is valuable in advanced Parkinson's disease, when medications cannot adequately control motor symptoms. There is now more experience using this approach in the elderly population, but older patients need to be very carefully screened for compromised cognitive function, as this may worsen after surgery. Although complications are rare, the risks of surgery need to be carefully weighed, and it is not used in other forms of parkinsonism. Cell-based transplant therapy and gene therapy techniques are now being explored as future potential treatments.

PSYCHOSOCIAL IMPLICATIONS

Parkinsonism has profound ramifications for patients, families, and caregivers. It affects ability to work and may lead to early retirement and changes in social roles. A multidisciplinary team approach can help patients, their families, and caregivers achieve the highest possible quality of life. This often means involving a neurologist closely collaborating with a primary care provider, skilled nurses, social workers, specialists in rehabilitation medicine, and professionals able to perform counseling and psychiatric evaluation. Individual counseling forms a large part of clinic visits, and support groups can be a highly effective forum for the exchange of information. Home care services are invaluable in managing more advanced patients. The role of telemedicine is also being actively explored to improve access to specialized care. Appropriate institutional care may be considered when the patient's needs are no longer safely met at home. Given the physical, psychological, and social complexities of parkinsonian syndromes, management for an individual with parkinsonism is optimized by developing a flexible, creative, and integrated approach to lifestyle, with patients, families, and health care professionals operating as a team.

Harini Sarva and Claire Henchcliffe

Abeliovich, A., & Rhinn, H. (2016). Parkinson's disease: Guilt by genetic association. *Nature, 533*(7601), 40–42.

Bajaj, N., Hauser, R. A., & Grachev I. D. (2013). Clinical utility of dopamine transporter single photo emission CT (DaT-SPECT) with (^{123}I) ioflupane in diagnosis of parkinsonian syndromes. *Journal of Neurology, Neurosurgery, and Psychiatry, 84*, 1288–1295.

Chaudhuri, K. R., Odin, P., Antonini, A., & Martinez-Martin, P. (2011). Parkinson's disease: The nonmotor issues. *Parkinsonism & Related Disorders, 17*(10), 717–723.

Cummings, J. L., Henchcliffe, C., Schaier, S., Simuni, T., Waxman, A., & Kemp, P. (2011). The role of dopaminergic imaging in patients with symptoms of dopaminergic system neurodegeneration. *Brain: A Journal of Neurology, 134*(Pt. 11), 3146–3166.

Fox, S. H., Katzenschlager, R., Lim, S. Y., Ravina, B., Seppi, K., Coelho, M., ... Sampaio, C. (2011). The Movement Disorder Society evidence-based medicine review update: Treatments for the motor symptoms of Parkinson's disease. *Movement Disorders, 26*(Suppl. 3), S2–S41.

Jellinger, K. A. (2012). Neuropathology of sporadic Parkinson's disease: Evaluation and changes of concepts. *Movement Disorders, 27*(1), 8–30.

Kieburtz, K., & Wunderle, K. B. (2013). Parkinson's disease: Evidence for environmental risk factors. *Movement Disorders, 28*, 8–13.

Koga, S., Aoki, N., Uitti, R. J., van Gerpen, J. A., Cheshire, W. P., Josephs, K. A., ... Dickson, D. W. (2015). When DLB, PD and PSP masquerade as MSA: An autopsy study of 134 patients. *Neurology, 85*, 404–412.

Kumar, A., Greggio, E., Beilina, A., Kaganovich, A., Chan, D., Taymans, J.-M.... Cookson, M. R. (2010). The Parkinson's disease associated LRRK2 exhibits weaker in vitro phosphorylation of 4E-BP compared to autophosphorylation. *PLoS One, 5*, e8730.

Kumar, K. R., Djarmati-Westenberger, A., & Grünewald, A. (2011). Genetics of Parkinson's disease. *Seminars in Neurology, 31*(5), 433–440.

Markham, A. (2016). Pimavanserin: First global approval. *Drugs, 76*(10), 1053–1057.

Pagonabarraga J., Martinez-Horta S., Fernández de Bobadilla R., Pérez J., Ribosa-Nogué R., Marín. J., ... Kulisevsky, J. (2016). Minor hallucinations occur in drug-naive Parkinson's disease patients, even from the premotor phase. *Movement Disorders, 31*, 45–52.

Pahwa, R., Factor, S. A., Lyons, K. E., Ondo, W. G., Gronseth, G., Bronte-Stewart, H., ... Weiner, W. J.; Quality Standards Subcommittee of the American Academy of Neurology. (2006). Practice parameter: Treatment of Parkinson disease with motor fluctuations and dyskinesia (an evidence-based review): Report of the Quality Standards Subcommittee of the American Academy of Neurology. *Neurology, 66*(7), 983–995.

Pringsheim, T., Jette, N., Frolkis, A., & Steeves, T. D. (2014). The prevalence of Parkinson's disease: A systematic review and meta-analysis. *Movement disorders, 29*(13), 1583–1590.

Seppi, K., Weintraub, D., Coelho, M., Perez-Lloret, S., Fox, S. H., Katzenschlager, R., ... Sampaio, C. (2011). The Movement Disorder Society evidence-based medicine review update: Treatments for the non-motor symptoms of Parkinson's disease. *Movement Disorders, 26*(Suppl. 3), S42–S80.

Strassheim, V., Newton, J. L., Tan, M. P., & Frith, J. (2016). Droxidopa for orthostatic hypotension: A systematic review and meta-analysis. *Journal of Hypertension, 34*, 1933–1941. doi:10.1097/HJH .0000000000001043

Tanner, C. M. (2010). Advances in environmental epidemiology. *Movement Disorders, 25*(Suppl. 1), S58–S62.

Web Resources
American Parkinson Disease Association, Inc.: http:// www.apdaparkinson.org
Michael J. Fox Foundation for Parkinson's Research: https://www.michaeljfox.org
National Parkinson Foundation, Inc.: http://www .parkinson.org
Parkinson's Disease Foundation: http://www .parkinsonsfoundation.org

PARTICIPANT-DIRECTED CARE

PRINCIPLES OF PARTICIPANT-DIRECTION

Participant-direction (PD) is a service model based on the philosophy that individuals who need long-term support should have choice and control over the supportive services they receive. PD is also referred to as *consumer-direction* or *self-direction* and is similar to independent living in the disability community and self-determination in the developmental disabilities field. The goal of PD services is to empower the individual to live a full life in the community—to work if desired, carry on family life, attend functions and use facilities in the community, get further education, or pursue other personal interests (Benjamin & Snyder, 2003; Robert Wood Johnson Foundation, 2013; Simon-Rusinowitz & Hofland, 1993). PD long-term services and supports reflect a shift from the traditional paradigm of the agency-administered model as it transfers the focus of decision making from the service provider to the participant and the family.

HOW PD WORKS

PD entails a continuum of approaches based on the degree of choice, control, and management responsibilities the participant wants to assume (Benjamin & Snyder, 2003). The essence of a PD program is the control the participant has over the employment terms of the caregiver or personal assistant who provides supportive services. Generally, personal assistance involves persons or devices that help individuals with disabilities perform the everyday tasks they would perform by themselves if they did not have disabilities, including bathing, dressing, using the toilet, eating, and taking medications, as well as other personal care, household, and community activities (Benjamin & Snyder, 2003; Simon-Rusinowitz & Hofland, 1993). Participants may be responsible for selecting, hiring, training, and firing caregivers and negotiating their work schedule and duties. Many PD programs allow the participant to hire friends and relatives as caregivers (Simon-Rusinowitz, Loughlin, Ruben, Garcia, & Mahoney, 2010); however, states often do not allow a spouse, parent, or legal guardian to be a paid worker (Sciegaj et al., 2014). More detailed information on PD programs is available through the National Resource Center for Participant-Directed Services (NRCPDS), Applied Self-Direction, and the Robert Wood Johnson Foundation.

CASH AND COUNSELING DEMONSTRATION AND EVALUATION

Cash and Counseling, one PD model, allows participants to manage a monthly budget, which they can use to purchase personal assistance services and a broad range of other services and products they determine appropriate, including assistive technology or home modifications (Simon-Rusinowitz, Loughlin, Ruben, & Mahoney, 2010). Conducted from 1998 to 2003, three states participated in Cash and Counseling Demonstration and Evaluation (CCDE), which compared traditional Medicaid personal-assistance services to a PD cash option for a diverse sample of participants: elders as well as adults and children with physical and cognitive disabilities. Program supports included counseling and bookkeeping services to help participants manage their monthly budget and employer responsibilities. Participants could choose a representative—a relative or friend—if they wanted or needed more help with these tasks.

The CCDE found that PD group members expressed significantly more satisfaction with the services received than those receiving agency workers (Schore, Foster, & Phillips, 2007). PD group members had fewer adverse health outcomes, expressed fewer unmet needs, and experienced reduced nursing facility usage than those in the agency-directed group (Carlson, Foster, Dale, & Brown, 2007; Dale & Brown, 2006). When faced with the option of hiring their caregivers of choice, more than half of the participants opted to hire relatives, including parents or spouses in some states. The participants' caregivers expressed less physical and financial stress and strain (Foster, Dale, & Brown, 2007). Despite policy makers' concerns about fraud and abuse, there were no major instances among the PD groups (Simon-Rusinowitz, Loughlin, Ruben, Garcia, & Mahoney, 2010). Initially, total Medicaid costs were higher among the PD group in each state and age group. These higher costs were largely related to the increased delivery of authorized care foregone in the agency group (Dale & Brown, 2007). However, the program has produced significant long-term savings in some cases. The Arkansas Cash and Counseling program saved $5.6 million over a

9-year period, excluding potential additional savings from reductions in nursing home use (Doty, Mahoney, & Sciegaj, 2010).

CASH AND COUNSELING REPLICATION

In 2004, given the evidence in support of Cash and Counseling, 12 additional states replicated the model. O'Keeffe (2009) conducted a process evaluation of the replication states, and examined states' experiences during planning, design, and implementation. She also captured state challenges, responses to challenges, and lessons learned.

During the planning and design stages, states found it was essential to differentiate between the traditional case manager role and the role of Cash and Counseling counselors. It was important to create distinct roles and ensure sufficient staffing to fulfill the duties of both roles. States also found designing financial management services (FMS) and obtaining FMS providers a challenge. Evaluation findings indicate that it was important to allocate sufficient time and resources to select the best FMS providers and obtain FMS technical assistance. Based on these challenges, the Cash and Counseling National Program Office developed FMS training programs and a national FMS conference (www.NRCPDS.org).

It was also challenging to design the individual budget component of the Cash and Counseling program, especially in light of pressures for cost neutrality relative to traditional services. States must consider the trade-off between the potentially higher short-term financial costs of Cash and Counseling relative to the potential for long-term savings and greater delivery of authorized services to beneficiaries (O'Keeffe, 2009). During the implementation stage, states agreed that it was beneficial to pilot or phase in their Cash and Counseling programs, then refine them before full implementation. It was also important to communicate sufficient information to all eligible and potentially eligible individuals to help them determine whether to enroll (O'Keeffe, 2009). Impact evaluation of the Cash and Counseling replication states indicate that total enrollment across participating states was 6,620 as of December 2008, significantly higher than the combined target enrollment of 4,786 as of September 2008.

CASH AND COUNSELING FOR VETERANS

In 2009, the Veterans Administration (VA) launched the Veteran-Directed Home and Community-Based Services Program (VD-HCBS). The program incorporates the Cash and Counseling design by providing veterans with a budget and the flexibility to purchase the goods and services that best meet their needs as well as the authority to hire and supervise workers (Robert Wood Johnson Foundation, 2013). As of October 2016, the VD-HCBS program has served more than 3,600 veterans across 35 states, the District of Columbia, and Puerto Rico. At the same time, 68 Veterans Affairs Medical Centers have partnered with Aging and Disability Network agencies, including state units on aging, Aging & Disability Resource Centers, area agencies on aging, and centers for independent living, to offer the program (www.acl.gov).

FUTURE OF PD CARE

Faced with a booming aging population and a caregiver workforce shortage, policy makers view PD long-term services and supports as a strategy to increase the direct-care labor force, reduce unmet needs, and address cultural-diversity issues in a cost-effective way (Infeld, 2004; Sciegaj et al, 2014; Simon-Rusinowitz, Loughlin, Ruben, Garcia, & Mahoney, 2010). The number of individuals in PD programs increased from approximately 486,000 in 2002 (Doty & Flanagan, 2002) to 815,000 in 2013 (NRCPDS, 2014). These programs have expanded to include individuals of all ages and various types of disabilities. Among PD programs targeting a single population, over half served either veterans (41%) or elders and adults with physical disabilities (18%) (Sciegaj et al., 2014). Every state now has at least one PD program, 44 states have an option that allows participants to direct their own budget, similar to Cash and Counseling (Mahoney, Doty, Simon-Rusinowitz, & Burness, 2016). In addition, states such as Massachusetts have enacted legislation that all people with developmental disabilities be offered self-directed budget options each time they are reassessed (Mahoney et al., 2016).

Continuing research seeks to understand additional populations that may benefit from PD programs, including the behavioral health population (i.e., mental health and substance use disorders). An environmental scan of self-direction in behavioral health, completed in February 2013, identified conditions that could facilitate or impede the development of PD programs for this population and found strong interest in self-direction. Among a sample of 50 directors of behavioral health program, 64% indicated that they were "very interested" in implementing a self-directed program (NRCPDS, 2013). Based on these findings, a multistate demonstration and evaluation of self-direction in behavioral health programs are underway. It will be completed in 2019 (Human Services Research Institute, 2017).

Amidst growth, there are some uncertainties. As findings from Cash and Counseling and subsequent work informed the Patient Protection and Affordable Care Act's (PPACA) emphasis on person-centered and participant-directed services, the future of the PPACA and potential replacement may impact the future of participant-directed services. Without further information about these impending steps, we must wait to determine the impact. The growth of managed long-term services and supports (MLTSS) also has the potential to influence the future of PD services.

Nevertheless, proliferation is forecast because Cash and Counseling is now being utilized by Australia's new National Disability Insurance Scheme. This program offers flexible budgets to all at the highest level of need (Mahoney et al., 2016). The appeal of PD services, including flexibility, potential for cost-effectiveness, and support for participant independence, seems likely to ensure continued expansion.

See also Autonomy.

Lori Simon-Rusinowitz,
Ronke E. Adawale, and Raphael Gaeta

Benjamin, A. E., & Snyder, R. E. (2003). Consumer choice in long-term care. In J. R. Knickman & S. L. Isaacs (Eds.), *Robert Wood Johnson Foundation anthology: To improve health and health care* (pp. 1–17). Princeton, NJ: Robert Wood Johnson Foundation.

Retrieved from http://www.rwjf.org/content/dam/farm/books/books/2002/rwjf37787

Carlson, B. L., Foster, L., Dale, S. B., & Brown, R. (2007). Effects of cash and counseling on personal care and well-being. *Health Services Research, 42*(1, Pt. 2), 467–487.

Dale, S., & Brown, R. (2006). Reducing nursing home use through consumer-directed personal care services. *Medical Care, 44,* 760–767. doi:10.1097/01.mlr.0000218849.32512.3f

Dale, S., & Brown, R. (2007). How does cash and counseling affect costs? *Health Research and Educational Trust, 42*(1), 488–509.

Doty, P., & Flanagan, S. (2002). *Highlights: Inventory of consumer-directed support programs.* Washington, DC: U.S. Department of Health and Human Services. Retrieved from https://aspe.hhs.gov/system/files/pdf/72981/highlght.pdf

Doty, P., Mahoney, K. J., & Sciegaj, M. (2010). New state strategies to meet long-term care needs. *Health Affairs, 29*(1), 49–56.

Foster, L., Dale, S., & Brown, R. (2007). How caregivers and workers fared in cash and counselling. *Health Services Research, 42,* 510–532. doi:10.1111/i.1457-6773.2006.00672.x

Human Services Research Institute. (2017). *Demonstration and evaluation of self-direction in behavioral health.* Cambridge, MA: Health Services.

Infeld, D. L. (2004). *States' experiences implementing consumer-directed home and community-based services: Results of the 2004 survey of the state administrators, opinion survey and telephone interviews.* Washington, DC: National Association of State Units on Aging and The National Council on Aging.

Mahoney, K. J., Doty, P., Simon-Rusinowitz., & Burness, A. (2016). Alchemy: Research turns into policy. *Public Policy and Aging Report, 26*(4), 129–133.

National Resource Center for Participant-Directed Services. (2013). *An environmental scan of self-direction in behavioral health: Summary of major findings.* Chestnut Hill, MA: Boston College, Graduate School of Social Work. Retrieved from http://web.bc.edu/libtools/details.php?entryid=392&page=2&topics=&types=&keyword=self%20direction

National Resource Center for Participant-Directed Services. (2014). *Facts and figures: 2013 national inventory survey on participant direction.* Chestnut Hill, MA: Boston College.

O'Keeffe, J. (2009). Implementing self-direction programs with flexible individual budgets: Lessons learned from the cash and counseling replications states. Retrieved from http://www.nasuad.org/sites/nasuad/files/hcbs/files/153/7636/CC_Replication_Report_final.pdf

Robert Wood Johnson Foundation. (2013). Cash and counseling. Retrieved from https://www.rwjf.org/en/library/research/2013/06/cash---counseling.html

Schore, J., Foster, L., & Phillips, B. (2007). Consumer enrollment and experiences in the Cash and Counseling Program. *Health Services Research* 42(1), 446–466.

Sciegaj, M., Mahoney, K. J., Schwartz, A., Simon-Rusinowitz, L., Selkow, I., & Loughlin, D. M. (2016). An inventory of publicly funded participant-directed long-term services and supports programs in the United States. *Journal of Disability Policy Studies*, 26(4), 245–251.

Simon-Rusinowitz, L., & Hofland, B. F. (1993). Adopting a disability approach to home-care services for older adults. *The Gerontologist*, 33(22), 159–167.

Simon-Rusinowitz, L., Loughlin, D. M., Ruben, K., Garcia, G. M., & Mahoney, K. J. (2010). The benefits of consumer-directed services for elders and their caregivers in the cash and counseling demonstration and evaluation. *Public Policy & Aging Report*, 20(1), 27–31. doi:10.1093/ppar/20.1.27

Simon-Rusinowitz, L., Loughlin, D. M., Ruben, K., & Mahoney, K. J. (2010). What does research tell us about a policy option to hire relatives as caregivers? *Public Policy & Aging Report*, 20(1), 32–37. doi:10.1093/ppar/20.1.32

Web Resources
Applied Self-Direction: http://www.appliedselfdirection.com

Clearinghouse for Community Living Exchange Collaboration: http://www.hcbs.org

National Association of States United for Aging and Disability: http://www.nasuad.org

National Resource Center for Participant-Directed Services: http://www.bc.edu/schools/gssw/nrcpds

Robert Wood Johnson Foundation: http://www.rwjf.org/en.html

U.S. Department of Health and Human Services, Office of the Assistant Secretary for Planning and Evaluation, Office of Disability, Aging, and Long-Term Care Policy: https://aspe.hhs.gov/office_specific/daltcp.cfm

U.S. Department of Veterans Affairs: http://www.va.gov/GERIATRICS/Guide/LongTermCare/Veteran-Directed_Care.asp

PATIENT–PROVIDER RELATIONSHIPS

A strong patient–provider relationship is based on open and clear communication between the patient and provider. Historically, a provider-centered model was primarily used; providers then were much more likely than today to make unilateral decisions. This former model of patient–provider relationships has been criticized as overly paternalistic and has been increasingly replaced by a more collaborative model in which patients are partners with their providers in a discussion that, ideally, combines evidence-based decision making with a more nuanced understanding of the patient's values and goals.

One of the central roles of the ongoing patient-provider relationship is the sharing of treatment decisions (Matthias, Salyers, & Frankel, 2013). The Informed Medical Decisions Foundation defines *shared decision making* as a collaborative process that allows patients and their providers to make health care decisions together, taking into account the best scientific evidence available, as well as the patient's values and preferences. Thus although the provider is no longer the sole source of health care information—increasingly the case in this era of unprecedented access to multiple streams of health information as well as misinformation—the provider's role in presenting objective advice and education necessary for making a truly informed decision remains critical.

At the center of shared decision making, especially among those who have chronic illnesses, is the patient–provider partnership. A partnered patient–provider relationship has been shown to increase patient satisfaction and treatment adherence, reduce the number of malpractice claims, and to lead to better treatment outcomes (Matthias et al., 2013). Shared decision making also emphasizes the importance of excellent communication and providing support for patients (Elwyn et al., 2012) which is part of any healthy relationship.

Connectedness is an essential component of meaningful relationships and patient–provider connectedness is thought to positively affect patient health outcomes (Phillips-Salimi, Haase, & Kooken, 2012). Attributes of connectedness include caring, empathy, trust, and reciprocity (Phillips-Salimi et al., 2012) which are important for rapport and trust building and enable patients and providers to communicate effectively and be partners in health care decisions.

Decisions made in the patient–provider relationship are influenced by more than simply the cognition of the patient and provider. Affect, intuition, and interpersonal relationships are just as important as cognitive reasoning. These concepts are described by Epstein (2013) as "shared mind" and embody the idea that we are not simply rational beings living in a vacuum but that our emotional attunement to the world around us influences our decisions. This indeed suggests a deeper understanding of shared decision making in the patient–provider relationship. In fact, the emotional attunement of the provider to the patient creates an environment of trust and connectedness, facilitating a therapeutic alliance which enhances the shared decision-making process.

SHARED DECISION MAKING

The patient–provider relationship has special relevance in the health care of older adults for several reasons. First, older people frequently face multiple health challenges, leading to increases in health care encounters and decisions. Second, the process of aging potentially involves functional impairment and cognitive decline that can complicate communication between the patient and provider. Third, health care decisions involving older patients often involve the perspective and input of third parties such as friends and family. Finally, health care problems generally increase in complexity and severity with age, requiring explicit discussion of end-of-life issues.

Older age has been predictive of a passive decision-making style (Lechner et al., 2016). However, sociodemographic factors likely explain only part of the variability. Other factors should be considered in understanding reasons for some patients' limited interest in shared decision making. For instance, cohort

effects of higher levels of deference to authority figures may explain part of the lower interest level in participatory decision making among older adults. Other factors may be age related, such as severity or complexity of illness and current quality of life. Although older patients appear to differ in the degree of interest in shared decision making, almost all continue to value open discussion of treatment options and personal values. Moreover, despite the varying level of patient interest in actively participating in decision making, it is incumbent on providers to consider patients' values and preferences in the context of treatment goals—information ideally obtained through the patient–provider relationship.

Cognition and Shared Decision Making

Increased age is a risk factor for cognitive impairment, which in turn may affect the abilities necessary for adequate decision-making capacity. On the other hand, mild cognitive deficits do not always imply impaired decision-making capacity. Thus many patients who have cognitive deficits are able to participate at some level in the shared decision-making process. Increasingly, it is recognized that decisional capacity can be optimized or enhanced through techniques as simple as repetition and checks for understanding. With more complex decisions, special care should be taken to explain concepts carefully, assess for understanding, and involve support systems such as family or caregivers. Even when patients lack the capacity to participate in some decisions, they may continue to possess the capacity to participate in decisions dealing with less complex issues and to express basic values and preferences.

Role of Third Parties

Although the Western model of patient care emphasizes autonomous decision making by the individual, patient care rarely occurs in a vacuum of a single individual acting independently. Older patients often rely on family members, friends, or caregivers for support in medical decision making. As persons presumably familiar with an individual's interests and values, third parties often serve as sources of information that can complement information from the patient. The dilemma for the provider is in balancing the strengths supplied by the additional perspectives of those involved in a patient's social system against the potential for conflict with multiple parties whose interests and values may differ from the patient's and provider's. The extent to which surrogate decision makers' choices accurately reflect the wishes or preferences of the patient remains in question (Combs, Rasinski, Yoon, & Curlin, 2013). In extreme cases such as emergent end-of-life care or cognitive impairment, in which the direct input of the patient may be unavailable, providers should help families reflect on the values and preferences of the patient. The provider can then discuss the family's values in the context of the patient's personal values and assist in reaching a consensus on goals. The final decisions should be the result of collaboration, not the victory of one party's viewpoint over that of others'.

End-of-Life Decision Making

The majority of aging patients are confronted at some point by important end-of-life decisions. Although serious illnesses bring these decisions into stark relief, the issues raised—such as defining desired treatment outcomes and developing advance care plans—are certainly not unique to those approaching the end of their life.

In developmental terminology, the key task of the last stage of life is to integrate one's life viewpoint and experience with the realization of personal mortality. This developmental process is facilitated by patient–provider communication that is open to discussion of mortality and end-of-life issues, preferences, and goals. Patients, families, and even providers, are often unable to accept the terminal nature of an illness. Discussion of patients' preferences regarding end-of-life care may be postponed until the final stages of a disease. Patients may conceal their distress and concerns, patients and families may remain optimistic despite medical futility, and there may be cultural prohibitions against open discussions of end-of-life issues. A frank discussion with the provider, beginning at the time of initial diagnosis, is necessary, so that patients and families can adequately prepare for these difficult matters. The provider has a duty to take an active role in leading these discussions which, above all, require a patient-centered shared decision-making model (Billings & Krakauer, 2011).

Barriers to implementation of this model of end-of-life decision making include time constraints, leading to discussion mainly of immediate clinical concerns with limited attention devoted to discussion of patient preferences, family members' concerns, and other aspects of end-of-life care. Moreover, it is often difficult to identify the locus of responsibility for conducting end-of-life discussions because multiple disciplines, specialties, and sites are commonly involved in the care of the terminally ill (Billings & Krakauer, 2011). Ideally, a multidisciplinary approach should be taken to end-of-life issues, integrating not only medical, but also cultural, familial, social, psychological, and spiritual perspectives.

CONCLUSION

A successful patient–provider relationship is a connected partnership with the patient and family members that allows for open discussion of the patient's values and treatment goals. The aging patient population faces increasingly complex choices requiring a patient–provider relationship that is collaborative. An empathic, emotionally attuned provider, who takes time to build rapport and trust, will more successfully allow for shared decision making that supports and honors patient's preferences.

See also Advance Directives; Autonomy; Competency and Capacity.

Lara Wahlberg and Nicholas Sollom

Billings, J. A., & Krakauer, E. L. (2011). On patient autonomy and physician responsibility in end-of-life care. *Archives of Internal Medicine, 171*(9), 849–853.

Combs, M. P., Rasinski, K. A., Yoon, J. D., & Curlin, F. A. (2013). Substituted judgment in principle and practice: A national physician survey. *Mayo Clinic Proceedings, 88*(7), 666–673.

P

P

Elwyn, G., Frosch, D., Thomson, R., Joseph-Williams, N., Lloyd, A., Kinnersley, P., ... Barry, M. (2012). Shared decision making: A model for clinical practice. *Journal of General Internal Medicine, 27*(10), 1361–1367.

Epstein, R. M. (2013). Whole mind and shared mind in clinical decision-making. *Patient Education and Counseling, 90*(2), 200–206. doi:10.1016/j.pec.2012.06.035

Lechner, S., Herzog, W., Boehlen, F., Maatouk, I., Saum, K., Brenner, H., ... Wild, B. (2016). Control preferences in treatment decisions among older adults—Results of a large population-based study. *Journal of Psychosomatic Research, 86*, 28–33. doi:10.1016/j.jpsychores.2016.05.004

Matthias, M., Salyers, M., & Frankel, R. (2013). Rethinking shared decision-making: Context matters. *Patient Education and Counseling, 91*(2), 176–179. doi:10.1016/j.pec.2013.01.006

Phillips-Salimi, C. R., Haase, J. E., & Kooken, W. C. (2012). Connectedness in the context of patient–provider relationships: A concept analysis. *Journal of Advanced Nursing, 68*, 230–245. doi:10.1111/j.1365-2648.2011.05763.x

Web Resources

American Medical Association: Code of Medical Ethics. Ch. 1—Opinions on patient–physician relationships: http://www.ama-assn.org/ama/pub/physician-resources/medical-ethics/code-medical-ethics.page

Informed Medical Decisions Foundation: http://www.informedmedicaldecisions.org/

National Institute on Aging: End of life: Helping with comfort and care—Care options at the end of life: https://www.nia.nih.gov/health/publication/end-life-helping-comfort-and-care/care-options-end-life

Office of Veteran Affairs: Geriatrics and extended care: Shared decision making overview: http://www.va.gov/GERIATRICS/Guide/LongTermCare/Shared_Decision_Making.asp

Patient Decision Aids: The Ottawa Hospital Research Institute: https://decisionaid.ohri.ca

Society for Medical Decision Making: http://www.smdm.org

PATIENT SAFETY

Patient safety and quality of care have received global recognition in the delivery of health care. Services that provide unsafe and poor quality health care lead to subpar outcomes and harm to patients. Concerns about the safety of American health care were described in 2000, when the Institute of Medicine (IOM) published the landmark report, *To Err is Human* in 1999. This report provided data about the safety of our health care system and is the roadmap for rapid improvements in quality and safety for patients. The IOM estimates that 98,000 patients die every year as a result of preventable medical errors, which costs $29 billion annually. The IOM executive summary states, "More people die in a given year as a result of medical errors than from motor vehicle accident, breast cancer or AIDS" (Kohn, Corrigan, & Donaldson, 2000, p. 1).

DEFINITIONS

There are multiple definitions of *patient safety*. The IOM defines it as "freedom from accidental injury; ensuring patient safety involves the establishment of operational systems and processes that minimize the likelihood of errors and maximizes the likelihood of intercepting them when they occur" (Kohn, Corrigan, & Donaldson, 2000, p. 211), whereas the WHO defines it as "the prevention of errors and adverse effects to patients associated with health care" (WHO, 2016). Emanuel et al. (2008) define patient safety as "a discipline in the health care professions that applies safety science methods toward the goal of achieving a trustworthy system of health care delivery" ("Abstract"). The National Patient Safety Foundation (NPSF) definition includes, "the prevention of healthcare errors, and the elimination or mitigation of patient injury caused by healthcare errors" (NPSF, n.d.). The NPSF believes that unintended health care outcomes can be caused by errors of commission, omission, or execution.

HISTORY

The tenet of any health care profession is to provide safe, quality, and culturally sensitive person-centered care. Specifically, the Hippocratic Oath for physicians and the Nightingale Pledge for nurses both include a version of "do no harm." Vowing to do no harm and aligning practice with any of the patient safety definitions are well intended. Outcomes must supersede intentions. Therefore focus must adapt to a new measurement.

In 1998, the IOM created the Committee of Quality of Healthcare in America. The committee developed a four-tiered approach to improving safety in health care. The areas included are creating leadership and protocols, identifying and learning from errors, raising standards, and creating safety systems (Kohn, Corrigan, & Donaldson, 2000). The first recommendation from this committee included the establishment of a Center for Patient Safety within AHRQ to set national patient safety goals and to set a research platform to identify, evaluate, prevent, and fund dissemination and communication activities that improve patient safety.

The IOM release of *To Err is Human* set forth the roadmap for improving patient safety through recommendations for the design of safer health care systems (IOM, 2000). Rather than point the blame at professionals who make honest mistakes, the report encourages open reporting and root cause analysis to prevent similar events in the future. Historically, medical errors were discussed behind closed doors and typically laid the blame for medical error on the health care provider. This is the time where less punitive and more preventive objectives to problem solving began. The IOM report suggested that systems must be and can be improved if safety processes are designed into processes of care (IOM, 2000). This shift is much like the shift from infection control to infection prevention.

Standards for health care professionals are set through national and state accrediting and credentialing programs. Before the IOM report, legislation instituted many organizations to develop and monitor standards to keep the public safe. The U.S. Food and Drug Administration (FDA), whose role is to protect and promote citizens health, can be traced back to 1846. In 1970, the Occupational Safety and Health Act was enacted to define safety and health standards. Many of the organizations whose job it is to keep patients safe have lacked focus on patient safety issues. For example, the FDA can approve a new

drug or innovative technology with strict standards on design and production but fails to standardize the products' safe use. The Health Care Financing Administration (HCFA) that is now known as the Centers for Medicare & Medicaid Services (CMS) enacted the Health Insurance Portability and Accountability Act (HIPAA) in 1996 to protect the privacy of individually identifiable health information. HIPAA set national standards for protecting health information and confidentiality provisions for patients. Congress created the Occupational Safety and Health Administration (OSHA) in 1970 to ensure safe and healthful working conditions for men and women and to enforce safety standards. Despite the plethora of committees, the government provided and enacted standards for safety; many have virtually lacked a focus on patient safety and provide no incentives for organizations to want to improve quality until recently.

SYSTEM QUALITY REPORTING

Health care reform efforts to improve quality and safety are now structured with financial incentives for organizations that meet standard quality and safety standards. There are many examples of quality initiatives that aim to reward hospitals for quality care. The Patient Protection and Affordable Care Act (PPACA) mandated the Value-Based Purchasing Incentive. This mandate includes processes of care and mortality outcome measures on which to base future payments and includes patient experience scores. The CMS Premier Hospital Quality Incentive Demonstration project was designed to determine whether financial incentives were effective in improving the quality of inpatient care. Hospital quality incentive payments were based on six clinical conditions. Hospital's volunteered to be included in the project and publicly shared their quality outcomes through 2003 to 2009. This project was successful in improving quality within each clinical area by 18.6% over the project's 6 years (Ryan, 2009). In 2008, CMS announced that it will no longer pay for eight complications it deems are preventable (Downey, Boussard, Banka, & Morton, 2012). Patient safety indicators (PSIs), established by the Agency for Healthcare Research and Quality

P

(AHRQ) to assist in monitoring potentially preventable events for patients treated in hospitals, are another example of a hospital being penalized for what AHRQ deems as preventable events. The indicators are measures that screen for potentially adverse events to hospitalized patients that are likely preventable by changes in system design or provider level (Downey et al., 2012).

Each year, patient safety issues are published and noted. In 2016, Barnet, Green, and Punke published the top-10 patient safety issues: (a) medication errors, (b) diagnostic errors, (c) discharged practice to post-acute, home care, (d) workplace safety, (e) hospital facility safcty, (f) reprocessing issues, (g) sepsis, (h) health care–acquired infections (HAIs), (i) cyber insecurity of medical devices, and (j) transparency with quality data.

NURSES' ROLE

Nurses partner with physicians and other key health care professionals in delivering safe care to patients Moreover, nurses play a critical role in patient safety (AHRQ, 2016). Nurses' assessment and critical thinking skills enable early identification and prevention of harm to patients (Kim, Lyder, McNeese-Smith, Leach, & Needleman, 2015). Nurse-sensitive indicators are markers of quality nursing care such as preventing falls and pressure injuries. The nurses' working environments include nursing skill mix, care hours, the quality of the practice environment (staffing ratios, respect of others), and turnover.

Nurses' abilities to integrate and coordinate care delivered by other health professionals across multiple systems provide quality safe care to the patients (Hughes, 2008).

SUMMARY

Patient safety is considered the biggest challenge in health care. Patients trust the health care system and expect that they will be safe when seeking care. Providing a safe environment for patients requires systems thinking, a safe reporting culture, process change, and national political awareness. Value is based on quality patient outcomes and is tied to financial incentives. Health care institution must be able to integrate the patient experience with quality and safety measures to thrive financially in the current state.

Nurses' role is key to patient safety. Further research and measurements for patient safety are needed. Policy and financial system alignment is important to achieving improvements in quality and safety.

See also Injury and Trauma.

Mimi Lim

Agency for Healthcare Research and Quality. (2016). Patient safety primers. AHRQ Patient Safety Network. Retrieved from https://psnet.ahrq.gov/primers

Barnet, S., Green, M., & Punke, H. (2016). 10 top patient safety issues for 2016. *Becker's Clinical Leadership & Infection Control.* Retrieved from https://www.beckershospitalreview.com/quality/10-top-patient-safety-issues-for-2016.html

Downey, J. R., Boussard, T. H., Banka, G., & Morton, J. M. (2012). Is patient safety improving? National trends in patient safety indicators. *Health Science Research, 47*(1 Pt. 2), 414–430.

Emanuel, L., Berwick, D., Conway, J., Combes, J., Hatlie, M., Leape, L., … Walton, M. (2008). What exactly is patient safety: A definition and conceptual framework. In K. Henriksen, J. B. Battles, M. A. Keyes, & M. L. Grady (Eds.), *Advances in patient safety: New directions and alternative approaches* (Vol. 1). Rockville, MD: Agency for HealthCare Quality and Research, Advances in Patient Safety. Retrieved from https://www.ncbi.nlm.nih.gov/books/NBK43629

Hughes, R. (2008). Patient safety and quality: An evidence-based handbook for nurses. Retrieved from https://archive.ahrq.gov/professionals/clinicians-providers/resources/nursing/resources/nurseshdbk/nurseshdbk.pdf

Kim, L., Lyder, C. H., McNeese-Smith, D., Leach, L. S., & Needleman, J. (2015). Defining attributes of patient safety through a concept analysis. *Journal of Advanced Nursing, 71*(11), 2490–2503. doi:10.1111/jan.12715

Kohn, L. T., Corrigan, J. M., & Donaldson, M. (Eds.). (2000). *To err is human: Building a safer health system.* Washington, DC: National Academies Press. Retrieved from https://www.ncbi.nlm.nih.gov/books/NBK225179

National Patient Safety Foundation. (n.d.). Patient safety dictionary. Retrieved from http://www.npsf.org/?page=dictionaryae

Ryan, A. M. (2009). Effects of the premier hospital quality incentive demonstration on Medicare patient mortality and cost. *Health Services Research, 44*(3), 821–842. doi:10.1111/j.1475-6773.2009.00956.x

World Health Organization. (2016). Patient safety. Retrieved from http://www.who.int/patientsafety/about/en

Web Resources

Agency for Healthcare Research and Quality (AHRQ): https://www.ahrq.gov

Association of Perioperative Registered Nurses: https://www .aorn.org

Centers for Disease Control and Prevention (CDC): https://www.cdc.gov

Centers for Medicare & Medicaid Services: https://www.cms.gov

Hospital Compare: https://www.medicare.gov/hospital compare/search.html

Institute for Healthcare Improvement (IHI): http://www.ihi.org/Pages/default.aspx

Institute for Safe Medication Practice (ISMP): http://www .ismp.org

Institute of Medicine (IOM): http://www.national academies.org/HMD

National Database of Nursing Quality Indicators (NDNQI): http://www.pressganey.com/solutions/clinical-quality/nursing-quality

National Patient Safety Foundation (NPSF): http://www.npsf.org

National Quality Forum: http://www.qualityforum.org/Home.aspx

The Joint Commission (TJC): https://www.jointcommission.org

WHO: http://www.who.int

PENSIONS AND FINANCING RETIREMENT

Nearly all workers hope to retire, but nearly all face the challenge of a financially secure retirement. Throughout the 20th century, retirement was financed through a combination of government retirement programs and employer pensions. Recently, the mix has changed to include personal savings and continued work in retirement.

Most Americans are neither saving enough for retirement nor investing saved funds the right way. To increase the chances of financial security in retirement, the prescription is simple. First, starting at age 25 years or earlier, an employee and employer should put 15% to 20% of an employee's gross income every year into a retirement fund. Second, that money should be invested in a diversified portfolio of stocks and bonds. Third, on retirement, no more than 5% of the current market value of retirement savings should be withdrawn in any year. Although simple, it is hard to maintain the discipline needed, and thus Munnell, Hou, and Webb (2014) report that more than half of workers are at risk of a falling standard of living in retirement.

SOME DEMOGRAPHIC TRENDS

People are living longer and retiring earlier, a bad combination for those concerned about retirement financing. Most Americans now retire between the ages of 65 and 67 years and live into their 80s. This means that nearly a third of adult life must be financed by lifetime savings and pensions.

In nearly all developed countries, there will be a significant increase in those older than 65 years of age relative to the size of the working population, primarily caused by declining birth rates and increased life spans. This implies that public pension systems will be under enormous pressure in the next 20 years to either raise taxes on workers to pay current retirement benefits, to decrease promised benefits, or both. In part, this uncertainty about future benefits has put further importance on supplemental ways to finance retirement.

SOURCES OF FUNDS FOR FINANCING RETIREMENT

Traditionally, retirement income consisted of what is sometimes called the *three-legged stool* of income from government retirement programs, employer pensions, and accumulated savings. Increasingly a fourth "leg" has emerged with increased reliance on earned income. Each "leg" has been under stress in recent years—each for different reasons.

Government retirement programs, such as the U.S. Social Security program, have been around since the 1930s. They are generally funded through taxes on worker earnings. Retirement benefits are then paid out of these tax receipts to qualified recipients. Benefits are based on lifetime earnings but, on average, the U.S. Social Security system attempts to replace about 40% of preretirement earnings. During the 20th century, this was the bedrock of retirement income, greatly reducing poverty rates of the elderly.

Although historically the U.S. Social Security system has run a surplus, there are strong demographic pressures on the solvency of the program. Citing reductions in birth rates and increased longevity, the Social Security Trustees (Board of Trustees, 2016) estimate that by 2034 the accumulated savings in the Social Security Trust Fund will be exhausted, meaning that Social Security tax revenues will cover only 79% of promised benefits. There are no painless solutions to the problem (e.g., the Center for Retirement Research's *Social Security Fix-it Book*, last updated in 2014), since it will only be achieved by a tax increase, a benefit reduction, or both. All paths, however, will result in lower income.

The second source of retirement funds is employer pensions. There are two main types of pensions. Defined benefit (DB) pensions, the traditional pension of the 20th century, involve promises by employers to fund an annuity, which is generally dependent on years of service at the firm and final salary. These pensions benefit from economies of scale in investing by the firm but do place the risk of funding retirement benefits on employers and are not portable if a worker is separated from the firm. The second type of pension, which became much more popular in the late 20th century, is the defined contribution (DC) pension (like the popular 401[k] plan). In these types of pensions, employees designate part of earnings to a tax-sheltered account, sometimes with additional monies added by the employer. Employees have the responsibility to invest wisely to generate money available during retirement. Although these types of pensions allow for more flexibility

in investing and portability, they shift the risk of adequate funding and smart investing to the worker.

The third source is accumulated savings to fill in gaps between income from government and employer pensions and a target standard of living in retirement. Unfortunately, research shows that there are significant shortfalls in savings among the near retired (Munnell et al., 2014), even with tax-favorable savings instruments like IRAs.

One of the largest recent changes is the increase in earned income in retirement. Obviously, this is limited by health and other constraints, but with the uncertainty in public and private pensions and the low level of accumulated savings, income from employment can be useful in accumulating more resources and/or a reduced reliance on other income sources for some retirement years. Experts expect postretirement employment to become increasingly important in the future.

In sum, research such as Munnell, Webb, and Golub-Sass (2011) suggests that retirees need about 80% of preretirement income, meaning that an average worker should save about 18% of yearly earnings above what is paid to Social Security. This 18% is a mixture of employer pensions and/or personal savings, so it falls on individuals to manage this portfolio of retirement funds.

MANAGING RETIREMENT FUNDS

With increased reliance on accumulated savings and the shift from employer-funded DB to self-directed DC pensions, people are increasingly trying to manage complex financial instruments. In an ideal world, managing a retirement portfolio is a job for financial professionals because most individuals have little experience or training in portfolio management. Regardless of who manages the money, workers should make a couple of key selections for investment instruments that do not have to be changed very often and should audit any professional advice that they get. That audit should see that funds are at least tracking the total return of an appropriate market index (such as the S&P 500 Index) over a

3- to 5-year period. The audit should also make sure all the costs are reasonable. Some mutual funds provide total management for under 0.60% of the value of the funds managed (particularly if they are linked to market indices). Any arrangement that costs more than a yearly fee of 1.5% should be closely scrutinized.

There is nothing more important than having a diversified portfolio, which means owning a mixture of bonds and stocks, including domestic and international stocks and stocks from firms of all sizes. It is unwise to (a) invest more than 5% of any retirement portfolio in the stock of the employer; (b) invest substantial funds in CDs or money market funds unless retirement is just a few years away; and (c) invest in high-risk financial instruments (e.g., hedge funds, option funds, currencies, and commodity funds). Professionals can provide advice on how much to put in stocks versus bonds, but a common rule of thumb is to have greater exposure to stocks early in the career and less exposure when approaching retirement. Major mutual fund organizations now offer target-date, retirement-type portfolios. For example, an individual who expects to retire in 2035 may have a mixture of 70% stocks and 30% bonds for the first 5 years, then switch to 65% stocks and 35% bonds for the next 5 years. The mix can be changed every few years until it is 30% stocks and 70% bonds just before retirement.

To encourage personal saving for retirement, the federal government has created a variety of incentive programs that offer tax breaks to the participants. Some of these programs (e.g., Keogh plans for small businesses or individual retirement accounts [IRAs]) are designed to benefit those who do not have employer retirement savings programs and permit pretax deductions from earnings for funding the program. Other types of IRAs are available to employees who want to make after-tax contributions to fund their retirement. All types have some degree of tax incentives. However, even if there were no tax benefits offered, it is important to increase personal saving for future retirement needs. As Munnell et al. (2011) show, regular savings, starting as early as possible and working as long as possible, are much more effective in generating a secure retirement than chasing higher returns.

Financing retirement is an important part of family budgeting. It is not something that can be put off until a few years before retirement, but rather, it is something that needs to start early in one's career. In the 21st century, financing retirement is not a task that can be fully left to others (be it the government or employers) to do. Just as people pay their utility bills every month, so too they must pay their "retirement account bill" every month to have a well-financed retirement.

Keith A. Bender

Board of Trustees. (2016). *The 2016 annual report of the Board of Trustees of the federal old-age and survivors insurance and federal disability insurance trust funds*. Washington, DC: U.S. Social Security Administration. Retrieved from https://www.ssa.gov/oact/tr/2016/index.html

Center for Retirement Research. (2014). *The Social Security fix-it book*. Newton, MA: Boston College. Retrieved from http://crr.bc.edu/special-projects/books/the-social-security-fix-it-book

Munnell, A. H., Hou, W., & Webb, A. (2014). *NRRI update shows half still falling short* [Issue-In-Brief No. 14-20]. Newton, MA: Boston College Center for Retirement Research. Retrieved from http://crr.bc.edu/briefs/nrri-update-shows-half-still-falling-short

Munnell, A. H., Webb, A., & Golub-Sass, F. N. (2011). *How much to save for a secure retirement* [Issue-In-Brief No. 11–13]. Newton, MA: Boston College, Center for Retirement Research. Retrieved from http://crr.bc.edu/briefs/how-much-to-save-for-a-secure-retirement

Web Resources

AARP: http://www.aarp.org

Board of Trustees, Social Security Administration: http://www.ssa.gov/oact/tr

Center for Retirement Research, Boston College: http://crr.bc.edu

Forbes: http://www.forbes.com

Money: http://www.money.cnn.com

Pension Research Council, University of Pennsylvania: http://www.pensionresearchcouncil.org

TIAA-CREF Institute: http://www.tiaa-crefinstitute.org/institute/index.html

PERIPHERAL ARTERIAL DISEASE

P

PREVALENCE AND RISK

Atherosclerosis is the most frequent cause of chronic peripheral arterial occlusive disease (PAD). This disease process involves both large and small arteries. By definition, PAD includes the carotid, renal, and gastric arteries. This discussion focuses on disease of the lower extremities.

It is estimated that approximately 8 million people in the United States are affected by PAD. The prevalence of PAD rises sharply with age and affects 12% to 20% of individuals older than 60 years. For more symptomatic, severe PAD, the prevalence is higher in men than in women and disproportionately affects more Blacks (Allison et al., 2007).

The risk factors for PAD are the same as those for coronary and cerebrovascular disease: cigarette smoking, diabetes, hypertension, hyperlipidemia, and obesity (Criqui & Aboyans, 2015). Other risk factors include, black ethnicity, decreased renal function, increased levels of fibrinogen, C-reactive protein, and homocysteine. The implications of these findings are obvious, especially because many of the events result in long-term, often devastating, disability.

HISTORY AND CLINICAL MANIFESTATIONS

Symptoms of lower-extremity arterial insufficiency are local manifestations of a generalized disease process. Intermittent claudication, one of the most characteristic symptoms of PAD, is usually described by patients as exercise-induced pain in the lower extremity (i.e., calf, thigh, or buttock) or as profound fatigue that is quickly relieved by rest. Symptoms appear distal to the site of occlusive lesions. Often, symptoms of claudication can be confused with those of spinal stenosis. Classically, the pain of spinal stenosis is relieved with bending forward, not by rest alone. Ischemic rest pain develops when the blood supply is severely compromised and is inadequate even at rest. Patients may describe burning or pain that is exacerbated by elevation of lower extremities and relieved by slow walking or by keeping the foot in a dependent position. The differential diagnosis of PAD includes peripheral neuropathy, spinal nerve-root compression, venous claudication, chronic compartment syndrome, and inflammatory arthritis of the knees, feet, hip, and back. Determining the actual cause of lower-extremity pain can be difficult, but the American College of Cardiology/American Heart Association (ACC/AHA) guidelines for the diagnosis of PAD outline specific maneuvers and characteristics of each (Hirsch et al., 2006).

Physical examination of the lower extremities should include careful inspection of both legs, checking for discoloration, shiny appearance, alopecia, nail or skin atrophy, dependent rubor, and ulceration. The clinician should palpate the femoral, posterior tibial, and dorsalis pedis arteries and auscultate the femoral arteries for bruits. The dorsalis pedis pulse is absent in 5% to 8% of normal subjects, but the posterior tibialis pulse should be present (both are absent in only 0.5% of patients). As disease advances, mottling in a fishnet pattern can occur. The feet become cold and ulcers heal poorly. The classic 5 Ps can be kept in mind when critical limb ischemia occurs: pain, pallor, pulselessness, paresthesia, and paralysis. Gangrene occurs when arterial flow is inadequate to maintain viability of the tissues.

SCREENING

The U.S. Preventive Services Task Force (USPSTF) does not recommend screening with ankle-brachial index (ABI) for asymptomatic adults with no known diagnosis of cardiovascular disease (CVD) or diabetes, concluding that there is insufficient evidence to "determine the balance of benefits and harms of screening for PAD with ABI to prevent future CVD outcomes" (Moyer & USPSTF, 2013, p. 348). However, the ACC/AHA recommends screening with resting ABI for detection of PAD in adults who are at increased risk: adults aged 65 years or older, adults aged 50 years or older with a history of diabetes or smoking, and adults younger than

50 years with diabetes and an additional CVD risk factor (Anderson et al., 2013). As of 2017, Medicare covers a one-time screening ultrasound for abdominal aortic aneurysm for beneficiaries who have a family history of aortic aneurysm or who are men between ages 65 and 75 years and have smoked 100 cigarettes.

DIAGNOSTIC TESTING

An absence or decrease in the force of the pedal pulses is an indication for obtaining a resting ABI, a simple method of identifying the degree of vascular insufficiency. Normally, distal blood pressures are higher than brachial blood pressures. Normal ABI noncompressible values are 1.00 to 1.40, borderline are 0.91 to 0.99, and abnormal are 0.90 or less (Anderson et al., 2013). In diabetic patients and those with end-stage renal disease, the ABI can be falsely elevated because of tibial artery calcification. Ischemic wounds and ankle surgery may interfere with pressure measurements.

Another useful test in assessing PAD with ABI measurement is segmental limb pressures, which are obtained by placing cuffs at different levels on the lower extremities. A discrepancy of 20 to 30 mmHg between extremities is indicative of occlusion proximal to the cuff in the extremity with decreased pressure. A decrease in pressure of more than 20 mmHg in two consecutive levels in the same extremity suggests a disease process at the level proximal to the cuff (Gerhard-Herman et al., 2006).

Pulse-volume recordings are another qualitative test for identifying occlusive lesions. These are plethysmographic tracings that demonstrate changes in blood flow through a lower extremity. Attenuation of the waveform (which is normally a rapid systemic upstroke) is indicative of PAD. This test may not be accurate in distal segments or in patients with low cardiac output. Other tests include toe systolic pressure measurements, duplex ultrasonography, and transcutaneous oximetry.

Patients referred to vascular laboratories for "noninvasive studies" have ABI, segmental pressures, and pulse-volume recordings performed. Other studies must be specified by name. Treadmill exercise testing with or without

ABIs is also a helpful tool for differentiating claudication from pseudoclaudication (i.e., spinal stenosis) and to following progression of symptoms.

Angiography is an invasive method that outlines the vessel diameter and thus identifies the level and anatomy of the occlusion. Angiography is necessary if the clinician is contemplating surgery or interventional radiographic procedures. Risks of the procedure include allergic reaction to the contrast material, renal failure (especially in the setting of diabetes), and damage to the arteries or limb.

CT and MR angiography (MRA), noninvasive techniques, can assist in the diagnosis of advanced disease, especially when surgery or intervention is being contemplated. MRA may be particularly useful for selecting patients for surgical revascularization and should be performed with gadolinium. CT angiography is widely available, but uses vascular contrast and may expose the patient to a significant contrast load and radiation, specifically considering that many have renal disease and diabetes. If revascularization is considered, conventional arteriography should be undertaken concomitantly (Anderson et al., 2013). Providers should become familiar with the capabilities of the cardiovascular and interventional radiology experts at their site of practice.

TREATMENT

Exercise, together with smoking cessation, remains the most important conservative therapy for intermittent claudication. In fact, the 2013 ACC/AHA update recommends all patients with PAD to stop smoking and to have behavioral and pharmacological treatment (varenicline, bupropion, nicotine-replacement therapy). Supervised exercise programs should last 30 to 45 minutes at least 3 times a week for a minimum of 12 weeks. Aggressive treatment of all cardiovascular risks is indicated, including blood pressure control (goal of 140/90 mmHg for those without diabetes and less than 130/80 mmHg for those with diabetes and chronic renal disease), management of diabetes (A1c goal of less than 7.0), and strict lipid lowering with the use of a statin (low-density lipoprotein

[LDL] lowered to less than 100 mg/dL for all patients with PAD and to less than 70 mg/dL for PAD patients who are at very high risk of ischemic events). The use of angiotensin-converting enzyme (ACE) inhibitors should be considered for overall cardiovascular risk, especially in patients with diabetes (Anderson et al., 2013).

Aspirin (daily doses of 75–325 mg) or clopidogrel (75 mg/day), as an alternative antiplatelet therapy to aspirin, are also recommended to decrease the risk of myocardial infarction (MI), stroke, and vascular death in patients with symptomatic lower-extremity PAD, including those with claudication, prior lower-extremity revascularization, or prior amputation for lower-extremity ischemia. A combination of aspirin and clopidogrel may be considered for some patients with symptomatic atherosclerotic lower-extremity PAD (including those with intermittent claudication or critical limb ischemia, in those before endovascular or surgical revascularization, or in those before amputation for lower-extremity ischemia), and for those who are not at increased risk of bleeding but are considered at high cardiovascular risk (Anderson et al., 2013).

Cilostazol (100 mg by mouth twice a day), a phosphodiesterase inhibitor that inhibits platelet aggregation and acts as a vasodilator, can increase walking distance, improve subjective quality of life, and improve ABIs (Beebe et al., 1999). Cilostazol is contraindicated in patients with congestive heart failure because of the risk of cardiac arrhythmia and hypotension. Pentoxifylline (400 mg by mouth three times a day) reduces blood viscosity and improves red blood cell deformability. It is approved for the treatment of intermittent claudication, but its overall efficacy is questionable. The 2013 ACC/AHA guidelines suggest consideration of pentoxifylline as a second-line therapy to cilostazol for intermittent claudication because its clinical effectiveness is not well established.

Invasive modalities include percutaneous transluminal angioplasty, placement of intraluminal stents, bypass surgery, and amputation. These remain the major options for patients whose claudication symptoms significantly interfere with their work and lifestyle activities despite exercise and drug therapy and who have a reasonable likelihood of symptomatic improvement through surgery. Surgery is not used as a prevention method for limb-threatening ischemia in patients with intermittent claudication.

Angioplasty has a good long-term patency rate in the common iliac artery and is further improved by the use of vascular stents: 86% patency at 1 year and 74% at 4 years (Hirsch et al., 2006). Patency rates are poorer in the superficial femoral artery, particularly with longer lesions, femoropopliteal patency reaching only 62% at 1 year. In most reported series, the use of intravascular stents below the inguinal ligament has not added significantly to long-term patency. Research is focusing on methods to prevent restenosis, including evaluation of the long-term effectiveness of coated stents, atherectomy, thermal devices, and cutting balloons.

CLINICAL IMPLICATIONS

Arteriosclerosis of limb arteries is associated with coronary and cerebral atherosclerosis. Diagnosis of PAD should help identify patients who are at increased risk of cardiovascular events such as stroke and MI. Most patients with peripheral arterial disease die of acute cardiac events or stroke. Atherosclerotic disease of the lower extremities causes pain and can lead to limb loss. Early identification and careful interventions may improve outcomes and quality of life.

Chin Hwa (Gina) Dahlem and Chin Suk Yi

Allison, M. A., Ho, E., Denenberg, J. O., Langer, R. D., Newman, A. B., Fabsitz, R. R., & Criqui, M. H. (2007). Ethnic-specific prevalence of peripheral arterial disease in the United States. *American Journal of Preventive Medicine, 32*(4), 328–333. doi:10.1016/j.amepre.2006.12.010

Anderson, J. L., Halperin, J. L., Albert, N. M., Bozkurt, B., Brindis, R. G., Curtis, L. H., … Shen, W.-K. (2013). Management of patients with peripheral artery disease (compilation of 2005 and 2011 ACCF/AHA guideline recommendations): A report of the American College of Cardiology Foundation/American Heart Association task force on practice guidelines. *Circulation, 127*(13), 1425–1443. doi:10.1161/CIR.0b013e31828b82aa

Beebe, H. G., Dawson, D. L., Cutler, B. S., Herd, J. A., Strandness, D. E., Bortey, E. B., & Forbes, W. P. (1999). A new pharmacological treatment for intermittent claudication: Results of a randomized, multicenter trial. *Archives of Internal Medicine, 159*(17), 2041–2050.

Criqui, M. H., & Aboyans, V. (2015). Epidemiology of peripheral artery disease. *Circulation Research, 116*(9), 1509–1526. doi:10.1161/CIRCRESAHA .116.303849

Gerhard-Herman, M., Gardin, J. M., Jaff, M., Mohler, E., Roman, M., Naqvi, T. Z., . . . Society for Vascular Medicine and Biology. (2006). Guidelines for non-invasive vascular laboratory testing: A report from the American Society of Echocardiography and the Society for Vascular Medicine and Biology. *Vascular Medicine, 11*(3), 183–200.

Hirsch, A. T., Haskal, Z. J., Hertzer, N. R., Bakal, C. W., Creager, M. A., Halperin, J. L., . . . White, R. A. (2006). ACC/AHA 2005 practice guidelines for the management of patients with peripheral arterial disease (lower extremity, renal, mesenteric, and abdominal aortic): A collaborative report from the American Association for Vascular Surgery/Society for Vascular Surgery, Society for Cardiovascular Angiography and Interventions, Society for Vascular Medicine and Biology, Society of Interventional Radiology, and the ACC/AHA task force on practice guidelines (writing committee to develop guidelines for the management of patients with peripheral arterial disease): Endorsed by the American Association of Cardiovascular and Pulmonary Rehabilitation; National Heart, Lung, and Blood Institute; Society for Vascular Nursing; TransAtlantic Inter-Society Consensus; and Vascular Disease Foundation. *Circulation, 113*(11), e463–e654. doi:10.1161/ CIRCULATIONAHA.106.174526

Moyer, V. A., & U.S. Preventive Services Task Force. (2013). Screening for peripheral artery disease and cardiovascular disease risk assessment with the ankle-brachial index in adults: U.S. Preventive Services Task Force recommendation statement. *Annals of Internal Medicine, 159*(5), 342–348. doi:10.7326/0003-4819-159-5-201309030-00008

Web Resources

American Heart Association: http://www.heart .org/HEARTORG/Conditions/More/Peripheral ArteryDisease/Peripheral-Artery-Disease-PAD_ UCM_002082_SubHomePage.jsp

Vascular Disease Foundation: http://vasculardisease .org

Vascular Web: http://www.vascularweb.org

P

PERSONALITY DISORDERS IN THE ELDERLY

According to the *Diagnostic and Statistical Manual of Mental Disorders* (5th ed.; *DSM-5*; American Psychiatric Association, 2013), personality disorders are a class of mental disorders characterized by an enduring, inflexible, and pervasive pattern of inner experiences and behaviors that are exhibited across many contexts and deviate markedly from those accepted by the individual's culture. Personality disorders have been associated with a failure of adaption, an impaired sense of self-identity, and failure to develop effective interpersonal functioning. Those diagnosed with a personality disorder may experience difficulties in cognition, emotiveness, or impulse control. These patterns of behavior and functional problems typically are recognized in adolescence and the beginning of adulthood and, in some unusual instances, childhood (APA, 2013).

In the *DSM-5* (APA, 2013) personality disorders are subdivided into 10 types or domains along three clusters: Those that are characterized as odd or eccentric (Cluster A) include paranoid, schizoid, and schizotypal types (the last of which is now also classified as a schizophrenia-spectrum disorder); Cluster B is associated with dramatic, emotional or erratic behaviors and includes antisocial personality disorder, borderline personality disorder, histrionic personality disorder, and narcissistic personality disorder; and Cluster C is associated with anxious and fearful behavior, which includes avoidant personality disorder, dependent personality disorder, and obsessive-compulsive personality disorder. Each of these personality disorders can be scored on a dimensional scale (1–5, with a score of 4 or 5 constituting the threshold for categorical diagnosis) for severity of symptoms. Although personality disorders generally persist into late life, more recent research suggests that the symptoms associated with personality disorders may improve over time with corrective life experiences or effective treatment (Gutierrez, 2014). In addition, because the *DSM-5* is descriptive, rather than theoretically based, it is seen by some as of limited value as a guide to treatment and research (Tsou, 2015).

Older adults with personality disorders often pose a challenge in treatment, particularly when they have multiple medical conditions. Patients with personality disorders have long-standing difficulties in certain aspects of functioning, often experiencing chaotic interpersonal relationships, problems maintaining a stable sense of self, and deficits in coping with strong emotions. As a result, elderly persons with personality disorders may present with additional needs but have greater difficulty in accepting or making use of available resources.

ASSESSMENT IN THE ELDERLY

Diagnosing personality disorders in the elderly is a complex task because of the need to demonstrate the early age of onset and the difficulty in teasing apart functional impairments related to personality and those related to physiological and environmental aspects of aging and medical illnesses associated with aging. The *DSM-5* does include personality change because of another medical condition to represent personality changes secondary medical compromise, such as Alzheimer's disease and related dementias. Although tools for assessing personality disorders exist, there has been, to date, no ideal assessment instrument for geriatric personality disorders. Most instruments tend to be lengthy, structured interviews that can overwhelm elderly subjects, and none of these instruments has been validated for elderly subjects.

Another question has been the relevance of some of the traditional personality disorder criteria to elders' life experiences (Abrams, 1991). Older individuals have fewer opportunities to manifest recklessness or impulsivity, and dependency can be misinterpreted in the setting of real functional impairment. Younger adults with developmental tasks of separating from parents,

establishing relationships, and functioning in the workplace differ from elders coping with loss and retirement. Difficulties in applying Axis II criteria have been suggested as the explanation for an unexpectedly large number of "Not Otherwise Specified" personality disorders in some elderly samples (Abrams, 1991).

PREVALENCE IN THE ELDERLY

The prevalence of late-life (age 55 years and older) personality disorders using the *Diagnostic and Statistical Manual of Mental Disorders*, fifth edition (5th ed.; *DSM-5*; American Psychiatric Association, 2013) criteria has been reported to be as high a 14.53%, with the highest prevalence in the 55 to 64 years old group (18.14%): 13% (Reynolds, Pietrzak, El-Gabalawy, Makenzie, & Sareen, 2015). Personality disorders at all ages appear to be concentrated among mood disorder patients. However, subsyndromal personality disorders may affect a larger segment of the elderly population than is presently appreciated (Zweig & Agronin, 2011). Rates of personality disorder in geriatric studies appear to be highest in depressives, about 31% among those with either major depression or dysthymia (Devanand, 2000).

COMORBIDITY WITH DEPRESSION AND ANXIETY

In mixed-age depressives, comorbid personality disorders have been associated with younger age of depression onset, multiple depressive episodes, and longer duration of episodes. Anxiety disorders have been associated with some Cluster C traits, such as avoidance and dependence (Bienvenu & Brandes, 2005).

PHARMACOLOGICAL TREATMENT OF OLDER ADULTS WITH PERSONALITY DISORDERS

Because personality disorders represent a range of phenomena, psychopharmacological treatments have tended to target individual symptoms rather than whole entities. Thus clinicians often prescribe second-generation antipsychotics when psychosis is present, mood stabilizers for affective fluctuations, and serotonin-enhancing antidepressants for low mood, suicidality, aggression, or obsessionality. These approaches appear to have had some success in moderating individual symptoms.

PSYCHOTHERAPY OF OLDER ADULTS WITH PERSONALITY DISORDERS

Psychotherapy with patients who have personality disorders is often complex, affectively charged, and difficult work, and this is no different with elderly patients. In fact, because of increased dependence, declining health, and the significant environmental changes that are often associated with aging, the elderly are perhaps more likely to have strong emotional reactions to their psychotherapist. Often the task of the therapist is to develop an alliance with patients, with the goal of looking collaboratively at ways in which they contribute to their own difficulties. In elderly patients with no prior experience in psychotherapy, this may feel confusing, demanding, or even unfair.

Although traditional psychotherapies can be effective for elderly outpatients, the trend has been in favor of treatments using cognitive-behavioral approaches. Studies of these therapies in the elderly have mostly involved depressed patients, however, and their applicability to older adults with personality disorders has not been specifically evaluated.

As people age, changes in their health, their surroundings, and their relationships put increased demands on their coping mechanisms. Whatever these normative challenges of aging may be, patients with personality disorders have greater difficulty managing these problems and using available resources effectively. Although overt self-destructive behavior such as self-mutilation is rare in this population, deficits in interpersonal skills and coping skills intersect with medical and psychiatric illness to accentuate the challenges of aging. Recognizing and treating underlying personality disorders in the elderly is an important aspect of providing useful and effective care to those who are most in need.

Steven L. Baumann

Abrams, R. C. (1991). The aging personality. [Editorial.] *International Journal of Geriatric Psychiatry, 6*, 1–3.

American Psychiatric Association. (2013). *Diagnostic and statistical manual of mental disorders* (5th ed.). Arlington, VA: American Psychiatric Publishing.

Bienvenu, J., & Brandes, M. (2005). The interface of personality traits and anxiety disorders. *Primary Psychiatry, 12*, 35–39.

Devanand, D. P., Turret, N., Moody, B. J., Fitzsimons, L., Peyser, S., Mickle, K., … Roose, S. P. (2000). Personality disorders in elderly patients with dysthymic disorder. *American Journal of Geriatric Psychiatry, 8*, 188–195.

Gutierrez, F. (2014). The course of personality pathology. *Current Opinion in Psychiatry, 27*, 78–83.

Reynolds, K., Pietrzak, R. H., El-Gabalawy, R., Makenzie, C. S., & Sareen, J. (2015). Prevalence of psychiatric disorders in U.S. older adults: Findings from a nationally representative survey. *World Psychiatry, 14*, 74–81.

Tsou, J. Y. (2015). DSM-5 and psychiatry's second revolution: Descriptive vs. theoretical approaches to psychiatric classification. In S. Demazeux & P. Singy (Eds.), *The DSM-5 in perspective: Philosophical reflections on the psychiatric babel* (pp. 43–62). New York, NY: Springer Publishing.

Zweig, R. A., & Agronin, M. E. (2011). Personality disorders. In M. E. Agronin & G. J. Maletta (Eds.), *Principles and practice of geriatric psychiatry* (2nd ed., pp. 523–544). Philadelphia, PA: Lippincott Williams & Wilkins.

Web Resources

American Association for Geriatric Psychiatry: http://www.aagpgpa.org

American Journal of Geriatric Psychiatry: http://ajgponline.org

Borderline Personality Disorder Resource Center: http://www.bpdresourcecenter.org

International Journal of Geriatric Psychiatry: http://www3.interscience.wiley.com/cgi-bin/jhome/4294

National Institutes of Health/MedlinePlus Personality Disorders page: http://www.nlm.nih.gov/medlineplus/personalitydisorders.html

P

Pet Ownership Among Older Adults

According to the American Veterinary Medicine Association's 2012 statistics, 36.5% of American households have dogs, 30.4% have cats, 3.1% have birds, and 1.5% have horses, composing over 155 million households (American Veterinary Medical Association, 2016). According to the U.S. Bureau of the Census, the projected U.S. population of 314 million in 2015 comprises 55 million older adults, or approximately 15% of the U.S. population (Ortman, Velkof, & Hogan, 2014). With a conservative estimate of a 50% pet ownership incidence rate, approximately 22 million older adults are pet owners. Given these potential numbers of older adult pet owners, health care providers are likely to work with this population. Knowledge of the benefits and drawbacks of pet ownership is important in assessing and planning health care for older adults.

PSYCHOSOCIAL BENEFITS

Numerous studies have indicated that having a companion animal is associated with physical, psychological, and health advantages (Matchock, 2015; Smith, 2012). Dogs in particular have been found to be social lubricants; people have been viewed more positively by others and more likely to be approached when they are accompanied by a dog than if they are alone. Pets have commonly been viewed as "members of the family," often enjoying sleeping locations with their owners, receipt of gifts for holidays, and inclusion in one-sided conversations. Older adult pet owners have been found to be less likely to feel depressed than non–pet owners (Rhodes, Murray, Temple, Tuokko, & Wharf, 2012). Having a pet has been associated with decreased loneliness in older adults (Stanley, Conwell, Bowen, & Van Orden, 2014). Living with a companion animal can involve older adults in thinking outside of themselves, provide a focus for conversation with others, and facilitate invaluable physical activity.

PHYSICAL BENEFITS

Older adult pet owners have been found to exercise more and to have fewer patient-initiated primary care visits than non–pet owners (Rhodes et al., 2012). Older adult dog owners who owned pets were more likely to have positive health effects than non–pet owners (Cherniack & Cherniack, 2014). In one study, older adults who were walking a dog had beneficial health outcomes (Ulz, 2014). Another study showed that older adults who walked a dog 5 days/week for 12 weeks had a 28% increase in normal walking speed (Johnson, 2013). These physical benefits may enable older adults to remain functionally independent for longer periods.

ISSUES ASSOCIATED WITH PET OWNERSHIP

Owning a pet involves making a commitment to providing the animal with proper veterinary care, food, grooming, interaction, love, and exercise. This can result in significant annual costs, which may be particularly challenging for older adults who are on a fixed income. One reason cited by older adults for not owning a pet was associated costs. Given the benefits of pet ownership to older adults, financial support of pet care can be a meaningful contribution made by family members who do not live nearby their older adult loved one.

Another concern is that as older adults experience limitations in physical or cognitive capacity, they may need help with pet caregiving. Unfortunately, a common response to this scenario is for the older adult to give up the pet. This "solution" to the issue can be inhumane for both the older adult and the pet, which may also be older. Pet ownership can be supported through some regular assistance with caregiving, leaving the beneficial interaction intact between older adults and their pets.

Senior housing options that include pets are increasingly common. An example of a housing option that is not only pet tolerant, but also pet encouraging, is the TigerPlace retirement residence in Columbia, Missouri. A collaborative venture between the University of Missouri Sinclair School of Nursing and Americare, Inc., TigerPlace is an aging-in-place facility. There, older adults receive needed support with pet ownership through the TigerPlace Pet Initiative (Johnson, 2013). The program assists older adults who do not have pets, but who would like one, to locate a pet that is a good match for them. It includes a pet care assistant (PCA) who visits each pet owner as needed (generally every 1–2 days) to provide caregiving assistance such as walking dogs, administering medications to pets, delivering pet food, or bathing pets. The program also engages a veterinarian (a faculty member from the College of Veterinary Medicine), who makes monthly house calls with each pet and owner for early identification of health or behavior problems. Pets' vaccination records are tracked and health or behavior problems managed through the help of the PCA. In addition, a veterinary medical examination room within the facility makes on-site health care for uncomplicated issues possible. The TigerPlace Pet Initiative also provides funds to support foster care of pets (until adoption occurs) when their owners pass away or can no longer take care of them. To date, this has not occurred within the facility because non–pet owning typically know the animal and want to adopt the bereaved pets. The program provides emotional support to older adults when their pet dies and, if they express readiness for another pet, helps to locate a pet meeting their preferences that will be a good match for them.

Nurses working in areas that do not have facilities that provide services like those at TigerPlace, may need to look to community resources to help older adults maintain pet ownership. These include veterinary medical practices, auxiliary or volunteer groups willing to help older adults, or nearby college or university programs in which students do service-learning or other volunteer activities. Other resources may be local pet enthusiast organizations such as kennel clubs, dog training organizations, Future Farmers of America (FFA), Boy or Girl Scouts, community service organizations, or animal shelters providing services to community residents.

Mary Shelkey

American Veterinary Medical Association. (2016). U.S. pet ownership statistics. Retrieved from https://www.avma.org/KB/Resources/Statistics/Pages/Market-research-statistics-US-pet-ownership.aspx

Cherniack, E. P., & Cherniack, A. R. (2014). The benefit of pets and animal-assisted therapy to the health of older adults. *Current Gerontology and Geriatrics Research, 2014*, 623203. doi:10.1155/2014/623203

Johnson, R. A. (2013). Promoting one health: The University of Missouri Research Center for Human Animal Interaction. *Missouri Medicine, 110* (3), 197–200.

Matchock, R. L. (2015). Pet ownership and physical health. *Current Opinion in Psychiatry, 28*(5), 386–392.

Ortman, J. M., Velkof, V. A., & Hogan, H. (2014). *Current population reports. U.S. Census reports, An aging nation: The older population in the United States.* Washington, DC: U.S. Census Bureau. Retrieved from https://www.census.gov/prod/2014pubs/p25-1140.pdf

Rhodes, R. E., Murray, H., Temple, V. A., Tuokko, H., & Wharf, H. (2012). Pilot study of a dog walking randomized intervention: Effects of a focus on canine exercise. *Preventive Medicine, 54*(5), 309–312.

Smith, B. (2012). The "pet effect": Health related aspects of companion animal ownership. *Australian Family Physician, 41*(6), 439–442.

Stanley, I. H., Conwell, Y., Bowen, C., & Van Orden, K. A. (2014). Pet ownership may attenuate loneliness among adult primary care patients who live alone. *Aging & Mental Health, 18*(3), 394–399.

Utz, R. (2014). Walking the dog: The effect of pet ownership on human health and health behaviors. *Social Indicators Research, 116*(2), 327–339.

Web Resources

Pets for the Elderly Foundation: http://www.petsfortheelderly.org

Purina Adoption Program for People 55+: http://www.animalhumanesociety.org/adoption/purinapetsfor55plus

P

P

PHARMACISTS

Medications are probably the single most important factor in improving the quality of life of older adults. However, these same medications can cause adverse effects, and older adults are at particular risk for medication-related problems. Consultant pharmacists have traditionally cared for older patients residing in nursing homes. Because most older adults continue to reside in the community and in assisted-living facilities, the role of the pharmacist in geriatrics (or senior care) has expanded beyond the nursing home. The term *senior care pharmacist* was coined by the American Society of Consultant Pharmacists (ASCP) to describe pharmacists who care for older adults and have specialized knowledge about the use of medications in older adults. These pharmacists are advocates for their senior patients, wherever they reside.

EDUCATION AND TRAINING

Since 2000, the entry-level degree into the profession of pharmacy has been the 6-year Doctor of Pharmacy (PharmD) degree. Previously, the program of study was a 5-year bachelor of science in pharmacy.

Although there is no nationally required geriatric content in the pharmacy curriculum, several older surveys found that essentially all colleges of pharmacy contain some geriatric content, either in required courses or electives (Linnebur et al., 2005; Odegard, Breslow, Koronkowski, Williams, & Hudgins, 2007). More than 90% of the colleges responding to the surveys offer experiential rotations in geriatrics or long-term care pharmacy practice. To help colleges identify geriatric topics for the curriculum, ASCP published the *Geriatric Curriculum Guide*. Now in its third edition, the guide can be used for all levels of geriatric training: students (didactic and experiential), pharmacy residents, and pharmacists who are seeking guidance in their professional development in the area of geriatrics. The guide covers foundational principles of aging, essential competencies for the practice of geriatric care, and the approach to practice and care of seniors.

Postgraduate training programs exist for pharmacists interested in specializing in geriatric pharmacy practice. In 2016, there were 20 post-graduate year (PGY)-2 residency programs in geriatric pharmacy practice. Most of these training programs are based in university hospitals, ambulatory care clinics, or long-term care settings. The American Society of Health-System Pharmacists (ASHP) has established standards and learning objectives for these specialized residencies in geriatric pharmacy practice. Some PGY-1 pharmacy residencies, particularly in the Veterans Affairs system, provide a focus in geriatrics. A survey of PGY-1 residencies found that 21% of responding programs had a required rotation in geriatrics and 47% offered an elective rotation. (Niehoff & Jeffery, 2016) For practicing pharmacists, the ASCP Foundation offers intensive traineeships in various areas of geriatric pharmacy practice (e.g., Parkinson's disease, pain management). Pharmacists may also participate in courses offered by federally funded geriatric education centers (GECs).

LICENSURE AND CERTIFICATION

After graduating from an accredited college of pharmacy, the individual must pass a state licensure examination. Every registered pharmacist must annually obtain a required amount of continuing education credits to renew and maintain the license. A few states require additional continuing education focused on geriatric care for pharmacists involved in long-term care consultant practice.

In 1997, ASCP voted to create the Commission for Certification in Geriatric Pharmacy (CCGP) to oversee a certification program in geriatric pharmacy practice. Candidates are required to pass a 150-question examination and are then entitled to use the designation, *certified geriatric pharmacist* (CGP). As of July 2016, there were more than 3,000 *certified geriatric pharmacists*, most of them in the United States. CGPs can be found in 20 countries. Certification is good for 5 years and recertification is through examination or a series of special continuing education programs.

PRACTICE SETTINGS AND ROLES

Pharmacists care for older adults in various settings: community, hospitals, long-term care facilities, assisted-living facilities, home care, and hospice (Spinewine, Fialova, & Byrne, 2012). They are an essential member of the health care team caring for an elderly patient. They provide drug information to other members of the team, monitor drug therapy, and provide patient education. Through regular review of the patient's medication regimen, the pharmacist can ensure appropriate choice of medication and appropriate dosing based on organ function, screen for drug interactions and adverse effects, and recommend the discontinuation of unnecessary medications. Pharmacists are involved in clinical research in many patient settings and within the pharmaceutical industry. A review of studies of the effects of pharmacists' interventions on patient care found a positive effect on therapeutics, safety, hospitalizations, and adherence outcomes in older adults (Lee et al., 2013).

The role of the pharmacist in medication therapy management (MTM) in community-dwelling older adults was expanded with the implementation of the Medicare outpatient drug benefit, Medicare Part D. Pharmacists are involved in MTM counsel and otherwise assist enrollees with multiple chronic diseases, multiple medications, and high drug costs. The objective of MTM programs is to optimize therapeutic outcomes while minimizing adverse effects.

PROFESSIONAL ORGANIZATIONS AND PUBLICATIONS

ASCP is the international professional association that provides leadership, education, advocacy, and resources for pharmacists caring for older patients. The ASCP Foundation funds research and educational projects in geriatric pharmacy practice. One of its major initiatives was the Fleetwood Project, a three-phase study documenting the value of pharmacists' services in long-term care facilities. The final report of the Fleetwood Project was published in 2006. ASCP has expanded its student programming to increase interest in geriatrics among pharmacy students. Other pharmacy organizations,

including ASHP, American Association of Colleges of Pharmacy (AACP), and American College of Clinical Pharmacy (ACCP), have special interest groups for pharmacists involved in geriatric practice. The American Geriatrics Society (AGS) has an active pharmacists section that sponsors medication-related sessions at the AGS annual meeting.

Two journals focus on geriatric pharmacotherapy. ASCP's journal, *The Consultant Pharmacist*, is a monthly peer-reviewed publication that publishes practice-based research and review articles. *Drugs & Aging* is a quarterly journal also covering a wide range of geriatric drug topics. ASHP has published a book, *Fundamentals of Geriatric Pharmacotherapy*, which can be useful to all health professionals providing care to older adults.

RESOURCES FOR PATIENTS AND HEALTH CARE PROFESSIONALS

A common question is "How does one find a pharmacist specializing in geriatric care?" Two websites list pharmacists specializing in geriatric practice. The ASCP website has a senior care pharmacist locator function which provides a geographical listing of pharmacists who voluntarily join the site. Pharmacists provide a description of their practice and specialty areas (e.g., psychopharmacy, patient education) and contact information. On the CCGP website, all current CGPs are listed geographically with their contact information. Patients and health professionals are invited to visit these websites to find a senior care pharmacist.

See also Medication Adherence; Psychotropic Medication Use in Long-Term Care.

Judith L. Beizer

Lee, J. K., Slack, M. K., Martin, J., Ehrman, C., & Chisholm-Burns, M. (2013). Geriatric patient care by U.S. pharmacists in healthcare teams: Systematic review and meta-analyses. *Journal of the American Geriatrics Society, 61*(7), 1119–1127.

Linnebur, S. A., O'Connell M. B, Wessell, A. M., McCord, A. D., Kennedy, D. H., DeMaagd, G., ... Sterling, T. (2005). Pharmacy practice, research, education and advocacy for older adults. *Pharmacotherapy, 25*(10), 1396–1430.

Niehoff, K. M., & Jeffery, S. M. (2016) Geriatric pharmacy training requirements: A survey of residency programs. *American Journal of Health-System Pharmacy, 73*(4), 229–234.

Odegard, P. S., Breslow, R. M., Koronkowski, M. J., Williams, B. R., & Hudgins, G. A. (2007). Geriatric pharmacy education: A strategic plan for the future. *American Journal of Pharmaceutical Education, 71*(3), 47.

Spinewine, A., Fialova, D., & Byrne, S. (2012). The role of the pharmacist in optimizing pharmacotherapy in older people. *Drugs & Aging, 29*(6), 495–510.

Web Resources

American Society of Consultant Pharmacists: https://www.ascp.com

Commission for Certification in Geriatric Pharmacy: http://ccgp.org

PHYSICAL AND MENTAL HEALTH NEEDS OF OLDER LESBIAN, GAY, BISEXUAL, TRANSGENDER, AND QUEER ADULTS

NEEDS OF OLDER LESBIAN, GAY, BISEXUAL, TRANSGENDER, AND QUEER ADULTS IN SOCIAL–POLITICAL–HISTORICAL CONTEXT

Although the exact number of lesbian, gay, bisexual, transgender, and queer (LGBTQ) older adults is unknown because of a lack of research on this historically underserved and invisible population, estimates suggest that there are approximately 9 million LGBTQ persons in the United States (Gates, 2011) and an estimated 2.4 million LGBTQ older Americans aged 50 years or older (Choi & Meyer, 2016). Similar to the general aging population, LGBTQ older adults experience common age-related health issues such as multimorbidity and geriatric syndromes and have complex care and transition care needs. What sets LGBTQ adults apart from the heterosexual population, however, is the historical prejudice that they have experienced. Research suggests that structural, population, and individual-level discrimination results in negative physical and mental health outcomes (Choi & Meyer, 2016; Healthy People 2020, 2016; Institute of Medicine [IOM], 2011); the current cohort of older adults has been particularly affected by stigma, marginalization, and victimization during the course of their lives. In the United States, "homosexuality" was listed as a mental health diagnosis until 1973, when it was removed from the *Diagnostic and Statistical Manual of Mental Disorders* (*DSM*) by the American Psychological Association. Before this time, society viewed being gay or lesbian as disordered or immoral and illegal. Many people lost jobs or were ostracized by family and friends when their sexual identity became known. Considering this social and historical context is essential when thinking about the origin of LGBTQ population and individual health disparities.

In the fast-changing world of LGBTQ civil rights, the younger cohort of LGBTQ older adults (ages 55–70 years) has had a vastly different life experience than their older cohorts, witnessing celebrities "coming out" and living publicly as LGBTQ, the repeal of the "Don't Ask, Don't Tell" law allowing LGBT persons to serve openly in the military, and the legal recognition of same-sex marriages in the United States. Younger LGBT adults have also seen more social services that are specifically designed for LGBTQ adults and their families. As they age, they will be able to openly define themselves as LGBTQ and seek services that, if not solely identified as targeted for LGBTQ persons, are at least sensitive to their needs.

THEORETICAL FRAMEWORK FOR ADDRESSING HEALTH NEEDS OF LGBTQ OLDER ADULTS

Minority stress theory holds that sexual and gender minorities experience chronic psychosocial stress as a result of being subjected to systemic and individual-level stigma (Meyer, 2003; Quinn & Chaudoir, 2009). The theory acknowledges the reality of discordant values between minority individuals and the dominant societal framework and posits that the resultant conflict is responsible for a host of stress-related health outcomes. In LGBT populations, this often contributes to an increase in mental health problems, such as depression, anxiety, and suicidality, and a possible increase in physical health problems, including cardiovascular disease and certain malignancies (Fredriksen-Goldsen, Kim, Barkan, Muraco, & Hoy-Ellis, 2013; IOM, 2011; Meyer, 2003). Because many chronic and serious health issues appear in the second half of life, it is possible that older LGBTQ adults are more vulnerable to the ill effects of minority stress than their younger counterparts. Furthermore, minority stress has been implicated in the increased tendency of LGBTQ individuals to engage in detrimental behaviors, including avoidance of medical care because of fear of prejudice or discrimination from health care providers (Dorsen, 2012); increased engagement in polysubstance abuse; and greater sexual risk-taking behaviors (Choi & Meyer, 2016; Healthy People 2020, 2016).

MENTAL HEALTH

Older lesbian, gay, and bisexual adults experience significant stress, anxiety, depression, and suicidal ideation/attempts as compared with heterosexuals, much of it because of the experience of systematic discrimination, concealment of one's identity, and/or increased rates of victimization and violence (Healthy People 2020, 2016). Although little research has been done specifically on the mental health of older transgender adults, that which does exist suggests that older transgender men and women have among the highest rates of depression, anxiety, and suicidality of any population in the United States (Fredriksen-Goldsen et al., 2014).

LGBTQ older adults are twice as likely to live alone and four times likely not to have adult children than heterosexuals. This is associated with social isolation and poorer health outcomes. In 2015, the U.S. Supreme Court ruled that the Defense of Marriage Act (DOMA) was unconstitutional, paving the way for federal recognition of same-sex marriage and extension of federal benefits to same-sex couples and families. Research is needed to examine the impacts that this expansion of rights will have on the mental and physical health of LGBTQ adults.

CHRONIC DISEASE

There is limited research on the role of sexual orientation and gender identity in the development and management of chronic diseases. Existing research suggests that LGBT older adults may be at high risk for cardiopulmonary diseases and certain cancers as a result of increased prevalence of smoking, obesity, and alcohol and drug use within the LGBTQ community compared with the general population (Fredriksen-Goldsen et al., 2013; Healthy People 2020, 2016). Further investigation is warranted, especially regarding the major causes of morbidity and mortality among U.S. older adults, including cardiovascular disease, cancer, cerebrovascular disease, and dementia (Grant, Koskovich, Frazer, & Bjerk, 2010). The increased risks of morbidity and mortality among older LGBTQ adults are compounded by decreased access to and use of preventive health care services and routine screening for chronic diseases. LGBTQ adults consistently report concerns about discrimination in health care settings, mistrust of health care providers, lack of knowledge of increased risk, and decreased rates of adequate of health care coverage (Ard & Makadon, 2009).

SUBSTANCE ABUSE

The prevalence of substance use and abuse (alcohol, tobacco, and illicit drugs) is higher among LGBTQ populations than in the general population (Choi & Meyer, 2016; Healthy People 2020, 2016). For example, whereas the national rate of smoking is declining, smoking rate within the LGBT community is approximately double to that in the general population (American Lung Association, 2010). Smoking is associated with higher rates of preventable conditions such as stroke and coronary artery disease (CAD) among LGBTQ older adults (Lee, Griffin, & Melvin, 2009). LGBTQ elders may also have higher rates of problematic alcohol consumption than their heterosexual peers (Fredriksen-Goldsen et al., 2013). Although empirical data on illicit drug use among LGBTQ older adults are scant, research suggests that rates of illicit drug use are higher in some LGBTQ subgroups, including men who have sex with men and transgender persons than in general populations (Hughes & Eliason, 2002).

Public health researchers believe tobacco, alcohol, and drug use disparities are caused by interactions with social and environment factors, including minority stress, peer pressure, and aggressive marketing among LGBTQ by the tobacco and alcohol industries (American Lung Association, 2010; Lee et al., 2009). Likewise, researchers have hypothesized that increased rates of tobacco and alcohol use may be due, in part, to the increased use of bars as safe social gathering spots for LGBTQ persons (Harley & Hancock, 2015).

HIV/AIDS

As AIDS mortality declines, the prevalence of HIV infection among people older than 50 years is increasing (Gleason, Luque, & Shah, 2013). In 2013, people aged 55 years and older accounted for about one quarter (24%) of the estimated 1.2 million people living with HIV infection and 18% of new HIV diagnosis in the United States (Centers for Disease Control and Prevention [CDC], 2016), HIV infection and lifelong antiretroviral therapy has been noted to increase risk for cardiovascular diseases such as CAD, myocardial infarction, peripheral arterial disease, and chronic heart failure (Esser et al., 2012). Older adults with AIDS are particularly at risk for polypharmacy because of multimorbidity (Gleason et al., 2013). HIV-positive LGBT elders have worse overall mental and physical health, disability, poorer health outcomes, and a higher likelihood of experiencing barriers to care than HIV-negative peers (Choi & Meyer, 2016). Despite these disparities, there are few HIV/AIDS prevention programs targeted to older adults or LGBT elders (IOM, 2011).

PALLIATIVE CARE AND END-OF-LIFE CARE

A paucity of literature has investigated the unique needs that LGBTQ elders may have related to palliative and end-of-life care. Many areas of health care disparities, including decreased access to and use of preventive care

services, increased rates of smoking, increased alcohol and drug use, increased incidence of heart disease and certain cancers, and increased rates of depression, anxiety, and suicidality, may put them at higher risk for serious and/or life-threatening illnesses. LGBTQ persons are less likely to have a primary caregiver who is a legal relative, and lack traditional sources of informal support (Croghan, Moone, & Olson, 2014). LGBTQ persons also report fears of discrimination in health care encounters and in health care settings such as hospitals and long-term care facilities, causing distress regarding accessing care and/or the need to "re-enter" the closet in these environments. Last, LGBTQ patients and providers may be confused about their rights, such as partnership and marriage equality policies, particularly as they relate to health care and advance care planning.

SPECIAL ISSUES FOR TRANSGENDER ELDERS

Transgender persons are considered to be the most vulnerable of the LGBTQ populations (Healthy People 2020, 2016). Although there is increasing research on LGB health-related issues, there is still very little known on the specific issues of older transgender persons. Existing data suggest that transgender elders may be at risk for numerous negative health outcomes and are at higher risk for poor physical health, disability, and mental health problems, including depressive symptoms and suicidality, than heterosexual adults (Choi & Meyer, 2016). Long-term estrogen use may increase the risk for blood clots, hypertension, hyperglycemia, and water retention, and long-term testosterone use may pose a risk of liver damage (Gay and Lesbian Medical Association [GLMA], 2012; IOM, 2011). Transgender persons also have significantly high rates of tobacco use and smoking-related diseases (American Lung Association, 2010) and the highest rates of HIV infection in the United States (Choi & Meyer, 2016).

Poor health care service utilization by transgender individuals is a major concern that is partly explained by a lack of health insurance and high rates of poverty or inability to afford health care (Healthy People 2020, 2016). Discrimination by health care providers is a major deterrent for accessing health resources among transgender persons. The National Center for Transgender Equality and National Gay and Lesbian Task Force transgender health study found that 20% of the respondents reported being denied medical care because of their transgender status and 50% of those surveyed reported having to teach their medical providers about transgender care needs (Grant et al., 2011).

CONCLUSION

The world of LGBT elders differs from that of their non-LGBT peers. In many areas of life, this population faces unique barriers and challenges. However, they share many of the same fears about growing old as all aging adults. They continue to show resilience, which results in improved conditions for themselves and younger cohorts of LGBT adults. Current political uncertainties, because of forces in society today that seek to undo these improved conditions, may remind older generations of their past experiences, possibly reinforcing a fear being open in their dealings with institutionalized systems. Service providers need to be cognizant of these unique dynamics and of continuing disparities in health and health care among LGBT elders.

As more research emerges, the health needs of LGBTQ older adults will be better understood. It must be noted that racial/ethnic minorities within the LGBTQ population are more vulnerable to the cumulative negative effects of persistent racism and the stigma attached to their sexual orientation and gender identity (IOM, 2011). Sexual minorities living in high-prejudice communities have on average a shorter life expectancy by approximately 12 years compared with sexual minorities living in nonprejudiced communities (Hatzenbuehler et al., 2014). To provide patient-centered, culturally competent care, providers must be aware that each distinct group has their own unique needs in spite of being lumped together within the LGBTQ acronym.

Given their distinct health care needs, LGBTQ persons were identified as a population of concern in Healthy People 2010 and the improvement of health, safety and well-being of LGBTQ people is a goal in Healthy People 2020

(Healthy People 2020, 2016). The Outing Age 2010 report provides detailed discussions on key issues unique to LGBTQ older adults within the domains of health care delivery, policy, and research. Providers working with LGBTQ older adults are encouraged to use this resource, as well as other resources listed here, to provide the highest quality care to this dynamic, evolving, and often underserved population.

Fidelindo Lim and Caroline Dorsen

American Lung Association. (2010). Smoking out a deadly threat: Tobacco use in the LGBT community. Retrieved from http://www.lung.org/ assets/documents/publications/lung-disease -data/lgbt-report.pdf

Ard, K. L., & Makadon, H. J. (2009). *Improving the health care of lesbian, gay, bisexual and transgendered (LGBT) people: Understanding and eliminating health disparities.* Boston, MA: The Fenway Institute. Retrieved from https://www.lgbthealtheducation .org/wp-content/uploads/Improving-the -Health-of-LGBT-People.pdf

Centers for Disease Control and Prevention. (2016). HIV among people aged 50 and over. Retrieved from http://www.cdc.gov/hiv/group/age/old eramericans/index.html

Choi, S., K., & Meyer, I. H. (2016). LGBT aging: A review of research findings, needs, and policy implications. Retrieved from http://williams institute.law.ucla.edu/wp-content/uploads/ LGBT-Aging-A-Review.pdf

Croghan, C. F., Moone, R. P., & Olson, A. M. (2014). Friends, family, and caregiving among midlife and older lesbian, gay, bisexual, and transgender adults. *Journal of Homosexuality, 61*(1), 79–102.

Dorsen, C. (2012). An integrative review of nurse attitudes towards lesbian, gay, bisexual, and transgender patients. *Canadian Journal of Nursing Research, 44*(3), 18–43.

Esser, S., Gelbrich, G., Brockmeyer, N., Goehler, A., Schadendorf, D., Erbe, L. R., … Reinsch, N. (2012). Prevalence of cardiovascular diseases in HIV-infected outpatients: Results from a prospective, multicenter cohort study. *Clinical Research in Cardiology, 102*(3), 203–213. doi:10.1007/ s00392-012-0519-0

Fredriksen-Goldsen, K. I., Cook-Daniels, L., Kim, H., Erosheva, E. A., Emlet, C. A., Hoy-Ellis, C. P., … Muraco, A. (2014). Physical and mental health of transgender older adults: An at-risk and underserved population. *The Gerontologist, 54*(3), 488– 500. doi:10.1093/geront/gnt021

Fredriksen-Goldsen, K. I., Kim, H. J., Barkan, S. E., Muraco, A., & Hoy-Ellis, C. P. (2013). Health disparities among lesbian, gay, and bisexual older adults: Results from a population-based study. *American Journal of Public Health, 103*(10), 1802–1809. doi:10.2105/AJPH.2012.301110

Gates, G. J. (2011). *How many people are lesbian, gay, bisexual, and transgender?* Los Angeles: The Williams Institute, University of California, Los Angeles, School of Law. Retrieved from http://williams institute.law.ucla.edu/wp-content/uploads/Gates-How-Many-People-LGBT-Apr-2011.pdf

Gay and Lesbian Medical Association. (2012). Top ten things transgender persons should discuss with their healthcare care provider. Retrieved from http://www.glma.org/index.cfm?fuseaction=Page.viewPage&pageID=692

Gleason, L. J., Luque, A. E., & Shah, K. (2013). Polypharmacy in the HIV-infected older adult population. *Clinical Interventions in Aging, 8,* 749–763. doi:10.2147/CIA.S37738

Grant, J. M., Koskovich, G., Frazer, S., & Bjerk, S. (2010). *Outing age 2010: Public policy issues affecting gay, lesbian, bisexual and transgender elders.* Washington, DC: National Gay and Lesbian Task Force Policy Institute.

Grant, J. M., Mottet, L. A., Tanis, J., Harrison, L., Herman, J., & Keisling, M. (2011). *National transgender discrimination survey report on health and health care.* Washington, DC: National Center for Transgender Equality and National Gay and Lesbian Task Force.

Harley, D. A., & Hancock, M. T. (2015). Substance use disorders intervention with LGBT elders. In D. A. Harley & P. B. Teaster (Eds.), *The handbook of LGBT elders* (pp. 473–490). Cham, Switzerland: Springer Publishing.

Hatzenbuehler, M. L., Bellatorre, A., Lee, Y., Finch, B. K., Muennig, P., & Fiscella, K. (2014). Structural stigma and all-cause mortality in sexual minority populations. *Social Science and Medicine, 103,* 33–41. doi:10.1016/j.socscimed.2013.06.005

Healthy People 2020. (2016). *Lesbian, gay, bisexual, and transgender health.* Washington, DC: U.S. Department of Health and Human Services, Office of Disease Prevention and Health Promotion. Retrieved from http://www.healthy people.gov/2020/topicsobjectives2020/overview.aspx?topicid=25.

Hughes, T., & Eliason, M. (2002). Substance use and abuse in lesbian, gay, bisexual and transgender populations. *Journal of Primary Prevention, 22*(3), 263–298.

Institute of Medicine. (2011). *The health of lesbian, gay, bisexual, and transgender people: Building a foundation for better understanding.* Washington, DC: National Academies Press.

Lee, J. G., Griffin, G. K., & Melvin, C. L. (2009). Tobacco use among sexual minorities in the USA 1987 to May 2007: A systematic review. *Tobacco Control, 18*(4), 275–282. doi:10.1136/tc.2008.028241

Meyer, I. H. (2003). Prejudice, social stress, and mental health in lesbian, gay, and bisexual populations: Conceptual issues and research evidence. *Psychological Bulletin, 129,* 674–697.

Quinn, D. M., & Chaudoir, S. R. (2009). Living with a concealable stigmatized identity: The impact of anticipated stigma, centrality, salience, and cultural stigma on psychological distress and health. *Journal of Personality and Social Psychology, 97,* 634–651.

Web Resources

AARP: http://www.aarp.org/relationships/friends-family/aarp-pride

Centerlink—The Community of LGBT Centers: http://www.lgbtcenters.org

Center of Excellence for Transgender Health: http://www.transhealth.ucsf.edu/trans?page=home-00-00

Centers for Disease Control and Prevention (CDC)—Lesbian, Gay, Bisexual and Transgender Health: http://www.cdc.gov/lgbthealth/index.htm

Gay and Lesbian Medical Association (GLMA): http://glma.org

Healthcare Equality Index: Creating a national standard for equal treatment of lesbian, gay, bisexual and transgender patients and their families: http://www.hrc.org/hei

MedlinePlus—Gay, Lesbian and Transgender Health: http://www.nlm.nih.gov/medlineplus/gaylesbi anandtransgenderhealth.html

National Coalition for LGBT Health: http://www.healthhiv.org/sites-causes/national-coalition-for-lgbt-health

PHYSICAL THERAPISTS

The Office of the Surgeon General established the physical therapy profession during World War I through the Division of Special Hospitals and Physical Reconstruction. More than 2,000 "reconstruction aides" restored function to patients with poliomyelitis and other disabilities (Murphy, 1995). Today, conditions that limit an individual's physical function affect one in seven Americans, with the cost of care approaching more than $170 billion annually. Physical therapists (PTs) are an integral component of an interdisciplinary care team dedicated to meeting the needs of elders with impairments, functional limitations, and participation restrictions.

According to the U.S. Bureau of Labor Statistics (2015), there were 209,690 PTs and 81,230 physical therapy assistants (PTAs), practicing who provided care to more than 1 million clients per day in the United States in 2015. Employment of PTs is projected to grow 34% from 2014 to 2024, considerably faster than the average for all occupations, which is 7%.

PTs are educated at the university or collegiate level and are required to be licensed in the state in which they practice. Licensure examinations are state administered. The doctor of physical therapy (DPT) is the required degree for all entry-level PT educational programs. PT education programs are accredited by the Commission on Accreditation in Physical Therapy Education (CAPTE). There are over 233 accredited physical therapy programs and 29 programs in development in 2016 in the United States. The American Physical Therapy Association (APTA) is the national professional organization that represents over 80,000 PTS and PTAs. The APTA established the specialist certification program in 1978 to provide formal recognition for PTs with advanced clinical knowledge, competence, and skills in a special area of practice. According to the American Board of Physical Therapy Specialists (ABPTS), "Specialization is the process by which a physical therapist builds on a broad base of professional education and practice to develop a greater depth of knowledge and skills related to a particular area of practice" (ABPTS, 2017, para. 1).

In 1992, 14 PTs became the first geriatric clinical specialists (GCGs) in the field and by 2016, there were 2,133 clinical specialists practicing in the field of geriatrics in the country. Clinical specialization in geriatric physical therapy responds to a specific patient population and requires advanced knowledge, skill acquisition, and clinical experience exceeding that of an entry-level PT, concomitant with a unique skill set to practice in a geriatric setting. GCSs are PTs who are specialists in the treatment of older adults and are boarded by the ABPTS. To become a GCS, the PT must have a minimum of 2,000 hours of direct patient care or must successfully complete a postprofessional clinical residency program in geriatrics from a credentialed, APTA-accredited program and pass a written examination. To maintain certification, candidates must hold a current license, log a minimum number of patient-care hours in the specialty, and complete a competency assessment.

The PTA works under the direction and supervision of a PT. According to the U.S. Bureau of Labor Statistics, employment of PTAs is expected to grow 40% between 2014 and 2024. According to the APTA, in 2016 there were 353 PTA programs accredited by the CAPTE, and 41 programs in development across the country. Licensure or certification is required for PTAs in all states. An associate's degree from a program accredited by the CAPTE is the minimum educational qualification to become a PTA. The PTA's scope of practice and supervision requirements are defined by the PTA practice act in each state.

The settings in which PTs who treat older adults is quite diverse. They include acute care hospitals, home health, physical therapy private practice, outpatient clinics, acute rehabilitation centers, nursing homes, hospices, fitness centers, integrative care centers, adult day-care centers geriatric sports centers, and academic and research facilities. The myriad of settings reflect the versatility of the skill and knowledge base that a PT has when treating the older adult. PTs who work in geriatrics typically utilize a comprehensive treatment approach when caring for the older adult with acute or chronic illnesses that limit function, impair mobility, and restrict activity participation. PTs use an evidence-based approach to the overall management of these difficult and complex patients by establishing an individualized treatment plan and plan of care.

Physical therapy, as defined by each state's practice act and adopted by the APTA, involve examining patients with impairments, functional limitations, and disabilities in which the

PT determines a physical therapy diagnosis, prognosis, treatment intervention, and individualized plan of care. Patient-directed goals may include, but are not limited to, alleviating impairments and functional limitations by designing, implementing, and modifying therapeutic interventions, as well as preventing injuries and disability, including the promotion and maintenance of fitness, health, and quality of life, through education, and evidenced based practice.

Major sources of reimbursement for physical therapy in the geriatric population are health maintenance organizations (HMOs), Medicare, and Medicaid. Both managed-care companies and Medicare cap the number of PT visits, depending on diagnoses. Every state, the District of Columbia, and the U.S. Virgin Islands have direct access to PTs. This means that the physician referral mandated by state law is removed to access physical therapy services for evaluation and treatment. According to the APTA (2016), "many states continue to impose arbitrary restrictions on direct access, or only allow for treatment without referral under very limited circumstances" ("Directly Benefiting Patients")

It is projected that by 2020, between 9.7 and 13.6 million older people will have moderate to severe functional disability. PTs provide care through direct intervention to individuals who may benefit from such professional consultation with the goal of optimizing physical function.

PTs examine and perform a comprehensive evaluation based on the patient's past medical history, current diagnosis, functional impairment, disability, and review of relevant systems. Specific tests provide baseline data regarding the patient's cardiovascular, neurological, pulmonary, and musculoskeletal systems. Evaluations performed by a PT may include, but are not limited, to motor function, joint integrity and mobility, range of motion, muscle performance, posture, gait and balance, pain, neuromotor development, sensory integration, and aerobic endurance; interventions are likely to produce improvement in the patient's condition. The patient, PT, and other members of the health care team (e.g., occupational therapist,

geriatrician, social worker, geriatric nurse practitioner) determine the plan of care and goals of treatment. The model of physical therapy is an evidence-based practice approach that uses clinical experience, external evidence such as research reports, clinical practice guidelines, and quality indicators.

See also Physical Therapy Services; Rehabilitation.

Sandy B. Ganz

American Board of Physical Therapy Specialists. (2017). Specialist certification. Retrieved from http://www.abpts.org/Certification
American Physical Therapy Association. (2014). *Guide to physical therapist practice 3.0.* (2014). *Table of contents.* Alexandria, VA: Author. Retrieved from http://guidetoptpractice.apta.org
American Physical Therapy Association. (2016). FAQ: Direct access at the state level. Retrieved from http://www.apta.org/StateIssues/DirectAccess/FAQs
Murphy, W. (1995). *A history of physical therapy and the American Physical Therapy Association.* Washington, DC: American Physical Therapy Association.
U.S. Bureau of Labor Statistics, U.S. Department of Labor. (2015). *Occupational outlook handbook, 2016–17 edition.* Retrieved from http://www.bls.gov/ooh/home.htm

Web Resource
APTA Section on Geriatrics: http://geriatricspt.org

PHYSICAL THERAPY SERVICES

Physical therapy is a service provided by physical therapists and physical therapy assistants to assess and treat functional impairments, activity limitations, and participation restrictions that result from disability relating to musculoskeletal, neuromuscular, cardiovascular, pulmonary, or integumentary systems. According to the *Guide to Physical Therapist Practice,* "Physical Therapy is a dynamic profession with an established theoretical and scientific base and widespread clinical applications in the restoration, maintenance, and promotion of optimal physical function" (American Physical Therapy Association [APTA], 2014, para. 4).

The physical therapy treatment of older adults is a challenging endeavor because these individuals often present with a myriad of clinical issues. The goals of physical therapy are to (a) minimize or alleviate pain; (b) reduce or prevent the onset and progression of physical impairments of specific body structures; (c) diminish the functional limitations and disability that result from disease or injury; and (d) restore, maintain, and promote general physical fitness, health, and quality of life (APTA, 2014).

The physical therapist obtains information pertaining to a patient's health status, both past and present, and identifies specific complaints, along with health-risk factors and concomitant problems that have implications for therapeutic intervention. Data obtained from a patient history may include general demographics, social history, occupation or employment, medications, living environment, history of current condition, functional status and activity level, laboratory and diagnostic tests, and past medical, and surgical history. It should also include a family history, self-reported health status, and cognitive and communication ability (APTA, 2014).

SYSTEMS REVIEW

The system review encompasses a brief physical examination of the following systems: (a) cardiovascular/pulmonary system to obtain heart rate, respiratory rate, and blood pressure; (b) integumentary system to assess skin integrity; (c) musculoskeletal system to assess gross range of motion, strength; and (d) neuromuscular system to assess upper- and lower-extremity coordination, balance, transitions from one surface to another (i.e., transfer ability), and motor control. Communication is assessed by patients' ability to follow simple and complex commands and make their needs known; language ability; orientation to person, place, and time; and assessment of learning barriers.

Information obtained during the systems-review assists therapists in determining whether issues that need addressing are within the scope of physical therapy practice or whether the patient needs to be referred to another health care professional. The physical therapist formulates a diagnosis, prognosis, plan of care, and appropriate therapeutic interventions.

Specific Tests and Measures

After synthesizing all pertinent information from the history and systems review, the physical therapist utilizes an evidenced-based approach to determine which tests and measures will be used during the initial evaluation. The purpose of administering specific tests and measures is to enable to physical therapist to rule in or rule out causes of impairment leading to activity limitations and participation restrictions.

Therapists select particular tests and measures based on their psychometric properties (i.e., validity and reliability, sensitivity to change, responsiveness to identifying the minimal detectable change over time). Based on the evaluation the physical therapist determines whether self-report or performance-based measures should be administered to the individual.

There are 26 categories in which physical therapists can select the tests and measures they will use. The categories are aerobic capacity/endurance, anthropometric characteristics, assistive technology, balance, circulation, community, cranial and peripheral nerve integrity, education life, environmental factors, gait, integumentary, joint integrity and mobility, mental function, mobility, motor function, muscle performance, pain, posture, range of motion, reflex integrity, self-care and domestic life, sensory integrity, skeletal integrity, ventilation and respiration, and work life (APTA, 2014). Common tests and measures that are used to assess gait and balance impairments are the Timed Up and Go (TUG) Test (Podsiadlo & Richardson, 1991), Tinetti Gait and Balance test (Tinetti, 1986), Functional Reach Test (Duncan, Weiner, Chandler, & Studenski, 1990), 2-Minute Walk Test (Stewart, Burns, Dunn, & Roberts, 1990), Five Times Sit to Stand

P

Test (Csuka & McCarty, 1985) (see Measuring Physical Function for test descriptions).

The tests and measures that are chosen during the initial assessment provide the clinician with a baseline measurement and ongoing status to determine the effect of the physical therapy intervention. Examples would be the Shoulder Pain and Disability Index (SPADI), which is utilized for patients with shoulder pathology (Breckenridge & McAuley, 2011); the Lower Extremity Functional Scale (LEFS), used for patients with lower-extremity pathology (Binkley, Stratford, Lott, & Riddle, 1999); and the Oswestry Disability Index, utilized for patients with spinal pathology (Fairbank & Pynsent, 2000).

DIAGNOSIS AND PROGNOSIS

Physical therapists use a systematic procedure, also known a *differential diagnosis*, to determine an appropriate diagnostic category. The therapist then synthesizes and integrates the information obtained during the examination to determine the prognosis and individualized plan of care that addresses the patient's impairments and functional limitations. The prognosis is the predicted optimal level of improvement in physical function at various intervals during the course of physical therapy and the amount of time required to reach that level.

INTERVENTION

Physical therapy intervention is broken down into nine categories. The categories are patient instruction (utilized with every patient); airway-clearance techniques; assistive technology; biophysical agents; functional training in self-care, work, community, and social life; integumentary repair and protection techniques; manual therapy techniques; and motor function training and therapeutic exercise.

OUTCOMES

Functional outcomes demonstrate the results of the implementation plan. Measures at the level of pathology, body function, and body structure indicate the success or failure of therapeutic interventions that were administered during an episode of care. The results of the outcome measures demonstrate the value of physical therapy intervention in assisting individuals to achieve both long- and short-term goals.

Sandy B. Ganz

American Physical Therapy Association. (2014). *Guide to physical therapist practice 3.0*. Alexandria, VA: Author. Retrieved from http://guidetoptpractice.apta.org

American Physical Therapy Association. (2017). The physical therapist scope of practice. Retrieved from http://www.apta.org/ScopeOfPractice

Binkley, J. M., Stratford, P. W., Lott, S. A., & Riddle, D. L. (1999). The Lower Extremity Functional Scale (LEFS): Scale development, measurement properties, and clinical application. *Physical Therapy*, 79(4), 371–383.

Breckenridge, J. D., & McAuley, J. H. (2011). Shoulder Pain and Disability Index (SPADI). *Central West Orthopedics & Sports Physiotherapy*, 57(6), 197.

Csuka M., McCarty D. J. (1985). Simple method for measurement of lower extremity muscle strength. *American Journal of Medicine*, 78, 77–81.

Duncan, P. W., Weiner, D. K., Chandler, J., & Studenski, S. (1990). Functional reach: A new clinical measure of balance. *Journal of Gerontology*, 45A(6), M192–M197.

Fairbank, J., & Pynsent, P. (2000). The Oswestry Disability Index. *Spine*, 25, 2490–2953.

Podsiadlo, D., & Richardson, S. (1991). The timed "up and go": A test of basic functional mobility for frail elderly persons. *Journal of the American Geriatrics Society*, 39(2), 142–148.

Stewart, D. A., Burns, J. M. A., Dunn, S. G., & Roberts, M. A. (1990). The two-minute walking test: A sensitive index of mobility in the rehabilitation of elderly patients. *Clinical Rehabilitation*, 4(4), 273–276.

Tinetti, M. E. (1986). Performance-oriented assessment of mobility problems in elderly patients. *Journal of American Geriatrics Society*, 34(2), 119–126.

Web Resource
Rehabilitation Measures Database: http://www.rehabmeasures.org

PHYSICIAN AID IN DYING, PHYSICIAN-ASSISTED SUICIDE, AND EUTHANASIA

Physician aid in dying (PAD) and euthanasia are contentious issues in the United States. In this discussion, *euthanasia* refers to *voluntary active euthanasia*—that is, the intentional termination of life at the person's request as performed by someone other than the patient. Euthanasia is illegal in all states of the United States. PAD, on the other hand, requires that the patient perform the final act of taking a lethal dose of medication that has been prescribed by a physician. *Physician-assisted suicide* (PAS) is another term that has been used for PAD. Indeed, so controversial are these topics that there is disagreement about what to name them. Proponents refer to this practice as *physician aid in dying* and assert, without strong evidence, that only opponents of the practice use the phrase *physician-assisted suicide*. We will use PAD in this article for convenience, without endorsing a particular view of the practice.

In 1997, Oregon became the first state to legalize PAD through the Oregon Death with Dignity Act (DWDA). Vermont, Washington, and California have since passed legislation legalizing PAD; Montana legalized PAD through a court ruling. Although a New Mexico court legalized PAD in Bernalillo County in 2014, this decision was overturned in 2015.

ARGUMENTS FOR AND AGAINST PAD

Autonomy is the primary ethical principle used to support PAD. Proponents of PAD argue that an individual's right to govern personal medical decisions, based on personal beliefs, values, and choices, extends to include requests for PAD. Proponents argue that allowing PAD could alleviate unbearable pain and suffering at the end of life, as well as support a terminally ill patient's desire to control the time of death and avoid burdening the family. In *Vacco v. Quill*, a case that ultimately went to the U.S. Supreme Court, advocates for PAD presented an equity argument. They noted that some patients may facilitate their dying by simply refusing a life-sustaining treatment, such as a ventilator or dialysis. Other patients who are gravely ill may simply refuse a treatment. These patients, it was argued, ought to be offered the option of aid in dying. The Supreme Court determined that there is no constitutional right to assisted suicide but permitted states to draft legislation to support the practice, as several have done.

Opponents of PAD highlight several ethics-based concerns. Opponents argue that legalization of PAD may lead to a slippery slope, resulting in involuntary euthanasia. Second, legalization might result in tiered care, with vulnerable and marginalized patients opting for assisted death because of cost concerns from the medical establishment or weary family members. Third, some argue that PAD violates both the sanctity of human life and physicians' obligations to support life. Finally, opponents contend that a patient's suffering can, almost always, be addressed by palliative care measures.

OREGON

Oregon's DWDA authorizes certain individuals whose death is expected within 6 months to end their lives by taking self-administered lethal medications prescribed by a physician for this purpose. The individual must meet the following additional criteria: be a resident of the state (Oregon), 18 years or older, and capable of making and conveying personal health care decisions. Of note, the requirement for decision-making capacity will likely impede persons with dementia from successfully requesting PAD. Physician participation in the Oregon DWDA is voluntary; physicians who do participate must be an MD or Doctor of Osteopathy (DO) licensed in the state of Oregon.

To obtain a prescription for lethal medications, qualifying individuals must make two separate oral requests to a willing physician, at least 15 days apart, and submit a written request to the physician signed by two witnesses, only one of whom can be related to the patient. The patient must wait 48 hours from the time of their written request to fill the prescription.

The physician, along with a consulting physician, must confirm the individual's diagnosis and prognosis, and ability to make independent health care decisions. If either physician is concerned that the patient may have impaired judgment, referral for a psychological evaluation is required. The physician must also inform the patient of alternatives to PAD, including hospice care and pain control.

The attending physician can request (but not require) that the individual notify his or her next-of-kin of the prescription request. Physicians can decide which medication to prescribe; to date, most patients have received a prescription for oral barbiturates. All requests for PAD must be reported to the Oregon Department of Human Services, which publishes yearly statistics about the DWDA.

An individual can rescind the request at any time. The physician must offer an opportunity for the individual to cancel the request 15 days after the first request is made. Since Oregon's DWDA was passed via referendum in November 1997 and through 2015, 1,545 people have obtained prescriptions for lethal medications; 991 individuals have died after ingesting prescribed medications (Oregon Public Health Division, 2016). In Oregon, patients who participated in PAD were more likely to be middle aged or older (55 years or older), White, married, with a baccalaureate degree or higher. Approximately 9 of 10 patients were enrolled in hospice, and all but 1.5% had health insurance. Most informed their family of the decision to take lethal medications and most died at home (Oregon Public Health Division, "Death with Dignity Act: 2015 data summary").

Since Oregon's DWDA was passed, percentages of participation in PAD have been highest among patients with malignancies, followed by amyotrophic lateral sclerosis (ALS), respiratory disease, heart disease, and HIV/AIDS. End-of-life concerns that contributed to patient requests for aid in dying include loss of autonomy (91.5%), a decreasing ability to participate in activities that make life enjoyable (89%), and loss of dignity (79%). During 2014 and 2015, prescriptions written under the Oregon DWDA increased by an average of 24%, and during 2015, 38.6 per 10,000 deaths resulted after taking prescribed medications. (Oregon Public Health Division, "Death with Dignity Act: 2015 data summary").

WASHINGTON

The Washington DWDA passed via referendum in 2008 and was implemented in 2009. The requirements for individuals requesting PAD are the same as those for Oregon, except individuals making a request must be residents of Washington State. The physician protocols for aiding a patient in their request are also the same as in Oregon, and physicians must report all requests for PAD-related prescriptions to the Department of Health, which publishes yearly reports related to use of the DWDA.

Since Washington's DWDA was passed in 2009 and through 2015, 938 individuals have received prescriptions for lethal medications; 917 have died after taking prescribed medications. In 2015, of the participants who died, 72% had cancer, 8% had a neurodegenerative disease, and 20% had other illnesses, including heart and lung disease; 98% were White, an equal percentage (47%) were married versus widowed/divorced, and 74% had at least some college education. Also in 2015, concerns of patients who participated in Washington's DWDA included loss of autonomy (86%), less ability to participate in enjoyable activities (86%), and loss of dignity (69%) (Washington State Department of Health, 2015).

MONTANA

In 2009, the Montana Supreme Court decided in *Baxter v. Montana* that physicians who prescribe lethal medications to terminally ill, mentally competent individuals would violate no Montana state law. This ruling, cited Montana's Rights of the Terminally Ill Act, shields physicians from prosecution for assisting in suicides requested by a consenting patient; this act finds little difference between removal of life support and prescribing lethal medication to a patient. The Montana court ruling, while providing common-law support for the practice of PAD, provides few guidelines to patients and providers who wish to pursue PAD.

VERMONT

In 2013, Vermont's DWDA—The Vermont Patient Choice and Control at the End of Life Act—was passed. It is very similar to the DWDAs in Oregon and Washington. Although Oregon and Washington passed their acts through referenda, Vermont is the first state to pass a DWDA through the legislative process.

CALIFORNIA

In June 2016, the California End of Life Option Act, modeled after Oregon's DWDA, went into effect. The highly publicized case of Brittany Maynard, a 29-year-old Californian with terminal brain cancer who moved to Oregon in 2014 for PAD, helped spur legislative approval for PAD in California.

REQUESTS FOR AID IN DYING

Despite legal prohibition of PAD in most of the United States, national surveys reveal that approximately one in five physicians have received at least one request to assist a terminally ill individual with dying. Approximately 3% to 18% of physicians who receive requests go on to honor such requests (Meier, Emmons, Litke, Wallenstein, & Morrison, 2003). Requests for aid in dying made to U.S. nurses in various practice settings are also common (Ersek, 2004).

Patients' reasons for requesting hastened death seem to be multifactorial and varied. Some requests are related to the physical, psychological, existential, and social components of suffering (Dees, Vernooij-Dassen, Dekkers, & van Weel, 2010). Depression is correlated with the interest in hastening death, although in the United States, it is unclear whether depression is more prevalent in patients whose request is honored (Levene & Parker, 2011). A person's personality, prior experiences, and level of spirituality/religiosity may also play a role in the request for assistance in dying. Fears about loss of personal dignity or control and becoming a burden to family are other commonly cited reasons (Quill & Arnold, 2008b).

RESPONDING TO REQUESTS

A request for aid in dying should be regarded as an expression of great distress, and should prompt further discussion with the patient (Meier et al., 2003). By eliciting the reasons behind an individual's request, the provider will better understand the patient's perspective and can subsequently provide optimal treatment and support.

When exploring a patient's request for aid in dying, a provider may want to consider clarifying the patient's question (i.e., is the patient asking for the provider's assistance in dying now?); assessing the patient's decision-making capacity; evaluating and treating potential contributing factors (i.e., pain, existential suffering, spiritual distress); and offering ongoing support and commitment to finding a mutually agreeable solution to the request. Providers might find it helpful to discuss a request for aid in dying with trusted colleagues; palliative care and ethics consultants may provide helpful input. Finally, providers should work diligently with the patient and family to explore alternative options to PAD, carefully balancing the commitment to patient autonomy with the integrity of personal moral principles (Quill & Arnold, 2008a).

Hospice and palliative care programs should be discussed with patients and caregivers who request PAD. Palliative care focuses on pain and symptom management for patients with serious illness while also addressing emotional, spiritual, and existential suffering that may be present. Palliative-care providers also provide support for patients' caregivers and are helpful in establishing goals of care based on patients' stated wishes. A patient can receive palliative care while still undergoing active treatment for an underlying disease. Hospice is a benefit of Medicare and many private insurers and provides palliative care in the home (as well as other settings) to patients with life-limiting illness.

When health care providers receive requests for aid in dying, it is imperative to focus on the suffering of patients and on interventions that can help alleviate suffering. In so doing, patients will receive support to live their remaining days

P

with dignity and an acceptable quality of life—one in which euthanasia and assistance in dying are not seen as the only options.

See also Autonomy; Palliative Care; Suicide in Late Life.

Melissa Kurtz and Tia Powell

Dees, M., Vernooij-Dassen, M., Dekkers, W., & van Weel, C. (2010). Unbearable suffering of patients with a request for euthanasia or physician-assisted suicide: An integrative review. *Psycho-Oncology, 19,* 339–352.

Ersek, M. (2004). The continuing challenge of assisted death. *Journal of Hospice and Palliative Nursing,* 6(1), 46–59.

Levene, I., & Parker, M. (2011). Prevalence of depression in granted and refused requests for euthanasia and assisted suicide: A systematic review. *Journal of Medical Ethics, 37,* 205–211.

Meier, D. E., Emmons, C. A., Litke, A., Wallenstein, S., & Morrison, R. S. (2003). Characteristics of patients requesting and receiving physician-assisted death. *Archives of Internal Medicine, 163*(13), 1537–1542.

Oregon Public Health Division. (2016). Oregon Death with Dignity Act: 2015 data summary. Retrieved from http://www.worldrtd.net/sites/default/files/newsfiles/Oregon%20report%202015.pdf

Quill, T., & Arnold, R. M. (2008a). Evaluating requests for hastened death #156. *Journal of Palliative Medicine, 11*(8), 1151–1152.

Quill, T., & Arnold, R. M. (2008b). Responding to a request for hastening death #159. *Journal of Palliative Medicine, 11*(8), 1152–1153.

Washington State Department of Health. (2015). Washington State Department of Health 2015 Death with Dignity Act report: Executive summary. Retrieved from https://slide.world/view/JlmAGGb-VnAJ

Web Resources

Death with Dignity National Center: California: http://californiadeathwithdignity.org

Death with Dignity National Center: Montana: https://www.deathwithdignity.org/states/montana

Death with Dignity National Center: Vermont: http://www.deathwithdignity.org/states/vermont

Death with Dignity National Center: Washington: http://www.deathwithdignity.org/states/washington

Education in Palliative and End-of-Life Care (EPEC): http://www.epec.net

Legal Encyclopedia: Death with dignity in Montana: http://www.nolo.com/legal-encyclopedia/death-with-dignity-montana.html

National Hospice and Palliative Care Organization: Hospice and palliative care: http://www.nhpco.org/about/hospice-and-palliative-care

Oregon Health Authority: Oregon revised statute: https://public.health.oregon.gov/ProviderPartnerResources/EvaluationResearch/DeathwithDignityAct/Pages/ors.aspx

Oregon Public Health Division: Oregon Death with Dignity Act: 2015 data summary: http://public.health.oregon.gov/ProviderPartnerResources/EvaluationResearch/DeathwithDignityAct/Pages/index.aspx

Vacco v. Quill, 117 S. Ct. 2293 (1997): https://www.law.cornell.edu/supct/html/95-1858.ZS.html

Washington State Department of Health: Washington State Department of Health 2015 Death with Dignity Act Report: Executive Summary: http://www.doh.wa.gov/portals/1/Documents/Pubs/422–109-DeathWithDignityAct2012.pdf

PIONEER NETWORK

Pioneer Network is a 501c(3) organization formed in 1997 by professionals in long-term care and aging services to advocate for transforming care environments and organizational culture to support person-directed care. This group called for a radical change in the culture of aging so that when one moves to a nursing home or receives support in another community-based setting, it is to thrive, not to decline. This movement—away from institutional, task-oriented models to more humane consumer-driven models that embrace flexibility and self-determination—has come to be known as the long-term care *culture change* movement. Pioneer Network's partners and audience are primarily engaged in some aspect of long-term care services and supports, including long-term care chief executive officers and administrators, consumers and family caregivers, physicians and nurses, direct caregivers, and others who care about, and care for, the aging.

Now in its 20th year, Pioneer Network has earned a reputation as the voice of the culture change movement for the transformation of long-term care services and supports and is considered the national convener for essential dialogue in the culture change movement. As such, it has contributed strategic and substantive work in the field of aging and care of elders. As a national convener, Pioneer Network maintains a relationship with state and federal policy makers, including the Centers for Medicare & Medicaid Services (CMS). In April 2008 and in February 2010, CMS cosponsored with Pioneer Network two national symposia, Creating Home in the Nursing Home I and II, to promote discussion, dispel barriers, and coordinate action that supports culture change in nursing home environments. The symposia and follow-up efforts were extensive, including:

1. Revisions to the Guidance to Surveyors (often referred to as Interpretive Guidelines) for several regulatory requirements related to quality of life and physical environment. These changes add clarifications to assist surveyors in determining compliance with these requirements and have ground-breaking implications for resident choice, the physical environment, and quality of life.
2. Revisions to the National Fire Protection Association (NFPA) 2012 edition of the Life Safety Code that remove unintended barriers and support creation of the home in the nursing home (recommended by a Pioneer Network–convened task force with funding from the Hulda B. and Maurice L. Rothschild Foundation).
3. Development of new Dining Practice Standards through a Pioneer Network–convened task force (with funding from the Hulda B. and Maurice L. Rothschild Foundation) and endorsed by CMS.

With support from The Commonwealth Fund, Pioneer Network convened a medical advisory panel to discuss and create core competencies of culture change for medical directors. The panel developed competency statements related to each of the existing "function and task" guidelines of the AMDA—The Society for Post-Acute and Long-Term Medicine. A person-directed task force of AMDA medical directors then further refined the list to create a ninth function with six task statements to promote the medical director's role in person-directed care in

long-term care settings. Also, with support from The Commonwealth Fund, Pioneer Network convened a core group of expert gerontological nurses to develop core competencies specific to nursing home culture change. Ten competencies were finalized after extensive input from nurses throughout the country. These 10 competencies are deemed most relevant and critical for nurses to be successful in creating and sustaining person-directed care in nursing homes.

Pioneer Network is committed to studying how adoption of culture change practices translates into outcomes and quantifiable metrics and to benchmarking those metrics with national data. Outcomes to support the efficacy of culture change are documented through anecdotal accounts, qualitative evaluation, and empirical studies and can be categorized into four broad impact areas:

1. Organizational impact in areas such as increased levels of occupancy, increased percentage of private pay census, reduction in the use of agency staff, and increases to operating margins and improved market position
2. Quality-of-care impact through reductions in the use of restraints, weight loss, falls, agitation, pressure injuries, medication use, and re-hospitalizations
3. Staffing impact through reductions in turnover, low or no use of agency staff, and increased levels of staff satisfaction
4. Life-engagement impact as measured through improved levels of resident well-being, especially in residents with chronic health conditions or dementia (measured by minimum data set [MDS] 3.0).

Through collaborative partnerships with other like-minded national organizations, Pioneer Network's impact is evident in hundreds of organizations and for individuals that have collaborated with and benefitted from its commitment to creating humane environments for older Americans to interact with and in which to live and flourish. Over 10,000 individuals are connected with Pioneer Network to receive updates on culture change innovation through a national network of stakeholders. Pioneer Network believes that the quality of life and living for America's elders is rooted in a supportive community and cemented by relationships that respect each person as an individual regardless of age, medical condition, and physical or cognitive limitations.

Lynda Crandall and Ruta Kadonoff

Web Resource
Pioneer Network: https://www.pioneernetwork.net

PODIATRIC MEDICINE

The American Podiatric Medical Association defines podiatrists as qualified doctors who diagnose and treat conditions of the foot, ankle, and related structures of the leg (APMA, 2017).

Podogeriatrics as a special area of practice focuses on the prevention, education, and treatment of diseases and disorders of the foot, ankle, and related structures including focal diseases, disorders, disabilities, deformities, and complications of systemic diseases associated with aging. Foot conditions may be focal in etiology or result from complications associated with multiple chronic diseases such as diabetes mellitus, peripheral arterial disease, neurological deficits, and various forms of arthritis, as well as changes associated with the aging process itself. Given that older persons tend to react to illness, deformity, and disease differently from younger persons, caring for geriatric patients must include an understanding of both the specific syndromes that older patients experience and team skills (Helfand, 2003).

Foot problems occur universally. By age 65 years, almost 90% of the population has had one or more foot problems that caused some level of discomfort, pain, ambulatory dysfunction, or functional disability and that negatively impact quality of life and reduces the activities and instrumental activities of daily living. Some factors contributing to the development of foot and related problems in older patients include ambulatory dysfunction, prior hospitalization, pedal manifestations of systemic disease, mental status change, increased drug sensitivity, and increased susceptibility to local infection because of neurovascular impairment. Older patients and those with chronic diseases such as diabetes mellitus, peripheral arterial insufficiency, and the various forms of arthritis exhibit foot complaints. Many chronic systemic diseases are first manifest by foot symptoms (Arenson et al., 2009; Armstrong & Lavery, 2005; Halter et al., 2009).

The ability to walk pain-free enhances an active lifestyle in older and chronically ill patients. Concern about the prevention and early detection of disease, deformity, and disability, as well as the ability to stratify risk, reduces the prevalence of foot disability in later life. Programs for older patients must focus on prevention—primary, secondary, and tertiary—and offer comprehensive services and access based on patient need, with the goals of providing quality care and maintaining the quality of life.

EDUCATION

Doctors of Podiatric Medicine are licensed to practice in all states and the District of Columbia. Attaining this degree requires 4 years of academic study at a school or college of podiatric medicine accredited by the Council on Podiatric Medical Education of the American Podiatric Medical Association, preceded by preprofessional undergraduate degree education and followed by podiatric medical and surgical residencies with added qualifications in reconstructive rear-foot and ankle surgery in the majority of programs (3 years), specialty fellowships, and continuing education, that are compatible with and supportive to programs in the other health professions. The educational program in podiatric medicine is competency based and includes education, training, licensure, certification, and credentialing processes.

Primary training in clinical geriatrics occurs during the first professional degree and subsequent residency education. Continuing education programs provide additional training and fellowships that enhance clinical knowledge by focusing on academic elements. Many podiatrists are in solo or small group practices, but interdisciplinary team care and health system-based programs are expanding.

The basic education at the nine schools or colleges of podiatric medicine provides a core curriculum in the basic medical sciences, similar to those in the medical, dental, and osteopathic medical programs. In addition, the basic clinical aspects of podiatric and medical care include biomechanics, pathomechanics, medicine, gerontology, and clinical podiatric medicine and surgery. Didactic clinical education includes medical areas such as peripheral vascular disease, neurology, dermatology, radiology, orthopedics, general and podiatric surgery, public health, preventive medicine, jurisprudence, ethics, and the psychosocial aspects of patient management. Practical clinical education includes ambulatory clinical care, inpatient hospital care, clerkships, and institutional externships, including long-term care. Segments of clinical education are enhanced through affiliations with the Department of Veterans Affairs, university, and community hospitals, ambulatory community care health systems, and long-term care and rehabilitation programs.

The core program prepares new practitioners for their roles as primary providers of foot and ankle care and prepares students for educational programs beyond the first professional degree, such as residencies, fellowships, graduate education, and continuing education. Specific areas include podiatric surgery, podiatric medicine, and orthopedics, leading to board certification in these specialized areas of care. Each state defines the scope of practice and prescribes the requirements for licensure, which may include examinations provided by the National Board of Podiatric Medical Examiners or appropriate examinations or endorsements provided by the various state licensing agencies. The scope of podiatric medical and surgical practice is defined by each state law, as is the case for all health disciplines.

PODIATRIC MEDICAL MANAGEMENT

Care provided by podiatric physicians includes services for ambulatory patients, hospitalized patients, and patients in post-acute and long-term care settings. Education, preventive services, and assessment may also be provided as a part of community, agency, and public health programs. In general, care components include the history,

physical examination, assessment, risk stratification, imaging and radiographs, laboratory studies, and other special diagnostic tests, such as those related to biomechanics, pathomechanics, and neurological and vascular analysis (Helfand, 2006, 2007; Helfand & Jessett, 2012; Menz, 2008; Turner & Merriman, 2005; Yates, 2008).

Neurological, vascular, musculoskeletal, dermatological, onychial, and other related conditions should be managed primarily, with appropriate consultation, as indicated. Debridement, pathomechanical, orthopedic, biomechanical, imaging, radiographic, orthotic, surgical, primary podiatric medical, and dermatological procedures are elements of total patient management. Conservative and surgical management are within the purview of podiatry. Health education, preventive services, assessment, and surveillance, as well as continuing education, should be a major component of care for older patients.

REIMBURSEMENT

Third-party reimbursement for podiatric services is similar to that for Medicare and private insurance. In 1967, podiatrists were included in the Medicare regulations and considered physicians with respect to the services they are legally authorized to perform by the state (§1861r, Social Security Act). Certain types of treatment or foot care are excluded, whether performed by a doctor of medicine, doctor of osteopathic medicine, or doctor of podiatric medicine. These exclusions are generally defined as routine foot care in the absence of systemic and localized illness, injury, or symptoms involving the foot and related structures. Services are covered when systemic conditions such as metabolic, neurological, or peripheral vascular disease result in vascular compromise or areas of diminished sensation in the feet or legs and evidence documents that inappropriate care would be hazardous for the patient because of underlying systemic disease. Examples of covered diseases include peripheral arterial disease, diabetes mellitus, peripheral neuropathy, and multiple sclerosis. The U.S. Department of Veterans Affairs, however, takes a more enlightened prevention-oriented view of eligibility for basic foot care and includes patients who are visually or cognitively impaired, who may have severe arthritis or chronic low back pain, or who are on anticoagulant therapy.

Pain alone may not be an indication for coverage. Patients must be under active care of a primary care physician or specialist for the covered medical conditions and have clinical findings, known as *class findings*, such as nontraumatic amputation, edema, absent pulses, claudication, trophic changes in hair growth, thickened toenails, skin changes, decreased temperature, cyanosis, and/or clinical findings associated with neurosensory deficits. Because the majority of foot problems in older patients are chronic and related to other diseases, disorders, and systemic diseases, it is important that management includes continuing surveillance, assessment, and care. Other risk factors include visual impairment, physical impairment, neuromuscular diseases such as Parkinson's disease, arthritis with deformity, spinal disc disease, cognitive dysfunction, mental illness, anticoagulant therapy, chronic edema, dialysis, obesity, the inability to bend, and long-term institutionalization.

The 1981 White House Conference on Aging in its Recommendation #148 stated, "Comprehensive foot care should be provided for the elderly in a manner equal to care provided for other parts of the body." This key position speaks to the need and right of foot care for all. The inclusion of appropriate podiatric services in care programs for the elderly often produce dramatic effects. Immobility can be replaced by activity. Quality of care translates into improved quality of life. Support and encouragement can be directed to independence and a strong sense of personal identify and worth. Isolation can be replaced by interaction. When the quality of life decreases because of disease, disability, or age, those precious aspects must be restored to a maximum level by those who care for patients. Because ambulation is an important catalyst for quality of life, podiatric care can help regain some of the lost dignity by keeping patients walking and moving so that they can live life to the end with the dignity of age.

See also Foot Problems.

Arthur E. Helfand and Jeffrey M. Robbins

American Podiatric Medical Association. (2017). What is a podiatrist? Retrieved from https://www.apma.org/learn/content.cfm?ItemNumber=992&navItemNumber=558

Arenson, C., Bubby-Whitehead, J., Brummel-Smith, K., O'Brien, J. G., Palmer, M. H., & Reichel, W. M. (2009). *Reichel's care of the elderly: Clinical aspects of aging* (6th ed.). New York, NY: Cambridge University Press.

Armstrong, D. G., & Lavery, L. A. (2005). *Clinical care of the diabetic foot.* Alexandria, VA: American Diabetes Association.

Halter, J. B., Ouslander, J. G., Tinetti, M. E., Studenski, S., High, K. P., & Asthana, S. (2009). *Hazzard's geriatric medicine and gerontology* (6th ed.). New York, NY: McGraw-Hill.

Helfand, A. E. (2003). Clinical podogeriatrics: Assessment, education, and prevention: *Clinics in Podiatric Medicine and Surgery, 20,* xvii–xxiii.

Helfand, A. E. (2006). *Public health and podiatric medicine: Principles and practice* (2nd ed.). Washington, DC: American Public Health Association Press.

Helfand, A. E. (2007). *Foot health training guide for long term care personnel.* Baltimore, MD: Health Professions Press.

Helfand, A. E., & Jessett, D. F. (2012). Foot problems in the elderly. In A. J. Sinclair, J. E. Morley, & B. Vellas (Eds.), *Pathy's principles and practice of geriatric medicine* (5th ed., pp. 1111–1130). Oxford, UK: John Wiley.

Menz, H. B. (2008). *Foot problems in older people—assessment and management.* Philadelphia, PA: Churchill Livingstone Elsevier.

Turner, W. A., & Merriman, L. M. (2005). *Clinical skills in treating the foot* (2nd ed.). London, UK: Churchill Livingstone Elsevier.

White House Conference on Aging. (1981). *Final report, the 1981 White House Conference on Aging.* Washington, DC: Author.

Yates, B. (2008). *Merriman's assessment of the lower limb* (3rd ed.). London, UK: Churchill Livingstone Elsevier.

Web Resource
National Institute on Aging: http://www.niapublications.org/engagepages/footcare.asp

POLYPHARMACY

Persons aged 65 years and older are prescribed the highest proportion of medication in relation to the percentage of the U.S. population. Approximately 13% of the U.S. population is age 65 years and older. This group purchases 33% of all prescription drugs. These figures are expected to increase. The U.S. Census Bureau reported that between 2010 and 2050, the United States is projected to experience rapid growth in its older population. In 2050, the number of Americans aged 65 years and older is projected to be 88.5 million, more than double its population of 40.2 million in 2010 (Campanelli, 2012).

Older adults are at risk of encountering polypharmacy because they have multiple comorbidities and have various health care providers. Several important pharmacological and nonpharmacological issues influence the safety and effectiveness of drug therapy in geriatric patients. Awareness of pharmacodynamics principles is key when treating older adults with multiple comorbidities. Adverse drug reactions occur about twice as often in older as younger patients. Inappropriate prescribing occurs when the risk of medication outweighs the benefits. Therefore understanding pharmacodynamics, risks, benefits, and consequences of drug therapy in older patient is very important.

Pharmacologic treatment among elderly patients is complex. *Pharmacodynamics* refers to the effect the drug has on an individual at the organ site. The physiological changes that accompany aging affect the pharmacologic processes of absorption, distribution, metabolism, and excretion. There is little change in absorption with increasing age. It is important to remember that some medications can affect the absorption of other medications. Some factors that alter absorption in the elderly include drug–drug interaction, drug–food interaction, and drug–disease interaction. There is a reduction in lean body mass with aging and an increase in body fat, thus resulting in a reduction in total body water. Drugs, such as digoxin, are considered hydrophilic and have a lower volume of distribution. Their concentration is higher, so when prescribing these medications, one may need to use lower doses. On the other hand, lipophilic drugs have a longer half-life, and their volume of distribution is high. Metabolism is affected by aging. Most drugs' metabolism takes place in the liver. There is a decrease in the size, mass, and blood flow of the liver with aging, which reduces drug metabolism. It may also decrease the rate of biotransformation of some drugs. Most drugs are excreted through the kidney; in general, renal function is reduced with advancing age, although there is marked individual variation.

It is crucial for all providers to perform medication reconciliation and include vitamins, herbal preparations, and over-the-counter medications. The prevalence of complementary and alternative medication is increasing among older adults. Over-the-counter medications or alternative medications have been associated with adverse events. Likewise, important drug interactions between these types of medications and conventional drug therapies have been described. Therefore it is imperative to perform a complete medication history in older adults. Maintaining an active medication list is one of the objectives listed in the Centers for Medicare & Medicaid Services (CMS) meaningful use of the electronic medical record.

Concerns about polypharmacy should not deprive patients of needed medications. Although elders' excessive use of medications is well documented, the underuse of clinically indicated medications is also receiving attention. Several studies have reported substantial levels of undertreatment of chronic conditions in the elderly. Rates of undertreatment have been reported to be as high as 60% for management of some chronic conditions, including osteoporosis, hypertension, and depression. Thus it is critical when managing polypharmacy that health care providers optimize medication management, avoiding both the underuse of beneficial medications and the excessive and inappropriate use of drugs.

Prescribing the appropriate medications is important for the delivery of safe and quality care. Polypharmacy, however, can lead to patient nonadherence, adverse drug reactions, and inappropriate prescribing. The risk for polypharmacy increases with age, and approximately half of hospitalized patients are prescribed more medications on discharge than they were taking 1 month before admission.

Comprehensive geriatrics assessment can be used as an intervention for polypharmacy.

Patients' medications should be assessed regularly and reconciled in the electronic medical record. Collaboration with pharmacists is important. Pharmacists can review drug inconsistencies and can help address difficulties with adherence to medications. Pharmacists can foresee inappropriate prescribing, potential side effects, and drug–drug interactions. Many electronic medical record systems can likewise be programmed to alert prescribers of potential drug–drug interactions.

Improving the quality of life for patients should be the focus when adding or withdrawing a medication. Adverse drug events are associated with inappropriately prescribed medications, drug-drug interactions, or drug–disease interactions. To decrease the risk of adverse drug events, prescribers should attempt to decrease the number of medications, especially potentially inappropriate medications (PIMs). Staff education with an academic focus is an effective intervention in nursing homes.

The Beers criteria can be used to identify PIMs. The Beers criteria list is an important evidence-based tool, but it does not cancel clinical judgment or override patient's values and preferences (Campanelli, 2012).

The Beers criteria were developed to decrease the use of inappropriate medications in nursing homes. Potential inappropriate prescribing can occur when risks outweigh benefits; as a result, the Beers list was expanded to primary care and inpatient settings and has been revised multiple times. The Beers list should always be reviewed and updated because medication prescription is always changing. Beers criteria were updated in 2015 to incorporate new evidence on current PIMs for older adults, grading the strength and quality of each PIM based on level of evidence and strength of recommendation, and to make the criteria more individualized in clinical practice and settings (AGS, 2015).

The 2015 updated criteria added new medications, dose adjustments for new medications for those with kidney impairment, and added selected drug–drug interactions. The criteria also include a quality of evidence and strength of recommendation. Recent changes of the 2015 criteria include a revision to nitrofurantoin use; it can be used with relative safety and efficacy with a creatinine clearance of greater than or equal to 30 mL/min versus the 2012 guidelines of not to use if creatinine clearance less than 60 mL/min. The recommendation to avoid classes 1a, 1c, and III antiarrhythmic drugs for atrial fibrillation were removed. Several updates were added to the criteria, including (a) any prescription of proton pump inhibitors not exceeding 8 weeks without justification because of association with *Clostridium difficile* infection, bone loss, and fractures; (b) avoidance of desmopressin for nocturia or nocturnal polyuria because of risk of hyponatremia; (c) avoidance of benzodiazepine receptor agonist hypnotics and non-benzodiazepines for persons with cognitive impairment; and (d) avoidance of opioids for those with a history of falls.

Drug–drug interactions were added to the criteria, such as prescribing peripheral alpha-blockers used with loop diuretics, prescribing three or more central nervous system-active drugs together, prescribing angiotensin-converting enzyme inhibitors (ACEIs) with potassium-sparing diuretics, and prescribing lithium with an ACEI or a loop diuretic. Non–anti-infective medications were added to the list of PIMs to be avoided based on kidney function. The American Geriatrics Society (AGS) publication contains a list of the all updated criteria (AGS, 2015).

In the 2015 updated AGS Beers criteria, it is important to mention the rational to avoid antipsychotics in older adults. The rational was modified to "avoid antipsychotics for behavioral problems unless nonpharmacologic options have failed or are not possible, and the older adult is threatening substantial harm to self or others" (AGS, 2015, p. 15). Beers criteria encourage the use of nonpharmacologic interventions in older adults with delirium or dementia.

Patients should be educated about the medications that they are prescribed. For each medication they should know the generic and brand name, the disease or problem it is intended to treat, the way to take it, any important food or drug interactions, its desired responses or therapeutic goals, and commonly encountered side effects. This information should be provided verbally and in writing and individualized for each patient. The electronic medical record can provide an automated summary of all of medications at the end of each outpatient visit. A strategy called *teach back* may be helpful in reviewing whether the patient understands the instructions.

Patients with complicated medication regimens (or those with cognitive impairment) may have difficulty remembering all the necessary information about their medications. Such patients may benefit from keeping a written list of their medications or having a caregiver maintain a pillbox for them. Some persons with cognitive impairment require additional support for taking medications.

See also Geriatric Consultation.

Jonny A. Macias Tejada
and Laila M. Hasan

American Geriatrics Society. (2015). Updated Beers criteria for potentially inappropriate medication use in older adults. *Journal of the American Geriatrics Society*, 63(11), 2227–2246.

Boparai, M. K., & Korc-Grodzicki, B. (2011). Prescribing for older adults. *Mount Sinai Journal of Medicine*, 78(4), 613–626.

Campanelli, C. M. (2012). American Geriatrics Society updated Beers criteria for potentially inappropriate medication use in older adults: The American Geriatrics Society 2012 Beers Criteria Update Expert Panel. *Journal of the American Geriatrics Society*, 60(4), 616.

Duthie, E. H. (2006). Geriatrics. *Journal of the American Geriatrics Society*, 54(10), 1628–1629.

Gokula, M., & Holmes, H. M. (2012). Tools to reduce polypharmacy. *Clinics in Geriatric Medicine*, 28(2), 323–341.

Landefeld, C. S., Palmer, R. M., Johnson, M., Johnston, C. B., & Lyons, W. L. (2004). *Current geriatric diagnosis and treatment*. New York, NY: Lange Medical Books/McGraw-Hill.

Pacala, J. T., & Sullivan, G. M. (Eds.). (2010). *Geriatrics review syllabus: A core curriculum in geriatric medicine* (7th ed.). New York, NY: American Geriatrics Society.

Sergi, G., De Rui, M., Sarti, S., & Manzato, E. (2011). Polypharmacy in the elderly: Can comprehensive geriatric assessment reduce inappropriate medication use? *Drugs & Aging*, 28(7), 509–518.

Terrey, C., & Nicoteri, J. (2016). The 2015 American Geriatrics Society Beers criteria: Implications for nurse practitioners. *Journal for Nurse Practitioners*, 12(3), 192–200.

Web Resource
American Geriatrics Society: Updated Beers criteria for potentially inappropriate medication use in older adults: http://www.americangeriatrics .org/files/documents/beers/2012BeersCriteria_ JAGS.pdf

POLYPHARMACY: DRUG–DRUG INTERACTIONS

Polypharmacy can be defined as the use of five or more chronic medications, although the administration of more medication than is clinically indicated is another definition (Patterson et al., 2014). Older people take more prescription and over-the-counter (OTC) medications than younger people. Although those 65 years and older constitute only 14.5% of the population, they consume 34% of all prescribed drugs and 30% of OTC drugs. In 2010, 39% of people older than 65 years were taking five or more medications, an increase from 13% 20 years earlier (Charlesworth, Smit, Lee, Alramadhan, & Odden, 2015). Some medications are absorbed, distributed, metabolized, and excreted (pharmacokinetics) differently in older adults, and the action of drugs (pharmacodynamics) may be exaggerated or diminished. Of special significance in the older population, different drugs interact with one another either by pharmacokinetic inhibition or induction of drug metabolism or by pharmacodynamic potentiation or antagonism. Knowledge of these pharmacological pathways has a profound impact on the quality of medical care.

Polypharmacy mishaps in older adults occur for numerous reasons (AGS, 2015). Older patients often have multiple providers, who may be unaware of one another's new prescriptions or medication changes, especially after hospitalization (Brown, Hutchison, Li, Painter, & Martin,

P

2016). Older patients may have visual and cognitive impairments that may likewise lead to errors in self-administration. Older patients who are unable to afford to take all of their medicines consistently may be too embarrassed to tell their providers and may overdose when they take all medicines as prescribed (e.g., when a patient is admitted to the hospital from home). Functional illiteracy, which is not uncommon among older individuals, makes adherence to a medical regimen difficult. Finally, the average clinician is not knowledgeable about the vast number of possible drug interactions. Computer databases may not reflect all interactions or may display too many, making it difficult to identify the clinically important ones.

Although changes in drug metabolism in healthy older persons are often minimal and not clinically significant, the clinical impact of these changes in those with kidney or liver disease can be considerable. Adverse drug reactions are two to three times more likely to occur in older patients. In general, drug absorption is complete in older persons, although it often occurs at a slower rate. Bioavailability, the fraction of an oral drug reaching the systemic circulation, depends on absorption and first-pass metabolism. Some drugs have increased bioavailability (e.g., labetalol, levodopa, nifedipine, omeprazole) in the elderly.

Drug distribution can change because of age-related alterations in body composition. Weight is reduced, percentage of body fat is increased, and total body water and lean mass are decreased. Hydrophilic drugs have a higher concentration because they are distributed in a smaller volume of body water. Lipophilic drugs have a larger volume of distribution and a longer half-life because they are distributed in a larger volume of fat. Decreased albumin and other binding proteins may or may not affect the active drug (free) concentration (Wooten, 2012).

Hepatic metabolism varies greatly among individuals based on age, sex, lifestyle, hepatic blood flow, presence of liver disease, and other factors. Although enzymes are usually unchanged by aging, many drugs are metabolized more slowly in older people because of a reduction in hepatic blood flow. Renal excretion

of drugs diminishes by 35% to 50% because of decreased glomerular filtration rate (GFR). However, because of decreased muscle mass, measurement of serum creatinine does not reflect GFR. Furthermore, many formulas for estimating creatinine clearance (based on age, weight, and creatinine) are inaccurate. Obtaining a 24-hour urine collection for creatinine clearance is the most accurate way of calculating the GFR. The approach to medication dose reduction for older patients is similar to that for patients with kidney dysfunction.

These age-related pharmacokinetic changes result in a longer drug half-life, a diminished clearance, and a longer time to reach a steady state. This is reflected in different serum levels for a given dose. Because of age-related pharmacodynamic changes, drugs have a different effect at the same serum level. For example, opioids have a greater analgesic effect, benzodiazepines have a greater sedative effect, and anticoagulants are associated with a higher risk of bleeding. Beta-blockers, in contrast, are less effective in older patients.

DRUG–DRUG INTERACTIONS

When more than one drug is taken, age-related pharmacokinetic and pharmacodynamic considerations may complicate drug interactions (Lavan, Gallagher, & O'Mahony, 2016). Some interactions result in less drug being available through the mechanisms of impaired absorption, induced hepatic enzymes, and inhibition of cellular uptake. Impaired absorption can be because of binding by a concurrently administered drug, such as cholestyramine-binding digoxin and thyroxine. Administering these drugs 2 hours apart helps minimize this interaction.

Certain drugs induce hepatic metabolic enzymes in the cytochrome P450 (CYP) system. It may take weeks for these enzymes to become maximally active. Increased enzyme supply breaks down the active drug and causes less drug delivery. This occurs with drugs such as phenobarbital, rifampin, and phenytoin. Smoking and chronic alcohol use can induce similar effects. Hepatic enzyme induction results in lower levels of warfarin, quinidine, verapamil, cyclosporine, methadone, and many other medications. Inhibition of cellular uptake or binding may produce less drug availability. The interaction of clonidine and tricyclic antidepressants occurs through this mechanism, diminishing the efficacy of both drugs.

Interactions that result in more drug availability include inhibition of metabolic enzymes and inhibition of renal excretion. Inhibition of metabolism leads to increased half-life, accumulation of the drug, and potential toxicity. Inhibition, unlike induction, can occur immediately. The mixed-function oxidase system and its isoforms allow prediction of potential interactions. For example, CYP3A metabolizes cyclosporine, quinidine, lovastatin, warfarin, nifedipine, lidocaine, erythromycin, methylprednisolone, carbamazepine, and triazolam. Many of these medications are also inhibitors of the same CYP oxidase system. Cyclosporine can reach toxic levels if administered with erythromycin. CYP2C19 is inhibited by omeprazole and decreases the conversion of clopidogrel to its active metabolite, which makes clopidogrel less effective as an antiplatelet agent. Inhibition of renal excretion causes more drug availability. For example, probenecid inhibits the excretion of penicillin. Clinicians can utilize this interaction to prolong the half-life of penicillin.

The drug efflux transporter P-glycoprotein (P-gp) can be inhibited or induced by drug interactions. Drugs that affect CYP3A4 are likely to affect P-gp. Many drugs, including digoxin, non-sedating antihistamines, cyclosporine, some protease inhibitors, and some anticancer drugs require this transporter in the gastrointestinal tract, liver, and kidney for excretion to occur. The role of other drug transporters in drug–drug interactions is an area of active research.

Pharmacodynamic interactions are those in which the actions of different drugs affect the same end point. Warfarin and aspirin interact by increasing the likelihood of bleeding through separate pathways. Similarly, warfarin and nonsteroidal anti-inflammatory drugs (NSAIDs) make gastrointestinal bleeding more likely. NSAIDs also raise blood pressure and may undermine the action of antihypertensive agents.

MANAGING A PATIENT ON MULTIPLE MEDICATIONS

With careful attention to the drug regimen, physicians, nurses, pharmacists, and older patients themselves can reduce the risk of serious drug–drug interactions.

- Be aware of all medications the patient is taking, including OTCs, vitamins, and herbal remedies. One method is to ask patients to bring all their medications to each office visit ("the brown paper bag"). The practitioner may be surprised by the medications other providers have prescribed, by old prescriptions still being refilled at the pharmacy, and by the range of OTC drugs the patient is using. Another approach for avoiding polypharmacy is to provide older patients with a "medication passport" that lists all medicines they are taking. The patient shows this list to subspecialists and to the primary provider at each visit.
- Start all new medications at low doses and increase the strength slowly ("start low, go slow"). Limit the number of medications to as few as necessary, and routinely review all drugs. Attempt to withdraw ("deprescribe") any unnecessary agents and consider non-drug therapy. Continue to monitor effects of medications and be alert to the development of adverse drug effects at any time during therapeutic use, not just when initiating treatment (Lavan et al., 2016).
- Be cautious with newly released medications. Report any adverse reactions, working closely with pharmacists, drug manufacturers, and public health departments. Investigate all complaints, as they may point to drug–drug interactions. Drug toxicity and drug interactions should be part of the differential diagnosis for altered mental status, fatigue, incontinence, gait disorder, and other geriatric syndromes (Lavan et al., 2016).
- Institute plans to monitor drug-treatment programs on a regular basis in institutional settings.
- In the home setting, use reminders, pillboxes, and other memory aids to reduce errors

and enhance compliance. Attention to the patient's individual needs, with compensation for any specific functional or cognitive impairment, is critical. Family members and personal caregivers should be trained to monitor medication adherence and to report any difficulties.

- Use computer databases and drug-interaction software to check for known interactions. The pharmacy should have a record of all the medications the patient is taking, even those supplied elsewhere. The patient and health care provider should also have this updated record of medications, including OTC and herbal treatments. Some websites allow easy creation of such a record.
  - Avoid giving a medication to counter the effects of another medication (e.g., giving antiparkinsonian medication to treat the rigidity caused by antipsychotics or metoclopramide). The best approach is to lower the dose or substitute another agent for the offending one.
  - Check for food–drug interactions, such as grapefruit juice potentiating buspirone or simvastatin, among many others.

Barrie L. Raik

American Geriatrics Society. (2015). Updated Beers criteria for potentially inappropriate medication use in older adults. *Journal of American Geriatrics Society, 63,* 2227–2246.

Brown, J. D., Hutchison, L. C., Li, C., Painter, J. T., & Martin, B. C. (2016). Predictive validity of the Beers and Screening Tool of Older Persons' Potentially inappropriate Prescriptions (STOPP) criteria to detect adverse drug events, hospitalizations, and emergency department visits in the United States. *Journal of the American Geriatrics Society, 64,* 22–30.

Charlesworth, C. J., Smit, E., Lee, D. S. H., Alramadhan, F., Odden, M. C. (2015). Polypharmacy among adults aged 65 years and older in the United States: 1988–2010. *Journals of Gerontology: Medical Science, 70*(8), 989–995.

Lavan, A. H., Gallagher, P. F., & O'Mahony, D. (2016). Methods to reduce prescribing errors in elderly patients with multimorbidity. *Clinical Interventions in Aging, 11,* 857–866.

Patterson, S. M., Cadogan, C. A., Kerse, N., Cardwell, C. R., Bradley, M, Ryan, C., & Hughes, C. (2014). Interventions to improve the appropriate use of polypharmacy for older people. *Cochrane Database of Systematic Reviews, 10,* CD008165. doi:10.1002/14651858.CD008165.pub2

Wooten, J. M. (2012). Pharmacotherapy considerations in elderly adults. *Southern Medical Journal, 105*(8), 437–445.

Web Resources

Center for Education and Research on Therapeutics: Drug interaction and medication list generator resource: http://www.azcert.org

Commercial Site (user friendly to check drug interactions): http://www.drugs.com/drug_interactions.html

Flockhart, D. A. (2007). Drug interactions: Cytochrome P450 drug interaction table. Indiana University School of Medicine: http://medicine.iupui.edu/clinpharm/ddis/table.aspx

Preventable Adverse Drug Reactions (professional presentation): http://www.fda.gov/Drugs/DevelopmentApprovalProcess/DevelopmentResources/DrugInteractionsLabeling/ucm110632.htm

University-Based Drug Interaction Tool: http://umm.edu/health/medical/drug-interaction-tool

U.S. Food and Drug Administration Center for Drug Evaluation and Research: http://www.fda.gov/Drugs/ResourcesForYou/ucm163354.htm

POST-ACUTE CARE

Post-acute care (PAC) is provided to patients who require ongoing medical management, rehabilitation, palliative care, or skilled nursing care, in some cases instead of a stay in an acute care hospital (American Hospital Association, 2015). This care is provided in long-term acute care hospitals (LTACHs), inpatient rehabilitation facilities (IRFs), skilled nursing facilities, and at home through home health agencies (HHAs). Research suggests that patients who receive PAC following a major health event experience greater and more rapid clinical improvements compared with patients discharged to their homes without follow-up (Research Triangle Institute, 2009). PAC services are covered by Medicare and other public and private payers;

a 2013 Institute of Medicine (IOM) report identified the sector as the source of 73% of the variation in Medicare spending (IOM, 2013).

Data from a Medicare claims file for 30% of beneficiaries with an acute hospital-initiated episode in 2008 indicated that 38.7% of beneficiaries were discharged to a PAC setting (Morley, Bogasky, Gage, Flood, & Ingber, 2014). The most common Medicare Severity Diagnosis Related Group (MS-DRG) by volume of discharges to PAC is major joint replacement of lower extremity, with 94.2% of beneficiaries in this MS-DRG discharged to PAC. The second most frequent MS-DRG among PAC users is intracranial hemorrhage, with 75% of beneficiaries discharged to PAC. The next most common MS-DRGs are hip and femur procedures, kidney and urinary tract infections, and simple pneumonia and pleurisy, with 95.4%, 36.3%, 43.9% of beneficiaries in these MS-DRGs discharged to PAC, respectively.

There are no established standards for guiding the selection of the appropriate type of PAC setting, as described in the following. Factors considered include the availability of social support; home environment; patient functional status, comorbidity, medical acuity, and preference; and coverage rules of the payer (AHA, 2015).

1. LTACHs provide long-term, intensive services posthospitalization for medically complex patients. The LTACH may be a freestanding hospital, typically 50 to 90 beds, located on its own property, or it may be located on the grounds or on a wing of an existing hospital, typically 30 to 40 beds. The patients in this setting have the highest overall severity of illness compared with other LTAC settings. Examples of conditions commonly cared for include multisystem organ failure, severe postsurgical wounds, and ventilator dependence. Medicare payment rules require that the average length of stay at LTACHs be greater than 25 days (Medicare Payment Advisory Commission, 2016a).
2. IRFs provide the care of specialty physicians, registered nurses, rehabilitation therapists, social workers, and other interdisciplinary team members under a plan of care approved by a rehabilitation physician. The rehabilitation interventions are rigorous and extensive; at least 3 hours of direct rehabilitation therapy is provided per day. The most commonly treated condition is stroke (20% admissions); other leading diagnoses include brain and spinal cord injury, major joint replacement of the lower extremity, and traumatic injury (Medicare Payment Advisory Commission, 2016b).
3. Skilled nursing facilities (SNFs) are used by those who do not require or cannot tolerate the intensity of LTACHs. The SNF is the most commonly used PAC setting; 2006 Medicare claims data indicate that almost half of all Medicare PAC users received SNF care (Research Triangle Institute, 2009). These facilities treat a broad range of patients; respiratory, kidney, and other infections are common diagnoses among SNF patients, as are joint replacements (Medicare Payment Advisory Commission, 2016b).
4. HHA patients typically have fewer acute medical needs than patients in other PAC settings but require ongoing support to acquire or maintain clinical or functional gains or to ensure a good clinical outcome. To qualify for care from a HHA, a patient must require significant effort and assistance to leave the home. Some of the services provided include physical, speech, and occupational therapy; wound care; education regarding medication management; and assistance with personal hygiene. Some 37% of Medicare beneficiaries who receive PAC are discharged from a general acute care hospital to an HHA, and 60% of all PAC users ultimately receive some home health care (Morley et al., 2014).

See also Home Health Care; Hospital-Based Services; Medicaid; Medicare; Nursing Homes; Rehabilitation.

Marie Boltz

American Hospital Association. (2015). The role of post-acute care in new care delivery models. *Trendwatch*. Retrieved from http://www.aha .org/ research/reports/tw/15dec-tw-postacute.pdf

Institute of Medicine. (2013). *Variation in health care spending: Target decision making, not geography.* Washington, DC: National Academies Press.

Medicare Payment Advisory Commission. (2016a). Long-term care hospital services. In *March 2016 report to the Congress: Medicare payment policy* (pp. 273–296). Washington, DC: Medpac. Retrieved from http://www.medpac.gov/docs/default-source/reports/chapter-10-long-term-care-hospital-services-march-2016-report-.pdf?sfvrsn=0

Medicare Payment Advisory Commission. (2016b). Post-acute care. In *June 2016 a data book: Health care spending and the Medicare program* (pp. 107–128). Washington, DC: Medpac. Retrieved from http://www.medpac.gov/docs/default-source/data-book/june-2016-data-book-section-8-post-acute-care.pdf?sfvrsn=0

Morley, M., Bogasky, S., Gage, B., Flood, S., & Ingber, M. J. (2014). Medicare post-acute care episodes and payment bundling. *Medicare & Medicaid Research Review, 4*(1), E1–E12. doi:10.5600/mmrr.004.01.b02

Research Triangle Institute. (2009). *Examining post-acute care relationships in an integrated hospital system.* Waltham, MA: Author. Retrieved from http://aspe.hhs.gov/health/reports/09/pacihs/report.shtml

Web Resources

American Medical Directors Association (AMDA): http://www.amda.com

Medicare Payment Advisory Commission: http://www.medpac.gov

POVERTY

Although the poverty rate has decreased over the last three decades, poverty is a major concern for the elderly. For purposes of determining the federal poverty level, *income* is defined as all cash payments received by an individual or family from earnings, government benefits, or any other source. For a family unit of one, the poverty threshold is $11,770; for a family of two, $15,930 (Federal Poverty Guidelines, 2016). This poverty line is adjusted upward each year as the cost of supporting a family rises. Longer life, higher costs for medical care, smaller and more distant families, and greater needs for daily living support constitute the poverty scenario for elders. Generally, elders prefer to maintain their dignity by hiding their financial needs rather than asking for help or burdening their caregivers. Even when elders agree to accept financial aid, they need to be guided through the intricacies of the application process. It is estimated that over 25 million Americans aged 60 years and older live at or below 250% of the federal policy level (National Council on Aging, 2016).

Certain groups of elders have higher levels of poverty. Older age, gender, widowhood, and race/ethnicity all impact financial status. The poverty rate of elderly women is nearly twice the level of elderly men. However, Social Security keeps many women out of poverty. Even though women's total Social Security contributions are 38% of total contributions, because of income levels and years of work, women receive 53% of total benefits (Center on Budget and Policy Priorities, 2016). The poverty rate of elderly African Americans (17%) and Hispanics (21%) is more than twice the level of elderly Whites in the United States (AARP, 2012). A lifetime of low wages predisposes minority elderly to poverty. Elderly legal immigrants are not eligible for safety-net programs such as supplemental security income (SSI), food stamps, and Medicaid. However, some states have adopted laws that maintain the previous coverage for legal immigrants (National Immigration Law Center, n.d.).

Social Security and SSI are a safety net for older adults. Social Security provides the majority of the cash income for 61% of older Americans. For one third, it provides 90% or more of their income (Center on Budget and Policy Priorities, 2016). It is the major financial antipoverty program and successfully reduces the severity or impact of poverty among this group. With the introduction of SSI in the mid-1970s, the face of poverty changed. Elders who are not eligible for Social Security because of a limited work history may now access a minimum level of financial aid through SSI. In addition, SSI recipients receive state medical, prescription, and transportation services. However, even after receiving federal benefits, 14.7% of women and 8.2% of men remain impoverished. SSI, Social Security, and private pensions kept the elderly poverty rate in the United States at 10% in 2016 (Center on Budget and Policy Priorities, 2016). Elders can access a variety of services through local and regional service providers. Agencies use a computer program that includes a comprehensive listing of federal and state programs. When workers enter a client's financial, medical, and social needs, the program matches the person to appropriate resources and services.

The elderly are the most underrepresented group receiving food stamps. Many elders do not participate because they assume they will only receive the minimum, do not know how to apply, have difficulty completing the required paperwork, and are reluctant to accept any help from government sources (Food Research and Action Center, 2012). The poverty among rural elders is higher than urban areas.

Financial safety-net programs have strict eligibility guidelines that leave many individuals ineligible for assistance. These are the near-poor, or "tweeners"—those who, because they have some income and assets, are ineligible for many assistance programs. The near-poor income level is 25% above the poverty threshold. The proportion of elderly at this income level (16.2%) is higher than the percentage of poor in the general population (Hokayem & Heggeness, 2014). Widowed middle-class women who lose spousal pensions when their husbands die also find themselves in this financial situation.

Several programs exist to help the near-poor. Elders who are house rich and cash poor can apply for reverse-mortgage programs. These programs allow homeowners to receive monthly checks based on the equity in their home; more elders are relying on the value of their home to be their retirement plan. Banks are familiar with the rules and regulations. Medicare Part D prescription drug plans were created for all Medicare-eligible participants in 2006. However, drug benefits are available for low-income elders throughout the country. Some states also offer to pay Medicare premiums for near-poor elders. The Medicare assistance program pays all or part of the Medicare premium based on an elder's monthly income and total assets. The Medicare office can assist with the application and processing (Centers for Medicare & Medicaid Services, 2016). The Senior Community Service Employment Program (SCSEP) is a federal workforce initiative that offers job training to individual's aged

55 years or older that meet low-income guidelines. Supported by the U.S. Department of Labor, the SCSEP provides retraining, employment, and community service opportunities for eligible elders. Salaries are subsidized for work performed in nonprofit agencies.

Securing a place to live is a challenge for many elders because of the declining availability of affordable housing and the loss of medical-subsidy programs for the poor and near-poor. The U.S. Department of Housing and Urban Development Section 8 housing and voucher programs reduce the rate of poverty among older adults. Although the number and types of housing subsidies and vouchers are decreasing, opportunities for public-housing units are still available. Eligibility requirements for services differ for each authority. The local, county, or state housing authority can be contacted for information. Homeless elders living on the street have difficulty accessing services; they avoid shelters for fear of being victimized by other residents. Homeless elders often have untreated medical conditions, suffer more than other homeless persons, and need assistance in negotiating the eligibility processes to obtain services. Some states provide limited subsidies for assisted-living facilities for the poor and near poor. Waiting lists for subsidized housing are long. The state department of aging can be contacted for information and assistance regarding assisted-living initiatives.

Legal Counsel for the Elderly, an affiliate of the AARP (www.aarp.org), offers legal aid for low-income elders regarding landlord–tenant problems, eligibility for benefits, pension disagreements, and employment discrimination. This service is available to nonmembers. The U.S. Department of Veterans Affairs offers medical, pharmaceutical, residential, and social supports for veterans and their families. The Gray Panthers (graypanthers.org), a social action group, and Services & Advocacy for GLBT Elders (SAGE; sageusa.org) are also valuable resources.

See also Access to Care; Aging Agencies: City and County Level; Aging Agencies: Federal Level; Aging Agencies: State Level; Homeless Elders Meals on Wheels; Medicaid.

Elizabeth A. Capezuti

AARP. (2012). Poverty more likely as adults age. Retrieved from blog.aarp.org

Center on Budget and Policy Priorities. (2016). *Social Security*. Washington, DC: Author. Retrieved from http://www.cbpp.org

Centers for Medicare & Medicaid Services. (2016). *Medicare & you*. Baltimore, MA: Author.

Federal Poverty Guidelines. (2016). Retrieved from http://inequality.stanford.edu/sites/default/files/Pathways-SOTU-2016.pdf

Food Research and Action Center. (2012). Seniors and food stamp programs. Retrieved from http://www.frac.org

Hokayem, C., & Heggeness, M. L. (2014). Living in near poverty in the United States: 1966–2012. *Current Population Reports*. Retrieved from https://www.census.gov/prod/2014pubs/p60-248.pdf

National Council on Aging. (2016). Economic security for seniors facts. Retrieved from https://www.ncoa.org/news/resources-for-reporters/get-the-facts/economic-security-facts

National Immigration Law Center. (n.d.). Guide to immigrant eligibility for federal programs. Retrieved from https://www.nilc.org/issues/economic-support/overview-immeligfedprograms

Web Resources

AARP: http://www.aarp.org

Administration on Aging: http://www.aoa.dhhs.gov

Center for Advocacy for the Rights and Interests of the Elderly: http://www.carie.org

Center on Budget and Policy Priorities: http://www.cbpp.org

Gray Panthers: http://www.graypanthers.org

National Council on Aging: https://www.ncoa.org/news/resources-for-reporters/get-the-facts/economic-security-facts

Senior Action in a Gay Environment: http://www.sageusa.org

Senior Corps: http://www.seniorcorps.org/medicare/how-does-a-green-card-holder-become-eligible-for-medicare

Pressure Injury Prevention and Treatment

As of April 2016, the National Pressure Ulcer Advisory Panel (NPUAP) is using the term *pressure injury* to replace the term *pressure ulcer*. This was done to clarify the fact that pressure ulcer staging included a stage of ulcer in which the skin was not broken and lead to confusion. Pressure injuries may be referred to as *pressure ulcers, bedsores,* and *decubitus ulcers* in the care setting.

The NPUAP also revised the definition of *pressure injury,* clarified the definitions of *medical device injury* and *mucosal pressure injury,* and delineated the six stages of pressure injury. A summary of the evidence and teaching point for these changes, along with the results of the consensus voting for different items, has been published as an open-access article (Edsberg et al., 2016). *Pressure injury* is now defined as localized damage to the skin and/or underlying soft tissue, usually over a bony prominence or related to a medical or other device. The injury can present as intact skin or an open ulcer and may be painful. The injury occurs as a result of intense and/or prolonged pressure or pressure in combination with shear. The tolerance of soft tissue for pressure and shear may also be affected by microclimate, nutrition, perfusion, comorbidities, and condition of the soft tissue (www.npuap.org). Common sites affected are the sacrum, coccyx, heels, ischial tuberosities, shoulders, elbows, cranium, and trochanters (VanGilder, Amlung, Harrison, & Meyer, 2009).

Pressure injuries increase hospital costs significantly. In the U.S., pressure injury care is estimated to approach $11 billion (USD) annually, with a cost of between $500 (USD) and $70,000 (USD) per individual pressure ulcer. (Haesler, 2014)

EPIDEMIOLOGY

Pressure injuries are a significant issue for older patients, critically ill patients, and patients with physical impairments. Pressure injuries are considered by the Centers for Medicare & Medicaid Services (CMS) to be a preventable consequence, and as of 2008 their regulations indicate that hospitals will not receive further funding when patients develop a stage 3 or 4 injury (www.cms.gov). Health care providers may need to develop more effective prevention strategies; however, many experts in the field believe that not all pressure injuries can be avoided even with good practice (Thomas, 2003).

The incidence of pressure injuries in acute care has been reported to range from 2.8% to 9% (Goldberg, 2012). Prevalence in a large national survey has reported prevalence rates as 13.5% in 2008 (*N* = 90,398) and 12.3% in 2009 (*N* = 92,408; VanGilder et al., 2009). Facility-acquired pressure injuries were reported as 6% in 2008 (*N* = 90,398) and 5% in 2009 (*N* = 92,408; VanGilder et al., 2009). In the United States, approximately 3 million pressure injuries are treated each year with great mortality, morbidity, and health care costs (Saha et al., 2013). In long-term care, CMS data from the minimum data set (MDS) 3.0 reports a pressure injury prevalence rate of 7.3% for the first quarter of 2016 (CMS, 2016).

RISK FACTORS

Risk factors for developing pressure injuries may include the following:

- Old age
- Male gender
- Dry skin over bony prominences
- Incontinence
- Difficulty turning in bed
- Residing in a nursing home
- Prior hospitalization in the last 6 months
- Poor nutritional status (Baumgarten et al., 2006).

In the Lyder et al. (2012) study, 16.7% of individuals who acquired a pressure injury during hospitalization were non-White, were aged 75 to 84 years, and had higher rates of congestive heart failure (CHF), chronic obstructive pulmonary disease (COPD), cardiovascular disease (CVD), diabetes mellitus, obesity, and use of corticosteroids (Lyder et al., 2012). Predictors of heel pressure injuries in hospitalized patients were Braden scores equal to or less than 18, diabetes mellitus, vascular disease, and immobility (Delmore, Lebovits, Suggs, Rolnitzky, Ayello, 2015) In home care patients, a study of OASIC-C data found that the key risk factors for pressure injury risk were bowel incontinence and immobility (Bergquist-Beringer & Gajewski, 2011).

PREVENTION

Prevention is key to reducing the morbidity, mortality, and costs associated with pressure injuries (Tran, McLaughlin, Li, & Phillips, 2016). One illustrative analysis found that prevention and surveillance methods resulted in a net savings of $127 per patient (Spetz, Brown, Aydin, & Donaldson, 2013). The Agency for Healthcare Research and Quality (AHRQ) has a free toolkit available on their website as a resource to assist hospitals in preventing and reducing pressure injuries (www.ahrq.gov/professionals/systems/long-term-care/resources/pressure-ulcers/pressureulcertoolkit/index.html). Elements of successful pressure injury–reduction initiatives in hospitals and long-term care (Delmore, Lebovits, Baldock, Suggs, & Ayello, 2011; Niederhauser, VanDeusen-Lukas, & Parker, 2012; Stotts, & Wu, 2007; Tran et al., 2016) include:

- Incorporation of pressure injury prevention practices into everyday care and use of enablers
- Skin champions on each unit
- Skin and pressure injury risk assessment on admission and reassessment frequency depending on care setting and patient acuity
- Risk assessment level or status as part of patient handoff
- Education for the patient, education for the caregivers, education for the families (Haesler, 2014)

Effective methods recommended for the prevention of pressure injuries include:

- Frequently repositioning of patients (Haesler, 2014):
  - Use of a turn team (Harmon, Grobbel, & Palleschi, 2016)
  - Regularly scheduled clinical rounding with the interprofessional team (Anderson et al., 2015)
- Use of specifically designed support surfaces (Saha et al., 2013; Smith et al., 2013)
- Patient nutrition (Dorner, Posthauer, & Thomas, 2009; Posthauer, Banks, Dorner, & Schols, 2015)

P

- Management of moisture and incontinence issues (Haesler, 2014)

Repositioning patients is commonly recommended for the prevention of pressure injuries. In the 2014 NPUAP/EPUAP/PPPIA clinical practice guidelines (www.npuap.org), a new recommendation regarding individualized time to reposition patients is based on patient comorbidity and type of support surface, rather than the standard indicating repositioning every 2 hours for everyone. For example, the guideline states that an individual should be repositioned with greater frequency on a non–pressure-redistributing mattress than on a viscoelastic foam mattress (Haesler, 2014). Consensus recommendations for turning and repositioning the critically ill patient with hemodynamic instability have also been proposed (Brindle et al., 2013). The "turn" study has provided some additional evidence that the traditional every-2-hours repositioning schedule may not be the only option for repositioning some elderly patients. (Bergstrom et al., 2013). In this randomized controlled trial of 942 long-term care (LTC) residents, there was no difference in pressure injury occurrence between 2-, 3- and 4-hour repositioning schedules (2 hours [2.5%]; 3 hours [0.6%], 4 hours [3.1%], $P = .68$; Bergstrom et al., 2013). In a small pilot study of nine residents in LTC, Wong (2011) found no statistical differences in local oxygenation or skin temperature and concluded that this raised concerns about the efficiency of the every-2-hour turning interval. In another study on elderly persons in a nursing home in the United Kingdom, researchers found that despite being marginally more clinically effective alternating every 2 hours and every 4 hours repositioning, it is not cost effective (Mardsen et al., 2015). The length of time a person should remain in a position is unclear; however, it has been demonstrated that skin erythema occurs in healthy adults in less than 2 hours when on a standard mattress (Knox, Anderson, & Anderson, 1994). Different support surfaces are available including foam mattresses, special pads, mattresses of air, water or gel, air flotation beds, and air fluidized beds (McInnes, Jammali-Blasi, Bell-Syer, Dumville, & Cullum, 2011). There is reasonable

evidence that patients at high risk for pressure injuries should use higher-specification foam mattresses than the standard hospital foam mattresses, that medical grade sheepskins may decrease pressure injury formation, and that gel pads may be helpful in the operating room (McInnes et al., 2011, 2015). A recent systematic comparative effectiveness review found that more advanced static support surfaces are more effective than standard mattresses for preventing injuries in higher-risk populations (Chou et al., 2013).

Nutritionally depleted patients should be assessed by a dietician and have their nutritional status monitored (Dorner et al., 2009; Posthauer et al., 2015). It is not possible to draw firm conclusions about the use of enteral feeding for preventing or treating injuries at this time (Chou et al., 2013; Langer & Fink, 2014).

Moisture can cause breakdown of the skin. Urine and feces are very caustic to the surface of the skin, and attempts to protect the skin from these elements should be made by limiting exposure. The evidence to support the use of prophylactic dressings to prevent pressure injuries has recently been summarized (Reid, Ayello, & Alavi, 2016).

EVALUATION

Once present, pressure injuries first need to be assessed for stage, size (length, width, depth), sinus tracts, necrotic tissue, exudates, and infection. Patient-centered concerns, including pain assessment and management, are important (Sibbald, Elliott, Ayello, & Somayaji, 2011). The revised staging definitions were presented at a meeting of more than 400 professionals in Chicago on April 8–9, 2016 and released April 13, 2016. The staging numbers are now Arabic instead of Roman (Edsberg et al., 2016). The NPUAP (www.npuap.org) now classifies pressure injuries in six stages:

Stage 1 Pressure Injury: Nonblanchable erythema of intact skin: Intact skin with a localized area of nonblanchable erythema, which may appear differently in darkly pigmented skin. The presence of blanchable erythema or changes in sensation, temperature, or firmness may precede visual changes. Color changes do not include purple or maroon discoloration; these may indicate deep tissue pressure injury.

Stage 2 Pressure Injury: Partial-thickness skin loss with exposed dermis: Partial-thickness loss of skin with exposed dermis. The wound bed is viable, pink or red, and moist and may also present as an intact or ruptured serum-filled blister. Adipose (fat) and deeper tissues are not visible. Granulation tissue, slough, and eschar are not present. These injuries commonly result from adverse microclimate and shear in the skin over the pelvis and shear in the heel. This stage should not be used to describe moisture-associated skin damage (MASD), including incontinence-associated dermatitis (IAD), intertriginous dermatitis (ITD), medical adhesive-related skin injury (MARSI), or traumatic wounds (skin tears, burns, and abrasions).

Stage 3 Pressure Injury: Full-thickness skin loss: Full-thickness loss of skin, in which adipose (fat) is visible in the ulcer and granulation tissue and epibole (rolled wound edges) are often present. Slough and/or eschar may be visible. The depth of tissue damage varies by anatomical location; areas of significant adiposity can develop deep wounds. Undermining and tunneling may occur. Fascia, muscle, tendon, ligament, cartilage, or bone is not exposed. If slough or eschar obscures the extent of tissue loss, this is an unstageable pressure injury.

Stage 4 Pressure Injury: Full-thickness skin and tissue loss: Full-thickness skin and tissue loss with exposed or directly palpable fascia, muscle, tendon, ligament, cartilage, or bone in the ulcer. Slough and/or eschar may be visible. Epibole, undermining, and/or tunneling often occur. Depth varies by anatomical location. If slough or eschar obscures the extent of tissue loss, this is an unstageable pressure injury.

Unstageable Pressure Injury: Obscured full-thickness skin and tissue loss—dark eschar Full-thickness skin and tissue loss in which the extent of tissue damage within the ulcer cannot be confirmed because it is obscured by slough or eschar. If slough or eschar is removed, a stage 3 or stage 4 pressure injury is revealed.

Stable eschar (i.e., dry, adherent, intact, without erythema or fluctuance) on an ischemic limb or the heel should not be removed.

Deep Tissue Pressure Injury: Intact or nonintact skin with a localized area of persistent nonblanchable, deep red, maroon, or purple discoloration, or epidermal separation revealing a dark wound bed or blood-filled blister. Pain and temperature change often precede skin color changes. Discoloration may appear differently in darkly pigmented skin. This injury results from intense and/or prolonged pressure and shear forces at the bone–muscle interface. The wound may evolve rapidly to reveal the extent of tissue injury or may resolve without tissue loss. Visible necrotic tissue, subcutaneous tissue, granulation tissue, fascia, muscle, and other underlying structures indicate a full-thickness pressure injury (unstageable, stage 3, or stage 4). The term *deep tissue pressure injury* should not be used to describe vascular, traumatic, neuropathic, or dermatological conditions.

Two types of pressure-related injury were given their own definitions, as follows:

Medical Device-Related Pressure Injury: These injuries result from the use of medical devices designed for therapeutic or diagnostic purposes. These injuries may conform to the shape or pattern of the device used by the clinician to provide care. They should be staged using the NUPAP staging system.

Mucosal Membrane Pressure Injury: These are pressure injuries found on the mucous membranes with a history of use of a medical device and are not staged.

The reasons for the changes were to help with accuracy of identifying the type of pressure injury (www.npuap). The Joint Commission and the National Database of Nursing Quality Indicators (NDNQI) have adopted the new NPUAP terminology and staging definitions.

MANAGEMENT

Wound bed preparation (WBP) is a model that provides clinical guidance for the treatment of persons with chronic wounds such as pressure injuries (Sibbald et al., 2011, 2015). Key to managing pressure injuries is to first identify the underlying issues and correct them if possible. Then the classification of the wound, whether it is healable, maintenance, or nonhealable must be determined, which drives treatment options (Sibbald et al., 2011, 2015).

Pressure injuries are mainly caused by increased pressure or shear forces (issues extrinsic to the patient). A multidisciplinary team is usually needed to address the needs of the patient. Off-loading by ensuring appropriate distribution of weight over a large surface by the use of an off-loading surface (bed, wheelchair seat, or booties) is the first step. Moisture issues such as incontinence and sweating need to be addressed because moisture-damaged skin needs less external pressure break down (Haesler, 2014). Sometimes, a patient may need to have a catheter or bowel-management system while the pressure injury heals. Shear and friction issues should be addressed, and steps need to be taken to minimize these forces. Proper transferral of the patient must occur to decrease these forces. Other extrinsic issues include cost of treatment if prohibitive, lack of resources (i.e., wound care specialists), and ability to adhere to treatment.

There is evidence for the use of air-fluidized beds to help with the healing of ulcers compared with the use of standard hospitalized beds (Saha et al., 2013; Smith et al., 2013). Other support surfaces and cushions have not been adequately studied to recommend the use of one surface brand or type over the other (Smith et al., 2013). The Wound, Ostomy and Continence Nurses (WOCN) Society has published an algorithm for support surface selection (McNichol, Watts, Mackey, Beitz, & Gray, 2015). Repositioning the patient seems logical in the treatment of pressure injuries, but the effect of repositioning has not been adequately studied to conclude whether or not it affects healing rates (Moore & Cowman, 2015).

The patient should be assessed for intrinsic issues that may affect wound healing (Ayello, 2017). These include comorbid conditions such as diabetes mellitus (hemoglobin A1c [HbA1c] level), anemia, deficient nutritional status, peripheral vascular disease, and illnesses requiring certain medications (Ayello, 2017). Once these are optimized, the patient is more likely to heal. Heel pressure injuries are very susceptible to issues within the arterial system (Delmore et al., 2015). Vascular status must be assessed before any debridement can occur. A recent systematic comparative effectiveness review found a greater reduction in size of ulcers with protein supplementation compared to without but did not show more wound healing (Smith et al., 2013). Low-strength evidence revealed that supplementation with vitamin C did not show benefits of wound healing. No conclusions about zinc supplementation could be drawn because of insufficient evidence (Smith et al., 2013).

If underlying issues, extrinsic or intrinsic, cannot be managed appropriately, the patient's wound is considered to be a maintenance wound; healing will not occur completely and the goal of treatment will be to maintain, the wound, monitor for infection, and keep the wound clean (Sibbald et al., 2011, 2015). Healable wounds are those in which all underlying issues are corrected and the prognosis is that the wound will heal. Nonhealable wounds usually have issues involving the arterial system and should be assessed for revascularization by a vascular surgeon, or the patient has other factors that prevent healing, such as those at life's end (Sibbald, Krasner, & Lutz, 2010).

The wound itself needs to be evaluated for the presence of infection, either deep or superficial. Mnemonics for identifying superficial and deep infection in chronic wounds have been validated to make the identification easier (Sibbald et al., 2011, 2015).

For superficial infections, NERDS: (Sibbald et al., 2015):

Nonhealing wounds
Exudative wounds
Red and bleeding wound-surface granulation tissue
Debris (yellow or black necrotic tissue) on the wound surface
Smell or unpleasant odor from the wound

For deep infection, think of STONEES: (Sibbald et al., 2015):

Size is bigger
Temperature is increased
Os probe to or exposed bone
New or satellite areas of breakdown
Exudate
Erythema, Edema
Smell

Superficial infections and critical colonization with bacteria can be treated with topical antiseptics such as povidone-iodine and biguanide-based products (Sibbald et al., 2015). Biofilms may form on the surface of the wounds and require surgical removal and application of a povidone/cadex; mer product. Debridement can occur surgically, autolytically, mechanically, biologically, or enzymatically to remove devitalized tissues. This may be needed serially.

An extensive description of the products available for wound care is available in the literature (Sibbald et al., 2015). Despite the wide variety of materials available, however, there are few studies comparing products. Most clinicians develop preferences based on familiarity with a limited number of products rather than research results. When the dressing is choosen, several principles must be considered, including the goal of care and the determination of whether it is a healable, maintenance, or nonhealable wound (Sibbald et al., 2015). For healable wounds, keeping the wound moist is important to promote moist wound healing; at the same time the exudate needs to be controlled, maintaining the surrounding intact skin dry. The wound must be protected from contamination by outside organisms. Removing the dressing should not cause trauma to the wound. In today's economic climate, it is also important to consider the cost of the dressings along with the cost of the time taken to dress the wound (Registered Nurses' Association of Ontario, 2016).

Adjunctive therapies, such as electromagnetic therapy or therapeutic ultrasound, have not been found different from sham treatment or standard care in wound-healing outcomes (Smith et al., 2013). There is some evidence that light therapy (Smith et al., 2013) and radiant heat dressings (Saha et al., 2013) may help with injury healing (Smith et al., 2013), although this is not a part of standard care. There is moderate evidence that electrical stimulation may help with healing (Haesler, 2014); however, further study needs to be done to determine the type and dosage (Saha et al., 2013). In general, most studies about pressure injury treatments are of poor quality with inadequate follow-up periods (Saha et al., 2013). This is an area where further good quality research is clearly needed.

Good wound care requires frequent assessment, pressure redistribution, pain management, adequate nutrition, cleanliness, and a readiness to try a different wound-care products if a regimen is not working. Reassessment of all factors must occur on a regular basis if the wound is not healing as predicted. Questions to entertain include the following. Is there sufficient pressure redistribution? Is the wound truly clean, or is there still dead tissue or bacterial colonization? Is the patient receiving adequate nutrition? Is the wound being dressed properly? Does this individual have end-of-life needs?

Although most patient's pressure injuries heal with proper care, their cost, pain, and functional consequences make prevention paramount.

See also Pressure Injury Risk Assessment.

Carol L. B. Ott and Elizabeth A. Ayello

Anderson, M., Guthie, P. F., Kraft, W., Reicks, P., Skay, C., & Beal, A. L. (2015). Universal pressure ulcer prevention bundle with WOC nurse support. *Journal of Wound, Ostomy, and Continence Nursing, 42*(3), 217–225.

Ayello, E. (2017). Predicting pressure injury risk. *Try This: Best Practices in Nursing Care to Older Adults,* (5). Retrieved from https://consultgeri.org/try-this/general-assessment/issue-5.pdf

Baumgarten, M., Margolis, D. J., Localio, A. R., Kagan, S. H., Lowe, R. A., Kinosian, B., ... Ruffin, A. (2006). Pressure ulcers among elderly patients early in the hospital stay. *Journals of Gerontology: Series A, Biological Sciences and Medical Sciences, 61*(7), 749–754.

Bergquist-Beringer, S., & Gajewski, B. J. (2011). Outcome and assessment information set data that predict pressure ulcer development in older

P

adult home health patients. *Advances in Skin and Wound Care, 24*(9), 404–414.

Bergstrom, N., Horn, S. D., Rapp, M. P., Stern, A., Barrett, R., & Watkiss, M. (2013). Turning for ulcer reduction: A multisite randomized clinical trial in nursing homes. *Journal of the American Geriatrics Society, 61*(10), 1705–1713.

Brindle, C. T., Malhotra, R., O'Rourke, S., Currie, L., Chadwik, D., Falls, P., ... Creehan, S. (2013). Turning and repositioning the critically ill patient with hemodynamic instability: A literature review and consensus recommendations. *Journal of Wound, Ostomy, and Continence Nursing, 40*(3), 254–267.

Centers for Medicare & Medicaid Services. (2016). MDS frequency report. Retrieved from https://www .cms.gov/Research-Statistics-Data-and-Systems/ Computer-Data-and-Systems/Minimum-Data -Set-3-0-Public-Reports/Minimum-Data-Set-3-0 -Frequency-Report.html

Chou, R., Dana, T., Bougatsos, C., Blazina, I., Starmer, A., Reitel, K., & Buckley, D. I. (2013). Pressure ulcer risk assessment and prevention. *Annals of Internal Medicine, 159*(1), 28–38.

Delmore, B., Lebovits, S., Baldock, P., Suggs, B., & Ayello, E. A. (2011). Pressure ulcer prevention program: A journey. *Journal of Wound, Ostomy, and Continence Nursing, 38*(3), 505–513.

Delmore, B., Lebovits, S., Suggs, B., Rolnitzky, L., & Ayello, E. A. (2015). Risk factors associated with heel pressure ulcers in hospitalized patients. *Journal of Wound, Ostomy, and Continence Nursing, 42*(3), 242–248.

Dorner, D., Posthauer, M. E., & Thomas, D. (2009). The role of nutrition in pressure ulcer prevention and treatment: National Pressure Ulcer Advisory Panel white paper. *Advances in Skin and Wound Care, 22*(5), 212–221. Retrieved from http://www.npuap.org/ wp-content/uploads/2012/ 03/Nutrition-White-Paper-Website-Version .pdf

Edsberg, L. E., Black, J. M., Goldberg, M., McNichol, L., Moore, L., & Sieggreen, M. (2016). Revised National Pressure Ulcer Advisory Panel staging system. *Journal of Wound, Ostomy, and Continence Nursing, 43*(6), 1–13.

Goldberg, M. (2012). General acute care. In B. Pieper (Ed.), *Pressure ulcers: Prevalence, incidence, and implications for the future* (p. 27). Washington, DC: National Pressure Ulcer Advisory Panel.

Harmon, L. C., Grobbel, C., & Palleschi, M. (2016). Reducing pressure injury incidence using a turn team assignment. *Journal of Wound, Ostomy, and Continence Nursing, 43*(5), 477–482.

Haesler, E. (Ed.). (2014). *Prevention and treatment of pressure ulcers: Clinical practice guideline.* Osborne Park, Western Australia: Cambridge Media.

Knox, D. M., Anderson, T. M., & Anderson, P. S. (1994). Effects of different turn intervals on skin of healthy older adults. *Advances in Wound Care, 7*(1), 48–52, 54–56.

Langer, G., & Fink, A. (2014). Nutritional interventions for preventing and treating pressure ulcers. *Cochrane Database of Systematic Reviews, 2015*(6), CD003216. doi:10.1002/14651858.CD003 216.pub2

Lyder, C. H., Wang, Y., Metersky, M., Curry, M., Kliman, R., Verzier, N. R., & Hunt, D. R. (2012). Hospital-acquired pressure ulcers: Results from the National Medicare Patient Safety Monitoring System study. *Journal of the American Geriatrics Society, 60*(9), 1603–1608.

Marsden, G., Jones, K., Neilson, J., Avital, L., Collier, M., & Stansby, G. (2015). A cost-effectiveness analysis of two different repositioning strategies for the prevention of pressure ulcers. *Journal of Advanced Nursing, 71*, 2879–2885.

McInnes, E., Jammali-Blasi, A., Bell-Syer, S. E., Dumville, J. C., & Cullum, N. (2011). Support surfaces for pressure ulcer prevention. *Cochrane Database of Systematic Reviews, 4*.

McInnes, E., Jammali-Blasi, A., Bell-Syer, S. E., Middleton V., Dumville, J. C., & Cullum, N. (2015). Support surfaces for pressure ulcer prevention. *Cochrane Database of Systematic Reviews, 2015*(9), CD0001735. doi:10.1002/14651858.CD001735 .pub5

McNichol, L., Watts, C., Mackey, D., Beitz, J. M., & Gray, M. (2015). Identifying the right surface for the right patient at the right time: Generation and content validation of an algorithm for support surface selection. *Journal of Wound, Ostomy, and Continence Nursing, 42*(11), 19–37.

Moore, Z. E. H., & Cowman, S. (2015). Repositioning for treating pressure ulcers. *Cochrane Database of Systematic Reviews, 1*, CD006898. doi:10.1002/ 14651858CD.006898.pub4

National Pressure Ulcer Advisory Panel. (2016, August 30). Governmental agencies and professional organizations support NPUAP's pressure injury staging system. Retrieved from http:// www.npuap.org/?s=Joint+commission+and+pre ssure+injury

National Pressure Ulcer Advisory Panel. (2016). National Pressure Ulcer Advisory Panel (NPUAP) announces a change in terminology from pressure ulcer to pressure injury and updates the stages of pressure injury. Retrieved from

http://www.npuap.org/national-pressure-ulcer
-advisory-panel-npuap-announces-a-change-in
-terminology-from-pressure-ulcer-to-pressure
-injury-and-updates-the-stages-of-pressure-injury

Niederhauser, A., VanDeusen-Lukas, C., & Parker, V. (2012) Comprehensive programs for preventing pressure ulcers: A review of the literature. *Advances in Skin and Wound Care, 25*(4), 167–188.

Posthauer, M. E., Banks, M., Dorner, B., & Schols, J. M. (2015). The role of nutrition for pressure ulcer management: National Pressure Ulcer Advisory Panel, European Pressure Ulcer Advisory Panel, and Pan Pacific Pressure Injury Alliance white paper. *Advances in Skin and Wound Care, 28*(4), 175–188.

Registered Nurses Association of Ontario. (2016). *Nursing best practice guidelines: Assessment and management of pressure injuries for the interprofessional team* (3rd ed.). Toronto, ON, Canada. (Original work published 2002.)

Reid, K., Ayello, E. A., & Alavi, A. (2016). Pressure ulcer prevention and treatment: Use of prophylactic dressings. *Chronic Wound Care Management and Research, 2016*(3), 117–121.

Saha, S., Smith, M. E. B., Totten, A., Fu, R., Wasson, N., Rahman, B., ... Hickam, D. H. (2013). *Pressure ulcer treatment strategies: Comparative effectiveness.* Comparative Effectiveness Review No. 90. (Prepared by the Oregon Evidence-based Practice Center under Contract No. 290-2007-10057-I.) AHRQ Publication No. 13-EHC003-EF. Rockville, MD: Agency for Healthcare Research and Quality. Retrieved from http://www.effectivehealthcare.ahrq.gov/reports/final.cfm

Sibbald, R. G., Elliott, J. A., Ayello, E. A., & Somayaji, R. (2015). Optimizing the moisture management tightrope with wound bed preparation 2015©. *Advances in Skin and Wound Care, 28*(10), 466–476.

Sibbald, R. G., Goodman, L., Woo, K. Y., Krasner, D. L., Smart, H., Tariq, G., ... Salcido, R. S. (2011). Special considerations in wound bed preparation 2011: An update. *Advances in Skin and Wound Care, 24*(9), 415–436.

Sibbald, R. G., Krasner, D. L., & Lutz, J. (2010). SCALE: Skin changes at life's end: Final consensus statement: October 1, 2009. *Advances in Skin and Wound Care, 23*(5), 225–236.

Smith, B. M. E., Totten, A., Hickam, D. H., Fu, R., Wasson, N., Rahman, B., ... Saha, S. (2013). Pressure ulcer treatment strategies. *Annals of Internal Medicine, 159*(1), 39–51.

Spetz, J., Brown, D. S., Aydin, C., & Donaldson, N. (2013). The value of reducing hospital-acquired pressure ulcer prevalence: An illustrative analysis. *Journal of Nursing Administration, 43*(4), 235–241.

Stotts, N. A., & Wu, H. S. (2007). Hospital recovery is facilitated by prevention of pressure ulcers in older adults. *Critical Care Nursing Clinics of North America, 19*(3), 269–275, vi.

Thomas, D. (2003). Are all pressure ulcers avoidable? *Journal of the American Medical Directors Association, 4*(2), 43–48.

Tran, J. P., McLaughlin, J. M., Li, R. T., & Phillips, L. G. (2016). Prevention of pressure ulcers in the acute care setting: New innovations and technologies. *Plastic and Reconstructive Surgery Journal, 138*(3S), 232S–240S.

VanGilder, C., Amlung, S., Harrison, B. A., & Meyer, S. (2009). Results of the 2008–2009 Internal National Pressure Ulcer Prevalence Survey and a 3-year, acute care, unit-specific analysis. *Ostomy Wound Management, 55*(11), 39–45.

Wong, V. (2011). Skin blood flow response to 2-hour repositioning in long-term care residents: A pilot study. *Journal of Wound, Ostomy, and Continence Nursing, 38*(5), 529–537.

Web Resources

American Academy of Wound Management: http://www.aawm.org

American Professional Wound Care Association: http://www.apwca.org

National Pressure Ulcer Advisory Panel: http://www.npuap.org

World Council of Enterostomal Therapists: http://www.wcetn.org

Wound Care Communications Network: http://www.woundcarenet.com

Wound, Ostomy, and Continence Nurses Society: http://www.wocn.org

PRESSURE INJURY RISK ASSESSMENT

The National Pressure Ulcer Advisory Panel (NPUAP), in April 2016, renamed *pressure ulcers* as *pressure injuries* so that it better includes the staging in which the skin is *not* broken (www.npuap.org). A *pressure injury* is now defined as "injury to the skin and/or underlying soft tissue *usually* over a bony prominence, or related to a **medical** or **other device**. The injury can present as intact skin or an open ulcer and may be painful. The injury occurs as a result of **intense** and/or **prolonged pressure** or **pressure** in **combination** with **shear**. The tolerance of soft tissue for pressure and shear may also be affected by microclimate, nutrition, perfusion, comorbidities and condition of the soft tissue" (Edsberg et al., 2016; NPUAP, 2016). For example, stage 1, or deep tissue, injuries are not well defined as ulcers because the skin is not broken. Pressure injuries are a serious health problem in older adults and occur in all health care settings. Hospital stays are almost three times longer for persons with pressure injuries compared with those without pressure injuries. Among older adults with a pressure injury who were hospitalized, 16.7% also developed other pressure injuries during their stay. A cohort of older patients who entered the hospital without a pressure injury developed one at an incidence rate of 4.5% (Lyder et al., 2012). In a large survey, pressure injury prevalence in acute care settings was 11.9%, facility-acquired rate was 5.0%, long-term care prevalence was 11.8%, and facility-acquired rate was 5.2% (VanGilder, MacFarlane, & Meyer, 2008). In the United States, pressure injury care is estimated to approach $11 billion dollars annually (Haesler, 2014). Therefore it is paramount that each patient be assessed for risk of developing pressure injuries and plans be put in place to reduce the risk of suffering to the patient and cost to the health care system.

RISK ASSESSMENT SCALES

Two commonly used validated prediction scales, the Norton and Braden Scales are available to identify those at high risk of developing pressure injuries. The Norton Scale uses a 1- to 4-point scoring system that rates patients in five subscales: physical condition, mental condition, activity, mobility, and incontinence. Scores less than 14 indicate that the patient is at high risk for developing pressure injuries. The Braden Scale rates patients in six areas: sensory perception, moisture, activity, mobility, nutrition, and friction/shear. The maximum score is 23, and scores below 18 indicate that a person is

at risk (Sibbald, Goodman, Norton, Krasner, & Ayello, 2012; www.bradenscale.com). Although these scales are widely used, there is growing evidence that other patient risk factors not found on these tools should be considered when performing a comprehensive assessment to determine a person's risk for pressure injury development (Haesler, 2014). Regardless of the tools or process used, health care professionals should know their patient's pressure injury risk and develop an interprofessional plan of care to address the patient's specific prevention needs. Rounding with wound ostomy and continence nurses has been shown to decrease pressure injuries in ICU patients (Anderson et al., 2015). Foam dressings applied prophylactically may reduce pressure injury occurrence (Haesler, 2014; Reid, Ayello, & Alavi, 2016). Harmon, Grobbel, and Palleschi (2016) report a reduction in pressure injury incidence when a "a turn team" was used. Tran, McLaughlin, Li, and Phillips (2016) have provided an extensive review of the literature pertaining to new innovations and technologies that can be used in the prevention of pressure injuries in the acute care setting.

The changes inherent in aging and/or darkly pigmented skin in Black and Latino patients require that scores be adjusted for these patient populations. The total risk assessment score provides a limited picture. Clinicians must also address any subscore with a low score (Centers for Medicare & Medicaid Services [CMS], 2004; Haesler, 2014) by providing appropriate measures to correct the problem area. The risk-assessment score is an adjunct to nursing judgment about when to implement pressure injury–prevention strategies. A review (Moore & Cowman, 2014) suggests that the scales themselves may not be better than nurses' clinical judgment. Further study needs to be done in this area.

RISK FACTORS BEYOND THE SCALES

Decreased mobility and bowel incontinence were predictors of pressure injury risk in a study of home care patients ($n = 5,375$) based on OASIS-C data with a finding of 1.3% incidence of pressure injuries (Bergquist-Beringer

& Gajewski, 2011). Based on a review of over 50,000 Medicare-insured, hospitalized elderly patients, those who had diabetes mellitus, heart failure, or chronic obstructive pulmonary disease (COPD), cardiovascular disease; who were on corticosteroids; or who were obese had increased risk of hospital-acquired pressure injuries (Lyder et al., 2012). Diabetes mellitus, vascular disease, immobility, and a Braden score of 18 or below were predictors of heel pressure injuries in hospitalized adults (Delmore, Lebovits, Suggs, Rolnitzky, & Ayello, 2015).

There is some evidence that subepidermal moisture may be a risk factor for pressure injury development in older persons with darkly pigmented skin (Bates-Jensen, McCreath, & Pongquan, 2009). There are some studies have looked at measuring skin temperature for changes as a pressure injury risk factor (Rapp, Bergstrom, & Padhye, 2009; Sprigle, Linden, McKenna, Davis, & Riordan, 2001; Wong, Stotts, Hopf, Dowling, & Froelicher, 2011).

RISK ASSESSMENT FREQUENCY

Clinical practice guidelines of the former Agency for Healthcare Research and Quality (www.guideline.gov/content.aspx?id=36059) recommend pressure injury risk assessment on admission to a facility and then periodically, based on the clinical setting and changes in the patient's condition. In acute care, reassessment typically occurs based on the patient's acuity level, either once every 24 hours or once every 12 hours for critically ill patients (such as those in the intensive care unit). Reassessment should also be done when major changes occur in the patient's condition. In long-term care, reassessment should occur weekly for the first 4 weeks after admission and then at a minimum each quarter. In home care, reassessment should be done at every visit by the nurse, based on the patient's illness severity (Ayello & Braden, 2002; CMS, 2004).

PREVALENCE AND ASSESSMENT OF STAGE 1 PRESSURE INJURIES

Several national surveys (Barczak, Barnett, Childs, & Bosley, 1997; vanGilder et al., 2008;

vanGilder, MacFarlane, Harrison, Lachenbruch, & Meyer, 2010; Whittington & Briones, 2004) support the idea that the largest percentage of pressure injuries are stage 1 or 2. Color, especially erythema, has been the gold standard used by clinicians to identify stage 1 pressure injuries. Erythema, however, is not adequate for detecting pressure injuries in individuals who have darker skin pigmentation, and thus other characteristics of stage 1 pressure injuries, such as temperature or touch, need to be assessed (Haesler, 2014). Patients with darkly pigmented skin have the lowest prevalence of stage I pressure injuries and a significantly higher prevalence of higher stage, full-thickness injuries. Because intact, darkly pigmented skin does not change color (i.e., does not blanch) when pressure is applied over a bony prominence, reliance on "nonblanchable erythema of intact skin" might account for missed identification of early skin injuries in persons with darkly pigmented skin. Color changes in stage 1 pressure injuries do not include purple or maroon discoloration; instead these colors may indicate deep tissue injury (DTI; Edsberg et al., 2016; NPUAP, 2016).

Rather than redness, the new indicator for assessing stage 1 pressure injuries in persons with darkly pigmented skin would be discoloration/darkening of the individual's skin tone from the usual color. Adequate light is essential when assessing patients with darkly pigmented skin. Natural or halogen light sources are better than fluorescent lights, which cast a bluish hue and can interfere with detection of pressure injuries. Clinicians should avoid wearing tinted glasses that alter their ability to make color assessments.

Clinicians also need to include factors other than color, such as the temperature of the skin over bony prominences, to ascertain differences from the surrounding skin. Initially, an area of early skin injury feels warmer. As the capillaries collapse as a result of pressure and the tissue dies, the skin temperature cools. Because pressure injuries occur most frequently on the sacrum and secondarily on the heels, clinicians should give particular attention to these areas (Haesler, 2014). Clinicians benefit from further guidance from the NPUAP about the concept of

DTI (Ankrom et al., 2005; Black & NPUAP, 2005; Doughty et al., 2006), as well as some emerging research (Honaker, Brockopp, & Moe, 2014; Sullivan, 2013).

Tissue consistency may also be an indicator of a stage 1 pressure injury. Clinicians should palpate for a firm or boggy feel. The revised NPUAP (2016) stage I definition also alerts clinicians to include sensation, temperature, and firmness as indicators. Sensation may present as pain or itching. Some researchers are investigating ultrasound as a way of detecting stage 1 pressure injury. Color changes such as purple or maroon discoloration indicates DTI (Edsberg et al., 2016; NPUAP, 2016).

As soon as a stage 1 pressure injury is suspected, the patient should be positioned so that there is redistribution of pressure on the area; in addition, an appropriate pressure-redistribution device must be placed beneath the patient. The WOCN algorithm can be used to identify the best support surface (McNichol, Watts, Mackey, Beitz, & Gray, 2015). Even when a patient is on a support surface, repositioning is essential (Haesler, 2014). The frequency of repositioning needs to be individualized for the patient's characteristics, comorbidities, goals of care, and support surface being used (Haesler, 2014). Although some studies have questioned the classic every-2-hour turning and repositioning schedule, clinicians need to individualize the schedule based on the patient's individual needs and tissue tolerance to pressure (Haesler, 2014). Pressure injury prevention guidelines as recommended by NPUAP (www.npuap.org) should be implemented. Prompt cleansing of soiled skin with appropriate protection from the detrimental effects of incontinence also helps prevent skin injury because moisture-damaged skin needs less pressure to break down (Haesler, 2014).

The NPUAP is currently reviewing the concept of DTI, which has posed a problem for clinicians in pressure injury staging, identification, prevention, and treatment. This is an emerging area of practice with little in the literature. The most current information on DTI can be obtained from the NPUAP website (www .npuap.org). This is one of the reason behind the name changes.

Stage 2 pressure injuries can be misidentified as moisture-associated skin damage (MASD). Excellent reviews of how to differentiate pressure injuries from MASD are noted in DeFloor et al. (2005), Gray et al. (2007, 2011), Wolfman (2010), and Zulkowski (2008).

NUTRITIONAL ASSESSMENT

Malnutrition and nutritional deficiencies have been linked to pressure injury formation (Dorner, Posthaurer, & Thomas, 2009). Guidelines recommend an abbreviated nutritional assessment at least every 3 months for patients at risk for malnutrition (Haesler, 2014). Clinically significant malnutrition is serum albumin less than 3.5 g/dL, total lymphocyte count less than 1,800/mm^3, or a decrease in body weight of more than 15%. Individuals should also be assessed for oral and cutaneous signs of vitamin and mineral deficiencies. For example, extreme transparency of the skin on the hands, cellophane or tissue-paper skin, and purplish blotches on lightly traumatized areas (because of capillary fragility and subepithelial hemorrhage) may reflect vitamin C deficiency. Superficial flaking of the epidermis may suggest a deficiency of essential fatty acids and, in nonpigmented skin, vitamin A deficiency. Dry, reddened skin around the nose and eyebrows is a sign of zinc deficiency. Adequate nutrition includes appropriate protein, calories, vitamins, minerals, and fluids and is important for older persons at risk of developing pressure injuries, as well as those for whom wound healing is the goal (Ayello, Thomas, & Litchford, 1999). Meta-analysis of studies in the literature, however, indicate that the exact role nutrition plays in preventing wounds is unclear (Langer & Fink, 2014).

The importance of accurate and regular assessment of an older person's weight and height cannot be overemphasized. Unintended weight loss of even 5% can affect a patient's ability to maintain skin or heal a pressure injury. A comprehensive plan of care must include assessment of the risks for developing pressure injury. The Braden Scale (www .bradenscale.com) is an example of a valid and reliable instrument that should be used as part of a comprehensive risk assessment that includes a head-to-toe skin assessment and review of other risk factors such as comorbidities (Haesler, 2014). Risk assessment should be done within 8 hours of admission or on first contact with a health professional and on a regular basis thereafter, based on the patient's condition (Haesler, 2014). Since patients with medical devices are also at risk for developing a pressure injury, the skin beneath the medical device should be assessed at least twice daily and more frequently if the person is having fluid shifts or localized or generalized edema (Haesler, 2014). Attention to nutrition is an important component of risk assessment of, and the treatment plan for, individuals at risk for pressure injuries. Patients who are immobilized for a long time before surgery, have long time in the operating room, have multiple hypotensive episodes or a low core body temperature during surgery, or have reduced immobility on the first postoperative day may be at increased risk for a pressure injury (Haesler, 2014).

See also Pressure Injuries Prevention and Treatment; Skin Issues: Bruises and Discoloration; Skin Tears.

Carol L.B. Ott and Elizabeth A. Ayello

Anderson, M., Guthie, P. F., Kraft, W., Reicks, P., Skay, C., & Beal, A. L. (2015). Universal pressure ulcer prevention bundle with WOC nurse support. *Journal of Wound, Ostomy, and Continence Nursing*, 42(3), 217–225.

Ankrom, M., Bennett, R., Sprigle, S., Langemo, D., Black, J. M., Berlowitz, D. R., ... National Pressure Ulcer Advisory Panel. (2005). Pressure-related deep tissue injury under intact skin and the current pressure ulcer staging systems. *Advances in Skin and Wound Care*, 18(1), 35–42.

Ayello, E. A., & Braden, B. (2002). How and why to do pressure ulcer risk assessment. *Advances in Skin and Wound Care*, 15(3), 125–132.

Ayello, E. A., Thomas, D. R., & Litchford, M. A. (1999). Nutritional aspects of wound healing. *Home Health Nurse*, 17(11), 719–729.

Barczak, C. A., Barnett, R. I., Childs, E. J., & Bosley, L. M. (1997). Fourth National Pressure Ulcer Prevalence Survey. *Advances in Wound Care*, 10(4), 18–26.

Bates-Jensen, B. M., McCreath, H. E., & Pongquan, V. (2009). Subepidermal moisture is associated with early pressure ulcer damage in nursing home residents with dark skin tones. *Journal of Wound, Ostomy, and Continence Nursing*, 36(3), 277–284.

Bergquist-Beringer, S., & Gajewski, B. J. (2011). Outcome and assessment information set data that predict pressure ulcer development in older adult home health patients. *Advances in Skin and Wound Care*, 24(9), 404–414.

Black, J. M., & National Pressure Ulcer Advisory Panel. (2005). Moving toward consensus on deep tissue injury and pressure ulcer staging. *Advances in Skin and Wound Care*, 18(8), 415, 416, 418–421.

Centers for Medicare & Medicaid Services. (2004). Tag F314: Pressure ulcers guidance for surveyors in long-term care. Retrieved from http://www .cms.gov/Regulations-and-Guidance/Guidance/ Transmittals/downloads/R5SOM.pdf

DeFloor, T., Schoonhoven, L., Fletcher, J., Furtado, K., Heyman, H., Lubbers, M., ... Soriano, J. V. (2005). Statement of the European Pressure Ulcer Advisory Panel—Pressure ulcer classification. *Journal of Wound, Ostomy, and Continence Nursing*, 32(5), 302–306.

Delmore, B., Lebovits, S., Suggs, B., Rolnitzky, L., & Ayello, E. A. (2015). Risk factors associated with heel pressure ulcers in hospitalized patients. *Journal of Wound, Ostomy, and Continence Nursing*, 42(3), 242–248.

Dorner, D., Posthauer, M. E., & Thomas, D. (2009). *The role of nutrition in pressure ulcer prevention and treatment: National Pressure Ulcer Advisory Panel white paper.* Retrieved from http://www.npuap.org/ wp-content/uploads/2012/03/Nutrition-White -Paper-Website-Version.pdf

Doughty, D., Ramundo, J., Bonham, P., Beitz, J., Erwin Toth, P., Anderson, R., & Rolstad, B. S. (2006). Issues and challenges in staging of pressure ulcers. *Journal of Wound, Ostomy, and Continence Nursing*, 33(2), 125–132.

Edsberg, L. E., Black, J. M., Goldberg, M., McNichol, L., Moore, L., & Sieggreen, M. (2016). Revised National Pressure Ulcer Advisory Panel staging system. *Journal of Wound, Ostomy, and Continence Nursing*, 43(6), 1–13.

Gray, M., Black, J. M., Baharestani, M. M., Bliss, D. Z., Colwell, J. C., Goldberg, M., ... Ratliff, C. R. (2011). Moisture-associated skin damage: Overview and pathophysiology. *Journal of Wound, Ostomy, and Continence Nursing*, 38(3), 233–241.

Gray, M., Bliss, D. Z., Doughty, D. B., Ermer-Seltun, J., Kennedy-Evans, K. L., & Palmer, M. H. (2007). Incontinence-associated dermatitis: A consensus. *Journal of Wound, Ostomy, and Continence Nursing, 34*(1), 45–54.

Harmon, L. C., Grobbel, C., & Palleschi, M. (2016). Reducing pressure injury incidence using a turn team assignment. *Journal of Wound, Ostomy, and Continence Nursing, 43*(5), 477–482.

Honaker, J., Brockopp, D., & Moe, K. (2014). Suspected deep tissue injury profile: A pilot study. *Advances in Skin and Wound Care, 27*(3), 133–140.

Langer, G., & Fink, A. (2014). Nutritional interventions for preventing and treating pressure ulcers. *Cochrane Database of Systematic Reviews, 2014*(6), CD003216. doi:10.1002/14651858.CD003216.pub2

Lyder, C. H., Wang, Y. C., Metersky, M., Curry, M., Kliman, R., Verzier, N. R., & Hunt, D. R. (2012). Hospital-acquired pressure ulcers; Results from the National Medicare Patient Safety Monitory System Study. *Journal of the American Geriatrics Society, 60*(9), 1603–1608.

McNichol, L., Watts, C., Mackey, D., Beitz, J. M., & Gary, M. (2015). Identifying the right surface for the right patient at the right time: Generation and content validation of an algorithm for support surface selection. *Journal of Wound, Ostomy, and Continence Nursing, 42*(11), 19–37.

Moore, Z. E. H., & Cowman, S. (2014). Risk assessment tools for the prevention of pressure ulcers. *Cochrane Database of Systematic Reviews, 2014*(2), CD006471. doi:10.1002/14651858.CD006471.pub3

National Pressure Ulcer Advisory Panel. (2016). NPUAP announces a change in terminology from pressure ulcer to pressure injury and updates the stages of pressure injury. Retrieved from http://www.npuap.org/national-pressure-ulcer-advisory-panel-npuap-announces-a-change-in-terminology-from-pressure-ulcer-to-pressure-injury-and-updates-the-stages-of-pressure-injury

Haesler, E. (Ed.). (2014). *Prevention and treatment of pressure ulcers: Clinical practice guideline.* Osborne Park, Western Australia: Cambridge Media.

Rapp, M. P., Bergstrom, N., & Padhye, N. C. (2009). Contribution of skin temperature regularity to the risk of developing pressure ulcers in nursing facility residents. *Advances in Skin and Wound Care, 22*(11), 506–513.

Reid, K., Ayello, E. A., & Alavi, A. (2016). Pressure ulcer prevention and treatment: Use of prophylactic dressings. *Chronic Wound Care Management and Research, 3*, 117–121.

Sibbald, R. G., Goodman, L., Norton, L., Krasner, D. L., & Ayello, E. A. (2012). Prevention and treatment of pressure ulcers. *Skin Therapy Letter, 17*(8), 4–7.

Sprigle, S., Linden, M., McKenna, D., Davis, K., & Riordan, B. (2001). Clinical skin temperature measurement to predict incipient pressure ulcers. *Advances in Skin and Wound Care, 14*(3), 133–137.

Sullivan, R. (2013). A two-year retrospective review of suspected deep tissue injury evolution in adult acute care patients. *Ostomy Wound Management, 59*(9), 30–39.

Tran, J. P., McLaughlin, J. M., Li, R. T., & Phillips, L. G. (2016). Prevention of pressure ulcers in the acute care setting: New innovations and technologies. *Plastic and Reconstructive Surgery Journal, 138*(3S), 232S–240S.

VanGilder, C., MacFarlane, G. D., Harrison, P., Lachenbruch, C., & Meyer, S. (2010). The demographics of suspected deep tissue injury in the United States: An analysis of the International Pressure Ulcer Prevalence Survey 2006–2009. *Advances in Skin and Wound Care, 23*(6), 254–261.

VanGilder, C., MacFarlane, G. D., & Meyer, S. (2008). Results of nine International Pressure Ulcer Prevalence Surveys: 1989–2005. *Ostomy Wound Management, 54*(2), 40–54.

Whittington, K. T., & Briones, R. (2004). National prevalence and incidence study: 6-year sequential acute care data. *Advances in Skin and Wound Care, 17*(9), 90–94.

Wolfman, A. (2010). Preventing incontinence-associated dermatitis and early stage pressure injury. *World Council of Enterostomal Therapists Journal, 30*(1), 19–24.

Wong, V. K., Stotts, N., Hopf, H. W., Dowling, G. A., & Froelicher, E. S. (2011). Changes in heel skin temperature under pressure in hip surgery patients. *Advances in Skin and Wound Care, 24*(12), 562–570.

Zulkowski, K. (2008). Perineal dermatitis versus pressure ulcer: Distinguishing characteristics. *Advances in Skin & Wound Care, 21*(8), 382–388.

Web Resources

American Academy of Wound Management: http://www.aawm.org

American Professional Wound Care Association: http://www.apwca.org

Braden Scale: http://bradenscale.com

National Pressure Ulcer Advisory Panel: http://www.npuap.org

Wound, Ostomy, & Continence Nurses Society: http://www.wocn.org

PRIMARY PALLIATIVE CARE

Palliative care is interdisciplinary health care for people with serious illnesses. "Palliative care is focused on providing relief from the symptoms and stress of a serious illness. The goal is to improve quality of life for both the patient and the family" (Center to Advance Palliative Care, 2017). One way to conceptualize the delivery of palliative care is to consider the degree of specialization needed by the providers. Palliative care provided by highly trained specialists is reserved for more complex cases in which there are unmet palliative care needs. All providers who care for patients with serious illnesses should have a basic competency in palliative care. Although palliative care specialists hold specific expertise in this field (specialty palliative care), the principles of palliative care can be readily applied within any treatment setting. *Primary palliative care* refers to the core set of skills rooted in the philosophy of palliative care that can be implemented by all health care providers.

As medical treatments advance and the population ages, the number of patients living with chronic diseases and comorbidities will increase. More than 65% of Medicare beneficiaries have two or more chronic illnesses. By 2020, the number of people with multiple chronic conditions is expected to increase to 81 million from 57 million in 2000. These patients benefit from careful attention to symptom management, care coordination, and advance care planning Studies to date have shown that palliative care reduces health care costs, improves patient quality of life, and may even increase survival (Temel et al., 2010).

Although access to palliative care for patients with serious illnesses has increased in the past 10 years, the number of palliative care specialists (in both the inpatient and the outpatient settings) is insufficient to meet the demand of the increasingly complex patient population. Primary care providers and other health care professionals who have continuity with patients are particularly well positioned to seamlessly integrate preventive and curative care alongside palliative care into their practices. With sufficient palliative care training, competency in core palliative care principles, and dedication of resources, all health care professionals, including doctors, nurses, health aides, social workers, and chaplains, should be able to provide primary palliative care appropriate to their role.

A primary palliative care approach is ideal for several reasons. Health care providers who know patients over time can initiate early goals of care and advance care planning conversations to ensure that patient preferences align with treatment decisions. Long-standing, trusting relationships may help facilitate communication around these difficult topics. Because these providers know the patient longitudinally, they can more effectively advocate and coordinate care for their patients. Last, following patients closely as they near the end of their life may help reduce the sense of abandonment some patients experience and can be very meaningful and rewarding for providers as well.

COMPONENTS

The main components of primary palliative care include coordination of care, symptom assessment and management, patient education, goals of care and advance care planning, skill in difficult conversations, support for caregivers, and referral to specialists in palliative care services. These components often need to be provided by a multidisciplinary team.

Coordination of Care

Patients and their families benefit from an enduring relationship with a health care provider who orchestrates care that often stretches across multiple treatment settings. As patients and families find themselves balancing visits to multiple specialists and coordinating a variety of treatments, the guidance of a health care provider can achieve smoother transitions from one physician's office to another, coordination of posthospitalization care, or facilitated access to community services for patient, family, or caregiver support. Coordination of care not only eases the stress and burden of patients and families, but also ensures continuity of care, and limits the risk of errors in follow-up. Providers can also consider additional strategies for improving continuity and coordination of care, the best evidence of which comes from referral to comprehensive and multidisciplinary teams that may include postdischarge support and case management (Lorenz et al., 2008).

Symptom Assessment and Management

One of the most fundamental applications of primary palliative care is the assessment and management of symptoms arising from advanced illness. Physical symptoms such as pain, shortness of breath, nausea, constipation, and others can severely impair a patient's quality of life, limit function, and preclude meaningful interactions with loved ones. The primary care provider must screen spiritual and emotional distress when assessing physical symptoms. The recognition that physical, emotional, and spiritual distress may each contribute to a patient's experience of pain is termed *total pain*, a concept initially proposed by Dame Cicely Saunders, one of the earliest champions of the hospice movement. This notion of total pain requires practitioners to screen equally for physical symptoms as well as psychological or spiritual distress and to work toward the relief of any identified symptoms in the hope of achieving global relief from suffering. The potential for a wide range of symptoms highlights the importance of multidisciplinary approaches to palliative care, capitalizing on the expertise of social workers, pain management specialists, chaplains, and mental health providers.

Patient and Caregiver Education

All health care providers are integral to providing education to patients experiencing serious illnesses and their families, particularly those with a long-standing knowledge of the patient. This is a particularly important aspect of primary palliative care, wherein clarification of a patient's diagnosis, risks, and benefits of potential treatment options, anticipated illness course, or prognosis provides a foundation for patients and their families to make health care decisions or navigate treatment options that are consistent with their values and health beliefs. Providers may have concern that exploring prognosis

and end-of-life issues may result in significant distress in their patients. However, this type of discussion has been associated with improved outcomes for patients, including a higher quality of life and less aggressive treatments at the last weeks of life, with no significant impact on depression or anxiety (Wright et al., 2008).

Goals of Care/Advanced Care Planning

The hallmark of patient-centered care is ensuring that patients are able to use medical information about their illness to inform treatment decisions that are consistent with their values and wishes, or their *goals of care*. To that end, primary palliative care promotes the active exploration of those priorities and values with each patient over the evolution of their illness. This process can begin at any point in a patient–physician relationship, is useful in guiding a patient's health care at any age and may change with new information about or changes in a patient's health. As patients age or their health status becomes tenuous, thorough knowledge of their values becomes increasingly urgent. *Advance care planning* is a process that allows patients to consider values and preferences that specifically relate to their end-of-life care (Detering, Hancock, Reade, & Silvester, 2010). This can include making decisions about surrogate decision makers, code status, artificial nutrition, or the aggressiveness of symptom management. These decisions can be documented in the form of an *advance directive* to ensure adherence to patients' wishes if they are too ill or otherwise unable to voice them. It is important for patients to understand the legal process and implications of completing advance directives.

Caregiver Support

An often under-recognized need is caregiver support. The management of complex and advanced illness frequently involves caregivers who have sometimes committed years to the care of their loved ones. The role of caregiver itself is associated with increased rates of illness and even death; caregivers benefit from awareness of this burden, recognition of their effort and need for self-care, education and guidance in the care of their loved one, and the provision of respite opportunities when possible. Referral should also be considered for disease-specific training and support programs for caregivers. An example for caregivers of people with dementia is the Resources for Enhancing Alzheimer's Caregiver Health II (REACH II) program, an individualized multicomponent home- and telephone-based intervention designed to enhance caregiver's coping skills and management of dementia-related behaviors. Availability of this program varies by community.

Referral to Specialized Palliative Care and Hospice

Although palliative care can be initiated by any health care professional, even among the most skilled providers a comprehensive palliative approach can be difficult to achieve. A patient's symptoms may not improve with attempted treatments. There may be factors limiting effective discussion of a patient's goals of care and thereby decision making around appropriate treatments. Or a patient may need resources—such as chaplains or social workers—who might not be available in the current health care setting. For these patients, a timely referral to specialist palliative care services is indicated, either to outpatient palliative care clinics or, if immediate evaluation is needed, to inpatient consulting teams.

For patients with an expected prognosis of less than 6 months whose primary focus is on preserving quality of life and symptom management, a referral to a community hospice program would provide them and their families with specialized palliative care. *Hospice* is a universal Medicare benefit for all eligible patients that provides an opportunity for more aggressive symptom management; access to interdisciplinary resources such as chaplains, social workers, nurses, and volunteers; and ongoing coordination of care. Hospice services can be provided either in the home or in a community facility, such as a residential hospice or a skilled nursing facility. Referring providers have the opportunity to continue their close involvement with patients and their families, with the added expertise of nursing and physician teams trained in palliative medicine.

Robert Smeltz

Center to Advance Palliative Care. (2017). What is palliative care? Retrieved from https://getpalliativecare.org/whatis

Detering, K. M., Hancock, A. D., Reade, M. C., & Silvester, W. (2010). The impact of advance care planning on end of life care in elderly patients: Randomised controlled trial. *British Medical Journal, 340*, 1345.

Lorenz, K. A., Lynn, J., Dy, S. M., Shugarman, L. R., Wilkinson, A., Mularski, R. A., ... Shekelle, P. G. (2008). Evidence for improving palliative care at the end of life: A systematic review. *Annals of Internal Medicine, 148*(2), 147–159.

Temel, J. S., Greer, J. A., Muzikansky, A., Gallagher, E. R., Admane, S., Jackson, V. A., ... Lynch, T. J. (2010). Early palliative care for patients with metastatic non-small-cell lung cancer. *The New England Journal of Medicine, 363*(8), 733–742.

Wright, A. A., Zhang, B., Ray, A., Mack, J. W., Trice, E., Balboni, T., ... Prigerson, H. G. (2008). Associations between end-of-life discussions, patient mental health, medical care near death, and caregiver bereavement adjustment. *Journal of the American Medical Association, 300*(14), 1665–1673.

Web Resources

Center to Advance Palliative Care (CAPC): http://www.capc.org

Education for Physicians on End-of-Life Care (EPEC): http://www.epec.net

End-of-Life Nursing Education Consortium (ELNEC): http://www.aacn.nche.edu/elnec

ePrognosis : http://eprognosis.org

GeriPal (a geriatrics and palliative care blog): http://www.geripal.org

Get Palliative Care: http://www.getpalliativecare.org

National Palliative Care Research Center: http://www.npcrc.org

PROGRAM OF ALL-INCLUSIVE CARE FOR THE ELDERLY (PACE)

The Program of All-Inclusive Care for the Elderly (PACE) values the idea that older adults with chronic care needs and their families are better served in the community whenever

P

possible. PACE is a capitated and coordinated care program that combines Medicare and Medicaid benefits to provide primary, acute, and long-term services and supports for the frail elderly. PACE serves individuals who are aged 55 years or older (the average age of individuals enrolled in PACE in 2016 was 76 years, according to the National PACE Association [NPA]; CalPACE, 2016) and certified by their state to need a nursing home (NH) level of care. Other eligibility criteria include being able to live safely in the community with the support of PACE at the time of enrollment, as well as living in a PACE service area. Enrollment is not affected by changes in health status (unless participant is no longer NH eligible) and continues as long as enrollees desire. PACE programs provide a comprehensive set of preventive, primary, acute, long-term, and end-of-life care, all specifically tailored to the needs of each enrollee. The PACE model of care can be traced to the early 1970s, when the Chinatown community of San Francisco saw the pressing need for long-term care services for the families whose elders had immigrated to the United States. A nonprofit corporation, On Lok senior health services, was formed to create a community-based system of care. By 1997, federal legislation authorized PACE as a permanent Medicare benefit and a Medicaid state plan optional service (Larson, 2002).

Given that PACE programs are financially responsible for all Medicare- and Medicaid-covered services, the program is designed to maintain enrollees health and safety in the community, avoiding high-cost institutional care (i.e., hospital and NHs) through proactive assessment and care management. The program closely monitors enrollees for the most subtle changes in health status and needs, which could lead to inappropriate and avoidable use of institutional care if left unattended. This approach not only ensures enrollees' wellness and satisfaction, but also provides a strong financial incentive for the PACE organization to identify and immediately respond to enrollees' health care needs (Gong & Aldrich, 2008). As a result, PACE enrollees spend significantly less time in hospitals compared with a cohort of similar high-care needs older adults living in the community (Meret-Hanke, 2011).

At the center of PACE services is the interdisciplinary team (IDT), which consists of professional and paraprofessional staff. Each PACE team includes a primary care physician, nurse, social worker, physical therapist, occupational therapist, recreational therapist or activity coordinator, dietician, PACE center supervisor, home-care liaison, health workers or aides, and drivers. The IDT brings together the viewpoints of different disciplines, as well as information obtained during interactions with the PACE enrollees in different settings over time. Mukamel et al. (2006) delved into the distinction between *formal* and *informal* communication of the IDT regarding each PACE participant. *Formal* communication occurs during regularly scheduled IDT meetings with all staff furnishing care to a participant in attendance. Conversely, *informal* communication regarding a participant's care occurs in everyday practice among staff (Mukamel et al., 2006). This ongoing communication structure ensures that staffs is well informed and equipped to address a participant's needs. To integrate care provision, the team assesses and periodically reassesses participants' needs; develops care plans encompassing all Medicare- and Medicaid-covered services (including institutional, home, community, and end-of-life care); and directly delivers all or most services. Social and medical services are delivered primarily in PACE's adult day health centers. Center-based services must include primary care services, nutritional counseling, recreational therapy, and meals. Oversight of progress and delivery of care is facilitated by PACE's emphasis on day-center attendance by enrollees, but congregate housing and in-home services have been developed and integrated into care planning and provision. Some PACE programs contract with independent (i.e., non-staff) community-based primary care physicians to allow them to continue to follow their patients who enroll in PACE. Under this arrangement, PACE provides enrollees and their physicians with all IDT services, including care coordination and nurse practitioners or physician assistants (Eng, 2005). Proposed changes to the PACE Regulation issued in August of 2016 provide opportunities for flexibility in the composition of the IDT—specifically, it introduces changes to the clinical provisions of care wherein one (qualified) health care professional can perform two distinct roles on the IDT (e.g., serve as an RN and a social worker). Furthermore, the proposed PACE Regulation seeks to allow primary care services to be furnished by a physician assistant, nurse practitioner, or community-based physician (without a need for a waiver) (The Office of the Federal Register, 2016). Traditionally, PACE organizations have been required to apply for waivers to allow care to be furnished by community-based physicians and nurse practitioners.

The financial underpinnings of PACE are complex, varied, and evolving. PACE programs represent a three-way partnership among providers, the state, and the federal government. The Centers for Medicare & Medicaid Services (CMS) pays the Medicare capitation, and each state establishes and pays the Medicaid capitation. In return, PACE programs assume complete financial responsibility for providing to enrollees all services covered by Medicare and Medicaid, and many providers offer added services (Petigara & Anderson, 2009). The capitation model gives PACE programs flexibility and incentive to provide preventive services that would not otherwise be covered by Medicare or Medicaid, if the IDT team determines that these services are appropriate for the enrollee. Since 2004, CMS has been using a risk-adjusted payment approach to calculate PACE payments on the basis of each enrollee's demographic, functional, and diagnostic characteristics. Under Medicaid, the monthly capitation is negotiated and annually contracted between the local PACE provider and the state. Generally, states base their payments on their reimbursements for a NH-eligible population, including both NH residents and community-based long-term care recipients. In 2016, combined Medicare and Medicaid dual-eligible capitation payments averaged approximately $5,951 per participant per month (NPA, n.d.). Typically, 39% of payment comes from Medicare and 61% from Medicaid. Medicare-eligible enrollees who are not eligible for Medicaid pay monthly premiums equivalent to the Medicaid capitation amount, but no deductibles, co-insurance, or other type of Medicare or Medicaid cost-sharing

applies. PACE providers assume full financial risk for enrollees' Medicare- and Medicaid-covered care without limits on amount, duration, or scope of services (Centers for Medicare & Medicaid Services, 2012).

As of August 2016, there were 120 PACE programs operating in 31 states. Most of these programs were sponsored by nonprofit healthcare providers, with the exception of 10 for-profit PACE programs. The NPA, a nonprofit trade association that exists to advance the efforts of PACE, has been developing strategies to reach new populations in need of comprehensive health care. As a result of NPA's work, PACE has been made available to diverse populations across the country. In 2006, the passage of the Community Options for Rural Elders (CORE) Act led to the creation start-up grants for the development of 15 PACE programs in rural areas, of which 11 remain in operation. Separate from the CORE Act, other PACE programs have been developed in rural areas. In 2008, Cherokee Elder Care started operations in Oklahoma, the first PACE program in the country sponsored by a Native American Tribe (Cherokee Elder Care, 2012). In 2015, NPA reported 14 PACE programs working in partnership with the Veterans Affairs Medical Centers (VAMCs) to provide comprehensive care to veterans—the U.S. Department of Veterans Affairs (USDVA) considers PACE as a type of home and community-based service, making PACE no longer a pilot program for the VA; rather, it is one of the community-based services that the VA has opted to offer its beneficiaries. Expansion of the PACE model has also garnered congressional support—in November 2015, the PACE Innovation Act (PIA) was signed into law. The PIA provides an opportunity for new populations to benefit from the PACE model of care; the range of potential populations includes: individuals younger than 55 years with a disability, as well as those who are medically complex and at risk of requiring an NH level of care. The PACE model has been considered the gold standard for community-based care for more than two decades, and with the expansion of the PACE model to new populations, more individuals will have access to all-inclusive, coordinated care.

P

See also Naturally Occurring Retirement Communities (NORCs); Nursing Homes.

Shawn M. Bloom and Asmaa Albaroudi

CalPACE. (2016). Program of all-inclusive care for the elderly. Retrieved from http://www.calpace.org/fileadmin/Fact_sheet_--_CalPACE_--_4-18-16_Final.pdf

Centers for Medicare & Medicaid Services. (2012). PACE benefits. Retrieved from http://www.medicaid.gov/Medicaid-CHIP-Program-Information/By-Topics/Long-Term-Services-and-Support/Integrating-Care/Program-of-All-Inclusive-Care-for-the-Elderly-PACE/PACE-Benefits.html

Cherokee Elder Care. (2012). FAQ sheet. Retrieved from http://eldercare.cherokee.org/FAQs.aspx

Eng, C. (2005). *Community primary care physicians in PACE: On Lok experience.* Presented at a NPA Teleconference Series.

Gong, J., & Aldrich, S. (2008). PACE is good business. *Advance for Long-Term Care Management, 16*(5), 7.

Larson, L. (2002). A better way to grow: The PACE model. *Trustee Magazine.* Retrieved from http://www.seniorjournal.com/NEWS/Eldercare/2–08-08PACE.htm

Meret-Hanke, L. A. (2011). Effects of the Program of All-Inclusive Care for the Elderly on hospital use. *The Gerontologist, 51,* 774–785.

Mukamel, D. B., Temkin-Greener, H., Delavan, R., Peterson, D. R., Gross, D., Kunitz, S., & Williams, T. F. (2006). Team performance and risk-adjusted health outcomes in the Program of All-Inclusive Care for the Elderly (PACE). *The Gerontologist, 46*(2), 227–237.

National PACE Association. (n.d.). PACE facts and trends. Retrieved from http://www.npaonline.org/policy-and-advocacy/pace-facts-and-trends-0

Petigara, T., & Anderson, G. (2009). Program of All-Inclusive Care for the Elderly. *Health Policy Monitor.* Retrieved from http://old.npaonline.org/website/download.asp?id=3034&title=PACE_-_HealthPolicyMonitor_-_2009

Web Resources

Centers for Medicare & Medicaid Services: http://www.medicaid.gov/Medicaid-CHIP-Program-Information/By-Topics/Long-Term-Services-and-Support/Integrating-Care/Program-of-All-Inclusive-Care-for-the-Elderly-PACE/Program-of-All-Inclusive-Care-for-the-Elderly-PACE.html

Office of the *Federal Register.* (2016): PACE proposed rule: https://www.federalregister.gov/articles/2016/08/16/2016-19153/medicare-and-medicaid-programs-programs-of-all-inclusive-care-for-the-elderly-pace

Psychological/Mental Status Assessment

It is generally acknowledged that the world's population is aging. It is also clear, although not always thought about, that psychological and mental health functioning is a critical part of healthy aging. Unfortunately, the risk of occurrence or reoccurrence of mental illness increases with age, and significant cognitive decline is common in the elderly. The ability to carry out a careful mental status assessment is an important skill for any health professional working with older adult.

Although it is true that the risk of significant cognitive decline increases with age and that mental illness is common in later life, it is not true that such changes and disorders are an inevitable consequence of aging. This is in fact a common myth that is part of the stigma associated with aging, or ageism. Despite their education, health professionals are not immune from this myth, and because they see mostly medically ill or functionally disabled older adults, this myth may be reinforced. There is a complex interplay of social, biological, and psychological factors involved in the aging process, which makes accurate diagnosis and effective treatment more elusive.

Although the format for mental status assessment of older adults does not differ significantly from that used with younger clients, the process needs to begin with an evaluation of the person's hearing, vision, and cognitive functioning, as well as primary language and linguistic heritage, health literacy and cultural background. The health professional takes a psychiatric history, including a history of the presenting complaint and the medical, psychiatric, personal, and family history. The mental status examination should include the usual areas of appearance, behavior, speech, mood and affect, form and content of thought, perception, sensorium and cognition, as well as insight and judgment. Nevertheless, it is important for clinicians to be mindful of age-related changes in physical and psychological capacities when assessing older adults, both to maximize the quality of care and to protect the validity of the assessment process. For older adults with hearing impairment, clinicians may need to modify the rate, pitch, and enunciation of their speech to encourage appropriate levels of understanding when communicating. Also, if a hearing-assistive device or hearing aid is used by the older adult it is important to ensure that it is available during the assessment and is working properly. Visual or written means of communication may be required, word-to-text apps for handheld devices are now available. Individuals with cognitive deficits or neurodiversity (different learning ability) may require simplified instructions or repetition to ensure understanding between clinician and client. A general slowing of the pace of the assessment may also be necessary to accommodate age-related reductions in processing speed. In addition, environmental accommodations such as conducting assessments in a well-lit room with minimal background noise may alleviate some difficulties related to sensory impairments. Finally, it is important for clinicians to ensure that the assessment tools they select are appropriate for use in older adults. The person's level of fatigue and motivation needs to be considered at the outset and monitored during the assessment. For the majority of factors, clinicians might wish to assess, there are instruments that have been specifically normed for use in older adult populations.

From a psychosocial perspective, clinicians should consider if elders are going through life transitions, such as retirement or bereavement, as well as their gender, cohort experiences, ethnicity, and legal status, all of which contribute to the presentation. As with geriatric assessment in general, collateral sources of information need to be explored, and the demonstration of abilities, when possible, is superior to an interview about them, even to family members who might

not have noticed the extent of the age- or disease-related changes.

PSYCHIATRIC INTERVIEW

The primary means of evaluation of an older adult, if it can be done, is the psychiatric interview (Blazer, 2015). The interview should be structured and begun with a review of the presenting symptoms, collateral information from the family (two generations if possible), and the medical record, ideally with permission of the patient. As in other areas of medicine, the standard questions regarding the presenting symptom or problem should be asked. When did it start? How long it has lasted? Has the severity changed over time? Likewise, what has the person tried to correct or deal with the symptoms, how did that work, and how does the symptom vary in the course of the day, week, or season (Blazer, 2015)? Important to identifying the correct diagnosis of a psychiatric disorder, according to the *Diagnostic and Statistical Manual of Mental Disorders* (5th ed.; *DSM-5*; American Psychiatric Association, 2013), is investigating the duration of the symptoms: more than 1 month and/or more than 6 months. Essential to *DSM-5* is how has these symptoms affected the person's functioning, including ability to work, carry out activities and ADL, and function socially.

Past psychiatric and medical history of the person is very important for accurate evaluation of the symptoms or problems. Has the health care provider diagnosed this condition before? How often? How long were the episodes? What, if anything, was used to treat it? How well did these approaches or medications work? Mood swings, excessive activity, and excessive alcohol intake are important, specific questions (Blazer, 2015). Family psychiatric history and general family assessment are important components of the evaluation of the mental health of the older adult. A genogram that contains both medical and major psychosocial events, such as when parts of the family moved away, is very important for understanding both something of the genetic vulnerability and psychosocial context of mental health changes. Periods of economic or environmental stressors should be included, if possible. What services the family provides for the patient and how this support is perceived are important, and the potential for excessive critical, conflictual, or abusive family interactions must be considered. The presence of other family members with psychiatric illness or disability should also be discussed.

Information about the person's current and past medications offers some evidence of conditions as viewed by previous health care providers. Verification of current medications by having the person bring in original pill bottles or list of medication often reveals discrepancies between what is prescribed and what is taken. Possible drug–drug and drug–alcohol interactions need to be considered.

The assessment of mental status of older persons is not unlike that of younger persons, although needed screening tools should be specific for older adults. Although the meaning of many assessment items are often different in later life, the areas are the same as those for younger persons: appearance, affect and mood, psychomotor activity, perception, disturbance of thought and processing, as well as suicidality (Blazer, 2015). The value of screening scales in mental health/mental status examination is very important to confirming the clinical impression and discussing the extent of the symptoms or problems with other clinicians, family, and caregivers. Various assessments for neurocognitive disorders, depression, and general assessment are available. One particular challenge in the assessment of older adults is the overlap of symptoms of delirium, dementia, and depression. Distinguishing among these clinical conditions can be difficult, particularly when two or more of them may be present; the approach and treatment for each is quite different (Zarit & Zarit, 2011).

See also Cognitive Instruments; Depression in Dementia; Depression Measurement Instruments; Mental Capacity Assessment; Neuropsychological Assessment.

Steven L. Baumann

American Psychiatric Association. (2013). *Diagnostic and statistical manual of mental disorders* (5th ed.). Arlington, VA: American Psychiatric Publishing.

Blazer, D. G. (2015). The psychiatric interview. In D. C. Steffens, D. G. Blazer, & M. E. Thakur (Eds.), *The American Psychiatric Publishing textbook of geriatric psychiatry* (5th ed., pp. 89–107). New York, NY: American Psychiatric Publishing. doi:10.1176/appi.books.9781615370054

Zarit, S. H., & Zarit, J. M. (2011). *Mental disorders in older adults: Fundamentals of assessment and treatment* (2nd ed.). New York, NY: Guilford Press.

Web Resources
ConsultGeri (assessment tools and how to use them): https://consultgeri.org
Gerocentral (geropsychology training, service provision, policy, and research): http://gerocentral.org

PSYCHOLOGY

As the average life expectancy improves, older adults are forming an increasing percentage of the population (U.S. Census Bureau, 2008). Many clinicians, no matter what age or level of experience, are aging. It's important for psychologists to reflect on how their own aging and/or medical illness affects their attitudes and clinical practice in working with this increasing and underserviced population (Schwartz & Schwartzberg, 2011).

MENTAL HEALTH ISSUES AND PSYCHOLOGICAL PRACTICE

Even though older adults have a lower prevalence of major depressive disorders than the younger adults (American Psychological Association [APA], 2009a), baby boomers are generally more psychologically minded, have higher rates of depression and have had a higher use of behavioral health services throughout their lifetimes (APA, 2009b). In all likelihood, there will be an increase in demand for psychological services with older adults in the years ahead. Although many older adults are resilient and lead active and productive lives, including remaining in the work force and delaying retirement, volunteering, or performing unpaid volunteer work involving grandchildren, they nonetheless face many challenges, such as increasing health problems and loss of loved ones. Older adults may need help facing the normal life transitions from the work world to retirement and make behavioral adaptations to loss of independence, financial challenges, changes in relationships, social isolation, and loneliness. Depressive symptoms may reflect coming to terms with physical decline and death. Suicide is a significant issue in older adults who are depressed, and suicide rates in older adult white males, in particular, are among the highest of any age group. Practitioners working with older adults must be vigilant about assessing for suicide risk (APA, 2014).

Alcohol abuse is one of the fastest growing and most underidentified health problems in the older adult population (Substance Abuse and Mental Health Services Administration [SAMSHA], 2008). All older adults are at increased risk for alcohol-related problems because of physiological changes. Use of illicit drugs and prescription pill abuse in this population is expected to increase as the baby boomers age (Institute of Medicine, 2012). Psychologists will also treat more older clients with queries or worries about their sexuality. Unfortunately, societal stereotypes continue to ignore the importance of sexual activity and intimacy with respect to quality of life and emotional well-being (Lee, Nazroo, O'Connor, Blake, & Pendleton, 2014). Studies show that a significant number of community-dwelling older adults retain interest in having sexual relationships, so it is essential that psychologists do not adopt ageist misconceptions (Lindau et al., 2007).

Clinicians must develop knowledge of the biological, psychological, cultural, and social contexts associated with normal aging. A life-span developmental perspective is important, with awareness of the positive psychological perspectives and maturation that can occur in late life. As a result of these considerations, the APA developed guidelines to provide practitioners with (a) a frame of reference for engaging in clinical work with older adults and (b) basic information and further references in the areas of attitudes, general aspects of aging, clinical issues, assessment, intervention, consultation,

and continuing education and training relative to work with older adults (APA, 2014).

DEMOGRAPHIC CHANGES AND CHALLENGES

The fastest growth in population in the United States is seen in the oldest old; estimates indicate that the number of centenarians will increase by a factor of close to eight, from 79,000 centenarians in 2010 to 601,000 by 2050 (U.S. Census Bureau, 2008). With a difference of perhaps seven generations between client and therapist, an understanding of differing social, cultural, and technological differences as well as age differences across generations is vital (Laidlaw & Pachana, 2009). This is especially relevant as the number of older adult racial/ethnic and gay minorities will increase and have their own unique cultural and mental health challenges (APA, 2014).

Aging women have a greater likelihood of being caregivers to frail husbands, becoming widows and being at increased risk for dementia and other illnesses associated with aging. Aging may be affected by other gender-related issues such as women marrying later, having smaller families, and outliving their spouses, meaning that many senior women will be challenged with the chores of caring for adult children and/or grandchildren and their increasingly dependent and frail parents (Laidlaw & Pachana, 2009).

Although there can be positive aspects to caregiving for a loved one, the caregiver's needs are often neglected, which can lead to physical decline and depression. Caregivers must address important psychological tasks to cope successfully with the caregiving experience (Jacobs, 2006).

PSYCHOTHERAPEUTIC INTERVENTIONS WITH OLDER ADULTS

Psychotherapy interventions with older clients may include individual, group, couple, and family work. Aging often leads to an increased recognition of the passing of time and of limited future prospects, which may lead older adults to seek psychotherapeutic intervention to focus on meaningful emotional goals and to concentrate

P

on relationships that have the most significance for them (APA, 2014). No single modality of treatment is preferable for all older adults (APA, 2014). An increasing number of studies suggest that older adults respond well to a variety of forms of psychotherapy and can benefit to a degree comparable with younger adults (Pinquart & Sorensen, 2001). The selection of the most appropriate treatment and mode of delivery depends on the nature of the problem, context, cohort of patients, clinical goals, immediate situation, and individual characteristics, preferences, and place on the continuum of care (APA, 2014).

Societal stereotypes of aging often lead to barriers hindering aging individuals from being referred or appropriately treated. Therapists must be on guard against having ageist attitudes, such as aging being associated with decline and loss, being ill, or being too old to change. Realistic therapeutic expectations guard against negative countertransference such as denial and despair. Some clinicians may avoid work with this population, for example, because it evokes discomfort or stirs up uncomfortable feelings in relation to the aging of one's family members (APA, 2014).

Most psychotherapeutic interventions need not be significantly altered for an older population. The main reason for adapting therapy approaches with the older adult has more to do with the particular setting and context of the therapy (APA, 2009b). Yet cognitive-behavior therapists can use this approach to challenge the evidence for and against that older clients have to support their fears, not so much that they have a restricted and limited time frame, but that their remaining life will be one of unhappiness and despair (Laidlaw & Pachana, 2009).

Group therapy is both an effective and cost-efficient treatment for older adults (American Group Psychotherapy Association, 2007). Group therapy is helpful with older adults who struggle with aging-related losses of interpersonal, emotional, social, physical, and cognitive capacities. Unfortunately, this clinical intervention remains underutilized as clinicians remain unaware of its benefits and the unique techniques required to work with this population (Schwartz, 2011).

An integration of relevant psychotherapy models in individual and/or group sessions, using developmental, cognitive-behavioral, interpersonal, and dynamic approaches, can be combined to create a unique model of psychological intervention. This intervention uses appropriate social, cognitive, and behavioral skills to cope with the experience of aging, illness, and dying. Psychotherapies delivered as part of integrative care models have been found to be effective in the treatment of depression in primary care settings (APA, 2014).

Couple and family work may often need to focus on providing both practical suggestions and emotional support. Issues relating to "role reversal" and undermining of the older parent's autonomy are common, placing the burden of care on adult children. Another issue relates to finances when older parents want to set limits on supporting a child. This creates conflict with the child and between spouses. Unfortunately, difficulty in setting up appropriate boundaries may also end up compromising the older couple's hard-earned financial security.

CONCLUSION AND FUTURE IMPLICATIONS

As the population ages, older adults struggle with mental health issues previously not resolved, as well as with present issues, both practical and existential, relating to loss of meaning and purpose, loss of loved ones, and mortality. There is an increasing need to train more clinicians who are knowledgeable about the life cycle, demographic change, and gerontological theories of aging. Also, research into the attitudes, motivation, and experiences of clinicians is required, so the ability and motivation of clinicians to work with the aging population is increased (Laidlaw & Pachana, 2009). Health policies must promote independence, dignity, and purpose with a need to move away from hospital and long-term care toward an approach assisting people to reside in the community, with the development of more caregiver programs and encouragement of individuals to make healthier life choices. Therapists must also remember that for many individuals aging may be a positive experience and that they may only see a small cohort of those whose experience of aging is associated with distress and loss (Laidlaw & Pachana, 2009). After all, aging and illness is not just what happens to individuals, but more important, it is what individuals do with their experience of aging and illness.

See also Coping with Chronic Illness; Validation Therapy.

Kenneth Schwartz and William Shapiro

American Group Psychotherapy Association. (2007). *Practice guidelines for group psychotherapy.* New York, NY: Author.

American Psychological Association. (2009a). Depression and suicide in older adults resource guide. Retrieved from http://www.apa.org/pi/aging/resources/guides/depression.aspx

American Psychological Association. (2009b). Psychotherapy and older adults resource guide. Retrieved from http://www.apa.org/pi/aging/resources/guides/psychotherapy.aspx

American Psychological Association. (2014). Guidelines for psychological practice with older adults. *American Psychologist*, *69*(1), 34–65.

Institute of Medicine. (2012). The mental health and substance abuse workforce for older adults: In whose hands? Retrieved from http://www.nationalacademies.org/hmd/reports/2012/the-mental-health-and-substance-use-workforce-for-older-adults.aspx

Jacobs, B. J. (2006). *The emotional survival guide for caregivers: Looking after yourself and your family while helping an aging parent.* New York, NY: Guilford Press.

Laidlaw, K., & Pachana, N. A. (2009). Aging, mental health and demographic change: Challenges for psychotherapists. *American Psychologist*, *40*(6), 601–608.

Lee, D., Nazroo, J., O'Connor, D. B., Blake, M., & Pendleton, N. (2016). Sexual health and wellbeing among older men and women in England: Finding from the English longitudinal study of ageing. *Archives of Sexual Behaviour*, *45*, 133–144.

Lindau, S. T., Schurnm, L. P., Laumann, E. O., Levinson, W. L., O'Muircheartaigh, C. A., & Waite, L. J. (2007). A study of sexuality and health among older adults in the United States. *New England Journal of Medicine*, *357*(8), 762–774.

Pinquart, M., & Sorenson, S. (2001). How effective are psychotherapeutic and other psychosocial interventions with older adults: A metaanalysis. *Journal of Mental Health and Aging*, *7*, 207–243.

Schwartz, K. (2011). Psychotherapy groups for long-term care residents: Intervention training manual. Retrieved from http://www.baycrest.org/publication

Schwartz, K., & Schwartzberg, S. L. (2011). Psychodynamically informed groups for elders: A comparison of verbal and activity groups. *Group*, *35*(1),17–31.

Substance Abuse and Mental Health Services Administration. (2008). *Substance abuse among older adults, treatment improvement protocol series.* Rockville, MD: Author. Retrieved from http://www.ncbi.nlm.nih.gov/books/NBK64419/pdf/Bookshelf_NBK64419.pdf

U.S. Census Bureau. (2008, August 14). *U.S. Census Bureau news: An older and more diverse nation by mid-century.* Washington, DC: U.S. Government Public Information Office. Retrieved from http://www.census.gov/newsroom/releases/archives/population/cb08-123.html

Web Resource
American Psychological Association: http://www.apa.org/practice/guidelines/older-adults.aspx

PSYCHOSIS IN LATE LIFE

Delusions and hallucinations are psychotic symptoms that usually represent problems with reality testing. By definition they involve beliefs that are unshakable and false but exclude widely accepted religious or cultural beliefs. It can also sometimes be difficult to distinguish delusions from unusually strong but equally dubious beliefs (e.g., about political conspiracies) that may be part of an individual's subculture. Shared beliefs of this nature are better construed as overvalued ideas than as delusions.

Most often, though not invariably, psychotic symptoms are a source of functional impairment and/or subjective distress. Psychotic symptoms in older persons are generally less bizarre than in younger adults, and their content often has some personal relevance to the individual experiencing them. As such, an observer who makes an effort to be empathic can often appreciate how they may be meaningful to the person

612 ■ PSYCHOSIS IN LATE LIFE

P

experiencing them, insofar as they may represent the patient's psychological sense of reality. Psychotic symptoms can sometimes be restitutional, meeting some need of the patient, such as when a sense of abandonment is associated with hallucinations of visitors. For example, a retired farmer, missing his work, feels comforted seeing cows outside his window. Likewise, a widower may intermittently see or think he hears his recently deceased wife. Neither of these cases requires treatment with a psychotropic medication. One who likely might, however, is an elderly music teacher living alone, barely able to manage because of cognitive impairment, who has become distressed by seeing intruders in her apartment and hearing a band play off-key outside the building.

EPIDEMIOLOGY AND ETIOLOGY

In community settings, up to 4% of older adults manifest generalized persecutory ideation, and another 0.2% to 0.9% suffer from schizophrenia. The prevalence of paranoid disorder in outpatient geriatric psychiatry clinics is about 15%. Up to 10% of older patients newly admitted to hospitals, and up to 20% of new admissions to nursing homes, have delusions.

Delusions and hallucinations can appear in many different kinds of clinical problems, including cognitive disorders such as delirium (e.g., because of medical problems, medications, toxins) and dementia (e.g., Alzheimer's, vascular, and Lewy body); mood disorders (e.g., depression, mania); substance abuse (either intoxication or withdrawal); and psychotic disorders, such as delusional disorder and schizophrenia (either early- or late-onset). In hospitalized older adults, the leading cause of psychotic symptoms is dementia, followed in descending order by psychotic depression, delirium, medical/medication problems, mania, and psychotic disorders.

RISK FACTORS

Older adults with acute, chronic, or progressive cognitive impairment are at higher risk for developing psychotic symptoms, as are those under significant environmental or interpersonal stress (e.g., bed bound, poor relationship with caregivers). Sensory impairment (especially in vision or hearing) and social isolation may also be predisposing factors.

ASSESSMENT

A sound understanding of late-life psychosis requires a fundamental appreciation of basic principles of geriatrics. These especially include an appreciation for the higher degree of variability in physical and mental health status stemming from physiological changes of aging (which vary by organ system), along with increased prevalence of age-associated diseases. The diagnostic and therapeutic challenges grow when these factors are combined with (a) the presence of multiple interacting problems, (b) more frequent side effects of medications, (c) atypical presentations of common illnesses, (d) the increased frequency of the same symptoms being caused by different factors simultaneously, and (e) the tendency of older patients to under-report symptoms. Hence one needs to consider medical conditions because psychotic symptoms are not infrequently attributed to psychiatric problems when, in fact, they are because of, or being aggravated by, some common undiagnosed but treatable concurrent medical conditions (e.g., unrecognized episodes of hypoglycemia). Like other psychiatric issues, psychotic symptoms are colored by each individual's unique personality, history of experiences, and personal values.

In situations involving an older adult with acute psychotic symptoms accompanied by severe agitation, the first task is to assess the dangerousness of the situation and to try to implement behavioral interventions. These include verbal redirection, reassurance, stimulus reduction, and possibly a change in the environment. Acute pharmacotherapy is warranted if there are significant imminent risks to self or others and if the behavioral interventions are not adequate to reduce these risks. Antipsychotic medication can be preferably given orally (e.g., dissolvable tablet) or intramuscularly in an emergency situation.

PSYCHOSIS IN COGNITIVE DISORDERS

Dementia

Psychotic symptoms constitute one set of the behavioral and psychological symptoms of dementia (BPSD). Delusions and hallucinations are common in dementia. They are found in approximately half of patients in clinical settings who suffer from Alzheimer's disease. They occur more frequently in advanced dementia, and correlate with poor prognosis (i.e., faster decline in cognitive abilities). It is important to remember that they may signal an underlying medical problem, especially if it is an acute onset/change (e.g., delirium). Common themes in the delusions of patients with dementia are theft, infidelity, abandonment, paranoia, and the belief that one's house is not one's own. Hallucinations in dementia tend to be visual more than auditory or tactile. No treatment is required if the delusions or hallucinations are benign (e.g., as with the example of the farmer seeing "cows"). Antipsychotics have a lower benefit/risk ratio for nonpsychotic disturbances in dementia (hence federal regulations regarding their use in long-term care settings; see entry on the use of psychotropic medications in nursing homes).

Determining appropriate, effective treatment of psychotic symptoms in patients with dementia, such as Alzheimer's disease or vascular dementia, is a special challenge. The pooling of multiple retrospective studies has revealed an increase in mortality in dementia patients treated with atypical antipsychotics compared with those treated with placebo. The risk is approximately 1.5 to 1.7 times higher, with the difference in absolute rates being about 4.5% versus 2.6%, respectively (i.e., a 1.9% higher risk; Steinberg & Lyketsos, 2012). Causes of mortality included heart failure, sudden death, other cardiac events, and infection (primarily pneumonia). There was some initial concern about an increase in risk for strokes as well, but the data for this are conflicting. Subsequent reviews of the use of typical antipsychotics for dementia-related psychosis revealed these drugs to have elevated mortality risks similar to the atypical antipsychotics.

For these reasons the U.S. Food and Drug Administration (FDA) has issued Black Box Warnings on the use of both atypical and typical antipsychotics for the treatment of dementia-related psychosis. Unfortunately, the likelihood of dementia patients developing psychotic symptoms over the course of the illness ranges from 25% to 45% (Chan, Lam, & Chen, 2011), which leaves suffering patients, their families, and other caregivers, as well as clinicians, in a quandary. Per the FDA, antipsychotics are not indicated for this specific use. It is important to note, however, that lack of an FDA indication for the use of a medication does not imply that its use is forbidden by the FDA. In other words, although using antipsychotic medication for dementia-related psychosis is not recommended by the FDA, using it for this reason is not prohibited, as the FDA has not declared that its use is contraindicated for this purpose.

Experts in geriatric psychiatry recommend reserving the use of antipsychotic medication for dementia-related psychotic symptoms that are severe and debilitating. This is done after carefully informing, obtaining, and documenting consent from the patient (to the extent feasible), family members, and where appropriate, the durable power of attorney for health care or the guardian. Informed consent needs to be based on a frank discussion of the possible risks and potential benefits of proceeding with the use of antipsychotic medication, of any adjunct and alternative interventions, and of the likely consequences of not using anti-psychotic medication at all (Devanand, 2013; Reus et al., 2016).

Delirium

Hallucinations and delusions, in which there is a disturbance of consciousness characterized by reduced ability to focus, sustain, or shift attention, frequently occur in delirium. Hyperactive or agitated delirium is usually quite evident, but a hypoactive ("quiet") delirium is less likely to be recognized or appropriately treated. Older patients are more vulnerable to delirium, especially if they already have a coexisting cognitive problem (e.g., mild cognitive impairment or dementia). Hence, it can often be more difficult to diagnose. Significant clues to look for include problems with attention, worsened memory or orientation; uncharacteristically disorganized thinking, changes in the sleep/wake cycle, atypical behaviors, and atypical psychotic symptoms. In a typical delirium, these usually develop over hours to days. Appropriate treatment encompasses the most effective medical and environmental interventions that address the conditions causing or aggravating the delirium. Antipsychotic medication, used cautiously, continues to be indicated for the treatment of severe psychotic symptoms or agitation in delirium that has significant potential for physical or psychological harm.

Mood Disorders

Major depressive episodes may have psychotic features (Andreescu & Reynolds, 2011). These can be categorized by the extent to which they match the patient's mood. Typical mood-congruent psychotic symptoms in depression include delusions of guilt, inadequacy, disease, death, nihilism, or deserved punishment, whereas those that are mood-incongruent include delusions of persecution, thought insertion, thought broadcasting, or of being under someone's or something's control. Episodes of bipolar affective disorder, a diagnosis sometimes overlooked in the elderly, may also have psychotic features, such as delusions of grandeur (Sajatovic & Chen 2011). The delusions and hallucinations in mania may also be either mood-congruent or mood-incongruent. Episodes of agitated depression or mania may mimic delirium or dementia.

Effective treatment consists of utilizing an antipsychotic in combination with an antidepressant for psychotic depression and a mood stabilizer for psychotic mania, along with appropriate psychosocial and environmental supports. Acute episodes of psychotic depression or psychotic mania may become highly risky because of intense psychomotor symptoms (severe hypoactivity or hyperactivity), especially in the face of intense psychotic symptoms, increasing physical frailty (e.g., inadequate oral intake of food and/or fluids), or imminent suicidality. In such situations, electroconvulsive therapy (ECT), which is done under general anesthesia with muscle relaxation, can be very effective (Bailine et al., 2010). Recourse to ECT may also be warranted in instances in which medications are ineffective (e.g., after at least three adequate trials) or their side effects are not tolerable.

PSYCHOSIS IN MEDICAL PROBLEMS

Delusions and hallucinations arising in the context of medical problems are sometimes referred to as *organic psychoses*. Drugs are frequent contributors to this class of psychotic symptoms. Medications with the potential to generate psychotic symptoms include analgesics, anti-inflammatory agents, anticholinergics, antihistamines, anticonvulsants, tricyclic antidepressants, antipsychotics, antiparkinsonians, hormones (e.g., steroids), stimulants, cimetidine (an OTC antacid), sedatives, tranquilizers, chemotherapeutic agents, and some cardiac drugs (e.g., digoxin).

In addition to the dementias, other general medical conditions that may give rise to psychotic symptoms include (a) endocrine disorders (e.g., hypoglycemia occurring in diabetes, hyperthyroidism or hypothyroidism, hyperparathyroidism or hypoparathyroidism, hyperadrenocorticism or hypoadrenocorticism), (b) metabolic disturbances (e.g., electrolyte problems in liver or kidney failure, hypoxia in severe lung disease), (c) neurological problems (e.g., seizure disorders; migraine), (d) nutritional deficiencies (e.g., vitamin B_{12}, folate, thiamine, niacin), (e) normal pressure hydrocephalus, (f) tumors (e.g., brain, pancreas), (g) toxicities (from heavy metals, pesticides, medications), (h) infections (e.g., bacterial, viral, fungal, parasitic, prion), (i) immune diseases (e.g., arteritis, multiple sclerosis); and (j) cerebrovascular problems (e.g., large- or small-vessel strokes). Appropriate treatment is dictated by the most effective ways of addressing the conditions from which the psychotic symptoms are emerging, reserving antipsychotic medication for adjunct use (Karim & Burns, 2011).

Severe impairment in vision, short of total blindness, is sometimes the cause of visual hallucinations. Called *Bonnet's syndrome*, it is characterized as an organic hallucinosis. Affected

P

individuals are aware of the unreal nature of these hallucinations but may be bothered by them to some degree or embarrassed to let on that they are experiencing them.

PSYCHOTIC DISORDERS

Schizophrenia

Schizophrenia in late life is as serious a chronic mental illness as it is with younger adults. In comparison with unaffected peers in the community, older adults suffering from schizophrenia are much less likely to meet the criteria for successful aging (Ibrahim, Cohen, & Ramirez, 2010), and more likely to die prematurely.

The symptoms of schizophrenia referred to as positive symptoms include delusions, hallucinations, disorganized speech (e.g., incoherent and derailment), and/or grossly disorganized/catatonic behavior. Those referred to as negative symptoms include blunted affect and loss of initiative (Cohen, Natarajan, Araujo, & Solanki, 2013). The diagnosis requires that these sets of symptoms be chronic and cause social/occupational dysfunction. The diagnosis is not made if the psychotic symptoms are secondary to a mood disorder or a medical problem. Older adults with this severe mental disorder have usually had it for decades. Early onset schizophrenia (EOS) typically starts for men in the late teens or early twenties, and in the mid to late twenties for women. For some, the schizophrenia has a late-onset, among those hospitalized because of this form of the illness, approximately 13% had it begin in their 50s, approximately 7% in their 60s, and approximately 3% in their 70s or even later.

The overall prevalence of schizophrenia in late life is approximately 0.3% (Iglewicz, Meeks, & Jeste, 2011). Social isolation and suspiciousness may mask its true prevalence, and the rates are confounded by varying inclusion/exclusion criteria. Some patients with EOS have only a few residual psychotic symptoms, which may be sufficiently mild as to not require antipsychotic medication. For others, however, severe psychotic symptoms may persist into late life. For these patients, continuation of treatment with antipsychotic medication and psychosocial

support is indicated. Care is further guided by an appreciation for the interventions that were effective in the past and the need to make adjustments according to aging changes while monitoring for the appearance of new medical problems.

Risk factors for EOS and late-onset schizophrenia (LOS) are somewhat different. These include a family history of schizophrenia, with the prevalence of affected first-degree relatives slightly higher in EOS versus LOS. Other factors that appear to be associated with an increased risk for LOS include relative sensory deprivation because of auditory or visual impairment and social isolation; a history of an abnormal personality ("eccentric"); lack of marriage or children; lower social class; and female sex. The prevalence of LOS is about 10 times greater in women than in men. Speculations to account for this striking difference include relative excess of D2 dopamine receptors in the brains of older women in contrast to men because women tend to lose these receptors more slowly than men. Another possibility involves questions about the role of declining estrogen levels in postmenopausal women. Neuroimaging of patients with LOS reveals changes in brain structure and functioning: deep white matter ischemic changes ("mini-strokes") and decreased cerebral blood flow in frontal/temporal lobes.

Assessing older adults with long-standing EOS who are acutely psychotic can be quite challenging. It is often assumed that the acute psychotic symptoms represent an exacerbation of the EOS itself, but sometimes, the exacerbation is because of an underlying medical problem that is presenting in an atypical manner. For example, a urinary tract infection or early pneumonia may develop in an older adult without causing the usual physical symptoms and signs but instead generates psychotic symptoms. Such clinical situations call for remembering the geriatric rule of thumb: to think diagnostically in terms of "both/and" instead of "either/or" and to consider whether the psychotic symptoms have a multifactorial origin. Carefully assessing the extent to which the acute psychotic symptoms are qualitatively and/or quantitatively different than the patient's usual psychotic symptoms may provide useful clues, and help avoid misdiagnosis. It is estimated that underlying medical problems are missed in older patients with chronic mental health problems at a rate of 25% to 40%.

In contrast to the usual symptoms of EOS, individuals with LOS are more likely to experience visual, olfactory, or tactile hallucinations, but less likely to shows signs of blunted affect or abnormal flow of thoughts. They are more likely to manifest delusions of persecution and of partition (e.g., that their walls, floors, ceilings, and doors are permeable to toxic substances or intruders; Iglewicz et al., 2011). They are also less functionally impaired; they may still be able to sufficiently manage their affairs, whereas individuals with EOS frequently require the assistance of community support programs. A common scenario in LOS involves an older woman, living alone, who is making frequent calls for help about perceived threats, much to the consternation of local emergency service providers but declining any sort of mental health referral. Because of the lack of insight about their delusions, they typically decline offers of treatment but may be open to some indirect care through their primary care provider. With appropriate interventions, including treatment with antipsychotic medication, outcomes are fairly good: Approximately 55% become symptom free, approximately 30% have some residual symptoms, and approximately 15% remain unchanged.

It is important to assess for cognitive changes in older adults. This can be particularly challenging in patients with either EOS or LOS. Cognitive impairment, especially problems with executive function, such as initiative, organization, and implementation of plans, is common in EOS. In fact, in the 19th century, schizophrenia was referred to as *dementia praecox* (i.e., precocious dementia). Crucial questions to ask in the event of cognitive changes include: How long have they been going on? How abruptly did they begin? Is the situation progressing? If so, how fast? Has the person's functional status changed? If the individual had some cognitive impairment to begin with, has there been any further decline from the previous baseline?

Schizoaffective Disorder

Schizoaffective disorder shares the features of both schizophrenia and mood disorders. As a consequence, when it occurs in older adults, it can be mistaken for bipolar disorder or major depression with psychotic features. What distinguishes schizoaffective disorder is that it is predominantly a psychotic disorder. Per the *Diagnostic and Statistical Manual of Mental Disorders* (5th ed.; *DSM-5*; American Psychiatric Association, 2013), the diagnosis requires not only the presence of both psychotic and mood symptoms, but also a period of 2 or more weeks of psychotic symptoms alone, without any significant co-occurring mood symptoms. Treatments for this disorder are fairly analogous to those for mood disorders with psychotic features.

Delusional Disorder

The diagnostic feature of delusional disorder is the presence of nonbizarre delusions. The typical types of delusions are grandiose, jealous, persecutory, somatic, erotomanic (i.e., that a famous person is in love with them), or some mixture of these. Older adults with this disorder, by definition, do not experience hallucinations. They also do not manifest cognitive or functional impairment, aside from consequences of their delusion; for example, they may make accusations against others for which there is no basis in fact; may fail to pay bills, believing that they are being exploited; or quarrel with spouses they claim are unfaithful. Treatment with antipsychotic medication can significantly reduce the intensity of the psychotic symptoms and associated behavioral problems, but only approximately a third of patients achieve full remission and regain clear insight.

Psychosis in Geriatric Substance Abuse

When older adults abuse and misuse substances, whether alcohol, prescription medications, or illicit drugs, they may start to exhibit hallucinations and/or delusions. When this occurs, the psychotic symptoms may appear subtle, present atypically, or mimic other illnesses. If unrecognized or unaddressed, substance abuse or misuse can exacerbate medical problems (e.g., hypertension, diabetes) and make them hard to treat. They can also cause or exacerbate cognitive impairment, ranging from mild forgetfulness to delirium/dementia, which may incorrectly be attributed to another problem (e.g., Alzheimer's). Psychotic symptoms may be part of intoxication with, or withdrawal from, substance use/misuse. These may persist even after patients achieve sobriety; confabulation (e.g., alcohol hallucinosis; flashbacks).

TREATMENT

The clinical complexities in working with older adults who have psychotic symptoms can seem daunting, especially in the face of less than complete clinical information. Diagnosis, treatment, and prognosis in geriatrics are each characterized by higher levels of ambiguity. In this setting, it is important to avoid the temptation to come to premature closure and to think in terms of both/and as opposed to either/or.

It is important to note that clinical guidelines for the use of psychotropic medications in the elderly are based on research involving groups of patients and that older adult populations are much more heterogeneous, with considerable variability from one individual to the next, based on differences in physiological status, personal experiences, and environmental conditions/exposures over decades. Hence, although these criteria apply to the population of older adults in general, they might not be appropriate for individual older adults who represent exceptions to the general rule.

An integrated ecological approach can help to reduce the uncertainties and avoid these pitfalls (Howell, 2015). In the context of these nearly unavoidable complexities inherent in assessing psychotic symptoms in older adults and providing them with effective geriatric care, it is helpful to work with an ad hoc interdisciplinary team, involving not only clinicians and patients, but also family and other caregivers. When working with older individuals who have psychotic symptoms or disorders, a care provider's priority needs to be to develop and maintain a resilient therapeutic alliance with patients. Including family members and others involved as members of an ad hoc team can be extremely helpful as well. Doing so calls for an enduring combination of both availability and respect for these patients and the things that make each of them unique as individuals. This open and nonjudgmental investment can foster the trust necessary to ensure accurate diagnoses and effective treatments.

When encountering patients' delusions or hallucinations, it important to be accepting of what they are reporting as their experiences. One need not agree to false notions or perceptions, but it helps to appreciate how these constitute the truth at that moment for those individuals and try to understand how and why they came to think and feel as they do. Given that delusions are by nature are often fixed beliefs, direct confrontational efforts to persuade patients otherwise will be fruitless and often counterproductive. Instead one can focus on learning what these symptoms mean to the patients and how they are trying to cope with them. Often, though not always, there are clues to this in the content of the delusion (e.g., the retired music teacher whose auditory hallucinations reflect her social isolation). The care provider can then begin to explore ways that these issues might be more effectively addressed. The use of traditional standardized guidelines which use either/or clinical algorithms or decision trees can be hazardous when approaching multifactorial problems.

Initial treatment of elderly patients with psychotic symptoms is guided by findings from careful physical and mental status examinations. These, together with appropriate laboratory testing, are crucial. Treatment begins with informing patients and caregivers about the potential advantages, possible risks, and alternatives to the proposed therapies. Choosing optimal pharmacotherapy is challenging in light of trade-offs between symptom relief and potential side effects. The well-informed and judicious use of antipsychotic medications, tailored to fit the unique biopsychosocial needs of each patient, can be quite effective and minimize risks.

P

Nonpharmacological Treatments

Psychotherapy and social interventions can be introduced as acute psychotic symptoms begin to subside. Psychological/social interventions in the stabilization phase can start with a meaningful skills evaluation by a geriatrics-trained occupational therapist. The results can increase the specificity and sensitivity of subsequent training in social skills (e.g., conflict resolution), stress management, problem solving, and development of more effective coping strategies (Cohen, Solanki, & Sodhi, 2013). These individualized interventions can be combined with further enhancement of patients' support networks. Social interventions that can contribute to the maintenance of stability include secure nonstigmatizing housing with access to private restful space, individualized supervision, or assistance with instrumental activities of daily living, and personally meaningful daily activities.

Providing support for family and other caregivers is another important component of overall treatment because psychosis in late life does not usually happen to just the patients. This can be accomplished through education about the causes and consequences of the delusions or hallucinations and coaching on how to effectively engage with the older individual experiencing such psychotic symptoms. As collateral sources, caregivers can be enormously helpful with numerous tasks: (a) enhancing the initial and ongoing diagnosis by providing clear, specific descriptions of events (particularly by noting social and/or environmental stressors); (b) tracking medications (e.g., adherence with those prescribed, and use of over-the-counter and "borrowed") drugs; (c) monitoring responses to interventions in terms of the frequency and severity of the psychotic symptoms; (d) observing for changes in symptoms resulting from medical problems (chronic, acute, or unsuspected) and/or other psychiatric problems or substance use/abuse; and (e) sharing background about personality traits, values, and usual coping strategies. Regular contact among members of the ad hoc team also facilitates monitoring for and addressing of caregiver burden.

Sustaining effectiveness in the treatment of late-life psychoses requires a continuous process of ongoing reassessments and adjustments. Where the response to interventions appears to have been successful, in that the psychotic symptoms have remitted altogether for at least 3 to 6 months, a gradual tapering of the antipsychotics medication can be attempted. When there is only partial improvement, however, persistent psychotic symptoms may need longer courses of treatment.

Antipsychotics for Older Patients

Antipsychotic medication is generally the first choice for psychotic symptoms. The judicious use of these medications with older adults, as with other psychotropic medications, is founded on basic principles of geriatric psychopharmacology. These include starting with low doses (e.g., 25% of usual adult dosage), titrating slowly according to the individual's response and tolerance, and taking care to neither undertreat nor overtreat. Older (first-generation) antipsychotics are usually referred to as *typical antipsychotics*, whereas newer (second generation) ones are called *atypical antipsychotics*. The following lists of these medications provide each one's generic name, accompanied in parentheses by the brand name commonly used to refer to it.

Typical antipsychotics can be categorized according to their degree of potency. High-potency antipsychotics include haloperidol (known familiarly as Haldol), thiothixene (Navane), fluphenazine (once known as Prolixin), and trifluoperazine (once known as Stelazine). Chlorpromazine (once known as Thorazine) and thioridazine (once known as Mellaril) are examples of low-potency antipsychotics. Middle or intermediate-potency antipsychotics include loxapine (known familiarly as Loxitane) and perphenazine (once known as Trilafon). The atypical antipsychotics include aripiprazole (Abilify), asenapine (Saphris), clozapine (Clozaril), iloperidone (Fanapt), lurasidone (Latuda), olanzapine (Zyprexa), paliperidone (Invega), quetiapine (Seroquel), risperidone (Risperdal), and ziprasidone (Geodon).

The transmission of electrical impulses in the circuits of the brain depends on the chemical release of molecules (called *neurotransmitters*) across the gaps (synapses) between individual nerve cells (neurons). These neurotransmitters work by interacting with receptors on the synaptic surfaces of the neurons, and scores of them have been identified, both in the brain and other parts of the body. A number of primary neurotransmitters are involved in the neurobiological processes that form the basis for perceptions, conceptions, emotions, behavior, and sleep. Acetylcholine sustains the functioning of cholinergic circuits, and norepinephrine, the adrenergic circuits. Serotonin, dopamine, and histamine are three other crucial neurotransmitters. Antipsychotic medications are presumed to work, at least in part, by blocking some of the receptors (primarily the D2 dopamine receptor in the middle part of the brain) for these neurotransmitters. Their effects and many of their common potential side effects can be classified by neurotransmitter. Most, but not all, side effects are dose dependent (i.e., the higher the dosage, the more likely to occur).

Anticholinergic side effects within the brain can result in confusion; blockage of acetylcholine receptors elsewhere in the body can result in blurred vision, dry mouth, constipation, urinary retention, and decreased perspiration (a risk in hot weather). Potential antihistaminic side effects include sedation and increased appetite (with subsequent weight gain). Alpha-adrenergic blockade can result in orthostasis (a drop in blood pressure with standing). Geriatric patients are more susceptible and more vulnerable than younger patients to each of these sets of side effects. Unlike the side effects from older typical antipsychotics, the side effects are less frequent with the newer atypical antipsychotics (except for clozapine, which has the side effect profile of a low-potency atypical antipsychotic). Among the typical antipsychotics, the less potent agents are more likely to cause these types of adverse drug reactions.

The so-called extrapyramidal side effects (EPSEs) stem from the blocking of dopamine receptors in a lower part of the brain that affect the extrapyramidal nerve tracts involved in the modulation of voluntary muscle activity throughout the body. These EPSEs include parkinsonism, akathisia, and dystonias (sustained muscle spasms). Their emergence tends to be less frequent with the newer atypical antipsychotics

than with the older typical agents and tends to become more likely to occur with increasing potency among typical antipsychotics.

Older adults are more likely than younger ones to develop parkinsonism, so-called because of its resemblance to the signs of Parkinson's disease: muscle rigidity, resting tremor, akinesia and hypokinesia (slowness in initiating and sustaining movements), and postural instability (with a tendency to fall backward). Parkinsonian side effects tend to occur several weeks or even months after beginning antipsychotics. Akathisia is manifested by a subjective sense of restlessness (especially in the legs) and an urge to pace (which characteristically provides some relief). It tends to occur within a few weeks of starting treatment, and elderly patients appear to be no more vulnerable to this side effect than younger ones. Akathisia may mimic the agitation commonly associated with psychotic symptoms; failing to recognize it as a medication side effect can mistakenly lead to a vicious cycle of increasing antipsychotic dosage and increasing agitation. Acute dystonic reactions usually occur in the first 1 to 2 weeks of treatment with antipsychotics. Older adults are less likely to experience these, presumably because muscle mass decreases as age increases.

Another class of antipsychotic side effects is dyskinesia. Dyskinesias consist of abnormal involuntary movements which may involve muscles in different regions of the body, most commonly the mouth and face (e.g., lip-smacking, puckering, grimacing); sometimes the trunk or limbs (e.g., rocking, twisting, gyrating), and rarely the diaphragm (e.g., irregular breathing, grunting). The abrupt discontinuation, or even relatively rapid tapering, of antipsychotic medication can precipitate withdrawal dyskinesias, which gradually remit over time. Similar dyskinetic movements that spontaneously emerge after many months to years of exposure to antipsychotics, however, can become a potentially irreversible side effect. After 3 years of treatment with typical antipsychotics, up to two thirds of older adults may develop what is called *tardive dyskinesia* (TD) because of its delayed-onset. Although the prevalence of TD is many times lower with the newer atypical antipsychotics, it may still occur. Hence, monitoring for signs of TD is now standard practice, utilizing a rating scale such as the Abnormal Involuntary Movement Scale (AIMS), which tracks the abnormal movements, the patient's awareness of movements, and the degree of incapacity because of the movements. Additional potential side effects of antipsychotics include falls, metabolic syndrome (increased likelihood of obesity, insulin resistance, dyslipidemia, hypertension, atherosclerosis), prolonged or abnormal conduction of electrical impulses through the heart, and sexual dysfunction.

See also Behavioral and Psychological Symptoms of Dementia; Bipolar Disorder in Later Life; Dementia: Special Care Units; Depression in Dementia; Psychotropic Medication Use in Long-Term Care.

Paula Lueras and Timothy Howell

American Psychiatric Association. (2013). *Diagnostic and statistical manual of mental disorders* (5th ed.). Arlington, VA: American Psychiatric Publishing.

Andreescu, C., & Reynolds, C. F. (2011). Late-life depression: Evidence-based treatment and promising new directions for research and clinical practice. *Psychiatric Clinics of North America, 34*(2), 335–55, vii.

Bailine, S., Fink, M., Knapp, R., Petrides, G., Husain, M. M., Rasmussen, K., ... Kellner, C. H. (2010). Electroconvulsive therapy is equally effective in unipolar and bipolar depression. *Acta Psychiatrica Scandinavica, 121*(6), 431–436.

Chan, W. C., Lam, L. C., & Chen, E. Y. (2011). Recent advances in pharmacological treatment of psychosis in late life. *Current Opinion in Psychiatry, 24*(6), 455–460.

Cohen, C. I., Natarajan, N., Araujo, M., & Solanki, D. (2013). Prevalence of negative symptoms and associated factors in older adults with schizophrenia spectrum disorder. *American Journal of Geriatric Psychiatry, 21*(2), 100–107.

Cohen, C. I., Solanki, D., & Sodhi, D. (2013). Interpersonal conflict strategies and their impact on positive symptom remission in persons aged 55 and older with schizophrenia spectrum disorders. *International Psychogeriatrics, 25*(1), 47–53.

Devanand, D. P. (2013). Psychosis, agitation, and antipsychotic treatment in dementia. *American Journal of Psychiatry, 170*(9), 957–960.

Ibrahim, F., Cohen, C. I., & Ramirez, P. M. (2010). Successful aging in older adults with schizophrenia: Prevalence and associated factors. *American Journal of Geriatric Psychiatry, 18*(10), 879–886.

Howell, T. (2015) The Wisconsin Star Method: Understanding and addressing complexity in geriatrics, In M. L. Malone, E. Capezuti, & R. M. Palmer (Eds.), *Geriatrics models of care: Bringing 'best practice' to an aging America* (pp. 87–94). Cham, Switzerland: Springer. doi:10.1007/978-3-319-16068-9_7

Iglewicz, A., Meeks, T. W., & Jeste, D. V. (2011). New wine in old bottle: Late-life psychosis. *Psychiatric Clinics of North America, 34*(2), 295–318, vii.

Karim, S., & Burns, A. (2011). Psychotic disorders in late life. In M. E. Agronin, & G. J. Maletta (Eds.), *Principles and practice of geriatric psychiatry* (2nd ed., pp. 465–475). Philadelphia, PA: Wolters Kluwer.

Reus, V., Fochtmann, M., Eyler, E., Hilty, D., Horvitz-Lennon, M., Jibson, M., ... Yager, J. (2016). The American Psychiatric Association practice guideline on the use of antipsychotics to treat agitation or psychosis in patients with dementia. *American Journal of Psychiatry, 175*(5), 543–546.

Sajatovic, M., & Chen, P. (2011). Geriatric bipolar disorder. *Psychiatric Clinics of North America, 34*(2), 319–33, vii.

Steinberg, M., & Lyketsos, C. G. (2012). Atypical antipsychotic use in patients with dementia: Managing safety concerns. *American Journal of Psychiatry, 169*(9), 900–906.

Web Resources

Agency for Healthcare Research and Quality (AHRQ): Comparative effective review for off-label use of atypical antipsychotics: An update (2011): http://effectivehealthcare.ahrq.gov/index.cfm/search-for-guides-reviews-and-reports/?pageaction=displayproduct&productid=786

Canadian Academy of Geriatric Psychiatry (Resources Section: Guidelines and Clinical Tools): http://www.cagp.ca

PSYCHOTROPIC MEDICATION USE IN LONG-TERM CARE

The residents of nursing homes in the United States have high rates of neurocognitive, medical, and other psychiatric problems, and as many as two thirds of them are on several psychotropic medications. This is despite the fact that, beginning in the 1970s, advocates for nursing home residents raised concerns, not only about the widespread use of physical restraints on patients in these facilities, but also about the inappropriate use of psychotropic medications as chemical restraints (i.e., for the convenience of staff, as disciplinary measures to control patients). Around the same time, the Institute of Medicine (IOM) also expressed concerns that depression was underdiagnosed and undertreated in nursing homes. These controversies culminated in congressional hearings and subsequent federal legislation, namely the Nursing Home Reform Act. This act was part of the Omnibus Budget Reconciliation Act of 1987, since commonly referred to as *OBRA regulations* (Kapp, 2009).

The Health Care Financing Administration (HCFA) issued interpretive guidelines to be used by federal and state quality-assurance inspectors to enforce these regulations, but these were initially very broad in scope and quite controversial. Hence, they underwent revision and were finalized in 1990. The HCFA has since been supplanted by the Centers for Medicare & Medicaid Services (CMS), which continues to update the guidelines on an ongoing basis.

A key OBRA regulation is that nursing home residents be free from unnecessary medications. These include any drugs that are administered at excessive doses, for excessive periods of time, without adequate indications for their use, without adequate monitoring for side effects, or despite adverse consequences. Hence, a long-term care resident being prescribed a psychotropic drug needs to have a specific diagnosis that warrants such a medication. Furthermore, that person must be followed to determine whether the medication is effective, adequately tolerated, and still required after a designated time. A record must be kept in the patient's clinical chart, with documentation of the diagnosis for which the psychotropic medication is indicated, the patient's response to this medication, any relevant side effects, and the rationale for continuing its use.

Health care providers who prescribe psychotropic medications sometimes chafe under the burden of these requirements, but following these rules not only benefits patients but also protects providers from medical liability should concerns be raised on any reviews of their clinical practice. One of the key goals of these OBRA regulations was the encouragement of better differential diagnoses of behavioral problems in long-term care facilities, with better identification of their underlying causes. Another goal was to prevent a long-standing over-reliance on treating these problems primarily with psychotropic medication, when identifying and addressing contributing psychosocial stressors, environmental factors, and/or medical problems could reduce or eliminate the need for such medication.

Many of the CMS guidelines are based on a list of drugs and on diagnosis–drug combinations, which are associated with significantly higher risks of adverse drug effects for patients aged 65 years or older. These lists are based on the Beers criteria, which were developed to help clinicians predict when the risks of using certain medications in older adults might outweigh their benefits (American Geriatrics Society, 2015). It is important to note that the Beers criteria are subject to periodic revisions (Gallagher, Barry, Ryan, Hartigan, & O'Mahony, 2008). It is also important to remember that the older adult population is a heterogeneous one, with considerable variability from one person to the next (Lavretsky, 2008). Although these criteria apply to the population of older adults in general, they might not be appropriate for specific individual older adults who represent exceptions to the general rule (Steinman et al., 2015). CMS guidelines do not preclude the use of psychotropic medications that may not adhere to those guidelines, so long as this use is judicious, it is consistent with the intent of the OBRA regulations, and the rationale for not following the guidelines is clinically reasonable and carefully documented.

There are a number of sets of guidelines for psychotropic medications, according to the class of psychoactive drugs to which the medication belongs. These include both long-acting and short-acting benzodiazepines and other antianxiety/sedative agents, hypnotics (medications used for sleep induction), and antipsychotic medications. Psychotropic medications are a class of drugs that are psychoactive; that is, they are designed to exert their effects on the brain. They and antipsychotic medications are not one and the same; antipsychotic drugs are a subclass within the class of psychotropic drugs.

Long-acting benzodiazepines include chlordiazepoxide, clonazepam, clorazepate, diazepam, lorazepam, halazepam, and quazepam. Short-acting benzodiazepines include lorazepam, oxazepam, alprazolam, and estazolam. Medications used to induce sleep include zolpidem, zaleplon, eszopiclone, temazepam, triazolam, estazolam, lorazepam, and oxazepam. Other drugs occasionally used for sedation, sleep induction, anxiety include diphenhydramine, hydroxyzine, and chloral hydrate. OBRA guidelines specify that these medications be used for anxiety only with patients who have been diagnosed with specific anxiety disorders (i.e., generalized anxiety disorder, panic disorder, specific psychiatric or medical disorders complicated by anxiety). Whether for anxiety or insomnia, they are to be used only if they are effective and are not to be used where there is evidence that the patient's distress or insomnia is because of factors that can be addressed nonpharmacologically. The use of long-acting benzodiazepines is limited to instances in which trials of short-acting benzodiazepines are ineffective.

Older hypnotics, sedatives, and antianxiety medications such as barbiturates, ethchlorvynol, glutethimide, meprobamate, methyprylon, and paraldehyde are still used on occasion for anxiety or sleep, but safer agents have, for the most part, replaced them. Nursing home residents should not be started on these medications for anxiety or sleep, and if they are receiving them at the time of admission to the long-term facility, plans should be made to gradually taper and discontinue them as feasible. Barbiturates, such as phenobarbital, are exempt from these guidelines if used to treat a seizure disorder.

Antipsychotic medications have been divided into two groups: first generation and second generation. More commonly used, first-generation antipsychotics are generally lower in potency; agents in this group are chlorpromazine, prochlorperazine, and thioridazine.

Second-generation antipsychotics are higher in potency; this group includes fluphenazine and haloperidol. Loxapine, perphenazine, thiothixene, and trifluoperazine are typical antipsychotics that are intermediate in potency. Low-potency antipsychotic medications tend to have higher degrees of side effects such as sedation, postural hypotension, and anticholinergic symptoms but have a lower degree of side effects such as acute dystonia, akathisia, and signs that mimic those of Parkinson's disease. High-potency antipsychotic medications tend to have side effect profiles that are the opposite of the low-potency antipsychotics, whereas intermediate-potency antipsychotics tend to lie somewhere in between. Long-term use of typical antipsychotics, regardless of their potency, is associated with an increasing risk of tardive dyskinesia.

The newer atypical antipsychotics include aripiprazole, asenapine, brexpiprazole, cariprazine, iloperidone, lurasidone, olanzapine, paliperidone, pimavanserin, quetiapine, risperidone, and ziprasidone. These medications are much less likely to cause tardive dyskinesia and somewhat less likely to cause the other kinds of side effects associated with the typical antipsychotics. Clozapine is a medication in a class by itself; although it is an older antipsychotic, it has the therapeutic properties of the newer atypical antipsychotics. Unfortunately, its side effect profile matches that of the lower-potency typical antipsychotics. Older adults are less likely to tolerate these side effects, so its use is usually limited to low doses for patients who have psychotic symptoms in the context of Parkinson's disease or Lewy body dementia. Clozapine also has the potential to reduce the level of white blood cells (needed to fight infections); its use requires the need for frequent blood testing for the first 6 months of, contributing to its rare use in nursing homes (Divac et al., 2016). OBRA guidelines specify that antipsychotic medications be used, with appropriate behavioral interventions for psychotic symptoms and/or severe agitation but only with patients who have been diagnosed with specific psychotic disorders. Appropriate clinical indications include schizophrenia, schizoaffective disorder, delusional disorder, psychotic depression or mania, acute psychotic episodes, atypical psychotic disorders, neurocognitive disorders complicated by psychotic symptoms, and certain neurodegenerative disorders characterized by abnormal motor function.

If these medications are used for agitation, the agitated behaviors must be severe enough that they interfere with the ability of staff to provide care to the patient and other residents or that staff is at significant risk of being harmed. The guidelines require that the specifics of the agitation, including physical and verbal aggression, be clearly documented. For psychotic symptoms not associated with physical agitation, antipsychotic medications are to be reserved for patients when nonpharmacological interventions are not adequately effective and their delusions, hallucinations, and paranoia are causing significant subjective distress or impairing their functional ability. In contrast to how they may have been used in the past, antipsychotic medications are not indicated for situations involving nonspecific restlessness, self-neglect, poor memory, wandering, lack of sociability, fidgeting, uncooperativeness, apathy, anxiety, nonpsychotic depression, insomnia, unspecified agitation, or other nondangerous behaviors.

Determining what constitutes appropriate, effective treatment of psychotic symptoms occurring in patients with dementia, such as Alzheimer's disease or vascular dementia, represents a special challenge. The pooling of multiple retrospective studies has revealed an increase in mortality in dementia patients treated with atypical antipsychotics compared with those treated with placebo (Steinberg & Lyketsos, 2012). The risk is approximately 1.5 to 1.7 times higher, with the difference in absolute rates being about 4.5% versus 2.6%, respectively (i.e., a 1.9% higher risk). Causes of mortality include heart failure, sudden death, other cardiac events, and infection (primarily pneumonia). There was some initial concern about an increase in risk for strokes, but the data for this have turned out to be conflicting. Subsequent reviews of the use of typical antipsychotics for dementia-related psychosis revealed these drugs to have elevated mortality risks similar to the atypical antipsychotics.

For these reason, the U.S. Food and Drug Administration (FDA) in 2005 and subsequently in 2008, issued Black Box Warnings on the use of both atypical and typical antipsychotics for the treatment of dementia-related psychosis. Unfortunately, the likelihood of patients with dementia developing psychotic symptoms over the course of the illness ranges from 25% to 40% or higher, which leaves suffering patients, their families, and other caregivers, as well as clinicians, in a quandary. Although using antipsychotic medications for dementia-related psychosis is not recommended by the FDA, their level of warning does not identify them as contraindicated. Experts in geriatric psychiatry recommend reserving the use of antipsychotic medication for when the dementia-related psychotic symptoms are severe and debilitating. They are prescribed after carefully informing, obtaining, and documenting consent from the patient (to the extent feasible), family members, and where appropriate, the activated durable power of attorney for health care or guardian. Informed consent needs to be based on a frank discussion of the possible risks and potential benefits of the use of antipsychotic medication, of adjunct and alternative interventions (both nonpharmacological and other pharmacological), and of the likely consequences of not using antipsychotic medication.

The guidelines for all these sets of psychotropic medications include recommended maximum daily doses for each medication. They also specify that daily use not exceed a certain number of unless attempts at gradual dose reduction are unsuccessful (i.e., result in the reemergence of the symptoms for which the medication was prescribed). The duration varies according to which class they belong. Attempts at reducing the dosage of benzodiazepines must be made every 4 months, and at least twice a year for antipsychotic medications, unless it has been established and documented that the patient's condition worsens in the face of such dosage reductions and remains improved with continuation of the medication. In general, the use of psychotropic medications on a PRN as-needed basis is discouraged.

Overall, use of nonpharmacological measures in nursing homes and periodic review of antipsychotic use can reduce antipsychotic use by 50% (Ballard et al., 2016). Integrating these interventions with social interaction can contribute to reductions in mortality in nursing home settings. Using multisensory stimulation rooms, massage chairs, and problem adaptation therapy can help control most neuropsychiatric symptoms and depression, respectively (Kiosses et al., 2015). Exercise is associated with a reduction in behavioral symptoms in nursing homes (Ballard et al., 2016; Forbes et al., 2015). Person-centered care, communication skills training for staff, resident activities and music therapy can also play significant roles in reducing dementia-associated agitation without the need for anti-psychotic medication (Livingston et al., 2014). A stepwise protocol for treating pain using acetaminophen, morphine, buprenorphine patch, and pregabalin has demonstrated the potential benefits of using acetaminophen for pain and resulting agitation secondary to pain (Sandvik, 2017). For nursing home residents with advanced dementia and challenging behaviors, behavioral training for staff resulted in improved behaviors and less psychotropic use, including antidepressant use (Pieper et al., 2016).

Some health care providers misinterpret OBRA guidelines for prescribing psychotropic medications, thinking that the use of certain medications is absolutely prohibited or that repeated dose reductions are mandatory. In fact, any psychotropic medication can be prescribed at clinically justifiable doses for any legitimate reason as long as there is a clear, well-documented rationale for doing so in terms of diagnosis, clinical justification, monitoring of response and side effects, and attempts at nonpharmacological interventions. Using medications with older adults in any setting optimally is a complex task (Scott, Gray, Martin, & Mitchell, 2012; Seitz, Gill, & Hermann, 2013; Steinman & Hanlon, 2010) and more effectively accomplished by an inter-professional team with a diversity of talents, experiences, and perspectives. A well-organized behavioral health team in the nursing home setting, working together with residents, their families, and other professional and informal care providers, can ensure that residents' behavioral problems are thoroughly assessed in terms of medication, medical, psychiatric, personal,

and social/environmental factors that may be interacting and contributing to those problems (Howell, 2015). Utilizing such comprehensive assessments, the team can then develop interventions that are not only sensitive and specific to the individual, but also effective and well tolerated.

See also Behavioral and Psychological Symptoms of Dementia; Depression in Dementia; Elder Mistreatment: Overview; Nursing Homes; Restraints; Psychosis in Late Life; Wandering and Elopement.

Satya Gutta and Timothy Howell

American Geriatrics Society 2015 Beers Criteria Update Expert Panel. (2015). American Geriatrics Society 2015 updated Beers criteria for potentially inappropriate medication use in older adults. *Journal of the American Geriatrics Society, 63*(11), 2227–2246.

Ballard, C., Orrell, M., Yong Zhong, S., Moniz-Cook, E., Stafford, J., Whittaker, R., … Fossey, J. (2016). Impact of antipsychotic review and nonpharmacological intervention on antipsychotic use, neuropsychiatric symptoms, and mortality in people with dementia living in nursing homes: A factorial cluster-randomized controlled trial by the Well-Being and Health for People with Dementia (WHELD) program. *American Journal of Psychiatry, 173*(3), 252–262. doi:10.1176/appi .ajp.2015.15010130

Divac, N., Stojanović, R., Savić Vujović, K., Medić, B., Damjanović, A., & Prostran, M. (2016). The efficacy and safety of antipsychotic medications in the treatment of psychosis in patients with Parkinson's disease. *Behavioural Neurology,* Article ID 4938154, 6 pages. doi:10.1155/2016/4938154

Forbes, S. C., Forbes, D., Forbes, S., Blake, C. M., Chong, L., Thiessen, E. J., … Rutjes, A. W. S. (2015). Exercise interventions for preventing dementia or delaying cognitive decline in people with mild cognitive impairment. *Cochrane Database of Systematic Reviews, 15*(4), CD006489. doi:10.1002/ 14651858.CD006489.pub4

Gallagher, P. F., Barry, P. J., Ryan, C., Hartigan, I., & O'Mahony, D. (2008). Inappropriate prescribing in an acutely ill population of elderly patients as determined by Beers' criteria. *Age and Ageing, 37*(1), 96–101.

Howell, T. (2015) The Wisconsin Star Method: Understanding and addressing complexity in geriatrics. In M. L. Malone, E. Capezuti, & R. M. Palmer (Eds.), *Geriatric models of care: Bringing 'best practice' to an Aging America* (pp. 87–94). Cham, Switzerland: Springer. doi:10.1007/978-3-319-16068-97

Kapp, M. B. (2009). Ethical and medicolegal issues. In W. E. Reichman & P. R. Katz (Eds.), *Psychiatry in long-term care* (2nd ed., pp. 465–483). New York: Oxford University Press.

Kiosses, D. N., Rosenberg, P. B., McGovern, A., Fonzetti, P., Zaydens, H., & Alexopoulos, G. S. (2015). Depression and suicidal ideation during two psychosocial treatments in older adults with major depression and dementia. *Journal of Alzheimer's Disease, 48*(2), 453–462.

Lavretsky, H. (2008). Neuropsychiatric symptoms in Alzheimer disease and related disorders: Why do treatments work in clinical practice but not in the randomized trials? *American Journal of Geriatric Psychiatry, 16*(7), 523–526.

Livingston, G., Kelly, L., Lewis-Holmes, E., Baio, G., Morris, S., Patel, N., … Cooper, C. (2014). Non-pharmacological interventions for agitation in dementia: Systematic review of randomized controlled trials. *British Journal of Psychiatry, 205*(6), 436–442.

Pieper, M. J., Francke, A. L., van der Steen, J. T., Scherder, E. J., Twisk, J. W., Kovach, C. R., & Achterberg, W. P. (2016). Effects of a stepwise multidisciplinary intervention for challenging behavior in advanced dementia: A cluster randomized controlled trial. *Journal of the American Geriatrics Society, 64*(2), 261–269.

Sandvik, R. K. N. M. (2017). Management of pain and burdensome symptoms in nursing home patients. Retrieved from http://bora.uib.no/bitstream/handle/1956/15473/dr-thesis-2017-Reidun-%20%20%20%20%20Norheim-Myhre-Sandvik.pdf?sequence=1&isAllowed=y

Scott, I. A., Gray, L. C., Martin, J. H., & Mitchell, C. A. (2012). Minimizing inappropriate medications in older populations: A 10-step conceptual framework. *American Journal of Medicine, 125,* 529–537.

Seitz, D. P., Gill, S. S., & Herrmann, N. (2013). Pharmacological treatments for neuropsychiatric symptoms of dementia in long-term care: A systematic review. *International Psychogeriatrics, 25*(2), 185–203.

Steinberg, M., & Lyketsos, C. G. (2012). Atypical antipsychotic use in patients with dementia: Managing safety concerns. *American Journal of Psychiatry, 169*(9), 900–906.

Steinman, M. A., Beizer, J. L., DuBeau, C. E., Laird, R. D., Lundebjerg, N. E., & Mulhausen, P. (2015). How to use the American Geriatrics Society 2015 Beers criteria—a guide for patients, clinicians, health systems, and payors. *Journal of the American Geriatrics Society, 63*(12), e1–e7.

Steinman, M. A., & Hanlon, J. T. (2010). Managing medications in clinically complex elders: "There's got to be a happy medium." *Journal of the American Medical Association, 304*(14), 1592–1601.

Web Resources
Alzheimer's Association: http://www.alz.org
American Association for Geriatric Psychiatry: http://www.aagponline.org
Centers for Medicare & Medicaid Services: https://www.cms.hhs.gov/manuals
Family Caregiver Alliance: https://www.caregiver.org
National Citizen's Coalition for Nursing Home Reform: http://www.nccnhr.org

REHABILITATION

Arguably, elements of the rehabilitation field have been in existence since the time of ancient Egyptians. However, the earliest incidence of a formal rehabilitation profession in the United States occurred in the early 1900s. The field of rehabilitation is unique among the medical disciplines because treatment targets an individual's function rather than their disease. In addition, rehabilitation can involve many different medical professionals. Consequently, for a long time, there was no unifying theory. The World Health Organization's International Classification of Functioning, Disability and Health (ICF) provides a framework that applies to rehabilitation professionals because it considers functioning as well as disease. Within the ICF framework, functioning is examined in the context of the body part, the individual as a whole, and the environment of the individual. Within each of these three contexts of functioning, there are the three domains of body functions and structures, activities, and participation. Disability in this model occurs if each of these three domains is affected.

During the first two decades of the 20th century, the individual rehabilitation fields in existence began to operate as a multidisciplinary team in response to rehabilitation needs following World War I and with the advent of workers' compensation. At that time, the focus of rehabilitation services was on injured soldiers and then workers affected by industrial injury and disability. Beginning in 1966 with the implementation of Medicare (a federally funded health insurance for adults aged 65 years and older and specified younger persons), the focus started to shift toward the rehabilitation of older adults and has

continued because of the increasing aging population and the prevalence of chronic conditions among older adults.

The first noted rehabilitation team in the 1920s comprised a physician and physical, occupational, and vocational therapists. This team has expanded over the decades and may now include a physiatrist, rehabilitation nurse, physical therapist, occupational therapist, speech pathologist, prosthetist, orthotist, respiratory therapist, dietician/nutritionist, music therapist, recreational therapist, social worker, or other ancillary staff. Each of these professionals serves different, but sometimes overlapping, roles in the rehabilitation of older adults. A brief description of each of the members of the rehabilitation team follows.

- *Physiatrist* (American Academy of Physical Medicine and Rehabilitation)
  - A medical doctor specializing in physical medicine and rehabilitation
  - Leads and coordinates the rehabilitation team and other medical professionals
  - Performs disability/impairment assessment and rehabilitation prescription
  - Performs specialized tests such as nerve conduction studies and nerve and muscle biopsies
  - Performs special procedures such as joint aspirations/injections or nerve blocks
- *Rehabilitation nurse* (Association of Rehabilitation Nurses)
  - A registered nurse who can become board certified as a rehabilitation nurse
  - Assists clients with disabilities/chronic illnesses to adapt to an altered life in a therapeutic environment
  - Coordinates nursing care in conjunction with other rehabilitation team members
  - Performs hands-on nursing care
  - Educates clients and family about pathology

- *Physical therapist* (American Physical Therapy Association)
  - A health care professional who helps patients maintain, restore, and improve movement, activity, and functioning
  - Examines, evaluates, diagnoses, prognosticates, and intervenes in pathologies affecting the musculoskeletal, neuromuscular, cardiovascular, pulmonary, and/or integumentary systems that may affect the ability to perform an action, a task, or an activity necessary for function
  - Performs manual therapy techniques, motor function training, or airway clearance techniques
  - Uses therapeutic exercise, assistive technology, and biophysical agents
- *Occupational therapist* (American Occupational Therapy Association, Inc.)
  - A health care professional who uses everyday activities to assist patients to do things they need or want to do
  - Performs individualized evaluations, customizes interventions to help patients in performing everyday activities, and evaluates the outcome of the intervention
  - Provides adaptive equipment recommendations and training, and advises on task modification to improve an individual's participation in a task or activity
- *Speech pathologist* (American Speech-Language-Hearing Association)
  - A health care professional who is involved in the prevention, assessment, diagnosis, and treatment of speech, language, communication (as a result of social or cognitive deficits), and swallowing disorders
  - Performs evaluation and training to use augmentative and assistive communication systems
  - Implements interventions to improve control of the vocal and respiratory systems
- *Prosthetist and orthotist* (American Board for Certification in Orthotics, Prosthetics & Pedorthics)
  - An allied health professional who is certified to design, fabricate, fit, educate patients on use, and monitor both prosthetic and orthotic devices based on a doctor's prescription

- A prosthetic is a device that replaces a body part. A prosthetist is a person who is only certified in the design, fabrication, and fitting of prosthetic devices (artificial limbs).
- An orthotic is a supportive device that is provided to patients with neuromuscular and/or musculoskeletal impairments that result in functional limitations. An orthotist is a person who is only certified in the design, fabrication, and fitting of orthotic devices.
- *Respiratory therapist* (American Association for Respiratory Care)
  - A health care professional who treats disorders affecting the cardiopulmonary system
  - Recommends treatments based on lung and breathing pathologies
  - Manages assistive breathing devices (e.g., ventilators)
- *Dieticians/nutritionist* (Academy of Nutrition and Dietetics)
  - A health care professional who uses food and nutrition to affect health and disease
  - Dieticians or dietician nutritionists complete a course of training approved by the Accreditation Council for Education in Nutrition and Dietetics (ACEND) and then complete an internship period followed by a national examination to be eligible to register to practice.
  - Nutritionists do not have to be health professionals, and those who do not use the designations "dietician" or "registered dietician" may practice without being registered in some states.
- *Music therapist* (American Music Therapy Association)
  - A health care professional trained in the use of music to treat the physical, emotional, cognitive, and social needs of individuals
  - Performs an assessment of the strength and needs of patients, then implements a treatment that includes creating, singing, moving to, and/or listening to music
  - Involved in the rehabilitation of speech, cognitive, pain, respiratory, sleep, motor function, and communication dysfunctions.
- *Recreational therapist* (American Therapeutic Recreation Association)

- A health care professional that uses recreation (sports, games) and other activities (arts, drama) to restore, remediate, or rehabilitate an individual's physical, psychological, social, and leisure needs
- Facilitates improved health through living active, satisfying lives
- *Social worker* (National Association of Social Workers)
  - A professional trained to assist individuals, families, or groups in need by restoring or improving their social functioning
  - Uses psychosocial services and advocacy to help people in need
  - Assists persons experiencing discrimination, physical illness, and disability

REHABILITATION SERVICES AND OLDER ADULTS

The settings where rehabilitation services are provided to older adults include acute care hospitals, inpatient rehabilitation facilities, skilled nursing facilities, custodial nursing facilities, outpatient facilities, and home. Because older adults are known to move between these setting as their condition or needs change, ensuring that transitions do not affect care quality is critical. The transition from acute care facilities has been the focus of attention because one in five Medicare beneficiaries are reported to be readmitted within 30 days of discharge. Because hospitals servicing Medicare and Medicaid patients with unacceptably high readmission rates face financial penalties under the Patient Protection and Affordable Care Act, addressing the readmission rate is a priority.

Among the factors associated with readmission are breakdowns in communication between providers, inadequate patient education, breakdowns in provider accountability, and impaired physical function (Falvey et al., 2016). Models of transitional care developed to address the aforementioned limitations include the Care Transitions Intervention (CTI), Better Outcomes for Older adults through Safe Transitions (BOOST), Geriatric Resources for Assessment and Care of Elders (GRACE), Geriatric Floating Interdisciplinary Transition Team (Geri-FITT), Transitional Care Model

(TCM), and Ideal Transition of Care (ITC). Despite a large number of TCMs, Falvey et al. (2016) lament the lack of involvement of rehabilitation professionals in such models, especially because functional deficits are a predictor of readmissions. Using the ITC TCM, Falvey et al. identified several areas where greater consideration of physical function can improve the transitional care of older adults and potentially result in lower post-acute care readmissions. The areas recognized as needing improvement include communication between inpatient and community health care personnel on the patient's physical function; providing physical function information during care planning, monitoring, and follow-up; including information on physical function in discharge summaries; ensuring that discharge summaries are clear and timely; discussing the effects of medication on function; and providing patient and family education on physical functioning.

In addition to improving transitional care, rehabilitative efforts to address hospital-associated deconditioning (HAD) may also be instrumental in reducing the rate of readmission of older adults to acute care facilities. Falvey, Mangione, and Stevens-Lapsley (2015) describe a conceptual model that can be implemented after hospitalization. The model by Falvey et al. advocates for a reconsideration of the rehabilitation paradigm for managing HAD, placing greater emphasis on general condition activities and "simple" activities of daily living (ADL), gait, and balance training, with relatively less emphasis on aerobic and resistance training. In the model by Falvey et al., the emphasis is on high-intensity resistance training, and moderate to high-intensity gait, balance, and ADL training. Moderate-intensity aerobic training and general condition activities play a much smaller role in the model by Falvey et al.

INTERVENTIONS

When implementing interventions for older adults, the health care provider must first consider that the recovery process tends to be slower than for their younger counterparts and that modification to the intervention may be necessary because of comorbidities and normal changes associated with aging (Paraschiv, Esanu, Ghiuru, & Gavrilescu, 2015). Interventions can include but are not limited to exercise, adaptive techniques, assistive technology, physical modalities, orthoses, and prostheses.

One of the most frequently used interventions by rehabilitation professionals is exercise/physical activities. The documented benefits of exercise/physical activities for older adults include improved executive function, fall prevention in those with or without dementia, improved functional abilities such as walking speed and chair-rise time, reduced joint pain from arthritis, increased bone density, improved posture and balance, increased lean body mass (muscle), and reductions in mortality (Burton et al., 2015; Daly, McMinn, & Allan, 2014; Hupin et al., 2015; Leung, Chan, Tsang, Tsang, & Jones, 2011; Mangione, Miller, & Naughton, 2010; Mansfield, Wong, Bryce, Knorr, & Patterson, 2015). Exercise also helps to prevent, remediate, or eliminate physical limitation in the presence of other disease or illness.

Current evidence also suggests that the sedentary behavior of older adults should be viewed as an independent risk factor for deficits in ADL and detrimental health outcomes (Biswas et al., 2015; Dunlop et al., 2015). That is, the time spent engaging in sedentary behaviors is associated with deficits in ADL and general health irrespective of physical activity. Therefore advising older adults to reduce the time spent in sedentary behaviors should also be incorporated into rehabilitation programs.

Performing self-care tasks safely and independently can involve learning adaptive techniques. For example, therapists may train an individual with hemiplegia due to a stroke to dress independently using only one arm. Adaptive techniques may involve assistive technologies—devices designed to support safe activity. Devices may be simple, such as raised toilet seats or canes, or may be complicated, such as modifications to the home (e.g., patient lifts, grab bars, handrails). However, even for simple devices, consultation with a rehabilitation professional may be necessary because improper equipment (by type or fit) is unlikely to maximize function and may even be dangerous.

Physical modalities use techniques that promote healing by reducing local inflammation, muscle spasm, or pain. Ultrasound, diathermy, transcutaneous electrical nerve stimulation (TENS), whirlpool, massage, and the application of heat or cold are a few examples. Efficacy for many of these physical modalities is unproved, but anecdotes often support their use in individual situations.

Both orthoses and prostheses can be critical elements in restoring function. Physicians and rehabilitation therapists assess need and prescribe these devices. Therapists also perform training to monitor equipment fit, especially with prostheses.

See also Activities of Daily Living; Assistive Technology; Deconditioning Prevention; Exercise; Gait Disturbances; Occupational Therapy Assessment and Evaluation; Physical Therapy Services; Post-Acute Care.

Sylvester Carter

Biswas, A., Oh, P. I., Faulkner, G. E., Bajaj, R. R., Silver, M. A., Mitchell, M. S., & Alter, D. A. (2015). Sedentary time and its association with risk for disease incidence, mortality, and hospitalization in adults: A systematic review and meta-analysis. *Annals of Internal Medicine, 162*(2), 123–132.

Burton, E., Cavalheri, V., Adams, R., Browne, C. O., Bovery-Spencer, P., Fenton, A. M., … Hill, K. D. (2015). Effectiveness of exercise programs to reduce falls in older people with dementia living in the community: A systematic review and meta-analysis. *Clinical Interventions in Aging, 10*, 421–434.

Daly, M., McMinn, D., & Allan, J. L. (2014). A bidirectional relationship between physical activity and executive function in older adults. *Frontiers in Human Neuroscience, 8*, 1044.

Dunlop, D. D., Song, J., Arnston, E. K., Semanik, P. A., Lee, J., Chang, R. W., & Hootman, J. M. (2015). Sedentary time in US older adults associated with disability in activities of daily living independent of physical activity. *Journal of Physical Activity & Health, 12*(1), 93–101.

Falvey, J. R., Burke, R. E., Malone, D., Ridgeway, K. J., McManus, B. M., & Stevens-Lapsley, J. E. (2016). Role of physical therapists in reducing hospital readmissions: Optimizing outcomes for older

R

adults during care transitions from hospital to community. *Physical Therapy, 96*(8), 1125–1134.

Falvey, J. R., Mangione, K. K., & Stevens-Lapsley, J. E. (2015). Rethinking hospital-associated deconditioning: Proposed paradigm shift. *Physical Therapy, 95*(9), 1307–1315.

Hupin, D., Roche, F., Gremeaux, V., Chatard, J. C., Oriol, M., Gaspoz, J. M., … Edouard, P. (2015). Even a low-dose of moderate-to-vigorous physical activity reduces mortality by 22% in adults aged ≥60 years: A systematic review and meta-analysis. *British Journal of Sports Medicine, 49*(19), 1262–1267.

Leung, D. P., Chan, C. K., Tsang, H. W., Tsang, W. W., & Jones, A. Y. (2011). Tai chi as an intervention to improve balance and reduce falls in older adults: A systematic and meta-analytical review. *Alternative Therapies in Health and Medicine, 17*(1), 40–48.

Mangione, K. K., Miller, A. H., & Naughton, I. V. (2010). Cochrane Review: Improving physical function and performance with progressive resistance strength training in older adults. *Physical Therapy, 90*(12), 1711–1715.

Mansfield, A., Wong, J. S., Bryce, J., Knorr, S., & Patterson, K. K. (2015). Does perturbation-based balance training prevent falls? Systematic review and meta-analysis of preliminary randomized controlled trials. *Physical Therapy, 95*(5), 700–709.

Paraschiv, C., Esanu, I., Ghiuru, R., & Gavrilescu, C. M. (2015). General principles of geriatric rehabilitation. *Romanian Journal of Oral Rehabilitation, 7*(1), 76–80.

Web Resources

Academy of Nutrition and Dietetics: Eatright: http://www.eatright.org

American Academy of Physical Medicine and Rehabilitation: What is a Physiatrist?: http://www.aapmr.org/about-physiatry/about-physical-medicine-rehabilitation/what-is-physiatry

American Association for Respiratory Care: http://www.aarc.org

American Board for Certification in Orthotics, Prosthetics & Pedorthics: https://www.abcop.org

American Music Therapy Association: http://www.musictherapy.org

American Occupational Therapy Association Inc.: About occupational therapy: http://www.aota.org

American Physical Therapy Association: http://www.apta.org

American Speech-Language-Hearing Association: http://www.asha.org

American Therapeutic Recreation Association: https://www.atra-online.com

Association of Rehabilitation Nurses: Role Descriptions: http://www.rehabnurse.org

RELOCATION STRESS

In their classic work, Litwak and Longino (1987) described three relocations that older adults commonly experience as they age, characterized by increasing need for assistance. These transitions have been expanded in subsequent work characterizing relocations as serial amenity moves, positioning moves, informal assistance moves, formal assistance moves, and dependency moves (Lovegreen, Kahana, & Kahana, 2010). It has been estimated that one third of older adults relocate after the age of 65 years (Wu, Prina, Barnes, Matthews, & Brayne, 2015). However, most relocations occur during the last year of life (Buurman et al., 2014). Community-residing older adults likely to move can be identified through a profile of vulnerability based on their concerns about their health problems, finances, and architectural features of their homes that may not be conducive to aging in place (Carpenter et al., 2007) and self-prediction that they will not be able to live independently within the next 2 years (Sergeant, Ekerdt, & Chapin, 2010) or that they have little time left to live (Beyer, Rupprecht, & Lang, 2016). Their comprehension that relocation is necessary has been associated with better outcomes (Gilbert, Amella, Edlund, & Nemeth, 2015). Furthermore, low education, low social class, and living in rural areas are associated with relocation, as has area deprivation (Wu et al., 2015). Thus individual preference for relocation may be preempted by economic, cultural, and political factors (e.g., need for safe, more economical housing; Portacolone & Halpern, 2016; Riley, Hawkley, & Cagney, 2016).

Many older adults must relocate due to declining functional ability or worsening health. For example, the inability to walk outside alone has been associated with the desire to relocate to more supportive housing (Matsumoto, Naruse, Sakai, & Nagata, 2016). Furthermore, older adults who experience a cerebrovascular accident, angina, or congestive heart failure have been found to be likely to relocate 1 year after such experiences (Lovasi et al., 2014). They are more likely to move if they are cognitively impaired and have limited assistance in their homes. Use of personal care services and senior center services is associated with the ability to remain living in the community (Chen & Thompson, 2010). Volunteering has been associated with reduced likelihood of relocation (Shen & Perry, 2014). Relocation to a long-term care facility occurs when care needs surpass the availability and capacity of community services and family caregivers. Older adults who have Down syndrome have an increased risk and higher incidence of placement in a nursing home (Patti, Amble, & Flory, 2010). Often older adults relocate to retirement residences offering aging-in-place. However, this concept may require relocation one or more times within the facility or to a new facility as care needs intensify. The TigerPlace residence founded by University of Missouri Sinclair School of Nursing is one of the few facilities where older adults remain in their apartments for the duration of their lives, with care added as it is needed (Rantz et al., 2008).

Nearly all professionals working with older adults have had the experience of trying to help older adults and their families make decisions about relocation. It can be challenging to assess and make recommendations. Relocation can be particularly challenging for older adults with neurocognitive impairment (Kaplan, Andersen, Lehning, & Perry, 2015). Relocation decision making may be one important situation where nurses can intervene to assist older adults.

IDENTIFYING RELOCATION STRESS

Two questions considered by those helping older adults through relocation follow: (a) Who is most vulnerable to the stress associated with relocation? (b) How is this stress identified? Relocation stress may occur with greater regularity and intensity when an older adult relocates precipitously, with limited choice or input into the decision. Involuntary moves in which there is little perceived improvement in living conditions may be especially stressful. Perhaps the most stressful situation, and ironically one of the most common, is when the relocation occurs in response to a health crisis. In this situation, the older adult may feel rushed into the relocation, and have little choice in the location of the new home, with minimal preparation time. The Pressure to Move Scale may be helpful to measure the extent to which the cognitively intact older adult feels pressure from others to move (Bekhet, Zauszniewski, & Nakhala, 2011). Several studies have reported that older adults may have minimal participation in relocation decision making (Falk, Wijk, & Persson, 2011; Fraher & Coffey, 2011). The decision to relocate is commonly made by the older adult's physician, adult child, or another family member (Johnson, Schweibert, & Rosenmann, 1994). Older adults' participation in relocation decision making may be less related to their capacity to participate than to their informal support systems (Johnson, Popejoy, & Radina, 2010). The situation may be especially stressful for ethnic elders who may fear discrimination when they relocate (Johnson & Tripp-Reimer, 2001). Patterns of relocation and adjustment outcomes differ significantly across cultures (Bekhet & Zauszniewski, 2014a, 2014b, Yeboah, 2015).

Any older adult who relocates, but particularly those in the most potentially stressful scenario (e.g., precipitous move; little choice, especially due to cognitive impairment; little preparation; and limited perceived improvement in living conditions), may show signs of depression, anxiety, withdrawal, and morbidity (Lutgendorf et al., 2001). Social isolation during and subsequent to relocation has been associated with cooccurring seasonal variation (Perry, 2014a). These may be accompanied by declines in the ability to perform basic activities of daily living (ADL) and instrumental activities of daily living (IADL; Chen & Wilmoth, 2004), weight loss, anorexia, poor nutrition, falls, a decline in self-perceived health, reduced social support, decline in sense of coherence (Johnson & Tripp-Reimer, 2001), intrusive thoughts, and decreased vigor (Lutgendorf et al., 2001). Any of these manifestations may occur during the process of relocation decision making, during the actual move, or within 3 months afterward, particularly if the older adult has an unhealthy relocation transition style (Rossen & Knafl, 2003). The first month following relocation may be the most difficult, and signs of stress may be most obvious. During the first week, older adults may experience elevated stress hormone levels (i.e., cortisol) that may begin to resolve by the fourth week (Hodgson, Freedman, Granger, & Erno, 2004). Within the first 3 months postrelocation, older adults may have lowered natural killer cell cytotoxicity that may make them vulnerable to infection (Lutgendorf et al., 2001).

Careful, multidisciplinary assessment during these periods is critical to identifying signs of relocation stress. Use of a well-tested instrument to assess depression and changes in functional status may assist in the early identification of relocation stress. The Index of Relocation Adjustment may be assistive in predicting early relocation stress syndrome (RSS; Bekhet & Zauszniewski, 2013). The theory of residential normalcy may provide a useful framework for assessing the likelihood of successful relocation (Golant, 2015). However, it is also necessary to assess the ability to perform ADL, signs of infection, nutritional status, engagement in social behavior, physical activity level, sleep, and morbidity. These areas are equally important to assess in those who are cognitively impaired.

PREVENTING SEVERE RELOCATION STRESS

As with most negative health situations, preventing severe relocation stress is a better approach than trying to minimize it once it is already present. The ability to control decision making regarding relocation has been identified as important in relocation outcomes (Brownie, Horstmanshof, & Garbutt, 2014). Ensuring the older adult's participation in making the decision to relocate is the earliest preventive measure. This is a multidisciplinary task for those helping the older adult in the situation preceding relocation. Clearly, not all older adults want to participate, nor should they be expected to do

so. Participation assumes some cognitive capacity and includes considering alternatives and exercising choice. Recognition that relocation is needed may not be as immediate for the older adult as for participating family members.

If the older adult has a companion animal, the decision may be particularly stressful because not all residential options allow pets. The importance of the bond formed between the older adult and the pet must be taken into account. Often older adults need some assistance with pet care that can enable them to keep their companion. Too often the most common response to this situation may be to "get rid of" the pet. This loss combined with the stress of relocation may result in negative outcomes. Options for pet care assistance should be investigated. Some facilities not only allow but also encourage and facilitate pet ownership among older adults because of the known benefits of the unconditional love, companionship, and motivation to remain active that have been found in older adult pet owners (Johnson, 2013; Johnson & Bibbo, 2014a). Dog walking has been found to be helpful in promoting health and health behavior (Curl, Bibbo, & Johnson, 2016).

Professionals working with families that are contemplating relocation need to ascertain the degree of difference in view, if any, between the older adult and family members. This is best done by interviewing them separately. Family members should not pressure the older adult into the decision but instead discuss the benefits of the new location in terms of how it may improve living conditions. Participation and choice in selecting the new residence may help prevent severe relocation stress. Relocation may even be viewed as "a gift" between the older adult and loved ones as the safety and care needs of the older adult can be better met (Perry, 2014b).

Beyond choice, careful preparation and assistance may minimize the stress of relocation. This also involves a multidisciplinary approach. For example, the case manager or social worker may facilitate contact between staff at the new residence, the older adult, and family for rapport development. The advanced practice nurse or primary care physician should conduct a thorough cognitive and functional assessment and transmit the results to those responsible for care of residents at the new location. A clinical practice guideline may be useful for this process (Hertz, Koren, Rossetti, & Tibbits, 2016). This may promote optimal care and decrease older adults' fears.

Unfortunately, hospitalized older adults often must relocate to the first available place (e.g., a nursing home) when their inpatient days have lapsed or to a place that they may have tentatively considered years earlier. Alternatively, they may have to relocate to an adult child's or other relative's house for home care. When precipitous relocation may seem to prevent choice and participation, however, even limited participation by the older adult in decisions can be helpful. Deciding which belongings to move, what new things are needed, and what will be done with belongings not taken may help minimize relocation stress, assuming that it is unhurried. The process of selling possessions and seeing their material value when "downsizing" may be helpful to the older adult in detaching from these objects (Ekerdt & Addington, 2015). Decisions about the new residence, such as room color and furniture arrangement, may help prevent severe relocation stress. This personalizing of the new living environment may facilitate adjustment (Perry, 2014c) because older adults must reconstruct their meaning of "home" (Johnson & Bibbo, 2014b).

Anticipatory planning involves visiting the new residence at different times of the day and week, meeting and visiting with residents and staff, having meals there, and viewing the new living space. It also includes asking and receiving answers to questions about policies, special services, programming, and events.

TREATING SEVERE RELOCATION STRESS

Although preventive strategies are the optimal approach, they may not always be used or be effective. Most relocating elders experience some degree of stress. This may facilitate adaptation because changes in behavior, attitudes, or both are necessary for older adults to adjust to a new residence. To minimize severe relocation stress, resourcefulness training (Bekhet & Zauszniewski, 2016), reminiscence therapy, massage, therapeutic touch, bibliotherapy, animal-assisted activity (Friedmann et al., 2015), active listening, prayer, music therapy, art therapy, social programming, and linking new residents with a "buddy" who is not a newcomer for social support may be helpful. Caregiving staff in facilities may need to keep in mind the perspectives of the older adults in relocating and the capacity of the staff to lessen the stress of the process (Ellis & Rawson, 2010). Pharmacological treatment for depression and anxiety may be needed in severe cases. Encouraging older adults to express their feelings may be assistive (Brownie et al., 2014). Continuing assessment of nutritional status, self-care, and social behavior is needed to monitor progress. Older adults and their family members should participate in assessment and intervention.

Despite more than three decades of research demonstrating the profound effects of relocation stress, precipitous, relatively unplanned, and involuntary relocation still occurs regularly. Professionals who work with older adults and their families should advocate for the older adults' choice, participation, and preparation to decrease the incidence of this largely preventable yet potentially damaging situation.

See also Discharge Planning; Transitional Care.

Rebecca A. Johnson

Bekhet, A. K., & Zauszniewski, J. A. (2013). Resourcefulness, positive cognitions, relocation controllability and relocation adjustment among older people: A cross-sectional study of cultural differences. *International Journal of Older People Nursing, 8*(3), 244–252.

Bekhet, A. K., & Zauszniewski, J. A. (2014a). Individual characteristics and relocation factors affecting adjustment among relocated American and Egyptian older adults. *Issues in Mental Health Nursing, 35*(2), 80–87.

Bekhet, A. K., & Zauszniewski, J. A. (2014b). Psychometric properties of the index of relocation adjustment. *Journal of Applied Gerontology, 33*(4), 437–455.

Bekhet, A. K., & Zauszniewski, J. A. (2016). The effect of a resourcefulness training intervention on relocation adjustment and adaptive functioning among older adults in retirement communities. *Issues in Mental Health Nursing, 37*(3), 182–189.

R

Bekhet, A. K., Zauszniewski, J. A., & Nakhla, W. E. (2011). Psychometric properties of the pressure to move scale in relocated American older adults: Further evaluation. *Issues in Mental Health Nursing, 32*(11), 711–716.

Beyer, A., Rupprecht, R., & Lang, F. R. (2016). Subjective time left in life and precautionary relocation planning in the last half of life. *Zeitschrift für Gerontologie und Geriatrie, 50*(3), 194–199. doi:10.1007/s00391-016-1025-1

Brownie, S., Horstmanshof, L., & Garbutt, R. (2014). Factors that impact residents' transition and psychological adjustment to long-term aged care: A systematic literature review. *International Journal of Nursing Studies, 51*(12), 1654–1666.

Buurman, B. M., Trentalange, M., Nicholson, N. R., McGloin, J. M., Gahbauer, E. A., Allore, H. G., & Gill, T. M. (2014). Residential relocations among older people over the course of more than 10 years. *Journal of the American Medical Directors Association, 15*(7), 521–526.

Carpenter, B. D., Edwards, D. F., Pickard, J. G., Palmer, J. L., Stark, S., Neufeld, P. S., . . . Morris, J. C. (2007). Anticipating relocation: Concerns about moving among NORC residents. *Journal of Gerontological Social Work, 49*(1–2), 165–184.

Chen, P. C., & Wilmoth, J. M. (2004). The effects of residential mobility on ADL and IADL limitations among the very old living in the community. *Journals of Gerontology: Series B, Psychological Sciences and Social Sciences, 59*(3), S164–S172.

Chen, Y. M., & Thompson, E. A. (2010). Understanding factors that influence success of home- and community-based services in keeping older adults in community settings. *Journal of Aging and Health, 22*(3), 267–291.

Curl, A. L., Bibbo, J., & Johnson, R. A. (2016). Dog ownership, walking, and bonding, and older adults' health and health behaviors. *The Gerontologist.* doi:10.1093/geront/gnw051

Ekerdt, D. J., & Addington, A. (2015). Possession divestment by sales in later life. *Journal of Aging Studies, 34*, 21–28. doi:10.1016/j.jaging.2015.03.006

Ellis, J. M., & Rawson, H. (2010). Nurses' and personal care assistants' role in improving the relocation of older people into nursing homes. *Journal of Clinical Nursing, 24*(13–14), 2005–2013. doi:10.1111/jocn.12798

Falk, H., Wijk, H., & Persson, L. O. (2011). Frail older persons' experiences of interinstitutional relocation. *Geriatric Nursing, 32*(4), 245–256.

Fraher, A., & Coffey, A. (2011). Older people's experiences of relocation to long-term care. *Nursing Older People, 23*(10), 23–27.

Friedmann, E., Galik, E., Thomas, S. A., Hall, P. S., Chung, S. Y., & McCune, S. (2015). Evaluation of a pet-assisted living intervention for improving functional status in assisted living residents with mild to moderate cognitive impairment: A pilot study. *American Journal of Alzheimer's Disease and Other Dementias, 30*(3), 276–289.

Gilbert, S., Amella, E., Edlund, B., & Nemeth, L. (2015). Making the move: A mixed research integrative review. *Healthcare, 3*(3), 757–774.

Golant, S. M. (2015). Residential normalcy and the enriched coping repertoires of successfully aging older adults. *The Gerontologist, 55*(1), 70–82.

Hertz, J. E., Koren, M. E., Rossetti, J., & Tibbits, K. (2016). Management of relocation in cognitively intact older adults. *Journal of Gerontological Nursing, 42*(11), 14–23.

Hodgson, N., Freedman, V. A., Granger, D. A., & Erno, A. (2004). Biobehavioral correlates of relocation in the frail elderly: Salivary cortisol, affect, and cognitive function. *Journal of the American Geriatrics Society, 52*(11), 1856–1862.

Johnson, R. A. (2013). Promoting one health: The University of Missouri Research Center for Human/Animal Interaction. *Missouri Medicine, 110*(3), 197–200.

Johnson, R. A., & Bibbo, J. (2014a). The utopia of Tiger Place: Older adults, relocation to a nursing home, and pet relinquishment. *Tijdschrift voor Ouderengeneeskunde (Journal of Geriatric Medicine, Netherlands), 1*, 28–30.

Johnson, R. A., & Bibbo, J. (2014b). Relocation decisions and constructing the meaning of home: A phenomenological study of the transition into a nursing home. *Journal of Aging Studies, 30*, 56–63.

Johnson, R. A., Popejoy, L. L., & Radina, M. E. (2010). Older adults' participation in nursing home placement decisions. *Clinical Nursing Research, 19*(4), 358–375.

Johnson, R. A., Schwiebert, V. B., & Rosenmann, P. A. (1994). Factors influencing nursing home placement decisions: The older adult's perspective. *Clinical Nursing Research, 3*(3), 269–281.

Johnson, R. A., & Tripp-Reimer, T. (2001). Relocation among ethnic elders. A review—Part 2. *Journal of Gerontological Nursing, 27*(6), 22–27.

Kaplan, D. B., Andersen, T. C., Lehning, A. J., & Perry, T. E. (2015). Aging in place vs. relocation for older adults with neurocognitive disorder: Applications of Wiseman's behavioral model. *Journal of Gerontological Social Work, 58*(5), 521–538.

Litwak, E., & Longino, C. F. (1987). Migration patterns among the elderly: A developmental perspective. *The Gerontologist, 27*(3), 266–272.

Lovasi, G. S., Richardson, J. M., Rodriguez, C. J., Kop, W. J., Ahmed, A., Brown, A. F., … Siscovick, D. S. (2014). Residential relocation by older adults in response to incident cardiovascular health events: A case-crossover analysis. *Journal of Environmental and Public Health, 2014,* Article ID 951971. doi:10.1155/2014/951971

Lovegreen, L. D., Kahana, E., & Kahana, B. (2010). Residential relocation of amenity migrants to Florida: "Unpacking" post-amenity moves. *Journal of Aging and Health, 22*(7), 1001–1028.

Lutgendorf, S. K., Reimer, T. T., Harvey, J. H., Marks, G., Hong, S. Y., Hillis, S. L., & Lubaroff, D. M. (2001). Effects of housing relocation on immuno-competence and psychosocial functioning in older adults. *Journals of Gerontology: Series A, Biological Sciences and Medical Sciences, 56*(2), M97–M105.

Matsumoto, H., Naruse, T., Sakai, M., & Nagata, S. (2016). Who prefers to age in place? Cross-sectional survey of middle-aged people in Japan. *Geriatrics & Gerontology International, 16*(5), 631–637.

Patti, P., Amble, K., & Flory, M. (2010). Placement, relocation and end of life issues in aging adults with and without Down's syndrome: A retrospective study. *Journal of Intellectual Disability Research, 54*(6), 538–546.

Perry, T. E. (2014a). Moving as a gift: Relocation in older adulthood. *Journal of Aging Studies, 31,* 1–9.

Perry, T. E. (2014b). Make mine home: Spatial modification with physical and social implications in older adulthood. *Journals of Gerontology: Series B, Psychological Sciences and Social Sciences, 70*(3), 453–461.

Perry, T. E. (2014c). Seasonal variation and homes: Understanding the social experiences of older adults. *Care Management Journals: Journal of Case Management; The Journal of Long Term Home Health Care, 15*(1), 3–10.

Portacolone, E., & Halpern, J. (2016). "Move or suffer": Is age-segregation the new norm for older Americans living alone? *Journal of Applied Gerontology, 35*(8), 836–856.

Rantz, M. J., Porter, R. T., Cheshier, D., Otto, D., Servey, C. H., Johnson, R. A., … Taylor, G. (2008). TigerPlace: A state-academic-private project to revolutionize traditional long-term care. *Journal of Housing for the Elderly, 22*(1–2), 66–85.

Riley, A., Hawkley, L. C., & Cagney, K. A. (2016). Racial differences in the effects of neighborhood disadvantage on residential mobility in later life. *Journals of Gerontology: Series B, Psychological Sciences and Social Sciences, 71*(6), 1131–1140.

Rossen, E. K., & Knafl, K. A. (2003). Older women's response to residential relocation: Description of transition styles. *Qualitative Health Research, 13*(1), 20–36.

Sergeant, J. F., Ekerdt, D. J., & Chapin, R. K. (2010). Older adults' expectations to move: Do they predict actual community-based or nursing facility moves within 2 years? *Journal of Aging and Health, 22*(7), 1029–1053.

Shen, H. W., & Perry, T. E. (2014). Giving back and staying put: Volunteering as a stabilizing force in relocation. *Journal of Housing for the Elderly, 28*(3), 310–328.

Wu, Y. T., Prina, A. M., Barnes, L. E., Matthews, F. E., & Brayne, C.; MRC CFAS. (2015). Relocation at older age: Results from the Cognitive Function and Ageing Study. *Journal of Public Health, 37*(3), 480–487.

Yeboah, C. A. (2015). Choosing to live in a nursing home: A culturally and linguistically diverse perspective. *Australian Journal of Primary Health, 21*(2), 239–244.

Web Resources

Housing alternatives and resources: http://www.eldercare.gov/Eldercare.NET/public/Resources/Brochures/docs/Housing_Options_Booklet.pdf

Importance of physical activity for older adults: http://www.cdc.gov/aging/pdf/community-based_physical_activity_programs_for_older_adults.pdf

Resources for older adults in the LGBT community: http://www.stonewallchico.org/resources/older-adults

Resources on types of housing alternatives: http://www.eldercare.gov/Eldercare.NET/Public/Index.aspx

R

RESPITE CARE

Respite care refers to short-term supervisory, personal, and nursing care provided to impaired older adults, typically those who cannot be left alone because of physical or mental disabilities. The purpose of respite care is to provide the informal caregivers of impaired older adults with temporary relief or respite from their caregiving responsibilities. Providing support to the caregivers of impaired elderly is an important strategy for well-being, although some studies have found that a relatively small number of caregivers utilize supportive services (Wolff, Spillman, Freedman, & Kasper, 2016). Of all the services designed for community-dwelling impaired older adults, respite care is the most firmly rooted in recognition of the social, primarily family, context within which caregiving occurs.

There are three primary forms of respite care: in-home respite care, temporary residential respite care, and adult day care. All three forms provide very different experiences for the care recipient. Adult day care is provided in a community setting to multiple impaired older adults. Depending on the caregiver's preference and ability to pay for the service, as well as the care recipient's illness severity, weekly day care schedules range from 1 to 5 days. The cost of adult day care varies, depending on location, but on average runs approximately $67/ day. In-home respite care is provided in the impaired older adult's home by a respite care worker. The length and frequency of in-home respite visits vary widely, from companionship to skilled care. Respite care workers are generally paid an hourly wage, and the median per day cost of in-home care is $126. Inpatient respite care involves a short-stay placement, usually 2 weeks, in a hospital or nursing home. Most respite care services are paid out of pocket, although some resources are available for low-income (e.g., Medicaid) households and may be a benefit provided by long-term care insurance.

The need for respite care services emerged primarily because of overwhelming research evidence that caregivers are at substantial risk for negative physical, emotional, and financial consequences (National Alliance for Caregiving [NAC] & AARP Public Policy Institute, 2015; Wolff et al., 2016). Research demonstrates that the older persons at greatest risk of nursing home placement are those without families and those whose families are no longer willing or able to tolerate the demands of home care. In some studies, caregivers' levels of burden predict institutionalization of the impaired relatives for whom they care (Eska et al., 2013). Thus respite care has the primary purpose of decreasing caregiver stress and permitting the impaired

elder to remain in the community and delay institutionalization, although recent reviews have not supported that link (Maayan, Soares-Weiser, & Lee, 2014; Vandepitte et al., 2016).

The number of respite care programs in the United States continues to grow. The greatest impetus for the growth of respite care was the reauthorization of the Older Americans Act (OAA) in 2000, which included the National Family Caregiver Support Program (NFCSP). As a result, states applying for funds to support services to older adults are required to implement respite care programs through local area agencies on aging. Further support for respite programs came from the Lifespan Respite Care Program that was authorized by Congress in 2006 to support coordinated systems of community-based respite care services for family caregivers. The intent, to develop infrastructures at the state and local level, was to increase efficiency and decrease duplication of services. Beginning in 2009, Congress appropriated approximately $2.5 million in funds to implement programs to fill the service gaps for respite and to develop outcome measures. In 2011, the legislation was due for reauthorization (Lifespan Respite Reauthorization Act of 2011 [H.R. 3266]) and was introduced and referred to the House Energy and Commerce Committee, where no action was taken. The bill was reintroduced in 2017 (H.R. 2535) for reauthorizations and is currently being considered by the Congressional Subcommittee on Health.

Research examining the impact of respite care services on caregiver and care recipient outcomes continues to expand. Research findings are inconsistent and many of the studies lack the rigorous design necessary to assess outcomes in relation to evidence-based practices (Kirk & Kagan, 2015; Maayan et al., 2014; Vandepitte et al., 2016). Despite the limitations of the research, respite care appears to provide some benefit to caregivers.

Much of the research has related to the use of respite care with cognitively impaired elderly. The use of adult day care is the type of respite care most investigated. Overall, adult day care seems to decrease caregiver burden and provide some positive effects on care recipient behavior. In a systematic review, Vandepitte et al. (2016)

noted that adult day-care services accelerate nursing home placement, but cautioned that this finding was likely because of multifactorial issues and concluded that multiple strategies should be implemented with respite to alleviate burden. It is difficult to conclude a causal relationship between respite care and institutionalization. A more likely scenario is that highly stressed caregivers are more likely to both increase the use of community-based services and subsequently seek institutional placement for the care recipient.

Evidence for the effectiveness of respite is more mixed. Nonetheless, recent evaluations of adult day care and in-home respite report some success in reducing caregiver burden or increasing caregiver well-being (Mason et al., 2007), but the effects of respite care on caregivers vary, depending on the specific outcome under investigation. Although temporary residential respite seems to have some positive health and well-being effects on the caregiver, care recipients often experienced more negative consequences (Vandepitte et al., 2016).

More recent research has focused largely on the factors that make respite care services more or less attractive to caregivers and the characteristics of caregivers who do and do not use respite care services. It is widely recognized that specific features of respite care programs can have significant effects on utilization. Much of the literature notes that respite services are underutilized (Neville, Beattie, Fielding, & MacAndrews, 2015; Phillipson, Jones, & Magee, 2014). Flexibility of respite schedules, cost of respite care, and the rapport established between respite workers and their care recipients, for example, affect caregivers' decisions to use respite care and the length and frequency of use. Demographic and social status factors also are related to respite care use. In general, high levels of education, income, and community involvement are related to greater utilization of respite serves. There also are racial/ethnic differences in patterns of respite utilization. African Americans often report "no need for" or are not aware of respite services more often than other ethnic groups (Casado, van Vulpen, & Davis, 2011). These findings may be related to cost, lack of access, cultural differences, or disparities in health literacy.

Recent recommendations for a research agenda on respite care (Kirk & Kagan, 2015) call for methodological rigor in design to assess impact. In addition, studies should address family outcomes, cost–benefit analysis, access to respite programs, and provider competency. There is general agreement among researchers and service providers that too few caregivers use respite care and that those who initiate use do so too late in the care receiver's illness or use too few services to make a sizeable reduction in caregiver burden.

See also Adult Day Services; Caregiver Burden.

Janet M. Bairardi

Casado, B. L., van Vulpen, K. S., & Davis, S. L. (2011). Unmet needs for home and community-based services among frail older Americans and their caregivers. *Journal of Aging and Health, 23*(3), 529–553.

Eska, K., Graessel, E., Donath, C., Schwarzkopf, L., Lauterberg, J., & Holle, R. (2013). Predictors of institutionalization of dementia patients in mild and moderate stages: A 4-year prospective analysis. *Dementia and Geriatric Cognitive Disorders Extra, 3*(1), 426–445.

Kirk, R., & Kagan, J. (2015). *A research agenda for respite care: Deliberations of an expert panel of researchers, funders and advocates.* ARCH National Respite and Research Center. Retrieved from http://archrespite.org/images/docs/2015_Reports/ARCH_Respite_Research_Report_web.pdf

Maayan, N., Soares-Weiser, K., & Lee, H. (2014). Respite care for people with dementia and their carers. *Cochrane Database of Systematic Reviews, 2014,* CD004396. doi:10.10002/14651858.CD004396.pub.3

Mason, A., Weatherly, H., Spilsbury, K., Golder, S., Arksey, H., Adamson, J., & Drummond, M. (2007). The effectiveness and cost-effectiveness of respite for caregivers of frail older people. *Journal of the American Geriatrics Society, 55*(2), 290–299.

National Alliance for Caregiving & AARP Public Policy Institute. (2015). *Caregiving in the US 2015.* Retrieved from http://www.caregiving.org/wp-content/uploads/2015/05/2015_CaregivingintheUS_Executive-Summary-June-4_WEB.pdf

Neville, C., Beattie, E., Fielding, E., & MacAndrew, M. (2015). Literature review: Use of respite by carers of people with dementia. *Health & Social Care in the Community, 23*(1), 51–53.

Phillipson, L., Jones, S. C., & Magee, C. (2014). A review of the factors associated with the non-use of respite services by carers of people with dementia: Implications for policy and practice. *Health & Social Care in the Community, 22*(1), 1–12.

Vandepitte, S., Van Den Noortgate, N., Putman, K., Verhaeghe, S., Verdonck, C., & Annemans, L. (2016). Effectiveness of respite care in supporting informal caregivers of persons with dementia: A systematic review. *International Journal of Geriatric Psychiatry, 31*(12), 1277–1288.

Wolff, J. L., Spillman, B. C., Freedman, V. A., & Kasper, J. D. (2016). A national profile of family and unpaid caregivers who assist older adults with health care activities. *JAMA Internal Medicine, 176*(3), 372–379.

Web Resources

Caregiving Help Guide: http://www.helpguide.org/home-pages/caregiving.htm

Elder Locator Respite Care: http://www.eldercare.gov/ELDERCARE.NET/Public/Resources/Factsheets/Respite_Care.aspx

Family Caregiver Alliance: http://www.caregiver.org/caregiver/jsp/home.jsp

National Adult Day Services: http://www.nadsa.org

National Alliance for Caregiving: http://www.caregiving.org

National Caregivers Library: http://www.caregivers library.org/caregivers-resources/grp-caring-for-yourself/hsgrp-support-systems/what-is-adult-day-care-article.aspx

National Family Caregiver Support Program: http://www.aoa.gov/aoa_programs/hcltc/caregiver/index.aspx

National Respite Network and Resource Center: http://archrespite.org

Older Americans Act 2016: http://www.acl.gov/News Room/NewsInfo/2016/2016_04_19.aspx

RESTRAINTS

A *physical restraint* is defined as "any action or procedure that prevents a person's free body movement to a position of choice and/or normal access to his or her body by the use of any method that is attached or adjacent to a person's body and that he or she cannot control or remove easily" (Bleijlevens, Wagner, Capezuti, & Hamers, 2016, p. 2309). Examples of physical restraints include vest restraints, belt restraints (materials attached to the waist), sleep suit (clothing that deters a person from undressing), special sheet (a fitted sheet that includes a coat and encloses a mattress), deep or overturned (wheel)chair, and devices attached to furniture (e.g., full-enclosure side rails, four half side rails, or wheelchairs with a locked tray table; Gulpers et al., 2011).

Physical restraints are applied in both long-term care (e.g., nursing homes) and acute care (e.g., hospitals) to manage difficult clinical situations (e.g., risk of falling), control behavior, and prevent interference with medical devices (Fariña-Lopez et al., 2014). To date, no studies have demonstrated that physical restraints effectively safeguard patients from injury, protect treatment devices, or alleviate behavioral symptoms such as wandering or agitation. In fact, several studies suggest that physical restraints are associated with falls, serious injuries, and decreased cognitive function (Capezuti et al., 2007, Gulpers et al., 2011, 2013). There is substantial evidence that physical restraints can cause considerable harm (Castle & Engberg, 2009; Möhler, Richter, Köpke, & Meyer, 2012). They reduce functional capacity because the person quickly loses muscle strength, steadiness, and balance when restricted to a bed or chair. Because of the immobilization that physical restraints cause, they are associated with contractures, functional incontinence, aspiration pneumonia, circulatory obstruction, cardiac stress, skin abrasions or breakdown, poor appetite, and dehydration and delirium. Attempting to physically restrain a frightened, delirious patient increases levels of panic and fear, producing angry, belligerent, or combative behavior. Other emotional responses include a sense of abandonment or desolation, loss of control, reduced self-esteem, depression, and withdrawal. A vicious cycle occurs when the harms of restraints are combined with the characteristics of persons likely to be restrained—usually those of advanced age who are physically and mentally frail, prone to injury and confusion, and experiencing invasive treatments.

Physically restrained persons may incur injuries when attempting to remove restraints or ambulating while restrained. These actions can lead to asphyxiation and even death, resulting from gravitational chest compression when the person is suspended by a vest restraint, inhibiting the ability to inhale, or is entrapped within rails. In response to the reports of restraint-related deaths, there are now mandates in some jurisdictions that all devices carry a warning label concerning potential hazards.

Nurses' attitudes toward physical restraint use in geriatric care are mainly negative. Nevertheless, many health care professionals and other caregivers see few alternatives to physical restraint use in some situations and experience perceived need for using these measures in clinical practice (Möhler & Meyer, 2014). In both acute and long-term care, there is little staff with expertise in aging or with the requisite skills for assessing and treating clinical problems specific to older adults. Fears about legal liability (albeit misplaced), lack of interdisciplinary discussions about decisions to restrain, and staff perceptions about resident behaviors and assumed risks to patients also influence restraint practices. Insufficient staffing levels and the costs associated with hiring additional employees have long been regarded as obstacles to reducing the use of physical restraints. Moreover, using a physical restraint is often provided as part of the treatment plan to maximize safety, despite the associated harms and lack of proven efficacy. A recent meta-synthesis revealed that concern about and responsibility for safety, unclear and inconsistent definitions of physical restraints, difficulties in the transition from acceptance to removal, lack of involvement in the decision-making process to remove restraints, and insufficient resources (alternatives for physical restraint use) and education are barriers to physical restraint reduction in long-term care (Kong, Choi, & Evans, 2017). Furthermore, in general, nursing staff in nursing homes have considered the use of physical restraints in clinical practice as appropriate. Bilateral side rails have been viewed as a moderate restrictive measure, and nursing staff do not feel much discomfort in using them. The use of belt restraints was rated as most restrictive and nurses have expressed pronounced discomfort in using such devices (Hamers et al., 2009).

It is now well established that physical restraint use, including side rails, in nursing homes can be significantly reduced without increasing fall incidents, serious injuries, or hiring more staff (Capezuti et al., 2007). This is accomplished through implementing alternative approaches to assessing, preventing, and responding to behaviors that routinely lead to physical restraint use. An example of such an approach concerns the expelling belt (EXBELT) program. EXBELT comprises four important components: a policy change by the nursing home management, with new use of belts prohibited and current use reduced; an intensive educational program offered by two nurse specialists (RNs with extensive experience in physical restraint reduction) to the nursing home staff; consultation from the two nurse specialists (who delivered the educational program) to individual nurses on the intervention wards; and availability of alternative interventions, with nursing home managers providing resident-centered alternative interventions, such as sensor mats, balance training, exercise, and low-height adjustable beds (Gulpers et al., 2011, 2013).

Such a change in approach requires a fundamental change in philosophy and attitudes at the institutional and caregiving levels. In settings where restraints have been reduced (or eliminated), there is strong emphasis on individualized, person-centered care; normal risk taking; rehabilitation and choice; interdisciplinary team practices; environmental features that support independent, safe functioning; involvement of family and community; and administrative and caregiver sanction and support for change (Köpke et al., 2012). It is also crucial to have involved professionals, particularly medical directors and expert nurses, with education, skill, and expertise in both geriatrics and individualized care.

Similarly, in hospitals, restraint standards developed by The Joint Commission have led to reductions in overall physical restraint use, as well as changes in patterns of use. Physical restraints tend to be used more to prevent treatment disruption than to avert falls and related injuries; thus arm/limb restraints are more frequently used than vest/waist restraints. Moreover, reduction of physical restraints use in acute care has been successfully implemented without increases in falls or patient-initiated discontinuation or dislodgment of therapeutic devices (Cosper, Morelock, & Provine, 2015; Enns, Rhemtulla, Ewa, Fruetel, & Holroyd-Leduc, 2014). When physical restraints are used, after all alternatives have been attempted, clinicians must provide continual individualized assessment and reevaluation of patients as long as they are restrained. Direct care staff must also be trained in the proper and safe use of restraining devices.

Approaches to restraint reduction vary along a continuum from promotion of individualized care, free of any restraints, to an attitude of tolerance for restraint use under certain circumstances. To some extent, successful (although incomplete) reduction of physical restraints in nursing homes underscores the need to achieve the same changes in hospitals, where disproportionately high incidences of iatrogenesis occurs, much of it exacerbated by the use of physical restraints and adverse reactions to psychoactive drugs. The resulting complications—especially delirium, pressure injuries, infections, and fall-related injuries—can add dramatically to loss of function, thus increasing the cost of care.

SIDE RAILS

Side rails are also considered physical restraints and they have been used primarily to prevent individuals from falling from bed. However, evidence suggests that raised side rails may actually cause falls when patients try to transfer over them or when patients can become trapped between the rails. Like other physical restraints, side rails can cause injuries and even death. Reducing their use is also associated with fewer bed-related falls and injuries (Capezuti et al., 2007). In March 2006, the U.S. Food and Drug Administration (FDA) issued design guidelines for hospital beds to reduce entrapment injuries (Center for Devices and Radiological Health, 2006). The guidelines also include recommendations for manufacturers of new hospital beds and suggest ways for health care facilities to assess existing beds.

CONCLUSION

Care that does not involve the use of any physical restraints is increasingly considered the standard of care for elders in all health care settings across the globe. Such a standard challenges professional caregivers to conduct comprehensive assessments of patients and residents to make sense of individual behaviors. These assessments, in turn, suggest a wide range of interventions that enhance physical, psychological, and social function as well as to acknowledge and affirm the uniqueness and dignity of the older person.

See also Contractures; Psychotropic Medication Use in Nursing Homes.

Michel H. C. Bleijlevens
and Laura M. Wagner

Bleijlevens, M. H. C., Wagner, L. M., Capezuti, E. A., & Hamers, J. P. H. (2016). Physical restraints: Consensus of a research definition using a modified Delphi technique. *Journal of the American Geriatrics Society, 64,* 2307–2310. doi:10.1111/jgs.14435

Capezuti, E., Wagner, L. M., Brush, B. L., Boltz, M., Renz, S., & Talerico, K. A. (2007). Consequences of an intervention to reduce restrictive side rail use in nursing homes. *Journal of the American Geriatrics Society, 55*(3), 334–341.

Castle, N. G., & Engberg, J. (2009). The health consequences of using physical restraints in nursing homes. *Medical Care, 47*(11), 1164–1173.

Center for Devices and Radiological Health. (2006). Guidance for industry and FDA staff: Hospital bed system dimensional and assessment guidance to reduce entrapment. Retrieved from https://www.fda.gov/MedicalDevices/DeviceRegulationandGuidance/GuidanceDocuments/ucm072662.htm

Cosper, P., Morelock, V., & Provine, B. (2015). Please release me: Restraint reduction initiative in a health care system. *Journal of Nursing Care Quality, 30*(1), 16–23.

Enns, E., Rhemtulla, R., Ewa, V., Fruetel, K., & Holroyd-Leduc, J. M. (2014). A controlled quality improvement trial to reduce the use of physical restraints in older hospitalized adults. *Journal of the American Geriatrics Society, 62*(3), 541–545.

Fariña-López, E., Estévez-Guerra, G. J., Gandoy-Crego, M., Polo-Luque, L. M., Gómez-Cantorna, C., & Capezuti, E. A. (2014). Perception of

Spanish nursing staff on the use of physical restraints. *Journal of Nursing Scholarship, 46*(5), 322–330.

Gulpers, M. J., Bleijlevens, M. H., Ambergen, T., Capezuti, E., van Rossum, E., & Hamers, J. P. (2011). Belt restraint reduction in nursing homes: Effects of a multicomponent intervention program. *Journal of the American Geriatrics Society, 59*(11), 2029–2036.

Gulpers, M. J., Bleijlevens, M. H., Ambergen, T., Capezuti, E., van Rossum, E., & Hamers, J. P. (2013). Reduction of belt restraint use: long-term effects of the EXBELT intervention. *Journal of the American Geriatrics Society, 61*(1), 107–112.

Hamers, J. P., Meyer, G., Köpke, S., Lindenmann, R., Groven, R., & Huizing, A. R. (2009). Attitudes of Dutch, German and Swiss nursing staff towards physical restraint use in nursing home residents, a cross-sectional study. *International Journal of Nursing Studies, 46*(2), 248–255.

Kong, E. H., Choi, H., & Evans, L. K. (2017). Staff perceptions of barriers to physical restraint-reduction in long-term care: A meta-synthesis. *Journal of Clinical Nursing, 26*(1–2), 49–60.

Köpke, S., Mühlhauser, I., Gerlach, A., Haut, A., Haastert, B., Möhler, R., & Meyer, G. (2012). Effect of a guideline-based multicomponent intervention on use of physical restraints in nursing homes: A randomized controlled trial. *Journal of the American Medical Association, 307*(20), 2177–2184.

Möhler, R., & Meyer, G. (2014). Attitudes of nurses towards the use of physical restraints in geriatric care: A systematic review of qualitative and quantitative studies. *International Journal of Nursing Studies, 51*(2), 274–288.

Möhler, R., Richter, T., Köpke, S., & Meyer, G. (2012). Interventions for preventing and reducing the use of physical restraints in long-term geriatric care—A Cochrane review. *Journal of Clinical Nursing, 21*(21–22), 3070–3081.

Web Resources

American Geriatrics Society: Falls prevention in older adults: http://www.americangeriatrics.org/health_care_professionals/clinical_practice/clinical_guidelines_recommendations/2010

Registered Nurses Association of Ontario: Clinical practice guideline, "Promoting safety: Alternative approaches to the use of restraints": http://rnao.ca/bpg/guidelines/promoting-safety-alternative-approaches-use-restraints

U.S. Food and Drug Administration, Hospital Bed Safety Workgroup: http://www.fda.gov/medicaldevices/productsandmedicalprocedures/generalhospitaldevicesandsupplies/hospitalbeds/default.htm

RETIREMENT

Retirement in the United States includes several interrelated issues: historical background, changes in the way retirement is conceptualized and experienced, income security, retirement planning, its impact on health, and retirement in the context of family relationships.

Retirement programs for some government employees—teachers, police officers, firefighters, and veterans—date back to the 19th century. These privileged few, along with the wealthy, were financially able to retire. However, the Social Security Act of 1935 established income security for older workers and their families and enabled a much greater percentage of the population to experience retirement. The age of eligibility for Social Security has widely become considered the age when retirement is expected to occur. This age is gradually being raised from 65 to 67 years by 2027.

Despite this widely held view about the typical age of retirement, the way that retirement is conceptualized and experienced continues to evolve. An individual can go from work to complete retirement (i.e., no paid employment) or can gradually retire by transitioning from full-time to part-time work or partial retirement. Individuals may continue working part-time for the rest of their lives, or may later transition to a state of complete retirement. Individuals can also transition to a state of "less retirement" by reentering the labor force after complete retirement, by going from partial retirement to working full time, or by subjectively no longer considering themselves to be retired. This diversity in retirement transitions suggests the need to view retirement status as a temporary state that could change depending on circumstances, rather than a permanent status.

Retirement transitions can also be more complex if individuals exit the labor force for other reasons, such as disability, unemployment, or provision of caregiving assistance and can represent different life course trajectories. They can reflect an alternative route to retirement, an interim status until a certain age or pension eligibility requirement is reached, a temporary status (e.g., returning to work after being unemployed or temporarily disabled), or a continuation of a lifetime pattern of discontinuous labor force involvement. Those who have exited the workforce unwillingly or unexpectedly may have more financial and adjustment issues in retirement.

According to an AARP study, most Baby Boomers expect to work for pay during their retirement, some because of the stimulation, enjoyment, or sense of accomplishment that they get from work and others because of economic necessity (Olen, 2016). Increased flexibility in terms of work and retirement may help people stay economically active. However, employment-related age discrimination against older workers sometimes occurs (U.S. Equal Employment Opportunity Commission, n.d.), and this can present challenges for older adults who want or need to continue working.

In addition to paid employment, during retirement, older adults often engage in other types of productive activities, including formal and informal volunteering and parental caregiving. These activities provide socioemotional benefits, such as feeling better about oneself, engaging in meaningful activities and productively using time, and engaging in a social activity. Productive engagement has also been linked with lower depressive symptomatology, better physical functioning, and lower risk of mortality (Matz-Costa, Elyssa Besen, James, & Pitt-Catsouphes, 2012).

RETIREMENT AND INCOME SECURITY

In the United States, the income security of adults aged 65 and older is derived through a variety of sources. According to the SSA most older adults receive Social Security retirement benefits, half receive income from assets (e.g., rental property), 27% receive private pensions, 15% receive government employee pensions,

and 26% receive employment earnings. Ideally, these sources of income are supplemented by personal savings. However, in reality, Social Security payments represent at least 50% of the total income for half of couples and three quarters of unmarried Social Security beneficiaries. For older minorities, there is an even greater reliance on Social Security. Social Security retirement benefits make up more than 90% of family income for 29% of older African Americans and 26% of older Hispanics (Caldera, 2010).

Income security has important health-related implications for older adults. For example, concerns about the cost of prescriptions can be a barrier to medication adherence. Furthermore, for those with employer-provided health insurance, retirement before becoming eligible for Medicare can result in individuals and families being faced with difficult choices regarding paying high health insurance premiums or going without health insurance (and paying the federal tax penalty for lacking health insurance, too).

RETIREMENT PLANNING

Although commonly viewed as a normal part of the life cycle since the passage of the Social Security Act, retirement is also a potentially life-altering process. Preparing for this transition has positive outcomes, such as greater wealth accumulation, improved psychological well-being and better role adjustment, and higher relationship satisfaction. This preparation can consist of formal planning activities, such as attending financial seminars and meeting with a financial planner.

An individual can also plan for retirement informally by talking with friends about their experiences, planning for activities once retired, and understanding some of the changes and opportunities that will result from retirement. Informal planning can lead to better retirement outcomes in areas such as adjustment and satisfaction. With a clearer understanding of the expectations associated with the role of retiree, people may experience more positive psychosocial outcomes when transitioning into this role than those who fail to plan.

RETIREMENT AND HEALTH

The impact of retirement on health can be influenced by a number of factors, including the way that retirement is measured, the length of time since retirement, occupation, and work-related stressors and rewards. These are only a few of the differences in measuring how retirement affects health, which helps explain the mixed results of longitudinal studies regarding the impact of retirement on health.

Health professionals should assess for changes in health and levels of activity between work and retirement. Someone who has been physically active on the job and then becomes more sedentary postretirement could experience worse health, whereas those who had a mostly sedentary job might become more physically active when they retire. Health-promotion efforts could also target recent retirees, who may be more open to changing health behaviors (e.g., exercise, smoking cessation) as they develop new routines during their transition to retirement.

RETIREMENT AND THE FAMILY

Retirement of a family member can influence the lives of everyone in the household. Particularly for married persons, retirement by either spouse has potential consequences for household income. It can affect a couple's daily schedules, the amount of leisure time they have, their health insurance coverage, and their marital quality. Life course transitions such as retirement occur within the context of a couple's shared past, including decision-making patterns, child rearing, gender role orientation, division of household labor, and work histories. All of these have impacted the household before retirement. It is no surprise that retirement may affect this balance and cause a readjustment period. Therefore retirement needs to be framed within the context of family and household, and to help families (not just the individual who retires) adjust to retirement.

Individuals or couples may seek counseling to help with symptoms such as depression and/or anxiety related to difficulty in adjusting to retirement. Geriatric mental health professionals should encourage patients to discuss their plans, fears, anxieties, and expectations about retirement with their spouse and others. They can also focus on possible changes in relationships within the patient's social network and provide information and referral to community-based services as needed.

CONCLUSION

The nature of retirement (and work) is expected to continue to evolve as Baby Boomers retire, life expectancy rates increase, and environmental factors vary (e.g., economic booms, recessions). Although policies and social structures often lag behind changes in individuals' everyday experiences practitioners can be advocates for social change regarding retirement policies and options. Preparing and recognizing the implications of the changing nature of work and retirement will benefit individuals and society as a whole.

See also Employment; Financing Retirement; Pensions and Financing Retirement; Poverty; Social Security; Volunteerism.

Elizabeth A. Capezuti

Caldera, S. (2010). *Social Security: A key retirement income source for minorities.* [Fact Sheet 201]. Washington, DC: AARP Public Policy Institute. Retrieved from http://assets.aarp.org/rgcenter/ppi/econ-sec/fs201-economic.pdf

Matz-Costa, C., Elyssa Besen, E., James, J. B., & Pitt-Catsouphes, M. (2012). Differential impact of multiple levels of productive activity engagement on psychological well-being in middle and later life. *The Gerontologist, 54*(2), 277–289.

Olen, H. (2016). You call this retirement? Boomers still have work to do, as the idea of the American retiree evolves, not so many will be hitting the links. *AARP The Magazine.* Retrieved from http://www.aarp.org/work/retirement-planning/info-2014/boomer-retirement-little-savings-means-working.html

U.S. Equal Employment Opportunity Commission. (n.d.). Age discrimination. Retrieved from http://www.eeoc.gov/laws/types/age.cfm

Web Resources
AARP (work and retirement): https://www.aarp.org/work

Center for Retirement Research at Boston College:
http://crr.bc.edu

National Bureau of Economic Research Retirement
Research Center: http://www.nber.org/programs/
ag/rrc/rrchome.html

Pension Research Council: https://www.pension
researchcouncil.org

Social Security Administration: https://www.ssa.gov

U.S. Department of Labor (retirement plans, benefits
& savings): https://www.dol.gov/dol/topic/
retirement/index.htm

University of Michigan Retirement Research Center:
http://mrrc.isr.umich.edu

RHEUMATOID ARTHRITIS

Rheumatoid arthritis is a progressive and disabling systemic disease that results in pain, joint
damage, and functional loss. As a result, it is associated with economic consequences in terms of lost
wages, disability benefits, hospital costs, nursing
home costs, home care costs, and professional and
medication expenses. Many patients with rheumatoid arthritis fear loss of independence, and
the disease has been associated with psychological distress, depression, and anxiety. Furthermore,
patients with rheumatoid arthritis are at risk for
other health complications such as osteoporosis,
fractures, obesity, cardiovascular disease, and
early death. A multidisciplinary approach to treating patients with rheumatoid arthritis, as well as
early initiation of treatment, may improve quality
of life and long-term outcomes.

EPIDEMIOLOGY

Among the general adult population, rheumatoid arthritis most commonly occurs in the
third to fifth decades, with a prevalence rate in
the population of approximately 1%. Although
the overall incidence of rheumatoid arthritis has tended to decrease over the last 25 to
50 years, recent evidence suggests a rise in the
incidence of rheumatoid arthritis over the past
5 to 10 years, possibly attributable to a continuing rise in the prevalence of obesity (Crowson,
Matteson, Davis, & Gabriel, 2013). Several

authors have divided this disease into two subsets: adult-onset rheumatoid arthritis (AORA)
and elderly onset (after age 60 years) rheumatoid arthritis (EORA), each with distinctive
characteristics. New cases of EORA have been
reported to account for 14% to 55% of rheumatoid arthritis cases. Before the age of 60 years,
women are more frequently affected than men,
with a ratio of 2:1 to 3:1; however, with advancing age, the relative incidence in men is greater,
with the ratio becoming closer to 1:1.

DIAGNOSIS

The diagnosis of rheumatoid arthritis in the
elderly is made when characteristic symptoms of
the disease are present. The majority of patients
may have an indolent onset of disease, with progressive pain, swelling, and morning stiffness
of characteristic joints: proximal interphalangeal joints, metacarpophalangeal joints, wrists,
elbows, shoulders, hips, knees, ankles, and meta-
tarsophalangeal joints. In a minority of patients,
the onset is acute, with an asymmetrical presentation. A complete history, physical examination,
and laboratory evidence are necessary to confirm
a diagnosis of rheumatoid arthritis. Swelling in a
large number of small joints, evidence of inflammation on laboratory tests, disease duration
greater than 6 weeks, and positive serologies are
suggestive of the diagnosis. Radiographs of the
hands and other involved joints with evidence of
periarticular osteopenia or marginal erosions also
support the diagnosis. A complete blood count,
chemistries, inflammatory markers (erythrocyte
sedimentation rate [ESR]), C-reactive protein
(CRP), and serologies such as rheumatoid factor,
antinuclear antibody, and anti-cyclic citrinullated
peptide (anti-CCP) antibody titers should also be
obtained. In early disease, evaluation for potential infectious causes, including tests for hepatitis
B and C, may be indicated.

There is high prevalence of rheumatoid factor positivity in up to 40% of healthy elderly
patients. Only 32% of elderly patients with rheumatoid arthritis demonstrate a positive rheumatoid factor, making this test of little diagnostic
utility. This compares with 80% rheumatoid factor positivity in AORA. Several authors describe
a milder presentation in elderly seronegative

patients, with symptoms suggestive of polymyalgia rheumatica and frequent axial (i.e., shoulder and hip) involvement. Constitutional symptoms such as weight loss and a functional decline may accompany these symptoms. In contrast to seronegative patients, those who are rheumatoid factor positive have been described as having more persistently active disease, greater functional decline, more radiographic erosions, and increased mortality.

Older patients with long-standing disease may have joint deformities, synovitis (swelling in the joints), nodules, and radiographic erosions. Laboratory tests such as ESR and CRP are often elevated. However, because advanced age can explain an elevated ESR in the setting of relative quiescent rheumatoid arthritis, this test should be used with careful consideration of the overall picture. Anemia is common in patients with active rheumatoid arthritis. Often the indices are consistent with anemia of chronic disease; however, a mixed etiology may be present and should be evaluated thoroughly.

Two other disease entities described in the elderly may be difficult to distinguish from seronegative rheumatoid arthritis. First, polymyalgia rheumatica needs to be considered when evaluating an elderly patient with an acute presentation of symmetrical shoulder and hip pain associated with elevated ESR and CRP. The distinction may be difficult to make, and treatment with corticosteroids is effective for both entities. Potential distinguishing features for rheumatoid arthritis are the presence of small joint swelling (or synovitis on imaging), the presence of anti-CCP antibodies, the presence of bone erosions on radiographs (or other imaging), and other extra-articular manifestations. An additional differential diagnosis is remitting seronegative symmetrical synovitis with pitting edema. This is a relatively rare disease described in elderly men, with a presentation similar to polymyalgia rheumatica but also associated with pitting edema of the dorsum of the hands. The edema is due primarily to tenosynovitis of the extensor and flexor tendons at the wrist and metacarpal heads. Ultrasound to identify tenosynovitis may therefore be an additional useful adjunct to physical examination to distinguish this entity from seronegative rheumatoid arthritis. Crystal arthropathies such as polyarticular gout and calcium pyrophosphate deposition disease are common in elderly patients and may present similarly to rheumatoid arthritis. Synovial fluid analysis and radiographs may help make the distinction.

It may often be difficult to quickly establish a diagnosis in elderly patients with new-onset disease, particularly when they have polyarticular joint involvement, myalgias, negative serologies, and constitutional symptoms. Other diagnostic possibilities include viral and bacterial infections, connective tissue disorders such as systemic lupus erythematosus and Sjögren's syndrome, metabolic disorders, and malignancy.

Although the differential diagnosis appears straightforward, diagnosis in the elderly may be hindered by multiple factors, including difficulty in obtaining information from cognitively impaired patients, the presence of multiple coexisting diseases and comorbid conditions, the high frequency of positive serologies and elevated inflammatory markers in elderly patients, and the difficulty of obtaining laboratory studies and radiographs in nonambulatory patients, who may not have the social and financial support to obtain appropriate medical care. Overcoming diagnostic challenges is critical because (a) risks of drug toxicity are not trivial in the elderly and (b) early initiation of appropriate therapy results in superior long-term outcomes.

TREATMENT

Guidelines for the management of rheumatoid arthritis have been published (Singh et al., 2016). However, while the treatment strategy for rheumatoid arthritis in the elderly is similar to that used for younger patients, treatment in this group at higher risk for complications is a greater challenge (Schwab & Albert, 2001). The goal of therapy is to relieve pain, diminish disability, prevent joint destruction, and improve quality of life and functional outcome without subjecting the patient to undue drug toxicities. The use of composite scores in clinical practice to quantify disease activity and guide therapeutic decisions is recommended because it has been shown to improve the attainment of clinical remission. Use of these scores should be a

R

guide only and should be tempered by the physician's appraisal of the risk–benefit ratio for additional therapy.

The risk of drug toxicity is greater in the elderly secondary to age-related alterations in pharmacokinetics and pharmacodynamics. Polypharmacy, often observed in the elderly, can also substantially increase the risk of drug interactions and adverse reactions. Multiple comorbid conditions may alter the metabolism and excretion of prescribed medications, suggesting lower initial doses for many older patients. Although the recently championed treat-to-target approach for rheumatoid arthritis posits aggressive management until a patient reaches low disease activity or clinical remission, a less strict definition of *low disease activity* may be appropriate in elderly subjects, in whom the risks of therapy may outweigh the potential morbidity from the disease. "Start low and go slow" is the general therapeutic guideline for drug dosages. Noninflammatory causes of pain and disability should always be considered to avoid overaggressive treatment in this population.

Other concerns such as cognitive dysfunction, financial constraints, and limited social support influence treatment decisions. For instance, a practitioner may decide on a less toxic treatment regimen for a patient with multiple comorbid conditions, especially if physician visits are infrequent and blood monitoring is not available. A multidisciplinary team approach may help diminish these obstacles.

Simple analgesics such as acetaminophen are usually ineffective. Nonsteroidal anti-inflammatory drugs (NSAIDs) are effective at relieving symptoms in patients with mild disease and may not be well tolerated in the elderly due to side effects such as gastrointestinal inflammation and ulceration, nephrotoxicity, hepatoxicity, volume overload, central nervous system effects, and hematological abnormalities. Cyclooxygenase-2 inhibitors (celecoxib) and nonselective NSAIDs may also help relieve symptoms; however, there remains concern regarding risk of cardiovascular events, and caution must be exercised when prescribing to older adults who may be at risk for cardiovascular disease. Furthermore, these agents do not modify the underlying disease and do not prevent the structural joint damage that may occur over time and results in permanent disability.

Corticosteroids are generally not preferred for treating rheumatoid arthritis in the elderly because of the increased risk of osteoporosis, diabetes, cataracts, glaucoma, anxiety, delirium, and atherosclerosis associated with their use. Corticosteroids are effective in reducing inflammation and might act to modify the disease and prevent structural damage. However, they should be used with caution and at the lowest effective dose in elderly subjects. Antiresorptive therapy, in addition to calcium and vitamin D supplementation, should be started simultaneously to diminish potential bone loss, given the high risk of osteoporotic fractures in this group (Grossman et al., 2010).

Disease-modifying antirheumatic drugs (DMARDs) have evolved to become the mainstay of therapy in rheumatoid arthritis. The current treatment strategy includes the early initiation of disease-modifying agents to retard damage and ultimately prevent long-term disability. The choice of DMARD for a particular person depends on the progression of the disease, the toxicity of the drug, and the individual's coexisting conditions. Although these drugs are as effective in the elderly as they are in younger persons, their toxicities may be more apparent because of pharmacokinetic and pharmacodynamic alterations, drug interactions, and comorbid conditions. Although the strategy for the use of DMARDs in the elderly should be similar to that for younger patients, decisions may be driven to a greater degree by comorbid conditions.

Hydroxychloroquine seems to be well tolerated in the elderly and may be effective for patients with mild disease. Side effects include gastrointestinal discomfort, rash, photosensitivity, and rarely, retinal toxicity. Patients should obtain biannual ophthalmological examinations, especially if they have coexisting ocular disease such as cataracts or macular degeneration. For many patients with more active disease, this medication is inadequate when used alone.

Other agents such as methotrexate and sulfasalazine appear to be well tolerated in the elderly. Methotrexate is often the agent of first choice because of its efficacy, early onset of action, and high efficacy-to-toxicity ratio. The primary toxicity of methotrexate is hepatic and hematological and requires frequent surveillance of hepatic transaminases and blood counts. Starting doses are often low in the elderly (5–10 mg weekly) and slowly titrated. The primary toxicity of sulfasalazine is gastrointestinal problems; liver function and hematological abnormalities are rare. Leflunomide, an inhibitor of pyrimidine biosynthesis, has also been shown to be effective as a DMARD alone or in combination with other DMARDs. Side effects include rash, liver transaminase abnormalities, alopecia, weight loss, and gastrointestinal symptoms. Combination therapy with multiple DMARDs can safely and more effectively reduce signs and symptoms of rheumatoid arthritis, but this approach should be weighed against the potential for the noted increased risk of toxicity in this group.

In the last 20 years, targeted biologic therapies have been developed, which are highly effective at reducing the signs and symptoms of the disease and preventing structural joint damage with low toxicity. These agents include a number of monoclonal antibodies and fusion molecules targeted at proinflammatory pathways. A number of agents target the inflammatory cytokine tumor necrosis factor-alpha (TNF-α; infliximab, etanercept, adalimumab, certolizumab pegol, golimumab). Serious infections such as tuberculosis, atypical mycobacterial infections, and other opportunistic infections have been rarely described. A screening tuberculin skin test should be performed on all subjects before initiating therapy with these agents. Despite concerns about an increased risk of infection, studies have shown that anti-TNF therapy is safe and effective in the elderly (Migliore et al., 2009) and should be considered early in the management of patients with severe disease or in patients who show poor response to initial DMARD therapy.

Rituximab is a B cell-depleting monoclonal antibody approved for the management of rheumatoid arthritis and can be effective in anti-TNF failures (Emery et al., 2006). Rituximab can be associated with infusion reactions and infections and may result in poorer responses to immunizations. Patients should be evaluated to ensure that they are up to date on immunizations before receipt of the drug. Abatacept, a selective costimulation modulator that inhibits full T-cell activation, has also been approved for use as first- or second-line therapy in rheumatoid arthritis and has been shown to have similar safety and efficacy as anti-TNF therapy (adalimumab). Tocilizumab, targeted against anti-interleukin-6, has also been shown to be effective in rheumatoid arthritis and may also be considered.

Overall, biologic therapies have revolutionized the care of rheumatoid arthritis and may be desirable for many elderly subjects, given their stable pharmacodynamics and relative lack of medication interactions. The risk of infection appears to be comparable with other nonbiologic DMARDs such as methotrexate. However, it may be appropriate to avoid these drugs among elderly patients with a history of recurrent infections (Dubin Kerr, 2011). Furthermore, as these therapies are injectable only, they may also be a poor choice for elderly subjects who live alone and are unable to perform injections or routinely come in for intravenous infusions.

Tofacitinib, an oral Janus-kinase inhibitor, may be considered for subjects who cannot receive other DMARDs or biologic agents, particularly among those who cannot give themselves injections. The long-term safety profile of tofacitinib, particularly in elderly subjects, has not been fully established. Although the drug generally appears to be well-tolerated in clinical trials, monitoring for cytopenias, liver enzyme elevations, increases in lipids, and infections (including opportunistic infections) is recommended.

See also Osteoarthritis.

Joshua F. Baker and Edna P. Schwab

Crowson, C. S., Matteson, E. L., Davis, J. M., III, & Gabriel, S. E. (2013). Contribution of obesity to the rise in incidence of rheumatoid arthritis. *Arthritis Care & Research, 65*(1), 71–77. doi:10.1002/acr.21660

Dubin Kerr, L. (2011). Biologic use in the elderly. *Drug Safety Quarterly, 2*(1), 1–2.

Emery, P., Fleischmann, R., Filipowicz-Sosnowska, A., Schechtman, J., Szczepanski, L., Kavanaugh, A., ... Shaw, T. M. (2006). The efficacy and safety of rituximab in patients with active rheumatoid arthritis despite methotrexate treatment: Results of a phase IIB randomized, double-blind, placebo-controlled, dose-ranging trial. *Arthritis and Rheumatism, 54*(5), 1390–1400.

Grossman, J. M., Gordon, R., Ranganath, V. K., Deal, C., Caplan, L., Chen, W., ... Saag, K. G. (2010). American College of Rheumatology 2010 recommendations for the prevention and treatment of glucocorticoid-induced osteoporosis. *Arthritis Care & Research, 62*(11), 1515–1526.

Migliore, A., Bizzi, E., Laganà, B., Altomonte, L., Zaccari, G., Granata, M., ... Galluccio, A. (2009). The safety of anti-TNF agents in the elderly. *International Journal of Immunopathology and Pharmacology, 22*(2), 415–426.

Schwab, E. P., & Albert, D. (2001). Arthritis in the elderly. In M. Weisman & M. E. Weinblatt (Eds.), *Treatment of rheumatic diseases* (2nd ed.). Philadelphia, PA: W. B. Saunders.

Singh, J. A., Saag, K. G., Bridges, S. L., Akl, E. A., Bannuru, R. R., Sullivan, M. C., ... McAlindon, T. (2016). 2015 American College of Rheumatology guideline for the treatment of rheumatoid arthritis. *Arthritis & Rheumatology, 68*(1), 1–26.

Web Resources

American College of Rheumatology: http://www.rheumatology.org/publications/dsq
American College of Rheumatology: http://www.rheumatology.org/public/factsheets/ranew.asp
Arthritis Foundation: http://www.arthritis.org
Medline Plus: http://www.nlm.nih.gov/medlineplus

RISK ASSESSMENT AND IDENTIFICATION IN OLDER ADULTS

Risk assessment allows clinicians to target services by identifying older adults who are more vulnerable to declines in health. This has the potential to increase access to high-quality geriatric services for individuals who are most likely to benefit, resulting in improved outcomes and efficient resource use. Risks are not necessarily fixed; an individual's risk may change over time as conditions evolve or the environment changes.

Risk assessment may be particularly helpful at the time of care transitions. Vulnerability is more than the sum of existing medical conditions and is influenced by current function and adverse environmental conditions that increase the risk of functional decline or death.

Clinical teams can use clinical and demographic characteristics to identify elders at increased risk for functional decline or death. Risks have immediate or intermediate impact—typically less than 5 years and are important for interdisciplinary team assessments and care planning. The risk factors that contribute to important health outcomes can be divided into four groups: demographics and socioeconomic status (SES); function; health behaviors; and diagnoses, conditions, and associated treatments.

GROUP I: DEMOGRAPHIC AND SOCIOECONOMIC DOMAINS

Age influences response to disease and chances of functional recovery, decline, and death, even after accounting for other risk factors. Gender and marital status, especially recent loss of a spouse, have been associated with differences in health outcomes. Measures of caregiver availability and social support are important for identifying risk and predicting future needs.

Effective communication is important for interpreting an individual's needs. Ethnicity has been associated with differences in health beliefs and behaviors. Language accessibility, education, health literacy, and income are important influences on health outcomes and service use. Notably, difficulty with comprehending basic health-related written information is associated with increased mortality and can mediate the relationship between SES and health (Baker et al., 2007). Lower health literacy relates to poorer health outcomes and a higher prevalence of chronic diseases, including heart disease, stroke, and diabetes (Bostock & Steptoe, 2012).

GROUP II: FUNCTIONAL STATUS

Many widely accepted health models emphasize function over disease and define important disability as the functioning of individuals within their environments. Table R.1 lists markers of functional status associated with risk for functional decline, institutionalization, and death. The three groups of functional status measures are physical function or functional limitation, instrumental activities of daily living (IADL), and basic activities of daily living (BADL). Whereas physical function can be self-reported, the direct assessment of functional limitations also can be an important and simple part of the geriatric physical examination. Mobility and ability to rise from a chair unaided can be quickly observed and identify individuals at high risk for decline and falls.

IADL and BADL represent tasks important to independent living and self-maintenance. Although concerns have been raised about IADL applicability across gender groups, these items have been shown to have equal relationships to disability for both men and women (Saliba, Orlando, Wenger, Hays, & Rubenstein, 2000). For individuals, it is important that the majority with IADL or BADL limitations remain stable over 2 years, and a significant percentage have a decrease in the number of dependencies on follow-up. Staging by groups of IADL and BADL limitations may be more helpful in predicting resource needs and outcomes compared with a simple count of the number of limitations (Stineman et al., 2012).

GROUP III: HEALTH BEHAVIORS

Tobacco use strongly influences health and ability to recover from injury or illness. Knowledge of level of alcohol and drug use is important, in part because of their potential interaction with prescribed medications. Physical activity and diet are important predictors of health outcomes. Poor health practices (e.g., tobacco use, substance abuse, lack of exercise) not only contribute to the development of many conditions, but also affect condition management and can be independent risk factors for functional decline or death. Smoking, alcohol use, and decreased physical activity are also associated with low health literacy (Bostock & Steptoe, 2012).

GROUP IV: DIAGNOSES, CONDITIONS, AND ASSOCIATED TREATMENTS

Medical conditions and syndromes that are important risk factors for functional decline,

Table R.1
MARKERS OF FUNCTIONAL STATUS ASSOCIATED WITH INCREASED RISK OF DEATH OR DECLINE

Functional Limitation	*Instrumental Activities of Daily Living*	*Basic Activities of Daily Living*
Difficulty With Physical Function, Including	*Difficulty or Needing Help With*	*Difficulty or Needing Help With*
Doing heavy work around the house	Using telephone	Bathing
Walking ½ mile	Preparing meals	Walking across room
Climbing a flight of stairs	Maintaining house	Toileting
Standing for long periods	Taking own medications	Dressing
Lifting or carrying weights of 10 lb	Shopping for personal needs	Continence
Using hands or fingers	Doing laundry	Grooming/hygiene
Pulling or pushing large objects	Managing finances	Transferring
Stooping, bending, or kneeling	Driving car or using bus/taxi	Feeding
Reaching with either or both arms		
Picking up an object from the floor		
Rising from chair		
Standing on one foot		

R

institutionalization, and death include arthritis, cancer, cerebrovascular disease or stroke, chronic obstructive pulmonary disease, cognitive impairment, cardiovascular disease (e.g., myocardial infarction, heart failure, valvular heart disease, hypertension), depression and other psychiatric diagnoses, diabetes, falls, hip fracture, malnutrition, and vision or hearing impairment. Several of these diagnoses and conditions are underdetected across clinical settings and can be screened for by interdisciplinary teams. Underdetected conditions that place elders at risk include cognitive impairment, depression, pain, delirium, and falls. On a population basis, a simple count of conditions, or a weighted summary of conditions, contributes to overall risk assessment. However, clinical risk assessment requires consideration of the severity of each condition, the interaction of conditions, and the impact on the individual.

Medication class and count provide important information about illness severity, risk of side effects and interactions, and quality of medical care. Past use of other medical services also may identify persons at increased risk for future utilization and decline.

CHALLENGES IN RISK ASSESSMENT

The list of potential risk factors is considerable and presents potential measurement challenges for providers and patients. Comprehensive geriatric assessment (CGA) is thorough with many advantages; however, it is time-consuming and requires experienced staff to complete it. Simple screening approaches have been developed to help identify older adults who are most at risk and most likely to benefit from more detailed risk assessment.

Individual's rating of his or her own health as "fair" or "poor" is a strong and consistent risk factor for future decline or death. Self-rated health may be so effective because of its ability to capture unmeasured disease severity, unmeasured functional impairment, and difficult-to-measure factors such as self-efficacy or locus of control.

Formal risk assessment tools vary in the number of items included, domains covered, and outcomes assessed. One available tool is

the Vulnerable Elders 13-item Survey (VES-13; Saliba et al., 2001). The VES-13 was developed as a parsimonious approach for identifying older adults at significant risk for functional decline or death to facilitate better targeting of evaluations and care. Table R.2 shows the 13 items that address age, physical function, self-rated health, and IADL/BADL. Any interdisciplinary team member can administer the VES-13 in person or over the telephone in fewer than 5 minutes. Several health care systems use the VES-13 to identify elders warranting referral for CGA. VES-13 scores have been shown to predict (a) functional decline and death at 1, 2, and 5 years (Min et al., 2009, 2011); (b) functional impairment and outcomes in persons with cancer and therefore needing full CGA (Carneiro, Sousa,

Table R.2
VULNERABLE ELDER = INCREASED RISK FOR DEATH OR DECLINE OVER NEXT 2 YEARS

Measured by VES-13 Score	
Age	
75–84	+1
85+	+3
Self-rated health	
Fair or poor	+1
Physical function limitation[a]	
If one limitation	+1
If two or more limitations	+2
Functional disability[b]	
Need help or unable to do any of five IADL/ADL	+4

Note: Vulnerable elder = total points 3 or higher.
[a] Physical function limitation.
A lot of difficulty with or unable to do: (1) stooping, crouching, or kneeling; (2) lifting or carrying objects as heavy as 10 lb; (3) reaching or extending arms above shoulder level; (4) writing or handling and grasping small objects; (5) walking ¼ mile; and (6) heavy housework such as scrubbing floors or washing windows.
[b] Functional disability.
Receive help or don't do because of health: (1) shopping for personal items (e.g., toilet items or medicines); (2) managing money (e.g., keeping track of expenses or paying bills); (3) walking across the room (use of cane or walker is okay); (4) bathing or showering; and (5) doing light housework (e.g., washing dishes, straightening up, or light cleaning).
ADL, activities of daily living; IADL, instrumental activities of daily living; VES-13, Vulnerable Elders 13-item Survey.

Azevedo, & Saliba, 2015; Luciani et al., 2010; Ramsdale et al., 2013; Soubeyran et al., 2014); (c) complications and death in elders with traumatic injury (Min et al., 2011); and (d) functional deficits and risks of health deterioration in hospitalized elders with multiple comorbidities (Kroc, Socha, Soltysik, & Kostka, 2016). Scores range from 0 to 10, with higher scores indicating increasing vulnerability.

If an individual is classified as increased risk using a brief screener such as the VES-13, then a more in-depth assessment is warranted. This assessment should consider the breadth of factors that can place an individual at risk and should tailor interventions based on individualized risk assessments and personalized goals. If an individual is identified as needing CGA, an interdisciplinary team approach is particularly well suited, efficient, and cost-effective for assessing, identifying, and integrating the multiple factors needed for this more thorough risk assessment.

See also Measurement.

Debra Saliba and Susan D. Leonard

Baker, D. W., Wolf, M. S., Feinglass, J., Thompson, J. A., Gazmararian, J. A., & Huang, J. (2007). Health literacy and mortality among elderly persons. *Archives of Internal Medicine, 167*(14), 1503–1509.

Bostock, S., & Steptoe, A. (2012). Association between low functional health literacy and mortality in older adults: Longitudinal cohort study. *British Medical Journal, 344*, e1602.

Carneiro, F., Sousa, N., Azevedo, L. F., & Saliba, D. (2015). Vulnerability in elderly patients with gastrointestinal cancer—translation, cultural adaptation and validation of the European Portuguese version of the Vulnerable Elders Survey (VES-13). *BMC Cancer, 15*, 723.

Kroc, L., Socha, K., Soltysik, B. K., Kostka, T. (2016). Validation of the Vulnerable Elders Survey-13 (VES-13) in hospitalized older patients. *European Geriatric Medicine, 7*(5), 449–453. doi:10.1016/j.eurger.2016.03.008

Luciani, A., Ascione, G., Bertuzzi, C., Marussi, D., Codeca, C., Di Maria, G., ... Foa, P. (2010). Detecting disabilities in older patients with cancer: Comparison between comprehensive geriatric assessment and Vulnerable Elders Survey-13. *Journal of Clinical Oncology, 28*(12), 2046–2050.

Min, L., Ubhayakar, N., Saliba, D., Kelley-Quon, L., Morley, E., Hiatt, J., ... Tillou, A. (2011). The Vulnerable Elders Survey-13 predicts hospital complications and mortality in older adults with traumatic injury: A pilot study. *Journal of the American Geriatrics Society, 59*(8), 1471–1476.

Min, L., Yoon, W., Mariano, J., Wenger, N. S., Elliott, M. N., Kamberg, C., & Saliba, D. (2009). The Vulnerable Elders-13 Survey predicts 5-year functional decline and mortality outcomes in older ambulatory care patients. *Journal of the American Geriatrics Society, 57*(11), 2070–2076.

Ramsdale, E., Polite, B., Hemmerich, J., Bylow, K., Kindler, H. L., Mohile, S., & Dale, W. (2013). The Vulnerable Elders Survey-13 predicts mortality in older adults with later-stage colorectal cancer receiving chemotherapy: A prospective pilot study. *Journal of the American Geriatrics Society, 61*(11), 2043–2044.

Saliba, D., Elliott, M., Rubenstein, L. Z., Solomon, D. H., Young, R. T., Kamberg, C. J., ... Wenger, N. S. (2001). The Vulnerable Elders Survey: A tool for identifying vulnerable older people in the community. *Journal of the American Geriatrics Society, 49*(12), 1691–1699.

Saliba, D., Orlando, M., Wenger, N. S., Hays, R. D., & Rubenstein, L. Z. (2000). Identifying a short functional disability screen for older persons. *Journals of Gerontology: Series A, Biological Sciences and Medical Sciences, 55*(12), M750–M756.

Soubeyran, P., Bellera, C., Goyard, J., Heitz, D., Curé, H., Rousselot, H., ... Rainfray, M. (2014). Screening for vulnerability in older cancer patients: The ONCODAGE Prospective Multicenter Cohort Study. *PLOS ONE, 9*(12), e115060.

Stineman, M. G., Xie, D., Pan, Q., Kurichi, J. E., Zhang, Z., Saliba, D., ... Streim, J. (2012). All-cause 1-, 5-, and 10-year mortality in elderly people according to activities of daily living stage. *Journal of the American Geriatrics Society, 60*(3), 485–492.

Web Resource
National Institute on Aging: http://www.nia.nih.gov

RURAL ELDERLY

The world's population has migrated from rural settings to urban settings over the past several decades, and in 2014, approximately

R

half of the world's population lived in urban settings (United Nations, 2014). In the United States, about 17% of the population lives in rural settings, and rural communities are disproportionately older than urban or suburban communities (Hall & Owings, 2014). Individuals aged 65 years or older make up 17.2% of rural communities, as opposed to 12.8% of the population in urban areas (U.S. Census Bureau, 2011).

DEFINING RURAL

Defining the concept of rurality or what constitutes rural is complex and difficult. There has been a continuing lack of consistency in definitions of what is "rural" among policy makers and researchers. Clear and replicable definitions of *rurality* are necessary to develop and inform policy decisions related to rural development initiatives, and to conduct important epidemiological and health care research aimed at improving the health of rural elders. The U.S. government has developed several definitions of rural that are widely used to inform policy, direct development initiatives, and guide health care research. The U.S. Census Bureau, the White House Office of Management and Budget (OMB), and the U.S. Department of Agriculture (USDA) Economic Research Service (ERS) develop the most widely used federal definitions. Federal and state governments use these official definitions to allocate funds, set standards, and implement programs.

RURAL COMMUNITIES

There is wide agreement that rural populations have distinctive characteristics regarding their susceptibility to health problems, overall health status, and access to services. Rural elders face challenges related to health care and economic prosperity, and rate their overall health as poorer than their urban counterparts. They also face persistent poverty, have lower levels of education (USDA, 2016), and have higher rates of obesity and smoking compared with their urban counterparts (Institute of Medicine [IOM], 2005). Rural elders have a lower life expectancy (76.7 years vs. 79.1 years) than urban elders, with

heart disease, unintentional injuries, chronic obstructive pulmonary disease, lung cancer, stroke, suicide, and diabetes contributing to this disparity (Agency for Healthcare Research and Quality [AHRQ], 2014). In addition, rural communities are experiencing a significant outmigration of young adults to more urban settings, depleting the rural workforce and hurting economic development (Carr & Kefalas, 2009).

Rural hospitals face challenges due to their small size, lack of specialists (e.g., pharmacists), and low volume of procedures. At the same time, avoidable hospitalizations are more frequent in rural hospitals. Over half of all hospital inpatient admissions are older adults, and the number of discharges in rural hospitals for those aged 85 years or older is almost double that of urban hospitals (Hall, Owings, & Shinogle, 2006). Approximately half (51%) of residents hospitalized in rural hospitals are over the age of 65 years compared with only 37% of those hospitalized in urban hospitals (Hall & Owings, 2014). Furthermore, over half (53%) of hospitalized rural patients use Medicare as their primary source of payment (Hall & Owings, 2014). Rural hospitals are, however, more likely to offer hospice services (14.5% vs. 9.5%) and home health services (31.3% vs. 19.2%) than urban hospitals (Freeman, Thompson, Howard, Randolph, & Holmes, 2015). As the percentage of hospitalized rural elderly increases, health care solutions focused on the unique needs of this population need to be prioritized.

Rural communities make up 68% of areas with noted shortages in health care professional workers (U.S. Department of Health and Human Services [USDHHS], 2010). Rural communities often have difficulty recruiting and retaining qualified health care professionals, such as nurses and physicians (IOM, 2005). Approximately 17% of the U.S. population lives in rural areas, but fewer than 10% of physicians have practices in these areas. Primary care physicians are less prevalent in rural areas, with 39.8 per 100,000 population versus a ratio of 53.3/100,000 in metropolitan settings (Hing & Hsiao, 2014). Interestingly, the use of nurse practitioners or physician assistants in physician primary care offices is higher in less urban settings (Hing & Hsiao, 2014). Utilization of geriatric trained nurse practitioners and physician assistants may be an innovative approach for increasing and improving geriatric care in rural areas. Multidisciplinary, integrative care models such as the rural Program of All-Inclusive Care of the Elderly (PACE) have been shown to enhance the lives and improve the health of rural elders who are aging-in-place (USDHHS, 2011).

POVERTY

Poverty represents a greater problem among rural populations and frontier states (states where the majority of counties have low population density; USDA, 2016). In general, farming communities and mining industrial communities have higher incomes than nonfarming areas. Elderly rural men and women living in poverty have more disabilities, and consequently, are less likely to be employed. The nature of work in many rural areas is more physically demanding and puts adults at risk for serious physical injuries. Throughout their lifetime, they are likely to be without insurance and have less access to formal homecare and rehabilitative services. The main burden of care of disabled and frail elders falls on female informal caregivers. Older rural men share many of the same issues of health as women. In addition, retirement or job loss with stigmatization and few alternative opportunities is associated with higher incidences of depression and suicide and major addictions including alcoholism. Mental health services in many rural areas are woefully absent and providers specializing in geriatric mental health nearly nonexistent. In several frontier states, the majority of counties are designated *mental health shortage areas*. The most severe barriers to accessing those services that do exist are cost and availability.

SOLUTIONS

People in U.S. rural communities view connectivity and access to the Internet as necessary rather than merely desirable, and recent advances in adoption of electronic health records and telehealth technologies are improving care.

Technology and telehealth help remove the obstacle of distance, isolation, and lack of services, especially in the areas of mental health, critical care, and stroke for rural communities. Reimbursement for telehealth services has recently increased, and many interstate professional issues are in the process of being resolved. The use of home monitoring has increased contact of chronically ill elders with providers. Rural families and communities now have new and better means of communication and knowledge about health through the Internet. The rural elderly and their providers increasingly depend on the community to build and maintain the infrastructure to underpin new growth and find the resources they need.

Rural communities and universities need to be leaders in interdisciplinary and collaborative initiatives to build and strengthen services for the rural elderly. Universities can and should work within rural communities to maximize their resources, design newer approaches to care, and implement applied research programs. Universities are implementing more rural placements for students, creating initiatives to bring continuing education and health education to providers and rural residents, and partnering with states and communities to gather health data and disseminate it to agencies and communities for policy-making decisions and program planning. A key organization in connecting universities and health care providers to rural and underserved areas are the Area Health Education Centers (AHEC; National AHEC Organization, 2017). AHEC across the country bring rural communities, university faculty, and health care professional students together to improve health and quality of care in rural settings.

Available and appropriate financial resources are paramount to changes in rural health at the federal, state, and local levels. However, the most innovative solutions come from the communities in which the problems are encountered. With some resources already in place, communities need to assess and strategically place additional financial resources to support needed services.

The field of gerontology is growing steadily and knowledge about the care needs of rural elders is improving. The direction of future programming in rural areas depends on wise use of resources to enhance the lives of rural elderly and the communities in which they live. Researchers, practitioners, and policy makers have an obligation to be strong advocates to ensure that rural elderly receive high-quality health care and have the option to age in place.

See also Caregiver Burden; Caregiver Burnout; Poverty; Transportation.

Daniel D. Cline

Agency for Healthcare Research and Quality. (2014). *2014 National healthcare quality and disparities report chartbook on rural health care.* AHRQ pub. no. 15-0007-9-EF. Retrieved from https://www.ahrq.gov/sites/default/files/wysiwyg/research/findings/nhqrdr/2014chartbooks/ruralhealth/2014nhqdr-ruralhealth.pdf

Carr, P. J., & Kefalas, M. J. (2009). *Hollowing out the middle: The rural brain drain and what it means for America.* Boston, MA: Beacon Press.

Freeman, V. A., Thompson, K., Howard, H. A., Randolph, R., & Holmes, G. M. (2015). *The 21st century rural hospital: A chartbook.* North Carolina Rural Health Research Program. Cecil G. Sheps Center for Health Services Research. Retrieved from http://www.shepscenter.unc.edu/wp-content/uploads/2015/02/21stCenturyRuralHospitalsChartBook.pdf

Hall, M., & Owings, M. (2014). *Rural residents who are hospitalized in rural and urban hospitals: United States, 2010* [National Center for Health Statistics Data Brief, no. 19]. Hyattsville, MD: National Center for Health Statistics.

Hall, M., Owings, M., & Shinogle, J. (2006). Inpatient care in rural hospitals at the beginning of the 21st century. *Journal of Rural Health, 22*(4), 331–338. doi:10.1111/j.1748–0361.2006.00054.x

Hing, E., & Hsiao, C. (2014). *State variability in supply of office-based primary care providers: United States, 2012* [National Center for Health Statistics Data Brief, no. 151]. Hyattsville, MD: National Center for Health Statistics.

Institute of Medicine. (2005). *Quality through collaboration: The future of rural health.* Committee on the Future of Rural Health Care. Washington, DC: National Academies Press.

National AHEC Organization. (2017). About us. Retrieved from https://www.nationalahec.org/about/AboutUs.html

United Nations. (2014). *Population facts no. 2014/3.* Department of Economic and Social Affairs Population Division. United Nations. Retrieved from http://www.un.org/en/development/desa/population/publications/pdf/popfacts/PopFacts_2014-3.pdf

U.S. Census Bureau. (2011). *The older population: 2010. 2010 census briefs.* Retrieved from http://www.census.gov/prod/cen2010/briefs/c2010br-09.pdf

U.S. Department of Agriculture. (2016). *Rural America at a glance, 2015 edition.* Economic Research Service [Economic Information Bulletin Number 145]. Retrieved from https://www.ers.usda.gov/webdocs/publications/44015/55581_eib145.pdf?v=42397

U.S. Department of Health and Human Services. (2010). *The 2010 report to the secretary: Rural health and human services issue.* National Advisory Committee on Rural Health and Human Services. Retrieved from http://www.hrsa.gov/advisorycommittees/rural/2010secretaryreport.pdf

U.S. Department of Health and Human Services. (2011). *Report to Congress: Evaluation of the rural PACE provider grant program.* Centers for Medicare & Medicaid Services. Retrieved from http://www.npaonline.org/member-resources/special-initiatives/rural-pace/rural-pace%C2%AE-provider-grant-program

Web Resources

Center for Rural Affairs: http://www.cfra.org

Economic Research Service: http://www.ers.usda.gov

Health Resources and Service Administration (HRSA): http://www.hrsa.gov/ruralhealth

National Association for Rural Mental Health: http://www.narmh.org

Rural Development: http://www.rurdev.usda.gov/Home.html

Rural Information Hub: https://www.ruralhealthinfo.org/topics/aging

United States Department of Agriculture: http://ric.nal.usda.gov

World Health Organization: http://www.who.int/hrh/retention/guidelines/en/index.html

SELF-RATED HEALTH

Global self-ratings of health are the responses to the single question, "How would you rate your health?" The usual response categories are excellent, very good, good, fair, or poor. This question is often used to open a series of more specific questions relating to health in epidemiological surveys, or it may be the only measure of health status in an employment or opinion survey. For these reasons, it appears in many contexts and is therefore familiar and easy for respondents to answer. There are a large number of variants of the item, some of which include a specific age comparison (Compared with other people your age, how would you rate your health?), but all of them appear to tap similar content (Bjorner, Fayers, & Idler, 2005). Because the question is so widely used, and because it has proved to provide valuable information on the health status of populations, particularly elderly populations, it has been the focus of a large and still-growing body of research that goes back to the 1950s.

Self-ratings or self-assessments of health have been a particularly powerful research tool in elderly populations. Early research in the Duke Longitudinal Studies of Normal Aging compared elderly respondents' self-ratings to physician ratings for the same individuals, finding that older individuals often tended to be more optimistic about their health than physicians were and that self-ratings were good predictors of future health (Maddox & Douglass, 1973). Self-rated health is associated cross-sectionally with medical diagnoses, physical function, physical symptoms, pain, mental health, vital exhaustion, and possibly some biomarkers such as body mass index, total to high-density lipoprotein (HDL) cholesterol ratio, norepinephrine, and high-sensitivity C-reactive protein (Bjorner et al., 2005; Jylhä, 2009). Given the higher burden of chronic illness in aging populations, poor and fair ratings increase in prevalence with age.

Self-ratings of health are frequently used to track changes in population health over time or to make international comparisons. The National Center for Health Statistics has included the self-rated health question in its surveys, such as the National Health Interview Survey (NHIS) and the National Health and Nutrition Examination Survey (NHANES) for decades. Trends show that perceived health status among the older U.S. population has improved over the past 25 years. In 1982, 35.1% of the age-adjusted 65 years and older population rated their health as fair or poor; this has declined rather dramatically to just 21.7% in 2014 (www.cdc.gov/nchs). Similarly, the United Nations' World Health Survey (WHS) uses self-ratings of health as a comparative indicator of population health; among 21 countries in Europe, Latin America, Sub-Saharan Africa, and Asia, Ukrainian adults aged 18 years and older had the highest percentage reporting their health as fair/poor, and Uruguayans had the lowest (Van Ginneken & Groenewold, 2012).

The utility of self-ratings of health as an indicator of health status in populations was increased beginning in 1982 with a Canadian study that showed self-rated health to be a strong predictor of mortality in a large sample of elderly persons. Men and women who rated their health as poor were three times as likely to die as those who rated their health as excellent, even when sociodemographic factors and Manitoba Health Services data on diagnoses, physician visits, hospitalizations, and self-reports of conditions were included in the analysis. Respondents who rated their health as fair and even good also had significantly higher risks of mortality compared with those who

S

rated their health as excellent, even after adjustment for age, gender, and health status. Since this initial publication, there have been more than 100 such studies appearing in the international literature, almost all of which have had similar findings. The continuous outpouring of such studies is demonstrated by the frequency with which the self-rated health item is included in health surveys with longitudinal follow-up of mortality; these are by their nature secondary analyses of existing data with long follow-up periods. More than half of these studies have used samples of older persons (Benyamini & Idler, 1999; Idler & Benyamini, 1997). Thus self-ratings of health have proved to be a useful indicator of the present health status of populations and are also valid predictors of mortality over follow-up periods as long as 12 or more years.

More recent longitudinal studies have reported a range of other outcomes, including onset of coronary heart disease, withdrawal from the labor force (Bjorner et al., 2005), functional disability (Kaplan, Strawbridge, & Camacho, 1993), and health services utilization and expenditures (DeSalvo, Fan, McDonell, & Fihn, 2005). Another new direction for this research is the employment of self-ratings of health in clinical care settings, for the purpose of assessing quality-of-life outcomes in specific patient groups (www.patienteducation .stanford.edu/research/generalhealth.html and www.sf-36.org). A related area is the assessment of the quality-of-life of family caregivers who are coping with the needs of their cognitively or physically impaired elderly family members. An increasing body of research shows the health impact of caregiving and the need for assessments in which self-ratings of health of the caregivers themselves play a central role (www.caregiving.org/pdf/research/ Alzheimers_Caregiving_Costs_Study_FINAL .pdf). It is likely that there exist continuous new applications and analyses of the concept of self-rated health as a single item, or embedded in multidimensional quality-of-life measurements, in representative population samples of elderly persons, in patient samples, and in caregiver samples.

Self-ratings of health are driven by several processes that make them particularly interesting for older populations. Comparisons of the self-ratings of health and physical health status of older and younger respondents find that older persons tend to rate their health more positively, relative to younger persons at any given level of health status. This difference could be due to an effect of aging and adjustment to chronic illness over time and researchers have identified a "response shift" in how older persons evaluate their health (Sprangers & Schwartz, 1999). It could also be due to more stable cohort differences deriving from factors such as hardship or health disadvantage in early life (Schnittker & Bacak, 2014), or it could be due to selective survival of those with better self-ratings of health (Zajacova & Woo, 2015). Research shows support for all three explanations (Idler, 1993). Such research tends to dispel the stereotype of hypochondriasis among elderly persons; older persons are more likely to be under-reporters of health complaints than over-reporters.

CONCLUSION

Self-rated health is a widely used indicator of health status in cross-sectional population and clinical studies, and a predictor of mortality and other health outcomes in longitudinal studies. It is strongly associated with more objective measures of health status, such as physical function, diagnoses, and use of health services, but it appears to incorporate additional information beyond these indicators. Self-rated health may represent a higher order of integration of all information available to the respondent, as well as their trajectory and perceived prognosis. It may also represent a fundamental sense of health identity that underlies and colors new health events, that influences the reporting of symptoms, and motivates health behaviors resulting in measurable health outcomes. With its brevity and utility, it is likely to continue to stay in wide use in surveys and assessment instruments, which in turn lead to further research.

Ellen Idler

Benyamini, Y., & Idler, E. (1999). Community studies reporting association between self-rated health and mortality: Additional studies, 1995–1998. *Research on Aging, 21,* 392–401.

Bjorner, J. B., Fayers, P., & Idler, E. (2005). Self-rated health. In P. Fayers & R. Hays (Eds.), *Assessing quality of life in clinical trials* (2nd ed., pp. 309–323). New York, NY: Oxford University Press.

DeSalvo, K. B., Fan, V. S., McDonell, M. B., & Fihn, S. D. (2005). Predicting mortality and healthcare utilization with a single question. *Health Services Research, 40*(4), 1234–1246.

Idler, E. L. (1993). Age differences in self-assessments of health: Age changes, cohort differences, or survivorship? *Journal of Gerontology, 48*(6), S289–S300.

Idler, E. L., & Benyamini, Y. (1997). Self-rated health and mortality: A review of twenty-seven community studies. *Journal of Health and Social Behavior, 38*(1), 21–37.

Jylhä, M. (2009). What is self-rated health and why does it predict mortality? Towards a unified conceptual model. *Social Science & Medicine, 69*(3), 307–316.

Kaplan, G. A., Strawbridge, W. J., & Camacho, T. (1993). Factors associated with change in physical functioning in the elderly: A six-year prospective study. *Journal of Aging and Health, 5,* 140–153.

Maddox, G. L., & Douglass, E. B. (1973). Self-assessment of health: A longitudinal study of elderly subjects. *Journal of Health and Social Behavior, 14*(1), 87–93.

Schnittker, J., & Bacak, V. (2014). The increasing predictive validity of self-rated health. *PLOS ONE, 9,* e84933. doi:10.1371/journal.pone.0084933

Sprangers, M. A. G., & Schwartz, C. E. (1999). Integrating response shift into health-related quality of life research: A theoretical model. *Social Science & Medicine, 48,* 1507–1515.

Van Ginneken, J. K., & Groenewold, G. (2012). A single- vs. multi-item self-rated health status measure: A 21-country study. *Open Public Health Journal, 5,* 1–9. Retrieved from https://benthamopen.com/contents/pdf/TOPHJ/TOPHJ-5-1.pdf

Zajacova, A., & Woo, H. (2015). Examination of age variations in the predictive validity of self-rated health. *Journals of Gerontology: Social Sciences, 71*(3), 551–557.

Web Resources

Health Surveys (Optum): https://campaign.optum.com/optum-outcomes/what-we-do/health-surveys.html?gclid=CJCV0bLMuc4CFYgfhgodcJwLDQ

National Caregiving Alliance: http://www.caregiving.org/pdf/research/Alzheimers_Caregiving_Costs_Study_FINAL.pdf

National Center for Health Statistics: http://www.cdc.gov/nchs

Patient Education (Standford Medical Library): http://patienteducation.stanford.edu/research/generalhealth.html

World Health Organization: http://www.who.int/healthinfo/systems/sage/en/index3.html

SENIOR CENTERS

PURPOSE AND EVOLUTION

The purpose of senior centers is predicated on the philosophy that successful aging is active, and it is neither natural nor inevitable for people to disengage in late adulthood (Bengtson, 2009). The first senior centers were established in the 1940s, after World War II, to decrease the sense of isolation among the retired elderly, who were living longer and had little to do. The centers provided them with recreational, educational, and case management services to support their independence in the community. Since then, senior centers have evolved to serve as a venue of ongoing social activity, engagement, and integration for the elderly (Weill, 2014). Senior centers offer opportunities to develop supportive relationships, perform productive activities, access coping resources, and maintain high mental and physical functioning. These programs aim to help older adults maintain independence and integrity and to successfully age in place."

The Older Americans Act (OAA) directs senior centers to serve as community focal points for comprehensive service coordination and delivery at the local level. Thus senior centers not only provide services for older people, but also play important information and referral roles through links with a wide variety of other community organizations. Senior centers are often used by other agencies as delivery sites for programs such as congregate meals and health education.

Recently, increasing attention has shifted to preparing Baby Boomers' cohort's transition into older age, as senior centers have responded to the changing needs of a population that is living and working longer than previous generations. Many centers now provide self-enhancement programs in art, computers, language, exercise and wellness, and financial planning, among others. As more older adults have found themselves caring for aging parents, some senior centers have offered supportive resources around family caregiving (Weill, 2014). Overall, senior centers have had varied success in attracting newly retired individuals to their programs and face increasing competition from other service providers, especially for-profit businesses, and as the interests and activity patterns of older adults change.

Increasing demographic changes and diversity in race/ethnicity, culture, language, sexual orientation, and general needs among seniors have also created the need for initiatives and policies that support the delivery of diversified and competent senior center services. Several initiatives, policies, and practices have been instituted and infused throughout senior centers to respond to the diverse needs and interests that exists across the elderly who attend senior centers. To further advance the quality of senior centers nationwide and address the diverse needs of their participants, the National Institute of Senior Centers (NISC; National Council on Aging [NCOA], 2016) has developed nine standards of excellence for senior center operations that are used for accreditation, purpose, community, governance, administration, program planning, evaluation, fiscal management, records/reports, and facility. These standards serve as a guide for all senior centers to improve their operations and position themselves for the future.

Senior centers generally have multiple funding sources, including the OAA, state and local government funding, local business contribution, fundraising, in-kind donations, and participant contributions and volunteering. Larger senior centers have professional, paid staffs but also rely heavily on older people as volunteers.

DEMOGRAPHICS

According to the NCOA (2016), approximately 70% of senior center participants are women.

Half of them live alone. The average age of all participants is 75 years. Three-quarters (75%) of participants visit their centers 1 to 3 times per week. They spend an average of 3.3 hours per visit. Almost 50% of participants are Caucasian, followed by African Americans, Hispanics, and Asians, respectively. More than 60% of senior centers provide access to multiple services in one place.

ACTIVITIES AND SERVICES

Senior centers offer a range of diverse activities that vary according the geographic area, the size of the facility, the number of staff, the availability of resources, and the needs of the population being served. Activities and services can include transportation, meal and nutrition programs, recreational games, educational programs, discussion groups, art programs, trips, birthday activities, information and assistance, and health or mental health care programs. Many centers offer health screening and maintenance, health education, and nutrition education, and information and assistance services (e.g., consumer protection; housing; crime prevention; financial, tax, and legal aid; Social Security).

A taskforce of senior center directors and administrators from around the country was established in 2007 by the NISC to identify and define new, emerging models of senior centers in the country. The six models of innovative senior centers are as follows: community, wellness, lifelong learning/arts, continuum of care/transitions, entrepreneurial, and café (Pardasani & Thompson, 2012). The new models expand the continuum of services and many provide a coordinated and structured system of links to provide for community-dwelling older adults.

IMPACT ON PSYCHOSOCIAL WELL-BEING

The majority of research suggests that senior center users generally have higher levels of health, social interaction, and life satisfaction and lower levels of income than do nonusers (Turner, 2004). Senior center participants also tend to have more social contacts and friendships and fewer problems with activities of daily living, better psychological well-being, lower rates of depression, and reduced stress levels (Pardasani & Thompson, 2012; Turner, 2004).

Senior centers have grown and diversified over the years. Shifts in federal and state spending, evolving priorities in health and social services for the elderly, a greater focus on cost-containment and targeting those at risk, and changing demographics and retirement patterns present considerable challenges for senior center programming (Weill, 2014). Among the strengths of senior centers are their diversity and ability to serve different segments of the older population in many different ways. Senior centers do many things well with relatively few resources and are certainly capable of improving and expanding existing functions, given the appropriate resources and mission. Although clearly a part of the system of community-based services, their role in the long-term-care continuum is still evolving.

Ihab Girgis

Bengtson, V. L., Gans, D., Putney, N. M., & Silverstein, M. (2009). *Handbook of theories of aging* (2nd ed.). New York, NY: Springer Publishing.

National Council on Aging. (2016). Senior centers fact sheet. Retrieved from https://www.ncoa.org/resources/fact-sheet-senior-centers

Pardasani, M., & Thompson, P. (2012). Senior centers: Innovative and emerging models. *Journal of Applied Gerontology, 31*(1), 52–77.

Turner, W. K. (2004). Senior citizens centers: What they offer, who participates, and what they gain. *Journal of Gerontological Social Work, 43*(1), 36–47.

Weill, J. (2014). *The New Neighborhood Senior Center: Redefining social and service roles for the baby boom generation.* New Brunswick, NJ: Rutgers University Press.

Web Resources
American Society on Aging: http://www.asaging.org
Area Offices on Aging: http://www.aoa.gov
National Association of Area Offices on Aging: http://www.n4a.org
National Council on the Aging: http://www.ncoa.org
National Institute of Senior Centers: http://www.ncoa.org/national-institute-of-senior-centers

SENIOR HUNGER

It is conventional wisdom that a problem cannot be solved unless it is first recognized. It may provide a partial explanation to the tragic situation in which millions of our nation's older adults find themselves living today. We are speaking about the monumental, growing, and largely overlooked problem of senior hunger in the United States.

There had been a general lack of attention to the issue of senior hunger until a national research study demonstrated that in 2005 an excess of 5 million individuals—11.45% of all seniors, or almost one in nine—faced the threat of hunger (Ziliak, Gundersen, & Haist, 2008). The study also provided an important benchmark against which to measure our nation's progress in the fight against food insecurity among seniors. Regrettably, over the course of the last decade, the change in the number of seniors facing the threat of hunger is more aptly characterized as *regress* rather than *progress*. Nearly 16% of seniors were threatened with hunger (Feeding America, 2017). It translates into 10.2 million older individuals and marks an egregious milestone, namely the first time in our nation's history that more than 10 million seniors were adversely affected. This growth reflects a 119% increase in the number of the elders experiencing hunger's threat since 2001 and a 65% increase in the 7 years since the start of the Great Recession in 2007 (Ziliak & Gundersen, 2013). Furthermore, this growth cannot be explained away simply as a function of demographic changes because the increases in hunger threat exceed the rate of population growth for the older cohort.

The Ziliak, Gundersen, and Haist study was commissioned by the predecessor organization to the National Foundation to End Senior Hunger (NFESH). Two things are remarkable about this study. First, although attention has been focused for decades on hunger among particular subgroups of the population, such as children or the homeless, it was not until 2008 that any meaningful consideration was given to the matter as it related to older persons. Second, when that did occur, it was not Congress, the presidential administration, a federal agency, a university, a corporation, or a major think tank that took the initiative. Rather it was a small, and then little-known, nonprofit foundation that sponsored the research. The study received almost immediate attention from the academic community, and the media was not far behind in showing interest.

The NFESH was founded on the belief that raising public awareness about the issue of senior hunger is absolutely critical to the success of the foundation's mission to reduce, eliminate, and prevent it. The NFESH also understood, and continues to believe, that the manner in which the issue is described—that is, the words used to convey research findings to a broad audience that includes, but is not limited to, academics and policy makers—are just as critical as the facts themselves. Although professionals in the antihunger arena are conversant with terms such as *food insecurity*, most of the general public is not. Instead of finding the official nomenclature compelling, most people found it confusing; instead of bringing the fact of hunger to life, such terminology put it at a distance. Together with Drs. Ziliak and Gundersen, the terms *facing the threat of hunger*, *at-risk of hunger*, and *suffering from hunger* were devised to correspond to the U.S. Department of Agriculture's (USDA) terminology of *marginally food insecure, food insecure, and very low food security* and to describe the food insecurity continuum. The threat of hunger is the broadest measure, encompassing the whole spectrum of hunger and is the measure that NFESH typically uses to quantify senior hunger. Given the characteristics of the senior population, and their differences from the population as a whole, we were and continues to be, convinced that the broadest measure is the most appropriate to use. The fact that the media, corporate America, researchers, and other non-profit organizations routinely cite our research as the definitive source of senior hunger data is indicative of the fact that general agreement is coalescing around the belief that this is the appropriate measure and most accurate means of understanding the scope and breadth of the hunger problem among older people.

When it comes to issues related to hunger, seniors face unique challenges. Between 2007 and 2010, when food insecurity rates improved slightly in all other age cohorts and in the population as a whole, they worsened among those aged 60 years and older. We know from NFESH-commissioned and many other studies that being poor or near-poor places older adults at risk of hunger, and we also know that poverty should be measured differently for seniors. This is not simply an opinion on our part, and we are not alone in our view. In fact, in late 2011, the U.S. Census Bureau, the federal agency charged with calculating the official U.S. poverty rate, released the Supplemental Poverty Measure (SPM), an alternate measure to the official federal poverty index that takes into account additional factors, such as medical out-of-pocket expenses (MOOP), which affect older adults disproportionately. The SPM verified that there are many more poor seniors in the United States than have been recognized traditionally. According to the official poverty measure (2010), 9% of individuals aged 65 years and older fall below poverty; however, when calculated according to the SPM, that number rises to 15.9%, an astounding 76.7% increase over those found to fall below poverty according to the "official" poverty measure. As a result, it is not surprising that the majority of seniors facing the threat of hunger have incomes above the official federal poverty line. Close to a third have incomes between 100% and 200% of poverty, and nearly another quarter have incomes more than 200% of poverty, according to Ziliak and Gundersen's work, which is based on the official poverty measure and not the SPM. Of particular concern is the growth of the 200%+ of poverty cohort threatened by hunger, which has increased incrementally and steadily. This may, in fact, be more evidence of the SPM's veracity. Regardless of which measure is used, the number of individuals aged 60 years and older facing poverty is unacceptable and has significant deleterious consequences not only for the individuals affected, but also for the nation as a whole.

The risk of hunger has a staggering negative impact on a senior's overall quality of life. A senior at risk of hunger, for instance, has the same chance of a limitation in activities of daily living (ADL) as an individual who is 14 years older. Ziliak et al. (2008) found that hunger risk creates, in effect, a large disparity between actual chronological age and "physical" age so that a 69-year-old senior suffering from hunger is likely to have the ADL limitations of an 83-year-old. It is noteworthy that this hunger–aging–ADL connection was not found to be present in any cohort of those aged 59 years and younger. As the number of seniors afflicted by hunger-related ADL limitations continues to grow, national spending for in-home caregiving, nursing home, and other institutional care doubtless increases in tandem. Seniors at risk of hunger are also more likely than their peers to be in poor or fair health and are more likely to have lower intakes of major nutrients.

The primary focus of NFESH is to bring national attention to a national problem to solve it. However, we are keenly aware of the fact that national problems are also fundamentally local. They exist first and always in communities. Similar to most social and health problems, the incidence of the threat of senior hunger varies considerably from state to state. To determine just how significant the disparities were and to pinpoint states that were most severely affected, in 2009, NFESH commissioned Drs. Ziliak and Gundersen to provide a state-by-state profile, which has been, and will continue to be, updated annually. This information has been critical in assisting state and local hunger relief, social welfare, and health care organizations in developing more effective programs and strategies to address the problem. As has been true every year since the state-by-state information has been produced, in 2014 we saw widely discrepant rates among the states. The range for the threat of hunger spanned from 7.26 % in North Dakota to 24.85% in Arkansas (Ziliak & Gundersen, 2016). These rates and rankings shift from year to year, as noted by comparing the 2014 rankings with those of 2010, when the threat of hunger spanned from 5.52% in North Dakota to 21.53% in Mississippi (Ziliak & Gundersen, 2012). What is particularly disturbing, however, is that in 2014 only four states had rates less than 10%. Although it is helpful for the individual states to view their standing in a national context, NFESH believes that there is particular benefit to states in being able not only to evaluate the magnitude of its senior hunger

problem relative to other jurisdictions but also to gauge its own effectiveness, or lack thereof, in year-over-year self-comparisons.

The correlation between good nutrition and good health is well accepted, and the direct impact of proper nutrition on specific diseases, such as diabetes, hypertension, and certain types of cancers, is well recognized. Also documented by the Centers for Disease Control and Prevention (CDC) is the fact that obese individuals are at greater risk of these and other diseases than adults of healthy weight. Although it may seem counterintuitive that many individuals facing the threat of hunger are obese, it is frequently the case that they are. Obesity rates are high among those threatened with and at risk of hunger. Although the significant U.S. medical costs attributable to diseases associated with obesity have been well documented, the same attention has not been given to determining the national health care savings that could be realized by reducing the incidence of obesity through interventions designed to ensure that individuals at risk of hunger receive proper nutrition, not just food. We remain eager to engage partners, such as hospitals and insurers, within the health care community to work with us to gather and analyze this critical information. Regrettably, such partnerships are persistently rare for antihunger organizations.

Similarly, the connection between hunger and health, the connection between hunger and health care costs, and the issue of the place of meal provision and nutrition education in the emerging long-term services and support system (LTSS) remain relatively unexamined. Research in this area could assist in the development of public policies intended to improve health and reduce social and economic costs to the nation. For example, projects that test the integration of nutrition services as a standard element in the LTSS system could be a first step. Little progress has been made in this area.

Our own organization has recently begun to focus our attention on what we have termed "Two Problems, One Solution," namely the coexistence of hunger and food waste and wasted food in the United States. Stepping out into new areas of study and experimentation, like we did with commissioning of senior hunger research in 2008, NFESH has recently created the What A Waste (WAW) program. We originally developed WAW specifically for senior nutrition programs (SNPs) funded under Title III of the federal Older Americans Act (OAA) and administered by the states. The so-called Title III program is the flagship national food program for older adults that provides meals, rather than simply furnishing food or funds to purchase food. As the name *senior nutrition program* implies, it also seeks to emphasize the importance of nutrition and healthy eating as well as to make healthful meals available to those individuals aged 60 years and older who need them. All meals served with OAA funds must meet the standard of providing one third of the Dietary Reference Intakes (DRIs) as prescribed for the older population under the most current federal Dietary Guidelines for Americans. It has long been accepted that SNPs do an excellent job of serving these meals. Regrettably, serving healthful meals that meet the DRI standard does not necessarily achieve the goal of ensuring that seniors are getting the nutrition they need to remain healthy. Only if seniors consume the nutrients that the DRIs require does this occur. Before the introduction of WAW, there was no focus on this dichotomy and no means of determining whether the goal was being achieved.

Through nutrient analytics performed by NFESH based on the actual nutrient content of each specific meal, coupled with the exact daily measurement for food waste (from prepared foods not served, but discarded) and wasted food (from foods served on seniors' plates, but not eaten), WAW is providing SNPs the tools and resources necessary to evaluate just which and how much of each vital nutrient seniors in the SNPs are consuming. At the same time, it identifies which specific food items seniors most frequently forego so that menu substitutions, which NFESH recommends, can be made. In addition, WAW calculates the cost of waste to the specific SNP in terms of both dollars and meals lost, both of which are of critical importance in the context of the severely limited financial resources with which these SNPs typically operate. Learning to eliminate waste means recouping money and meals that can be leveraged to achieve the mission of reducing hunger by expanding nutrition services to additional seniors who need them.

The facts are clear and undeniable. As the U.S. population has grown older, it has become hungrier as well. From 2001 to 2014 the number of older persons facing the threat of hunger grew by 47%. The number of seniors aged 60 years and older has increased by 119% over the same period and by 65% between 2007 and 2014. The dimension of the problem defines it as a crisis in our lexicon; and the steady growth provides compelling evidence that the practices of the past and present have aged as well and are inadequate to effect any real improvement. They are not the solutions at all.

Having said that, we at NFESH are confident that the solutions—which likely require a rethinking of current practice and a cobbling together of an array of innovative initiatives—can be found. Our mission is to seek them and our hope and invitation is that the whole of the anti-hunger community as well as the healthcare sector, the aging network, the agricultural sector, the food industry, and government at all levels will commit, as we have, to creating and implementing programs and approaches to reverse the insidious trend and begin reducing the threat of hunger among some of the nation's most vulnerable and venerable citizens.

Enid A. Borden and Margaret B. Ingraham

Feeding America. (2017). Senior hunger fact sheet. Retrieved from http://www.feedingamerica.org/assets/pdfs/fact-sheets/senior-hunger-fact-sheet.pdf

Ziliak, J. P., & Gundersen, C. G. (2012). *The state of senior hunger in America 2010: An annual report.* Alexandria, VA: National Foundation to End Senior Hunger.

Ziliak, J. P., & Gundersen, C. G. (2013). *The state of senior hunger in America 2011: An annual report.* Alexandria, VA: National Foundation to End Senior Hunger.

Ziliak, J. P., & Gundersen, C. G. (2016). *The state of senior hunger in America 2014: An annual report.* Alexandria, VA: National Foundation to End Senior Hunger.

Ziliak, J. P., Gundersen, C. G., & Haist, M. (2008). *The causes, consequences and future of senior hunger in America*. Alexandria, VA: Meals on Wheels Association of America Foundation.

Web Resource
National Foundation to End Senior Hunger: https://www.nfesh.org/research

SENIOR SERVICE LINE

BACKGROUND

The concept and structure of service lines are based on the product line management model that began in the manufacturing industry after World War II. This was developed as a means of diversification into multiple lines of business, each focusing on a certain product and consisting of all the elements needed to develop, manufacture, sell, and service the product (Fligstein, 1985). Service lines began appearing in health care in the early 1980s within integrated delivery systems. There is no standard definition of a health care service line. There are, however, some common elements (Tesch & Levy, 2008): patient-centered care, coordination of care, multidisciplinary leadership, efficient care, enhanced patient experience, and clinical outcomes measures.

SERVICE LINE TYPES

The three main service line types can be categorized as specific disease or diagnosis focus (e.g., congestive heart failure [CHF], chronic obstructive pulmonary disease [COPD], cancer), procedure or interventions (e.g., joint replacements, cardiac), and population groups (e.g., seniors, children). Since 2012, service lines in health care have continued to grow, mostly along the disease/diagnosis and procedural lines that are driven by volumes and revenue. The new imperative, based on changing payment models, moves from silo service lines based on their own specialty to advancing integrated, interdisciplinary team-based care (Delaveris, 2015).

THE NEED

As the Centers for Medicare & Medicaid Services moves payment systems from fee for service to models of population health management, such as bundled payment, accountable care organizations (ACOs), value-based purchasing, and payment based on episodes of care, health care leaders are compelled to develop new models of care that meet patient needs across the continuum of care. Hospitals are finding that to do this, they need to identify strategic partners within the continuum of care and organize care around patients, not around buildings and departments. In this environment, service lines should be the vehicle for the evolution of programs to support care coordination and population health management (Delaveris, 2015).

The United States has an aging population along with a shortage of geriatricians and health care professionals with geriatric training to care for this aging population. U.S. Census data show that by the year 2030, there will be 72 million Americans aged 65 years and older. According to the American Geriatrics Society (2017), in 2016 there were fewer than 7,300 geriatricians in the United States. By 2030, the need increases to 30,000, and it is not likely that the need will be met. Medicare has become increasingly concerned about the rising cost of care for this burgeoning population. One example of the need for a senior service line is the effort to decrease the risk of rehospitalization of older patients.

SENIOR SERVICE LINE

America's growing senior population is living longer, often in the context of multiple chronic diseases, complex medication regimens, and behavioral health needs. This challenge presents an imperative for high-quality, efficient and coordinated care. Development of a senior service line can help accomplish this imperative. It also lends itself to an "integrated" service line structure, as seniors are often part of other diagnosis and procedure categories, such as heart failure, cancer, or joint replacement. The most common design considered a good fit for the senior service line is the matrix design. This model is a blend of traditional management structure with system-level leadership. The matrix design allows authority, accountability, and resource control to be balanced between system-level service line directors and local facility management level (Jain, Thompson, Kelley, & Schwartz, 2006). It is also imperative that a senior service line be multidisciplinary because of the complex and diverse needs of the senior population.

A good example of this structure is the Aurora Health Care System in Wisconsin. Aurora is a nonprofit integrated health care system of 14 hospitals, one psychiatric hospital, more than 150 clinics, 70 pharmacies, and a home care agency that serves their entire system's service area. They serve approximately 30,000 seniors aged 65 years and older in their hospitals each year. They have structured a senior service line that is interdisciplinary at the leadership level and that serves the entire system. The system leadership team includes a geriatrician, an administrative leader (background in geriatric social work and nursing home administration), and a board-certified geriatric clinical nurse specialist. They have a sanctioned system budget for senior service leaders, program support, and system geriatric education. They have responsibility for development, dissemination, and support of effective programs of care for seniors system-wide. They also have responsibility for tracking and reporting outcomes of care to system leaders, as well as site leaders. They work in a matrix reporting relationship to system vice presidents and through relationships with individual site team leaders. The main geriatric program that the senior service line leaders develop and support is the acute care for elders (ACE) program, across all hospital sites. They work with interdisciplinary teams at each site and involve local long-term care partners (Malone et al., 2010).

The system leaders work with each site to teach the principles of care, provide geriatric education and outcome measures, and develop and support site-level advisory teams. They develop and maintain good leadership support both at the system and site levels and develop positive relationships with local physician groups. It is imperative that each local site has a strong nursing leader and physician leader to champion the geriatric programs. Service line leaders manage both the business plan and the clinical leadership. They have strong collaboration skills both inside and outside the organization.

BENEFITS

One benefit of the service line approach for seniors is that there is a standard of care for this population across sites. Whether patients are in one of the urban teaching hospitals or one of the small rural hospitals, they have, for example, the same interdisciplinary team approach to care, the same assessment for delirium, and the same review for high-risk medications. Another benefit is that their care needs are addressed beyond the hospital episode, to home care, skilled nursing care, and/or outpatient follow-up. This meets the requirements of the new payment models based on episodes of care and population health management. Through this approach to care, seniors may also experience a better quality of life due to reduced rehospitalizations and fewer acute episodes that may bring them to an emergency department for care.

Documented positive outcomes and high patient satisfaction scores can be included in marketing campaigns for the hospital and health system. Partnering with long-term care and other community service providers can improve coordination of care and reduce avoidable hospital readmissions. There is also benefit as an integrated service line to partner with palliative care and hospice programs to improve end-of-life care. The latter can reduce treatment intensity (e.g., use of critical care services) and thus reduce costs, and more important, improve quality of life. In fact, several health systems have structured leadership for geriatrics and palliative care under one service line.

KEY SUCCESS FACTORS

There are several key ingredients to a successful service line: health system priority of excellence in senior care, physician and nursing identification of the importance of senior care, credible expertise in geriatrics, and the ability to identify and improve the quality and safety of health care.

Finding the right leaders for the senior service line is also imperative for success. The leaders must have a clear vision for the service line, and must have clinical credibility through both their credentials and practice. They must also be well-versed in public policy and payment models and be open-minded. It is important to have a strong physician leader to get buy-in from physicians in the system. When the physician leader is focused on research-guided and evidence-based clinical models of care, physician support is more easily obtained. Equally important is a strong nurse leader who has advanced practice skills. This leader acts as both formal and informal educator and consultant for geriatric clinical excellence. The nurse leader also influences program development and management. This is imperative for obtaining support from nursing administrators throughout the system. This is essential because nursing is the largest 24/7 department of care for hospital patients. The third important leadership team member is the service line director with solid administrative skills for budgeting, planning, legal contracts, collaboration, development, and reporting outcomes. This leader must also understand the senior population, market trends, and overall hospital operations and have a commitment to quality improvement. All leaders need to be team players.

Tracking, managing, and reporting outcomes are also needed for success. The leaders should identify their outcomes dashboard and structure regular data extraction and reporting. If they are unable to demonstrate quality and favorable cost outcomes, there is a risk of losing the service line and programs. There is also an increased risk of losing buy-in and momentum from the front-line staff. In the population health payment environment, it is important to show improved outcomes for the population group cost reduction/savings.

Service lines must be patient-centered to be successful. Improving patient satisfaction should be an objective of any service line model. For a senior service line, patient satisfaction, specifically for the population aged 65 years and older, should be tracked (King & Jenkins, 2008). Patient focus groups should be conducted if there is a specific focus area for improvement. Adding a patient or family community member to the hospital advisory teams provides invaluable input.

The senior service line must be multidisciplinary; seniors often have complex health issues and needs. It takes the entire team to meet these needs.

See also Acute Care for Elders; Hospice; Hospital-Based Services; Palliative Care.

Marsha Vollbrecht

American Geriatrics Society. (2017). Geriatrics workforce by the numbers. Retrieved from http://www.americangeriatrics.org/geriatrics-profession/about-geriatrics/geriatrics-workforce-numbers

Delaveris, S. L. (2015). At your service line. *Physician Leadership Journal, 2*(1), 34–35.

Fligstein, N. (1985). The spread of the multidivisional form among large firms, 1919–1979. *American Sociological Review, 50,* 377–391.

Jain, A. K., Thompson, J. M., Kelley, S. M., & Schwartz, R. W. (2006). Fundamentals of service lines and the necessity of physician leaders. *Surgical Innovation, 13*(2), 136–144.

King, J., & Jenkins, J. (2008). Information management: Why it's vital to effective service line operation. *Healthcare Financial Management, 62*(4), 76–80.

Malone, M. L., Vollbrecht, M., Stephenson, J., Burke, L., Pagel, P., & Goodwin, J. S. (2010). Acute care for elders (ACE) tracker and e-geriatrician: Methods to disseminate ACE concepts to hospitals with no geriatricians on staff. *Journal of the American Geriatrics Society, 58*(1), 161–167.

Tesch, T., & Levy, A. (2008). Measuring service line success: The new model for benchmarking. *Healthcare Financial Management, 62*(7), 68–74.

Web Resources
Advisory Board Company: https://www.advisory.com
Medicare: https://www.medicare.gov
Institute for Healthcare Improvement: http://www.ihi.org

SEXUAL HEALTH

Human sexuality has biological, affective, motivational, and cognitive aspects that can be

S

expressed as part of erotic, nurturing, or pathological relationships. Although not universally true, sexual activity generally becomes less frequent in later life, mostly not only because of reduced ability, but also because of less interest (Gentili & Mulligan, 2013). Sexual behavior involves the genitalia and erogenous zones. Sexuality is the dynamic outcome of physical capacity, motivation, attitudes, and the potential for intimate partnership (Waite, Laumann, Das, & Schumm, 2009). Age-related changes associated with sexual health and sexuality include biological, pharmacological, and psychosocial factors. Often, one or more of these factors may lead to sexual dysfunction. The incidence of many sexual disorders increases with advancing age. For healthy community-dwelling older men, there is a clear decline in sexual function, with erectile dysfunction (ED) as the main complaint. Female sexual dysfunction also increases with age. Common dysfunctions in older women include declining lubrication and desire, symptoms that increase mainly during menopause and thereafter.

Many older individuals enjoy healthy sexual lives despite a number of barriers. One is lack of a partner. Of those aged 75 to 85 years of age, 38% of men and 17% of women report that they have had sex with a partner in the last year (Waite et al., 2009). Clinician reluctance to query patients about their sexual activity is based, in part, on the societal norm that sexuality and sexual behavior are private. Although clinicians may express reluctance in discussing sexual issues with their older patients, most men and women want their physicians to inquire. In addition, people frequently differ on what is meant by *sex*. The term is often used interchangeably to refer to a person's gender; to kissing or caressing; and to oral, vaginal, and anal intercourse. Hence, an accurate history is often difficult to obtain if clinicians or patients are unwilling to use the appropriate terms.

Sexual dysfunction (e.g., impotence, premature ejaculation, anorgasmy) or simply the inability to appreciate or want an intimate physical experience is often driven by notions of physical attractiveness and societal, religious, and cultural norms about appropriate elders' sexual behavior. Sex education for senior citizens has not been a high-priority health issue; few elderly are

knowledgeable about changes in sexual response associated with aging or ways to compensate for them. Information might help elders avoid fear, ridicule, and, in some cases, anxiety and depression. In addition, the teaching of safe sexual practices, such as the use of condoms, is crucial to help prevent sexually transmitted diseases and the spread of HIV. This is especially important in light of the Centers for Disease Control and Prevention (CDC, 2014) report that adults aged 55 years and older accounted for 24% (288,700) of those living with HIV.

SEXUAL RESPONSE CYCLE

In general, more time is needed by older sexually active men and women to be sexually aroused, complete intercourse, achieve orgasm, and be aroused in comparison to younger sexually active individuals. Testosterone decrease, a normal age-related change in men, reduces the tone of erectile tissue. Changes in collagen and the vascular endothelium may impair erection stiffness or frequency. Erection can take longer to achieve, be less full, and less likely to result in ejaculation than in younger men. The force of the ejaculation is decreased; the volume of seminal fluid is less; and there are fewer contractions with orgasm, rapid loss of erection, and a longer refractory period.

Women also experience fewer orgasmic contractions; vasocongestion reduces more rapidly in older than in younger women. Fatty tissue loss in the pelvic area may predispose the clitoris to becoming more easily irritated. Vaginal estrogen cream or water-based lubricants can be applied directly to the vagina to treat such irritation. Diminished libido is more likely related to increased age, dyspareunia, body-image change secondary to breast or gynecological surgery, and psychosocial factors rather than to the physiology of menopause. Hormone replacement alone is not sufficient to restore flagging libido or loss of interest in sexual activity.

DISEASES AND DIAGNOSTICS ASSOCIATED WITH SEXUAL DYSFUNCTION

Various endocrine, vascular, neurological, and psychological diseases and their pharmacological treatments can affect sexual health. Medications that may cause ED include the selective serotonin reuptake inhibitors (SSRIs), tranquilizers, anticholinergics, and antipsychotics (Lindau, Schumm, & Laumann, 2007). Bupropion is less likely to cause sexual side effects than the SSRIs. In addition, almost all antihypertensive drugs have been implicated in sexual dysfunction. These include diuretics, sympatholytics such as alpha-methyldopa, beta-blockers, alpha-blockers, vasodilators, calcium channel blockers, and angiotensin-converting enzyme (ACE) inhibitors (Lindau et al., 2007).

Postmenopausal estrogen deficiency causes changes in the entire pelvic region, including reduction in the length of the vaginal vault, atrophy of the vaginal epithelium, and reduced amount and acidity of vaginal secretions, all of which predispose to infections and can cause dyspareunia. Urinary incontinence and irritation of the bladder and urethra because of thinning of the vaginal wall may also discourage a woman from having sexual relations. For older men, ED is the most common of sexual dysfunction, with vascular disease being the most common cause. It is associated with many medications, prior surgical procedures, and disease processes. Emotional factors associated with ED include anxiety, depression, alcohol use, and fatigue. Treatment approaches include self-injection of intracavernosal medications that are smooth muscle relaxants (i.e., prostaglandin E, papaverine, and phentolamine in a combined low dose); oral ingestion of phosphodiesterase inhibitors, including sildenafil citrate (Viagra), vardenafil (Levitra), and tadalafil (Cialis); external vacuum devices; implants or prostheses; and revascularization. The phosphodiesterase inhibitors should not be taken more than once daily and are contraindicated in patients who are on nitrates. Vacuum devices are the least invasive; newer models reduce ejaculatory pain associated with earlier devices.

Certain diseases and medical conditions are associated with sexual side effects. For example, after a stroke, men can have erectile and ejaculatory difficulties, and women may experience reduced vaginal secretions. Parkinson's disease is associated with loss of sexual desire and other sexual dysfunctions. L-Dopa improves sexual performance because it elicits a richer sense of well-being and increased mobility. Men and women with diabetes mellitus may have a variety of sexual difficulties at earlier ages than other individuals. Men may experience ED and decreased libido, and women may develop clitoral nerve damage and vascular damage (Lindau et al., 2007). Three months after a myocardial infarction (MI), if the patient can climb two flights of steps without chest pain, sexual activity can be resumed.

INTERVENTIONS FOR AND PREVENTION OF SEXUAL DYSFUNCTION

Lifestyle changes in midlife, such as regular exercise, reduced-fat diet, and smoking cessation, increase the probability of remaining potent and sexually active. Interventions and prevention strategies must, of necessity, be contingent on careful assessment and identification of contributing factors. Clinicians and caregivers may need time to recognize and understand their own feelings about sexual activity, the source of their attitudes, and the range of options for older people.

Those who are isolated by location, finances, lack of a partner, or language proficiency may require counseling and community-based support services. Recently there has been increased attention on the value of sexual relationships in long-term care facilities and encouraging dating in senior centers, as well as online matchmaking services for seniors. Clinicians must address chronic medical conditions, including pain, and must address the benefit, burden, and consequences of each treatment option. Appropriate physical fitness programs for cardiac patients can moderate the physical signs and anxiety associated with sexual activity. Those suffering from arthritis can achieve sexual pleasure with a combination of effective arthritis-management strategies and sexual-position change.

Clinicians should assess the older patient's sexuality, validate and reassure age-related sexuality changes, counsel and educate patients who must cope with altered body image and age effects, and refer patients for special diagnostics and therapy when indicated. This requires sensitivity to the culture, constraints, language, and sexual interests of the patients. A therapeutic environment between provider and patient recognizes the embarrassment, for some, associated with sexual topics and language. The clinician must balance support of an older person's possible lack of interest in sexual activity while dispelling the myths and stereotypes that reduced physical intimacy is a natural consequence of aging.

See also HIV, AIDS, and Aging; Physical and Mental Health Needs of Older LGBT Adults; Social Isolation; Social Supports (Formal and Informal).

Steven L. Baumann

Centers for Disease Control and Prevention. (2014). *HIV surveillance report* (Vol. 26). Retrieved from http://www.cdc.gov/hiv/library/reports/surveillance

Gentili, A., & Mulligan, T. (2013). *Disorders of sexual function* (pp. 488–494). Geriatric Review Syllabus Book 1. New York, NY: American Geriatrics Society.

Lindau, S. T., Schumm, L. P., & Laumann, E. O. (2007). A study of sexuality and health among older adults in the United States. *New England Journal of Medicine, 357,* 762–774.

Waite, L. J., Laumann, E. O., Das, A., & Schumm, P. (2009). Sexuality: Measures of partnerships, practices, attitudes, and problems in the national social life, health, and aging study. *Journals of Gerontology: Series B, Psychological Sciences and Social Sciences, 64B*(Suppl. 1), i56–i66.

Web Resources
Helpguide: Lifelong Sexuality: http://www.helpguide.org/elder/sexuality_aging.htm
National Institute on Aging: Sexuality in later life: http://www.nia.nih.gov/health/publication/sexuality-later-life

SIGNAGE

Signs are a way of compensating for an unfamiliar environment and would be unnecessary if other forms of wayfinding were adequate (Calori & Vanden-Eynden, 2015). It is ironic that hospitals and large residential institutions are some of the most unfamiliar environments (Marquardt, 2011), yet the people who have to interact with these environments may have the most difficulty reading or understanding signs.

The ability to navigate independently through an environment enhances autonomy. An environment that is difficult to navigate can make people feel confused, anxious, irritable, or frustrated. They may lose confidence or form a poor image of the institution. Staff may become frustrated by visitors frequently asking them how to find their destination.

Older adults tend to be of smaller stature than younger adults some may have a slight forward head tilt. Poor eyesight and cognitive dementia, more common in older adults, can make reading and understanding signs difficult. Age-related vision changes include opacities in the central lens (i.e., cataracts), opacities in the periphery of the lens, changes in the vitreous (resulting in an increased scattering of light), deterioration in visual acuity (even in the absence of cataracts), yellowing of the lens, and decreased upward gaze in some people. These changes may cause difficulty reading small writing or indistinct lettering, unevenness in the perception of color, and sensitivity to glare. Sensitivity to glare becomes even more problematic in bright light or environments with bright surfaces. Glaucoma, if present, can constrict peripheral vision. The effects of dementia that can affect a person's ability to recognize signs are a decreased ability to read, interpret abstract symbols, reason or problem-solve, and make a mental map of a building or space; elders can also have an unreliable memory of recent events.

SIGN ATTRIBUTES

Signs should be easily seen, easily understood, and attractive. They should be designed primarily for people unfamiliar with the environment, such as visitors or people with poor memory, rather than for staff. The lettering should be clear and simple. Generally, a sans serif font is easier to read for short signs. A combination of uppercase and lowercase is preferable because the use of all upper case letters removes the word's "shape" and decreases legibility.

Dark lettering on a light background with minimal use of different colors is easiest to read. Blue can be difficult to differentiate from black. Red on black is difficult for color-blind people. Yet, certain colors are internationally associated with safety. Red indicates prohibition or stop. Yellow indicates caution or risk of danger, such as where infectious or hazardous materials are present. Blue indicates some mandatory action, such as, "Break glass in case of fire." Green indicates a safe action or safe condition, such as a fire exit (www.iso.org). Conventions in current practice may not carry the same meaning for people from a different culture (Hashim, Alkaabi, & Bharwani, 2014) or for different age-cohorts or people with cognitive decline due to memories of an earlier time (Calkins, 1988).

The size of a sign should be determined by its location and the target population. The minimum recommended letter height for the general population is that capital letters should be 1 in. high for every 30 feet of viewing distance (or 3-cm high for every 10-m viewing distance; McLendon & Blackistone, 1982). The size should be larger for an elderly population.

Images can enhance comprehension but should be used in addition to words, not as a replacement for them (Gross et al., 2004; Hashim et al., 2014). The image should be realistic rather than abstract. People with dementia find a realistic picture of a toilet more recognizable than the international symbol of a male or female stick figure. Potential images should be tested on the target population (Hashim et al., 2014; Wilkinson, Henschke, & Handscombe, 1995).

To the extent possible, language should be in "plain English" and use natural speech, such as would be used when talking to a friend. Depending on the local culture, *toilet* is usually preferable to *rest room, lavatory, bathroom,* or *powder room. X-ray Department* is more easily understood by laypeople than *Department of Medical Imaging* or *Radiology*. People understand *ear, nose, and throat* more easily than *otorhinolaryngology*. The language should be friendly and positive. For example, *No Parking* can be made more positive by erecting an arrow and sign to the *Visitors' Car Park*.

LOCATION AND ENVIRONMENT

Sign location is best determined by assuming the role of a visitor coming to the building for the first time. Every point throughout the building that requires a decision by the visitor should have a sign. Signs protruding perpendicular to a wall may be more visible in some situations, but they should not be placed too high.

In a complex environment, a hierarchy of signs can be helpful (Calori & Vanden-Eynden, 2015; Gibson, 2009). Directions can be given to a general area and, as a person approaches the desired destination, more specific directions can be given. Ideally, a sign should provide only enough information to allow someone to reach the next decision point. The more information provided, the longer it takes to read and the harder it is to remember. Signs intended for staff use can be differentiated from those intended for public use. Signs for staff can be smaller, in a different color, and placed below those for the public.

Lighting should be sufficient but should not create glare. Signs placed in a "puddle" of darkness between two bright areas are harder to see and less likely to be regarded as important. Glare comes not only from inappropriate lighting but also from shiny or polished surfaces.

Signs are not just written labels or symbols. Latent clues, such as placing chairs outside a room designed for sitting, are a form of sign that may be more comprehensible than writing. Labeling of some areas, such as toilets, may require a combination of sign clues. Some people may follow a clearly written sign, some may recognize a bright canopy above the door, some may be guided by the door color, and others may need personal guidance. Ensuring that all toilet doors are a particular color, all exit doors are a different color, and all cupboard doors are the same color as the walls are important indicators of their function. A reception area is more recognizable if it is in an open, accessible space, has a counter with someone behind it, and is well lit.

Signs should be considered in the overall design of a building rather than as an afterthought. The environment should be as self-explanatory as possible and should not rely on the people being able to remember where they are or how they got there (Judd, Marshall, &

Phippen, 1998). Signs are necessary when there has been a failure or inability to achieve this. They should avoid unnecessary detail and be simple, attractive, clearly written, well placed, and designed with the first-time visitor in mind.

See also Environmental Modifications: Home, Institutional; Vision Changes and Care.

Tim J. Wilkinson

Calkins, M. P. (1988). *Designing for dementia: Planning environments for the elderly and the confused.* Owings Mills, MD: National Health Publishing.

Calori, C., & Vanden-Eynden, D. (2015). *Signage and wayfinding design: A complete guide to creating environmental graphic design systems* (2nd ed.). Hoboken, NJ: John Wiley.

Gibson, D. (2009). *The wayfinding handbook: Information design for public places.* New York, NY: Princeton Architectural Press.

Gross, J., Harmon, M. E., Myers, R. A., Evans, R. L., Kay, N. R., Rodriguez-Charbonier, S., & Herzog, T. R. (2004). Recognition of self among persons with dementia: Pictures versus names as environmental supports. *Environment and Behavior, 36*(3), 424–454.

Hashim, M. J., Alkaabi, M. S., & Bharwani, S. (2014). Interpretation of way-finding healthcare symbols by a multicultural population: Navigation signage design for global health. *Applied Ergonomics, 45*(3), 503–509.

Judd, S., Marshall, M., & Phippen, P. (1998). *Design for dementia.* London, UK: Hawker Publications.

Marquardt, G. (2011). Wayfinding for people with dementia: A review of the role of architectural design. *Health Environments Research & Design Journal, 4*(2), 75–90.

McLendon, C. B., & Blackistone, M. (1982). *Signage: Graphic communications in the build world.* New York, NY: McGraw-Hill.

Wilkinson, T. J., Henschke, P. J., & Handscombe, K. (1995). How should toilets be labelled for people with dementia? *Australian Journal on Aging, 14,* 163–165.

Web Resources
ADA Accessibility Guidelines for Buildings and Facilities (ADAAG): https://www.access-board.gov/guidelines-and-standards/buildings-and-sites/about-the-ada-standards/background/adaag

Alzheimer's Australia. Dementia Care and the Built Environment: Position Paper 3. 2004: https://fightdementia.org.au/files/20040600_Nat_NP_3DemCareBuiltEnv.pdf

Keane-Cowell, S. Signs of the times: https://www.architonic.com/en/story/simon-keane-cowell-signs-of-the-times/7000779

Project for Public Spaces: http://www.pps.org/reference/signage_guide

SKIN ISSUES: BRUISES AND DISCOLORATION

General health, diet, heredity, activity, and environmental exposure influence the rate at which age-related skin changes occur. Changes in the function and appearance of the skin because of aging alone, known as *intrinsic aging*, include decreased wound healing, decreased elasticity and tensile strength, diminished ability to respond to injury, decreased mechanical protection and insulation, and diminished ability to thermoregulate (Kane, Ouslander, Abrass, & Resnick, 2013; Yaar & Gilchrest, 2012).

Most age-related skin changes are not the result of aging alone but because of a combination of aging and chronic environmental exposure, primarily sun exposure, which causes the most damaging and cosmetically compromising effects on the skin (Yaar & Gilchrest, 2012). This process, *photo aging*, is responsible for wrinkling and yellowing of the skin and thickening of the epidermis on sun-exposed areas. In addition, sebaceous glands enlarge, blood vessels become dilated and tortuous, and skin pigmentation becomes mottled. The physiological consequences of the intrinsic aging result in the characteristic features commonly observed in the skin of older adults, such as fragility, tears, discoloration, and bruising. However, discoloration and bruising may be accelerated or exacerbated by the effects of photo aging.

Although it is commonly believed that the epidermis thins with advanced age, research shows flattening of the dermal–epidermal junction because of retraction of the papillae that connect the dermis to the epidermis. The result is a reduction in the surface area of the skin rather than an actual thinning of the epidermis; it leads to poor adhesion among these two layers and an overall decrease in the resilience of the skin. The combination of these factors results in the separation of these layers and the likelihood of skin tears. Older adults are therefore more susceptible to bruises, blistering, and abrasions from mechanical stress or shear-type injuries.

Changes in the pigmentation, or coloration, of the skin, also are noticeable with age. Melanocytes in the epidermis show some decline in function; the remaining cells may be unevenly distributed and not functioning normally. As a result, the skin becomes blotchy and unevenly pigmented, with areas of brown, spotty pigmentation frequently occurring on the scalp, neck, face, arms, and hands. These benign macular lesions are commonly referred to as *age spots*. A decrease in melanocytes also reduces tanning, and the ability of the remaining melanocytes to shield the underlying dermis from ultraviolet rays is diminished (Kane et al., 2013; Yaar & Gilchrest, 2012). Thus older adults are at increased risk for sun exposure skin damage, predisposing to both benign and malignant skin changes.

The density, cellularity, and vascularity of the dermis progressively diminish with aging, resulting in the loss of elasticity and turgor and less "give" under stress. The characteristic pale, thin, paper-like quality of the skin further contributes to tear-type injuries. Vascular changes in the dermis predispose older adults to *petechiae*, or minor bruising. The thin-walled, fragile blood vessels lose their connective tissue support. Following minor trauma, petechiae develop, because of the fragile nature of the skin and increased capillary fragility. Areas of ecchymosis subsequently develop. These well-defined, red-brown macules, termed *senile purpura*, vary in size from a few millimeters to several centimeters (Yaar & Gilchrest, 2012). They occur most commonly on the exposed surfaces of the forearms and hands but can occur elsewhere as well.

Minor bruising is a normal and common finding in older adults. Women usually bruise more easily than men, and a tendency to bruise easily may be hereditary. Bruising from minor injuries is common in the forearms, hands, legs, and feet. Age-related changes in the skin, coupled with the damaging effects of sun exposure, cause blood vessels to break easily, leading to bruising. Bruising also may be an indicator of a pathological process, such as acute leukemia or Cushing's syndrome (Valente & Abramson, 2006). Other comorbid conditions that can preclude bruising include cardiac valve disorders, hypothyroidism, liver disease, renal disease, autoimmune disease, a myeloproliferative neoplasm, and lymphoproliferative disease (Rydz & James, 2012). In addition, a number of pharmacological agents can induce purpuric bleeding; these include sulfa drugs, aspirin, nonsteroidal anti-inflammatories, clopidogrel, thiazides, procaine penicillin, phenytoin, methyldopa, barbiturates, and anticoagulants such as heparin, warfarin, or novel oral anticoagulants such as dabigatran. Bleeding ceases when the drug is withdrawn. Of note, corticosteroids can thin the skin, increasing the likelihood of bruising from minor trauma. In addition, some dietary supplements such as fish oils, ginkgo biloba, ginger, and garlic have a blood-thinning effect, reducing the blood's ability to clot, thereby allowing enough blood to leak into the tissues to cause bruising. Also, deficiencies in vitamins B_{12}, C, and K or folic acid may increase the frequency of bleeding (Rydz & James, 2012).

Mosqueda, Burnight, and Liao (2005) studied the life cycle of bruises in 100 older adults aged 65 years and older (mean age = 83). Although a system of dating bruises may be helpful as a general guide, they concluded that the age of a bruise could not be reliably predicted by its color. They found that the period when bruises were visible varied from 4 to 41 days (mean = 11.73 ± 7.13 days). Half of the bruises (54%) resolved by day 6 and most (81%) resolved by day 11. Interestingly, contrary to the perception that yellow indicates an old bruise, 16 bruises were predominately yellow on the first day of observation, and 30 bruises were largely purple on the 10th day of observation. Although some research supports that a yellow color occurs significantly faster in individuals aged 65 years and older, it is clear that further research is necessary to learn more about bruising in this population. Nash and Sheridan (2009), as well as Mosqueda et al. (2005) noted that determining the age of a bruise primarily by its color in older adults is problematic and not the best practice. Although they indicate that there is more evidence on dating bruises in the pediatric population, this is not the case in the geriatric population.

The presentation of a bruise is influenced by many factors, including the amount of force and area of injury, the health status of the older adult, the condition of the skin, and medications known to induce purpuric bleeding. Major bruising can occur in individuals who have coagulation deficiencies, liver disease, and a warfarin overdose. Often, laboratory studies such as platelet count, bleeding time, prothrombin time, and partial thromboplastin time are performed when there is a question about the extent and amount of bruising present.

A thorough history and careful examination of the skin can provide important information about the health status of the older adult and possibly serious problems, such as falls, neglect, and abuse. Multiple bruises in various stages of healing may alert the clinician to problems of physical abuse, alcoholism, or self-neglect. Bruises that are larger than 5 cm, on the head and neck, lateral and anterior arms (especially the right arm), or posterior torso are suggestive indicators of physical elder abuse and should warrant further assessment (Rosen et al., 2016; Wiglesworth et al., 2009; Ziminski, Wiglesworth, Austin, Phillips, & Mosqueda, 2013). Clinical evaluation is based on a thorough understanding of the normal skin changes associated with aging. This knowledge is essential for distinguishing changes that may signal the presence of a more serious problem requiring further evaluation.

Maintaining skin integrity and preventing injury are important goals for clinicians working with older adults. Miller (2012) offers some helpful tips on skin care. Strategies to promote healthy skin include a diet with adequate amounts of vitamins A and C and fluids. Humidification and the application of emollient lotions at least twice a day, particularly after bathing, help prevent dryness, which makes the skin more susceptible to tears. Mild soaps such as Dove unscented, Cetaphil Restoraderm, CeraVe, or Aveeno should be used when bathing. Daily bathing (i.e., complete bath or shower) should be discouraged for those with dry skin. Suggestions on bathing patterns in this population vary from a partial daily bath to a complete bath two to three times per week (Miller, 2012). Restricting the amount of time in the shower or bath and using cool or lukewarm water is also recommended (Adis Medical Writers, 2015). In addition, skin-care products that contain alcohol or perfumes should be avoided because of their drying effect.

Exposure to ultraviolet radiation leads to free radical formation, which causes cell damage and death, leading to skin aging. Incorporating antioxidants into the diet in the form of vitamins A, C, D, and E and carotenoids, such as beta-carotene, lycopene, and lutein, helps fight against free radical formation and keeps the skin healthier. A diet rich in fruits and vegetables is the best way to accomplish adequate antioxidants for this purpose (Pappas, Liakao, & Zouboulis, 2016). Application of topical retinoids is effective and safe for managing photo-damaged skin and reducing the signs of skin aging for older adults. Clinical improvements include the reduction of coarse wrinkling, skin roughness, and appearance of skin discolorations and increased smoothness of the skin (Darlenski, Surber, & Fluhr, 2010; Kang, Valerio, Bahadoran, & Ortonne, 2009; Riahi, Bush, & Cohen, 2016).

Older adults can avoid sun damage by wearing sun visors, wide-brimmed hats, and long-sleeved cotton shirts while in the sun. A broad-spectrum sunscreen with an SPF of at least 30 should frequently be applied to protect against UVA and UVB rays. Older adults should be encouraged to avoid sun exposure during the late morning and early afternoon.

Frequent changes in position are important for older adults who have an activity or mobility limitations. Skin breakdown is more likely to occur in the presence of impaired circulation and external pressure. Many pressure-relieving appliances are useful in maintaining skin integrity. Proper positioning in bed, with the head of the bed elevated and the knees flexed and supported, helps prevent shearing of the skin against the bed surface.

Environmental factors such as cluttered rooms; poor lighting; slippery floors; throw rugs; low, soft furniture; small animals; and sharp-cornered objects are the cause of many accidental injuries. These potential hazards can be avoided by creating an environment that is safe, well-lit, comfortable, and stimulating for the older adult. Home assessments to reduce fall risks is an important part of caring for the older adult. Prevention plays a key role in maintaining skin integrity and reducing potential problems.

See also Pressure Injury; Skin Tears.

Barbara J. Edlund and Kathy VanRavenstein

Adis Medical Writers. (2015). Manage chronic pruritus in the elderly with various agents depending on the pathophysiology and aetiology of the condition. *Drugs and Therapy Perspectives, 31*(9), 302–306.

Darlenski, R., Surber, C., & Fluhr, J. W. (2010). Topical retinoids in the management of photodamaged skin: From theory to evidence-based practical approach. *British Journal of Dermatology, 163*(6), 1157–1165.

Kane, R., Ouslander, J. G., Abrass, I., & Resnick, B. (2013). *Essentials of clinical geriatrics* (7th ed.). New York, NY: McGraw-Hill.

Kang, H. Y., Valerio, L., Bahadoran, P., & Ortonne, J. P. (2009). The role of topical retinoids in the treatment of pigmentary disorders: An evidence-based review. *American Journal of Clinical Dermatology, 10*(4), 251–260.

Miller, C. A. (2012). *Nursing of wellness in older adults*. Philadelphia, PA: Lippincott Williams & Wilkins.

Mosqueda, L., Burnight, K., & Liao, S. (2005). The life cycle of bruises in older adults. *Journal of the American Geriatrics Society, 53*(8), 1339–1343.

Nash, K. R., & Sheridan, D. J. (2009). Can one accurately date a bruise? State of the science. *Journal of Forensic Nursing, 5*(1), 31–37.

Pappas, A., Liakou, A., & Zouboulis, C. C. (2016). Nutrition and skin. *Reviews in Endocrine & Metabolic Disorders, 17*(3), 443–448. doi:10.1007/s11154-016-9374-z

Riahi, R. R., Bush, A. E., & Cohen, P. R. (2016). Topical retinoids: Therapeutic mechanisms in the treatment of photodamaged skin. *American Journal of Clinical Dermatology, 17*(3), 265–276.

Rosen, T., Bloemen, E. M., LoFaso, V. M., Clark, S., Flomenbaum, N. E., & Lachs, M. S. (2016). Emergency department presentations for injuries in older adults independently known to be victims of elder abuse. *Journal of Emergency Medicine, 50*(3), 518–526.

Rydz, N., & James, P. D. (2012). Why is my patient bleeding or bruising? *Hematology/Oncology Clinics of North America, 26*(2), 321–344, viii.

Valente, M. J., & Abramson, N. (2006). Easy bruisability. *Southern Medical Journal, 99*(4), 366–370.

Wiglesworth, A., Austin, R., Corona, M., Schneider, D., Liao, S., Gibbs, L., & Mosqueda, L. (2009). Bruising as a marker of physical elder abuse. *Journal of the American Geriatrics Society, 57*(7), 1191–1196.

Yaar, M., & Gilchrest, B. A. (2012). Aging skin. In L. Goldsmith, S. Katz, B. Gilchrest, A. Paller, D. Leffell, & K. Wolf (Eds.), *Fitzpatrick's dermatology in general medicine* (pp. 1213–1226): New York, NY: McGraw-Hill.

Ziminski, C. E., Wiglesworth, A., Austin, R., Phillips, L. R., & Mosqueda, L. (2013). Injury patterns and causal mechanisms of bruising in physical elder abuse. *Journal of Forensic Nursing, 9*(2), 84–91; quiz E1.

Web Resources

American Academy of Family Physicians: Bleeding and Bruising: http://www.aafp.org/afp/2016/0215/p279.html

Clinical Evaluation of Bleeding and Bruising in Primary Care POGOe: https://www.pogoe.org

Elder Mistreatment Assessment: https://consultgeri.org/try-this/general-assessment/issue-15

Medline Plus: http://www.nlm.nih.gov/medlineplus/ency/article/003235.htm

SKIN TEARS

Skin tears are a common injury among older adults, particularly those who are institutionalized. The prevalence of skin tears was found to be 3.3% to 22% in hospital patients and 5.5% in home-care clients (Strazzieri-Pulido, Picolo Peres, Campanili, & Conceicao de Gouveia Santos, 2015). It is widely believed that skin tears are significantly underreported because of their perceived low risk. Since April 2012, the Centers for Medicare & Medicaid Services (CMS) has required long-term care facilities to record the skin tears in section M 1.040 G. (www.cms.gov) and reports a prevalence rate of ranging from a low of 4.7% to a high of 5.4% over 2012 to 2016. Costs for care of skin tears have been estimated at $10 per day for up to 30 days, for an estimated annual expense of $4.5 billion (Stephen-Haynes, Callaghan, Bethell, & Greenwood, 2011). A skin tear can be a source of pain and disfigurement, as well as a site for infection; it is important that facilities have detailed, evidence-based protocols in place for consistent care.

DEFINITION AND CLASSIFICATION

Over the years the definition of a skin tear as an acute wound (either partial or full thickness) has evolved (LeBlanc & Baranoski, 2011; LeBlanc, Baranoski, Christensen, et al., 2013; Payne & Martin, 1990). The International Skin Tear Advisory Panel (ISTAP) currently defines *skin tears* as:

A wound caused by shear, friction, and/or blunt force resulting in separation of skin layers. A skin tear can be partial-thickness (separation of the epidermis from the dermis) or full thickness (separation of both the epidermis and dermis from underlying structures). (LeBlanc et al., 2016, pp. 34–35)

There are several classification systems for skin tears used around the world. The Payne–Martin system was developed in 1990 and revised in 1993. The system consists of three categories and two subcategories:

Category I: Skin tear without loss of tissue. The epidermal flap either completely covers the dermis or covers the dermis to within 1 mm of the wound margin.
 Ia: Linear type
 Ib: Flap type
Category II: Skin tears with partial tissue loss
 IIa: Scant tissue loss (25% or less)
 IIb: Moderate to large loss of tissue (more than 25% loss of the epidermal flap)
Category III: Skin tears with complete tissue loss (Payne & Martin, 1993)

The STAR Skin Tear Classification system resulted from a study that aimed to gain consensus from wound experts in Australia on classification and testing reliability. It is a refined version of the Payne–Martin Classification system commonly used in Australia.

Category Ia: A skin tear where the edges can be realigned to the normal anatomical position (without undue stretching) and the skin or flap color is not pale, dusky, or darkened.
Category Ib: A skin tear where the edges can be realigned to the normal anatomical position (without undue stretching) and the skin or flap color is pale, dusky, or darkened.
Category IIa: A skin tear where the edges cannot be realigned to the normal anatomical position and the skin or flap color is not pale, dusky, or darkened.
Category IIb: A skin tear where the edges cannot be realigned to the normal anatomical position and the skin or flap color is pale, dusky, or darkened.
Category III: A skin tear where the skin is completely absent (Carville et al., 2007).

A more simplified classification system with only three categories has been proposed (LeBlanc & Baranoski, 2011; LeBlanc, Baranoski, Christensen, et al., 2013) and validated for intra- and inter-rater reliability (LeBlanc, Baranoski, Holloway, & Langemo, 2013). This ISTAP Skin Tear Classification (Figure S.1) is as follows:

Type 1: No skin loss. Linear or flap tear can be repositioned to cover the wound bed.
Type 2: Partial flap loss. Partial flap loss that cannot be repositioned to cover the wound bed.
Type 3: Total flap loss. Entire wound bed is exposed.
(LeBlanc & Baranoski, 2011; LeBlanc, Baranoski, Christensen, et al., 2013; LeBlanc et al., 2016).

Some 80% of skin tears occur in the upper extremities, particularly in the forearms, elbows, and hands. Other sites include the shin, back, and buttocks. Skin tears over bony prominences should not be mistaken for Stage 2 pressure injuries, which have a different etiology and treatment.

CAUSES

There are many causes of skin tears (Baranoski, LeBlanc, & Gloeckner, 2016). Families and patients often perceive skin tears as the result of poor care or rough handling. Skin tears can occur as the result of a fall, and are captured on the CMS MDS 3.0 under section J (www.CMS.gov); skin tears from other causes are captured under section M1040G. Providers should assess patients with skin tears for risk of abuse or neglect. Recurrent skin tears may also be predictive of more serious health problems, such as delayed healing. More than half of reported skin tears have no apparent cause. Wheelchair injuries account for 25% of skin tears, accidental bumping into objects in the room for 25%, transfers for 18%, and falls for about 135% of skin tears (McGough-Csary & Kopac, 1998).

Skin tears originate with both intrinsic and extrinsic risk factors (see Table S.1; Baranoski, LeBlanc, & Gloeckner, 2016). Intrinsic factors include the normal dermal and subcutaneous tissue loss associated with aging, as well as the loss of tensile strength and elasticity. Slow production of sebum causes the skin to be drier. The rete pegs, which are the structures responsible for the adherence of the epidermis to the dermis, shorten with aging, making separation of the layers more likely with the application of directional force (e.g., friction, shear). Other factors increasing a patient's risk for skin tears include diminished sensation, cognitive decline, polypharmacy, chronic disease, poor nutrition, systemic steroid therapy, falls, stiffness and spasticity, limited vision, dementia, polypharmacy,

and history of previous tears (Ayello, 2003). ISTAP has a comprehensive tool kit and a skin tear risk-assessment pathway, as well as a guide to risk reduction program (www.skintears.org).

Extrinsic factors include impaired mobility, history of falls, lifts and transfers, repositioning, bathing frequency and type of soap, and use of assistive devices (such as wheelchairs). Furniture arrangement, clutter, and room lighting also contribute to skin tear risk (Baranoski, 2000; LeBlanc & Baranoski, 2011; LeBlanc, Baranoski, Christensen, 2013; LeBlanc et al., 2016). Most of the skin tear prevention literature is based on expert opinion (LeBlanc et al., 2016).

DOCUMENTATION

The wound should be described on discovery, including the exact location, size in centimeters, direction of the skin tear flap (if still present), appearance, associated pain, drainage type/amount, treatment measures, and circumstances leading to the injury, if known. Following the wound bed preparation model, begin with the identification and treatment for the cause. If the cause was lift-related, for example, the care plan should be amended to include lifting precautions. Individual facilities may require an incident report. It is advisable to notify the

Table S.1
FACTORS ASSOCIATED WITH INCREASED RISK OF SKIN TEARS

Intrinsic Factors	Extrinsic Factors
• Female sex	• Inadequate nutritional intake
• White race	• Polypharmacy
• Immobility	• Using assistive devices
• Presence of ecchymosis	• Application and removal of stockings
• History of previous skin tears	• Removal of tape or dressings
• Long-term corticosteroid use	• Blood draws
• Dependence for ADL	• Transfer and falls
• Altered sensory status	• Prosthetic devices
• Cognitive impairment	• Skin cleansers
• Limb stiffness and spasticity	
• Neuropathy	
• Very young (neonate) or very old (more than 75 years of age)	
• Vascular problems	
• Cardiac problems	
• Pulmonary problems	
• Visual impairment	
• Incontinence, MASD	

ADL, activities of daily living; MASD, moisture-associated skin damage.
Source. Baranoski, LeBlanc, and Gloeckner (2016).

patient's family or significant others; such notification may be mandated. The wound should be assessed and described at least weekly in documentation. Collection of data on skin tears can lead to process quality improvement in a facility (Baranoski, 2000). Use of the new ISTAP classification system should be considered for identifying the three types of skin tears and the skin tear decision algorithm for selection of care interventions (Figure S.1).

TREATMENT

Recommendations for skin tear prevention and treatment are based on expert opinion and emerging evidence (Figure S.2; Baranoski, Ayello, Levine, Leblanc, & Tomic-Canic, 2016; LeBlanc & Baranoski, 2011; LeBlanc, Christensen, Orstead, & Keast, 2008; LeBlanc et al., 2016; Pennsylvania Safety Authority Skin Tear Initiative, 2006; Ratliff & Fletcher, 2007). The skin tear should be gently irrigated with sterile normal saline, clean/potable water, or a pH-balanced wound cleanser at a low pressure of less than 8 psi to remove drainage, blood, and debris (LeBlanc & Baranoski, 2011; LeBlanc

et al., 2008; Pennsylvania Safety Authority Skin Tear Initiative, 2006). ISTAP recommends the use of topical antiseptic solutions for non-healing or skin tears where bacterial burden outweighs healing (LeBlanc et al., 2016). If necrotic tissue is in the skin tear, debridement when there is adequate blood flow is indicated (LeBlanc et al., 2016). Tetanus toxoid should be given before debridement as exotoxin may be released with tissue manipulation (LeBlanc et al., 2016).

If the edges of the skin flap can be approximated over the wound (category or type 1), the flap is replaced on the wound edges using sterile technique. ISTAP no longer recommends that edges of the skin flap be affixed to the surrounding skin with wound-closure strips (e.g., SteriStrips) because it can prevent additional trauma to the periwound skin and skin tear flap). Rather, the health care provider should consider using 2-octyl cyanoacrylate topical bandage (skin glue; LeBlanc et al., 2016). Category or type 2 skin tears should have the partial skin flap straightened and approximated over the wound (Baranoski et al., 2012; LeBlanc & Baranoski, 2011).

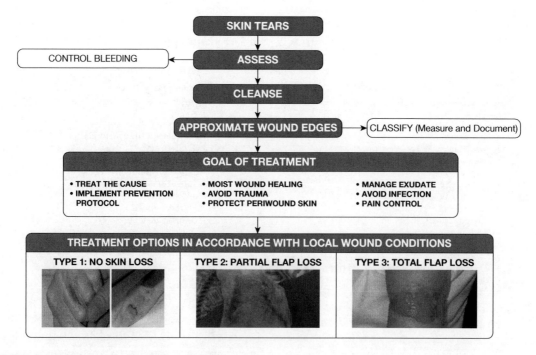

FIGURE S.1 Skin tear decision algorithm.

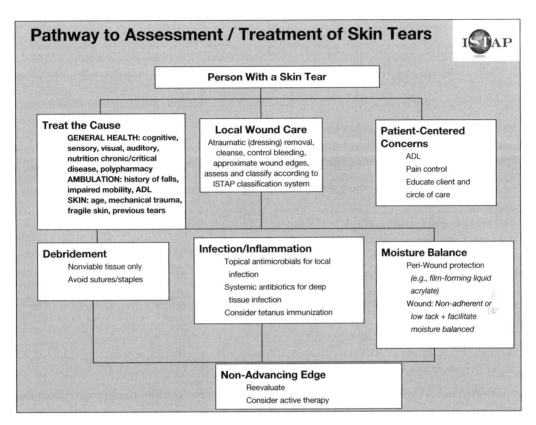

FIGURE S.2 Pathway to assessment/treatment of skin tears.

ADL, activities of daily living; ISTAP, International Skin Tear Advisory Panel.

Source: Adapted from Sibbald et al. (2008). Modified from LeBlanc, Christensen, Orstead, and Keast (2008). © ISTAP 2016.

Type of dressing should be matched to the category of the skin tears (LeBlanc & Baranoski, 2011; LeBlanc et al., 2016). Dressings that provide a moist wound-healing environment but do not cause further tearing or damage to the skin should be chosen (LeBlanc et al., 2016). Various experts and protocols suggest covering the skin tear with a nonocclusive, nonadherent, dressing such as nonadherent mesh dressings, foam dressings, hydrogels, alignate, hydrofiber, and acrylic dressings. The dressing should not stick to the wound bed. Some clinicians are reporting good results with nonadherent silicone dressings, which can be removed to visualize the wound and then replaced. Absorptive dressings, such as gauze 4 × 4s or rolled gauze, can be applied over the nonadherent to absorb drainage and to keep the dressing in place. The dressing should be changed as often as necessary to keep it clean and dry. Dressings should be held in place using stocking-like products or gauze wraps rather than tape (LeBlanc et al., 2016). For infected skin tears, ISTAP recommends using methylene blue, gentian violet, or silver dressings (LeBlanc et al., 2016). For skin tears that are located on lower limbs, management of peripheral edema by compression therapy needs to be part of the treatment plan (LeBlanc et al., 2016). Pain medications administered on a regular basis may be necessary for the patient to continue with daily activities and/or dressing changes (Ayello, 2003).

S

TREATMENTS TO AVOID

Although common treatment for skin tears in the past has included the use of transparent occlusive film dressings, ISTAP does not recommend their use because they may cause injury to the skin on removal (LeBlanc et al., 2016). Accumulation of exudate at the wound site can lead to maceration of healthy tissue. Removal of these very adherent dressings can cause additional skin trauma (White, Karam, & Cowell, 1994).

If a patient is admitted with a transparent dressing already in place over a skin tear, it may be better to leave it in place rather than cause further injury by changing the dressing. If an area of liquefied blood appears under the dressing, it can be left alone unless the site appears infected (Baranoski, 2000). To remove a transparent film dressing, the skin should be gently pushed away from the dressing rather than removing the dressing from the skin. Dressings that are not nonadherent, such as gauze, should not be placed directly over the skin tear. Tape should not be applied to at-risk skin. Antimicrobials such as hexachlorophene, povidone/iodine, and chlorhexidine are not recommended as these wounds are usually clean and free from bacteria.

PREVENTION

Assessment of risk is an important step in preventing skin tears. The Skin Integrity Risk Assessment Tool (White et al., 1994) is not well known. Patients dependent on others for all activities of daily living (ADL) are at greatest risk, with tears occurring during lifting, positioning, transferring, dressing, and bathing. Independently ambulating patients have the second highest number of skin tears, occurring mostly on the lower extremities. The third highest category of patients with skin tears are sight impaired, who sustained their injuries from bumping into furniture and equipment (White et al., 1994). Skin tears can result from falls, so implementing a fall-reduction protocol may help prevent skin tears (LeBlanc & Baranoski, 2011). ISTAP recently conducted a review of the literature and has compiled a list of factors associated with increased risk of skin tears (see Table S.1; Baranoski, LeBlanc, & Gloeckner, 2016).

Caregivers should be knowledgeable about proper positioning, lifting, and transferring techniques and devices to reduce friction and shear. The use of a gait belt under the axillae can help the caregiver lift without using the patient's arms. Hard surfaces in the patient environment, such as wheelchair arms, leg supports, and bed rails can be padded. Clearing a safe, well-lit path for sight-impaired elders is also helpful. If agreeable, the patient should wear long sleeves and pants (White et al., 1994). Patients at risk should be bathed less often, no more than three times weekly, with an emollient soap. The use of adherents such as tape to secure dressings and tubes should be avoided.

See also Skin Issues: Bruises and Discoloration.

Elizabeth A. Ayello and Carol L. B. Ott

Ayello, E. A. (2003). Preventing pressure ulcers and skin tears. In M. D. Mezey, T. Fulmer, I. Abraham, & D. A. Zwicker (Eds.), *Geriatric nursing protocols for best practice* (2nd ed., pp. 165–184). New York, NY: Springer Publishing.

Baranoski, S. (2000). Skin tears: The enemy of frail skin. *Advances in Skin and Wound Care, 13*, 123–126.

Baranoski, S., Ayello E. A., Levine, J. M., LeBlanc, K., & Tomic-Canic, M. (2016). Skin: An essential organ. In S. Baranoski & E. A. Ayello (Eds.), *Wound care essentials: Practice principles* (4th ed., pp. 52–81). Philadelphia, PA: Wolters Kluwer.

Baranoski, S., LeBlanc, K., & Gloeckner, M. (2016). Preventing, assessing and managing skin tears: A clinical review. *American Journal of Nursing, 116*(11), 24–30. Retrieved from http://www.nursing center.com/cearticle?an=00000446-201611000 -00025&Journal_ID=54030&Issue_ID=3847557

Carville, K., Lewin, G., Newall, N., Haslehurst, P., Michael, R., Santamaria, N., & Roberts, P. (2007). STAR: A consensus for skin tear classification. *Primary Intention, 15*(1), 18–28.

Centers for Medicare & Medicaid Services. (2012). MDS 3.0 RAI manual. Retrieved from http:// www.cms.gov/Medicare/Quality-Initiatives -Patient-Assessment-Instruments/NursingHome QualityInits/MDS30RAIManual.html

LeBlanc, K., & Baranoski, S. (2011). Skin tears: State of the science: Consensus statements for the prevention, prediction, assessment, and treatment of skin tears. *Advances in Skin and Wound Care, 24*(9, Suppl. 1), 2–15.

LeBlanc, K., Baranoski, S., Christensen, D., Langemo, D., Sammon, M. A., Edwards, K., ... Regan, M. (2013). International Skin Tear Advisory Panel: A tool kit to aid in the prevention, assessment, and treatment of skin tears using a simplified classification system. *Advances in Skin and Wound Care, 26*(10), 459–476.

LeBlanc, K., Baranoski, S., Holloway, S., & Langemo, D. (2013). Validation of a new classification system for skin tears. *Advances in Skin and Wound Care, 26*(6), 263–265.

LeBlanc, K., Baranoski, S., Christensen, D., Langemo, D., Edwards, K., Holloway, S., ... Woo, K. Y. (2016). The art of dressing selection: A consensus statement on skin tears and best practice. *Advances in Skin & Wound Care, 29*(1), 32–46.

LeBlanc, K., Christensen, D., Orstead, K., & Keast, D. (2008). Best practice recommendations for the prevention and treatment of skin tears. *Wound Care Canada, 6*(8), 14–32.

McGough-Csary, J., & Kopac, C. (1998). Skin tears in institutionalized elderly: An epidemiological study. *Ostomy Wound Management, 44*, 14S–24S.

Payne, R. L., & Martin, M. (1990). The epidemiology and management of skin tears in older adults. *Ostomy Wound Management, 26*, 26–37.

Payne, R. L., & Martin, M. L. (1993). Defining and classifying skin tears: Need for a common language. *Ostomy Wound Management, 39*(5), 16–20, 22–24, 26.

Pennsylvania Safety Authority Skin Tear Initiative: PA-PSRA Patient Safety Advisory. (2006). Skin tears: The clinical challenge. *PA PSRS Patient Safety Advisory, 3*(3), 1, 5–10. Retrieved from http://www.patientsafetyauthority.org/ADVISORIES/AdvisoryLibrary/2006/Sep3%283%29/Pages/01b.aspx

Ratliff, C. R., & Fletcher, K. R. (2007). Skin tears: A review of the evidence to support prevention and treatment. *Ostomy Wound Management, 53*(3), 32–42.

Sibbald, R. G., Woo, K. Y., & Ayello, E. (2008). Wound bed preparation: DIM before DIME: Wound care. *Wound Healing Southern Africa, 1*(1), 29–34.

Stephen-Haynes, J., Callaghan, R., Bethell, E., & Greenwood, M. (2011). The assessment and management of skin tears in care homes. *British Journal of Nursing, 20*(11 Suppl.), S12–S22.

Strazzieri-Pulido, K. C., Picolo Peres, G. R., Campanili, T. C. G. F., & Conceicao de Gouveia Santos, V. L. (2015). Skin tear prevalence and associated factors: A systematic review. *Revista da Escola de Enfermagem da USP, 49*(4), 674–680. doi:10.1590/S0080-623420150000400019

White, M., Karam, S., & Cowell, B. (1994). Skin tears in frail elders: A practical approach to prevention. *Geriatric Nursing, 15*(2), 95–99.

Web Resources

Challenge of skin tear poster: http://www.patient safetyauthority.org/EducationalTools/PatientSafetyTools/skin_tears/Pages/poster.aspx

Challenge of skin tears in acute care video: http://www.patientsafetyauthority.org/EducationalTools/PatientSafetyTools/skin_tears/Pages/skintears_video.aspx

National Guideline Clearinghouse: Preventing Pressure Ulcers and Skin Tears: http://www.guideline.gov

Sample policy on skin tear management: http://www.patientsafetyauthority.org/EducationalTools/PatientSafetyTools/skin_tears/Pages/mgmt_policy.aspx

Sample policy on skin tear prevention: http://www.patientsafetyauthority.org/EducationalTools/PatientSafetyTools/skin_tears/Pages/mgmt_policy.asp

Skin Integrity, Immobility, and Pressure Ulcers in Class III Obese Patients: http://www.patientsafetyauthority.org/ADVI-SORIES/AdvisoryLibrary/2013/Jun;10%282%29/Pages/50.aspx

Skin Tears.org: http://www.skintears.org/Consensus-Statements/References.aspx

Wound, Ostomy and Continence Nurses Society: http://www.wocn.org

SLEEP DISORDERS

GLOSSARY OF SLEEP TERMS

- *Apnea*: Cessation of breathing for 10 or more seconds during sleep.
- *Hypopnea:* Decrease in breath amplitude of more than 30% for at least 10 seconds, associated with 3% oxygen desaturation.
- *Excessive daytime sleepiness*: Increased propensity to fall asleep; sleepiness in a situation wherein the person would be expected to be awake and alert.
- *Insomnia*: Difficulty initiating sleep, maintaining sleep, or awakening too early in the morning, accompanied by daytime dysfunction.
- *Non-REM (NREM) sleep:* Sleep stages that progress from light (stage N1) to deep sleep (stage N3).
- *Phase advance:* A change in the circadian cycle of wake/sleep in which the individual falls

S

asleep early in the evening and awakens earlier than desired the following morning.

- *Polysomnography*: A study of the physiological characteristics of sleep; it includes, at a minimum, EEG, electro-oculography (EOG) eye movements, and chin electromyography (EMG) to determine sleep stages. It may also include EKG, respiratory parameters, measurements of leg movements, and other parameters, depending on the goals of the study.
- *REM sleep:* The stage of sleep characterized by muscular twitching, irregular breathing, irregular heart rate, and increased autonomic activity when dreaming occurs.
- *Sleep efficiency:* The percentage of time in bed that one is asleep is calculated as follows: total sleep time divided by time in bed multiplied by 100.
- *Sleep fragmentation*: Disruption of sleep characterized by arousals or abrupt transitions to a lighter stage of sleep.
- *Sleep hygiene:* Behaviors, routines, and activities that influence the quality and quantity of sleep.
- *Sleep latency:* Duration of time that it takes from lights out to sleep onset.
- *Sleep maintenance:* Ability to sleep consistently throughout the desired sleep interval.
- *Wake after sleep onset:* Time awake after sleep onset.
- *Zeitgeber*: An environmental or social cue that results in entrainment of the circadian rhythm. Examples include light and dark, regularly scheduled meals, and exercise.

NORMAL SLEEP

Sleep and wakefulness are regulated by the homeostatic sleep–wake process and the intrinsic circadian biological clock, an internal mechanism that regulates the 24-hour sleep–wake cycle. The circadian rhythm is controlled by the *suprachiasmatic nucleus* (SCN) of the hypothalamus (Borbely & Ackermann, 2005). Light enters the eye and travels via the optic nerve to the SCN, where the function and timing of this biologic clock are reset on a daily basis.

The homeostatic sleep drive, or propensity to fall asleep, depends on the degree of sleep pressure, a factor that increases progressively as waking hours accumulate and decreases with an adequate amount of good quality sleep. The "two-process" model of sleep regulation includes both homeostatic and circadian processes.

Aging is associated with a flattened circadian rhythm, phase advance (earlier bedtime and early morning awakenings), decreased slow wave and REM sleep, and increased arousals (Redeker, 2011). Napping seems to be more common among older adults and increases with aging. Some 69% of people aged 75 years and older reported napping in a 2-week period (Driscoll et al., 2008). However, rates vary according to the evaluation methods, and the positive or negative health effects of napping are not completely known (Redeker, 2011). Naps may have a restorative effect, but napping may reduce the homeostatic sleep drive. Although some studies suggest that sleep times decrease with aging, a meta-analysis of healthy adults living in the community demonstrated little change in the median sleep time among older adults between the ages of 60 years and 75 years and older (Ohayon, Carskadon, Guilleminault, & Vitiello, 2004). Likewise, evidence of age-related changes in sleep latency is conflicting (Redeker, 2011).

Although many people believe that poor sleep quality is a normal part of aging, deterioration in sleep quality is often a sign of comorbid physical or mental health problems or treatable sleep disorders. In fact, a recent study suggested that good sleep is a marker of healthy aging (Driscoll et al., 2008). Therefore an important role for health professionals is clarifying perceptions about sleep and aging and evaluating potential contributors to poor sleep that are often treatable.

CIRCADIAN DISTURBANCES

Circadian phase advance (early bedtimes and early morning awakenings) is a common developmental change associated with aging. It is not pathological unless it interferes with the individual's preferred lifestyle (e.g., evening social activities). However, circadian disturbances may occur when there are changes in environmental cues (e.g., zeitgebers). These may include social isolation, lack of exposure to bright light that often occurs in long-term care facilities, visual impairment, and hearing deficits. Given that older adults already have more flattened circadian rhythms, they may be particularly vulnerable to these effects. Daytime napping may also decrease nocturnal sleep propensity and disrupt the normal circadian pattern. These problems are of particular concern in long-term care settings (Lorenz, Harris, & Richards, 2011). Conversely, exposure to bright light early in the morning and vigorous and engaging daytime activity and social activity may promote restful and satisfying sleep the following night. However, more research is needed on the effects of these interventions (Lorenz et al., 2011).

INSOMNIA

Insomnia is a disorder of initiating or maintaining sleep or waking too early in the morning. Primary insomnia occurs without an identified cause. Insomnia may be acute, short-term, or chronic. However, insomnia that is comorbid with other psychiatric or medical conditions or sleep disorders is far more common. Insomnia may be transient or chronic, and the perception of sleep duration does not consistently correspond with objective sleep measures, such as polysomnography. Insomnia may result from physiologic (e.g., hyperarousal), neurocognitive, and behavioral mechanisms. Spielman's "3P" model of sleep (Spielman, Caruso, & Glovinsky, 1987) postulates that predisposing (e.g., aging, genetics), precipitating (e.g., stressors, hospitalization, medical or psychiatric conditions, death of a loved one), or perpetuating (e.g., beliefs, attitudes, behaviors) factors contribute to insomnia. Insomnia is very common in people with acute and chronic conditions, such as cancer and heart failure and often occurs in hospital and long-term care settings.

The most efficacious treatments for insomnia include hypnotic medications and interventions focused on modifying sleep-related behaviors and cognitions (Cognitive Behavioral Therapy for Insomnia [CBT-I]). Although the treatment of psychiatric (e.g., anxiety, depression) or comorbid medical conditions may improve insomnia somewhat, these interventions usually do not result in complete elimination of insomnia.

Prescription hypnotic medications such as non-barbiturate hypnotics, benzodiazepines, and antidepressants and should not be prescribed if possible (e.g., trazodone may be used for insomnia among people with mild depressive symptoms). Although the use of hypnotics increases with advancing age and may improve nighttime sleep, older adults often report daytime dysfunction, such as drowsiness resulting from the use of these medications. This may result in falls or other events that cause injury. Many people, including older adults, use over-the-counter sleeping aids that contain diphenhydramine. There is little evidence of benefit from these aids that lead to daytime functional compromise and cholinergic effects. Melatonin is also often used and may benefit older adults because of the beneficial effects of circadian rhythmicity and lack of negative daytime effects. However, like other supplements, it is not approved by the U.S. Food and Drug Administration (FDA; Jungquist, 2011). Long-term use of hypnotic medications should be avoided.

CBT-I is a multimodal treatment that includes sleep hygiene, stimulus control (management of environmental stimuli), sleep restriction, and cognitive therapy focused on dysfunctional beliefs and attitudes about sleep. It may also include relaxation therapy. CBT-I is as efficacious as hypnotic medications, is more durable, and lacks the negative daytime effects associated with hypnotics in many populations, including older adults. It focuses on addressing the cognitive, perceptual, and behavioral factors that perpetuate insomnia. Although sleep hygiene focused on general guidelines about health practices (e.g., caffeine, exercise) is often used as a first-line intervention, it is not efficacious as a solo treatment for insomnia. However, modifying environmental factors, such as sound and lighting, may be helpful, especially in institutional settings, such as the acute care hospital or nursing home.

OBSTRUCTIVE SLEEP APNEA

Obstructive sleep apnea (OSA) is a condition that results from the intermittent pharyngeal obstruction that causes repetitive apneas and hypopneas, oxygen desaturation, sympathetic arousal, frequent awakenings (and/or brief EEG arousals that may not be associated with full awakening), and excessive daytime sleepiness. People with OSA usually, but not always, snore loudly and may demonstrate apneas when sleep is observed. Excessive daytime sleepiness and fatigue are common. OSA also contributes to cardiovascular (e.g., stroke, hypertension heart failure) and metabolic (e.g., diabetes) conditions, including increasing the likelihood that patients are refractory to effective treatment of these conditions. OSA may contribute to functional decline among older adults (Cole et al., 2009).

OSA is characterized as mild (5–15 apneas and/or hypopneas per hour of sleep); moderate (more than 15–30 per hour) and severe (more than 30 per hour). As many as 24% of adults aged 65 years and older have OSA (Ancoli-Israel et al., 1991), with prevalence, rather than severity increasing with advancing age (Bixler, Vgontzas, Ten Have, Tyson, & Kales, 1998). As many as 70% to 80% of long-term care residents who have dementia may have OSA, but it is often underdiagnosed (Martin & Ancoli-Israel, 2008; Martin, Mory, & Alessi, 2005).

Risk factors for OSA include obesity, male gender, and large neck size (greater than 16 in. for men, greater than 15 in. for women). The most efficacious treatment for OSA is nocturnal nasal continuous positive airway pressure. Weight loss is also efficacious but is difficult for many people to accomplish. Oral appliances that modify the position of the mandible, tongue and other oropharyngeal structures can be fitted by a dentist and are effective in treating mild to moderate OSA. A number of surgical treatments are available, but these do not have strong evidence of efficacy (Sawyer & Weaver, 2011).

SLEEP-RELATED MOVEMENT DISORDERS

Periodic limb movement disorder (PLMD) is associated with periodic repetitive limb movements (usually lower extremity). These include an extension of the big toe and partial flexion of the ankle, knee, or hip. Movements may also occur in the upper extremities. Severity is determined by the number of limb movements per hour, with 15/hour considered diagnostic in adults. PLMD is thought to be quite rare. However, the prevalence of periodic limb

movements (PLMs) increases with age, with as many as 34% of older adults experiencing PLMs.

Restless legs syndrome (RLS) is characterized by an almost irresistible urge to move the limbs, usually associated with disagreeable presleep leg sensations. These sensations often interfere with initiating and maintaining sleep, resulting in daytime sleepiness. Primary RLS is the result of dysfunction in brain iron storage and abnormalities in dopamine metabolism (Cuellar & Redeker, 2011). Genetics also play a role. RLS may also be caused by iron deficiency anemia, uremia, neurological lesions, diabetes, hypertension, Parkinson's disease, rheumatoid arthritis, and certain drugs (e.g., tricyclics, selective serotonin reuptake inhibitors, lithium, dopamine blockers, xanthines).

Treatment of RLS and PLMD includes behavioral and pharmacological interventions. Behavioral strategies include methods to promote restorative sleep and moderate exercise, as well as cognitive behavioral therapy. Dopaminergic drugs, benzodiazepines, opioids, and anticonvulsants in monotherapy or a combination therapy are also beneficial (Cuellar & Redeker, 2011).

ASSESSMENT AND TREATMENT

Given the high prevalence of sleep disorders among older adults and their deleterious consequences, screening and assessment should be a routine part of assessment and treatment in the primary care setting. Self-report and other assessment tools are readily available (Luyster et al., 2015). Promotion of adequate sleep and circadian patterning of activity and rest should also be included in institutional settings, such as acute and long-term care settings where older adults receive health care. Referral to a specialized sleep disorders program is recommended, especially when there is suspicion of a primary sleep disorder, such as disordered breathing. After specialized treatment of sleep disorders, providers in the primary care setting should follow up to ensure that the treatment regimen is followed and effective.

See also Daytime Sleepiness.

Nancy S. Redeker

Ancoli-Israel, S., Kripke, D. F., Klauber, M. R., Mason, W. J., Fell, R., & Kaplan, O. (1991). Sleep-disordered breathing in community-dwelling elderly. *Sleep, 14*(6), 486–495.

Bixler, E. O., Vgontzas, A. N., Ten Have, T., Tyson, K., & Kales, A. (1998). Effects of age on sleep apnea in men: I. Prevalence and severity. *American Journal of Respiratory and Critical Care Medicine, 157*(1), 144–148.

Borbely, A., & Ackermann, P. (2005). Sleep homeostasis and models of sleep regulation. In M. Kryger, T. Roth, & W. C. Dement (Eds.), *Principles and practice of sleep medicine* (4th ed., pp. 405–417). Philadelphia, PA: Elsevier Saunders.

Cole, C. S., Richards, K. C., Beck, C. C., Roberson, P. K., Lambert, C., Furnish, A., … Tackett, J. (2009). Relationships among disordered sleep and cognitive and functional status in nursing home residents. *Research in Gerontological Nursing, 2*(3), 183–191.

Cuellar, N., & Redeker, N. S. (2011). Sleep-related movement disorders and parasomnias. In N. S. Redeker & G. Phillips McEnany (Eds.), *Sleep disorders and sleep promotion in nursing practice* (pp. 121–139). New York, NY: Springer Publishing.

Driscoll, H. C., Serody, L., Patrick, S., Maurer, J., Bensasi, S., Houck, P. R., … Reynolds, C. F. (2008). Sleeping well, aging well: A descriptive and cross-sectional study of sleep in "successful agers" 75 and older. *American Journal of Geriatric Psychiatry, 16*(1), 74–82.

Jungquist, C. (2011). Insomnia. In N. S. Redeker & G. Phillips McEnany (Eds.), *Sleep disorders and sleep promotion in nursing practice* (pp. 71–94). New York, NY: Springer Publishing.

Lorenz, R. A., Harris, M., & Richards, K. C. (2011). Sleep in adult long term care. In N. S. Redeker & G. Phillips McEnany (Eds.), *Sleep disorders and sleep promotion in nursing practice* (pp. 339–354). New York, NY: Springer Publishing.

Luyster, F. S., Choi, J., Yeh, C. H., Imes, C. C., Johansson, A. E., & Chasens, E. R. (2015). Screening and evaluation tools for sleep disorders in older adults. *Applied Nursing Research, 28*(4), 334–340. doi:10.1016/j.apnr.2014.12.007

Martin, J. L., & Ancoli-Israel, S. (2008). Sleep disturbances in long-term care. *Clinics in Geriatric Medicine, 24*(1), 39–50, vi.

Martin, J. L., Mory, A. K., & Alessi, C. A. (2005). Nighttime oxygen desaturation and symptoms of sleep-disordered breathing in long-stay nursing home residents. *Journals of Gerontology: Series A, Biological Sciences and Medical Sciences, 60*(1), 104–108.

Ohayon, M. M., Carskadon, M. A., Guilleminault, C., & Vitiello, M. V. (2004). Meta-analysis of quantitative sleep parameters from childhood to old age in healthy individuals: Developing normative sleep values across the human lifespan. *Sleep, 27*(7), 1255–1273.

Redeker, N. S. (2011). Developmental aspects of normal sleep. In N. S. Redeker & G. Phillips McEnany (Eds.), *Sleep disorders and sleep promotion in nursing practice* (pp. 19–32). New York, NY: Springer Publishing.

Sawyer, A. M., & Weaver, T. E. (2011). Sleep-related breathing disorders. In N. S. Redeker & G. Phillips McEnany (Eds.), *Sleep disorders and sleep promotion in nursing practice* (pp. 121–140). New York, NY: Springer Publishing.

Spielman, A. J., Caruso, L. S., & Glovinsky, P. B. (1987). A behavioral perspective on insomnia treatment. *Psychiatric Clinics of North America, 10*(4), 541–553.

Web Resources
American Academy of Sleep Medicine: http://www.aasmnet.org
National Center on Sleep Disorders Research: http://www.nhlbi.nih.gov/health/public/sleep/index.htmhttp://www.nhlbi.nih.gov/health/prof/sleep/index.htm
National Sleep Foundation: http://www.sleepfoundation.org
New Abstracts and Papers in Sleep (NAPS): http://www.websciences.org/bibliosleep/NAPS
Restless Legs Syndrome Foundation: http://www.rls.org

S

SOCIAL ISOLATION

Social isolation is an aspect of health that may be underassessed, but at the same time cannot and should not be ignored. Numerous facets of social isolation are known, including risk factors, assessment, and the negative outcomes of older adults who are socially isolated. Because social isolation is strongly correlated with myriad costly negative outcomes, interventions provide an opportunity to restore health to older adults while preserving resources. Social isolation is specifically defined as "a state in which the individual lacks a sense of belonging socially, lacks engagement with others, has a minimal number of social contacts, and they are deficient in fulfilling and quality relationships" (Nicholson,

2009, p. 1346). Family members, caregivers, health care providers, and older adults themselves would benefit greatly from a swift recognition of the risk factors of social isolation

RISK FACTORS

Social isolation impacts the lives of numerous older adults around the globe. The prevalence of social isolation in older adults has been shown to be between 10% and approximately 50% (Ibrahim, Abolfathi Momtaz, & Hamid, 2013; Nicholson, 2012). Social isolation may increase as adults age, which underscores the importance of early detection, effective intervention, and continued follow-up. To properly identify older adults who are impacted by social isolation, it is essential to recognize its common risk factors.

These health factors, which have support in the literature as leading to social isolation, come from many facets of an older adult's life. The physical health of individuals who are overweight, as well as those who smoke, may promote an increased risk of social isolation. Likewise, depression as well as the psychological perception of not having opportunities to engage in social activities are both antecedents for social isolation.

The risk for social isolation goes beyond physical and psychological health. The socioeconomic status of older adults is an important risk factor for social isolation (Shankar, McMunn, Demakakos, Hamer, & Steptoe, 2017). In addition, personal factors, such as the death of a partner or a relative who is close puts an individual at a higher risk for social isolation (Beer et al., 2016), as does disconnection from the family. Finally, the location where an older adult lives is an important component leading to social isolation; urban settings have been shown to be more associated with social isolation (Ibrahim et al., 2013).

NEGATIVE OUTCOMES

Despite several theories on the mechanism/ pathway, exactly how and why social isolation influences health and well-being are not well understood. Nevertheless, research supports a relationship between social isolation and poor physical, psychological, and social outcomes.

Older adults who are socially isolated have negative physical health outcomes. They often have poor nutrition, are more sedentary, and are at a greater risk for falls. In fact, older adults who are socially isolated are at higher risk of all-cause mortality (Nicholson, 2012). When compared with adults of the same age with more relationships with relatives, friends, and the community, socially isolated older adults are two to four times more likely to die.

Psychological health is also a major concern in socially isolated older adults. Social isolation is associated with dementia and cognitive decline (Franck, Molyneux, & Parkinson, 2016). This may be because of later diagnosis and treatment, but more data are necessary. In addition to memory concerns, socially isolated older adults are at a greater risk of depression and depressive symptoms (Franck et al., 2016; Nicholson, 2012). This is especially concerning, considering the increased risk of death by suicide, particularly in socially isolated older men. Two additional outcomes of social isolation are heavy alcohol consumption and subjective feelings of loneliness.

In addition to increased physical and psychological health concerns, social isolation in older adults is associated with negative social outcomes. Older adults who are socially isolated are four to five times more likely to be rehospitalized within 1 year of an initial hospitalization (Nicholson, 2012). This is particularly costly, considering cutbacks in Medicare reimbursements to hospitals for readmissions. Socially isolated older adults are also at an increased risk of institutionalization.

Socially isolated older adults are at heightened risk of death, depression, and death by suicide. They are also costlier to care for because of rehospitalization and institutionalization. Therefore it is important to identify older adults who are isolated or at risk of isolation.

ASSESSMENT

The multitude of negative outcomes of social isolation highlights the importance of identifying this phenomenon in older adults. There are many barriers to the assessment of social isolation, such as lack of time in clinical settings, lack of understanding of the phenomenon, and lack of an ideal instrument. An ideal instrument would be quick, psychometrically tested to be both valid and reliable in older adults, theory-based, sensitive to change, and able to measure the construct of social isolation as defined without ambiguity. One measure that is widely used in the literature to measure social isolation is the Lubben Social Network Scale (LSNS; Lubben et al., 2006). The LSNS has several versions; however, the 6-item version (LSNS-6) may be the most appropriate for screening in the clinical setting. The LSNS-6 measures emotional, tangible, and actual network size relating to family and friends of the respondent. Although this measure has limitations, the LSNS-6 has demonstrated some success in assessing older adults in clinical settings.

WHAT TO DO IF SOCIAL ISOLATION IS DETECTED/INTERVENTIONS

Important interventions strategies include providing activities, support, and home visits in group or one-to-one settings. Using technology to reduce social isolation is a new, but promising, intervention strategy. Although research supports a number of strategies, the measurement of effectiveness is inconsistent and therefore it is difficult to compare results.

Groups

Participation in activity groups appears to be beneficial in reducing social isolation in older adults (Franck et al., 2016). Older adults who participated in a reminiscence therapy group showed improvement in loneliness and depressive symptoms. Those who participated in indoor gardening programs reported lower rates of loneliness, increased life satisfaction, and increased socialization.

Support groups also show promise for improvement in social isolation. Women who participated in a breast cancer support group reported increased satisfaction with social support, a reduction in feelings of loneliness, and

an increased number of confidants (Dickens, Richards, Greaves, & Campbell, 2011). Similarly, participation in a bereavement support group resulted in increased socialization and reduction in depression.

One-To-One

There is some evidence that one-to-one intervention activities may also reduce social isolation, but the results are less robust. Older adults who participated in foster grandparent programs reported developing new relationships, but there was no impact on loneliness (Dickens et al., 2011). On the other hand, older adults who played an interactive video game with an undergraduate research assistant reported lower rates of loneliness (Franck et al., 2016). Those who were visited by a volunteer home-visiting program reported increased feelings of worth and social integration (Dickens et al., 2011).

Technology

New interventions are being developed to reduce social isolation in older adults using information and communication technology (ICT). Most ICT interventions use the Internet or other web-based apps on a computer. Others use telephones, smartphones, tablets, video game systems, and visual pet companion apps. ICT interventions allow older adults to remain connected with family and friends and to reconnect with old hobbies. Most ICT interventions purported a reduction in loneliness and an increased social support, social connectedness, and social contacts.

When considering interventions for social isolation, service providers need to consider the diversity of their older clients, including differences in race, cultural background, socioeconomic status, home settings, and general functioning. Many communities have a comprehensive network of senior centers, opportunities for volunteerism, and recreational activities; however, they may not be user-friendly for older adults who are frail, belong to ethnic minority groups or require specialized transportation.

S

S

CONCLUSION

Numerous negative outcomes of social isolation may be costly regarding financial resources and increased disability in the older adult population. An understanding of those who have increased risk factors for social isolation is an important first step. Using available measures to assess social isolation is an important next step in mitigating the impact on older adults. Family members, caregivers, health care providers, and older adults look to limit disability related to social isolation. Numerous evidence-based interventions provide a cost-effective opportunity to restore health holistically to older adults needing assistance.

See also Aging Agencies: City and County Level; Autonomy; Life Review; Rural Elders.

Nicholas R. Nicholson, Jr. and
Stephanie A. Jacobson

Beer, A., Faulkner, D., Law, J., Lewin, G., Tinker, A., Buys, L., … Cessman, S. (2016). Regional variations in social isolation amongst older Australians. *Regional Studies, Regional Science, 3*(1), 170–184. doi:10.1080/21681376.2016.1144481

Dickens, A. P., Richards, S. H., Greaves, C. J., & Campbell, J. L. (2011). Interventions targeting social isolation in older people: A systematic review. *BMC Public Health, 11,* 647.

Franck, L., Molyneux, N., & Parkinson, L. (2016). Systematic review of interventions addressing social isolation and depression in aged care clients. *Quality of Life Research, 25*(6), 1395–1407.

Ibrahim, R., Abolfathi Momtaz, Y., & Hamid, T. A. (2013). Social isolation in older Malaysians: Prevalence and risk factors. *Psychogeriatrics, 13*(2), 71–79.

Lubben, J., Blozik, E., Gillmann, G., Iliffe, S., von Renteln Kruse, W., Beck, J. C., & Stuck, A. E. (2006). Performance of an abbreviated version of the Lubben Social Network Scale among three European community-dwelling older adult populations. *The Gerontologist, 46,* 503–513.

Nicholson, N. R. (2009). Social isolation in older adults: An evolutionary concept analysis. *Journal of Advanced Nursing, 65*(6), 1342–1352.

Nicholson, N. R. (2012). A review of social isolation: An important but underassessed condition in older adults. *Journal of Primary Prevention, 33*(2–3), 137–152.

Shankar, A., McMunn, A., Demakakos, P., Hamer, M., & Steptoe, A. (2017). Social isolation and loneliness: Prospective associations with functional status in older adults. *Health Psychology, 36*(2), 179.

Web Resources
Connect2Affect (AARP Foundation): http://connect2affect.org
Home for the Holidays Campaign: http://www.n4a.org/h4h2016

SOCIAL SECURITY

The national pension system of the United States is officially called Old-Age, Survivors, and Disability Insurance (OASDI). The general term *Social Security* is used to describe this program.

The Social Security Act of 1935 initially provided monthly benefits only to retired workers aged 65 years and older. Starting in 1956 in the case of women and 1961 in the case of men, Congress permitted eligible workers to claim actuarially reduced retirement benefits between the age of 62 years and 64 years. "Auxiliary" Social Security benefits are provided to the eligible dependents of Social Security pensioners. Disability insurance benefits were added to Social Security in 1956. In 1983, the normal retirement age was raised for workers born in 1938 and later. Retirement age is currently 66 years and will reach 67 years in 2027 for workers born in 1960 and later years. The early retirement ages will not change, but the benefit reductions for claiming an early pension will be larger percentages of the worker's primary insurance amount.

The benefit formula provides a pension increase, known as a delayed retirement credit, for workers who defer claiming a pension until after the normal retirement age. For workers who attained the normal retirement age before 1990, the increase reached the normal retirement age in 1990, and later, the increases became progressively larger.

Eligibility for benefits depends on having the required number of earnings credits. In 2016, credit is given for each $1,260 of earnings, up to a maximum of four credits per year. For retirement and survivor benefits, no more than 40 credits are required for benefit eligibility. To qualify for disability benefits, disabled workers must ordinarily have 20 credits in the past 10 years. The amount of earnings required for credit is increased from year to year in proportion to the percentage change in economy-wide average wages.

INCOME TAXATION OF OASDI BENEFITS

Beginning in 1994, OASDI benefits became taxable for some taxpayers who had incomes above these thresholds. Up to 85% of OASDI benefits are considered taxable income for income tax purposes for single people who have total incomes, including half of their OASDI benefits, more than $34,000 a year and married couples with incomes more than $44,000 a year. Unlike many elements of the OASDI program, the threshold amounts used to calculate income tax liabilities on Social Security benefits do not change in line with either prices or economy-wide average wages. In most states, OASDI benefits remain exempt from state and local income taxes.

Financing OASDI

Income flowing into the Social Security system is deposited into two reserve funds, the Old-Age and Survivors Insurance (OASI) Trust Fund and the Disability Insurance (DI) Trust Fund. The benefits and administrative expenses of the OASDI program are paid out of these trust funds. The income of the trust funds consists of payroll tax revenues, interest earnings on trust fund investments, and since 1984, most of the receipts collected from imposing income taxes on OASDI benefits.

From the inception of Social Security until the 1980s, the basic financing concept of OASDI rested on the idea that the program should be supported by scheduled payroll taxes and investment income earned on reserves. Congress sometimes made exceptions to this rule, using general revenues to pay for benefits to some old people who would not otherwise qualify for them. The 1983 amendments indirectly

introduced general revenue financing. Since 1984, the Social Security program has derived part of its revenues from income taxes imposed on OASDI benefits.

By law, the reserves held in the trust funds must be invested in securities guaranteed as to principal and interest by the federal government. As a practical matter, the reserves have been almost entirely invested in U.S. Treasury securities. Congress has never seriously considered allowing investments in private securities because it would then be subject to greater year-to-year variability. Treasury securities can be redeemed at any time at face value, although marketable securities are subject to the forces of the open market and may suffer a loss, or enjoy a gain if sold before maturity.

Problems Facing Social Security

In the early 1980s, the OASDI system faced both short- and long-term financing problems. The balance in the OASI trust fund was falling rapidly and would have been exhausted if Congress had not enacted legislation that permitted interfund borrowing. At the same time, the Social Security Actuary estimated that expected program outlays in the subsequent 75 years would be significantly higher than anticipated income.

The long-term problem was the more serious one. Declines in the U.S. birth rate and increases in Americans' life span have gradually increased the ratio of Social Security beneficiaries to Social Security payroll taxpayers. The ratio of beneficiaries to taxpayers has begun to rise sharply since 2010, since the post–World War II baby boom generation has begun to retire. The change in the ratio of beneficiaries to contributors would pose no special problem if Social Security were financed on a purely advance-funded basis. In that case, future benefits would be paid out of the accumulated reserves of the system, and future taxpayers would face only small tax increases associated with gains in their longevity compared with earlier generations. However, the reserves built up in the Social Security trust funds were comparatively small in the early 1980s. Nearly all of the payroll tax contributions collected through 1983 had been paid out as benefits or used up in administering

S

the system. In the absence of a large financial reserve, the rapid increase in the expected number of pensioners beginning in 2010 will likely lead to either a rise in payroll taxes or a cut in pension payments to keep the program solvent. According to the June 22, 2016, Social Security Board of Trustees annual report, the combined assets of the OASDI Trust Funds are projected to become depleted in 2034, with 79% of benefits still payable at that time (Board of Trustees, Federal Old-Age and Survivors Insurance and Federal Disability Insurance Trust Funds, 2016). The DI Trust Fund will become depleted in 2023, with 89% of benefits still payable. It should be noted that the DI Trust Fund has been supplemented by the tax rate reallocation enacted in the Bipartisan Budget Act of 2015.

The unfavorable actuarial forecast does not mean that OASDI is doomed to collapse. Rather, Congress can gradually make a sequence of small changes in the program that would prevent this from occurring. For example, benefit costs can be reduced over the long run by speeding up and extending increases in the normal retirement age that were put into law in 1983. Similarly, small and gradual increases in the OASDI tax rate can be phased in before the trust-fund reserves are exhausted.

Administration of OASDI

The OASDI program is administered principally by the Social Security Administration (SSA). In 2016, the cost of administering the program was 0.08% of total expenditures. Before April 1995, the SSA was part of the Department of Health and Human Services, but since then, it has been an independent agency. The U.S. Department of the Treasury collects OASDI payroll taxes, manages the OASDI trust funds, and prepares monthly benefit checks. Determinations of worker disability are made by state agencies, usually a state vocational rehabilitation agency.

Possible Future Developments

It is unlikely that significant benefit changes will be made to the OASDI program in the next few years unless the change is part of a broad package to resolve the long-range financing problems, especially because the reallocation enacted in the Bipartisan Budget Act of 2015, have significantly benefitted the DI Trust Fund. Two kinds of changes have been widely discussed in recent years: means-testing Social Security benefits and privatizing part or all of the Social Security system.

The critics of Social Security believe that it is too costly. Even if the program is affordable today, many believe it will become unaffordable after the baby boom generation is fully retired in 2030. To make the program more affordable, some people propose means-testing benefits by reducing or eliminating the benefits paid to high-income retirees. This proposal can be viewed from several perspectives. The United States is one of a handful of the richest countries in the world. Comparison with the public retirement systems of other rich countries, the U.S. Social Security program provides below-average replacement rates, especially to workers who earn high wages throughout their careers. As a result, the United States spends a smaller proportion of its national income on public pensions than other rich countries, and this is likely to remain true even when the baby boom generation is fully retired.

One objection to means-testing OASDI benefits is that it discourages workers from saving for their retirement, either in employer-sponsored pension plans or personal savings accounts. When workers know they cannot obtain Social Security benefits if they receive non-OASDI income more than a threshold amount, say, $20,000 a year, some middle-income workers may refrain from saving in their behalf. In a sense, the redistributive formula for OASDI benefits already accomplishes one goal of means-testing by limiting the wage-replacement rates available to workers who have high lifetime earnings. As noted, the OASDI benefit formula provides monthly pensions that are more generous about earnings for low-wage than for high-wage workers. In addition, retired workers who have high retirement incomes also have a bigger percentage of their OASDI benefits included in taxable income. Taxing benefits is redistributive because marginal and average income tax rates rise with household income.

Congress has never subjected OASDI benefits to a straightforward means test. In adopting and consistently following this principle, Congress almost certainly raised the long-term cost of Social Security, but it also increased the program's political acceptability and appeal. Social Security is widely regarded as a middle-class program, one that provides benefits to middle-income and affluent elders, as well as to the poor. The link between workers' OASDI contributions and benefits encourages contributors to regard their Social Security benefits as an earned right. If a large percentage of workers were required to contribute to the program but were then denied benefits in old age, the program's broad political appeal would suffer.

Starting in the mid-1990s, many proposals were offered with the goal of privatizing Social Security in whole or in part. A privatized pension system is one in which the workers build their retirement savings in an account, over which they exercise some control. With restrictions, they would be able to invest their savings as they chose and would pay for part or all of their retirement consumption from funds accumulated in their accounts.

One reason that Social Security critics favor privatization is their view that workers could obtain a better rate of return on their contributions if they were placed in a private account. This view is partly true, but it is misleading. It is true that individual workers can find investment opportunities that offer better-expected returns than their contributions to Social Security. However, a large percentage of current OASDI contributions is used to pay for current benefit payments. Only a small portion of current payroll taxes is available for investment in financial markets. The part of OASDI contributions available for investment is invested in U.S. Treasury securities. Collectively, workers can obtain somewhat better returns than those available on Treasury securities, but higher returns would also require workers to accept a greater risk because investments sometimes perform poorly. The only way that workers can collectively obtain a significantly higher return on their OASDI contributions is to reduce OASDI payments to current retirees, which would free up more of their contributions for immediate investment. However, no serious proponent of privatization suggests that the government should immediately and substantially cut benefits to workers who are already retired. If the benefits of current retirees are fully protected and if the total contribution rate for retirement programs remains unchanged, privatization could at best produce a very small improvement in the return on workers' contributions.

The debate over privatization is, in essence, a debate over the proper division of responsibility for financing Americans' retirement and managing the risks associated with pension financing. The traditional Social Security system provides a government guarantee of a modest retirement income that is scaled in proportion to a worker's previous earnings. Workers who wish to obtain a more comfortable standard of living when they retire must save on their own or find jobs with employers who offer good pensions. In 2016, the SSA estimated that Americans aged 65 years and older, 48% of married couples, and 71% of unmarried people receive 50% or more of their income from OASDI. Almost all of the remainder is derived from private-income sources, including employer-sponsored pensions, current earnings, and investment income from personal savings. The government-guaranteed Social Security pension has provided reliable income protection in old age. The pension is largely protected against the risk of inflation, and it lasts as long as the retired worker or the worker's dependent spouse continues to live.

Occupational pensions and personal savings accounts offer less protection. Employer-sponsored pensions are only rarely increased in line with inflation after a worker retires. This poses important risks to workers who live for many years after they begin collecting a pension. Retirement consumption that can be financed from a personal savings account depends on the workers' ability to save consistently and invest prudently. Even a worker who meets these challenges may be unlucky in reaching retirement age at a time when financial markets are in turmoil or inflation is high. A worker who does not convert personal savings into an annuity may be "unlucky" in living a very long life, possibly exhausting retirement savings. A sensibly designed privatization plan can reduce some of these risks. For example, if a fixed percentage of every paycheck is automatically deposited in a worker's retirement account, workers would face little risk of reaching old age with an empty savings account. If workers' investment alternatives were tightly restricted, if workers were offered an investment alternative with a minimum guaranteed rate of return, and if workers were compelled to convert some of their pension savings into an inflation-protected annuity when they retired, there would be less risk that retirees would suffer serious deprivation.

Social Security faces an uncertain future. All plausible long-term forecasts suggest that the program will eventually begin to pay out more benefits than it collects in taxes and earns on its investments. Once benefit payments begin to exceed revenues, the difference between outgo and income steadily rise until the trust-fund reserve is exhausted. When this occurs, probably in the coming four decades, the program will collect only enough payroll taxes to pay for 75% of currently promised benefits.

Not surprisingly, the public now has less confidence in the program than it had in the 1960s, when the financial future of the system seemed secure. At the beginning of the 21st century, many Americans lacked confidence that the OASDI program would still exist and be capable of paying retirement benefits in the future. The nation's experience during the first seven decades of Social Security demonstrates, however, that the program is highly adaptable. Successive Congresses and presidential administrations have made timely adjustments in the program to reflect changing demographic, economic, and political conditions. For this reason, it has always seemed likely that Social Security in some form will endure.

However, in the extremely volatile and mercurial political climate that exists today, the future of Social Security and all federal programs on aging is murky at best.

See also Medicaid; Medicare; Pensions and Financing Retirement.

William T. Lawson, III

Board of Trustees, Federal Old-Age and Survivors Insurance and Federal Disability Insurance Trust Funds. (2016). 2016 annual report of the board of trustees. Retrieved from https://www.ssa.gov/OACT/TR/2016/tr2016.pdf

Web Resources
Center for Retirement Research at Boston College: http://crr.bc.edu
Social Security Administration: Fact sheet: https://www.ssa.gov/oact/FACTS
University of Michigan Retirement Research Center: http://www.mrrc.isr.umich.edu
U.S. Social Security Administration: http://www.ssa.gov

SOCIAL SUPPORTS: FORMAL AND INFORMAL

Demographic trends suggest that both informal and formal supports to the elderly will be increasingly important in the future. The growing elderly population is heterogeneous, with elderly who are poor or in ill health most at risk for a lack of social support.

The population of Americans aged 65 years and older, 14.5% of the total population in 2014, is anticipated to increase rapidly in the coming decades such that by 2050, it will represent 22.1% of the U.S. population (U.S. Census Bureau, 2016a, 2016b). Although the overall rates of elderly poverty in the United States have been declining, there are considerable differences in the rates of poverty among subgroups of elderly persons by living status, race, and gender. For example, the poverty rate for elderly individuals who live alone is almost double that for elders overall. The poverty rate for Black elderly and elders of Hispanic origin is more than twice as high as the poverty rate for White elders (U.S. Census Bureau, 2015). Older women of color are especially likely to be living in poverty, with Black or Hispanic elderly women having close to a 25% poverty rate (AARP, 2010).

Informal social support is provided to the elderly by family members, friends, neighbors, clergy, and coworkers. Formal support is the broad array of social, welfare, health, and mental health services.

INFORMAL SUPPORT SYSTEMS: BURDENS AND GRATIFICATIONS

Family members provide extensive support to the elderly and represent the elderly's most significant social resource (Johnson & Wiener, 2006). According to findings from a national study on social support of the elderly, the majority of older people (59.6%) receive emotional support from family members only (White, Philogene, Fine, & Sinha, 2009). Adult children provide substantial amounts of support, with children of frail elders assuming an even larger share of activities necessary to meet the elders' care needs. Noninstitutionalized elderly receive most medically related personal care services from their children.

Friends and neighbors are also significant providers of social support for the elderly because of their physical proximity. Community groups and associations are important to the well-being of the elderly, although elders participate to a lesser degree than other age groups. The maximum participation in voluntary organizations by the elderly is either church or synagogue related.

A small but significant number of the elderly population is socially and physically isolated, with few, if any, significant others to turn to for help and assistance. These elderly are at a greater risk for health and mental health problems and institutionalization. They are also at a greater risk for mortality and functional limitations (Luo, Hawkley, Waite, & Cacioppo, 2012; Udell et al., 2012). Formal care providers must assess the needs of this at-risk population group and provide or arrange for needed formal supports.

Many families report that caregiving is an emotional, physical, social, and, at times, financial burden that can impact caregivers' physical health as well as increase the risk of mortality. Caregiving burden can also affect caregivers' mental health. A study comparing psychological outcomes between elderly Alzheimer caregivers and non-caregivers found that caregiving is associated with depressive symptoms (Mausbach, Chattillion, Roepke, Patterson, & Grant, 2013). Care-recipient behavioral problems and caregiver burden may be major factors in the decision to institutionalize an elderly parent.

It has also been noted that caregiving can have positive aspects for the caregiver as well, although this research has been far more limited than examinations of the costs of caregiving. Caregivers report satisfaction, enjoyment, and benefits and rewards from caregiving.

Increasing attention has been given to the role of race/ethnicity in caregiving. Although the impact of caregiving on the quality of life does not differ significantly by race/ethnicity (Lahaie, Earle, & Heymann, 2012), non-White caregivers are more likely to experience high caregiving burden compared with White caregivers (Reckrey, DeCherrie, Kelley, & Ornstein, 2013). Non-White dementia caregivers also experienced more positive aspects of caregiving than their White counterparts (Roth, Dilworth-Anderson, Huang, Gross, & Gitlin, 2015). Regarding help-receiving patterns, a recent study that compared White, Hispanic, African American, and Asian American caregivers found that Asian American caregivers were most likely to receive help from informal sources only, White caregivers most likely to receive help from formal sources only, and African American caregivers most likely to rely on a combination of formal and informal support (Chow, Auh, Scharlach, Lehning, & Goldstein, 2010).

For informal support systems to be most effective, links are needed among family caregivers, neighbors, friends, clergy, and other helpers. However, this often does not occur because of the fragmentation of helping networks.

BARRIERS TO THE USE OF FORMAL SERVICES

Studies of service-utility patterns indicate that many older people eligible for service programs, especially racial/ethnic minorities, do not use them. A variety of barriers to the use of health, mental health, and social services by at-risk older people has been identified in the literature (Biegel & Leibbrandt, 2006). These barriers are often the greatest for elders in poverty, minority elderly, those with physical or mental disabilities, and those whose service needs span both the aging network and other more specialized service-delivery systems.

Effective interventions for addressing the needs of the elderly who may be underusing formal services must define the barriers and identify their locus or source. The latter is especially important because strategies for addressing them must be tailored to their specific locus to be most effective. Barriers can be conceptualized on system, staff, community, or individual levels (Biegel & Leibbrandt, 2006).

System-level barriers refer to deficits at the service-agency and agency-network level that are impacted by political, economic, and social forces that shape the development of agency services and funding for such services. Such barriers include availability and cost, availability of transportation, hours of service, auspices of services, provision of information about services to potential referral agents and users of services, appropriateness of services, and links with formal and informal service systems and providers.

Staff-level barriers are the levels of knowledge, skills, attitudes, and behaviors of agency staff. Such barriers include lack of knowledge of specific problems and needs of subgroups of older people, negative attitudes by professionals about aging, and lack of a culturally competent staff.

Community-level barriers refer to negative attitudes and behaviors toward professional service use by informal helpers and community-based organizations. Such barriers include lack of knowledge of agency services by informal helpers, lack of relationships between informal helpers and agency service providers, and an unwillingness to recognize problems of the elderly (Biegel & Leibbrandt, 2006).

Individual-level barriers refer to personal and family attitudes and behaviors toward service use. These barriers include lack of knowledge about services in general; lack of understanding of how services can be helpful; lack of knowledge about where to go for help with specific problems or issues; lack of linguistic acculturation; negative attitudes toward formal services and unwillingness to accept help; and the role of family members in discouraging or preventing service use (Hansen & Aranda, 2012; Keith, Wacker, & Collins, 2009). In studies of ethnic minority elderly individuals, stigma attached to illness/mental illness and distrust of service systems are also identified to be barriers to service use (Guzman, Woods-Giscombe, & Beeber, 2015; Sun, Mutlu, & Coon, 2014). Other barriers relate to the health status characteristics of the elderly and may include health problems such as chronic illnesses or physical mobility problems and activity restrictions.

STRENGTHENING SUPPORT SYSTEMS OF THE ELDERLY

To strengthen support systems of the elderly, a multidimensional approach targeting all four-barrier levels—system, staff, community, and individual/family—required. One of the greatest barriers to service delivery, affecting in particular at-risk is elderly (e.g., poor, older women, racial/ethnic minorities, the rural elderly) is the lack of knowledge about the problems and needs of elders, at both the system and staff levels. This barrier is significant because it contributes to the development and delivery of services that do not adequately meet the needs of this population. A second barrier, at the staff level, involves the provision of services by professionals who lack the specialized knowledge and skills needed to attend to the needs of at-risk older adults.

Strengthening the informal and formal social networks of at-risk elderly people requires a thorough psychosocial assessment and a specific focus on the strengths and weaknesses of elderly individuals' informal and formal social support systems. Specific attention should be given to unmet needs and elders whose support systems are adequate at present but have a tenuous future.

See also Caregiver Burden; Caregiver Burnout; Caregiver Relationships; Caregiving Support Groups; Cultural Competence and Aging; Family Care for Frail Elders.

David E. Biegel and Ching-Wen Chang

American Association of Retired Persons. (2010). *Older Americans in poverty: A snapshot*. Washington, DC: Author.

Biegel, D. E., & Leibbrandt, S. (2006). Social work practice with elders living in poverty. In B. Berkman & S. Ambruoso (Eds.), *Handbook of social work in health and aging* (pp. 167–180). New York, NY: Oxford University Press.

Chow, J., Auh, E., Scharlach, A., Lehning, A., & Goldstein, C. S. (2010). Type and sources of support received by family caregivers of older adults from diverse racial and ethnic groups. *Journal of Ethnic & Cultural Diversity in Social Work, 19*, 175–194.

Guzman, E. D., Woods-Giscombe, C. L., & Beeber, L. S. (2015). Barriers and facilitators of Hispanic older adult mental health service utilization in the USA. *Issues in Mental Health Nursing, 36*(1), 11–20.

Hansen, M. C., & Aranda, M. P. (2012). Sociocultural influences on mental health service use by Latino older adults for emotional distress: Exploring the mediating and moderating role of informal social support. *Social Science & Medicine, 75*(12), 2134–2142.

Johnson, R. W., & Wiener, J. M. (2006). *A profile of frail older Americans and their caregivers: The Retirement Project, occasional paper number 8*. Washington, DC: The Urban Institute.

Keith, P. M., Wacker, R., & Collins, S. M. (2009). Family influence on caregiver resistance, efficacy, and use of services in family elder care. *Journal of Gerontological Social Work, 52*(4), 377–400.

Lahaie, C., Earle, A., & Heymann, J. (2012). An uneven burden: Social disparities in adult caregiving responsibilities, working conditions, and caregiver outcomes. *Research on Aging, 35*(3), 243–274.

Luo, Y., Hawkley, L. C., Waite, L. J., & Cacioppo, J. T. (2012). Loneliness, health, and mortality in old age: A national longitudinal study. *Social Science & Medicine, 74*(6), 907–914.

Mausbach, B. T., Chattillion, E. A., Roepke, S. K., Patterson, T. L., & Grant, I. (2013). A comparison of psychosocial outcomes in elderly Alzheimer caregivers and noncaregivers. *American Journal of Geriatric Psychiatry, 21*(1), 5–13.

Reckrey, J. M., DeCherrie, L. V., Kelley, A. S., & Ornstein, K. (2013). Health care utilization among homebound elders: Does caregiver burden play a role? *Journal of Aging and Health, 25*(6), 1036–1049.

Roth, D. L., Dilworth-Anderson, P., Huang, J., Gross, A. L., & Gitlin, L. N. (2015). Positive aspects of family caregiving for dementia: Differential item functioning by race. *Journals of Gerontology: Series B, Psychological Sciences and Social Sciences, 70*(6), 813–819.

Sun, F., Mutlu, A., & Coon, D. (2014). Service barriers faced by Chinese American families with a dementia relative: Perspectives from family caregivers and service professionals. *Clinical Gerontologist, 37*, 120–138.

Udell, J. A., Steg, P. G., Scirica, B. M., Smith, S. C., Ohman, E. M., Eagle, K. A., … Bhatt, D. L.; REduction of Atherothrombosis for Continued Health (REACH) Registry Investigators. (2012). Living alone and cardiovascular risk in outpatients at risk of or with atherothrombosis. *Archives of Internal Medicine, 172*(14), 1086–1095.

U.S. Census Bureau. (2015). *Income and poverty in the United States: 2014*. Washington, DC: U.S. Government Printing Office. Retrieved from http://www.census.gov/content/dam/Census/library/publications/2015/demo/p60-252.pdf

U.S. Census Bureau. (2016a). *Facts for features: Older Americans month: May 2016*. Washington, DC: U.S. Government Printing Office. Retrieved from http://www.census.gov/content/dam/Census/newsroom/facts-for-features/2016/cb16-ff08_older_americans.pdf

U.S. Census Bureau. (2016b). *An aging world: 2015*. Washington, DC: U.S. Government Printing Office. Retrieved from https://www.census.gov/content/dam/Census/library/publications/2016/demo/p95-16-1.pdf

White, A. M., Philogene, G. S., Fine, L., & Sinha, S. (2009). Social support and self-reported health status of older adults in the United States. *American Journal of Public Health, 99*(10), 1872–1878.

Web Resources

American Association of Retired Persons: http://www.aarp.org

National Alliance for Caregiving: http://www.caregiving.org

U.S. Census Bureau: https://www.census.gov

SOUTH ASIAN ELDERS

HISTORIC AND CULTURAL CONTEXT

Older adults from the Indian subcontinent represent a large and highly diverse population regarding ethnicity, culture, language, and faith. The U.S. Census Bureau (2012) categorizes people from India, Pakistan, Bangladesh, and Sri Lanka as being of South Asian descent. Other sources, including the United Nations Economic and Social Commission for Asia and the Pacific (2017), include people from Afghanistan, Bhutan, Nepal, and Maldives. Approximately 1.7 billion live in South Asia, and an estimated one of every four people throughout the world have roots there (United Nations Economic and Social Commission for Asia and the Pacific,

S

2017). Despite the diversity and differences among this population, many share cultural values and practices that make aging distinct. Asian Indians are the largest group of subcontinental older adults living in the United States.

According to the 2010 census, 3.2 million South Asian Indians (referred to as such by the Census, to distinguish them from Native American "Indians") live in the United States. Representing just under 1% of the population, Indians are the third largest group of Asians in the United States, following individuals of Chinese and Filipino descent (U.S. Census Bureau, 2012). Approximately 5% of Indians living in the United States are 65 years of age or older. Indian older adults in the United States belong to two groups: those who immigrated around 1965 and have since settled in the United States and those who have come to join or visit their families living in the United States. These two groups greatly differ demographically and face different issues as they continue to live in the United States. The former tends to be more acculturated, affluent, and independent, whereas the latter may find it harder to acclimatize to Western ideologies because of language and cultural differences. The older adults who came to join their family may face new challenges and barriers as they strive to adjust to the new environment.

Indians have been in the United States since the late 18th century, initially as unskilled laborers or agricultural immigrants. Although immigration was curtailed in 1917 by the passage of the Barred Zone Act, it was initiated again in 1946 with the passage of a bill allowing a small quota of Indians to annually immigrate and become naturalized. The passage of the Immigration and Nationality Act (INA) of 1965 and subsequent policies allowing family reunification allowed for a surge in the immigration of Asian Indians who were highly educated and skilled (Alagiakrishnan & Chopra, 2004). The Asian Indian population grew steadily through the 1970s and 1980s, and then there was a second surge heralded by the information technology boom in the 1990s.

HEALTH AND HEALTH BELIEFS

Indians have high prevalence and incidence of coronary artery disease, hypertension, diabetes mellitus, and hyperlipidemia (Ivey, Khatta,

& Vedanthan, 2002; Mohanty, Woolhandler, Himmelstein, & Bor, 2005). Contributing to these conditions are genetic predispositions to altered transport of cholesterol, endothelial dysfunction, and inflammation; increased insulin resistance; metabolic syndrome; and lifestyle factors. Traditional Indians diets are high in carbohydrates, as well as tropical oils, butter, and ghee (clarified butter). In addition, many Asian Indian elders do not exercise regularly, increasing their cardiovascular risk. Asian Indian women tend to be at a high risk for cancer and osteoporosis (American Cancer Society, 2016).

Many Indians traditionally believe mental illness is a sign of possession of the "evil eye"; as such, mental disorders carry a great deal of stigma among Indian elders, and symptoms are often concealed as somatic complaints. Treatment of mental and emotional disorders by Western allopathic means is frowned upon. Many older adults do not agree to counseling or social work services, because personal issues are kept in the family and not discussed outside that tight circle (Alagiakrishnan & Chopra, 2004).

Many older Indians practice traditional medicine such as homeopathy or Ayurveda (Periyakoil & Dara, 2010). Ayurvedic medicine has existed for 5,000 years, and it is believed to prevent and cure illness. Ayurveda is derived from two Sanskrit words *Ayu* and *veda*, meaning 'life" and "knowledge of," respectively. Ayurveda is also a science that explains the imbalance in the three universal energies (i.e., *tridosha*) that regulate all natural processes: *pitha* (i.e., bile), *vatha* (i.e., wind/air), and *kapha* (i.e., phlegm). The *tridosha* are related to the soul, mind, senses, and body functioning (Alagiakrishnan & Chopra, 2004). Many older Asian Indians may take Ayurvedic herbs or other alternative treatments in conjunction with or instead of traditional, Western allopathic treatments.

The majority of Asian Indians are Hindu. Karmic law—a principle by which actions of the past (in this life or a previous life) have consequences in this life or future lives—is a central tenet of Hinduism, as well as Buddhism, Jainism, and Sikhism (Deshpande, Reid, & Rao, 2005). Illness and its accompanying symptoms, including pain, are a result of karma. Many older Indians are accepting of death as a part of the life cycle and tend not to fear it. They may view this stage of their life as preparation of their soul for death and the afterlife. Older Indians have very low prevalence rates of completed advanced directives and end-of-life planning.

IMPLICATIONS FOR PRACTICE

Traditionally, Indians and other South Asians strongly value families and family caregiving. It is important that health care providers be familiar with the influence of the family structure and health beliefs as strong determinants of decision making about health. For instance, in the close-knit family, older adults hold an esteemed position, where they are respected and seen as the link to Indian culture, heritage, and religion (Periyakoil & Dara, 2010). Older Indians come from a culture that respects physicians and expects physicians to have all the answers and to make all health care decisions. Indians tend to view themselves as part of a family unit, and the concept of patient autonomy may not be familiar; medical discussions and decision making require family involvement. Women are more passive in the Indian culture, and men pay a major role in health care decisions.

It is important for providers to be aware of certain customs practiced among Indian elderly patients to avoid culturally insensitive remarks or behaviors. For instance, older women fast frequently as part of a religious belief that it improves the welfare of the family. Providers should be mindful of special attire and clothing which have multiple meanings; the attire may be sacred and should not be removed without permission. Older women may wear a *mangalsutra* necklace (a combination of black and gold beads) indicating that they are married. Widows often wear only white (the color of mourning), whereas the Indian men may wear a sacred string around their wrist or across their trunk. Sikhs often wear a steel bracelet (*karha*). Modesty is paramount when examining women, and many women prefer a female health care provider. Older men may be nonexpressive of pain, and providers need to attend to nonverbal behavior.

Although many older Indians are well educated and speak English, access to a translator or translating service should be available to ensure informed communication. Attention needs to be given to food preferences and religious restrictions, scheduling of procedures/tests (i.e., accounting for auspicious/inauspicious dates and times), clothing (i.e., ensuring appropriate hygiene and coverage), and gender of the health care provider. Many South Asian elders prefer to die at home, and families are most likely to place an elder in a nursing home only as a last resort. When older Indian patients die, it is important to ascertain from the family what practices and rituals are considered important and allow them some privacy. Interfering with premortem and postmortem rituals can be offensive for Indian families. Most Asian Indians do not readily agree to organ donation or postmortem examinations.

Margaret Salisu

Alagiakrishnan, K., & Chopra, A. (2004). Health and health care of Asian Indian American elders. Retrieved from https://web.stanford.edu/group/ethnoger/asianindian.html

American Cancer Society. (2016). *Asian Americans & cancer.* Retrieved from http://www.cancer.org/acs/groups/content/@midwest/documents/document/acspc-029976.pdf

Deshpande, O. M., Reid, M. C., & Rao, A. S. (2005). Attitudes towards end-of-life care among Asian Indian Hindus. *Journal of the American Geriatrics Society, 53*(1), 131–135.

Ivey, S. L., Khatta, M., & Vedanthan, R. (2002). Cardiovascular disease, a brown paper: The health of South Asians in the United States. Retrieved from http://www.sapha.net

Mohanty, S. A., Woolhandler, S., Himmelstein, D. U., & Bor, D. H. (2005). Diabetes and cardiovascular disease among Asian Indians in the United States. *Journal of General Internal Medicine, 20,* 474–478.

Periyakoil, V. J., & Dara, S. (2010). *Health and health care of Asian Indian American older adults.* Retrieved from http://geriatrics.stanford.edu/wp-content/uploads/downloads/ethnomed/asian_indian/downloads/asian_indian.pdf

United Nations Economic and Social Commission for Asia and the Pacific. (2017). Subregional Office for South and South-West Asia. Retrieved from http://www.unescap.org/subregional-office/south-south-west-asia

U.S. Census Bureau. (2012). *2010 Census briefs: The Asian population.* Retrieved from http://www.census.gov/prod/cen2010/briefs/c2010br-11.pdf

S

Web Resources
Ethnomed: http://ethnomed.org
National Aging Pacific Center on Aging (NAPCA): http://napca.org
National Indo-American Association of Senior Citizens: http://www.niaasc.org
Stanford University Geriatric Education Center Ethnogeriatric Resources: http://geriatrics.stanford .edu/ehtnomed/asian_indian

SPEECH AND LANGUAGE PROBLEMS

As the population of older adults in the United States continues to increase, providing health care services to this population can be enhanced by having a better understanding of the age-related changes in language and communication skills in this population.

Gradual changes in speech, language, and communication skills are observed in the lifetime. Cumulative effects of exposure to noise for several decades may result in hearing loss. Presbycusis is an age-related sensorineural hearing loss that is common among older adults. Sensory loss can contribute to changes in speech and language decline. Decreased hearing sensitivity directly and negatively affects communication and language abilities. For example, hearing loss can hinder the perception of speech sounds, particularly high-frequency sounds such as [s] and [th]. Difficulty hearing in noisy environments can limit social exchanges. In terms of language skills, many older adults report declines in their ability to comprehend and use language. Changes in cognition that accompany aging include attention, working memory capacity, and executive function. Multitasking, a common demand of modern day life, requires attention to two or more sets of information (usually from different sources) at the same time. Despite hands-free devices, talking on the phone and driving at the same time is an example of multitasking. As one ages, the ability to meet these demands becomes more challenging. A common complaint of older adults is the struggle to find words in conversational exchanges. The experience of having the word "on the tip of the tongue" is more prevalent in older adults. The ability to understand and produce grammatically complex sentences also declines with age. For example, a sentence like, "The student who graded the teacher's essay left the school after distributing report cards to the fifth graders," is difficult because of the number of relative clauses and phrases. It is also difficult because of the incongruent relationship among the words "student" and "teacher" in the sentence. With reduced processing speed, older adults struggle with working memory demands, where they temporarily hold information and then manipulate the information to make sense of what is being said.

Physiological changes in the larynx and vocal fold tissues over time result in voice changes. The American Academy of Otolaryngology—Head and Neck Surgery describes these changes as lower vocal pitch for men's voices and higher vocal pitch for women's voices; reduced loudness and the ability to project the voice; and reduced vocal endurance and difficulty being heard in noisy situations. Along these lines, aging also affects how safely one can swallow liquid and solid foods. Although most swallowing difficulties are attributable to medical conditions, including stroke and postoperative status in head–neck surgeries, approximately 20% of otherwise healthy older adults experience some form of swallowing difficulties. These can arise from changes in vocal cord sensitivity (ability to protect the airway), reduced strength of the tongue and throat to safely and effectively move food from the mouth to the esophagus, and reduction in the size of the opening of the esophagus that leads to a feeling of food being "stuck." Other factors, including use of medication (which may lead to dry mouth sensations), missing teeth, postural changes in cases of osteoarthritis, and even changes in the senses of taste and smell, may contribute to changes in the ability to swallow. Healthy adults continue to communicate and swallow effectively throughout their lifetime, despite changes to the systems that support these functions.

Changes in speech, language and communication may result from medical conditions.

Aphasia, dementia, dysarthria, apraxia, and dysphagia are the most common disorders of these systems.

APHASIA

Aphasia is an acquired language disability resulting from stroke; in fact, 25% to 40% of stroke survivors demonstrate some form of aphasia. Other causes of aphasia include head trauma, brain tumors, and other neurological insults. Aphasia affects one's ability to manage language modalities, including listening comprehension, oral expression, reading, and/or writing. It is *not* a form of impaired cognition or a type of mental illness. Patients can demonstrate a wide range of aphasia, from very mild to global aphasia (in which all four modalities are severely affected). In any case, compromised ability to express wants and needs negatively affects quality of life, even more severely than cancer and Alzheimer's disease (Lam & Wodchis, 2010).

Aphasia can be described as fluent and nonfluent. In nonfluent aphasia, the damage is in the third frontal convolution of the left temporal lobe, known as *Broca's area*. Broca's area makes up the lower part of the premotor cortex (Brookshire, 2003). Damage to this area results in speech that is halting, labored, and telegraphic. Reduction in use of grammatical words (*and, the, a, of, is, are*) and reduced sentence complexity are hallmark features of nonfluent aphasia. In some cases, verbal output may include unintended syllables or words. An example of a *paraphasia* is saying *pronunciate* for *pronunciation*. In addition, nonfluent patients can have difficulty repeating words and sentences. Articulation is impaired so their speech may be difficult to understand. Comprehension is relatively spared, although it is *not* perfect. As result, patients may *appear* to understand what is being said when they really do not. In fluent aphasia, the damage is in the posterior portion of the temporal lobe, known as *Wernicke's area*. Lesions are found near Heschl's gyrus, which is the primary auditory cortex (Brookshire, 2003). Damage to this area results in poor comprehension of spoken and written words. Word meaning and word finding are severely affected, although grammar, prosody, and rate of speech are relatively intact, resulting in natural sounding output that carries little meaning (Table S.2).

DEMENTIA

The term *dementia* refers to a set of symptoms associated with memory loss and reasoning skills. Alzheimer's disease is one form of dementia. Receptive and expressive language skills are affected, as are language skills. For example, patients demonstrate problems in finding words and following conversational exchanges, organizing information for narrative productions, executing multistep commands, recalling information, and sustaining focus and attention. McKhann et al. (2011) established key criteria for the diagnosis of dementia, wherein many of these features

---

Table S.2

Nonfluent Aphasia Sample	Fluent Aphasia Sample
(Describing a Cinderella picture) "…uh…this…sh…sh…say…shoe…oh my god…hard…this…shoe…slip…slip…girl…dammit"	(Responding to questions about what brought the patient to the hospital) "Is this some of the work that we work as we did before?…all right…from when wine [why] I'm here. What's wrong with me because I…was myself until the taenz took something about the time between me and my regular time in that time and they took the time in that time here and that's when the time took around here and saw me around in it's started with me no time and I began work of nothing else that's the way the doctor find me that way…"

Source: Adapted from Obler and Gjerlow (1999).

S

either directly or indirectly involve language skills:

1. Problems acquiring and retaining new information
2. Reduced reasoning and judgment and difficulty executing complex tasks
3. Poor word-finding skills
4. Writing errors

DYSARTHRIA

Dysarthria is a collective term referring to speech disruptions involving muscle control following brain damage; it does not affect a patient's language skills. Stroke, brain tumors, and neurological conditions, including Lou Gehrig's disease, or amyotrophic lateral sclerosis (ALS), can cause facial paralysis and affect the muscle coordination required for speech production. Symptoms include slow and labored speech, reduced loudness or speaking too loudly, rapid rate of speech, nasal quality, drooling, and difficulty moving the tongue and facial muscles. Patients with aphasia may also show symptoms of dysarthria.

APRAXIA

Apraxia is a motor speech disorder in which messages from the brain to the articulators are disrupted. An individual with apraxia struggles to plan and to coordinate the muscles movements needed for speech production, even though the muscles for these gestures are physiologically intact and functional. Because this difficulty, individuals with apraxia know what they want to say but may produce different or even made-up words (e.g., *pimteno* instead of *pimento* or saying *chicken* for *kitchen*). Symptoms also include difficulty imitating and producing speech sounds, inconsistent speech sound errors, groping of the articulators to make specific sounds, reduced speech rate, and impaired rhythm/prosody. Apraxia is caused by damage to areas of the brain needed for motor planning. Common causes include stroke, traumatic brain injury (TBI), dementia, brain tumors, and progressive neurological diseases. Apraxia can occur with other speech,

language, and communication difficulties, including aphasia and dysphagia.

DYSPHAGIA

Dysphagia is difficulty in the movements needed for safely and effectively swallowing food and liquid. Dysphagia can result from several diseases, conditions, or surgical interventions. General symptoms of dysphagia include coughing during eating or drinking; extra effort or time needed to chew and swallow, food/liquid leaking from the mouth during eating, recurring pneumonia, and weight loss/dehydration from not being able to consume enough food. Dysphagia can be caused by damage to the nervous system, such as stroke, TBI, spinal cord injury, Parkinson's disease, ALS, Alzheimer's disease, or multiple sclerosis. Problems in the head and neck can also result in dysphagia; these include cancer of the mouth, throat, or esophagus; injury of or surgery in the area; and decayed/missing teeth. Dysphagia may also occur with other speech and language challenges, including aphasia, dysarthria, and apraxia.

CONCLUSION

Given that older adults may have a wide range of speech, language, and communication challenges, nursing staff should be aware of these difficulties to best serve the patient. Some suggestions follow for working with patients who exhibit speech, language, and swallowing difficulties:

- Minimize background noise to ensure the patient's attention
- Use a reduced rate of speech
- Simplify the structure of sentences, but do not undermine the patient's comprehension abilities
- Give the patient time to develop and produce responses
- Provide drawings or writings to support spoken communication
- Offer alternative means of communication (i.e., writing or typing) for the patient, if needed

- If symptoms develop or worsen, refer the patient for a speech and language evaluation

Nancy Eng and Christina Oros

Brookshire, R. (2003). *Introduction to neurogenic communication disorders* (6th ed.). St. Louis, MO: Mosby.

Lam, J. M., & Wodchis, W. P. (2010). The relationship of 60 disease diagnoses and 15 conditions to preference-based health-related quality of life in Ontario hospital-based long-term care residents. *Medical Care, 48*(4), 380–387.

McKhann, G. M., Knopman, D. S., Chertkow, H., Hyman, B. T., Jack, C. R., Kawas, C. H., … Phelps, C. H. (2011). The diagnosis of dementia due to Alzheimer's disease: Recommendations from the National Institute on Aging-Alzheimer's Association workgroups on diagnostic guidelines for Alzheimer's disease. *Alzheimer's & Dementia, 7*(3), 263–269.

Obler, L. K., & Gjerlow, K. (1999). *Language and the brain.* New York, NY: Cambridge University Press.

SPIRITUALITY

Spirituality is an important component of an individual's identity and well-being and may be expressed through external behaviors such as participation in organized religion or through internal activities such as reflection and meditation (American Society on Aging, 2016). Research positively correlates well-being with improved health status and encourages health care providers to recognize and address the connection between spirituality and health in their practices (Miller & Thoresen, 2003). It is even more important that health care professionals caring for older adults promote spiritual caregiving as their patients and their families grapple with social change (i.e., retirement, loss of significant others), chronic or terminal illness, and/or quality- and/or end-of-life issues (Krause, 2003; Wink & Scott, 2005).

Gerontologists have attempted to understand how older peoples' involvement in religious and spiritual practices affects physical and mental health outcomes (Coleman, 2005). Although most research is descriptive, there appears to be a positive correlation between religiosity, spirituality, and improved health status (Dyer, 2007). One study of community-dwelling elders, for example, found that individuals who reported greater spirituality had higher perceptions of overall health status than individuals with lower spirituality scores (Daaleman, Perera, & Studenski, 2004). Another study found that older adults in long-term care facilities reported a higher quality of life after using religious and spiritual coping strategies (Vitorino et al., 2016). Regular participation in religious activities, such as attending weekly religious services, reading spiritual writings regularly, and engaging in routine prayer, also decreases markers of cumulative physiologic dysfunction, such as cortisol levels, blood pressure, waist–hip ratio, and epinephrine levels, resulting in lower stress and depression levels and reduced mortality in older adults (Maselko, Kubzansky, Kawachi, Seeman, & Berkman, 2007; Teinonen, Vahlberg, Isoaho, & Kivelä, 2005). The positive influences of spirituality on the quality of life in older people with dementia have also been noted in several studies (Toivonen, Stolt, & Suhonen, 2015).

Newer research is examining the use of secular approaches to spiritual care. The use of mindfulness as an accepted form of spiritual care for nonreligious older adults is gaining popularity (Stevens, 2016), as is the use of spiritual reminiscence in older adults with mild to moderate dementia (Mackinlay & Trevitt, 2010; Wu & Koo, 2016). Whether older adults are formally affiliated with organized religion, research supports the need for individuals to express their spiritual concerns and needs in the context of their life histories.

Previous research also supports the need to better integrate spiritual care into the overall care of older adults, recognizing that spiritual needs may change across contexts (e.g., home, hospital, long-term care setting). Indeed, Monod and Spencer (2010) argue that spirituality is a dynamic aspect of well-being, deserving an ongoing assessment in geriatric patient populations. Promoting such integration, however, requires appropriate assessment of spirituality and interventions to address spiritual issues.

Caregivers' failure to assess spiritual needs has been associated with numerous factors, including the ambiguous meaning of spirituality, provider discomfort with spirituality, inadequate educational preparation to provide spiritual care, patient reluctance to share spiritual concerns, and lack of clinical time to devote to patients' spiritual needs (Rushton, 2014; Wu, Tseng, & Liao, 2016). Few practice models operationalize spiritual assessment and care into clinical practice or measure clinical outcomes of the older person's spiritual well-being. Attempts to quantify spirituality through pretested instruments measuring various parameters of spirituality have often been flawed or statistically insignificant (Monod et al, 2011). Nonetheless, many researchers and clinicians agree that spirituality is important to older adults and suggest that providers include spiritual assessment as part of routine practice. Nurse and social work educators, in particular, are encouraged to prepare future nurses and social workers to incorporate spirituality into a holistic care paradigm.

First, providers need to respect elders' religious or spiritual articles and practices that symbolize individual faith and values. Certain religiously based dietary restrictions or care philosophies, for example, may not coincide with Western medical thought but should be considered in a patient's overall care plan. Second, health care providers need to provide an atmosphere in which expressions of spirituality are accepted and encouraged. Providers must also recognize that not all individuals express their spirituality in a religious framework and should encourage them to express their spirituality through other means, such as sharing life stories or personal perspectives on life meaning (Jackson, Doyle, Capon, & Pringle, 2016). Finally, providers could engage with patients in spiritual practices, such as prayer, meditation, or healing modalities in accordance with their own degree of comfort. Providers need to explore their own spiritual perspectives and practices to offer adequate spiritual interventions in situations in which they are most needed.

For many older adults, religious commitment and a sense of spirituality are important aspects of how they age and approach the end of life. Future research in spirituality and aging must assess outcomes of spiritual care, explore the meaning of spirituality across diverse groups of elders, and demonstrate clear educational and practice goals for nurses, physicians, social workers, and others caring for older patients. Only then can health care providers understand how older adults across the care continuum experience the religious and spiritual dimensions of later life.

Barbara L. Brush and Laura E. Gultekin

American Society on Aging. (2016). Forum on religion, spirituality, and aging. Retrieved from http://www.asaging.org/forum-religion -spirituality-and-aging-forsa

Coleman, P. G. (2005). Spirituality and ageing: The health implications of religious belief and practice. *Age and Ageing, 34*(4), 318–319.

Daaleman, T. P., Perera, S., & Studenski, S. A. (2004). Religion, spirituality, and health status in geriatric outpatients. *Annals of Family Medicine, 2*(1), 49–53.

Dyer, J. (2007). How does spirituality affect physical health? A conceptual review. *Holistic Nursing Practice, 21*(6), 324–328.

Jackson, D., Doyle, C., Capon, H., & Pringle, E. (2016). Spirituality, spiritual need, and spiritual care in aged care: What the literature says. *Journal of Religion, Spirituality & Aging, 28*(4), 281–295. doi:10.1080/15528030.2016.1193097

Krause, N. (2003). Religious meaning and subjective well-being in late life. *Journals of Gerontology: Series B, Psychological Sciences and Social Sciences, 58*(3), S160–S170.

Mackinlay, E., & Trevitt, C. (2010). Living in aged care: Using spiritual reminiscence to enhance meaning in life for those with dementia. *International Journal of Mental Health Nursing, 19*(6), 394–401.

Maselko, J., Kubzansky, L., Kawachi, I., Seeman, T., & Berkman, L. (2007). Religious service attendance and allostatic load among high-functioning elderly. *Psychosomatic Medicine, 69*(5), 464–472.

Miller, W. R., & Thoresen, C. E. (2003). Spirituality, religion, and health: An emerging research field. *American Psychologist, 58*(1), 24–35.

Monod, S., Brennan, M., Rochat, E., Martin, E., Rochat, S., & Büla, C. J. (2011). Instruments measuring spirituality in clinical research: A systematic review. *Journal of General Internal Medicine, 26*(11), 1345–1357.

Monod, S., & Spencer, B. (2010). The spiritual needs model: Spirituality assessment in the geriatric hospital setting. *Journal of Religion, Spirituality, & Aging, 22*(4), 271–282.

Rushton, L. (2014). What are the barriers to spiritual care in a hospital setting? *British Journal of Nursing, 23*(7), 370–374.

Stevens, B. A. (2016). Mindfulness: A positive spirituality for ageing? *Australia Journal of Ageing.* doi: 10.1111/ajag.12346

Teinonen, T., Vahlberg, T., Isoaho, R., & Kivelä, S. L. (2005). Religious attendance and 12-year survival in older persons. *Age and Ageing, 34*(4), 406–409.

Toivonen, K., Stolt, M., & Suhonen, R. (2015). Nursing support of the spiritual needs of older adults living with dementia: A narrative literature review. *Holistic Nursing Practice, 29*(5), 303–312.

Vitorino, L. M., Lucchetti, G., Santos, A. E., Lucchetti, A. L., Ferreira, E. B., Adami, N. P., & Vianna, L. A. (2016). Spiritual religious coping is associated with quality of life in institutionalized older adults. *Journal of Religion and Health, 55*(2), 549–559.

Wink, P., & Scott, J. (2005). Does religiousness buffer against the fear of death and dying in late adulthood? Findings from a longitudinal study. *Journals of Gerontology: Series B, Psychological Sciences and Social Sciences, 60*(4), P207–P214.

Wu, L. F., & Koo, M. (2016). Randomized controlled trial of a six-week spiritual reminiscence intervention on hope, life satisfaction, and spiritual well-being in elderly with mild and moderate dementia. *International Journal of Geriatric Psychiatry, 31*(2), 120–127.

Wu, L. F., Tseng, H. C., & Liao, Y. C. (2016). Nurse education and willingness to provide spiritual care. *Nurse Education Today, 38*, 36–41.

Web Resources

American Society on Aging, Forum on Religion, Spirituality, and Aging (FORSA): http://www .asaging.org/forum-religion-spirituality -and-aging-forsa

California Lutheran Homes Center for Spirituality and Aging: http://www.spiritualityandaging.org

Journal of Religion, Spirituality, and Aging: http:// www.tandfonline.com/toc/wrsa20/current

STAFF DEVELOPMENT

To prepare health care professionals for a constantly evolving clinical environment with a focus on quality and safety, educational strategies for students and professionals must reflect the realities of patient care. This transformation needs to occur in professional schools and the workplace. Risk reduction and prevention of adverse outcomes are critical priorities, which become the foundation for what is taught and how. When designing education, important components include generic competencies in the context of the changing health care environment, specific competencies focused on the care of the elderly, and teaching methods for the enhancement of interprofessional learning.

GENERIC COMPETENCIES

Patient safety is a prominent theme in health care. *To Err is Human: Building a Safer Health System* (Kohn, Corrigan, & Donaldson, 1999) launched a national campaign for patient safety goals. In 2002, The Joint Commission for Accreditation for Healthcare Organizations (TJC) formalized this concern by creating six National Safety Patient Goals (NSPGs). The Joint Commission (Chassin & Loeb, 2013) continues this theme of patient safety with the term *high-reliability organization* and describes opportunities for synergy, collaboration, and innovation to result in a culture of safety. In response to the paradigm shift of the patient experience, health care professionals are redefining their roles and relationships with one another and with their patients.

Health care professionals need to have a systems orientation, interdisciplinary collaborative skills, and the ability to produce data that address multiple and diverse stakeholders. The educational environment must move beyond the convenient skill/knowledge/task model of content education to one that includes concepts triggering the use of decision support and the application of the best evidence- and outcomes-based results. The exponential growth in knowledge makes it impossible to focus teaching based on content only, but teaching must help learners think conceptually. Concepts are the building blocks of learning. Nurses are practicing in varied settings where knowledge, technology, and innovation changes at an astonishing rate (Benner, Sutphen, Leonard, & Day, 2010), so self-directed, lifelong learning is critical to navigating the complexities of health care in the 21st century. The Institute of Medicine (IOM, 2010) report, *The Future of Nursing: Leading Change, Advancing Care,* recommends not only that nurses achieve higher levels of education but suggests new ways of continuing education to prepare better nurses to meet the diverse needs of population health across the life span, with emphasis on chronicity, aging, and obesity. The IOM Report on the Future of Nursing (2015) states that no single profession working alone can meet the complex needs of patients and communities. Nurses must continue to develop skills and competencies in leadership, innovation, and collaboration with other professions to improve health care practices and health system redesign.

Clinical experiences have broadened to include acute, rehabilitative, palliative, ambulatory, subacute, home, community, medical home, accountable, and long-term care. Consequently, all providers need to learn the goals of health care embedded in each of these settings. Knowledge about the Patient Protection and Affordable Care Act (PPACA) passed in March 2010, and upheld by the Supreme Court in June 2012 and July 2015 in two separate decisions, is key in understanding the varied regulatory changes that have been made to the U.S. health care system. The PPACA is the most significant regulatory overhaul of U.S. health care since Medicare and Medicaid in 1965. The entire health care team needs to be prepared for initiatives introduced to better manage care for a greater population of people with improved cost management, less variation, and ability to track and trend quality outcomes. Consistent communication among all levels of the care team and reliance on the evidence become strategic ingredients for patient safety and performance improvement. Consequently, the educational implications for understanding and functioning within this multidimensional, interdisciplinary model of health care complicate teaching in many ways. Myriad clinical experiences that promote diversity and independence become necessary for accomplishing this task. This new paradigm of education for nurses as a key member of the health care team is best described by Benner et al. (2010) with their claim that "redesigning nursing education is an urgent societal agenda: a call for radical transformation" (p. 45).

Patient-centered care is a perspective of accountability that relies on customer service skills as well as a health systems orientation to transitions. The "hand off" between practitioners or the "read back" between providers and patients can be a critical point of distinction between success and failure for clinical outcomes. Learning to appreciate the complexity of communication and transitions is a foundation of expert practice. Allowing for communication that offers the opportunity for sharing relevant data and asking questions to challenge the integrity of the process are key. Patient-centered care also requires that the clinician focus on the patients' experience and satisfaction with their care.

Planning comprehensive care also requires collaboration and negotiation among members of the health care team to make the right choices for patients and populations. When working together, seamless outcomes to complex solutions are facilitated. Collaboration is a clinician's priority and brings home the point that a group of people with complementary skills can experience more success than an individual alone. Interdisciplinary teamwork is not intuitive and not always learned in school or on the job. Interprofessional education models can diminish the silo approach to learning, thus encouraging shared exchanges rather than parallel, discipline-specific work flows. The additional transition to transdisciplinarity further reinforces a unity of knowledge beyond disciplines and the need for professional members to come together to practice collectively from the beginning.

Quality improvement and use of the best evidence are expectations of performance and act as the foundation for health care. They are necessary for alignment with regulatory requirements, mandated federal government clinical core measures, and subsequent financial integrity of the health care organization. The use of data and evidence to monitor outcomes of care processes serves to put into action continuous performance improvement. Minimizing the risk of harm to patients are key activities to high reliability in a health care organization. According to Chassin and Loeb (2013), Robust Process Improvement (RPI) methodologies are needed inclusive of Lean, Six Sigma and change management. RPI is a quality-improvement method developed in industry and imported into health care and has become more effective than the traditional PDCA (Plan, Do, Check, Act) because RPI has a distinctive focus on systematic attention to uncovering specific causes of failure. It is critical to teach these process-improvement methods to students and professionals to dramatically enhance commitment to high-quality and safe patient care.

Technology is an integral part of health-system operations that incorporates clinical, research, and informational aspects of care, although significantly altering the way health care providers and patients interact and control outcomes. The use of information technology assists in communication, education, management of knowledge, and mitigation of errors and provides a platform for decision support. Informatics education is a relevant staff-development investment in that it is the best tool for keeping pace with the information explosion and the need for self-directed learning.

SPECIFIC COMPETENCIES

The specific competencies necessary for the care of an older adult reflect four main themes: complexity, fragility, functionality, and vulnerability. The Silver Tsunami has invaded the world's nations. In 2020, it will become the first time in history that older people outnumber children younger than 5 years. As the number of senior people rises, the role of caregivers and models for quality health care need to evoke a myriad of care designs. According to Meier (2016) the *new* view of health care is for the patient to remain independent and functional, followed by symptom relief and preservation of life. The *current* view of health care is just the opposite, with a priority for the patient to stay alive, followed by symptom relief and patient independence and preservation of function.

Managing primary health problems while controlling a variety of coexisting conditions is a challenge for the novice, as well as the experienced professional. Theories of aging, age- related changes, generational and cultural diversity, and the competencies of palliative care can be discussed in workshops or through online learning options. In reality, the interdisciplinary health care team presents the

opportunity for the fusion of clinical expertise with planning and functionality because the needs of elders are often complicated by comorbidity, special needs, discharge challenges, and end-of-life decisions.

Familiarity with risk-assessment tools and concentration of health promotion and maintenance is key to quality care of the older adult. Common assessment tools include the evaluation of risk for falls, loss of skin integrity, and cognition issues; screening for dementia, depression, and delirium; and management of pain and mobility. Incorporating these tools into staff education is fundamental to "defensive practice" and the promotion of quality of life for the elderly. The vulnerability of the older adult means that the professional caregiver is the "watchful eye" for concerns such as age-related responses to care, elder mistreatment, insurance scams, education overload, bureaucratic confusion, and polypharmacy. Finally, the need for primary palliative care practice, which centers on individualized patient comfort and support, includes communication and specialized knowledge and skills (Gawande, 2014). Learning how to create a culture of safety in this vulnerable population is a complex but necessary exercise for the professional learning environment.

TEACHING METHODOLOGIES

Experiential learning is one of the strengths of nursing education, yet the need to integrate knowledge into practice context is vital. Teaching must shift from a focus on isolated content to one emphasizing teaching with a sense of salience, situated cognition, and action in particular situations (Benner et al., 2010). It is through simulation, case studies, and learning that nurses can be prepared to meet the challenges of increasingly complex clinical practice settings (Vezina & Paguirigan, 2015). For example, simulation embraces real-life scenarios with a no-risk approach. Debriefings, particularly if done in an interprofessional environment, increases comprehension and clinical reasoning. Engaging in an educational dialogue rather than listening to a lecture expresses this shift in the educational process. Learning experts report that students retain only 20% of what they hear and even less of what they read. There is up to 80% to 90% retention when individuals are involved in learning. Educators, both in schools and in institutions of work, can benefit by integrating small-group learning, simulation, and interactive approaches to education. Active learning invokes higher-order thinking skills. The "safety" of the classroom may be sacrificed for the experience of learning while working. Team teaching is another powerful strategy for role modeling to actualize interdisciplinary collaboration. Having faculty engaged in these exercises is motivating and provides teaching from a stance of clinical practice, not the didactic classroom.

Strategies for information-age education include avatar experiences in which learning can be safe yet participatory and supported by outcome-based responses; case-based-learning encouraging reflection and reasoning, resulting in planning care that makes a difference in patients' lives. Using failure-mode investigation or an exercise in root cause analysis may also prove instrumental in teaching the prevention and/or successful rescues of practice errors (Clarke & Aiken, 2003).

Focusing on competencies and teaching strategies to be prepared for practice in the 21st century of health care realigns nursing education and staff development with the changing environment in which health care professionals live and work. Nurses play an essential role in creating quality patient care, high reliability, and safety, thus prompting the need to manage what they learn and how they learn it.

See also Cultural Change; Future of Care; Hospital-Based Services; Patient Safety.

Maria L. Vezina

Benner, P., Sutphen, M., Leonard, V., & Day, L. (2010). *Educating nurses: A call for radical transformation.* San Francisco, CA: Jossey-Bass.

Chassin, M. R., & Loeb, J. M. (2013). *High reliability healthcare: Getting there from here.* Oakbrook Terrace, IL. The Joint Commission.

Clarke, S. P., & Aiken, L. H. (2003). Registered nurse staffing and patient and nurse outcomes in hospitals: A commentary. *Policy, Politics, & Nursing Practice, 4,* 104–111.

Gawande, A. (2014). *Being mortal.* New York, NY: Metropolitan Books, Henry Holt.

Institute of Medicine. (2010). *The future of nursing: Leading change, advancing care.* Washington, DC: Author.

Institute of Medicine. (2015). *Assessing progress on the Institute of Medicine report: The future of nursing.* Washington, DC: Author.

Kohn, L., Corrigan, J., & Donaldson, M. (Eds.). (1999). *To err is human: Building a safer health system: Committee of Quality of Healthcare.* Washington, DC: Institute of Medicine.

Meier, D. (2016). *"Many faces of pain": "Beyond mortality: Neuropalliative care and the quality of life."* New York, NY: Icahn School of Medicine at Mount Sinai Continuing Education Program.

Vezina, M., & Paguirigan, M. (2015). Concept based learning. In M. J. Smith, R. Carpenter, & J. Fitzpatrick (Eds.), *Encyclopedia of nursing education.* New York, NY: Springer Publishing.

Web Resources
American Association of Colleges of Nursing: http://www.aacn.nche.edu

Carnegie Foundation for the Advancement of Teaching: http://www.carnegiefoundation.org

Essentials of Baccalaureate Education for Professional Nursing Practice: http://www.aacn.nche.edu/education-resources

Hartford Institute for Geriatric Nursing: http://www.hartfordign.org/roles/staffDevEd.html

Institute of Medicine: Assessing Progress on the Institute of Medicine Report: *The Future of Nursing:* http://www.jonascenter.org

Institute of Medicine Report: Future of Nursing: Focus on Education: http://www.iom.edu/Reports/2010/The Future of Nursing

Institute of Medicine Report: The Future of Nursing: Leading Change, Advancing Health: http://nationalacademies.org/hmd/reports/2010/the-future-of-nursing-leading-change-advancing-health.aspx

The Joint Commission: http://www.jointcommission.org

SUBSTITUTE DECISION MAKING

With few exceptions, a health care or human services provider may not do anything to an adult patient without first obtaining voluntary, informed consent. Consent may be expressed (put into words) or implied by the conduct of the patient. Ordinarily, the provider must discuss all pertinent information and negotiate the details of any intervention directly with the patient, who is presumed to possess the capacity to understand and manipulate that information and engage in negotiations with the service provider. In some situations, however, the individual is not cognitively and emotionally able to assimilate the relevant facts and take part meaningfully in a rational decision-making process regarding proposed and alternative plans of action. This situation is especially likely to materialize in the case of older people whose mental capacities have been compromised because of dementia, depression, organic brain syndrome, or other age-related mental disorders.

Autonomous decision making cannot occur in the absence of a decision maker who is capable of exercising autonomy. Nonetheless, when the individual fails to have sufficient decisional capacity, the service provider still has the duty to obtain informed consent before intervening in the individual's life. This duty must be fulfilled by working with someone else who is willing and able to act as a substitute decision maker (a surrogate or proxy) on behalf of the patient.

A substantial percentage of older persons who lack adequate capacity to make and express their own legally valid decisions may be capable of some level of assisted or supported decision making and therefore should be encouraged and helped to participate in the decision-making process with family members or friends (Burke, 2016; Kohn, Blumenthal, & Campbell, 2013). Even when the decisionally impaired older person can participate, to some limited extent, in the decision-making process, a substitute decision maker ultimately is turned to by the health care team or institution to obtain legally valid decisions consenting to or declining particular medical interventions.

To maximize one's autonomous control, one may use legal advance planning instruments to take steps, while still mentally capable, to anticipate and prepare for later incapacity by voluntarily delegating or directing future power over major decisions. The durable power of attorney consists of a written document in which an

individual (the principal) may appoint an agent, sometimes termed the "attorney-in-fact" but who need not be an attorney-at-law, to make specified types of future choices for the principal. Every American jurisdiction has enacted one or more statutes that expressly permit the use of the durable power of attorney to empower an agent to make specified decisions on the principal's behalf, should the principal no longer possess adequate decision-making ability.

Use of the durable power of attorney mechanism is consistent with important ethical principles. Autonomy means that individuals should have control and integrity over what happens to themselves. To act autonomously, one requires information about reasonable alternatives and their possible consequences. For mentally incapacitated persons, autonomy is best promoted by informing the surrogate (ideally someone whom the incapacitated person had previously designated) of the principal's wishes and then expecting the surrogate to make particular choices based on the principal's substituted judgment. Substituted judgment is choosing what the principal would choose if able to make and express personal own decisions (i.e., standing in the shoes of the principal).

Durable powers of attorney fall into two categories. First, an immediate power becomes effective the minute an agent is designated. By contrast, a springing power allows the legal authority to move (spring) from the principal to the agent only when some specified future event, such as two physicians examining the principal and agreeing that the principal is decisionally incapacitated, materializes. An individual should be told by health care and human service providers when they have decided to proceed by substitute decision making rather than by the patient's informed consent; such information would give the principal a chance to contest the agent's power if so desired.

A durable power of attorney may be used in tandem with a living will or another instruction directive. Among other things, a living will assists an agent named under a durable power of attorney to exercise the individual's substituted judgment more accurately.

Some individuals who become decisionally incapacitated have not executed an instruction directive or appointed a decision-making agent. A majority of states have statutes that empower family members and specified other individuals to make certain choices for incapacitated persons (Wynn, 2014). In states that have enacted surrogate default legislation, the approved procedure usually entails documenting unanimous agreement among professional service providers, specified relatives, and sometimes others who are enumerated in a particular priority order. Even in states that lack surrogate default legislation, the courts (on the very rare occasions that they become involved) uphold as a matter of common law or a state's own constitution the family's power to exercise the incapacitated person's decision-making rights.

When no durable power of attorney has been appointed, there are no applicable surrogate default statute or judicial precedent authorizing family members or others to decide, and/or family members vehemently and irreconcilably disagree among themselves about the best course of care for the decisionally impaired individual, establishing a guardianship or conservatorship may be advisable. The guardianship or conservatorship order (terminology varies among different jurisdictions) has the effect of formally transferring decision-making when strategies such as mediation, referral to an institutional or organizational ethics committee, or supported decision making have failed in attempting to reconcile the conflicting positions of the interested stakeholders.

The guardianship/conservatorship process involves the appointment, generally in response to a petition filed by the family or a caregiver, by a state court with proper jurisdiction of a surrogate (the guardian or conservator), who is permitted to make certain decisions for a decisionally incapacitated person (the ward). The appointed guardian/conservator most frequently is a family member, but it could also be a private professional or a public agency (Cashmore, 2014) when no suitable family member is willing or available. The petition for court action ordinarily is supported by an affidavit or live testimony of a physician—and often other professionals and laypersons—who are familiar with the proposed ward.

In the majority of cases, guardianship/conservatorship is sincerely intended for the benefit of the ward. The state may intervene under its inherent *parens patriae* deprivation of an individual's fundamental decision-making rights, the least restrictive/least intrusive alternate doctrine argues for a partial or limited guardianship of only temporary duration, whenever such is feasible. That doctrine is based on the proposition that the state should interfere with individual rights only in the least restrictive or least intrusive way possible, consistent with the legitimate social goal of safeguarding the individual against harm. As part of this doctrine, courts have the authority to limit the guardian's decision-making power to only those particular kinds of choices that the ward personally, in fact, cannot rationally make, and only for as long a period as necessary.

Historically, the guardian as a fiduciary or trust agent has been entrusted to make decisions in line with the guardian's view of the ward's best interests. A number of jurisdictions still require guardians to be guided from the outset by this purportedly objective best interests standard. The more modern trend in substitute decision making, however, is toward recognition of and a preference for a substituted judgment standard. Under this autonomy-driven paradigm, the guardian is expected to make choices that the incapacitated person would make subjectively, according to the incapacitated person's values (to the extent that they can be accurately identified), if that person were able to make and communicate personal own autonomous decisions (English, 2016).

There are times that appointment of a guardian would be advisable but there are no obvious candidates for the job. An increasing number of individuals are growing older and unable to make their own autonomous decisions but are without family or friends who are willing and able to act as substitute decision makers for them. Developing dependable systems of substitute decision-making that protects the rights and interests of these "unbefriended" or "unfamilied" individuals presents a significant social, ethical, and legal challenge for the coming years (Connor, Elkin, Lee, Thompson, & Whelan, 2016; Pope, 2015).

See also Advance Directives; Guardianship and Conservatorship.

Marshall B. Kapp

Burke, S. (2016). Person-centered guardianship: How the rise of supported decision-making and person-centered services can help Olmstead's promise get here faster. *Hamline Mitchell Law Review, 42*, 873–896.

Cashmore, E. B. (2014). Guarding the golden years: How public guardianship for elders can help states meet the mandates of Olmstead. *Boston College Law Review, 55*, 1217–1251.

Connor, D. M., Elkin, G. D., Lee, K., Thompson, V., & Whelan, H. (2016). The unbefriended patient: An exercise in ethical clinical reasoning. *Journal of General Internal Medicine, 31*(1), 128–132.

English, D. M. (2016 Spring). Amending the Uniform Guardianship and Protective Proceedings Act to implement the standards and recommendations of the Third National Guardianship Summit. *NAELA Journal, 12*, 33–55.

Kohn, N. A., Blumenthal, J. A., & Campbell, A. T. (2013). Supported decision making: A viable alternative to guardianship. *Penn State Law Review, 117*, 1111–1157.

Pope, T. M. (2015). Adult orphans and the unbefreinded: Making medical decisions for unrepresented patients without surrogates. *Journal of Clinical Ethics, 26*, 180–188.

Wynn, S. (2014, September–October). Decisions by surrogates: An overview of surrogate consent laws in the United States. *Bifocal, 36*, 10–14.

Web Resources

American Association of Daily Money Managers: http://www.aadmm.com

Family Caregivers Alliance: http://www.caregiver.org

International Guardianship Network: http://www.international-guardianship.com

National Guardianship Association: http://www.guardian ship.org

National Resource Center for Supported Decision-Making: http://supporteddecisionmaking.org

Suicide in Late Life

Understanding the problem of suicide in late life is a complex challenge, whether considering the risks for a specific older adult or the elderly population as a whole. Suicide is a phenomenon that emerges from a web of causal factors ranging from genetics and neurochemistry to medical and psychiatric problems to socioeconomic and cultural environments and even to geography and weather.

EPIDEMIOLOGY

In the United States, approximately 37,000 people commit suicide each year, and another 650,000 people are seen in an emergency room after suicide attempts. The number of suicide attempts ranges from 10 to 40 times the number of completed suicides. Suicide is the 10th leading cause of death worldwide. These figures, however, may underestimate the true rates because legal issues or social stigma may result in suicidal deaths being misclassified. The suicide rate in older adults (more than 64 years of age) in the United States is 15 per 100,000 (U.S. Burden of Disease Collaborators, 2013). This rate is higher in the baby boomers as they age (Curtain, Warner, & Hedegaard, 2016). Approximately onefifth of suicide victims have a history of previous attempts, and approximately onesixth have alcohol-associated problems. Firearms are the most prevalent means of committing suicide in the United States, followed by hanging for men and overdosing for women. Approximately three fourths of individuals who commit suicide have contact with a primary care provider within a year of their death, as opposed to one third having had contact with a mental health service provider. Twice as many have contact with their primary care providers as with their mental health providers in the month before suicide.

RISK FACTORS

Many factors that raise the risks of suicide have been identified. With older adults, these risk factors can be thought of in two important ways. One is the usual approach to assessing whether these risk factors represent a motive for older individuals to kill themselves. Another is to construe them as masking an opportunity to detect indications of elevated suicide risk. Instead of trying to achieve the goal of eliminating suicides altogether, a more realistic strategy is reducing the number of missed opportunities for interventions to prevent suicide. Both these tasks are challenging in working with the elderly, because older adults are much more different from one another in multiple ways—physiologically, psychologically, experientially, and socially—than younger adults, which makes generalizing about them more hazardous (Bishop, Simons, King, & Pigeon, 2016; Conwell, Van Orden, & Caine, 2011; Curtain et al., 2016; Fässberg et al. 2016; Fiske & O'Riley, 2016; Mills, Watts, Huh, Boar, & Kemp, 2013; O'Dwyer, Moyle, Zimmer-Gembeck, & De Leo, 2016; Sachs-Ericsson, Rushing, Stanley, & Sheffler, 2016; Stanley, Hom, Rogers, Hagan, & Joiner, 2016; U.S. Burden of Disease Collaborators, 2013).

Social/Environmental/Demographic Factors

Age: The risk of completed suicide increases with age; older individuals are less likely to report distressing symptoms.

Sex: For women, the risks increase over the lifetime course until middle age and then levels out, whereas for men the risks keep climbing, even up until the ninth decade of life; men are less likely to report relevant symptoms.

Ethnicity: The rates are higher in the United States for Whites as opposed to Blacks and other minorities; in the United States, the suicide rate for elderly White men older than 74 years of age is the highest of all, at 42.4 per year per 100,000 population.

Marital and family status: Suicide risk increases in proportion to a decrease in the degree of connection with others, with the risk being lowest in those married with children, followed by married without children, divorced, separated, widowed, and highest of all in those who were never married.

Socioeconomic status: The lower such status, the higher the risks; risks for suicide are higher in those who are having significant financial difficulties, are unskilled, and/or have been unemployed; a notable exception to this is that clinicians appear to have a higher risk of suicide (and higher for female clinicians than for male clinicians); and those with military service.

Social environment: Risk is higher with social isolation, recent loss of a significant other or of a meaningful activity, marital discord, a family member with psychiatric or substance use disorder or legal problems (e.g., incarceration), exposure to violence or political

coercion, social discrimination against members of minority groups (e.g., based on ethnicity or sexual orientation); all of these factors can reduce the likelihood of risk factors being detected.

Economic: Suicide risk increases in the presence of personal financial crisis (including loss of health insurance), as well as economic recessions and depressions.

Physical environment: There is higher risk with easier access to firearms or medications that are lethal when taken in excessive quantities.

Geographic: Suicide risk is higher for those living in a rural environment.

Cultural: Stigma associated with mental illness, suicide, and seeking psychiatric assistance; high emphasis in prevailing culture or subculture on autonomy, independence, and achievement; and religious values emphasizing life and prohibiting suicide can all be protective.

Systems: Suicide risk increases with lack of access to mental health resources and time constraints in current health care delivery organizations.

Neurobiological/Genetic Factors

Neurotransmitters: Serotonin may play a role, along with other neurotransmitters, in the modulation of the kinds of impulsive behavior associated with attempted and completed suicides.

Family history of suicide: The risk of suicide is up to six times higher for individuals who have had a first-degree relative commit suicide; it is not clear whether the hereditary risk is primarily for the underlying psychiatric disorder or the suicide itself; twin studies have revealed both genetic and environmental components to elevated suicide risk.

Medication/Substance Factors

Alcohol: Misuse of alcohol significantly raises the risk of suicide.

Sedatives: Misuse of benzodiazepines may be associated with behavioral disinhibition, thereby raising the risk of suicide.

Pharmacotherapy: Nonadherence to prescribed medication (both psychiatric and nonpsychiatric) medications increases risk.

Psychiatric/Behavioral Factors

History of previous suicide attempts: A history of suicide attempts can increase the likelihood of another attempt by a factor of five to six times; this risk is greatest in patients with schizophrenia, unipolar depression, and bipolar disorder. Older adults who have never made a previous suicide attempt, however, make up the majority of completed suicides.

Psychiatric disorders: Patients with depression, bipolar disorder, substance abuse, schizophrenia, anxiety disorders, and personality disorders and patients with more than one co-occurring psychiatric disorder appear to be at higher risk of suicide, especially those with a combination of depression and anxiety or any psychiatric disorder and with the misuse of alcohol or drugs.

Psychiatric symptoms: In older adults, mood symptoms may sometimes be milder and harder to detect.

Biological symptoms of depression: Some of the biological symptoms (loss of appetite, fatigue, insomnia) are nonspecific and may also stem from co-occurring medical problems; if they are attributed primarily to the medical problems, they may be missed as clues to depression. Insomnia is associated with an elevated risk.

Psychological symptoms: Feelings of worthlessness, helplessness, and/or especially hopelessness (undue pessimism about the future); a sense of losing control over one's life, existential despair; a sense that one's life no longer has meaning or purpose; impulsivity.

Psychotic symptoms: These include delusions, hallucinations, and paranoia.

Suicidal ideation: The greater the specificity of the suicidal ideation, the higher the risk; when one has a specific plan, the intention to act on that plan is associated with increased risk, as is the likely lethality of the means for killing oneself (e.g., shooting, hanging, and jumping are much less reversible than overdosing).

Behaviors possibly suggestive of suicidality: These may include uncharacteristic actions such as making a clinical appointment for no readily apparent reason, giving away personally significant items, or atypical calmness after a period of turmoil. Some older adults who lack effective interpersonal skills may use suicidal language as a means to influence others around them, others who have led a long and full life may express a readiness or wish to die but have no intention of hastening the end of their lives, such expressions need not be considered abnormal.

Health Factors

Medical problems: Debilitating physical illnesses that compromise functional capacities, including the ability to perform activities of daily living and/or instrumental activities of daily living, may include such problems as congestive heart failure, chronic obstructive pulmonary disease, sleep disorders, severe arthritis, as well as any condition associated with chronic pain; professional care providers and family members may focus primarily on addressing significant and challenging medical problems but overlook pertinent psychiatric and social factors.

Personal Factors

Adverse life experiences: Risk is increased among those with emotional, physical, sexual, financial, or other abuse or neglect, either as a child or an adult; recent loss of a significant other; loss of the ability to perform especially meaningful activities (e.g., severe arthritis in the hands of a concert pianist; loss of vision for a painter).

Personality traits: In general, risk is elevated with individual personality traits that are either too strong or too weak and/or too rigid or too flexible, such that the individual's abilities to cope with stressors (resilience) is compromised (e.g., individuals whose personality styles are keen on autonomy, control, independence, self-reliance); risks have been noted to be higher with certain specific traits, including low openness to experience and low extraversion, both of which tend to be associated with lower levels of perceived support and smaller support networks.

Time Factors

Certain times are riskier, including (a) in the days and weeks after a significant stressor such as the loss of a spouse, a psychiatric hospitalization, surgery, and the diagnosis of a severe or terminal illness (e.g., cancer, dementia); (b) on the anniversary of a major loss; and (c) warmer seasons (e.g., spring, summer).

ASSESSMENT

The presence of suicidal ideation or unusual, suggestive behaviors in an older adult calls for careful assessment. This can be particularly challenging, given the complexity of the issues in combination with the tendencies of older adults and their family members to under-report relevant factors. An adequate evaluation includes consideration of relevant risk and protective factors with physical and mental status examination and assessment of the individual's support network.

Caregivers, whether professional or family, are sometimes concerned that inquiring about suicide may increase the risk. Almost always, however, the opposite is the case—the individual contemplating suicide is at some level usually appreciative of the fact that somebody cared enough to ask and, generally, will share such thoughts and concerns. Older adults, in particular, may not verbalize their suicidal ideation without being prompted.

The ability to predict who is likely to attempt or commit suicide is limited, especially given the number and complexity of risk factors in suicidal older adults, which overlap with those who are not suicidal. A number of standardized instruments have been developed to evaluate suicidal risk, but none have been shown to have high levels of either sensitivity or specificity, and thus to be of significant practical value in assessing the likelihood of suicide.

The initial step in the assessment of suicidal older adults is to determine the content and duration of their suicidal ideations, including how these may have been developing and changing and how well they have been coping with them. Starting with more general questions, such as whether they have felt as if life was no longer worth living, and then moving on to more specific inquiries about whether they have considered actively ending their own life, can facilitate a candid assessment. It is important to determine the extent to which they have developed a suicide plan. This includes the specific method, location, and timing, as well as the degree of intent (including lack of fear) about implementing this plan.

Inquiring, for example, whether they have been changing wills, writing a suicide note, and acquiring lethal means (e.g., gathering pills for an overdose, obtaining a gun) can provide useful clues, as can asking about how they view the future, what they anticipate would be the effect of their death on others, and the degree to which they feel hopeless and/or worthless. Further assessment includes how they have access to the means being considered, how lethal they consider these means to be (as well as their likely actual lethality), and how likely they are of being rescued after using these means.

Exploring these factors can help determine what the suicidal individuals' situations mean to them, as opposed to other people. Dialoguing to establish a clear and distinct understanding of such meaning, which is unique for each person, is critical. Meaning mutually shared by both the suicidal individual and care provider is essential, not only for diagnostic and prognostic purposes, but also as the basis for establishing a genuine therapeutic alliance. This is perhaps the most crucial element in achieving an effective outcome.

MANAGEMENT

Interventions for Suicidal Individuals

Management of suicidality in older adults includes reducing immediate risks, addressing contributing risk factors, and ensuring adequate monitoring and follow-up. If the risks of suicide are judged to be acute and high, hospitalization is warranted, as is contacting social supports (e.g., family or friends) and care providers. Regulations regarding patient confidentiality allow for this in situations that are life-threatening. If such an acutely suicidal older adult does not agree to hospitalization on a voluntary basis, it may be necessary to implement this option with the assistance of crisis intervention staff and/or police.

In situations that are less severe but still with significant risk, development of a proactive safety plan is critical. This includes firmly establishing (a) a connection between the suicidal older adult and another person who can reliably act as a "lifeline"; (b) a safe environment from which potential means of self-harm have been removed; and (c) initiation of interventions to address identified problems involving medical (e.g., pain or other discomfort), psychiatric (e.g., depression), personal (e.g., lack of meaningful activities), and/or social (e.g., isolation, other stressors) issues.

There is little evidence for the effectiveness of using formal or informal "no harm contracts" between care providers and suicidal patients in reducing suicide. Such contracts or agreements may provide clinicians with a false sense of security. Establishment and maintenance of a therapeutic alliance over time are considered much more effective.

For individuals identified as suffering from symptoms of major depression, treatment with antidepressants has been demonstrated to be effective in reducing the risk of suicide, as has treatment of bipolar disorder with lithium. In recent years, there has been a concern that the initiation of antidepressant therapy increased the risk of suicide, but this is not the case with older adults. For those with severe depression (e.g., psychotic depression) whose risk of suicide remains high even in the safety of a hospital and cannot wait the weeks required for medication to become effective, electroconvulsive therapy (ECT) can be lifesaving. ECT is also a consideration with suicidal older adults for whom antidepressant medication is not effective or associated with side effects that are difficult to tolerate.

Combining medication with some form of psychotherapy for late-life depression tends to be more effective than either alone, especially when psychosocial stressors have been identified. Such therapy may include individual and/or group counseling (e.g., cognitive or dialectical behavioral therapy [CBT/DBT], interpersonal therapy, and problem-solving or supportive therapy). Psychosocial interventions, which also engage

members of patients' families, community, and religious organizations, can enhance the support network of suicidal patients and reduce their sense of hopelessness. For older adults with some degree of functional impairment, a meaningful skills evaluation by an occupational therapist can provide clinical information for developing interventions that are more sensitive and specific to their unique needs and help restore a sense of control, meaning, and purpose in their lives.

Adequate monitoring and follow-up of at-risk patients are essential, especially as the risk for suicide may wax and wane. These involve a number of proactive measures on the part of care providers, including an increase in the frequency of contact with the patient, along with communication of a genuine commitment to stay engaged. These are essential components for the formation of a therapeutic alliance, which is the foundation for establishing a resilient lifeline for the patient. Monitoring includes tracking patients' response to interventions, their adherence to medication regimens and follow-up appointments, and an ongoing assessment of medication and therapy side effects, their degree of understanding of situations and interventions, and their appreciation for the consequences of their choices.

Interventions for Survivors of Suicide

There are different forms of individual counseling or group meetings designed to help care providers, family, and friends cope with the losses precipitated by completed suicide. These may help participants to understand better why the older person in their lives committed suicide, to deal with unwarranted feelings of responsibility or guilt over the person's death, and thereby help with their process of grieving.

PREVENTION

Prevention strategies can be directed toward the identification and treatment of at-risk individuals and populations. Both involve efforts to reduce risk factors, enhance protective factors, and make adequate services more available.

To date, there continues to be no definitive evidence that routine screening for suicidal ideation is effective (or not) in reducing attempted or completed suicide. The U.S. Preventive Services Task Force conducted a systematic review of screenings for suicide and determined that the evidence was insufficient to determine whether such screening was beneficial. The Canadian Task Force on Preventive Health Care came to similar conclusions as to the evidence for and against routine evaluation of suicide risk.

Environmental interventions such as dispensing medications in lower dosage forms, in more limited quantities, and/or in blister packs may be helpful for patients who are at risk of overdosing. Programs restricting access to suicidal means (e.g., control of analgesics, access to hot-spots for suicide by jumping) have demonstrated some effectiveness (Zalsman et al., 2016). Community programs that provide outreach to older adults at risk for suicide (e.g., by attempting to reduce social isolation) have had limited success. This appears likely because of the interference by both personal and cultural values involving autonomy, independence, and self-reliance. Older men are less likely to participate in such programs, and many have been noted to consistently decline offers of assistance or opportunities to become engaged in activities (Conwell et al., 2011). With a steadily increasing population of older adults, there are critical needs at the systems level not only for sustained efforts at enhancing education of clinicians and the general public, but also for increased numbers of resources that at-risk older adults can access, the number of adequately trained staff to assist them, and the number of ways for them to access timely help during crises. Given the complexities of suicide in late life, it is most likely that no single intervention prove significantly effective. Instead, a combination of integrated interventions, at the individual and the system levels, likely needs to be developed.

See also Anxiety Disorders; Bipolar Affective Disorder; Euthanasia; Physician-Assisted Suicide, Physician Aid in Dying, and Euthanasia; Social Isolation.

Timothy Howell

Bishop, T. M., Simons, K. V., King, D. A., & Pigeon, W. R. (2016). Sleep and suicide in older adults: An opportunity for intervention. *Clinical Therapeutics, 38*(11), 2332–2339.

Conwell, Y., Van Orden, K., & Caine, E. D. (2011). Suicide in older adults. *Psychiatric Clinics of North America, 34*(2), 451–468, ix.

Curtain, S. C., Warner, M., & Hedegaard, H. (2016). Increase in suicide in the United States, 1999–2014. *NCHS Data Brief, 241*, 1–8.

Fässberg, M. M., Cheung, G., Canetto, S. S., Erlangsen, A., Lapierre, S., Lindner, R., … Wærn, M. (2016). A systematic review of physical illness, functional disability, and suicidal behaviour among older adults. *Aging & Mental Health, 20*(2), 166–194.

Fiske, A., & O'Riley, A. A. (2016). Toward an understanding of late life suicidal behavior: The role of lifespan developmental theory. *Aging & Mental Health, 20*(2), 123–130.

Mills, P. D., Watts, B. V., Huh, T. J., Boar, S., & Kemp, J. (2013). Helping elderly patients to avoid suicide: A review of case reports from a National Veterans Affairs database. *Journal of Nervous and Mental Disease, 201*(1), 12–16.

O'Dwyer, S. T., Moyle, W., Zimmer-Gembeck, M., & De Leo, D. (2016). Suicidal ideation in family carers of people with dementia. *Aging & Mental Health, 20*(2), 222–230.

Sachs-Ericsson, N. J., Rushing, N. C., Stanley, I. H., & Sheffler, J. (2016). In my end is my beginning: Developmental trajectories of adverse childhood experiences to late-life suicide. *Aging & Mental Health, 20*(2), 139–165.

Stanley, I. H., Hom, M. A., Rogers, M. L., Hagan, C. R., & Joiner, T. E. (2016). Understanding suicide among older adults: A review of psychological and sociological theories of suicide. *Aging & Mental Health, 20*(2), 113–122.

U.S. Burden of Disease Collaborators. (2013). The state of US health, 1990–2010: Burden of diseases, injuries, and risk factors. *Journal of the American Medical Association, 310*(6), 591–606.

Zalsman, G., Hawton, K., Wasserman, D., van Heeringen, K., Arensman, E., Sarchiapone, M., … Zohar, J. (2016). Suicide prevention strategies revisited: 10-year systematic review. *Lancet: Psychiatry, 3*(7), 646–659.

Web Resources
American Association of Suicidology: http://www.suicidology.org
American Foundation for Suicide Prevention: https://afsp.org
Canadian Association for Suicide Prevention (CASP): https://www.suicideprevention.ca

S

International Association for Suicide Prevention (IASP): https://www.iasp.info

National Center for Injury Prevention and Control: https://www.cdc.gov/ncipc/wisqars/default.htm and https://www.cdc.gov/ncipc/factsheets/suifacts.htm

Suicide Prevention Resource Center: http://www.sprc.org

World Health Organization: Health Topics–Suicide: http://www.who.int/topics/suicide/en

SUNDOWNING

Sundowning (i.e., sundown syndrome) is the term that is used to describe a set of behavioral symptoms associated with neurocognitive disorders common in older adults, which become more evident late in the afternoon, evening, or night. Although sundowning is not included in the *Diagnostic and Statistical Manual of Mental Disorders* (5th ed.; *DSM-5*; American Psychiatric Association [APA], 2013), it is associated with the neurocognitive disorders that are part of the *DSM-5*. Sundowning occurs in many, but not all, institutionalized and elders with neurocognitive disorders. The name is derived from the time at which the behaviors begin (the afternoon, evening, and nighttime hours) and suggests that persons with delirium, dementia, and other sensory losses are sensitive to reduced light, fatigue, and other environmental changes, that most people accommodate to without difficulty. Sundowning is a clinical phenomenon based on disruptive behaviors, confusion, disorientation, agitation, aggression, pacing, wandering, resistance to redirection, screaming, and yelling. These behaviors may be related to underlying dementia or sleep disturbances. Other clinical features that may be present are mood changes, increased demands, suspiciousness, and visual or auditory hallucinations occurring late in the day.

Associated terms include acute confusion, altered mental state, dementia, and delirium. Delirium is a neuropsychological syndrome characterized by a disturbance of attention and awareness that develops over a short time (APA, 2013). It is an impaired environmental awareness and cognitive change, including altered memory, disorientation, and language disturbance or a perceptual disturbance that cannot be accounted for by preexisting dementia. Delirium is associated with neurochemical or medical etiology. In cases without mental illness, delirium is an emergent condition, and a physical or mental cause should be diagnosed as its etiology (e.g., urinary tract infection, pneumonia, untoward effects of medications and alcohol) and then promptly treated. Delirium also may be associated with sleep–wake disturbances and the altered psychomotor behavior of sundowning. Sleep disturbances are common in people with sundowning. Those with delirium may fall, remove their medical equipment, and vocalize by moaning, cursing, complaining, and screaming and may exhibit aggressive behavior. These behaviors have been found to be associated with a person's expression of physical pain or discomfort and emotional anguish. Nocturnal delirium is referred to as *sundown syndrome*.

ETIOLOGY

First described in 1941 by Cameron, sundowning has received research and clinical attention, particularly because it is as frustrating for caregivers as it is recurrent and difficult to treat effectively. Sensory deprivation, including visual and hearing impairments and inadequate exposure to light during the day, is associated with confusion and sundowning. Circadian rhythm disturbances related to sundowning include sleep–wake cycle changes in which dreams occur earlier; frequent, sudden awakenings; and increased motor activity at night. Circadian rhythms influence several physiological processes that regulate body functions and behavior. The suprachiasmatic nucleus and melatonin are involved in the pathophysiology of Alzheimer's disease and related dementia and regulate circadian rhythmicity. Melatonin is produced by darkness and sleep. Circadian rhythms are observable in 24-hour-cycle changes in core body temperature, hormonal secretions, red blood cell production, and other physiological processes. Individuals with Alzheimer's disease (AD) are more likely from those without AD to exhibit more activity at night and the later times of peak activity and temperature rhythms associated with sundown syndrome.

Sleep disturbances, common in people with all forms of dementia, include sleep apnea, sleep fragmentation, daytime napping, and restless legs syndrome. Medications, such as antidepressants, antipsychotics, hypnotics, benzodiazepines, anticholinergic agents, and analgesics may worsen sundowning.

DIAGNOSIS

Differential diagnosis is important when sundown syndrome is suspected. The most probable underlying disorders to be considered are delirium, neurocognitive disorders, and depression. *Acute confusion* is the term preferred to describe altered cognition and behavior until more definitive diagnoses can be established. The most frequent precipitating factor of any of these altered mental states is medication, especially antidepressants, antipsychotics, narcotics, and other drugs with psychotropic effects.

Differentiating delirium, neurocognitive disorders, and depression is important, and a method for identifying delirium is the confusion assessment method (CAM). The course of delirium fluctuates in 24 hours, whereas depression and dementia have more stable signs and are worse in the morning and during stressful situations. Delirium has a shorter course than either depression or dementia, with global rather than specific attentional disturbances, affect lability that varies from flat to excitable, impaired orientation, and incoherent speech. In depression, the affect is flat, and orientation is normal, with distractible attention and slowed speech. Disturbed sleep is common in both delirium and depression, but the usual pattern of daytime sleep and late wakefulness in depression is a significant indicator. In dementia, the affect is usually stable and may vary from disinhibited to vegetative, with task completion muddled by the inability to plan a sequence of steps, self-monitor, and adapt to cues. The mechanics of speech are normal, although there may be an inability to find or recall words.

As mentioned earlier, delirium is always related to the altered physiological or psychological processes associated with either drug ingestion/withdrawal or general medical conditions. Delirium is caused by diseases of the body systems other than the brain, inflammation, poisons, fluid/electrolyte or acid/base disturbances, and other serious, acute conditions. Peripheral infections such as urinary tract infections or pneumonia are now known to cross the blood–brain barrier, triggering delirium in individuals with preexisting cognitive vulnerabilities. Delirium is embodied by rapid changes such as from lethargy to agitation and from somnolence to euphoria with attention disruption, disorganized thinking, disorientation, and changes in sensation and perception. The multiple etiologies of delirium are described in Delirium.

INTERVENTIONS

The most important intervention is accurate and comprehensive assessment and documentation of altered mental states so that a differential diagnosis can be made and appropriate treatment can begin. When sundown syndrome is not related to an underlying medical condition, environmental interventions are appropriate. The patient's physical and social environment should be assessed for zeitgebers, or time providers such as lighting appropriate to the time of day and sleep needs, window shades that may be open or closed, structured meal and activity periods, suitable visitors and visiting hours, and morning and bedtime routines. The caregiver should monitor and modulate noises that are intrusive and use music or other sensory salves to soothe before bedtime. Opportunities for daytime activity and exposure to sunlight should be provided, and access to caffeinated beverages should be limited. Melatonin is available in health food stores and may promote nighttime sleep if administered before bedtime. Of note, melatonin is not approved by the U.S. Food and Drug Administration for safety, effectiveness, or purity. Of special concern are caregivers who need education and support in managing sundowning.

See also Depression Measurement Instruments; Sleep Disorders; Vascular and Lewy Body Dementia.

Steven L. Baumann

American Psychiatric Association. (2013). *Diagnostic and statistical manual of mental disorders* (5th ed.). Arlington, VA: American Psychiatric Publishing.

Web Resources
ICU Delirium and Cognitive Impairment Study Group: http://www.icudelirium.org/delirium
National Guideline Clearinghouse: http://www.guideline.gov/summary/summary.aspx?doc id=1804
Society of Critical Care Medicine: http://www.learn icu.org/SiteCollectionDocuments/Pain,%20 Agitation,%20Delirium.pdf

SUPPORT GROUPS

Support groups are a type of interpersonal network that, depending on objectives, initiation, leadership, and composition, may be variously described as self-help, mutual support, or treatment groups. The social and emotional bonding of individuals into networks of people, who perceive a shared fate and affirm mutual responsibilities for one another and are perceived to be experienced in the solution of challenging problems of living, is a basic process observed in all stable social groups. Kinship groups are prototypic mutual-support networks that are intended to provide timely and appropriate information, practical services, and emotional support when needed. In complex, socially differentiated societies, kinship-like interpersonal networks appear in large numbers and great variety, apparently to compensate in part for the attenuation of traditional kinship ties and the limited capacity of kin groups to provide needed support in a timely way.

In psychosocial terms, the essence of support groups is the reliable availability of interpersonal networks in which participants perceive themselves to be accepted and understood, as well as an expectation of timely information and supportive assistance in mastering problems of everyday life. Specifically, support groups provide (a) models of emotional mastery in responding to potentially traumatic events and circumstances; (b) guidance in cognitive interpretation and comparison of one's response to these events and circumstances with other members of the group perceived to be successful; (c) consensual validation of self-esteem or reinvention of the self in the face of significant challenges or loss; and (d) instrumental, palpable, practical help in securing and using resources required to cope and to adapt to one's new situation following a challenge or loss.

A growing body of evidence indicates that professional-led support groups can lead to beneficial health-related outcomes. Seçkin (2011) found that older women with cancer participated more often in online support groups and reported feeling less stressed in coping with cancer than younger women. Logsdon et al. (2010) reported that a nine-session support group for individuals with early stage memory loss resulted in a significantly better quality of life and improved mood. Although research has increasingly documented the extent and variety of support groups and their benefits, the level of evidence is limited.

Support groups are observed worldwide, but this kind of informal provision of informal care, particularly for aging populations, is especially common in the United States. The actual number and variety of support groups, although very large, is a matter of conjecture. In the 1980s, for example, an estimated 500,000 organized support groups involving millions of people existed. The Alzheimer's Association in the 1980s published principles for creating support groups and currently has 296 chapters and more than 4,500 support groups in all 50 states. The website of the National Library of Medicine, National Institutes of Health, lists 70 links to formal support groups by disease and condition and suggests that this is a partial list that can be supplemented by consulting local libraries, health care providers, and the Yellow Pages under "social services organizations."

Support groups have been shown to be the most widely implemented strategy of augmenting, specializing, or extending support for people in stressful situations. Conceptually, support groups are a component of the more general phenomena of social networking and social integration, both of which are considered to have positive implications for emotional well-being, life satisfaction, and happiness (Schultz & Albert, 2009).

Although support groups appear typically to produce benign or beneficial effects, systematic research is limited in specifying which kinds of support are beneficial for which individuals under which circumstances. The fluidity of membership in support groups and the complex number of variables that remain uncontrolled make definitive research difficult. Additional research continues to be required to refine decisional rules for professionals regarding whether and how to use support groups to assist patients. Of particular importance is knowledge about the limits of using support groups effectively and how to enhance the complementarity of formal and informal care services for older adults and their families.

Valerie T. Cotter

Logsdon, R. G., Pike, K. C., McCurry, S. M., Hunter, P., Maher, J., Snyder, L., & Teri, L. (2010). Early-stage memory loss support groups: Outcomes from a randomized controlled clinical trial. *Journals of Gerontology: Series B, Psychological Sciences and SocialSciences, 65*(6), 691–697.

Schultz, R., & Albert, S. M. (2009). Psychosocial aspects of aging. In J. B. Halter, J. G. Ouslander, M. E. Tinetti, S. Studenski, K. P. High, & S. Asthana (Eds.), *Hazzard's geriatric medicine and gerontology* (pp. 97–102). New York, NY: McGraw-Hill.

Seçkin, G. (2011). I am proud and hopeful: Age-based comparisons in positive coping affect among women who use online peer-support. *Journal of Psychosocial Oncology, 29*(5), 573–591.

Web Resources

Alzheimer's Association: http://www.alz.org/apps/findusall.asp

National Library of Medicine: http://www.nlm.nih.gov/medlineplus/ency/article/002150.htm

SURGERY IN THE ELDERLY

Elderly people undergo higher rates of surgical procedures than younger people. Therefore addressing elderly-specific perioperative needs must ensure optimal outcomes and quality of surgical care.

SURGICAL OUTCOMES OF OLDER ADULTS

Several studies have shown that rates of postoperative complications and mortality are higher in elderly adults. A study by Hamel, Henderson, Khuri, & Daley (2005) examined patients aged 80 years and older who underwent major noncardiac surgery and found that patients aged 80 years and older had higher mortality than younger patients (8% vs. 3%, p <.001). Using multivariate analysis, they found a 5% increase in mortality risk for each year age 80 years and older (i.e., a 90-year old has a 50% greater risk of 30-day mortality than an 80-year-old). A study by Gadjos et al. (2013) reinforced these findings and showed that increased age was associated with higher rates of postoperative mortality in nonemergent major general surgeries (1.7% in those aged 60 to 69 years vs. 24% in those aged 80 years and older; p <.001). In addition, they showed that the incidence of postoperative complications increased with age.

Recent literature has also focused on surgical outcomes in nursing home residents. Finlayson, Wang, Landefeld, & Dudley (2011) found that nursing home residents suffered higher operative mortality and more frequently required invasive interventions (e.g., mechanical ventilation) postoperatively compared with non–nursing home residents. Finlayson et al. (2012) also examined the outcomes after colectomy for nursing home patients and found a 53% mortality rate and 24% rate of sustained functional decline 1 year after surgery. Similarly, Oresanya et al. (2015) revealed poor outcomes in a population of nursing home residents undergoing lower extremity revascularization (63% died or were nonambulatory 1 year after surgery). These data on worse postoperative outcomes for elderly patients (especially nursing home residents) are important to consider and discuss during decision-making conversations with older adults undergoing surgery.

OPTIMIZING ELDERLY SURGICAL OUTCOMES: BEST-PRACTICE GUIDELINES

In 2012, the American College of Surgeons National Surgical Quality Improvement

Program (ACS NSQIP) and the American Geriatrics Society (AGS) collaborated to create best-practices guidelines for optimizing preoperative assessment for geriatric surgery patients (Table S.3). In 2016, ACS NSQIP and AGS provided recommendations for immediate preoperative, intraoperative, and postoperative periods (Table S.4; Mohanty et al., 2016). These guidelines, which represent both expert opinion and current evidence, have the potential to significantly improve the quality of perioperative care for older adults.

IMPORTANT ISSUES FOR ELDERLY PATIENTS UNDERGOING SURGERY

Frailty Assessment

Preoperative assessments (e.g., American Society of Anesthesiologists [ASA] Physical Status Classification System) are commonly used to predict postoperative outcomes. However, these traditional scores account for organ function rather than physiological reserve. Decreased reserve, or frailty, is also an important factor in predicting an individual's resilience postoperatively.

The association between frailty and worse postoperative outcomes has been demonstrated. A systematic review by Fagard et al. (2016) examining the impact of frailty on postoperative outcomes in elderly patients undergoing colorectal cancer surgery found that frail patients had a higher risk of developing postoperative complications, longer length of stay, higher rate of readmission, and decreased long-term survival. Similarly, Makary et al. (2010) showed that frailty is a predictor of worse postoperative outcomes and that frailty had considerable predictive capability over known indices of perioperative risk (e.g., ASA Physical Status

Table S.3

ACS NSQIP & AGS Best Practice Guidelines for the Optimal Preoperative Assessment of the Geriatric Surgical Patient

Area of Preoperative Assessment	Assessment Tools
Cognitive impairment and dementia	Mini-Cog.
Decision-making capacity	Four legally relevant criteria.
Depression	Patient Health Questionnaire-2.
Risk factors for postoperative delirium	Assess for cognitive or metabolic disorders, comorbidities, functional impairment.
Alcohol and substance abuse	Modified CAGE questionnaire.
Cardiac	ACC/AHA algorithm.
Pulmonary	Identify patient and surgery-related risk factors.
Functional status	ADL/IADL; deficits in vision, hearing, swallowing; fall risk; Timed Up and Go Test.
Frailty	Criteria include shrinkage, weakness, exhaustion, low physical activity, slowness.
Nutritional status	BMI, albumin, unintentional weight loss.
Medication management	Identify medications that should be started, continued, or stopped before surgery. Adjust doses for renal function. Consider polypharmacy.
Patient counseling	Discuss advance directive, treatment goals, postoperative course and potential complications, family/social support.
Preoperative testing	Hemoglobin, renal function, albumin for all geriatric surgery patients.

ACC/AHA, American College of Cardiology/American Heart Association; ACS NSQIP, American College of Surgeons National Surgical Quality Improvement Program; ADL/IADL, activities of daily living/instrumental activities of daily living; AGS, American Geriatrics Society; BMI, body mass index; CAGE, a questionnaire for alcoholism.

Source: Adapted from Mohanty et al. (2016).

Table S.4

ACS NSQIP & AGS Best Practice Guidelines for the Optimal Perioperative Management of the Geriatric Surgical Patient

Area of Preoperative Management	Guidelines
Immediate Preoperative Management	
Patient goals, preferences, and advance directives	- Discuss patient goals, treatment preferences, expected outcomes prior to surgery. - Document advance directive, health care proxy.
Preoperative fasting	- Minimize length of preoperative fast (e.g. 2 hours from clear liquids).
Antibiotic prophylaxis and venous thromboembolism prevention	- Preoperative antibiotics within 60 minutes of surgical incision. - Stratify for VTE and bleeding risk.
Medication management	- Discontinue nonessential and continue essential medications. - Consider polypharmacy.
Intraoperative Management	
Anesthesia in the older adult	- No single "best" anesthetic plan for elderly patients—consider individual comorbidities and role for regional anesthesia.
Perioperative analgesia in the older adult	- Educate personnel on effective and safe use of analgesic medications. - Multimodal analgesic plan individualized to patient based on pain history and physical.
Perioperative nausea and vomiting	- Assess risk factors for PONV; use appropriate prophylactic medications in the elderly.
Patient safety	- Ensure proper positioning.
Intraoperative strategies to prevent postoperative complications and hypothermia	- When possible, use epidural, laparoscopy; avoid intermediate- and long-acting neuromuscular blockers, ensure adequate recovery of neuromuscular function before extubation. - Monitor core temperature; use forced air warmers and/or warmed fluids.
Fluid management and targeting physiological parameters	- No single strategy recommended for fluid management; consider individual comorbidities and medications.
Postoperative Management	
Postoperative delirium	- Assess for delirium risk factors; consider daily postoperative screening. - Implement strategies for delirium prevention. - Evaluate delirious patients for precipitating conditions. - Treat delirious patient with nonpharmacological interventions first.
Pulmonary complication prevention	- Implement aspiration precautions, use of incentive spirometer, chest physical therapy, deep breathing exercises.
Fall risk assessment and prevention	- Utilize universal fall precautions in all older adult patients. - Patients with risk factors should receive targeted fall prevention.
Nutrition in the postoperative period	- Daily evaluation of adequate nutrition intake and fluid status. - Ensure patients with dentures have them available.
Urinary tract infection prevention	- Implement strategies to prevent UTI. - Attempt catheter removal as soon as possible.
Functional decline	- Implement structural characteristics (handrails), staffing requirements (education, multidisciplinary rounds), and patient-based interventions (early mobilization and physical therapy) to prevent functional decline.

(continued)

Table S.4

ACS NSQIP & AGS BEST PRACTICE GUIDELINES FOR THE OPTIMAL PERIOPERATIVE
MANAGEMENT OF THE GERIATRIC SURGICAL PATIENT   (*continued*)

Area of Preoperative Management	Guidelines
Pressure ulcer prevention and treatment	- Assess pressure ulcer risk. - Implement multicomponent interventions to prevent and treat pressure ulcers.
Care transitions	- Assess patient's social support and need for home health. - Assess nutrition, cognition, ambulation, functional status and presence of delirium prior to discharge and plan follow-up accordingly. - Include caregivers in discharge planning. - Detailed discharge instructions including new medications, pending tests, studies, and follow-up appointments. Assess understanding with repeat-back technique. - Communicate with patient's primary care doctor.

ACS NSQIP, American College of Surgeons National Surgical Quality Improvement Program; AGS, American Geriatrics Society; PONV, postoperative nausea and vomiting; UTI, urinary tract infection; VTE, venous thromboembolism.

Source: Adapted from Mohanty et al. (2016).

Classification System). Stoicea et al. (2016) reviewed six frailty scales and emphasized the importance of developing a universal frailty assessment tool. The authors recommended further investigation into the Edmonton Frail Scale (EFS) and the FRAIL scale (Fatigue, Resistance, Ambulation, Illnesses, and Loss of weight) given the relative ease of use. Future research should prioritize identifying a universal frailty assessment tool given the clear evidence that frailty is a predictor of worse postoperative outcomes in elderly patients.

Postoperative Delirium

The most common postoperative complication in the elderly is delirium (incidence 5%–50%), and 40% of episodes are preventable. Delirium is not only distressing to the patient and caregivers, but it can also lead to other complications such as increased length of stay, loss of functional independence, reduced cognitive function, and even death. Gleason et al. (2015) examined postoperative complications in 566 patients aged 70 years and older who underwent elective surgery and found that delirium exerted the highest attributable risk compared with all other adverse events.

In 2015, the AGS organized an interdisciplinary, multispecialty panel of experts and published a best-practice statement for postoperative delirium in older adults. It includes guidelines for the diagnosis and screening of delirium, intraoperative measures to prevent delirium, medications to avoid to prevent delirium, and pharmacological and nonpharmacological treatment of postoperative delirium. This statement represents an important first step to preventing postoperative delirium and appropriately treating this complication when it does occur.

CONCLUSION

With the aging of the population, it is imperative that physicians understand surgical outcomes specific to the elderly, best-practice guidelines for optimizing perioperative care, and the impact of frailty and postoperative delirium on outcomes. Significant improvements have been made but further work is needed to better understand this vulnerable population so that high-quality care and postoperative outcomes can be optimized.

Amy L. Lightner and Marcia M. Russell

American Geriatrics Society Expert Panel on Postoperative Delirium in Older Adults. (2015). Postoperative delirium in older adults: Best practice statement from the American Geriatrics Society. *Journal of the American College of Surgeons, 220,* 136–148.

S

Fagard, K., Leonard, S., Deschodt, M., Devriendt, E., Wolthuis, A., Prenen, H., ... Kenis, C. (2016). The impact of frailty of postoperative outcomes in individuals aged 65 and over undergoing elective surgery for colorectal cancer: A systematic review. *Journal of Geriatric Oncology, 7*(6), 479–491. doi:10.1016/j.jgo.2016.06.001

Finlayson, E., Wang, L., Landefeld, C. S., & Dudley, R. A. (2011). Major abdominal surgery in nursing home residents: A national study. *Annals of Surgery, 254,* 921–926.

Finlayson, E., Zhao, S., Boscardin, W. J., Fries, B. E., Landefeld, C. S., & Dudley, R. A. (2012). Functional status after colon cancer surgery in elderly nursing home residents. *Journal of the American Geriatrics Society, 60, 967–973.*

Gadjos, C., Kile, D., Hawn, M. T., Finlayson, E., Henderson, W. G., & Robinson, T. N. (2013). Advancing age and 30-day adverse outcomes after nonemergent general surgeries. *Journal of the American Geriatrics Society, 61,* 1608–1614.

Gleason, L. J., Schmitt, E. M., Kosar, C. M., Tabloski, P., Saczynski, J. S., Robinson, T., ... Inouye, S. K. (2015). Effect of delirium and other major complication on outcomes after elective surgery in older adults. *JAMA Surgery, 150,* 1134–1140.

Hamel, M. B., Henderson, W. G., Khuri, S. F., & Daley, J. (2005). Surgical outcomes for patients aged 80 and older: Morbidity and mortality from major noncardiac surgery. *Journal of the American Geriatrics Society, 53,* 424–429.

Makary, M. A., Segev, D. L., Pronovost, P. J., Syin, D., Bandeen-Roche, K., Patel, P., ... Fried, L. P. (2010). Frailty as a predictor of surgical outcomes in older patients. *Journal of the American College of Surgeons, 210,* 901–908.

Mohanty, S., Rosentham, R. A., Russell, M. M., Neuman, M. D., Ko, C. Y., & Esnaola, N. F. (2016). Optimal perioperative management of the geriatric patient: A best practices guideline from the American College of Surgeons National Surgical Quality Improvement Program and the American Geriatrics Society. *Journal of the American College of Surgeons, 222,* 930–947.

Oresanya, L., Zhao, S., Gan, S., Fries, B. E., Goodney, P. P., Covinsky, K. E., Conte, M. S., & Finlayson, E. (2015). Functional outcomes after lower extremity revascularization in nursing home residents: A national cohort study. *JAMA Internal Medicine, 175,* 951–957.

Stoicea, N., Baddigam, R., Wajahn, J., Sipes, A. C., Arias-Morales, C. E., Gastaldo, N., & Bergese, S. D. (2016). The gap between clinical research and standard of care: A review of frailty assessment scales in perioperative surgical settings. *Frontiers in Public Health, 4,* 150. doi:10.3389/fpubh.2016.00150

Web Resources

American Geriatrics Society: Geriatrics for Specialists Initiative: http://www.specialists.americangeriatrics.org/

Coalition for Quality in Geriatric Surgery: https://www.facs.org/quality-programs/geriatric-coalition

Sinai Hospital: http://www.lifebridgehealth.org/GeriatricSurgery/Resources1.aspx

U.S. Census Bureau: https://www.census.gov/prod/2014pubs/p25-1140.pdf

SWALLOWING DISORDERS AND ASPIRATION

Swallowing is a complex mechanism that requires the intricate coordination of several cranial nerves and a very large number of muscles of the face, mouth, pharynx, and esophagus. This enables the important physiological task of transporting liquids and firm food (i.e., the bolus) from the mouth into the esophagus while crossing a complicated anatomical region that is not only involved in swallowing but also in respiration and speech. The main causes of swallowing disorders are acute and chronic neurological conditions (e.g., stroke), local structural abnormalities (e.g., Zenker's diverticulum), and motility disorders of the upper esophageal sphincter (UES).

Swallowing disorders occur in all age groups and can be produced by a wide variety of pathologies (i.e., neurological and medical problems or structural abnormalities). The resulting impairment may range from very mild to life-threatening. It is, however, necessary to distinguish the effect of usual aging changes from the effects of specific diseases or degenerative changes. Indeed, nondysphagic elderly may have altered function without impairment. With increasing age, several changes can be observed such as increased stiffness of the UES, reduced upward movement of the hyoid, and shortening of the duration of the laryngeal closure, among others. These changes are congruent with a general impression that aging per se does not lead to pathology but that it puts the aging person at risk for swallowing problems if some pathology is present. As such, aspiration is likely to be caused by pathology and not because of normal aging.

Dysphagia (i.e., difficulty in swallowing) is a surprisingly common symptom and one that spans all ages. It is helpful to divide dysphagia into two types: oropharyngeal and esophageal. Dysphagia secondary to a lesion above or proximal to the esophagus is called *oropharyngeal dysphagia*. This symptom is often characterized as a transfer problem; the patient has trouble transferring food from the mouth into the pharynx and esophagus. Patients with esophageal dysphagia have difficulty transporting food down the esophagus once the bolus has been successfully transferred through the pharynx. In many cases, dysphagia occurs in the setting of other symptoms, but it may also occur solitarily.

A patient who complains about difficulties in swallowing certain foods or liquids may have a swallowing disorder. The globus sensation (a feeling of a lump in the throat) is usually not related to swallowing and should not be confused with dysphagia. Regurgitation, or the return of undigested food or liquid, may have different causes; delayed regurgitation of undigested food is suggestive of Zenker's diverticulum. Odynophagia, or painful swallowing, is most commonly because of acute disorders such as pharyngitis. *Aspiration* is defined as food (i.e., liquids or solids) entering the airway below the level of the true vocal cords (Logemann, 1998; Lundy et al., 1999). Coughing usually indicates that liquid or food has entered the airway, but some patients do not cough when they aspirate (i.e., silent aspiration). A voice quality that sounds like a gurgle after swallowing indicates that food remains in the larynx.

EVALUATION

Investigation of a swallowing disorder requires a multidisciplinary approach. It should always start with a proper history taking and a careful clinical evaluation, preferably by a speech–language pathologist.

Radiological imaging is central to evaluating, diagnosing, guiding the management of, and assessing the interventions for, swallowing disorders (Jones & Donner, 1991). A modified barium swallow/videofluorographic study of swallowing (Logemann, 1998) provides vital information for the management of patients with aspiration. The moment of aspiration in relation to the pharyngeal stage of deglutition (before, during, or after deglutition; Logemann, 1998) seems to be crucial.

Fiberoptic Endoscopic Evaluation of Swallowing with Sensory Testing (FEESST) can provide important information concerning the safety of deglutition. The main advantages of a FEEST are that it can be performed bedside, offers direct visualization of structures and sensory testing, and carries no radiation exposure. During the pharyngeal phase of swallowing, however, the view is obscured. It should be considered complementary to a radiological examination.

High-resolution manometry, in combination with impedance measurement and video fluoroscopy, offers the most complete information concerning the pathophysiology of swallowing; automated impedance manometry (AIM) analysis measures different swallow variables, defining bolus timing, intrabolus pressure, and contractile vigor and bolus presence. These parameters can be combined to derive a Swallow Risk Index (SRI) predicting the presence of aspiration (Omari et al., 2011). The UES nadir impedance seems to correlate with the opening diameter of the UES during bolus flow, and this offers perspectives for the evaluation of the opening of the UES, even in the absence of a video fluoroscopy (Omari et al., 2012).

MANAGEMENT

Once a clear insight into the patient's swallowing problem in terms of anatomical or physiological abnormalities has been obtained, treatment can be considered. This involves a team approach and an individualized treatment plan (Leonard & Kendall, 1997; Logemann, 1999). Some general rules when caring for older patients who have swallowing problems are as follows:

- Never attempt to feed orally unless the patient is fully alert. Maintain a calm environment because the patient should not become distracted.
- Sit beside the patient, at the same height, and ensure that the food is placed in the visual field. An upright position is best with the head in the midline.
- Allow sufficient time.
- Provide small quantities.
- Observe the patient and assist when necessary. Self-feeding sometimes improves swallowing.
- Offer another spoonful or forkful of food only when the previous one is swallowed. Do not presume that another spoonful will help move the previous one. Place the food in the mouth centrally or at the best side (i.e., left side if there is a right-sided paresis).
- Be sure that the patient's mouth and teeth (or dentures) are clean before eating; check for any oral residue after the meal.
- Do not encourage the patient to speak during mealtime. Do not initiate a conversation. Limit the talking to short clear messages such as "open your mouth" and "chew."
- Ask for advice concerning the utensils to use during eating

Attention should also be given to medication intake. Polypharmacy can be a major problem in the elderly. Some drugs (e.g., neuroleptics) may interfere with normal deglutition, whereas others pose a hazard when they are not at once transported into the stomach (e.g., iron tablets). Medications should therefore always be taken in an upright position with plenty of water.

Additional advice pertaining to medications includes the following:

- The patient should never swallow more than one pill at a time.
- Some water should be swallowed to moisten the mouth; then each pill should be taken with water. The process should end with a glass of water.
- Medication ordered for bedtime should be taken just before bedtime.
- Even a bedridden person should be placed in an upright position and kept in this position for at least 5 to 10 minutes after ingestion of the pill.

Oral medication is not always easy to swallow, and people often crush or open medication. Enteric-coated or extended-release forms cannot be crushed without losing their specific pharmacological properties. Medications mixed with food should always be given immediately after mixing to secure the integrity of the active component, or a so-called swallowing gel might be used. This gel surrounds the medication completely and enables it to be swallowed entirely. A medication lubricant, Gloup, designed to facilitate the swallowing of solid oral forms, has recently been introduced into the Australian and West European markets. It is intended to help those who have a psychological aversion to swallowing whole tablets and capsules (Jackson & Naunton, 2017). Further studies are required to determine whether it can also be recommended for use in dysphagics.

Liquid forms of medications may ease administration, but it is important when switching to a liquid form to check the dose. In some cases, effervescent and orally disintegrating tablets may also be available. Nonoral routes, such as transdermal preparations, are also important alternatives.

The interdisciplinary team should also recommend appropriate treatments such as compensatory measures, changes in food consistency, swallow maneuvers, exercises, medication, and endoscopic or surgical procedures. Postural changes can be regarded as compensatory measures. A chin-down position is recommended when delay in triggering the pharyngeal phase; when unilateral pharyngeal weakness is present, the head should be turned to the weaker side.

Patients should receive the food consistency best adapted to their situation. Mixed or pureed food is advisable if there is a chewing problem or if the patient is in the postoperative healing stages; liquids are indicated when there is an UES opening problem. In case of tongue and pharyngeal weakness, it may be necessary to alternate liquid and solid. A food thickener can be used in patients with a problem swallowing liquids.

Swallowing maneuvers require more cooperation and understanding from the patient. Among the most frequently used are as follows:

- The Mendelsohn maneuver, which prolongs the opening of the UES. In this maneuver, the patient is instructed to voluntarily elevate and hold the larynx in an upright position.
- The effortful swallow, which enhances the tongue thrust.
- The supraglottic technique, which teaches the patient to close the true vocal cords before and during the swallow and to clear any residue that may have entered the laryngeal vestibule. This technique is designed for patients with reduced laryngeal closure who are at risk of aspiration. It involves taking a deep breath, holding the breath while swallowing, and coughing immediately after the swallow. The super-supraglottic swallow is very similar to the supraglottic technique except that the patient bears down during breath-holding.
- Certain exercises, when performed on a regular basis, can also improve swallowing. Among these the most important is the so-called Shaker exercise, which is designed to improve the duration and width of the UES (Shaker et al., 1997). A second type consists of strengthening exercises for the tongue.

In rare cases, medication can improve swallowing (e.g., in patients with myasthenia gravis). Several surgical procedures can improve swallowing disorders. For significant cases of UES dysfunction, an extra mucosal myotomy of this sphincter may help correct the problem. Other therapeutic options may include an endoscopic dilation or a local injection of botulinum toxin. Zenker's diverticulum can be treated by a diverticulopexy with extramucosal myotomy; endoscopic treatment is also an alternative. Medialization of a paralyzed vocal cord can be performed through an injection or an implant technique. This intervention can be proposed to improve the voice and to avoid aspiration. In recent years a lot of work has been done concerning swallowing disorders after a stroke. It is now well established that sensory–stimulation techniques using both electrical and pharmacological stimuli can improve swallowing. In the near future, there might be a paradigm shift from compensatory strategies to the promotion of brain plasticity with the goal of obtaining recovery not only of swallow dysfunction, but also of brain-related swallowing dysfunction (Cabib et al., 2016).

If oral feeding places the patient at too great a risk, percutaneous endoscopic gastrostomy (PEG) should be considered as a temporary solution to allow recuperation and revalidation to take place without the burden of a nasogastric tube. PEG tubes are associated with risk of aspiration, so the patient's goals of care need to be reviewed. The overall prognosis may need to be assessed. Patients in end-of-life care may benefit from establishing a water protocol to prevent dehydration. It is important to maintain good oral hygiene for these patients.

See also Feeding: Non-Oral.

Eddy Dejaeger and Ann Goeleven

Cabib, C., Ortega, O., Kumru, H., Palomeras, E., Vilardell, N., Alvarez-Berdugo, D., … Clavé, P. (2016). Neurorehabilitation strategies for post-stroke oropharyngeal dysphagia: From compensation to the recovery of swallowing function. *Annals of the New York Academy of Sciences, 1380*(1), 121–138.

Jackson, S., & Naunton, M. (2017). Optimising medicine administration in patients with swallowing difficulties. *Australian Pharmacist, 36*(1), 28.

Jones, B., & Donner, M. W. (1991). *Normal and abnormal swallowing: Imaging in diagnosis and therapy.* New York, NY: Springer-Verlag.

Leonard, R., & Kendall, K. (1997). *Dysphagia assessment and treatment planning: A team approach.* Baltimore, MD: Singular Publishing.

Logemann, J. A. (1998). *Evaluation and treatment of swallowing disorders.* Austin, TX: Pro-Ed.

Logemann, J. A. (1999). Behavioral management for oropharyngeal dysphagia. *Folia phoniatrica et logopaedica, 51*(4–5), 199–212.

Lundy, D. S., Smith, C., Colangelo, L., Sullivan, P. A., Logemann, J. A., Lazarus, C. L., … Gaziano, J. (1999). Aspiration: Cause and implications. *Otolaryngology—Head and Neck Surgery, 120*(4), 474–478.

Omari, T. I., Dejaeger, E., van Beckevoort, D., Goeleven, A., Davidson, G. P., Dent, J., ... Rommel, N. (2011). A method to objectively assess swallow function in adults with suspected aspiration. *Gastroenterology*, *140*(5), 1454–1463.

Omari, T. L., Ferris, L., Dejaeger, E., Tack, J., Vanbeckevoort, D., & Rommel, N. (2012). Upper esophageal impedance as a marker of sphincter opening diameter. *American Journal of Physiology, Gastrointestinal and Liver Physiology*, *302*(9), G909–G913.

Shaker, R., Kern, M., Bardan, E., Taylor, A., Stewart, E. T., Hoffmann, R. G., ... Bonnevier, J. (1997). Augmentation of deglutitive upper esophageal sphincter opening in the elderly by exercise. *American Journal of Physiology*, *272*(6, Pt. 1), G1518–G1522.

Web Resources

American Speech-Language-Hearing Association: http://www.asha.org

Dysphagia Research Society: http://www.dysphagiaresearch.org

Dysphagia Resource Center: http://www.dysphagia.com

European Society for Swallowing Disorders: http://www.myessd.org

International Society for Diseases of the Esophagus: http://www.isde.net

TAX POLICY

Taxation is an increasingly important but often overlooked aspect of federal, state, and local policies for older adults. Beyond direct expenditures such as Social Security and Medicare, tax expenditures (credits, deductions, and exclusions) often embody governmental policies that affect older adults and are integral to their financial security.

At the federal level, very few tax provisions apply strictly by age, but certain applicable exclusions and deductions have particular significance for older taxpayers. State and local governments, in contrast, regularly deploy special "relief" provisions for older residents, especially older homeowners. Some of these provisions recognize the limited resources available to many older adults and accordingly are limited by a person's income. Other tax-relief provisions are aimed at older adults for the explicit purpose of attracting retirees.

FEDERAL TAX POLICY

The most important age-based federal tax provision is the additional standard deduction for taxpayers who are at least 65 years old and do not itemize their deductions. The amount of this deduction was $1,550 for a single person in 2016 and is adjusted annually for inflation. Because most older Americans do not itemize their deductions, this standard deduction is widely available, although its low limit diminishes its economic importance.

Other tax provisions are not age-based but have particular significance for older adults. For example, dividend income is subject to a maximum tax rate of 15% for all but the highest-bracket taxpayers, who owe 20% on such income. Both of these rates, however, are considerably lower than the tax rates that apply to wages, pension income, and interest receipts. Although this special dispensation for dividends (and long-term capital gains as well) applies to all taxpayers, older adults rely on dividends for a larger percentage of their income than younger people. Nonetheless, among taxpayers aged 50 years and older, dividend income is heavily concentrated for those with incomes more than $100,000 (Gist, 2003).

Of particular importance to older Americans, Social Security benefits are taxed according to the level of benefits received and the recipient's other income. A convoluted mechanism provides that an increasing percentage of a person's Social Security benefits is subject to income taxation as that person's income exceeds certain thresholds. The first tier of thresholds ($25,000 for singles and $32,000 for married persons) was enacted in 1983 and has not been adjusted for the intervening inflation. The second tier of thresholds ($34,000 for singles and $44,000 for married persons) was enacted in 1993 and is also not adjusted for inflation. As a result, the proportion of Social Security recipients who are affected by this particular taxing scheme has increased over time from one in eight to two in five (Kaplan, 2012).

A tax provision that is not restricted to older adults but has particular significance for them is the exclusion of gain from the sale of a principal residence. This provision has existed in various forms since the earliest days of the income tax, but its present iteration dates from 1997. Homeowners who have owned and used a home as their principal residence during at least 2 of the 5 years preceding its sale may exclude from taxation the first $250,000 of gain per owner. A married couple is allowed to exclude $500,000 of gain if both the husband and wife lived in the home during the testing period, although only one of them owned the home.

These dollar-based limitations are not adjusted for inflation or local costs of living, so the significance of this exclusion varies greatly depending on where the homeowners live. However, the bottom line is that most long-term homeowners, including older adults, can dispose of their residence without owing any income tax on the transaction.

Another tax provision that is available to taxpayers regardless of age but that has special significance for older adults is the deduction for medical expenses. Although most older Americans are enrolled in the federal government's Medicare program, this program covers only about half of the beneficiaries' medical costs. A dizzying array of deductibles and co-payment obligations combine with monthly premiums for Medicare Part B (physician charges), Medicare Part D (prescription drugs), and supplemental "Medigap" insurance to produce substantial out-of-pocket medical costs. In this connection, it should be noted that Medicare does not have an annual stop–loss provision that caps a beneficiary's personal outlays.

Moreover, many older adults are at risk for substantial long-term care costs, most of which are not covered by Medicare. Some older people have long-term care insurance, but that insurance typically excludes the costs of care during an "elimination" or "waiting" period, which can be 90 days or longer. Elders without such insurance may need to pay for home health aides, assisted-living facilities, or nursing homes. Other people pay for ramps, first-floor bathrooms, and other home modifications to enable them to stay in their residences as their abilities decline. All of these expenditures are medical expenses for purposes of this tax deduction (Kaplan, 2005).

One of the largest tax expenditures in the entire tax code pertains to pensions and salary-reduction plans under section 401(k) and individual retirement savings plans, such as Keoghs and Individual Retirement Accounts. Contributions to these plans can be deducted from present tax obligations by employers and by future elders. The amount of these contributions is limited, but workers aged 50 years and older may make additional "catch-up" contributions. On withdrawal of funds from these plans, the retiree owes tax at ordinary income rates, regardless of whether the amounts withdrawn represent dividends or capital gains, which would otherwise be eligible for lower tax rates (Kaplan, 2012).

Finally, the federal estate tax was made substantially less onerous at the end of President Obama's first term. This tax is imposed at rates as high as 40% but only after excluding the first $5,450,000 in 2016. The amount of this exemption is increased for inflation and applies only after deducting a decedent's medical expenses, the costs of administering the estate, and charitable bequests. Moreover, married couples are allowed to carry over the "unused" portion of the exemption when one spouse dies to augment the exemption that is available to the surviving spouse. As a result, only two of a thousand decedents owe any federal estate tax.

STATE AND LOCAL TAX POLICIES

State and local governments have enacted an array of tax policies that affect the income of older adults. As might be expected, great variations exist among the states, especially in income tax policy; seven states have no personal income tax, whereas two tax only interest and dividend income; 36 states and the District of Columbia exclude at least some pension income; and 27 states and the District of Columbia provide a full exclusion for Social Security benefits (National Conference of State Legislatures, 2015).

Property taxes are the focus of much attention regarding age-based relief efforts with every state except two having special provisions for homeowners who are 65 years old, although several states use younger ages (60 years or 62 years) and three states require the age to be 70 years. The most common forms of such efforts are "circuit breakers" that lower state income taxes based on property taxes paid (29 states) and stipulated exemptions of tax otherwise due (28 states). Twenty-one states allow property taxes to be deferred until the homeowner disposes of the home, and 12 states "freeze" a residence's assessed value (Lincoln Institute of Land Policy & George Washington Institute of Public Policy, 2016).

Finally, most sales taxes exempt from their application or apply significantly reduced tax rates to the purchases of food and prescription drugs, features that disproportionately help older people who spend a higher proportion of their income on such items.

BASIC ISSUES ARISING FROM TAX PREFERENCES FOR OLDER ADULTS

Basic issues are raised by the use of tax expenditures, not the least of which is the difficulty of determining their cost. Moreover, many tax policies are implemented as exclusions or deductions rather than as tax credits and therefore are more valuable to upper-income than to lower-income older adults.

Other issues spring from the use of tax laws to promote the welfare of older adults who need help the most. For example, would an increase in direct spending on low-income older adults be more effective than relying on tax provisions? More generally, is age an appropriate basis on which to bestow tax relief? In fact, little is known about the effectiveness of many tax provisions in increasing the well-being of older adults. For example, do property tax breaks enable older adults to keep their homes and age-in-place or encourage them to stay in their homes at considerable financial and personal health risk?

Subnational policies to encourage retirees to relocate may be especially shortsighted. Although older adults place fewer demands on state and local governments regarding schools and law enforcement, when these newly arrived residents get older, they may increase demands for government-subsidized health care.

Tax policies can be an important means of achieving key policy objectives, such as increasing homeownership and reducing the cost of health care. As the Baby Boomer generation retires, however, these policies may come under increasing scrutiny, especially if tax-reform efforts eliminate societal objectives other than revenue-raising from the tax code.

Richard L. Kaplan

Gist, J. (2003). Repealing the tax on dividends: Benefits and costs. *PPI Data Digest, 84*, 1–6. Washington, DC: AARP Public Policy Institute.

Kaplan, R. (2005). Federal tax policy and family-provided care for older adults. *Virginia Tax Review, 25*(2), 509–562.

Kaplan, R. (2012). Reforming the taxation of retirement income. *Virginia Tax Review, 32*(2), 327–366.

Lincoln Institute of Land Policy & George Washington Institute of Public Policy. (2016). Significant features of the property tax: Residential property tax relief programs. Retrieved from http://www .lincolninst.edu/subcenters/significant-features -property-tax/Report_Residential_Property_Tax_ Relief_Programs.aspx

National Conference of State Legislatures. (2015). *State personal income taxes on pensions and retirement income: Tax year 2014.* Denver, CO: Author.

TECHNOLOGY

The world has never experienced a period in which technological advancements are occurring as rapidly as they are now, and this trend is likely to continue. Technology also crosses many domains and ranges from high-tech microprocessor chips embedded in appliances to "low-tech" solutions such as well-balanced footwear to minimize falls. The majority of older adults want to continue to live at home. An AARP Public Policy Institute (2015) study, for example, found that 89% of people older than 50 years stated that they wanted to remain at home, to age-in-place for the remainder of their lives.

This chapter focuses primarily on the technologies that enable aging-in-place. The Center for Technology and Aging (CTA) at the University of California, Berkeley, suggests a three-component framework for "connected" aging to support the whole person and especially to support aging-in-place at home and in the community: promoting health, wellness, and prevention; minimizing the impact of function limitations and managing chronic diseases; and maintaining social connectedness to family and friends. Furthermore, technologies may be designed to address interventions at any of the four different levels: body; home environment; community; or caregiving.

BODY-BASED TECHNOLOGIES

These devices can range from low-tech solutions such as hip-protector pads and weight scales to Internet-connected devices that monitor sleep and/or activity, such as the increasingly popular fitness tracking bands that track several different vital signs and energy expenditure. These devices may give information just to the individual wearing the device or can be set up to integrate with computer-based tracking and management programs to telehealth systems that automatically transfer the data to a health care provider. The CTA suggests a list of categories of devices that includes vital signs monitors, activity monitors, sleep monitors, mood/depression/emotion monitors, personal emergency response systems (some of which have GPS and/or automatic fall-detection capabilities), medication-adherence systems (reminders) and dispensers, and smart toilets that analyze physiological functioning automatically.

Some of these technologies are meant to be managed by the older adult, although others are managed by caregivers. Medication-management systems, for example, are often designed to allow a caregiver (family or professional) to fill and set the system so that the elder does not have to remember which medications to take at a given time. This works well for pills, but liquids and drops and other forms of medication delivery are not yet well-addressed with these systems. Similarly, systems that track the location of someone living with memory impairment are typically set up and managed by a caregiver. Some allow family caregivers to track location, whereas others rely on local first responders having the appropriate technology to locate the individual. Finally, continued use of technology can be an ongoing issue, there is often a significant reduction in appropriate use over time.

HOME ENVIRONMENT

Smart home technologies have been discussed for years as being the way of the future, with appliances that know when to turn on lights, change the temperature, order groceries, or lock one's car from 500 miles away. Although the term "Internet of Things" was coined in 1985 (Sharma, n.d.), the concept is just beginning to gain real traction. In 2016, more than 5.5 million *new* devices were "connected" every day, and predictions are that 20.8 billion devices will be connected worldwide by 2014 (Weber, 2016). Although many of these devices are appealing to young tech-savvy professionals, they can be particularly useful in helping elders manage their homes and lifestyles more easily and safely. Many are safety-related such as gas or carbon monoxide detectors that automatically send an alarm to the fire department.

It is possible to equip the home with a variety of person-related sensors that can track location, motion, and activity (e.g., flushing a toilet or opening the refrigerator) and use either preset settings or algorithms to assess patterns of behavior and alert when there is a deviation for normal patterns (no more sleeping late on Sunday mornings). Beyond body worn fall sensors, there are gait-based sensors that assess patterns and changes in gait, which may signal a change in the condition of an individual with Parkinson's or Alzheimer's disease. Some systems use video-based technology, so that remote caregivers can "look in" on a parent unobtrusively. Finally, there is an increasing array of robots designed to support both social interaction and functional activities.

COMMUNITY

The number of different platforms for social media continues to increase at a rapid pace. Younger users are constantly on the lookout to find the latest, fastest, way of connecting with peers, and increasing proportions of older adults are also using social media platforms such as Facebook, Skype, and e-mail to stay connected with families and friends. "Seniors aged 65 and over represent one of the fastest growing age groups to use social media" (Cornish, 2013). However, according to CTA, staying connected with friends and family is only one category of technology. Other technologies focus on physical and cognitive training and include both online and mobile apps, as well as exercise equipment that is connected and allow the person exercising be a part of a virtual community.

As with some of the devices described earlier, these can be connected to health monitoring programs or systems to track workouts and biometric data, which in turn may be integrated into an electronic health record. Another category of technology supports educational, vocational, and work (paid or volunteer) activities.

CAREGIVING

The final category in CTA's framework relates to caregiving systems, particularly health care, including professional or "formal" care and, increasingly, "informal" care provided by family and friends. Some health systems have connected electronic health records that track and integrate many aspects of a person's health care needs and activities, although others are less effective, particularly when the individual uses health care from multiple nonintegrated health care systems. With telemedicine, the focus is on transmitting medical information to health care providers who can, in turn, be more efficient in delivering care.

Many of the chronic conditions elders face need routine monitoring, which is currently typically provided by a home health nurse. In rural areas, in particular, this makes for inefficient care because staff may drive an hour or more for a 10-minute checkup. In urban areas, seniors may be uncomfortable using public transportation and thus delay routine check-ups, allowing potential unstable conditions to go unmonitored. By using cameras and various monitoring devices (e.g., blood glucose measurement, spirometry, ECG, blood pressure, respiration), information about a broad range of conditions can be efficiently and accurately relayed to medical professionals. There is some evidence that telehealth is more positively received by individuals living at home as opposed to those in assisted living (Grant, Rockwood, & Stennes, 2015).

One pervasive concern with many technologies, especially web-enabled devices and systems, relates to privacy and the ability to control who has access to information—social, personal, or health. Researchers have explored elders' perceptions of acceptability of different monitoring systems and conclude that people are willing to accept more invasive/personally identifiable monitoring, if it means the difference between being able to stay at home and relocating to assisted living or a nursing home (Caine, 2005; Caine, Fisk, & Rogers, 2006). Another issue relates to cost. Although some say the era of smart homes has arrived (CTI), a truly connected home is often sufficiently expensive that it is not available to a significant proportion of elders living on fixed incomes.

One main challenge to face in the coming decades is being able to afford high-quality care with a rapidly aging cohort. Although the baby boomers are healthier than previous generations, the aging process increases vulnerability to a range of functional and cognitive impairments that require medical attention. In the future, technologies are focused more on prevention than treatment and on staying home as opposed to relocating to shared residential settings. Another significant challenge is managing the interoperability of these different technologies in a meaningful way to derive the additive benefits of each for older adults as well as their caregivers and health providers.

See also Information Technology.

Margaret P. Calkins

AARP Public Policy Institute. (2015). *State of 50+ America survey*. Washington, DC: Author. Retrieved from http://www.aarp.org/content/dam/aarp/livable-communities/learn/housing/housing-policy-solutions-to-support-aging-in-place-2010-aarp.pdf

Caine, K. (2005). Privacy perceptions of an aware home with visual sensing devices. *Proceedings of the Human Factors and Ergonomics Society Annual Meeting, 49*(21), 1856.

Caine, K. E., Fisk, A. D., & Rogers, W. A. (2006, October). Benefits and privacy concerns of a home equipped with a visual sensing system: A perspective from older adults. *Proceedings of the Human Factors and Ergonomics Society Annual Meeting* (Vol. 50, No. 2, pp. 180–184). Los Angeles, CA: Sage.

Cornish, A. (2013). Why are seniors the fastest-growing demographic on social media. Transcript from All Things Considered. Retrieved from http://www.npr.org/templates/story/story.php?storyId=247220424

Grant, L. A., Rockwood, T., & Stennes, L. (2015). *Telemedicine and e-Health, 21*(12), 987–991. doi:10.1089/tmj.2014.0218

Sharma, C. (n.d.). Correcting the IoT history. Retrieved from http://www.chetansharma.com/IoT_History.htm

Weber, R. M. (2016). Internet of things becomes the next big thing. *Journal of Financial Service Professionals, 70*(6), 43–46.

Web Resources

AARP Health@Home 2.0: http://assets.aarp.org/rgcenter/health/healthy-home-11.pdf

AbleData: http://www.abledata.com

Georgia Tech Aware Home initiative: http://www.awarehome.gatech.edu/drupal/?q=content/research-areas-0

TELEHEALTH

Telehealth, also referred to as *telemedicine*, is defined as the exchange of medical information from one site to another via electronic communications to improve a patient's clinical health status (American Telemedicine Association, 2012). Telehealth technologies emerged in the late 1960s with the advent of the need of the National Aeronautics and Space Agency (NASA) to monitor the health status of astronauts in space. Remote monitoring was one of the earliest telehealth technologies that became available after the development of satellite technology. By the early 1990s, telehealth was used in a wide variety of settings and consisted of technologies such as remote monitoring, diagnostics, video conferencing, digital imaging, robotics and remote controls, store and forward technology, and simulation and training (Sorrells-Jones, Tschirch, & Liong, 2006). Today, the rising cost of health care and the shift toward higher quality and contained costs has triggered the search for alternative techniques to keep patients at home and out of the hospital, although, still being closely monitored by a health care professional or team of professionals.

To provide an overview of the current literature related to the use of telehealth technologies in chronic-condition, self-management programs, a number of systematic reviews have been undertaken. Bensink, Hailey, and Wootton (2006) note that evidence exists for the clinical effectiveness of home telehealth in diabetes, mental health, high-risk pregnancy, and cardiac disease. The majority of these studies have utilized the telephone as a simple, affordable, and easily accessible communication technique. A systematic review of telehealth technologies for disease management suggest the main points to consider when assessing the effectiveness of these programs are whether the technology improves education and self-control; improves quality of care; helps curb costs and exposure to the risk; and has high patient acceptability (Garcia-Lizana & Sarria-Santamera, 2007).

A systematic review of home telemonitoring for chronic conditions conducted by Pare, Jaana, and Sicotte (2007) examined 65 studies related to pulmonary conditions, diabetes, cardiac disease, and hypertension. The authors found that although patients readily comply with telemonitoring programs, the sustained impact and overall significance of its effects on patients' chronic conditions remains inconclusive. In their literature review of information technology systems to promote improved care for chronic conditions, Dorr et al. (2007) reviewed 109 articles that included more than 112 information systems. The researchers noted that 67% of studies reviewed reported positive outcomes, with components incorporating links to an electronic medical record and a personal health record, computerized prompts, population management, specialized decision support, and electronic scheduling options.

Despite the wide variations that exist in the design of telehealth programs, detailed documentation of the structural aspects, process measures of care, and outcome measures need to be further examined to draw more consistent conclusions about the effectiveness of care delivery in this alternative environment. The design of telehealth programs needs to incorporate systems that can accurately capture patient-level characteristics such as understanding of condition management, medication status, physician office visits, comorbid conditions, and episodic illness, for example. Systems that can incorporate baseline data of patients and changes in status aid in understanding the confounding factors that may have implications for clinical and utility outcomes. The importance of understanding the process of care in a telehealth program, as well as the factors taking place at the individual level, cannot be overlooked when evaluating the effectiveness of care delivered.

Implications for practice for health care providers include training and familiarity with the use of technology to remotely monitor and interact with patients with chronic conditions. Telehealth programs have produced a wide variety of interventions through a number of different modes of delivery. Variations in telehealth programs may have implications for how care is delivered and received, as well as how processes and outcomes of care are measured. Examples of variations in the programs might include differences between the relationships that patients have with each of the health care professionals working with them through the program and responding to their questions, patients' comfort with the remote monitoring process, and feasibility of daily monitoring, all of which may have individual effects on patient results. These variations, in addition to patient-level variables such as diet, exercise, medication regimen, and comorbid conditions, further compound how care is delivered, measured, and interpreted.

In the context of health care reform, telehealth offers significant opportunities to address inequalities in access to health care, inefficiencies in care delivery, and increasing costs. Although the primary focus on technology in the health care systems is devoted to the use of electronic health records to promote transparency and improved communication among the providers (Bashshur & Shannon, 2009), the role that telehealth plays in providing integral connections between patients and providers and in the early detection of complications in patients with chronic conditions is noteworthy.

See also Technology.

Jill Nocella

American Telemedicine Association. (2012). Telemedicine defined. Retrieved from http://www.american telemed.org

Bashshur, R. L., & Shannon, G. W. (2009). National telemedicine initiatives: Essential to healthcare reform. *Telemedicine & e-Health, 15*(6), 600–610.

Bensink, M., Hailey, D., & Wootton, R. (2006). A systematic review of success and failures in home telehealth: Preliminary results. *Journal of Telemedicine and Telecare, 12,* 8–16.

Dorr, D., Bonner, L. M., Cohen, A. N., Shoai, R. S., Perrin, R., Chaney, E., & Young, A. S. (2007). Information systems to promote improved care for chronic illness: A literature review. *Journal of the American Medical Information Association, 14,* 156–163.

Garcia-Lizana, F., & Sarria-Santamera, A. (2007). New technologies for chronic disease management and control: A systematic review. *Journal of Telemedicine and Telecare, 13,* 63–68.

Pare, G., Jaana, M., & Sicotte, C. (2007). Systematic review of home telemonitoring for chronic diseases: The evidence base. *Journal of the American Medical Informatics Association, 14*(3), 269–277.

Sorrells-Jones, J., Tschirch, P., & Liong, M. S. (2006). Nursing and telehealth. *Nurse Leader, 10,* 42–58.

Web Resources
American Telemedicine Association: http://www.americantelemed.org

Department of Veterans Affairs—Office of Telehealth Services: http://www.telehealth.va.gov/index.asp

International Society for Telemedicine and eHealth: http://www.isfteh.org

Telehealth Resource Centers: http://www.telehealth resourcecenter.org

THERAPEUTIC RECREATION SPECIALISTS AND RECREATION(AL) THERAPISTS

Therapeutic recreation or *recreation(al) therapy* (used interchangeably) is a process that uses purposeful, goal-directed recreation and other activity-based interventions to address the needs of individuals and to optimize psychological and physical health, recovery, happiness, and quality of life. Therapeutic recreation specialists or recreation(al) therapists (RTs) are bachelor's- or master's-level professionals with academic preparation in leisure and therapeutic recreation theory and practice. The PhD degree is available in the field at a limited number of universities, and these professionals teach and conduct research.

Geriatric-service settings that benefit from the expertise of RTs include long-term care, hospice, home care, medical home, assisted living, continuous-care retirement, dementia care, physical rehabilitation, respite care, adult day, geropsychiatric, senior citizens' activity, municipal recreation, faith-based, and intergenerational programs (Austin, Crawford, McCormick, & Van Puymbroeck, 2015; Carter & Van Andel, 2011). RTs are knowledgeable about physical, social, cognitive, and psychological problems commonly associated with aging; recognize the critical importance of health promotion and maintenance, and use meaningful recreation and leisure as both a means and an end for achieving a reasonable quality of life. RTs know how to assess behavior, design appropriate adaptations, and interventions that fit patients' needs and interests and evaluate their effectiveness. In setting serving older adults, the RT is an advocate who understands quality of life and its relationship to function and health status that changes over the life span. The RT also serves as a liaison who advocates for person-directed practices, where the voices of older adults and those working with them are respected (Austin et al., 2015).

Modalities common in therapeutic recreation programming for older adults include therapeutic expressive arts, movement and music, stress management, assertiveness training, physical exercise, cognitive retraining, sensory stimulation, reality awareness, reality orientation, remotivation, resocialization, reminiscence, behavior management, pet-assisted therapy, horticulture and therapeutic gardening, aquatics, travel, community service, special-interest groups (e.g., hobbies, collections), and computer-technology activities (Carter & Van Andel, 2011).

Approximately 22,400 individuals practice therapeutic recreation in the United States (U.S. Bureau of Labor Statistics, 2016). In 2014, the National Council for Therapeutic Recreation Certification (NCTRC), the credentialing agency, reported that 13,500 individuals hold the Certified Therapeutic Recreation Specialist (CTRS) credential (NCTRC, 2015). Candidates for testing and certification must have at least a bachelor's degree in therapeutic recreation or recreation with a specialization in therapeutic recreation, specific courses in recreation/leisure theory, therapeutic recreation theory, abnormal psychology, anatomy and physiology, growth and development, and other human service disciplines, as well as an academically verified 560-hour internship under a CTRS (NCTRC, 2015). A CTRS is not an *activities specialist* or *recreation specialist* who works in recreation programs who do not have a bachelor's degree or the CTRS credential.

Individuals with degrees in related fields can also qualify to take the NCTRC examination, but additional course work and experience are required. NCTRC is recognized by the National Commission for Certifying Agencies (NCCA) for compliance with high standards of quality and integrity in the certification and competency-assurance process that serves the interests of the public, employers, and certificants. The National Association of Activity Professionals, an industry-supported association, focuses on support and training for activities directors in nursing homes who lack a college degree or who have degrees in fields not specific to therapeutic recreation. Its membership is open to CTRSs as well. All associations have the same goal: to promote quality recreation programming for long-term care residents.

Nursing homes receiving Medicaid or Medicare funding must offer planned and organized recreation/activity services that address each resident's individual needs and interests. Resident-focused services include leisure assessments, participation in care planning, program depth and breadth, and documentation of residents' progress toward treatment goals. Federal regulations do not require recreational personal working in nursing homes to be baccalaureate prepared or nationally certified. Nursing home operators/administrators determine who is better prepared to provide recreational services to a particular patient population. State surveyors, using the Centers for Medicare & Medicaid Services (CMS) guidelines, hold the agency accountable for the quality of care.

Activities personnel contribute to the federally mandated comprehensive assessment and care plan. The American Therapeutic Recreation Association (ATRA) encourages the employment of CTRSs in long-term care, especially in agencies that also have subacute and rehabilitation services or specialized dementia care. CTRSs are required for the provision of therapy prescribed by the physician. If a facility is accredited by the Commission on Accreditation of Rehabilitation Facilities (CARF), the provision of services by a CTRS is a required standard.

The goal of assisted-living facilities is to help residents remain as active and independent as possible, providing supportive services as needed. Many assisted-living agencies also offer dementia care. Proposed industry standards for assisted living recognize the value of structured and organized recreation services based on a well-developed service plan that identifies, similar to treatment plans in long-term care, the needs of each resident. As in long-term care, assisted-living facilities are not required to hire a CTRS, but the same benefits given to the residents must apply and should be an incentive to hire qualified, well-prepared professionals in consultant or full-time positions.

The care of dementia patients in special units, day care, and general psychiatric hospitals requires professional skills well suited to therapeutic recreation specialists. Because the activity level of patients in the early and middle stages of Alzheimer's disease remains high, treatment should not overstimulate easily confused patients but instead should fully use all their residual strengths and cognitive abilities. Therapeutic recreation specialists understand the degenerative nature of dementia and provide structured and creative activities that tap into the residents' past interests, keep social connections with family and friends at their optimal level, and monitor cognitive functioning so that new adaptations to the environment can be made.

Recreation employees without specialized educational training may provide senior programming in community recreation settings, senior centers, and retirement communities. Under the purview of a CTRS, however, programs operate in a health-promotion/disease-prevention model. Activities are designed to maintain high levels of fitness, emotional well-being, intellectual stimulation, and social interaction. Drawing on research that elders continue to learn and expand their areas of interest, activities that stimulate new learning and maximize the use of existing skills are stressed.

Leisure education or counseling, a standard programming technique used by therapeutic recreation specialists, helps program participants to understand the value of leisure and recreation and to develop or maintain a healthy leisure lifestyle. Education and service-oriented activities complement social opportunities and physical activity to create a well-rounded, solid program foundation. The seniors in these settings are encouraged to contribute to the community at large and their peers in ways that support meaningfulness in later life. As *leisure* implies a level of personal freedom, motivation from inside, and a desire to deepen personal happiness and life satisfaction, the role of the therapeutic recreation specialist in promoting quality of life is essential.

See also Assisted Living; Leisure Programs; Nursing Homes.

Ellen Broach

Austin, D., Crawford, M., McCormick, B., & Van Puymbroeck, M. (2015). *Recreational therapy: An introduction* (4th ed.). Urbana, IL: Sagamore.

Carter, M. J., & Van Andel, G. (2011). *Therapeutic recreation: A practical approach* (3rd ed.). Long Grove, IL: Waveland Press.

National Council for Therapeutic Recreation Certification. (2015). *2014 NCTRC report on the international job analysis of certified therapeutic recreation specialists*. New York, NY: Author.

U.S. Bureau of Labor Statistics. (2016). *U.S. Department of Labor, occupational outlook handbook, 2016–17* edition, recreational therapists. Retrieved from http://www.bls.gov/ooh/healthcare/recreational-therapists.htm

Web Resources
American Therapeutic Recreation Society: http://www.atra-tr.org
Florida International University listing of U.S. Universities offering degrees in therapeutic recreation/recreational therapy: http://www2.fiu.edu/~rt/usa_ot_locator.html

National Association for Activity Professionals: http://www.thenaap.com

National Center for Assisted Living: http://www.ncal.org

National Commission for Certifying Agencies: http://www.credentialingexcellence.org/ncca

National Council for Therapeutic Recreation Certification: http://www.nctrc.org

U.S. Bureau of Labor Statistics: http://www.bls.gov/ooh/healthcare/recreational-therapists.htm

THYROID DISEASE IN THE ELDERLY

Thyroid disease is common in the elderly. Multiple comorbid states, atypical symptoms, age-related changes, and polypharmacy may cause diagnostic challenges. When a thyroid abnormality is suspected the first step is to measure the thyroid-stimulating hormone (TSH) level. The thyroid gland secretes two hormones, thyroxine (T_4) and triiodothyronine (T_3), which are regulated by TSH. Treatment options need to be determined based on thyroid function abnormalities. A careful review of patient's goals of care and comorbidities needs to be assessed because the risks of therapy may outweigh the benefits.

HYPOTHYROIDISM

Hypothyroidism is very common in patients aged older than 60 years and steadily increases with age. Unlike symptoms of hyperthyroidism, the symptoms of hypothyroidism may be nonspecific in all patients, even more so in the older patient. Symptoms and signs of hypothyroidism include weight gain, sleepiness, dry skin, constipation, fatigue, and memory impairment. However, a lack of these symptoms does not rule out the diagnosis. To make this diagnosis in the elderly patient, a doctor often needs a high index of suspicion, especially in woman and patients with family history of thyroid disease. Patients at high risk for hypothyroidism include those with a history of treatment for hyperthyroidism, history of extensive surgery and/or radiotherapy to the neck, use of high-risk medications

like lithium or amiodarone, or recent exposure to iodine-containing contrast for radiographic evaluation. Sometimes, acute nonthyroidal illness can alter the thyroid hormone level, but returns to normal without thyroid hormone supplements after underlying illness resolves (Mulholland et al., 2015).

A decision to treat the patient with a new diagnosis of hypothyroidism rests on several factors, including whether the patient is symptomatic from hypothyroidism or just has an elevated TSH. The presence or absence, as well as severity, of thyroid-related symptoms and coexisting diseases such as coronary artery disease or heart failure determine the dose of thyroid hormone replacement that is given. The patient and family members must be aware of a possible increase in angina, shortness of breath, confusion, and change in sleep habits. Therefore treatment may begin with levothyroxine (Synthroid) in a dose of 25 to 50 mcg daily, and the dose should be increased every 4 to 6 weeks until laboratory tests show a gradual return of blood thyroid hormone and TSH levels to the normal range. Patients who experience increased angina pectoris, symptoms of congestive heart failure, or mental changes such as confusion need to have their dose of levothyroxine decreased, then more gradually increased over several months.

HYPERTHYROIDISM

In hyperthyroidism, there is too much thyroid hormone, every function of the body tends to be in accelerated mode; however, the elderly patient may have only minimal symptoms. A French study published in 2016 confirmed that elderly patients have fewer symptoms of thyrotoxicosis than younger subjects but are at an increased risk of cardiac complications (Goichot, Caron, Landron, & Bouee, 2016). For example, there was only a sensation of heart fluttering and some chest discomfort on climbing stairs. Other symptoms include weight loss, poor appetite, diarrhea, and tremor.

Graves' disease is a common cause of hyperthyroidism; toxic nodular goiter is seen more frequently in the older patient. Transient hyperthyroidism may occur after viral or other infection because of an increased release of thyroid hormone into the circulation during inflammation. During therapy, the effects of changes in thyroid function on other body systems must be closely monitored, because of an increased likelihood of coexisting cardiac and central nervous system disease in older patients. Thyroid function is brought under control first with antithyroid drugs (propylthiouracil or methimazole [Tapazole]). The definitive treatment is with radioactive iodine. Surgery is rarely recommended because of increased risks in the older patient. During the initial phase of treatment, physicians observe cardiac function closely because of the effect of changing thyroid hormone levels on the heart. Symptoms of hyperthyroidism may be brought under control with adjunctive medications, such as beta-blockers. Beta-blockers, often administered to slow rapid heart rate, must be given with caution in the patient with coexisting congestive heart failure, and the dose should be reduced once thyroid function is in the normal range. Symptoms and signs of angina pectoris and heart failure must be treated along with hyperthyroidism.

SUBCLINICAL THYROID DISORDER

The development of sensitive assays for thyrotropin (TSH) has led many older patients to have abnormal TSH levels without other alterations in serum thyroid hormone levels; these conditions are termed *subclinical hypothyroidism* (isolated elevation of TSH levels) and *subclinical hyperthyroidism* (isolated decreased TSH levels). Subclinical hypothyroidism occurs in 5% to 10% of elderly subjects, more so in women. Subclinical hyperthyroidism is less common, affecting less than 2% of the elderly population. Potential risks of subclinical hypothyroidism in the elderly include progression to overt hypothyroidism, cardiovascular effects, hyperlipidemia, and neurological and neuropsychiatric effects. Potential risks of subclinical hyperthyroidism in the elderly include progression to overt hyperthyroidism, cardiovascular effects (especially atrial fibrillation), and osteoporosis. Decisions to treat elderly subjects with subclinical thyroid disease should be based on a careful assessment of these risks in the individual.

As per the review study published in the *Journal of American Geriatrics Society* (Hennessey & Espaillat, 2015), treatment of subclinical hypothyroidism in older individuals requires special consideration about thyroid hormone replacement therapy and expected clinical outcomes. Apart from individuals with persistent subclinical hypothyroidism, current evidence suggests that individuals with TSH levels greater than 10 mIU/L who test positive for antithyroid antibodies or are symptomatic may benefit from levothyroxine treatment to reduce the risk of progression to overt hypothyroidism, decrease the risk of adverse cardiovascular events, and improve quality of life. After the treatment is initiated, careful monitoring is essential (Boursi, Haynes, Mamtani, & Yang, 2015).

NODULAR THYROID DISEASE

Thyroid nodules remain asymptomatic and are usually discovered by either the patient or the physician during a physical examination or accidentally during imaging studies such as CT scan or ultrasound of the neck. Risk increases with age. Nodules are more common in women. Some of the factors that increase the risk of developing thyroid nodules include exposure to radiation, iodine deficiency, and Hashimoto's thyroiditis (one of the causes of hypothyroidism). Concerning symptoms include the rapidly increasing size of a nodule, hoarseness of voice, difficulty in swallowing or breathing, and neck pain or neck tenderness.

Tests to rule out thyroid malignancy are TSH and thyroid ultrasound. Fine-needle aspiration biopsy is done if there is high suspicion for malignancy based on clinical evaluation, laboratory results, and ultrasonography. A benign thyroid nodule requires follow-up based on its size and characteristics. Thyroid cancer can be of various types, such as papillary, follicular, anaplastic, or medullary. Surgery is required for malignancy depending on comorbid diseases.

Vidita Divan, Ariba Khan, and Saima T. Akbar

Boursi, B., Haynes, K., Mamtani, R., & Yang, Y. X., (2015). Thyroid dysfunction, thyroid hormone replacement and colorectal cancer risk. *Journal of* the National Cancer Institute, 107(6). doi:10.1093/jnci/djv084

Goichot, B., Caron, P., Landron, F., & Bouee, S., (2016). Clinical presentation of hyperthyroidism in a large representative sample of outpatients in France: relationships with age, aetiology and hormonal parameters. *Clinical Endocrinology, 84*(3), 445–451.

Hennessey, J. V., & Espaillat, R. (2015). Diagnosis and management of subclinical hypothyroidism in elderly adults: A review of the literature. *Journal of the American Geriatrics Society, 63*(8), 1663–1673.

Mulholland, G. B., Zhang, H., Nguyen, N.-T., Tkacyzk, N., Seikaly, H., O'Connell, D., ... Harris, J. R. (2015). Optimal detection of hypothyroidism in early stage laryngeal cancer treated with radiotherapy. *Journal of Otolaryngology: Head and Neck Surgery, 44.* doi:10.1186/s40463-015-0085-3

TRANSITIONAL CARE

Transitional care is described as a successful model of care that encompasses a broad range of services focused on preparing and implementing safe and timely passage from one environment to another; such care is typically delivered by nurses or advanced practice registered nurses (APRNs; Boult et al., 2009). It encompasses the movement of patients between health care practitioners, settings, and home as their condition and care need change (The Joint Commission [TJC], n.d.). Patients and residents can transition to and from hospitals, subacute and post-acute nursing facilities, home, primary and specialty care offices, and long-term care facilities. Transitional care, which encompasses both the sending and the receiving aspects of the transfer, is based on a comprehensive plan of care and includes logistical arrangements, education of the patient and family, and coordination among the health professionals involved in the transition (Coleman & Boult, 2003). Whether led by an APRN or a physician, transitional care requires specific interventions designed to ensure the coordination and continuity of care as patients transfer among different locations or different levels of care in the same location (Li et al., 2016).

NEED FOR TRANSITIONAL CARE

Since the publication of the landmark report, *Crossing the Quality Chasm: A New Health System for the 21st Century,* by the Institute of Medicine (IOM), the quality and safety of care delivery remain a subject of debate (Baker, 2001). The IOM report indicated that delivery of care is often overly complex and uncoordinated, requiring steps and patient "handoffs" that slow care and decrease, rather than improve, safety. Transitional care is at the core of these discussions. Lack of coordination and communication between hospitalists and primary care providers (PCPs) has been documented to be a major source of transitional care breakdown, leading to readmissions (Vedel & Khanassov, 2015). One fifth of the Medicare beneficiaries are readmitted in 30 days and more than one third in 90 days of hospital discharge (Jencks, Williams, & Coleman, 2009). In 2011, there were approximately 3.3 million readmissions in the United States across all payers, contributing $41.3 billion in total hospital costs (Hines, Barrett, Jiang, & Steiner, 2014).

The major impetus to develop, implement, and sustain dedicated high-quality transitional care is the fragmentation of care delivery across all settings (Coleman & Boult, 2003). The lack of coordination and communication among multiple providers has been noted to cause medical errors, inappropriate care, service duplication, limited access to services, and poor continuity of care that ultimately lead to costly rehospitalization (Coleman & Boult, 2003; Li et al., 2016). Consequently, these poor outcomes lead to patient-care experience dissatisfaction. Because Medicare and Medicaid reimbursements are matched with Hospital Consumer Assessment of Healthcare Providers and Systems (HCAHPS) survey scores, low scores resulting from breakdowns in care impact hospital revenues. Hospitals with unacceptably high readmission rates for Medicare and Medicaid patients face financial penalties (TJC, n.d.).

POPULATIONS AT RISK

The patient populations at risk for negative post-discharge outcomes are those with multiple comorbid conditions, functional deficits, cognitive impairment (dementia and delirium), mental health issues, and poor general health behaviors (Naylor et al., 2004). Chronic conditions that have been shown to benefit from transitional care programs include congestive heart failure (CHF; Naylor et al., 2004; Stamp, Machado, & Allen, 2014; Vedel & Khanassov, 2015) and dementia or cognitive impairment (Bradway et al., 2012). Complex care patients benefit if they have 1 of 11 diagnoses, including stroke, CHF, coronary artery disease, cardiac arrhythmias, chronic obstructive pulmonary disease, diabetes mellitus, spinal stenosis, hip fracture, peripheral vascular disease, deep venous thrombosis, and pulmonary embolism (Coleman, Parry, Chalmers, & Min, 2006). The major positive outcomes reported from transitional care models tested in randomized controlled trials involving these vulnerable patient populations is a reduction in the total number of rehospitalizations and decreased health care cost (Coleman et al., 2006; Li et al., 2016; Naylor et al., 2004). Transitional care demonstrates great potential to improve clinical outcomes and economic benefits to major stakeholders.

BEST PRACTICES

Transitional care best practices overlap with standard interventions in routine discharge planning, which typically concludes on patient's departure from the facility. Evidence suggests that successful transitional care should begin on admission and be sustained for up to 90 days after discharge (Naylor et al., 2004). Model transitional care programs provide interventions that go beyond discharge instructions. The provider often an RN or an APRN, assumes the role of a coach (Coleman et al., 2006), patient advocate, and care broker who coordinates tailored multidisciplinary care. Patient-specific interventions closely linked with assistance with medication self-management; an up-to-date record owned and maintained by the patient to facilitate cross-site information transfer; timely follow-up with primary or specialty care; and a list of "red flags" indicative of a worsening condition and instructions on how to respond to them are some of the key "pillars" in high-quality transitional care (Coleman et al., 2006).

Based on an extensive review of transitional care programs, successful models in transitional care of chronically ill older adults share the following characteristics: patient and caregiver involvement, interdisciplinary primary care, comprehensive care in hospitals, and nurse–physician teams in nursing home (Boult et al., 2009; Li et al., 2016). Core features of effective transitional care programs proved to reduce the cost of care and rehospitalization based on randomized control trials include the following (Coleman et al., 2006; Naylor et al., 2004):

- A comprehensive assessment of an individual's health goals and preferences; physical, emotional, cognitive, and functional capacities and needs; and social and environmental considerations
- Implementation of an evidence-based plan of transitional care
- Transition care that is initiated at hospital admission but that extends beyond discharge through a home visit and telephone follow-up
- Mechanisms to gather and appropriately share information across sites of care
- Engagement of patients and family caregivers in planning and executing the plan of care
- Coordinated services during and following the hospitalization by a health care professional with special preparation in the care of chronically ill people, preferably a master's-prepared nurse or APRN

The role of APRNs or clinical nurse specialists (Bryant-Lukosius et al., 2015) in innovative transitional care is essential in successful implementation. Health professionals' education programs need to fully integrate transitional care training and to immerse future workforce in planning, implementing, and evaluating transitional care interventions.

SUMMARY

The complex needs of the aging population demand cost-effective and evidence-based transitional care interventions. The development of new programs seeking to improve the quality of transitional care may seek guidance from the position statements by the American Geriatrics

Society Health Care Systems Committee (Coleman & Boult, 2003):

- Clinical professionals must prepare patients and their caregivers to receive care in the subsequent setting and actively involve them in decisions related to the formulation and execution of the transitional care plan.
- Bidirectional communication among clinical professionals is essential to ensuring high-quality transitional care.
- Policies should be developed that promote high-quality transitional care.
- Professional educational institutions, specialty certification boards, licensing boards, and quality improvement programs should seek to improve, evaluate, and monitor health professionals' ability to collaborate across settings to execute a common plan of care.
- Research should be conducted to improve the process of transitional care.
- Transitional care is not simply a novel intervention.

Transitional care needs to be considered as a core value in health care education, practice, research, and policy. The role of health information technology (HIT) in the seamless flow of information among providers is a vision yet to be realized.

See also Clinical Pathways; Discharge Planning; Home Health Care; Hospital-Based Services.

Fidelindo Lim and Brian Marquez

Baker, A. (2001). Crossing the quality chasm: A new health system for the 21st century. *British Medical Journal, 323*(7322), 1192. doi:10.1136/bmj.323.7322.1192

Boult, C., Green, A. F., Boult, L. B., Paccala, J., Snyder, C., & Leff, B. (2009). Successful models of comprehensive care for older adults with chronic conditions: Evidence for the Institute of Medicine's "Retooling for an Aging America" report. *Journal of the American Geriatrics Society, 57*, 2228–2237. doi:10.1111/j.1532-5415.2009.02571.x

Bradway, C., Trotta, R., Bixby, M. B., McPartland, E., Wollman, M. C., Kapustka, H., … Naylor, M. D. (2012). A qualitative analysis of an advanced practice nurse-directed transitional care model intervention. *The Gerontologist, 52*(3), 394–407. doi:10.1093/geront/gnr078

Bryant-Lukosius, D., Carter, N., Reid, K., Donald, F., Martin-Misener, R., Kilpatrick, K., … DiCenso, A. (2015). The clinical effectiveness and cost-effectiveness of clinical nurse specialist-led hospital to home transitional care: A systematic review. *Journal of Evaluation in Clinical Practice, 21*(5), 763–781. doi:10.1111/jep.12401

Coleman, E. A., & Boult, C. (2003). The American Geriatrics Society Health Care Systems Committee. Improving the quality of transitional care for persons with complex care needs. *Journal of the American Geriatrics Society, 51*, 556–557.

Coleman, E. A., Parry, C., Chalmers, S., & Min, S. J. (2006). The care transitions intervention: Results of a randomized controlled trial. *Archives of Internal Medicine, 166*, 1822–1828.

Hines, A. L., Barrett, M. L., Jiang, J., & Steiner, C. A. (2014). Statistical brief #172. Conditions with the largest number of adult hospital readmissions by payer—2011. Retrieved from http://www.hcup-us.ahrq.gov/reports/statbriefs/sb172-Conditions-Readmissions-Payer.pdf

Jencks, S. F., Williams, M. V., & Coleman. E. A. (2009). Rehospitalizations among patients in the Medicare fee-for-service program. *New England Journal of Medicine, 360*(14), 1418–1428. doi:10.1056/NEJMsa0803563

The Joint Commission. (n.d.). Transitions of care: The need for a more effective approach to continuing patient care. Retrieved from https://www.jointcommission.org/assets/1/18/Hot_Topics_Transitions_of_Care.pdf

Li, J., Brock, J., Jack, B., Mittman, B., Naylor, M., Sorra, J.; Project ACHIEVE Team. (2016). Project ACHIEVE—using implementation research to guide the evaluation of transitional care effectiveness. *BMC Health Services Research, 16*(70). doi:10.1186/s12913-016-1312-y

Naylor, M. D., Brooten, D. A., Campbell, R. L., Maislin, G., McCauley, K. M., & Schwartz, J. S. (2004). Transitional care of older adults hospitalized with heart failure: A randomized, controlled trial. *Journal of the American Geriatrics Society, 52*, 675–684.

Stamp, K. D., Machado, M. A., & Allen, N. A. (2014). Transitional care programs improve outcomes for heart failure patients: An integrative review. *Journal of Cardiovascular Nursing 29*(2), 140–154. doi:10.1097/JCN.0b013e31827db560

Vedel, I., & Khanassov, V. (2015). Transitional care for patients with congestive heart failure: A systematic review and meta-analysis. *Annals of Family Medicine, 13*(6), 562–571. doi:10.1370/afm.1844

Web Resources

Care Transitions Program: http://www.caretransitions.org

Centers for Medicare & Medicaid Services: Patient Discharge Checklist: https://www.medicaid.gov/medicaid-chip-program-information/by-topics/delivery-systems/institutional-care/downloads/hospital-discharge-checklist.pdf

National Transitions of Care Coalition: Transition Care Advocacy Group: http://www.ntocc.org

Nurses Improving Care for Healthsystem Elders: Transitional Care Models: http://www.nicheprogram.org/niche_encyclopedia-geriatric_models_of_care-transitional_models

Partnership for Clear Health Communication and National Patient Safety Foundation: "Ask Me 3" campaign: http://www.npsf.org/askme3

Reducing Avoidable Readmissions Effectively (RARE): http://www.rarereadmissions.org/areas/transcare_resources.html

The Joint Commission: "Speak Up" initiative: planning your follow-up care: http://www.jointcommission.org/assets/1/6/Speak%20Up_initiatives_11_%2009.pdf

Transition Care Model (TCM): http://www.nursing.upenn.edu/media/transitionalcare/Documents/Information%20on%20the%20Model.pdf

TRANSPORTATION

Evidence suggests that effective transportation arrangements help improve the quality of life for older adults by facilitating social interaction and community participation (Glasgow, 1998). To access goods and services and to pursue social and economic opportunities, older adults use a range of modes of transportation, including driving, ride sharing, public transportation, special senior transportation, and walking. As in many nations, driving is the primary means of transportation in the United States. Except those living in extreme poverty or dwelling in cities, there are few impediments to personal mobility until age-related changes prevent individuals from safely operating vehicles. Public transportation is available in major cities but is often limited to outlying suburban and rural areas. In addition, age-related functional or cognitive limitations may hinder the use of public

transportation. Special senior transportation services, funded by a range of federal programs, are available to address the mobility needs of older adults who can no longer drive or use public transportation.

POLICIES AND FUNDING

In 1964, Congress enacted the Formula Grant Program for Elderly and Persons with Disabilities. This landmark legislation was the first step toward addressing the transportation needs of older adults and people with disabilities and led to a significant increase of special transportation services (Straight, 2003; Wacker & Roberto, 2013). Nearly a decade later, the Rehabilitation Act of 1973 required transportation systems to modify their designs to address the needs of older individuals, which paved the way for discount fares during off-peak hours and the creation of paratransit systems—special door-to-door transportation services for older adults. The Intermodal Surface Transportation Efficiency Act of 1991 was later the impetus for better coordination of local and regional transportation systems by including them as an essential factor in funding decisions. This act also permitted the transfer of funds between highway and transit programs. Most significantly, the Americans with Disabilities Act of 1990 mandated wheelchair access to all new public vehicles and paratransit systems, which are comparable to fixed-route systems in services and fares (Wacker & Roberto, 2013).

A significant amount of capital equipment costs, operational expenses, and administrative costs of public and private nonprofit senior transportation providers are covered by the Federal Transit Administration (FTA). In 2005 the FTA implemented Safe, Accountable, Flexible, Efficient Transportation Equity Act: A Legacy for Users (SAFETEA-LU) legislation, which requires every county or region to prepare a locally developed, coordinated public transit-human services transportation plan as a prerequisite for receiving federal funds from three FTA programs that are targeted to older adults, people with disabilities, and those with lower incomes (AARP, 2012). A second important source of funds is the U.S. Department of

Health and Human Services (USDHHS), which administers funded authorized by the Older Americans Act (OAA), Title XIX of the Social Security Act (1965), and the Community Services Block Grant (Wacker & Roberto, 2013). Many state and local agencies receive their transportation funding through these programs.

The costs to the user of senior transportation services vary, depending on the services used. For example, door-to-door transportation services may cost up to twice the regular fare, whereas off-peak travel using regular public transportation costs half the usual fare. If a patient is going to a physician's visit and lacks individual transportation, Medicaid often covers the costs of transportation to the selected provider. Human-service organizations may charge a nominal fee for the use of their transportation services.

MODES OF TRANSPORTATION

Driving

One survey found that 89% of older adults in the United States rely on their personal vehicles such as a car, pick-up truck, van, or sports utility vehicle as their primary mode of transportation (Collia, Sharp, & Giesbrecht, 2003). According to the National Highway Traffic Safety Administration (2015), the number of licensed older drivers in 2008 was 32 million, a 20% percent increase from 1999, representing 15% of all licensed drivers. Driving is not only the most accessible and convenient mode of transportation, but for many older adults, it also represents independence, self-reliance, and the ability to participate in other meaningful occupations (Oxley & Whelan, 2008). Some consider driving to be a key instrumental activity of daily living (American Occupational Therapy Association [AOTA], 2014). The U.S. Department of Transportation (2006) states that it is in the best interest of an individual to prolong automotive mobility as long as possible (i.e., as long as a person can safely drive). Determining if and how to discontinue a person's driving privileges is a difficult task. Some states have attempted to address this issue by regulating the renewal of drivers' licenses. However, proposals to limit the driving privileges of older persons have

been criticized as ageist, because they are implemented solely based on age and do not account for years of experience or health-related accommodations (Straight, 2003).

However, older adults have raised concerns over the high financial costs of driving, health and functional problems that limit their driving ability, stigma related to being an older driver, external pressure to stop driving, and fear of losing their driver's license (Glasgow & Blakely, 2000). Some public agencies and private organizations have developed programs to facilitate safe driving skills into late adulthood. Some Veterans Administration programs, for example, have begun to offer driving-rehabilitation services. The goal of these programs is to instruct drivers on ways to manage their illness or disability in a manner that allows the participants to operate a motor vehicle safely. The programs often involve physical and occupational therapy to strengthen and maintain a person's physical driving capabilities (U.S. Department of Veteran Affairs, 2003).

Ride Sharing

When driving oneself is no longer feasible, older adults often turn to friends or family to get them where they need to go. Reliance on ride sharing tends to increase with age and among non-drivers. One survey found that 19% of adults aged 75 to 79 years, 16% of adults aged 80 to 84 years, and 40% of those aged 85 years and older used ride sharing as their primary mode of transportation (Ritter, Straight & Evans, 2002). Older adults who are dependent on rides from others tend to be much less mobile than those who are not dependent on others (Metz, 2000). However, ride sharing may be inconvenient for those with poor health and may result in concerns about dependency and imposing on others (Ritter et al., 2002).

Walking

An estimated 5% of people aged 75 years or older identify walking as their primary mode of transportation (French, 2003). Walking provides the added benefits of engaging in a healthy activity and supporting independence. Barriers to walking include health and functional limitations and environmental conditions, such as the absence of public bathrooms or benches on which to rest along one's route. Older adults in rural areas, where the distance between destinations tend to be longer and require more time, view walking less favorably than older adults in urban areas (Glasgow & Blakely, 2000). Indeed, the majority of older adults find walking less accessible than other modes of transportation.

Public Transportation

Older adults use public transportation at a significantly lower percentage than other modes. An estimated 5% of older adults aged 50 years and older use public transportation as their primary mode of transportation (AARP, 2012). Because of the rise of the automobile as the primary means of personal mobility, the United States is less connected by public transportation today than it was in the late 1920s (Wacker & Roberto, 2013). However, public transportation use is higher among adults aged 75 years and older than the younger age groups (Rosenbloom & Winsten-Bartlett, 2002). Although the provision of public transportation is appropriate for many older adults, those who do not drive and or who have disabilities are often dissatisfied with conventional modes of fixed-route public transport (Alsnih & Hensher, 2003).

Paratransit and Demand-Response Systems

Paratransit or personally responsive transportation systems are increasingly available to eligible subgroups such as older adults or those with disabilities (Rahman, Strawderman, Adams-Price, & Turner, 2016). These services are more flexible than public transportation, bringing a passenger from one specific location to another. An estimated 200,000 paratransit trips are made annually (U.S. Government Accountability Office, 2012). However, the use of special transportation among older adults with health complications is only 12% (Collia et al., 2003). Some demand–response systems operate on short notice, whereas others require up to 24-hour notice. The systems also differ in the extent of services rendered. Some providers stop only at the curb, whereas others come to the door or even inside a home to pick up a passenger.

Another subtype of service is incidental transit, such as van services that transport clients to and from an adult day care center. Incidental transit is provided by private human-service organizations for their clients.

TRANSPORTATION UTILITY AND ACCESS

As people age, their need for daily and long-distance travel tends to decline. According to the 2011 National Household Travel Survey, adults in the United States aged 66 to 70 years make an average of 3.8 trips per day, whereas those aged 71 years and older make an average of 3.1 trips per day (Sivak & Schoettle, 2011). Substantial research has examined the factors influencing the selection and accessibility of transportation alternatives. According to Rosenbloom (1988), both physical and environmental factors act as barriers to the effective use of driving alternatives. In addition, a number of sociodemographic factors such as income, education, and living alone influence transportation and patterns of travel.

One particularly important factor in transportation access is geography. Older adults in rural areas tend to live farther from potential destinations and thus make longer and more infrequent trips than their urban counterparts. Their access to public transportation also differs significantly. Pucher and Renne (2005) found that rural households make an average of 5% fewer trips per day than urban households. Income also influences transportation patterns. With declining income, trip and travel distance fall considerably both in rural and urban areas. However, the mobility of low-income older adults appears to be higher in rural areas; this may be explained by the dispersed location of destinations, which requires more travel, not necessarily because of higher accessibility in rural areas.

Gender can also affect the travel pattern of older adults. Older women are more likely to use public transportation (Siren & Haustein, 2013) than men. Women aged 65 years and older drive less than any other group and travel less frequently and for shorter distances than younger women (Alsnih & Hensher, 2003). As drivers age, changes in their health may compromise their ability to maneuver a vehicle safely. Cognitive, sensory, and physical changes such as visual attention, memory, and reaction time that take place during normal aging may affect driving performance. In addition, medical conditions such as dementia, cardiovascular disease, sleep apnea, schizophrenia, and Parkinson's disease may affect driving ability and increase crash risk (Crizzle, Classen, & Uc, 2012).

MEETING THE TRANSPORTATION NEEDS OF OLDER ADULTS

Procedures for assisting clients in accessing transportation services are quite varied. Typically, the process begins with an assessment of the client's individual physical and cognitive needs. Service providers should provide the client with information about the availability, eligibility, and costs of local transportation and senior transportation systems. Typical eligibility requirements are based on age or specific levels of disability or chronic illness, and a letter verifying the need for transportation from a physician might be needed. The older adult may require assistance in gathering the required documentation and completing an application. In addition, the practitioner should arrange for someone to accompany the patient the first time that senior transportation is used, if it appears to be necessary.

RECOMMENDATIONS

Changes in government funding priorities and the overall structure of transportation services need to be enacted to accommodate the projected increase in the number of older Americans in the coming several decades. A U.S. Department of Transportation report on transportation for older adults made several policy recommendations, including construction of safer highway systems; improvement of signage; development of systems that aid in identifying and evaluating when driving becomes problematic or unsafe; performance-aiding technology such as collision-warning and collision-avoidance systems; and redesigns of complex intersections (U.S. Department of Transportation, 2006). Research suggests that a combination of in-class and on-road sessions significantly increase

driving performance in later life (AOTA, 2016). In addition, there is an increased need to provide alternative transportation options for the aging population. The U.S. Department of Transportation (2006) recommended increasing support for providing transportation alternatives for non-driving seniors. One alternative is operating deviated- or fixed-route systems in which the driver may deviate to accommodate the requests of eligible riders.

Finally, research suggests that older adults are often not aware of the transportation options available to them (Kostyniuk & Shope, 2003). Education and outreach programs that increase awareness of the alternatives to driving and facilitation of older adult's planning and self-assessment of mobility needs and preferences should be encouraged (Alsnih & Hensher, 2003). Much of the research on the transportation needs of older adults and transportation services is from the early 2000s. Further research is needed, particularly around the special needs of aging baby boomers, who are entering older adulthood at increasing rates and may have very different transportation needs and preferences than other cohorts.

Angela Ghesquiere and Ariunsanaa Bagaajav

AARP. (2012). Meeting older adults' mobility needs: Transportation planning and coordination in rural communities. Retrieved from http://www.aarp.org/content/dam/aarp/livable-communities/learn/transportation/meeting-older-adults-mobility-needs-transportation-planning-and-coordination-in-rural-communities-2012-aarp.pdf

Alsnih, R., & Hensher, D. A. (2003). The mobility and accessibility expectations of seniors in an aging population. *Transportation Research Part A: Policy and Practice, 37*(10), 903–916.

American Occupational Therapy Association. (2014). Occupational therapy practice framework: Domain and process (3rd ed.). *American Journal of Occupational Therapy, 68*(Suppl. 1), S1–S48.

American Occupational Therapy Association. (2016). Research opportunities in the area of driving and community mobility for older adults. *American Journal of Occupational Therapy, 70*(4), 1–2.

Collia, D. V., Sharp, J., & Giesbrecht, L. (2003). The 2001 National Household Travel Survey: A look into the travel patterns of older Americans. *Journal of Safety Research, 34*(4), 461–470.

Crizzle, A., Classen, S., & Uc, E. (2012). Parkinson disease and driving: An evidence-based review. *Neurology, 79*, 2067–2074.

French, M. (2003). Walking and biking. *Transportation and Health for Older People, 27*(2), 74–75.

Glasgow, N. (1998). *Life course transitions and transportation mobility of rural older persons.* Presented at the annual meeting of the American Sociological Association, San Francisco.

Glasgow, N., & Blakely, R. M. (2000). Older nonmetropolitan residents' evaluations of their transportation arrangements. *Journal of Applied Gerontology, 19*(1), 95–116.

Kostyniuk, L. P., & Shope, J. T. (2003). Driving and alternatives: Older drivers in Michigan. *Journal of Safety Research, 34*(4), 407–414.

Metz, D. H. (2000). Mobility of older people and their quality of life. *Transport Policy, 7*(2), 149–152.

National Highway Traffic Safety Administration. (2015). Traffic safety facts: 2015. Retrieved from https://crashstats.nhtsa.dot.gov/Api/Public/Publication/812384

Oxley, J., & Whelan, M. (2008). It cannot be all about safety: The benefits of prolonged mobility. *Traffic Injury Prevention, 9*(4), 367–378.

Pucher, J., & Renne, J. L. (2005). Rural mobility and mode choice: Evidence from the 2001 National Household Travel Survey. *Transportation, 32*(2), 165–186.

Rahman, M. M., Strawderman, L., Adams-Price, C., & Turner, J. J. (2016). Transportation alternative preferences of the aging population. *Travel Behaviour and Society, 4*, 22–28.

Ritter, A., Straight, A., & Evans, E. (2002). Understanding senior transportation: A report and analysis of a survey of consumers age. Retrieved from http://www.aarp.org

Rosenbloom, S. (1988). The mobility needs of the elderly (Special Report No. 218). In Committee for the Study on Improving Mobility and Safety for Older Persons (Ed.), *Transportation in an aging society: Improving mobility and safety for older persons* (Vol. 2, pp. 21–71). Washington, DC: National Research Council, Transportation Research Board.

Rosenbloom, S., & Winsten-Bartlett, C. (2002). Asking the right question: Understanding the travel needs of older women who do not drive. *Transportation Research Record: Journal of the Transportation Research Board, 1818*, 78–82.

Siren, A., & Haustein, S. (2013). Baby boomers' mobility patterns and preferences: What are the implications for future transport? *Transport Policy, 29*, 136–144.

Sivak, M., & Schoettle, B. (2011). Recent changes in the age composition of U.S. drivers: Implications for the extent, safety, and environmental consequences of personal transportation. *Traffic Injury Prevention, 12*(6), 588–592.

Straight, A. K. (2003). Public policy and transportation for older people. *Generations, 27*(2), 44–49.

U.S. Department of Transportation. (2006). Older drivers. Available at http://safety.fhwa.dot.gov/older driver

U.S. Department of Veteran Affairs. (2003, February). Driver rehabilitation program report (RCS 10–0099). Retrieved from http://www1.va.gov/vhapublications

U.S. Government Accountability Office. (2012). ADA Paratransit Services (GAO-13-17). Retrieved from http://www.gao.gov/assets/660/650079.pdf

Wacker, R. R., & Roberto, K. A. (2013). *Community resources for older adults: Programs and services in an era of change.* Thousand Oaks, CA: Sage.

Web Resources

U.S. Administration on Aging: http://www.aoa.gov/prof/transportation/transportation.asp

U.S. Department of Transportation: http://www.nhtsa.dot.gov

TREATMENTS FOR COGNITIVE IMPAIRMENT IN DEMENTIA

The characteristic feature of dementia, as currently defined, is a decline in cognitive abilities from a previous baseline that results in significant increases in functional impairment. There are many different causes of dementia, all of which affect the brain. Problems with the brain, however, can have adverse effects not only on cognitive functioning but also the processes that constitute the neurobiological basis for emotions and behavior. They can also affect the contents of brain processing, namely perceptions, beliefs, moods, and specific actions.

NEUROBIOLOGY OF COGNITIVE IMPAIRMENT

Problems with memory and executive functioning have been the focus of research on the cognitive deficits in dementia. Much effort in dementia research has been dedicated to better understand the causes of deterioration in cognition and the mechanisms by which these causes work so that possible ways to reverse the declines can be discovered.

The transmission of electrical impulses in the brain's circuits depends on the release of molecules (neurotransmitters) across the gaps (synapses) among individual nerve cells (neurons). These neurotransmitters work by interacting with receptors on the synaptic surfaces of the neurons that are specific for each kind of receptor. Many have been identified, both in the brain and other parts of the body. A few appear to constitute the neurotransmitters involved primarily in the neurobiological processes that form the basis for cognitive functioning. Acetylcholine is one of these crucial molecules. The brain's cholinergic circuits are called this because they use acetylcholine as their neurotransmitter and they are necessary for sustaining adequate cognitive function. It has long been appreciated that drugs with anticholinergic side effects within the brain cause confusion, and even delirium. (Blockage of acetylcholine receptors elsewhere in the body can result in blurred vision, dry mouth, constipation, urinary retention, and decreased perspiration.) Early research revealed Alzheimer's disease to be characterized by significant anatomical and physiological problems with the brain's cholinergic system. It was discovered that a major decline in the brain's production of choline acetyltransferase, the enzyme that synthesizes acetylcholine, resulted in a marked reduction in the level of acetylcholine available in the synapses. Hence, a therapeutic strategy was adopted that focused on developing drugs to increase the amount of acetylcholine available in the synapses among neurons, improving and perhaps even restoring cognitive functioning in patients who have dementia. It was hoped that such a discovery would lead to as much therapeutic success as was achieved by the discovery that the drugs increase the levels of the neurotransmitter dopamine, which helped patients with Parkinson's disease. There have been some significant successes with this strategy, but the results have not been as dramatic as the implementation of dopaminergic treatment for the motor symptoms of Parkinson's disease.

COGNITIVE ENHANCERS

The pharmacological treatment of dementias consists primarily of medications to enhance the activity of acetylcholine in the brain circuits critical for cognitive functioning. These are known collectively as *cholinesterase inhibitors* because they work by interfering with the enzyme that metabolizes acetylcholine, thereby making this neurotransmitter more available to support cognitive functioning. One additional medication for dementias is memantine, which appears to work by protecting neurons from exposure to excessive levels of glutamate, another neurotransmitter involved in memory and learning processes (Tricco et al., 2015).

Cholinesterase Inhibitors

Four cholinesterase inhibitors are approved by the U.S. Food and Drug Administration (FDA) for the treatment of Alzheimer's dementia (AD). Tacrine, the first to be approved, is now infrequently used because of its potential to cause liver problems as a side effect. The others are donepezil, galantamine, and rivastigmine. Numerous studies of their use in patients with various types of dementia have found them to be equally effective, as well as fairly similar regarding their potential side effects. Because donepezil has relatively less effect on acetylcholine receptors outside of the brain, it is usually tolerated fairly well by patients with dementia. The most common side effects with galantamine are gastrointestinal (e.g., nausea, vomiting, or diarrhea). To minimize the likelihood of such symptoms, it is recommended that this medication be taken with food and that its dosage be very gradually titrated. Rivastigmine is also available in a transdermal patch, which is associated with significantly fewer gastrointestinal side effects (Reus et al., 2016).

For patients with mild to moderate AD, treatment with the cholinesterase inhibitors has been found to yield, on an average, modest benefits on measures of cognitive function and activities of daily living (ADL). Some patients (up to 20%) benefit more than others, and some (30%–50%) manifest no improvements at all. The ultimate effects of these cognitive enhancers in the long run are more unclear, both regarding reductions in disability and avoidance of patient placement in long-term care facilities. Results of cholinesterase inhibitor treatment in patients with severe AD are even more modest and again vary from patient to patient (Tricco et al., 2015).

Overall, the use of cholinesterase inhibitors is best guided on an individual basis according to the patients' responses and long-term goals of care. It is important to note that although these medications can have somewhat positive effects on the symptoms of cognitive impairment, they do not remedy the underlying disease processes. This accounts for the clinical phenomenon that sometimes occurs when cholinesterase inhibitors are discontinued. If the drug has had some effectiveness, stopping it can be associated with an apparent further decline in cognitive functioning. This, in fact is simply a reflection of the progression of underlying dementia that would have been apparent if the medication had not been used.

Study of the use of cholinesterase inhibitors in other types of dementia is more limited and has yielded similar results. Modest clinical benefits have been found when they are prescribed to patients with vascular dementia (VaD), mixed dementia (i.e., AD and VaD), and frontotemporal dementia. Cognitive benefits may be a little more robust for patients who have dementia with Lewy bodies (DLB), as well as for subgroups of patients with Parkinson's disease dementia and dementia because of traumatic brain injury (Rolinski, Fox, Maidment, & McShane, 2012).

Memantine

Glutamate is another neurotransmitter involved in learning and memory. Excessive stimulation of one of the receptors for glutamate, the N-methyl-D-aspartate (NMDA) receptor, can have disruptive effects. Memantine blocks the NMDA receptor and thus may protect neurons crucial to effective cognitive functioning. Although there is little evidence that it has much effect in mild AD (Tricco et al., 2015), it has been approved for use by the FDA in patients with moderate to severe AD. It is often used in combination with one of the cholinesterase inhibitors for these patients. In comparison to the cholinesterase inhibitors, its effectiveness is equally modest and usually associated with fewer side effects. The most common side effect is dizziness. On rare occasions, its use in the context of AD is associated with an increased confusion, agitation, or psychotic symptoms (hallucinations or delusions). Memantine has been found to have modest effectiveness for patients with VaD but problematic for those with DLB. Further research is needed to determine the extent to which memantine protects neurons and whether its long-term use may be of some benefit to patients with mild to moderate AD (Howard et al., 2012).

Other Pharmacological Treatments

A number of other pharmacological interventions have been attempted to address the cognitive impairment in dementia. These include anti-inflammatory drugs, hormones (e.g., estrogen), omega-3 fatty acids, vitamin B complex (folate, B_6, B_{12}) supplementation, ginkgo biloba, vitamin E, selegiline, and statins. Each of these is targeted at different biological mechanisms that play a role in brain functioning, with the goal of preventing and/or slowing, if not reversing, the progression of cognitive impairment. Although there appear to be some benefits for certain patients with each intervention, the overall results of the research have not demonstrated consistent and convincing evidence of clinically significant effect for any of them (Howard et al., 2012).

NONPHARMACOLOGICAL TREATMENTS

Cognitive rehabilitation is based on the principle of "use it or lose it." It involves helping patients in the early stages of a dementing illness to discover and practice ways to maintain their memory and executive functions as much as feasible and to compensate for deficits that cannot be remedied. Current research suggests that this approach can have some significant cognitive benefits (Woods, Aguirre, Spector, & Orrell, 2012), but it remains to be seen to what extent can these have a significant impact on ADL. In an analogous fashion, the growing appreciation for the link between cognitive health and cardiovascular health has spurred the use of exercise programs to enhance brain functions (Rolland et al., 2007). This approach appears to have some promise in slowing the decline in ADL for nursing home residents with dementia. For patients with mild to moderate dementia, occupational therapy (Graff et al., 2006), focusing on individualized ways to compensate for functional deficits, was found to yield significant improvement in both processing skills and ADL.

RECOMMENDATIONS

Given the complexities of the human brain, especially when it is malfunctioning, it is no surprise that there is no consensus about how to address the cognitive impairment of patients with dementia. In general, for patients with mild to moderate dementia, a trial with a cholinesterase inhibitor is warranted. The choice of which to use should be individualized according to the effectiveness of the drug and patient preference, and ability to tolerate the medication, as well as its cost. A trial of memantine for patients unable to tolerate one of the cholinesterase inhibitors is also warranted. For patients in whom dementia has progressed to a moderate to a severe level, adding memantine is a reasonable option (Howard et al., 2012). For those patients being treated with cognitive enhancers whose dementia has become severe, the cholinesterase inhibitors can be discontinued, unless doing so is temporally associated with a significant further drop in cognitive functioning. Continuation of memantine therapy at this point, to the extent that it may have some neuroprotective effects, may also be reasonable. Throughout any dementia, attention should be paid to the nonpharmacological therapies described earlier. These should be implemented on an individualized basis to assist patients in remaining engaged with others and their surrounding environments in ways that are personally meaningful to them.

See also Behavioral and Psychological Symptoms of Dementia; Vascular and Lewy Body Dementias.

Timothy Howell

Graff, M. J., Vernooij-Dassen, M. J., Thijssen, M., Dekker, J., Hoefnagels, W. H., & Rikkert, M. G. (2006). Community based occupational therapy for patients with dementia and their care givers: Randomised controlled trial. *British Medical Journal, 333,* 1196.

Howard, R., McShane, R., Lindesay, J., Ritchie, C., Baldwin, A., Barber, R., … Phillips, P. (2012). Donepezil and memantine for moderate-to-severe Alzheimer's disease. *New England Journal of Medicine, 366,* 893.

Reus, V., Fochtmann, L., Eyler A., Hilty, D., Horvitz-Lennon, M., & Jibson, M. (2016) The American Psychiatric Association practice guideline on the use of antipsychotics to treat agitation or psychosis in patients with dementia. *American Journal of Psychiatry, 173,* 543–546.

Rolinski, M., Fox, C., Maidment, I., & McShane, R. (2012). Cholinesterase inhibitors for dementia with Lewy bodies, Parkinson's disease dementia and cognitive impairment in Parkinson's disease. *Cochrane Database of Systematic Reviews, 3,* CD006504. doi:10.1002/14651858.CD006504.pub

Rolland, Y., Pillard, F., Klapouszczak, A., Reynish, E., Thomas, D., Andrieu, S., … Vellas, B. (2007). Exercise program for nursing home residents with Alzheimer's disease: A 1-year randomized, controlled trial. *Journal of American Geriatrics Society, 55,* 158–165.

Tricco, A. C., Ashoor, H. M., Rios, P., Hamid, J., Ivory, J. D., Khan, P. A., … Ho, J. (2015). *Comparative safety and effectiveness of cognitive enhancers for the treatment of Alzheimer's disease: A rapidly updated systematic review and network meta-analysis.* Toronto, ON, Canada: Ontario Drug Policy Research Network. Retrieved from http://odprn.ca/wp-content/uploads/2015/08/Cognitive-Enhancers-systematic-review-FINAL-CENSORED-aug-2015.pdf

Woods, B., Aguirre, E., Spector, A. E., & Orrell, M. (2012). Cognitive stimulation to improve cognitive functioning in people with dementia. *Cochrane Database of Systematic Reviews, 2,* CD005562. doi:10.1002/14651858.CD005562.pub2

Web Resources

Agency for Healthcare Research and Policy: https://www.ahrq.gov

Alzheimer's Association: https://www.alz.org

U

UNDUE INFLUENCE ASSESSMENT IN ELDER CARE

As elderly populations increase around the world, there is a concomitant increase in the concern about possible elder abuse and associated undue influence, especially as it relates to financial exploitation. Unlike *mental capacity*, *undue influence* is a legal construct that refers to a dynamic in a confidential relationship, wherein a dominant party exploits its influence or position of power over a weaker party, often for financial gain. The dominant party acts in such a way to distort the victim's assessment of risks and benefits and thus surreptitiously gains control over the victim's decision making. The perpetrator typically exploits the trust, dependency, and fear of the victim and uses a variety of tactics that heighten the victim's reliance and dependence to accomplish this goal. Common tactics include flattery, importunity, and deceit. Undue influence may be alleged in legal transactions, such as executing a will, entering a contract, or conveying property to another, as well as in cases of financial abuse, sexual abuse, and even homicide (American Bar Association [ABA] Commission on Law and Aging & American Psychological Association [APA], 2008). A proof of undue influence may be used to reverse or negate a previous transaction in civil or probate litigation or may be considered an aggravating factor in criminal prosecution. Although specific statutory definitions vary, in most legal systems, the core elements of an undue influence case are (a) existence of a confidential relationship, (b) suspicious circumstances, and (c) an adverse outcome. Cognitive impairment of the victim increases susceptibility and dependence, but it is not a necessary component of undue influence (ABA Commission on Law and Aging & APA, 2008).

The forensic psychiatric or psychological evaluation is frequently a central piece of evidence in these cases, despite the variation in legal definitions among countries and the fact that this is an emerging area of study with little empirical research to guide clinicians (ABA Commission on Law and Aging & APA, 2008). Despite the limitations, many clinical issues are considered to be important components of a thorough, professional assessment.

The first task for a psychiatric evaluator is to distinguish between a victim's vulnerability to undue influence versus whether the psychosocial conditions of undue influence exist. The former involves a more traditional clinical assessment, whereas the latter involves assessment using various accepted behavioral models of undue influence.

Assessment of a given person's vulnerability, or "susceptibility," to undue influence involves a classic biopsychosocial evaluation, meaning that the forensic evaluator should include the information usually referenced for a capacity assessment plus consider the psychological, social, and environmental factors that have contributed to the older adult's susceptibility. A variant of this approach relabels some social and environmental factors as "legal" but otherwise seems to be equivalent (Peisah et al., 2009). Common potential "vulnerability indicators" to consider are age, recent widowhood, geographical isolation, or victim's significant or unexplained emotional or behavioral changes (see Table U.1; Hall, Hall, & Chapman, 2005). Everyone—regardless of age, health, education, or experience—is susceptible to undue influence. Medical issues, whether physical or mental, make it easier for a perpetrator to manipulate or overwhelm a victim but are not

U

Table U.1
VICTIMS' AND PERPETRATORS' FEATURES

Victims	Perpetrators
Advanced age (older than 75 years)	Sociopathic or antisocial character disorder/traits
Female	Related to victim and often living with victim
Middle or upper income bracket	History of mental illness, substance abuse, or health problems
Financially independent without financial caretakers	History of unstable relationships
Unmarried/widowed/divorced	False credentials or embellished position
Living alone or with the abuser	Recurrent behavior
Estranged from family—socially isolated	
Physically, mentally, or emotionally disordered	

Source: Modified from Hall et al. (2005).

necessary and do not have to be present. Many neuropsychologists and psychiatrists do not understand this, focus primarily on a cognitive assessment, and do not consider a large amount of non–capacity-related behavioral research in forming their assessments. This mistaken approach creates unnecessary confusion and erroneous findings. We agree with the statement that "(t)he only factor that would require the expertise of a neuropsychologist would be whether the testator was vulnerable to undue influence due to the presence of cognitive impairment or other mental condition" (Mart, 2016). An attempt to address this issue has been made by Lichtenberg, Stoltman, Ficker, Iris, and Mast (2015). The Lichtenberg Financial Decision Making Rating Scale (LFDRS) considers undue influence and vulnerability to financial exploitation to be important "contextual factors" when evaluating financial capacity and contains a small number of self-report items to test for these concerns (Lichtenberg et al., 2015). However, the self-report primarily assesses duress-related forms of undue influence.

Because these evaluations are often requested after an older adult has died or has become incompetent, the contemporaneous assessment may not be possible or relevant, so only a retrospective evaluation can be performed. In all cases, medical and legal records should be reviewed and information obtained from collateral informants. It is often also helpful to develop a timeline of events.

After noting the factors that increase the given person's vulnerability, the forensic evaluator should then review the nature of the relationship with the beneficiary, the statements and behaviors of the beneficiary regarding both the supposed victim and the transaction(s) in question, and the consistency of the supposed victim's previous spending habits, financial transactions, or previous wills. The evaluator should also consider the degree to which the acts in question are consistent with the supposed "victim's" established values and beliefs (Restatement, 2003). This information, plus the vulnerability factors, are then analyzed to determine whether the psychological and behavioral indicia of undue influence are present. Many theoretical frameworks for undue influence have been proposed, but the five models described later are the most commonly used. Each has unique strengths and limitations; therefore, it is recommended that the evaluators use multiple methods of analysis for this determination to increase the overall accuracy.

Note: Because these models emphasize analysis of behaviors, they retain their usefulness in many Western hemisphere courts.

The five theoretical models are as follows:

1. SODR (The Restatement [Third] of Property, 2003): SODR is a model that is based on case law in the United States. It is defined as (a) the donor was susceptible to undue influence, (b) the alleged wrongdoer had an opportunity to exert undue influence, (c) the alleged wrongdoer had the disposition to exert undue influence, and (d) there was a result appearing to be the effect of the undue influence [The Restatement (Third) of Property (Wills & Don. Trans.) § 8.3 cmt. e].

2. SCAM (ABA Commission on Law and Aging & APA, 2008): SCAM is the behavioral

variant of SODR. The elements of this model are (a) susceptibility of the victim, (b) a confidential and trusting relationship between the victim and perpetrator, (c) active procurement of the legal and financial transactions by the perpetrator, and (d) monetary loss of the victim.

3. IDEAL (ABA Commission on Law and Aging & APA, 2008): This model was created in the 1990s primarily for use in cases involving elder financial abuse, although it is used in many types of cases involving excessive or inappropriate manipulation tactics. Five categorical factors are analyzed in this model, isolation, dependency, emotional manipulation and/or exploitation of weaknesses, acquiescence, and loss.

   Isolation: Isolation refers to isolation from pertinent information, friends, relatives, or advisors. Frequent causes include medical disorders, perpetrator interference, history of poor relationships with others, geographic changes (e.g., travel), and technological isolation (e.g., loss of telephone services).

   Dependency: Dependency refers to the victim's dependence on the perpetrator (e.g., for physical support, emotional intimacy, or information).

   Emotional manipulation or exploitation of weaknesses: Emotional manipulation usually manifests as promises, threats, or a combination of both and involves issues of safety and security, or companionship and friendship.

   Acquiescence: Acquiescence refers to the victim's apparent consent or submission. Such "consent" is based on the factors noted earlier—dependency on the perpetrator, emotional or other vulnerability factors, and exposure to inadequate, misleading, or inaccurate information.

   Loss: Loss refers to the loss, damages, or harm resulting from the claimed undue influence (such as inter vivos financial loss).

4. The Brandle/Heisler/Steigel Model (ABA Commission on Law and Aging & APA, 2008): This model is based on domestic violence relationships, stalking, and sexual assault. It assumes that undue influence parallels these other situations. This model is currently taught by the National College of District Attorneys and the National District Attorneys Association for use in criminal prosecutions, but it is also applicable in some civil or probate proceedings. There are eight factors:

   - Keep the victim unaware
   - Isolate the victim from others and information
   - Create fear
   - Prey on vulnerabilities
   - Create dependencies
   - Create lack of faith in own abilities
   - Induce shame and secrecy
   - Perform intermittent acts of kindness

5. The "Thought Reform" or "Cult" Model of Margaret Thaler Singer, PhD (ABA Commission on Law and Aging & APA, 2008): Dr. Singer's model of thought reform developed from her work on the tactics used by cults and cult leaders. The model is based on the following six stages: creating isolation, fostering a siege mentality, inducing dependency, promoting a sense of powerlessness, manipulating fears and vulnerabilities, and keeping the victim unaware and uninformed. The specific tactics are (a) to keep the person unaware of what is going on and what changes are taking place; (b) to control the victim's time and, if possible, physical environment; (c) to create a sense of powerlessness, covert fear, and dependency; (d) to suppress much of the person's old behavior and attitudes; (e) to instill new behavior and attitudes; and (f) to put forth a closed system of logic, allowing no real input or criticism.

All elder care professionals, but especially forensic psychiatrists and psychologists, who work with civil or probate courts should expect to encounter questions about the decision-making capacity and impact of potential undue influence on elders or those with serious or chronic illnesses. Effective assessment can prevent needless emotional and financial losses of the victims and help them maintain their financial independence.

R. Bennett Blum and
Esperanza L. Gómez-Durán

American Bar Association Commission on Law and Aging & American Psychological Association. (2008). *Assessment of older adults with diminished capacity: A handbook for psychologists* (pp. 115–117). Washington, DC: Authors.

Hall, R. C. W., Hall, R. C. W., & Chapman, M. J. (2005). Exploitation of the elderly: Undue influence as a form of elder abuse. *Clinical Geriatrics, 13*(2), 28–36.

Lichtenberg, P., Stoltman, J., Ficker, L., Iris, M., & Mast, B. (2015). A person-centered approach to financial capacity assessment: Preliminary development of a new rating scale. *Clinical Gerontologist, 38*, 49–67. doi:10.1080/07317115.2014.970318

Mart, E. (2016). Assessment of testamentary capacity and undue influence. *Archives of Clinical Neuropsychology, 31*(6), 554 561. doi:10.1093/arclin/acw048

Peisah, C., Finkel, S., Shulman, K., Melding, P., Luxenberg, J., Heinik. J., … Bennett, H.; International Psychogeriatric Association Task Force on Wills and Undue Influence. (2009, February). The wills of older people: Risk factors for undue influence. *International Psychogeriatrics, 21*(1), 7–15.

The Restatement (Third) of Property (Wills & Don, Trans.) § 8.3 cmt. c (2003).

Web Resources

National Center on Elder Abuse: http://www.ncea.aoa.gov

National Centre for the Protection of Older People: http://www.ncpop.ie/educationandtraining_onlinemodules

National Committee for the Prevention of Elder Abuse: http://www.preventelderabuse.org

URINARY INCONTINENCE

Urinary incontinence (UI) is defined as the involuntary leakage of urine. It is common in older adults, and it increases in incidence with age but is not considered a part of normal aging. The prevalence of UI is estimated to be 15% to 30% for women living in the community, 50% of homebound older women, and almost 70% of those living in nursing homes (DuBeau, 2014). The prevalence is considered three times more common in women than men until the age of 85 years, after which it becomes equivalent.

TYPES

Urgency incontinence is associated with a compelling or sudden urge to void, which is hard to defer. Environmental conditions or cues that may precipitate urge incontinence include the sight or sound of running water, going outside into the cold air, or even arriving home and unlocking the front door. Stress incontinence is the leakage of urine with physiological processes such as sneezing, coughing, laughter, or exertion. In this type of incontinence, the sphincter mechanism fails to retain urine. If the incontinence occurs immediately after such an activity, it often involves uninhibited detrusor contraction. Mixed incontinence refers to urine leakage involving both stress and urge features or mechanisms. Overflow incontinence is incontinence associated with impaired bladder emptying. In frail older adults, urge incontinence often involves detrusor hyperactivity with impaired contractility (DHIC) with an elevated postvoid residual volume (DuBeau, 2014). Functional incontinence occurs with an intact urinary system, but factors outside the lower urinary tract fail to prevent urine leakage; examples are fecal impaction, delirium, functional limitations, and changes in neurological function (Dunphy, Winland-Brown, Porter, & Thomas, 2011). Many classes of medications have effects that may increase the risk of UI in the older adult. Medications that are associated with coughing, sedation, sphincter or bladder outlet tone, polyuria, or fluid retention may result in UI (Parker & Griebling, 2015).

Urological function is affected by several age-related changes. These include a decreased disinhibition of bladder contractions, reduced bladder capacity, increased nocturnal fluid and sodium excretion, and increased postvoid residual volume. Decreased estrogen after menopause affects the competence of the internal and external sphincters. With age, women often have weaker pelvic muscles. In men, benign prostatic hyperplasia increases urethral resistance, resulting in urinary overflow phenomena (Dunphy et al., 2011). As men and women age, direct pelvic floor injury is less a factor in causing incontinence, although various medical conditions have a greater impact (Wu, Matthews, Vaughan,

& Markland, 2015). Urgency incontinence is the most common type of UI experienced by older adults, although stress incontinence is the most common form of UI in the overall female population (Parker & Griebling, 2015).

RISK FACTORS AND IMPACT

Functional impairment, environmental barriers to the toilet, certain medications, dementia, and obesity are risk factors for UI. Physical mobility, intact cognition, dexterity, and motivation are needed to use bathrooms facilities effectively (Durso & Sullivan, 2013). For women, higher parity, diabetes mellitus, White race, arthritis, higher body mass index, and oral hormone therapy are associated with an increased risk. For males, prostate cancer treatment including radiation treatment and radical prostatectomy are associated with UI (Vaughan, Goode, Burgio, Markland, 2011).

Heart failure and diuretic treatment contribute to urinary frequency and UI. Likewise, a stroke can impair motor neuron function or disrupt subcortical pathways, as well as reduce cognition, mobility, or the sensation to need to void. Parkinson's disease, diabetes mellitus, spinal cord injury, delirium, dementia, constipation, vitamin B12 deficiency, obstructive sleep apnea, spinal stenosis, musculoskeletal disease, alcoholism, hypercalcemia, peripheral venous insufficiency, and normal pressure hydrocephalus are some of the conditions that can increase the risk of UI (Durso & Sullivan, 2013). The impact of UI on older adults is significant, often contributing to social isolation and reduced life satisfaction. It is a risk factor for falls and fall related injuries, as well as nursing home placement. In many older adults, UI goes untreated (Vaughan et al., 2011).

EVALUATION AND DIAGNOSIS

Routine screening for UI is an essential part of effective elder care. Assessment should be made about how much UI bothers older adults. Infrequent UI is a risk factor for more frequent UI, and interventions may prevent this progression to frequent UI (Vaughan, Goode, Burgio, & Markland, 2011). The evaluation of UI should be multifactorial, including mobility, functional status, cognition, comorbidity, and medications. A complete history should include onset, frequency, precipitating, and ameliorating factors, other associated lower urinary tract symptoms, and fluid intake. The status and time line of medical conditions (and changes in medical conditions) and medications during the onset of UI should be noted (Durso & Sullivan, 2013). Screening for depression and functional status should be performed because motivation and mobility/functionality may be causative (DuBeau, 2014). There is a bidirectional association with UI and depression (Durso & Sullivan, 2013). Cognitive status should be included in the evaluation of UI and may impact the treatment plan (DuBeau, 2014).

Physical examination should focus on possible urogenital abnormalities. A pelvic examination should be included for women. At the same time, the provider should assess for any comorbid conditions that may be contributing to the UI. UI presenting suddenly with pelvic or suprapubic/lower abdominal pain is a red flag for a possible malignancy or a neurological condition, and these people should be referred promptly to a specialist. Evaluation should include a urinalysis and may also include a voiding diary (DuBeau, 2014).

MANAGEMENT AND TREATMENT

The older adult patient and caregivers should be involved in the management of UI. The goals of care, along with desired outcomes, should be discussed. Goals may vary from complete continence to avoidance of large-volume incontinence or may focus on skin integrity. A stepwise progression in treatment is recommended. Lifestyle modifications and treatment of obesity may be sufficient to reach treatment goals. Although there is no strong supporting evidence, limiting evening fluids and caffeinate beverages may help, and smoking cessation is often recommended (DuBeau, 2014). Addressing other contributing factors and medications that exacerbate UI should also be considered (Durso & Sullivan, 2013).

For older adults with UI, behavioral therapy is a first-line therapy. Bladder training and pelvic muscle exercises are evidence-based approaches for stress, urge, and mixed incontinence (Durso & Sullivan, 2013). Bladder training has two components. One is to keep the volume of urine in the bladder low. This is done by toileting at regular intervals, initially every 2 hours. Second, the older adult should try to sit or stand still when urgency occurs, and complete pelvic muscle contractions, as well as deep breathing techniques, until feeling more in control. A timing schedule is established and then adjusted based on the success of decreasing the episodes of UI. Pelvic muscle exercises work to improve the strength of the pelvic support muscles. Isolated pelvic muscle contractions are performed and held for several seconds. Then the pelvis is relaxed, and another contraction is performed. They are completed in sets, several times per week, for several weeks. The intensity and duration of the contractions may increase as the patient progresses. For cognitively impaired patients, prompted voiding is the only behavioral therapy with proven efficacy. An initial 3-day trial is suggested (DuBeau, 2014).

Medications can be effective for urge or mixed incontinence (when urge incontinence is dominant). They are usually indicated when there has been no or limited improvement with behavioral therapy. It is important to note that stress incontinence has no U.S. Food and Drug Administration-approved medication in the United States. Antimuscarinic agents have been moderately effective for urge incontinence (DuBeau, 2014). These agents relax the smooth muscle of the bladder, by targeting muscarinic receptors in the bladder muscle. Different medications in this class have similar efficacy, but they also have frequent side effects, including constipation and dry mouth. These drugs may also have a negative effect on cognition (Vaughan et al., 2011). The beta-3 agonist class of drugs was approved in 2012. They also prompt relaxation of the bladder, but they may increase blood pressure and should be used only at a low dose if there is severe renal or moderate hepatic insufficiency (DuBeau, 2014).

For older adults with refractory incontinence, some minimally invasive procedures are available. There may be some benefit from pessary placement if a bladder or uterine prolapse has occurred. Sacral nerve neuromodulation has shown some effect in the treatment of urge incontinence that has not responded to other treatments (Durso & Sullivan, 2013). Surgical procedures have shown the highest cure rates for stress incontinence in women, depending on the problem. Colposuspension and midurethral and bladder neck slings are also options for treatment. For men with sphincter damage after radical prostatectomy, artificial sphincters may be placed (Durso & Sullivan, 2013).

Mary C. Ballin

DuBeau, C. E. (2014). Urinary incontinence. In R. L. Ham, P. D. Sloane, G. A. Warshaw, J. F. Potter, & E. Flaherty (Eds.), *Ham's primary care geriatrics: A case based approach* (6th ed., pp. 269–280). Philadelphia, PA: Elsevier Saunders.

Dunphy, L. M., Winland-Brown, J. E., Porter, B. O., & Thomas, D. J. (2011). *Primary care: The art and science of advanced practice nursing*. Philadelphia, PA: F. A. Davis.

Durso, S. C., & Sullivan, G. M. (Eds.). (2013). *Geriatric review syllabus: A core curriculum in geriatric medicine* (8th ed.). New York, NY: American Geriatrics Society.

Parker, W. P., & Griebling, T. L. (2015). Nonsurgical treatment of urinary incontinence in elderly women. *Clinics in Geriatric Medicine, 31*, 471–485.

Vaughan, C. P., Goode, P. S., Burgio, K. L., & Markland, A. D. (2011). Urinary incontinence in older adults. *Mount Sinai Journal of Medicine, 78*, 558–570.

Wu, J. M., Matthews, C. A., Vaughan, C. P., & Markland, A. D. (2015). Urinary, fecal, and dual incontinence in older U.S. adults. *Journal of the American Geriatrics Society, 63*, 947–953.

Web Resources
American College of Obstetricians and Gynecologists: https://www.acog.org
National Association for Continence: https://www.nafc.org
National Kidney and Urologic Diseases Information: https://www.niddk.nih.gov
The Simon Foundation for Continence: https://simonfoundation.org
Urology Health from the American Urological Association: https://www.urologyhealth.org

V

VALIDATION THERAPY

Validation therapy (VT) emerged from psychological theory, which posits that coming to terms with strong emotions before death is a major developmental challenge of late life. It is based on certain premises (a) that long-standing emotions suppressed in late-life can fester and become toxic and (b) that through the sharing of such emotions with an empathic listener, older individuals can receive external validation and, thereby, experience meaningful relief. For older adults with dementia, VT uses both verbal and nonverbal communication techniques, as well as a method for forming validation groups (Feil & De Klerk-Rubin, 2012).

The goal of VT is to enhance the quality of life through empathic listening and dialogue, especially for older adults suffering from neurocognitive disorders, who have unmet psychological needs. For VT to be effective, it requires an attitude of respect for those whose cognitive capacities are deteriorating. Its implementation aims to restore dignity and foster well-being for patients throughout the progressive course of dementia, from the initial stage of "the maloriented," to that of the "time-confused," and finally to the "repetitive motion" phase (Feil, 2007). VT is by nature interdisciplinary, so it can be used, with appropriate training, by many kinds of care providers, including psychologists, social workers, nurses, occupational and physical therapists, and administrators, as well as family members.

Some studies have revealed significant improvements after 6 months of VT in populations whose dementia had a late onset (i.e., older than 65 years). Reported positive outcomes include increased communication between staff and patients and decreased frequency of agitation associated with reductions in the need for tranquilizing medications. In addition, an increase in family visits and a decrease in staff burnout have been noted. One review concluded that there was insufficient evidence to demonstrate whether VT is effective for individuals with dementia (Neal & Briggs, 2003). The other studies, however, have demonstrated that it is not ineffective and suggest that, for some patients, it may improve some behavioral and psychological symptoms of dementia, including agitation, apathy, irritability, and abnormal nocturnal behaviors (Deponte & Missan, 2007; Tondi, Ribani, Bottazzi, Viscomi, & Vulcano, 2007; Toseland et al., 1997).

VERBAL VT TECHNIQUES

"Phase One Resolution" is directed toward older individuals whose cognitive impairment is moderate (referred to as "the maloriented"). They retain their verbal skills, have no history of mental illness, and are for the most part well oriented to time and place. However, these individuals tend to repeat things that are untrue or make false accusations about others being the source of their frustrations. According to VT, they are engaged in expressing emotions that they were previously unable to share with the people who were important to them. According to the principles of VT, the older individual's hurtful remarks are not to be taken literally, but instead are taken as symbolic of past experiences and feelings—to understand that critical remarks about current people or things, in fact, refer to distressing people or events in the past (Feil & De Klerk-Rubin, 2012). Taking such situations literally and feeling hurt in response interfere with the ability of caregivers/therapist to listen empathically. The validating caregiver or therapist seeks to appreciate the symbolic nature of the complaints, to accept these individuals

V

where they are currently at from a developmental perspective, and to allow them to heal engaging with an empathic listener.

Phase one VT requires being more aware of, monitoring, and clarifying one's own emotions, thereby enabling the self to be open to the older individual's emotions and what they mean and thus be able to respond with genuine empathy. It helps for caregivers/therapists to place themselves in the older individual's shoes through the process of "centering." Phase one verbal VT techniques (Feil, 2007, pp. 797–798) include the following:

1. Breathing deeply: inhaling through the nose, then exhaling from the center of one's body.
2. Avoiding the use of "feeling" words; instead of asking nonthreatening questions about matters of fact: Who? What? Where? When? How? But avoiding asking why.
3. Listening carefully to the language used: picking up on the use of verbs, particularly the preferred tense, as well as key personal terms and the tones in which they are expressed.
4. Reflecting back the look in the individual's eyes.
5. Identifying the parameters of distress (e.g., "How bad?" or "How often?").
6. Paraphrasing back what has been heard not only to communicate that one is listening actively, but also to determine whether an accurate understanding has been reached.
7. Encouraging, through the ongoing dialogue, reminiscing about the circumstances (i.e., having the individual recollect and describe the details of past events to the extent feasible).
8. Discovering and then helping the individual to use a familiar, more effective way of coping.

The following dialogue (Feil, 2007, p. 798) exemplifies the use of phase one verbal VT techniques:

A nurse encounters an 85-year-old woman who does not appear to be in physical pain but has frequent somatic complaints (e.g., "My back hurts. My hips hurt. I have a pain in my neck. I wish I were dead."). The validating nurse, hypothesizing that the individual may be afraid of dying alone, seeks to verify this intuition. To

do so, the nurse helps the senior woman articulate her psychological pain, thereby building trust in the process.

Nurse (using a kinesthetic sense): Does it feel sharp like a knife in your back, or is it a dull pain?

Elderly Woman: Yes. Just like a knife. That's right.

Nurse (establishing the parameters of distress): When is the pain worse?

Elderly Woman: It hurts all the time, but at night, it's horrible.

Nurse (paraphrasing, testing the hypothesis, and inviting the individual to reminisce): Is the pain worse when you are alone, by yourself? Have you ever had this terrible pain before?

Elderly Woman (beginning to trust, feeling safer, and with her voice less harsh and shrill): I had the same pain in my back after my husband died.

Nurse (attempting to elicit a familiar coping method): What did you do after he died? How did you stand it?

Elderly Woman: I listened to the music we used to dance to. We loved dancing together. That's how I got through those nights.

Nurse: I can help you get you some of that music. When your back starts hurting again, turn on your music player. If you need me, I'll be here.

Elderly Woman: You're sweet. You can go now. You have other people to take care of. But you'll come back with that music?

The nurse keeps her promise, and over time the senior woman expresses fewer somatic complaints. Although not remedied altogether, over the course of multiple similar validating interactions, she trusts the nurse more, and her fear of dying alone gradually fades. In this way, VT, although requiring some energy, focus, and genuine caring, need not take up a significant amount of time. Validating exchanges such as these take about 5 minutes each. These limited investments of time and caring can pay significant dividends over time regarding less stress and more meaningful interactions for all involved.

NONVERBAL VALIDATION TECHNIQUES

"Phase Two Resolution" involves "the time-confused." These individuals manifest more deterioration in cognitive functioning. No longer able to keep track of time, they rely on old memories. Losing their previous social inhibitions, they are more emotionally labile and may withdraw into the past, according to VT principles, not just because of an inability to manage in the present, but also because of unmet needs for resolving distressing issues from the past (Feil, 2007). The challenge for the validating caregiver/therapist is to remain respectful despite such individuals' cognitive and emotional deterioration and to continue to address their underlying psychological needs, using both verbal and nonverbal techniques. Nonverbal VT validation methods include:

1. Observing distressed individuals' expressions of affect.
2. Reflecting their emotion with an analogous emotion.
3. Genuinely mirroring their movements.
4. Making close eye contact.
5. Occasionally touching the patient, using soft movements (e.g., the "mother's touch," a gentle, circular motion on the cheek).

The following dialogue (Feil, 2007, pp. 798–799) exemplifies the use of nonverbal validation techniques:

> *An 86-year-old woman* (shouting): Get out of my way! I need to see my mother!
> Occupational Therapist (mirroring the woman's anxiety and movements): What's happened with your mother?
> Elderly Woman: She's sick and all alone. I've got to help her!
> Occupational Therapist (gently touching the old woman on the upper cheek, and maintaining eye contact, mirroring the fear): Are you scared of losing her?
> Elderly Woman (hesitating, looking into the occupational therapist's eyes, and nodding her head): Yes. I've lost her. She's dead.

On a deeper level, although the woman is aware that her mother has died, she has buried this knowledge. Old herself now, she expresses her grief through a brief reliving of the loss of her mother. The occupational therapist shares in her grief. The senior woman's subsequent crying affords her some relief. In a few minutes, the time-confused woman smiles.

> Elderly Woman: You're nice. I like you.

The senior woman is validated with each recurrence of this scenario. After a few weeks, she ceases to look for her mother, her emotions having been sufficiently expressed. Through these repeated expressions of her grief, she has become more used to the pain of the loss.

"Phase Three Resolution" focuses on "repetitive motion" patients. These are individuals with severe dementia, who despite the loss of the ability to communicate through language, are still able to sense how others feel. They still retain the very human needs to express their feelings and feel safe. They may use a range of repetitive body movements (e.g., with lips, tongue, teeth, jaw, and/or body) to make their needs known to the caregivers. Nonverbal VT techniques in this phase include music and ambiguity. Music, especially songs from childhood that are personally significant and can evoke emotional memories, may help those in repetitive motion to express their feelings. Ambiguous responses provide safe options through vague pronouns and numbers. The following dialogue (Feil, 2007, p. 799) exemplifies the use of nonverbal VT techniques with an individual in this phase:

> 94-year-old Man: He bridled on the beach.
> Caregiver (using "how much" as an ambiguous amount and "him" as an ambiguous pronoun): How much did it hurt him?
> Elderly Man (laughingly): No. We brittled over.

The Elderly Man and the Caregiver laugh together, singing, "The Gang's All Here." The elderly man continues to communicate in this way and eventually passes away. The use of vague pronouns and numbers as substitutes for specific word combinations in phase three resolution helps maintain active interpersonal engagement with those who have become verbally inarticulate, thereby preventing their becoming socially withdrawn and isolated. By meeting their emotional needs as human beings, caregivers, as VT therapists, can help to preserve and sustain some meaningfulness and quality in the remaining lives of many who have advanced dementia.

Through her application of VT, Naomi Feil has observed and documented improved behavioral function in older adults with dementia. There has been criticism in the application of VT concerning possible deterioration in the ability of older adults to reorient when confused (Kaplan & Berkman, 2015). Mixed findings, including lack of evidence to substantiate efficacy, alongside anecdotal reports of positive behavioral changes in older adults persist. It cannot be assumed that VT is not helpful to older adults with dementia; rather it is an approach that merits further understanding and research.

See also Behavioral and Psychological Symptoms of Dementia.

Suzanna Waters Castillo and Timothy Howell

Deponte, A., & Missan, R. (2007). Effectiveness of validation therapy (VT) in group: Preliminary results. *Archives of Gerontology and Geriatrics, 44*(2), 113–117.

Feil, N. (2007). Validation therapy. In E. Capezuti, E. Siegler, & M. Mezey (Eds.), *The encyclopedia of elder care* (2nd ed., pp. 797–799). New York, NY: Springer Publishing.

Feil, N., & De Klerk-Rubin, V. (2012). *The validation breakthrough: Simple techniques for communicating with people with Alzheimer's and other dementias* (3rd ed.). Baltimore, MD: Health Professions Press.

Kaplan, D., & Berkman B. (Eds.). (2015). *Oxford handbook of social work in health and aging* (2nd ed.). New York, NY: Oxford University Press.

Neal, M., & Briggs, M. (2003). Validation therapy for dementia. *Cochrane Database of Systematic Reviews, 3*, CD001394. doi:10.1002/14651858.CD001394

Tondi, L., Ribani, L., Bottazzi, M., Viscomi, G., & Vulcano, V. (2007). Validation therapy (VT) in
nursing home: A case-control study. *Archives of Gerontology and Geriatrics, 44*, 407–411.

Toseland, R. W., Diehl, M., Freeman, K., Manzanares, T., Naleppa, M., & McCallin, P. (1997). The impact of validation group therapy on nursing home residents. *Journal of Applied Gerontology, 16*(1), 31–50.

Web Resources
The Cochrane Library: http://www.thecochranelibrary.com

Validation Training Institute: http://www.vfvalidation.org

VASCULAR AND LEWY BODY DEMENTIAS

Although Alzheimer's disease (AD), now known as a major neurocognitive disorder, has received considerable attention from the public, epidemiological studies have confirmed the importance of vascular dementia (VaD) or major vascular neurocognitive disorder. Moreover, conditions such as diabetes, coronary artery disease, hypertension, and arrhythmias contribute to the risk of both VaD and AD. Lewy body dementia (LBD) now called a major neurocognitive disorder with Lewy bodies (LBs), follows AD and VaD in prevalence, with other forms of dementia accounting for a small minority of cases. Just as cerebrovascular pathology is seen in the brains of people with AD, plaques and tangles may also be present in LBD (Walker, Possin, Boeve, & Aarsland, 2015). These overlapping pathologies may in part explain present difficulties with the identification of disease-modifying therapies for dementia. At the same time, they highlight the promise that vascular risk factor reduction holds for more than one dementia phenotype.

DIFFERENTIAL DIAGNOSIS

The primary neuronal degeneration of AD is characterized by insidious, progressive cognitive decline, with symptoms of depression and psychosis presenting later in the disease course;

the prevalence varies from 60% to 90% (Baquero & Martín, 2015). Cerebrovascular pathology often accompanies the amyloid plaques and neurofibrillary tangles of AD, and in vitro evidence suggests chronic brain ischemia resulting from an increased amyloid plaque deposition (Bou Khalil, Khoury, & Koussa, 2016). The secondary neuronal degeneration of VaD is because of angiopathic disorders, most commonly ischemic heart disease, arrhythmias, hypertension, and diabetes (Korcyn, Vakhapova, & Grinberg, 2012). The pathology of VaD is frequently mixed (i.e., cortical and subcortical), with diverse presentations in which the loss of brain volume, ventricular dilation, and cognitive deficits are difficult to distinguish from AD. Dementia is likely to be vascular when the onset is abrupt, the course fluctuates between periods of decline and relative stability, and there is a significant evidence of ischemic brain injury. Prominent executive dysfunction, hemiparesis, gait disorder, and other signs of past stroke also suggest VaD (Farooq & Gorelick 2013).

LBD overlaps with both Parkinson's disease (PD) and AD in the presentation and distribution of pathology. Neuropathological features of LBD include LB—round inclusion bodies found in the substantia nigra, limbic cortex, and neocortex. LBs are also found in PD without dementia. Both dopaminergic and cholinergic deficits are seen in LBD and may exceed those found in AD. Patients whose disease begins with cognitive impairment without the motor manifestations of PD are diagnosed with LBD. In contrast, when the illness first presents with a tremor and bradykinesia followed by impaired cognition, the more appropriate diagnosis is dementia of PD (Walker et al., 2015).

Symptoms of LBD include prominent visual or auditory hallucinations and signs of PD. However, the disabling element of LBD is cognitive in origin, whereas in PD, the disability is primarily because of the movement disorder. The course of LBD is characterized by lucid moments alternating with marked confusion and may be mistaken for delirium. Paranoid delusions, falls, autonomic instability, and depression may also characterize LBD. The REM sleep behavior disorder is a striking phenomenon wherein patients enact the content of their dreams. Injuries to the dreamer or a bed partner are common (Dugger et al., 2012). REM sleep behavior disorder has a nearly unique relationship to PD, LBD, and the multisystem atrophies that warrant its addition to supporting the diagnosis of LBD.

DIAGNOSTIC PROCEDURES

Brain imaging with CT or MRI is useful when VaD is suspected. However, the detection of white-matter brain changes (leukoaraiosis) is not necessarily indicative of dementia (Varghese et al., 2016) and does not necessarily distinguish VaD from AD. Nonetheless, brain imaging may confirm the clinical diagnosis based on the timing of cognitive decline, which has therapeutic and prognostic significance for the patient because of the differing courses of decline seen among these two common forms of dementia. Brain imaging also has some role in LBD. Patterns of gray matter atrophy often differ from AD, with LBD mainly affecting the posterior parietal lobes, although there may be an overlap (Watson & Colby, 2016). In addition, functional imaging such as single-photon emission CT (SPECT) and $_{18}$F-fluorodeoxyglucose PET (FDG-PET), which measure perfusion and glucose metabolism, respectively, are better at differentiating LBD from AD and VaD (Watson & Colby, 2016).

TREATMENT

At present, the most promising means of preventing dementia is to prevent the onset and progression of cardiovascular disease and diabetes. Weight control, exercise, lowering cholesterol, treating diabetes and hypertension, eliminating tobacco use, and minimizing alcohol intake represent good preventive health behaviors at any age. Specifically, aerobic exercise may preserve neuronal structural activity and gray matter volume (Cheng 2016). Likewise, for patients with diabetes or cardiovascular disease, medication and behavioral approaches, particularly exercise, should be optimized (Verdelho et al., 2012).

V

MEDICATIONS TO PALLIATE COGNITIVE IMPAIRMENT

Cholinesterase inhibitors are approved by the U.S. Food and Drug Administration (FDA) for AD and PD dementia. VaD may be less responsive to cholinesterase inhibitors than AD, but the two dementias are difficult to distinguish; some practitioners offer every patient a cholinesterase inhibitor. Although the 2012 Cochrane Review (Rolinski, Fox, Maidment, & McShane, 2012) found no compelling evidence that cholinesterase inhibitors benefit people with LBD, a recent meta-analysis suggests otherwise (Wang et al., 2015). Cholinesterase inhibitors may improve cognition, lessen decline in activities of daily living, improve psychological and behavioral disturbances (including psychosis), ameliorate caregiver burden, and forestall nursing home admission. Transient side effects of cholinergic enhancement include nausea, diarrhea, sweating, bradycardia, and insomnia (Mori, Ikeda, & Donepezil-DLB Study Investigators, 2012). A 90-day trial should be sufficient for the family caregivers to detect any benefit.

Memantine is a noncompetitive antagonist of *N*-methyl-D-aspartate (NMDA) receptors and is thought to be a neuroprotective agent in both neurodegenerative and vascular processes. It is FDA approved for the treatment of moderate to severe AD. Randomized placebo-controlled trials in VaD show small beneficial effects on cognition and agitation (McShane, Areosa Sastre, & Minakaran, 2006).

MANAGEMENT OF BEHAVIORAL AND PSYCHOLOGICAL SIGNS AND SYMPTOMS

A variety of pharmacological (Steinber & Lyketsos, 2012) and nonpharmacological (Brodaty & Arasaratnam, 2012) approaches may counter behavioral disturbances. The goal is to reduce rather than eliminate the problem behavior. Problem behaviors are often an expression of the caregiving context, the caregiver's capacities, and the patient's disease. The fluctuating course of both LBD and VaD make the certainty of benefits and ease of adjustments difficult. The three-point sequence of problematic behavior

remains the central management strategy (Teri et al., 1992):

- Identify the triggering events, such as changes in daily routine or the environment, interpersonal conflict, and emotional or physical stressors. Antecedents can then be removed or minimized as a preventive measure.
- Describe the "behavior" in detail, including frequency and circumstances. This observation period also refines recognition of antecedents and the ways that the problem behavior fits into other aspects of the patient's life.
- Identify the "consequences" of the behavior, the ways that the caregiver or others react to reinforce or deter the activity, and the outcomes when the activity ceases.

Guidelines suggest nonpharmacological approaches should be the first line and include caregiver training programs (Kales, Gitlin, & Lyketsos, 2015). When this approach to problems identified by the caregiver is used, interventions, introduced in 9 to 12 sessions at home, reduce caregiver burden, with effect sizes equal or superior to those achieved with medications (Brodaty & Arasaratnam, 2012).

DELUSIONS, HALLUCINATIONS, UNWARRANTED SUSPICIOUSNESS, AND FALLS

It is important to distinguish persistent false beliefs or perceptions from transitory illusions that result from impairments in vision, hearing, and cortical deficits. If the phenomenon does not interfere with care or distress the patient, intervention is unnecessary. However, when patients act on their delusions through seclusiveness, threats, or assault, an FDA-approved medication for dementia and nonpharmacological interventions should be applied. If psychotic symptoms continue to be disturbing to, or impede the care and safety of, the patient, antipsychotic medication may be necessary.

Gait disturbance because of apraxia, weakness, rigidity, and poor vision predispose the patient to falls, soft tissue injury, and fractures. Physical therapy and changes in medications may reduce, although not eliminate, the risk for falls (Walker et al., 2015). This dilemma should be discussed with the caregivers to reach a balance between safety and independence.

MEDICATIONS TO LESSEN BEHAVIORAL AND PSYCHOLOGICAL DISTURBANCES

Short-acting benzodiazepines can help the patient through procedures such as a CT scan but impair alertness and should be avoided otherwise. The FDA has issued a public health advisory about the off-label use of antipsychotic medications for the treatment of dementia-related behavioral disorders (Wang et al., 2005). This advisory, based on an analysis of placebo-controlled trials of aripiprazole, olanzapine, quetiapine, and risperidone in patients with dementia-related behavioral disorders, found a 1.6- to 1.7-fold increase in mortality rate for antipsychotic-treated compared with placebo-treated patients. Thus the use of atypical antipsychotic medications for the treatment of psychological and behavioral symptoms in dementia should be approached cautiously. In the informed consent process, it is prudent to discuss the increased mortality in addition to the other potential adverse effects, such as cerebrovascular events, metabolic syndrome, and an accelerated cognitive decline (Steinberg & Lyketsos, 2012). The American Psychiatric Association recently released treatment guidelines on the use of antipsychotics to treat agitation or psychosis in patients with dementia (Reus et al., 2016). Some important recommendations include the following:

- Type, frequency, severity, pattern, and timing of symptoms should be evaluated, and the presence of pain or modifiable contributors to symptoms should be assessed.
- Comprehensive treatment plan should be developed.
- Nonemergency antipsychotic medication should be given only in severe situations.
- Clinical response to nonpharmacological intervention should be reviewed before antipsychotics are started.
- Informed consent of potential risks and benefits should be discussed with the patient and/or surrogate decision maker.

- Minimal effective dose should be initiated and tapered up for a clinically meaningful benefit, with continuous monitoring of adverse effects.
- If there is no clinically meaningful response after 4 weeks on an adequate dose of an antipsychotic, the medication should be tapered.
- If the patient has a good response, discussion of tapering should begin with the patient or surrogate decision maker, and tapering should be attempted in 4 months of initiation.
- Haloperidol and long-acting injectable antipsychotic medication should be avoided.

Preferable for longer-term treatment, risperidone is a mild sedative with a low risk of hypotension. At low doses, it is superior to placebo for treating agitation (Devanand et al., 2012), although in higher doses extrapyramidal signs begin to appear. Olanzapine is less likely to induce extrapyramidal effects than risperidone but more likely to elevate serum lipids and glucose and to induce weight gain. It may cause somnolence and gait disorder but is rarely hypotensive. However, olanzapine and risperidone are poorly tolerated in patients with LBD. Clozapine has shown significant improvement in symptoms, but mandatory monitoring limits regular use (Stinton et al., 2015). Quetiapine is more sedating than olanzapine but unlikely to cause extrapyramidal effects, and as a result, it is preferable when the hallucinations of LBD are so disruptive that medication is required. As an alternative to antipsychotic use for agitation, a recent randomized-controlled trial of dextromethorphan hydrobromide–quinidine sulfate showed significant improvement in agitation/aggression scores on the neuropsychiatric inventory compared with placebo (Cummings et al., 2015).

In summary, the phenotype of VaD and LBD may differ from that of AD, but the therapeutic approach is similar both pharmacologically and behaviorally. Optimizing treatment of comorbid conditions, supporting the caregiver, judiciously using medications, and planning for end-of-life care are the cornerstones.

Mirnova Ceïde and Gary J. Kennedy

V

Baquero, M., & Martín, N. (2015). Depressive symptoms in neurodegenerative diseases. *World Journal of Clinical Cases, 3*(8), 682–693.

Bou Khalil, R., Khoury, E., & Koussa, S. (2016). Linking multiple pathogenic pathways in Alzheimer's disease. *World Journal of Psychiatry, 6*(2), 208–214.

Brodaty, H., & Arasaratnam, C. (2012). Meta-analysis of nonpharmacologic interventions for neuropsychiatric symptoms of dementia. *American Journal of Psychiatry, 169*, 946–953.

Cheng, S. T. (2016). Cognitive reserve and the prevention of dementia: The role of physical and cognitive activities. *Current Psychiatry Report, 18*(9), 85. doi:10.1007/s11920-016-0721-2

Cummings. J. L., Lyketsos, C. G., Peskind, E. R., Porstcinsson, A. P., Mintzer, J. E., Scharre, D. W., ... Siffert J. (2015). Effect of dextromethorphan-quinidine on agitation in patients with Alzheimer disease dementia: A randomized clinical trial. *Journal of the American Medical Association, 314*(12), 1242–1254.

Devanand. D. P., Mintzer, J., Schultz, S. K., Andrews, H. F., Sultzer, D. L., de la Pena, D., ... Levin, B. (2012). Relapse risk after discontinuation of risperidone in Alzheimer's disease. *New England Journal of Medicine, 367*, 1497–1507.

Dugger, B. N., Boeve B. F., Murray, M. E., Parisi, J. E., Fujishiro, H., Dickson, D. W., & Ferman, T. J. (2012). Rapid eye movement sleep behavior disorder and subtypes in autopsy-confirmed dementia with Lewy bodies. *Movement Disorders, 27*(1), 72–78.

Farooq, M. U., & Gorelick, P. B. (2013). Vascular cognitive impairment. *Current Athersclerosis Reports, 15*, 330. doi:10.1007/s11883-013-0330-z

Kales, H. C., Gitlin, L. N., & Lyketsos, C. G. (2015). Assessment and management of behavioral and psychological symptoms of dementia. *British Medical Journal, 350*, 369. doi:10.1136/bmj.h369

Korcyn, A. D., Vakhapova, V., & Grinberg, L. T. (2012). Vascular dementia. *Journal of Neurological Science, 15, 322*, 2–10.

McShane, R., Areosa Sastre, A., & Minakaran, N. (2006). Memantine for dementia. *Cochrane Database of Systematic Reviews, 19*(2), CD003154. doi:10.1002/14651858.CD003154.pub5

Mori, E., Ikeda, K., & Donepezil-DLB Study Investigators. (2012). Donepezil for dementia with Lewy bodies: A randomized, placebo-controlled trial. *Annals of Neurology, 72*(1), 41–52.

Reus, V. I., Fochtmann, L. J., Eyler, A. E., Hilty, D. M., Horvitz-Lennon, M., Jibson, M. D., ... Yager, J. (2016). The American Psychiatric Association practice guideline on the use of antipsychotics to treat agitation or psychosis in patients with dementia. *American Journal of Psychiatry, 173*(5), 543–546.

Rolinski, M., Fox, C., Maidment, I., & McShane, R. (2012). Cholinesterase inhibitors for dementia with Lewy bodies, Parkinson's disease dementia and cognitive impairment in Parkinson's disease. *Cochrane Database of Systematic Reviews, 14*(3), CD006504. doi:10.1002/14651858.CD006504.pub2

Steinberg, M., & Lyketsos, C. G. (2012). Atypical antipsychotic use in patients with dementia: Managing safety concerns. *American Journal of Psychiatry, 169*, 900–906

Stinton, C., McKeith, I., Taylor, J. P., Lafortune, L., Mioshi, E., Mak, E., ... O'Brien, J. T. (2015). Pharmacological management of Lewy body dementia: A systematic review and meta-analysis. *American Journal of Psychiatry, 172*(8), 731–742.

Teri, L., Truax, P., Logsdon, R., Uomoto, J., Zarit, S., & Vitaliano, P. P. (1992). Assessment of behavioral problems in dementia: The revised memory and behavioral problems checklist. *Psychology and Aging, 7*, 622–631.

Varghese, V., Chandra, S. R., Christopher, R., Rajeswaran, J., Prasad, C., Subasree, R., & Issac, T. G. (2016). Factors determining cognitive dysfunction in cerebral small vessel disease. *Indian Journal of Psychological Medicine, 38*(1), 56–61.

Verdelho, A., Madureira, S., Ferro, J. M., Baezner, H., Blahak, C., Poggesi, A., & Inzitari, D. (2012). Physical activity prevents progression for cognitive impairment and vascular dementia: Results from the LADIS (Leukoaraiosis and Disability) Study. *Stroke, 43*(12), 3331–3335. doi:10.1161/STROKEAHA.112.661793

Walker, Z., Possin, K. L., Boeve, B. F., & Aarsland, D. (2015). Lewy body dementias. *Lancet, 386*(10004), 1683–1697.

Wang, P. S., Schneeweiss, S., Avorn, J., Fischer, M. A., Mogun, H., Solomon, D. H., & Brookhart, M. A. (2005). Risk of death in elderly users of conventional vs. atypical antipsychotic medications. *New England Journal of Medicine, 353*, 2335–2341.

Wang, H. F., Yu, J. T., Tang, S.W., Jiang, T., Tan, C. C., Meng, X. F., ... Tan, L. (2015). Efficacy and safety of cholinesterase inhibitors and memantine in cognitive impairment in Parkinson's disease, Parkinson's disease dementia, and dementia with Lewy bodies: Systematic review with meta-analysis and trial sequential analysis. *Journal of Neurology, Neurosurgery, and Psychiatry, 86*(2), 135–143.

Watson, R., & Colby, S. J. (2016). Imaging in dementia with Lewy bodies: An overview. *Journal of Geriatric Psychiatry and Neurology, 29*(5), 254–260.

Web Resources
Alzheimer's Association: http://www.alz.org
Alzheimer's Research Forum: http://www.alzforum.org
Lewy Body Dementia Association: http://www
.lewybodydementia.org
National Institute of Neurological Disorders and
Stroke: http://www.ninds.nih.gov/disorders/
dementiawithlewybodies/dementiawithlewy
bodies.htm

VETERANS AND VETERAN HEALTH

The promise, "To care for him who shall have borne the battle, and for his widow and his orphan," was part of President Lincoln's second inaugural address in 1865. Today, the mission of the U.S. Department of Veterans Affairs (DVA) continues to fulfill this promise to serve America's veterans, the women and men who have been honorably discharged from U.S. military service, and their families. In the broadest of perspectives, DVA's responsibilities include the provision of health care, coordinated by the Veterans Health Administration (VHA); socioeconomic support and assistance, coordinated by the Veterans Benefits Administration; and burial services, coordinated by the National Cemetery Administration. The DVA is the second largest department in the U.S. government, with 324,000 employees, most working in the VHA, to serve our nation's veterans with health care needs and related services through the continuum of care.

As the largest integrated health care system in the United States and, perhaps, the world, the DVA consists of more than 1,700 hospitals, clinics, community living centers, domiciliaries, readjustment counseling centers, and other facilities. VA facilities are located in every state, Washington, DC, the Commonwealth of Puerto Rico, the American Virgin Islands, the Philippines, and Guam. The VHA also purchases health care for veterans in other government or private facilities and, in certain circumstances, finances care for dependents and survivors of veterans. The VHA is rooted in academic medicine and trains the majority of graduates from medical schools in the United States. As an academic health system, the VHA is a major contributor to health science and research; with more than 25,000 affiliate physician faculty and more than 76,000 active voluntary medical faculties. The VHA also serves as the backup to the U.S. Department of Defense medical services and supports the National Disaster Medical System during national emergencies.

As of 2011, it has been estimated that there were approximately 22 million veterans of service in the U.S. Armed Forces. About a third of the veterans are enrolled in the DVA health care system, qualifying for health care because of a service-connected disability, and/or low-income, or net worth (Kizer, 2012). Most VA enrollees, older than 65 years, are also covered by Medicare.

As of 2012, there were an estimated 22,328,000 veterans (National Center for Veterans Analysis and Statistics, 2011). Vietnam veterans (7.5 million) are the single largest period-of-service group in the veteran population, followed by Gulf War veterans (6.2 million), Korean conflict participants (2.3 million), and World War II veterans (1.4 million). Approximately 5.6 million veterans served only during peacetime. The veteran population is projected to decline to 15 million by 2030, under currently expected armed forces strength.

Although the overall American veteran population is declining, the number of women in the military has grown steadily, as has the number of women veterans and women reservists, from 9% in 2013 to a projection of over 16% by 2043. To meet the unique needs of women veterans the VA has identified new standards and capabilities for VA facilities and programs (VA, 2010). This has resulted in improving care and access for women veterans of all ages.

The population of veterans aged 65 years or older peaked at 10.0 million in 2000. In 2011, the median age of male veterans was 64 years (National Center for Veterans Analysis and Statistics, 2011). This median age continues to remain high as the Vietnam era cohort ages. As in the general U.S. population, those aged 85 years or older (the "old-old") are the fastest-growing segment of the veteran population, representing 3.0% of current veterans. By 2030,

15% of older veterans will be aged 85 years or older (1.0 million). Thus the VA will encounter a large cohort of potentially frail elderly veterans in the following 25 years.

To meet this challenge of an aging population, the VA has developed a broad continuum of geriatrics and extended health care services. In addition, it supports a diverse portfolio of aging-related research and provides aging-related education and training for staff and students from a wide range of medical and associated health disciplines. The Office of Geriatrics and Extended Care oversees the policy and implementation of VA's programs that provide geriatric and other long-term care programs and services. As such, they provide subject matter experts that are dedicated to overseeing the quality of care for aging and chronically ill veterans.

The VHA has developed an extensive continuum of health care services targeting the needs of this group. This includes an increased focus on home and community-based programs, as well as coordinated use of hospital and residential nursing home programs. Together, these programs provide preventive, acute, rehabilitative, and extended care on an outpatient and/or inpatient basis. Examples of VHA geriatrics and extended care programs include home-based primary care, homemaker/home health aide services, respite care, adult day health care, domiciliary care, geriatric primary care, specialty geriatric evaluation and management, specialized Alzheimer's and related dementia care, nursing home care, and hospice. In addition to the direct provision of care, the VHA also contracts for certain services (e.g., community-nursing home care) and participates in others through a grant program to State Veterans Homes (nursing home, domiciliary, and adult-day health care).

For more than 25 years, the VA has also provided leadership in research, training, and education in geriatrics and long-term care. The VHA funds a wide range of aging-related research on basic biomedical applied clinical, rehabilitation, and health services topics, as well as cooperative (multisite) studies. In 1975, the VA established centers of excellence in geriatrics called Geriatric Research, Education, and Clinical Centers (GRECCs). The mission of the GRECC is to improve the health and care of older veterans through research, education, and training and the development and evaluation of innovative models of care. GRECCs are widely recognized as having provided leadership in geriatrics and gerontology, both in the VA and throughout the nation. There are 22 GRECCs across the VA system, each with a specific programmatic focus, including among others, neuroscience, including dementia; endocrinology, especially diabetes; rehabilitation of stroke and other disorders; osteoporosis; falls and gait disorders; exercise; immunology; cardiovascular diseases; and palliative care. GRECCs, as well as selected other VA medical centers, provide physician fellowship training in geriatric medicine, constituting the largest source of trained geriatricians in the nation. In addition, the VHA pioneered the concept and practice of interdisciplinary team training in geriatrics and has developed advanced training programs in geriatrics for psychiatrists, neurologists, dentists, nurses, and psychologists. Students from multiple other health care disciplines (e.g., social work, pharmacy, optometry) gain geriatrics experience during their training rotations in VA clinical settings. The VHA also provides aging-related continuing education for professional staff from the VA and the community and mandatory online training for all front-line staff on a regular basis (VA GRECC, 2012).

VHA aging initiatives include the integration of geriatrics into primary care and mental health care. A variety of research and education activities are underway to identify best-practice models of integrated care and to disseminate this information to health care providers in outpatient and inpatient clinical settings. A systematic review of research comparing the quality of nonsurgical care in VA and U.S. non-VA settings, published between 1990 and August 2009, found that regarding the recommended processes of care, the VA performed better than non-VA comparison groups. The studies that assessed risk-adjusted mortality mostly found levels of equivalent quality provided to patients in VA and non-VA settings (Trivedi et al., 2011). More recently, a study comparing outcomes at VA hospitals versus non-VA hospitals reported that veterans who received care for heart attack, heart failure, or pneumonia had lower mortality rates for heart attack and heart failure and higher 30-day all-cause readmission rates, although differences among these two cohorts were minimal (Sudhakar et al., 2016).

Many VA facilities have achieved designation as Nurses Improving Care for Healthsystem Elders (NICHE) facilities. NICHE facilities are designated as such for their high-level dedication to exemplary family-centered geriatric care via the implementation of evidence-based protocols, aging-sensitive policies, and the achievement of improved outcomes (NICHE, 2017).

In 2008, the VA began an intensive effort to end homelessness among veterans. Since then, more than 111,000 homeless veterans were placed in supportive housing through a collaboration between the VA and the U.S. Department of Housing and Urban Development (HUD). The program provides rent vouchers and clinical support services to keep veterans in their home and assist in finding jobs (HUD VASH, 2016).

The VA programs care for many health conditions unique to veterans. Amputations and spinal cord injuries have spawned research that has resulted in advances in prosthetics and even an exoskeleton for veterans with paraplegia. ReWalk, a powered exoskeleton, was developed as a collaboration between researchers at the James J. Peters VA Medical Center in Bronx, New York, and a technology firm. It enables veterans with paraplegia to walk upright, even climbing stairs. In addition to psychosocial benefits, "Regular exoskeletal-assisted walking improves many of the secondary medical complications that are associated with immobility and paralysis from spinal cord injury" (Asselin, Avedissian, Knezevic, Kornfeld, & Spungen, 2016, p. 16).

Given a new administration and related anticipated changes in the executive branch of the federal government, it is unknown if there will be significant changes in the DVA. Still, the mission to provide care and services to veterans, caring for our nations heroes and their families, will remain.

Lynda Olender and Kathleen M. Capitulo

Asselin, P. K., Avedissian, M., Knezevic, S., Kornfeld, S., & Spungen, A. M. (2016). Training persons with spinal cord injury to ambulate using a powered exoskeleton. *Journal of Visual Experiments, 16*(112). doi:10.3791/54071

Kizer, K. W. (2012). Veterans and the Affordable Care Act. *Journal of the American Medical Association, 307*(8), 789–790.

National Center for Veterans Analysis and Statistics. (2011). Projected Veteran population 2013–2043. Retrieved from www.va.gove/vetdata/docs/quickfacts/Population_slideshow.pdf

NICHE Program. (2017). Nurses improving care for healthsystem elders. Retrieved from http://www.nicheprogram.org

Trivedi, A. N., Matula, S., Miake-Lye, I., Glassman, P. A., Shekelle, P., & Asch, S. (2011). Systematic review: Comparison of the quality of medical care in Veterans Affairs and non-Veterans Affairs settings. *Medical Care, 49*(1), 76–88.

U.S. Department of Housing and Urban Development & Veterans Administration Supportive Housing. (2016). HUD and VA team up to find permanent homes for 5,200 veterans experiencing homelessness. Retrieved from https://portal.hud.gov/hudportal/HUD?src=/press/press_releases_media_advisories/2016/HUDNo_16-082

Veterans Administration. (2010). Health care services for women veterans. Retrieved from http://www.womenshealth.va.gov

Veterans Administration Geriatric Research, Education, and Clinical Center. (2012). GRECC demographics and profiles. Retrieved from https://www.va.gov/GRECC/GRECC_Demographics_and_Profiles.asp

Web Resources
Geriatric Research Education and Clinical Centers: http://www.va.gov/GRECC/index.asp
My Health eVet: http://www.myhealthevet.va.gov
National Center for Veterans Analysis and Statistics: http://www.va.gov/vetdata/index.asp
Office of Personnel Management: http://www.opm.gov
U.S. Department of Veteran Affairs: http://www.va.gov
Veterans Benefits Administration: http://www.vba.va.gov

V

V

Veterans Hospital Administration Geriatrics and Extended Care Strategic Health Care Group: http://www.va.gov/geriatricsshg

VOLUNTEERISM

Volunteerism is considered a powerful force for engaging people in addressing development challenges, benefitting both societies at large and the individual volunteer by strengthening trust, solidarity, and reciprocity among citizens. Volunteerism has the potential to create opportunities for citizen participation at global, national, and local levels.

Diverse examples of significant volunteerism in contemporary society abound. At the local level, Jim Hamilton, an airport manager in Columbia, South Carolina, served as a volunteer bus driver for 15 years, escorting 96 female residents of a retirement home on weekly shopping trips (Maddock, 2016). In Lower Moreland Township, Pennsylvania, the Pine Road Elementary School invites fourth-grade students' grandparents and other older adult volunteers to be part of an intergenerational project. Students interview the older adults and gain valuable understanding of their life experiences, education, and occupations. Students then organize the interviews and present a life story book to each adult. Some older adult volunteers return year after year to participate with students without grandparents. At the national level, the Honor Flight Network, a nonprofit organization, has worked as an umbrella organization with local chapters and subgroups to transport surviving World War II and terminally ill veterans to visit various war memorials in Washington, D.C. (Honor Flight Network, 2016). A vast network of volunteer guardians escorts honored veterans on the flights and around Washington, exhibiting a powerful form of compassion and support. The organization plans to transition the volunteer effort to honor Korean and Vietnam War veterans.

In the aftermath of Hurricane Sandy, the NBC Nightly News segment, "Making a Difference," focused on the disrupted support networks of victims and the multitude of volunteers who generously reached out to assist in Staten Island, New York (November 2, 2012). The newscast described the "Angel of Water," an older volunteer who carried buckets of fresh water and supplied up several flights of stairs to stranded older adults in high rise residences. Across our nation, thousands of volunteers carry out collections for disaster victims, restock community food banks, and serve food when religious organizations sponsor holiday meal programs for indigent and homeless individuals.

It is clear that citizen volunteer and outreach efforts have dramatically emerged in recent years in the United States and other nations. Whether we foster conservative or more liberal perspectives toward programs and services for older adults, it is imperative that these finely constructed activities be creatively strengthened and vigorously maintained to meet the needs of this growing population. Volunteerism continues to evolve as an area of increased interest and research (Connors, 1995; Eliasoph, 2011; Midlarsky & Kahana, 1994; Sherr, 2008). Sherr (2008) has articulated a definition of volunteerism as "making a choice to act in recognition of need, with an attitude of social responsibility and without concern for monetary profit" (p. 11). Thoughtful philanthropic responsibility and public service remain deeply ingrained in the American character, irrespective of one's gender, age, religion, ethnicity, occupation, socioeconomic status, or educational attainment. Volunteer service simultaneously spans the fields of health and mental health, child welfare, education, politics, and aging, among others. Various community membership, mutual aid, social action, and advocacy organizations provide a continuing backdrop for people of all ages seeking opportunities for creative utility of increased leisure time. Data provided by the Bureau of Labor Statistics, U.S. Department of Labor (2016), indicate that 62.6 million people volunteered through an organization at least once between September 2014 and September 2015. It was noted that older volunteers were more likely to reach out to religious organizations than their younger counterparts. A report by the Sloan Center on Aging & Work at Boston

College (2010) concluded that older volunteers contribute their time to a broad range of secular and religious organizations, participating in activities such as mentoring, coaching, tutoring, office services, and management assistance. Indeed, older volunteers have emerged as a crucial part of the mission of many hospital settings, delivering compassionate care that often reduces the anxiety, stress, and confusion of patients and their families.

A significant impetus for volunteer service in the United States followed President Ronald Reagan's 1983 proclamation of a national year of volunteerism, urging citizens and organizations to strengthen voluntary structures and recruit additional people as contributors to America's rich tradition of community service. As financially pressed governments reduced funding for social programs and services during the past several decades, numerous individuals and organizations have found additional motivation to support new, innovative solutions to existing community problems. Neuberger (2009) strongly believes that voluntary organizations should reach out to older volunteers who often are caricatured as "bent over, leaning on sticks." Older adults often are viewed as a cost to society, forced from work into retirement and even from volunteering. Some organizations believe that it is "not worth it" to purchase insurance to cover older volunteers (p. 102). Although volunteers provide vital human services in many agencies and organizations, there are some who cautiously suggest that volunteers cannot always substitute for professional personnel with education and experience in the human service disciplines. Eliasoph (2011) suggests that agencies show caution in the utility of "plug-in volunteers," who may often sever helpful attachments with youth, who may feel abandoned by their mentors.

As the United States and other nations advance further into the 21st century, it is imperative that gerontologists, geriatricians, health care, and social service professionals sustain the vision and goal of successful, productive aging in response to the predicted growth of our older population (Rowe & Kahn, 1998). A vision of the positive aspects of aging must replace preoccupation with a disability, declining health, marital status, and social exclusion for millions of older adults who age-in-place or reside in the rapidly accumulating array of continuing-care facilities. A recent European research study investigated the impact of older volunteers' available human, social, and cultural capital on their motivational forces to volunteer (Principi, Schippers, Naegele, Di Rosa, & Lamura, 2016). The study indicates that low educational level, poor health, widowhood or widowerhood, and divorced or single status, are associated with a higher propensity to volunteer to enhance one's self-esteem, to avoid thinking of personal problems, and to have social interactions. The researchers believe the results have "important implications for policy makers and voluntary organizations if they want to enhance volunteering among older people with fewer resources, i.e., that are more at risk of social exclusion" (p. 144). The findings of this study suggest that voluntary organizations need to find ways to engage this largely overlooked population of potential older volunteers in creative forms of public service.

Accompanying the "graying of America" is the present trend toward earlier retirement of mature, older workers. For many years, retirement was viewed as a critical, voluntary life transition. Increasingly, gerontologists, geriatricians, economists, and social and behavioral scientists approach the subject of retirement as a highly anticipated life transition, linked to factors such as financial security, opportunity to begin long-delayed couple activities, expected intergenerational roles, and community service responsibility. In reality, the previously held theory of retirement as a single life transition has evolved as many mature individuals make the additional transition to "unretirement." Atchley and Barusch (2004) and Euster (2004) have described retirement satisfaction as affected by opportunities to learn and feel useful, including activities that provide autonomy and a sense of personal control.

For a growing number of retired older adults, commitment to volunteer community service allows for interpersonal continuity in comfortable social and work environments, use of lifelong competencies and skills, links with familiar people, and sources of social support. For many older adults, volunteer participation

V

generates feelings of inner success and mastery, strengthening and rewarding significant social interactions. For many others, after productive, successful careers, volunteer roles may ameliorate discontinuity and loneliness caused by retirement or the death of a spouse or partner. Many older adults become increasingly attached to volunteer roles, serving others with whom they have no familial or obligatory ties (Keith, 2003). A study of older adults who mentored at-risk youth concluded that these interventions allowed volunteers to renew positive emotions and reinforced meaning in their lives (Larkin, Sadler, & Mahler, 2005). The Experience Corps program in Baltimore, Maryland, using a critical mass of older adult volunteers, has provided promising findings of selective improvements in student academic achievement and classroom behavior (Rebok et al., 2004). It also has provided important, ongoing research findings supporting the use of volunteering in public schools as a physical activity intervention for older adults (Tan, Li Xue, Li, Carlson, & Fried, 2006). A subsequent pilot study of at-risk older adult participants in the Experience Corps program sought to determine whether the program "would improve age-vulnerable executive functions and increase activity in brain regions in a high-risk group through increased cognitive and physical activity" (Carlson et al., 2009, p. 1275). Using functional MRI, preintervention, and postintervention, researchers demonstrated "intervention-specific short term gains in executive function and the activity of prefrontal cortical regions in older adults at elevated risk for cognitive impairment" (p. 1245). In addition, the findings suggest that a broad range of cognitive and physical activities in social settings may enhance interactional motivation, problem-solving skills, and generativity among many older adults who volunteer to assist others.

Euster (1997), in an extensive study of community-service activities of retired professional athletes, concluded that their continuing volunteer roles reflected an altruistic "contract" with their respective communities. After successful careers as members of professional sports organizations, many retired athletes choose community service activities as productive substitutes for on-the-field and on-the court roles. These retirees often described their service activities as a means of "giving back" to their respective communities. The professionals engaged in volunteer training and management observed that many older adults who perform volunteer service tend to have an extensive understanding of the importance of community participation. Many people do not discard such activities as they grow older, viewing service activities as a form of reciprocity for acts of kindness they received throughout their lifetime.

It is widely recognized that older adults introduce a vast amount of experience, knowledge, creativity, and energy as they assume volunteer roles. Senior volunteers tend to have higher incomes, greater education, and fewer functional and physical impairments. Women tend to volunteer at a higher rate than men across all educational levels and other major demographic characteristics. The desire to help others, feel useful, and assume moral and social responsibility appear to be the major reasons for volunteering among people aged 60 years and older.

In recent years there has been a considerable variation in sponsorship of volunteer opportunities for older adults and the service settings in which they participate. The federal government helps support an administrative entity, the Corporation for National & Community Service. *Senior Corps* taps the valuable life experiences, skills, and talents of adults aged 55 years and older. The *Foster Grandparents* program uses citizens aged 60 years and older to provide interpersonal care to children with special and exceptional needs. Through this intergenerational program, assistance is offered to children who have been abused and neglected, troubled teenagers, young mothers, premature infants, and children with physical disabilities. The *Senior Companions* program recruits seniors to provide emotional support and assistance to frail and homebound elders. The program aims to help at-risk older adults remain in their homes and community. The *Retired Senior Volunteer Program (RSVP)*, engages older adults in community-defined and supported projects. Volunteers may provide services in such settings as hospitals, schools, libraries, nursing homes, and community-service agencies.

Volunteer activities may include home repair, shopping assistance, respite care, telephone reassurance, assistance with tax preparation, and youth tutoring. Other volunteers may offer aid to terminally ill people, support community-policing efforts, or teach English to recent immigrants.

For many years, the AARP has been committed to volunteer service and advocacy activities at the national, state, and local levels. AARP volunteers, through chapters in the United States, Puerto Rico, and the Virgin Islands, offer services such as food and clothing drives, safe-driving education, job-search assistance, and neighborhood cleanup projects. AARP volunteers are widely recognized for helping older citizens complete income tax returns. Some volunteers assist older people with low or moderate incomes to locate benefit programs that help pay for prescription medications and other necessities. In some communities, AARP volunteers collaborate with organizations such as Habitat for Humanity and Meals on Wheels. AARP chapters are strongly committed to the creation of coalitions supporting the expansion of health insurance for older adults.

In addition, older adults are increasingly identified with corporate retiree projects, adopt-a-school programs, and crime-watch activities. Volunteers often assist widowed persons through mutual-support groups, conduct life-long-learning instruction, and serve communities as museum docents and curatorial assistants. Many serve as food bank workers and drivers; others read materials for audio tapes for visually impaired persons. Increasingly, older adults volunteer or are recruited to serve as citizen representatives on state boards, advisory councils, and commissions.

Volunteer services for older citizens are well-established in most communities and is performed by people of all ages. Thousands of community volunteers offer assistance to Meals on Wheels and nutrition site programs; provide respite for family caregivers of homebound adults; and offer transportation/escort services for seniors unable to attend religious services or make health care appointments. Many churches and synagogues have developed "adopt-a-grandparent" programs for seniors without extended or supportive families. Numerous organizations have sponsored volunteers who bring companion animals to visit older people confined in continuing care facilities. Boy and Girl Scouts serve as visitors and pen pals to nursing home residents; church and synagogue youth groups often provide entertainment and recreational assistance to seniors confined to such facilities.

The steady growth of volunteerism in American communities appears to be an inevitable outcome of our nation's humanitarian spirit. For many people perceived only as recipients of medical, interpersonal, and other services, enhanced citizenship roles and participation may become effective tools for developing latent interests, skills, and motivation for continued growth and development. Growing evidence of the professionalization of volunteer management personnel provides hope that more effective programs will be and services by and on behalf of older citizens developed in the years ahead. It is clear that substantive staff and volunteer training programs are required to ensure that the remarkable efforts of volunteers of all ages are woven into the existing fabric of quality services to older citizens.

See also Employment; Hospital Elder Life Program; Retirement; Social Supports: Formal and Informal.

Gerald L. Euster

Atchley, R. C., & Barusch, A. S. (2004). *Social forces and aging: An introduction to social gerontology.* Belmont, CA: Wadsworth/Thomson.

Bureau of Labor Statistics, U.S. Department of Labor. (2016). Volunteering in the United States, 2015. Retrieved from https://www.bls.gov/news.release/volun.toc.htm

Carlson, M. C., Erickson, K. I., Kramer, A. F., Voss, M. W., Bolea, N., Mielke, M., … Fried, L. P. (2009). Evidence for neurocognitive plasticity in at-risk older adults: The experience corps program. *Journal of Gerontology: Series A, 64*(12), 1275–1282.

Connors, T. D. (Ed.). (1995). *The volunteer management handbook.* New York, NY: John Wiley and Sons.

Eliasoph, N. (2011). *Making volunteers: Civic life after welfare's end.* Princeton, NJ: Princeton University Press.

V

Euster, G. L. (1997). *Great heroes, great deeds: Volunteer service activities of retired professional athletes.* Columbia: University of South Carolina.

Euster, G. L. (2004). Reflections upon university retirement: With thanks and apologies to James Joyce. *Educational Gerontology, 30,* 119–124,

Honor Flight Network. (2016). In *Wikipedia.* Retrieved from https://en.wikipedia.org/wiki/Honor_Flight

Keith, P. M. (2003). *Doing good for the aged: Volunteers in an ombudsman program.* Westport, CT: Praeger.

Larkin, E., Sadler, S. E., & Mahler, J. (2005). Benefits of volunteering for older adults mentoring at-risk youth. *Journal of Gerontological Social Work, 44,* 23–37.

Maddock, A. (2016). Jim Hamilton and the 96 women of Christopher Towers. *Columbia Star, 53,* 40, 6.

Midlarsky, E., & Kahana, E. (1994). *Altruism in later life.* Thousand Oaks, CA: Sage.

NBC Nightly News. (2012). Making a Difference: The angel of water. Retrieved from http://www.nbcnews.com/video/nightly-news/49667346

Neuberger, B. J. (2009). What does it mean to be old? In P. Cann & M. Dean (Eds.), *Unequal ageing: The untold story of exclusion in old age* (pp. 101–122). Bristol, UK: The Policy Press.

Principi, A., Schippers, J., Naegele, G., Di Rosa, M., & Lamura, G. (2016). Understanding the link between older volunteers' resources and motivation to volunteer. *Educational Gerontology, 42*(2), 144–158.

Rebok, G. W., Carlson, M. C., Glass, T. A., McGill, S., Hill, J., Wasik, B. A., … Rasmussen, M. D. (2004). Short-term impact of experience corps participation on children and schools: Results from a pilot randomized trial. *Journal of Urban Health: Bulletin of the New York Academy of Medicine, 81,* 79–93.

Rowe, J. W., & Kahn, R. L. (1998). *Successful aging.* New York, NY: Pantheon.

Sherr, M. E. (2008). *Social work with volunteers.* Chicago, IL: Lyceum Press.

Sloan Center on Aging and Work at Boston College (2010). Trends in volunteerism among older adults. Retrieved from http://www.bc.edu/content/dam/files/research_sites/agingandwork/pdf/publications/FS03_TrendsVolunteerism.pdf

Tan, E. J., Li Xue, Q., Li, T., Carlson, M. C., & Fried, L. P. (2006). Volunteering: A physical activity intervention for older adults—the experience corps program in Baltimore. *Journal of Urban Health: Bulletin of the New York Academy of Medicine, 83,* 954–969.

Web Resources

AARP: https://www.aarp.org/aarp-foundation/get involved

Bureau of Labor Statistics, United States Department of Labor: https://www.bls.gov/news.release/volun.nr0.htm

Corporation for National and Community Service: https://www.nationalservice.gov

Generations United: http://www.gu.org

WANDERING AND ELOPEMENT

DEFINITION AND DIMENSIONS

Although there are a number of different definitions of wandering in the literature related to people with cognitive deficits, most researchers and health care providers agree that it is apparently an aimless ambulation and that it sometimes involves lapping or pacing (Cipriani, Lucetti, Nuti, & Danti, 2014). It is one of the most common and problematic dementia-related behavioral disturbances. It is also associated with considerable wandering-related adverse consequences across settings and is seen in all stages of dementia, although, its incidence increases with dementia severity (Ali et al., 2015; Cipriani et al., 2014). It is a source of considerable concern and stress for caregivers of people with dementia and/or delirium because of the risk of harm to the individual and liability to the institution.

Wandering in some cases involves seeking a place or a person or even unescorted exiting, which is usually referred to as *elopement* when it is from a health care facility (Connell, 2003). For people with dementia, elopement is considered a negative consequence of wandering. For example, in one United Kingdom policing region in a 4-year period, although getting lost was relatively unusual for people with dementia, 4.6% (13) of those who got lost sustained harm and 0.7% (2) were found dead (White & Montgomery, 2015, p. 227). The work of Bowen, McKenzie, Steis, and Rowe (2011) found few antecedents to missing incidents, with most occurring when individuals were engaged in usual activities that were normally completed without incident.

Algase, Beattie, Bogue, and Yao (2001) identified five dimensions of the ambulating behavior of people with dementia: frequency, pattern or quality, boundary transgressions, deficits in navigation or wayfinding, and temporal distribution. These dimensions formed the core of the Algase Wandering Scale (AWS), which was later modified (i.e., AWS-V2) with the addition of subscales for attention shifting and shadowing. Attention shifting refers to whether the individual can be distracted, interrupted, or redirected from the walking activity. Shadowing includes searching for another person and following or seeking others (Algase et al., 2004).

EPIDEMIOLOGY

Wick and Zanni (2006) reported that one in five people with some degree of dementia wanders. In a recent prospective longitudinal study of community-dwelling veterans with mild dementia, 49% of study participants had falls, fractures, or other injuries because of wandering behavior and 43.7% had elopement events (Ali et al., 2015). Sink, Covinsky, Newcomer, & Yaffe (2004) had found a higher prevalence of wandering in community-dwelling Blacks (67%) and Latinos (63%) than Whites (58%). They attributed this difference to their more advanced dementia and lower family income.

ETIOLOGY

The etiology of wandering remains unclear and is probably complex, involving biomedical, psychosocial, and person–environment interaction aspects (Cipriani et al., 2015). Neuropathological processes in various brain regions and pathways have been linked to wandering, as has various cognitive dysfunctions, such as deficits in spatial perception, memory, and visual attention. Psychosocial theories have proposed that unmet needs, personality, and premorbid patterns of physical activity contribute to wandering.

W

People with dementia who also have delusions are more likely to wander (Ali et al., 2015). Some individuals have a well-established pattern of walking for pleasure, as part of their occupation, or as a stress-relieving activity. Whatever the mechanism, health care providers have come to accept it as a common behavior among people with dementia that meets some needs and need not be interrupted. Rather, the current emphasis remains on efforts to meet the unexpressed needs and maintaining safety for the wanderer (Dewing, 2005).

INTERVENTIONS

Interventions should focus on the at-risk individual, the staff or family caregiver, and the setting (Futrell, Melillo, & Remington, 2010). The combination of persistent walking and poor gait increases the risk of wandering-related adverse consequences (Ali et al., 2015). An individualized approach considers whether wandering represents unmet needs that might be addressed. For example, if incontinent episodes follow a flurry of motor activity, caregivers should be alert for this activity and schedule toileting accordingly. For the person who has always been physically active, an individualized exercise/activity plan might be helpful. If excessive pacing interferes with mealtime, providing finger foods that can be eaten "on the run," rather than trying to force a sit-down meal, can be tried. If the individual is distressed, strategies to reduce that distress should be found. Some people respond to music, others to a comfort item such as a stuffed animal. If a person shows no signs of distress and presents no danger to the self or others, there is no reason to intervene with wandering, it does provide exercise and improves appetite.

The way in which caregivers respond to wandering can ward off problems or escalate them. In the nursing home setting, staff should use a friendly, gentle approach to redirect a resident away from exits, other residents' rooms, and the nurses' office. Distraction works well with many people with dementia. Simply striking up a conversation and inviting the person to come with you often is effective. Unless there is a real danger (e.g., walking into traffic), physical restraint may trigger panic and result in harm to the patient and the care provider.

The environment is an important consideration about wandering. The factors associated with higher levels of wandering include brighter lighting, varied sound levels, and a higher environmental engaging quality (Algase, Beattie, Antonakos, Beel-Bates, & Yao, 2010). One aspect of special care units in nursing homes that emerged in the 1980s was design that facilitated safe wandering. Resident care areas were designed for smaller groups of people with shorter halls that made it easier to monitor the activity of residents. More open layouts allowed residents to see their destinations more easily. Exit doors were positioned near staff work areas rather than at the end of hallways. Although safety codes required exit signs, painting the door the same color as the surrounding walls made it less inviting. Secure outdoor walking paths were incorporated with points of interest along the way. Systems were installed that sounded an alarm if a door from the controlled area was opened.

Technology has continued to advance the options for preventing elopement and at the same time has raised some questions about patient surveillance and privacy. Long-term care residents who are prone to elopement may be fitted with a device such as a bracelet that alerts the staff if the resident leaves specific areas. One sophisticated system locks the door when a resident wearing the device approaches and unlocks it when the resident moves away from the door. Motion and pressure sensors on floors or mattresses may alert the caregiver to the patient's movements. These devices are commonly used in hospitals for potential wanderers. These individuals should be located near the central area of the unit so that they can be readily observed. Family and friends often provide some supervision. Hired sitters are another option. Scheduled "bed checks" should be done and documented frequently. All staff, including housekeeping and other personnel, should be educated to observe individuals in unusual places or attempting to exit. A colored wristband might be used to inform all personnel of people prone to wandering and/or elopement. Last, every facility should have a response plan to put into action as soon as a patient is reported absent. Devices are available that use GPS technology to aid in locating a lost person. Caregivers in the home or assisted-living setting must be vigilant and creative to prevent harm to the person who wanders. Home caregivers should be taught to use the same strategies outlined for professionals. Some patients recognize signs such as "Do Not Enter" or red "stop" signs as a means of controlling exits. Placing new locks higher or lower than the usual door locks may be effective. In addition, the home must be examined for dangers such as basement stairs that might best be made inaccessible. Community-dwelling people with dementia should wear MedicAlert tags with a telephone contact number. The Safe Return program of the Alzheimer's Association issues enrollees an identification bracelet or necklace. Personal information and a photograph are kept on file. If the individual is missing, the Safe Return program initiates a community effort to locate the person. Project Lifesaver is a nationwide network that is activated to locate an individual using a watch-size bracelet that emits a silent, low-level radio frequency. Based on the Amber Alert system, some communities issue public Silver Alerts to help locate missing older adults. All of these systems raise questions about the privacy that cannot be ignored. Discussing them with the person in the early stage of dementia provides an opportunity to obtain consent.

See also Environmental Modifications: Home; Signage; Technology.

Steven L. Baumann

Algase, D. L., Beattie, E. R. A., Antonakos, C., Beel-Bates, C. A., & Yao, L. (2010). Wandering and the physical environment. *Current Topics in Research, 25*, 340–346.

Algase, D. L., Beattie, E. R. A., Bogue, E., & Yao, L. (2001). The Algase Wandering Scale: Initial psychometrics of a new caregiver reporting tool. *American Journal of Alzheimer's Disease and Other Dementias, 16*, 141–152.

Algase, D. L., Beattie, E. R. A., Song, J.-A., Milke, D., Duffield, C., & Cowan, B. (2004). Validation of the Algase Wandering Scale (version 2) in a cross cultural sample. *Aging and Mental Health, 8*, 133–142.

Ali, N., Luther, S. L., Volicer, L., Algase, D., Beatti, E., Brown, L. M., … Joseph, I. (2015). Risk assessment of wandering behavior in mild dementia. *International Journal of Geriatric Psychiatry, 31*, 371–378.

Bowen, M. E., McKenzie, B., Steis, M., & Rowe, M. (2011). Prevalence of and antecedents to dementia-related missing incidents in the community. *Dementia and Geriatric Cognitive Disorders, 31*, 406–412.

Cipriani, G., Lucetti, C., Nuti, A. & Danti, S. (2014). Wandering and dementia. *Psychogeriatrics, 14*, 135–142.

Connell, B. R. (2003, April). Why residents wander—And what you can do about it. *Nursing Homes: Long Term Care Magazine*, 50–55.

Dewing, J. (2005). Screening for wandering among older persons with dementia: Wandering and its related activity is a phenomenon engaged in by many persons with dementia. *Nursing Older People, 17*(3), 20–24.

Futrell, M., Melillo, K. D., & Remington, R. (2010). Evidence-based guideline: Wandering. *Journal of Gerontological Nursing, 36*(2), 6–16.

Sink, K. M., Covinsky, K. E., Newcomer, R., & Yaffe, K. (2004) Ethnic differences in the prevalence and pattern of dementia-related behaviors. *Journal of the American Geriatric Society, 52*, 1277–1283.

White, E. B., & Montgomery, P. (2015). Dementia, walking outdoors and getting lost: Incidence, risk factors and consequences from dementia-related police missing-person reports. *Aging & Mental Health, 19*, 224–230.

Wick, J., & Zanni, G. (2006). Aimless excursions: Wandering in the elderly. *The Consultant Pharmacist, 21*(8), 608–618.

Web Resources

Alzheimer's Association Safe Return Program: http://www.alz.org.Services/SafeReturn.asp#id

Alzheimer's and Dementia Caregiver Center: Wandering and Getting Lost: http://www.alz.org/care/Alzheimers-dementia-wandering.asp

Project Lifesaver: http://www.projectlifesaver.org

Hartford Institute for Geriatric Aging: https://hign.org/

W

Xerostomia

Saliva plays a major role in maintaining oral health, and alterations in salivary gland function may compromise oral tissues and functions. Reduction in salivary flow most commonly manifests as symptoms of oral dryness. The subjective complaint of dry mouth is termed *xerostomia*, although the objective alterations in salivary performance are termed *salivary gland dysfunction*. This semantic distinction is important because not all dry mouth complaints are the result of salivary dysfunction. The term *xerostomia* should be reserved for the symptoms of oral dryness only and should not be used for reduced salivary function.

Multiple functions of saliva have been detected. Saliva is important for taste, mastication, deglutition, digestion, maintenance of oral and soft tissues, control of microbial populations, voice, and speech articulation. Lubrication of the oral cavity is another important function of saliva. Adequate salivary flow enhances movement of the tongue and lips, which aids in cleansing the oral cavity of food debris and bacteria. Saliva also allows for proper tongue and lip movement necessary for clear articulation.

Dysphagia in the elderly can be caused by various factors such as neurologic, systemic, or psychologic conditions, the environment, and oral changes. Patients with salivary gland dysfunction often complain of difficulty in swallowing. The oral preparatory phase of swallowing requires mastication and the formation of a food bolus. Efficient mastication and bolus formation are dependent on a moist, lubricated oral mucosa and an intact dentition and periodontium, and fluid to wet the food. Transport during swallowing requires the lubrication and wetting properties of salivary secretions. Saliva also plays a role in digestion by helping the upper gastrointestinal tract rinse gastric secretions from the esophageal regions.

Patients with xerostomia often complain of problems with eating, speaking, swallowing, wearing dentures, and altered taste. Xerostomia can lead to increased dental caries, oral ulcerations, erythema, oral candidiasis, salivary gland infections, and halitosis. Patients with autoimmune-associated xerostomia may have persistent swollen salivary glands.

CAUSES OF SALIVARY GLAND DYSFUNCTION AND XEROSTOMIA

Xerostomia is most commonly associated with diminished salivary gland function. However, the subjective complaint of dry mouth does not always correlate with the objective finding of decreased measured salivary flow rates (Joanna & Thomson, 2015). Nonsalivary gland etiologies, including changes in the patient's cognitive state, psychological distress, mouth breathing, and sensory alterations in the oral cavity, may lead to the perception of dry mouth. Therefore it is important to determine whether salivary gland function is decreased using objective measuring techniques.

Medication use is the most common cause of decreased salivary gland function. Anticholinergic medications such as antihistamines are most likely to cause hypofunction. Multiple classes of medications are associated with xerostomia, although the exact mechanism is not understood. Sedatives, antipsychotics, antidepressants, and diuretics are common drugs that induce xerostomia. Medication-induced xerostomia is reversed if the medication is discontinued or it can be switched to one that causes less xerostomia.

Aside from medications, there are other iatrogenic causes of salivary gland dysfunction.

Head and neck cancer is frequently treated with ionizing radiation (Perry et al., 2010). Salivary glands are often in the field of radiation, and permanent salivary gland destruction occurs. Fibrosis of the muscles of mastication and pharyngeal muscles results in chewing and swallowing difficulties. Other iatrogenic causes include cytotoxic chemotherapy, internal radionuclides (iodine-131 [I^{131}]), and bone marrow transplantation. Salivary gland surgery may involve removal of the gland or may cause damage to the gland or its innervation. Surgery is often performed for tumor removal, infection, stone removal, or duct stricture.

Systemic disease is also a common cause of salivary gland dysfunction. Sjögren's syndrome (SS) is a chronic autoimmune disease with lymphocyte-mediated destruction of the salivary glands and other exocrine glands. This autoimmune disease primarily affects postmenopausal women with a 9:1 female-to-male ratio. However, SS has been reported in children and younger adults too. SS often occurs with other autoimmune diseases such as rheumatoid arthritis and systemic lupus erythematosus. It has been noted that a higher number of patients diagnosed with SS report xerostomia versus patients with sicca and incomplete SS (Billings et al., 2016). Other systemic conditions with prominent salivary involvement include cystic fibrosis, Bell's palsy, diabetes mellitus, amyloidosis, sarcoidosis, HIV, thyroid disease, malnutrition, dehydration, anorexia, and psychological factors (affective disorders).

Contrary to common belief, salivary gland function is well preserved with age in the healthy elderly. However, xerostomia is a common complaint found in up to 25% of institutionalized older adults and is often caused by systemic disease or its treatments (Crogan, 2011).

Hypersalivation is another common complaint in the geriatric patient population. However, salivary flow rates are frequently normal, but motor function has been compromised, leading to a decreased swallowing efficiency and the perception of increased salivary flow. Botulinum toxin injections to the parotids have been used for patients who have difficulty managing saliva and are at risk for aspiration or who experience uncontrolled drooling. Some medications can cause increased saliva production. Patients who wear dentures for the first time can experience a mild transient increase in salivary flow.

DIAGNOSIS

Several specific questions can help differentiate salivary gland hypofunction from the subjective complaint of dry mouth (Navazesh, 2017). These questions focus on oral activities that require adequate saliva production. Questions helpful in evaluating patients with complaints of dry mouth include:

1. Do you have difficulty swallowing dry foods?
2. Does your mouth feel dry while eating a meal?
3. Do you sip liquids to aid swallowing dry food?
4. Does the amount of saliva in your mouth most of the time seem to be too little, too much or you do not notice?

A positive response to questions 1 to 3 or the perception of too little saliva is significantly associated with reduced salivary gland function.

Saliva collection determines whether the salivary glands are producing in a normal range. Saliva collection is helpful with diagnosis and appropriate treatment. Dentists with advanced education in oral medicine are trained to perform salivary function evaluations. Salivary flow rates are essential for diagnostic and research purposes. Existing salivary gland function is determined by objective measurement techniques. Salivary flow rates can be determined individually from the major glands or all the glands (whole saliva).

Whole saliva is the mixed fluid contents of the mouth. The main methods of whole saliva collection include the draining method, spitting method, suction method, and absorbent (swab) method. The draining and spitting method are more reliable and reproducible for whole saliva collection. Stimulated whole saliva can also be obtained by having the patient chew on an inert material such as paraffin wax, unflavored gum base, or a rubber band.

X

The American–European Consensus Criteria for Sjögren's Syndrome uses whole unstimulated salivary flow as one of the diagnostic criteria. Whole unstimulated salivary flow less than or equal to 1.5 mL in 15 minutes is one of the diagnostic criteria for SS.

Individual gland collection is performed using Carlson–Crittenden collectors. Individual collectors are placed over the Stenson's duct orifices and held in place with gentle suction. Submandibular–sublingual individual gland collection uses a suction device or an alginate-held collector called a segregator. As saliva is produced, it flows through tubing and is collected in a preweighted vessel.

Stimulated individual gland saliva is obtained by applying 2% citric acid bilaterally to the dorsal surface of the tongue at 30 second intervals. The normal stimulated flow rate is approximately 1 mL/minute per gland.

Ultrasonography is a sensitive tool, and clinicians are using ultrasound of the salivary glands to supplement investigations. Several institutions are working to standardize and validate normal and abnormal ultrasound findings (Fox, 2016).

The specific mechanisms of most causes of hypofunction are not known. Irradiation results in a reduction in cell number, a decrease in gland size, and fibrosis of the glandular parenchyma. Autoimmune exocrine disease is associated with inflammation and eventual loss of acini. The anticholinergic properties of medications also result in decreased salivary function. The specific mechanisms leading to these alterations have not been fully described.

Even though the mechanisms of destruction are different, the result in each may be the same: decreased salivary gland function and compromised oral functions.

TREATMENT OF SALIVARY GLAND DYSFUNCTION AND XEROSTOMIA

Treatment for xerostomia is limited; therefore preventive measures must be emphasized.

Prevention

Proper shielding and positioning during radiation therapy to the head and neck region protect the salivary glands and other tissues. Radioprotective agents such as amifostine may protect the salivary glands during head and neck radiation therapy and allow less salivary gland destruction.

Patients with dry mouth have increased susceptibility to dental caries (Zero et al., 2016). Patients should be encouraged to brush and floss daily. A soft tooth brush with a toothpaste formulated for patients with xerostomia is recommended. Dentifrices containing sodium lauryl sulfate may contribute to aphthous ulcer formation. Biotène and Oralbalance dentifrices are available over-the-counter and contain salivary enzymes designed to activate the oral bacterial system.

Applying a topical fluoride has been shown to reduce caries and help preserve the dentition. Fluorides are available in several forms, including professionally applied fluoride varnishes, rinses, and higher-concentration gels. Fluoride varnishes are recommended for caries prevention in patients with xerostomia. Varnish is not used in patients with nut allergies or applied when oral ulcers are present. Fluoride varnishes are now available in clear solutions and are applied by a dentist every 3 months. If varnishes are not an option, fluoride gels can be applied by brush or in custom-made carriers that occlude the fluoride solution against the teeth. Patients must refrain from eating, drinking, or smoking for 30 minutes after topical fluoride gel applications. The frequency and mode of the application must be determined for each patient based on the extent of salivary hypofunction and caries activity. Stannous fluoride gel or neutral sodium fluoride gel is effective for caries prevention. Neutral sodium fluoride is recommended when the taste of stannous fluoride is not tolerated. Neutral sodium fluoride is also recommended for patients with multiple ceramic dental restorations. When coupled with increased attention to dental hygiene and frequent professional dental care (every 3–4 months), supplemental fluoride can protect against the dental decay that can accompany salivary dysfunction.

Chlorhexidine rinses may also be helpful in caries prevention by reducing *Lactobacillus* counts in the oral cavity. Dentures should be removed nightly and soaked overnight.

Xylitol-containing sugarless gum has a cariogenic property. Sometimes even with meticulous oral hygiene, patients may continue to have increased caries.

Patients with salivary gland dysfunction have an increased incidence of salivary gland infections, and preventive measures are helpful. Patients should be encouraged to milk their salivary glands daily using a gentle massage of the major glands. Adequate fluid intake and hydration are important for infection prevention. Sucking on sugarless candies, using xylitol-containing chewing gum, or wiping the oral cavity with glycerin swabs stimulate salivary flow and help prevent mucous plug formation and salivary gland infections. Patients with dry mouth also have an increased incidence of oral fungal infections. Because of the increased incidence of caries, sugarless antifungal agents such as nystatin powder or clotrimazole troches are recommended.

Dry, chapped, cracking lips is a common problem that patients report and is painful and often makes them feel uncomfortable socially. Lubricants such as vitamin E, Orajel, Vaseline, and glycerin swabs may relieve dryness, soreness, and mucosal trauma.

Patients who breath through their mouths may find some relief using an air humidifier at the bedside during the night.

Treatment

Salivary gland destruction is not reversible regardless of the method of damage. Potential treatments are active areas of research. Treatment for salivary gland dysfunction is limited to symptomatic treatments or systemic sialagogues. Saliva substitutes are available as rinses and gels; however, patients often prefer sipping water. The taste and mechanical stimulation of salivation from sugarless candy and chewing gum provide relief for some patients. Xylitol-containing sugarless gum has been shown to aid in the prevention of caries.

Several systemic sialagogues have been investigated. These agents are useful only for patients with remaining functioning salivary glands. Limited clinical trials have shown anethole trithione to be effective for mild medication-induced xerostomia. Clinical trials with the mucolytic agent bromhexine have been conducted but with varying results. Pilocarpine and cevimeline are the two U.S. Food and Drug Administration–approved systemic sialagogues in the United States. Pilocarpine hydrochloride and cevimeline are parasympathetic agonists with muscarinic M_3 action that increases salivary flow. They have been shown to be effective in radiation- and SS-induced hypofunction. Side effects are common but often tolerated. Pilocarpine should be used with caution in patients with a history of respiratory difficulty, heart disease, or glaucoma.

Clinical trials have been conducted in investigating autoimmune disease–related xerostomia and treatments with the antirheumatic medication hydroxychloroquine and with other disease-modifying antirheumatic agents such as prednisone. Patients with SS are frequently prescribed such systemic medications. Serological signs of disease activity improve, and there are reports of improved salivary gland function. However, the side effects of prednisone and other disease-modifying agents may be severe, and the effects on underlying salivary gland pathology have not been demonstrated. General medical health, along with xerostomia symptoms, are taken into consideration when evaluating the risks and benefits of systemic medications. Nonsteroidal anti-inflammatories have not been shown to reduce dry mouth symptoms or to improve salivary flow rates.

Repeated corticosteroid irrigations have been associated with increased salivary flow in patients with SS (Wu et al., 2017). This procedure is not performed in an acutely inflamed gland. Patients who experience repeated salivary gland swellings following radioactive iodine therapy may benefit from sialendoscopy. In this patient population, both salivary gland destruction and ductal strictures may play a role in repeated salivary gland enlargements (Wu et al., 2017).

Researchers are investigating the use of gene therapy as a treatment modality for patients with radiation- or autoimmune-related salivary gland destruction.

In a phase 1 clinical trial, with adenoviral-mediated aquaporin-1 complementary DNA (cDNA) transfer to a single irradiated parotid

X

gland was shown to be beneficial in treating patients with radiation-induced xerostomia (Alevizos et al., 2017). Researchers have discussed possible future clinical trials using gene therapy for SS-associated xerostomia.

Researchers have found a correlation between cell volume and unstimulated salivary flow. This technique measures the water content of saliva by measuring calcium channel signaling pathway and cell volume in salivary gland tissue from minor salivary gland biopsies. This technique is used in a research setting. It serves as a good indicator at the cellular level of whether a patient has low flow. This method is a future therapeutic target (Teos & Leyla, 2016).

CONCLUSION

Salivary gland hypofunction is not reversible. However, preventive measures and conservative treatments can avoid or limit mucosal breakdown, infections, and permanent damage to teeth. Symptomatic relief may be obtained with local measures and systemic secretagogues in many patients. As clinicians, we should establish clear diagnoses, make certain that patients understand the causes of their dry mouth, and deliver the most efficacious, preventive, and management techniques available.

The presence of saliva impacts daily activities. It is required for support of the basic functions of the oral cavity: alimentation and communication. Management of symptoms and increasing saliva output may help patients feel more comfortable and improve the quality of their lives.

See also Swallowing Disorders and Aspiration.

Margaret M. Grisius

Alevizos, I., Zheng, C., Cotrim, A. P., Liu, S., McCullagh, L., Billings, M. E., ... Danielides, S. J. (2017). Late responses to adenoviral-mediated transfer of the aquaporin-1 gene for radiation-induced salivary hypofunction. *Gene Therapy*, 24(3), 176.

Billings, M., Dye, B. A., Iafolla, T., Baer, A. N., Grisius, M., & Alevizos, I. (2016). Significance and implications of patient-reported xerostomia in Sjögren's syndrome: Findings from the National Institutes of Health Cohort. *EBioMedicine*, 12, 270–279.

Crogan, N. L. (2011). Managing xerostomia in nursing homes: Pilot testing of the Sorbet increases salivation intervention. *Journal of the American Medical Directors Association*, 12(3), 212–216.

Fox, R. I. (2016). Is salivary gland ultrasonography a useful tool in Sjögren's syndrome? *Rheumatology*, 55(5), 773–774.

Joanna, N. D. Y., & Thomson, W. M. (2015). Dry mouth—An overview. *Singapore Dental Journal*, 36, 12–17.

Navazesh, M. (2017). Salivary gland dysfunction and xerostomia. In J. Ferreira, J. Fricton, & N. Rhodus (Eds.), *Orofacial disorders* (pp. 89–94). Cham, Switzerland: Springer Publishing.

Perry, D. J., Chan, K., Wolden, S., Zelefsky, M. J., Chiu, J., Cohen, G., ... Lee, N. (2010). High-dose-rate intraoperative radiation therapy for recurrent head-and-neck cancer. *International Journal of Radiation Oncology, Biology, & Physics*, 76(4), 1140–1146.

Teos, L. Y., & Alevizos, I. (2017). Genetics of Sjögren's syndrome. *Clinical Immunology*, 82(9), 41–47.

Wu, W. J., Shao, X., Huang, M. W., Lv, X. M., Zhang, X. N., & Zhang, J. G. (2017). Postoperative iodine–125 interstitial brachytherapy for the early stages of minor salivary gland carcinomas of the lip and buccal mucosa with positive or close margins. *Head & Neck*, 39(3), 572–577.

Zero, D. T., Brennan, M. T., Daniels, T. E., Papas, A., Stewart, C., Pinto, A., ... Singh, M. (2016). Clinical practice guidelines for oral management of Sjögren disease: Dental caries prevention. *Journal of the American Dental Association*, 147(4), 295–305.

Web Resources
American Academy of Oral Medicine: http://www.aaom.com
American Cancer Society: http://www.cancer.org
Internet Resources for People With Sjögren's Syndrome: http://www.dry.org
National Institute of Dental and Craniofacial Research: http://www.nidcr.nih.gov
National Institutes of Health: http://www.nih.gov

INDEX

borderline personality
disorder, 555
Boston Naming Test, 156
Botulinum toxin injections, 773
Braden Scale, 432
Brandle/Heisler/Steigel
Model, 749
Brief Pain Inventory (BPI), 524
Brookdale Foundation Group, 336
Relatives as Parents Program
(RAPP), 336
bruises, 670–671. *See also* skin issues
indicator of pathological
process, 671
life cycle of, 671
presentation of, 672
BTE hearing aids, 354

calcitonin, 515
California End of Life Option
Act, 573
cancer
biological therapy, 113
biology and aging, 111
Comprehensive Geriatric
Assessment (CGA) for, 112
chemotherapy, 113
hormonal therapy, 113
in Latino elders, 361
management of older adults
with, 111–112
surgical intervention, 113
treatment modalities, 112–113
Candida albicans, 209
Candida infections, 298
capacity, of patients, 160–163
assessment, 161
decisional, 162
to drive, 162–163
Capacity to Consent to Treat
Instrument (CCTI), 451
carbidopa/levodopa, 536
care coordination and
management, 329
care management
long-term services, 114–115
Care Transition Intervention®, 141
Care Transitions Coach®, 141
Care Transitions Intervention
(CTI), 377, 628
caregiver burden, 117–120
assessment, 118–120
definition, 117
and depression, 123

supports and interventions, 120
telehealth interventions, 120
caregiver burnout, 122–125
healing interventions, 124
informal, 122–123
manifestations of, 123–124
professional, 123–125
caregiver support groups, 126–128
benefits of, 127
race and ethnicity, 127
caregiving conflicts, 286
caregiving relationships, 130–132
CASES approach, 264
Casey Family Programs, 336
Cash and Counseling
Demonstration and
Evaluation (CCDE), 540–541
Cash and Counseling program, 541
cataracts, 133–136
centenarians, 137–138
environmental and genetic
influences, 137
estimated population, 137
nutritional interventions, 138
The Center for Epidemiologic
Studies Depression
Scale, 119
Center for Epidemiologic Studies
Depression Scale (CES-D),
215–2196
Centers for Disease Control and
Prevention (CDC), 501, 661
Centers for Medicare & Medicaid
Services (CMS), 258, 427,
443, 483–484
central auditory processing
disorder (CAPD), 356–357
cerebral vascular accident
(CVA), 497
cerebrovascular accident, 309–310
Certified Geriatric Pharmacist
(CGP), 560–561
Certified in Aging-in-Place
(CAPS), 255
Certified Nursing Assistant
(CNA), 185
certified nutrition specialist
(CNS), 490
cervicogenic headache, 344
Charcot, J. M., 326
Children's Health Insurance
Program (CHIP), 24, 436
Child Welfare League of
America, 336

cholinesterase inhibitors, 744, 758
chondroitin sulfate, 511
Chronic Care Management (CCM)
Services, 144
chronic disequilibrium, 232–233
chronic illnesses, 143–146
approaches to deal with, 144
functional assessment, 145
functional interventions, 146
medical assessment, 144–145
medical interventions, 146
prevention interventions,
145–146
psychosocial assessment, 145
psychosocial interventions, 146
chronic pain, 522–523
assessment of, 523–524
definitions, 522–523
management of, 524–525
cilostazol, 554
circardian disturbances, 680–681
Clinical Assessment of Driving-
Related Skills (CADReS)
Older- Driver Screening
Tool, 234
clinical competencies, 158–159
and capacity, 160–163
clinical ethics consultation
competencies of, 264
evaluation of, 264
goals of, 262–263
issues addressed by, 263
methods of, 264
modes of, 262
role of consultant, 263
clinical pathways, 147–149
*The Clinicians Guide to Assessing
and Counseling Older Drivers,*
3rd edition, 234
Clock Drawing Executive Task
(CLOX1/ CLOX2), 450–451
clock drawing test (CDT), 155
Clostridium difficile colitis, 385
clozapine, 538, 618, 759
cognitive aging, 150–151
cognitive behavioral therapy, 61–62
cognitive-behavioral
techniques, 527
cognitive changes in aging, 149–152
communication skills, 151–152
self-reporting, 151
cognitive impairment in dementia
causes of, 743–744
characteristic feature of, 743

Lewy body dementia (DLB),
94, 756
behavioral and psychological
disturbances, 759
behavioral and psychological
signs and symptoms, 758
delusions, 758–759
diagnostic procedures, 757
differential diagnosis, 757
hallucinations, 758–759
management of, 758
medications, 758
symptoms of, 757
treatment, 757
unwarranted suspiciousness,
758–759
LFDRS. *See* Lichtenberg Financial
Decision Making
Rating Scale
LGBTQ. *See* lesbian, gay,
bisexual, transgender,
and queer
Lichtenberg Financial Decision
Making Rating Scale
(LFDRS), 748
Lichtenberg Financial Decision
Screening Scale (LFDSS),
449–450
life events, 421–422
biological processes, 423
evolution of, 422
in life course perspective, 423
mediators and moderators,
422–423
research areas, 422
life review, 423–424
evaluative process, 424
positive results of, 424
research and practices, 424–425
life-sustaining medical treatments
(LSMTs), 18
Lifespan Respite Care
Program, 636
Likert scales, 432
Liverpool Classification System for
diabetic ulcers, 296
living will, 162
location and environment, 668–670
long-term acute care hospitals
(LTACHs), 584
long-term care, 437
institutional care and HCBS,
426–427
insurance, 426

management, of rising
demand, 426
for people with disabilities, 427
quality in, 427
residential care, 427
workers and workforce, 427–428
Long-Term Care Ombudsman
Program (LTCOP), 466
care-planning sessions, 467
complaints, 466–467
data for, 467
mission of, 467
ombudsman activities, 467
long-term services and support
(LTSS), 426–427, 480
long-term services and support
system (LTSS), 661
long-term services care
management, 114–115
care planning, 115
community-based, 114
components of, 115
comprehensive assessment, 115
issues in, 115–116
service arrangement and care
coordination, 115
loss of protective sensation
(LOPS), 297
lower GI bleeding (LGIB), 313–315
low-dose computed tomography
(LDCT), 350
Low Income Subsidy program, 444
loxapine, 618
LTACHs. *See* long-term acute care
hospitals
LTCOP. *See* Long-Term Care
Ombudsman Program
lumboperitoneal (LP) shunts
therapy for normal pressure
hydrocephalus (NPH), 477
lung screening, 350
lurasidone, 618

MacArthur Competence
Assessment Tools
(MacCAT), 451
macrocytic anemia, 51
Magnet® Recognition Program, 45
Major Depressive Disorder, 212
mammograms, 350
managed care organizations
(MCOs), 479
managed long-term care
(MLTC), 481

managed long-term service and
supports (MLTSS), 481
Meals on Wheels
congregate meal programs, 429
home-delivered meal
programs, 429
objective of, 429
senior nutrition programs
(SNPs), 429
measurement
assessment tool, in geriatrics,
432–433
definition, 431
health care delivery system, 430
interpretation of numerical
values, 432
levels of, 431–432
Medicaid
beneficiaries, 437
costs of long-term care, 437–438
coverage of prenatal care, 436
enacted in, 436
expansion, 436, 438
income and assets for, 437
research in, 438
supplemental health
coverage, 437
Medicaid and Medicare, 24–25, 36
medical device-related pressure
injury, 591
medical nutrition therapy
(MNT), 492
medical out-of-pocket expenses
(MOOP), 660
Medicare, 297
Advantage plans, 441
beneficiaries, 440
enacted in, 439
expenditures in, 440
Federal Coordinated Health
Care Office, 442
federal entitlement program, 440
Fee Schedule, 441
Medigap plans, 441
programs of, 440
Medicare Advantage (MA) plans,
24, 442–443, 480
benefits of, 443
Centers for Medicare &
Medicaid Services
(CMS), 443
establishment, 443
types of, 443
Medicare Advantage program, 440